ALLE · ZEIT · WACH
1842

Intracranial Pressure VIII

Edited by
C.J.J. Avezaat J.H.M. van Eijndhoven
A.I.R. Maas and J.Th.J. Tans

With 244 Figures and 166 Tables

Springer-Verlag
Berlin Heidelberg New York London Paris
Tokyo Hong Kong Barcelona Budapest

Prof. Dr. C.J.J. Avezaat
Dept. of Neurosurgery
University Hospital Rotterdam
Dr. Molewaterplein 40
3015 GD Rotterdam
The Netherlands

Dr. ir. J.H.M. van Eijndhoven
Central Dept. of Automation and Informatics
University Hospital Rotterdam

Dr. A.I.R. Maas
Dept. of Neurosurgery
University Hospital Rotterdam

Dr. J.Th.J. Tans
Dept. of Neurology
Westeinde Hospital
Lijnbaan 32
2512 VA Den Haag
The Netherlands

ISBN-13: 978-3-642-77791-2 e-ISBN-13: 978-3-642-77789-9
DOI: 10.1007/978-3-642-77789-9

Library of Congress Cataloging-in-Publication Data. Intracranial pressure VIII / edited by C.J.J. Avezaat . . . [et al.]. p. cm. "Proceedings of the eighth International Symposium on Intracranial Pressure, held in Rotterdam, The Netherlands, June 16–20, 1991." Includes bibliographical references and index. 1. Intracranial pressure—Congresses. 2. Brain—Pathophysiology—Congresses. I. Avezaat, C. J. J., 1942– . II. International Symposium on Intracranial Pressure (8th : 1991 : Rotterdam, Netherlands) III. Title: Intracranial pressure 8. RC386.2.I583 1993 616.8—dc20 92-41420

Softcover reprint of the hardcover 1st edition 1993

Typesetting Best-set Typesetter Ltd., Hong Kong
25/3130/SPS-5 4 3 2 1 0 – Printed on acid-free paper

Proceedings of the Eighth International Symposium on Intracranial Pressure
Held in Rotterdam, The Netherlands, June 16–20, 1991

List of Contributors

You will find the addresses at the beginning of the respective contribution

Preface

The pioneering work by Pierre Janny and Nils Lundberg added a new tool to the investigative armamentarium of the neurosurgeon: continuous monitoring of intracranial pressure (ICP). A small group of basic and clinical scientists recognized the importance of this method and in 1972 an International Symposium was organized by Mario Brock in Hannover, Germany. The workers "of the first hour" had high expectations and thought that the problem of intracranial hypertension could finally be dealt with. The Symposium continued to grow during subsequent meetings in Lund (1974), Groningen (1976) and Williamsburg (1979). However, the advent of the modern imaging techniques of CT and MRI have dramatically changed the scene in clinical neurology and neurosurgery. These new methods as well as other monitoring techniques have put ICP in its proper place as just one of the many aspects, albeit an important one, in the management of patients with intracranial space-occupying lesions. The symposia in Tokyo (1982), Glasgow (1985) and Ann Arbor (1988) confirmed the steady interest in ICP recording, both as a research tool and as a clinical method, and yielded many new developments in the field of ICP.

This book comprises the proceedings of the Eighth International Symposium on Intracranial Pressure that was held in Rotterdam, The Netherlands, from June 16th to 20th, 1991. The symposium was, in the tradition of the previous meetings, characterized by an informal atmosphere, hard work and an open exchange of ideas. There were 71 oral and 186 poster presentations selected from the more than 300 abstracts that were received. A novelty were the afternoon panels during which new developments and major trends as disclosed from the papers and posters of the day were discussed by experts in the field. It is hoped that this volume will be a valuable addition to the unique series of books that reflect the up-to-date status of research and clinical application of intracranial pressure monitoring.

The help of the sponsors is gratefully acknowledged, in particular the generous support given by Bayer AG to the publication of these proceedings.

The Ninth International Symposium on Intracranial Pressure will be held in Nagoya, Japan, in 1994.

Rotterdam/Den Haag,
March 1993

The Editors

Contents

Session II: Experimental Aspects

Chairmen: A. Baethmann and K.G. Go

Edema

Blood-Brain Barrier

Session IV: Cerebrovascular Dynamics II

Chairmen: J.T. Hoff and C.J.J. Avezaat

Transcranial Doppler

Wave Form Analysis

Pressure Waves

Postural Changes

Panel 2: Cerebrovascular Dynamics

Bayer Round-Table Discussion on Methodology of Head Injury Trials

Session V: Head Injury

Chairmen: B. Jennett and D.A. Hovda

Experimental

Computerized Tomography and Magnetic Resonance Imaging

Session VII: CSF Dynamics

Chairmen: A. Marmarou and P. Janny

Models

CSF Outflow Resistance and Volume-Pressure Relationship

Session VIII: Hydrocephalus

Chairmen: H. Nagai and J. Ekstedt

Normal Pressure Hydrocephalus

Hydrocephalus Following Subarachnoid Haemorrhage

Session I: Methodology and Mass Lesions

Chairmen: M. Brock and J.W.F. Becks

Clinical Evaluation of the Camino Ventricular Bolt Pressure Monitoring System

I.R. CHAMBERS[1], P.J. KANE[2], M.S. CHOKSEY[2], and A.D. MENDELOW[2]

[1] Regional Medical Physics Department, and [2] Department of Neurosurgery, Newcastle General Hospital, Westgate Road, Newcastle upon Tyne, NE4 6BE, England

Introduction

Intracranial pressure (ICP) measurement is a routine part of the clinical management of severe head injury in many neurosurgical units. A variety of measurement techniques are available including ventricular and subdural catheters and subdural screws [4]. Recently the Camino fibre optic transducer inserted via a subdural screw, into the subarachnoid space has been shown to provide a reliable measurement of ICP [1, 2]. Using a ventricular catheter to measure ICP is perhaps the most reliable method and allows the drainage of CSF. A previously available ventricular catheter system using the Camino transducer was found to have practical limitations [3]. The aim of this study was to compare readings from a ventricular catheter and an external transducer with the new Camino ventricular bolt system and to assess the reliability of the system in clinical practice.

Material and Methods

The Camino ventricular bolt pressure monitoring system consists of a fibre optic transducer tipped catheter, a ventricular catheter assembly and a bolt. The bolt is screwed into a burr hole and the ventricular catheter is then inserted into the ventricle through this bolt and secured with a compression cap to provide a fluid seal. The fibre optic transducer is then inserted into the lumen of the ventricular catheter so that it lies within the tip of the ventricular catheter. The system has an additional Y-connector designed to enable CSF drainage.

Seven patients with recent severe head injury (GCS ≤ 8) who required ICP measurement as part of their clinical management had a Camino ventricular bolt inserted into a right frontal burr hole. The arm of the Y-connector designed for CSF drainage was connected via a 15 cm length of pressure tubing

Table 1. Linear regression analysis of Camino transducers

Number	Recording length (hrs)	Correlation coefficient	Gradient	Intercept
1	42.7	0.850	0.94	3.5
2	33.2	0.904	1.03	6.2
3	98.1	0.934	1.03	5.2
4	51.0	0.954	1.01	7.4
5	48.2	0.991	0.94	4.2
6	57.4	0.841	0.99	0.9
All data	330.6	0.976	0.93	5.2

to an external transducer permitting intraventricular ICP measurement via the ventricular catheter. The external transducer was calibrated at the level of the patient's ear and both transducers were calibrated at regular intervals throughout the monitoring period.

The two transducers were connected to a Quadriscope modular monitoring system (Simonsen and Weel Vickers Ltd, Sidcup England) and a permanent recording of both traces made on a pen recorder. Data collection was performed by a purpose built module which determined the systolic, diastolic and

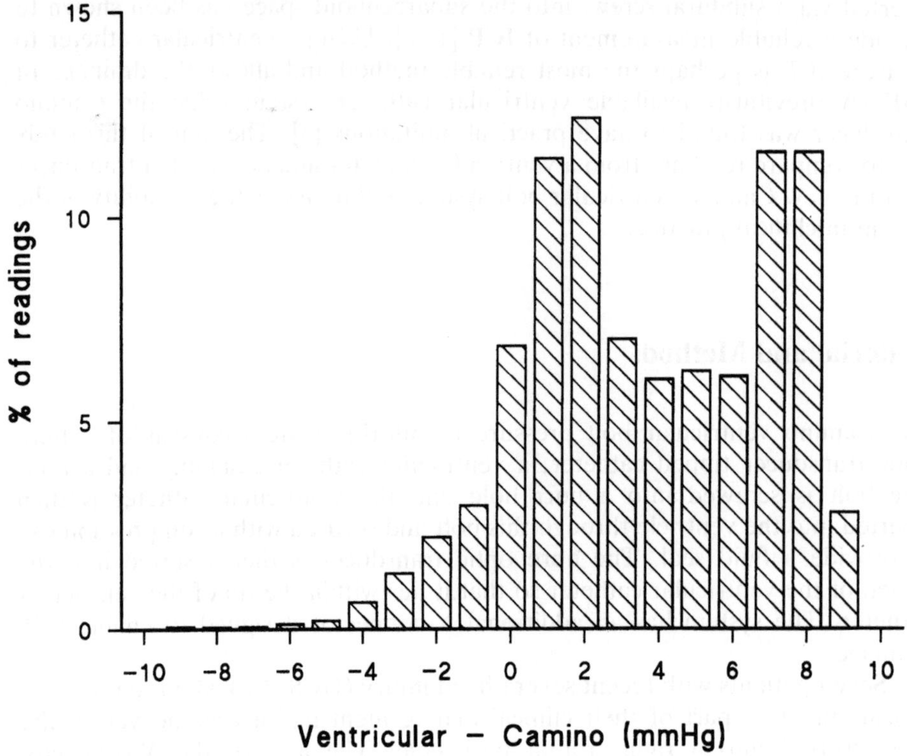

Fig. 1. Distribution of pressure differences

mean values of the pressure waveforms from the pressure channels and displayed them on a digital display. Additionally every two minutes comparative readings were taken and transmitted through a digital RS232 computer interface to a PSION II XP ORGANISER (TM) for the duration of the monitoring period. The sampled data was subsequently downloaded to a Personal Computer for analysis.

Results

The patients were studied over periods from 33.2 to 98.1 hours (Table 1). No complications related to the transducer placement or infection were encountered. In one case the fibre optic catheter failed within 30 minutes of insertion and was excluded from the analysis. In all the other cases measurements were made until removal of the ventricular catheter. The aggregate length of recording was 330.6 hours and ICP values were obtained over a wide range (0–97 mmHg). Within the total data recordings 36% of readings were within 2 mmHg and 97% within 10 mmHg (Fig. 1). Performing linear regression analysis the correlation coefficient from each transducer varied from

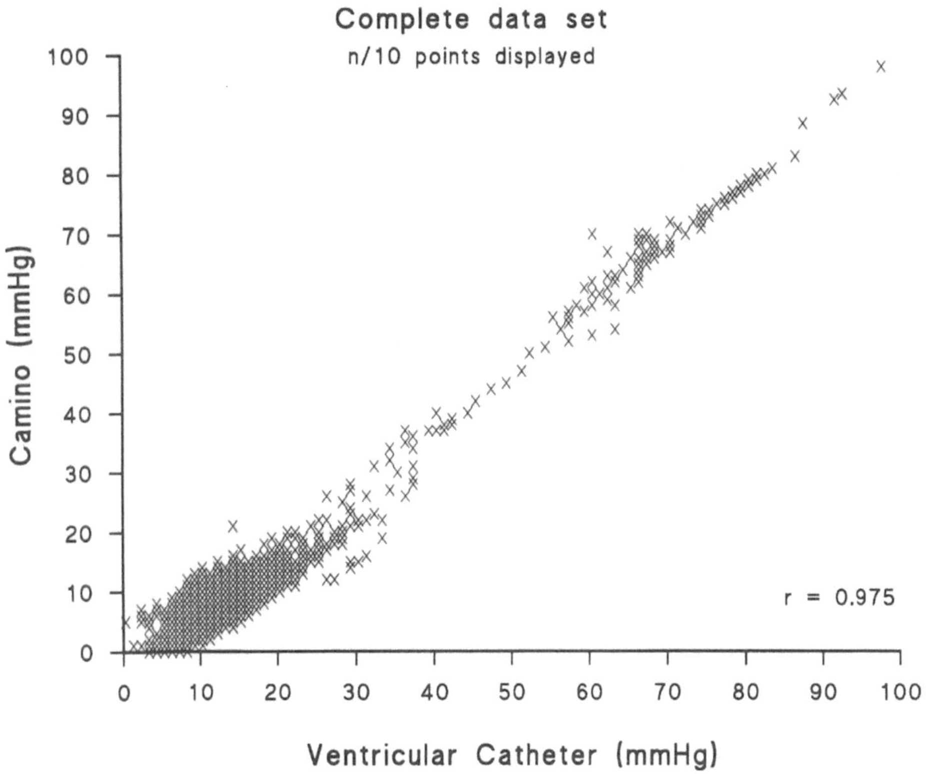

Fig. 2. Cumulative data from all transducers

0.841 to 0.991; Gradients from 0.94 to 1.03; and intercepts from 0.9 to 7.4 (Table 1). On the complete data set the correlation coefficient was 0.976 and gradient 0.93 and intercept 6.2 (Fig. 2). The average correlation coefficient was 0.921, gradient 0.99, and intercept 4.7.

Discussion

We have found the Camino ventricular bolt system easy to use and no instances of infection or other complications arose due to its use. The readings from the Camino transducer correlate very well with those obtained from a fluid-filled external transducer. This has been demonstrated over lengthy monitoring periods and over a wide range of ICP. On average there is a static pressure difference of 4.7 mmHg between readings obtained from an external transducer placed at the level of the patient's ear, which is due to the positional differences between the two transducer systems, the Camino tip lying above the zero line within the ventricle. Having the measuring device within the ventricle may be beneficial in studies of ICP waveform analysis. The ventricular Camino bolt may also prove useful in those patients where open ventricular access is needed in addition to ICP monitoring.

References

1. Bergenheim T, Blafors E, Rabow L (1989) Intraparenchymal brain pressure – clinical evaluation. In: Hoff JT, Betz AL (eds) Intracranial pressure VII. Springer, Berlin Heidelberg New York London Paris Tokyo Hong Kong, pp 66–68
2. Chambers IR, Mendelow AD, Sinar J, Modha P (1989) Clinical Evaluation of the Catheter Tipped Camino Transducer Inserted via a Subdural Screw. In: Hoff JT, Betz AL (eds) Intracranial pressure VII. Springer, Berlin Heidelberg New York London Paris Tokyo Hong Kong, pp 27–30
3. Chambers IR, Mendelow AD, Sinar J, Modha P (1989) A clinical evaluation of the camino subdural screw and ventricular monitoring kits. Neurosurgery 26:3, pp 421–423
4. North B, Reilly P (1990) Methods of measuring intracranial pressure. In: Raised intracranial pressure. A clinical guide. Heinemann Medical Books, Oxford, pp 42–62

A Clinical Evaluation of an Intraparenchymal Intracranial Pressure Transducer

P. Statham, S. Midgley, N.M. Dearden, C. McIntosh, and J.D. Miller

Department of Clinical Neurosciences, Western General Hospital, Edinburgh, UK

Introduction

The Camino pressure transducer is accurate experimentally over a range of clinically relevant intracranial pressures (ICPs). Three clinical studies have shown that intraparenchymal pressure mirrors intraventricular pressure. In two a different type of transducer was used, and one was a mixed animal and human study [3, 4, 2]. This study compares intraparenchymal pressure, measured with a Camino fibre-optic transducer, with intraventricular pressure, using a fluid filled catheter, in unconscious head injured patients and evaluates the clinical efficacy of the Camino system.

Patients and Methods

Unconscious head injured patients with a clinical indication for intracranial pressure monitoring were studied, after informed consent had been obtained from a relative. Zero and gain stability of the Camino transducer was ascertained in vitro. This and a ventricular catheter were then placed into the frontal lobe opposite to the side of predominant injury. Zero was taken at the tip of the Camino catheter. ICP was recorded daily from both systems for one hour periods at one minute intervals, with a ventricular catheter calibration check before and immediately after each recording epoch. The duration of monitoring was dictated by clinical considerations only. At the end of monitoring the zero drift and gain stability of the Camino catheter was rechecked. Statistical analysis was performed using correlation regression, the Altman and Bland analysis for ranked comparison studies [1] and paired and unpaired Students' t tests.

Results

Thirteen patients were entered into the study. In one patient compression of the ventricles prevented cannulation after 3 attempts, whilst in another ventricular catheter obstruction compromised dual monitoring. The remaining 11 patients were monitored for between one and eleven days (median 4 days),

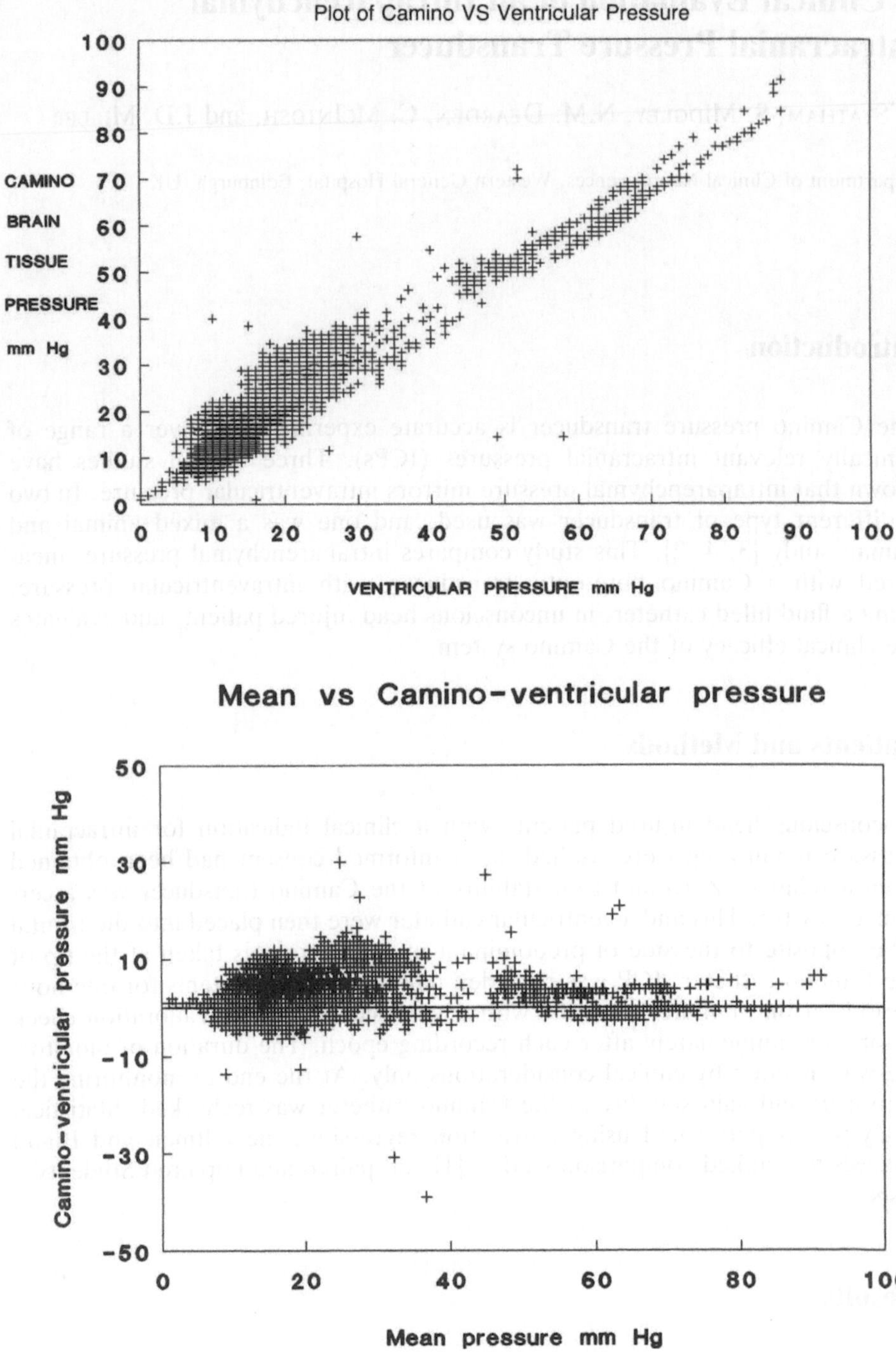

Fig. 1. The relationship between Camino and ventricular pressure

Table 1. Variation in agreement with pressure range, time and individual catheter

	r	p	limits of agreement (mmHg)		mean bias (mmHg)	confidence interval of bias (mmHg)		paired t test
Pressure range (mm Hg)								
0–10	0.41	0.0001	−4.05	10.9	3.45	3.22	3.67	30.2
11–20	0.60	0.0001	−5.85	10.5	2.33	2.17	2.48	29.5
21–30	0.41	0.0001	−5.71	15.10	4.69	4.23	5.14	20.3
31–40	0.40	0.0001	−8.51	10.45	0.97	−0.14	2.08	1.72
41–60	0.71	0.0001	−4.72	10.83	3.05	2.65	3.45	14.9
60–90	0.95	0.0001	−5.10	4.27	0.42	−0.73	−0.10	−2.6
Day of monitoring								
1	0.98	0.0001	−5.25	11.3	3.04	2.83	3.25	28.6
2	1.00	0.0001	−4.42	4.60	0.09	−0.05	0.23	1.27
3	0.86	0.0001	−2.93	14.15	5.61	5.32	5.90	38.2
4	0.77	0.0001	−9.84	13.97	2.25	1.80	2.69	9.84
5	0.95	0.0001	−1.30	6.23	2.46	2.14	2.78	15.3
7	0.97	0.0001	−1.35	5.96	2.30	1.99	2.61	14.6
8	0.93	0.0001	1.19	4.71	2.96	2.81	3.09	41.2
10	0.88	0.0001	−1.16	10.1	4.47	4.04	4.90	20.3
11	0.99	0.0001	0.84	6.02	3.43	3.12	3.73	22.1
Individual catheter								
A	0.83	0.0001	−3.67	8.17	2.24	2.07	2.42	24.8
B	0.95	0.0001	3.69	8.65	6.17	6.05	6.28	102.6
C	0.97	0.0001	−4.50	5.82	0.66	0.42	0.89	5.39
D	0.77	0.0001	0.29	16.72	8.51	8.21	8.80	56.4
E	0.93	0.0001	−1.25	7.19	2.97	2.76	3.17	28.1
F	0.85	0.0001	−4.30	4.43	0.07	−0.09	0.23	0.83
G	0.68	0.0001	−4.15	3.08	−0.53	−0.72	−0.34	−5.39
H	0.81	0.0001	−5.67	2.95	−1.36	−1.55	−1.17	−14.1
I	0.44	0.0001	−1.21	10.44	4.61	4.15	5.07	19.6
J	0.76	0.0001	−1.76	6.55	2.39	1.84	2.94	8.44
K	0.78	0.0001	8.08	12.08	10.08	9.82	10.35	75.8

r, correlation coefficient; p, probability

enabling 5116 comparative datapoints to be obtained over a range of venticular pressures from zero to 88 mmHg. Strong correlation ($r = 0.976$, $p < 0.0001$) was found between paired ICP measurements overall. Mean Camino ICP exceeded average ventricular ICP by 2.73 mmHg (95% confidence limits of agreement; −5.68 to 11.2 mmHg, 95% confidence interval of bias 2.61 to 2.85 mmHg). Correlation and difference in ICP (Camino − ventricular) compared with mean (Camino+ventricular/2) is shown in Fig. 1. The data with respect to pressure range, day of monitoring and individual catheter is summarised in Table 1.

Over the period of monitoring the mean zero drift of the Camino catheter was 0.16 mmHg (range 0–4 mmHg). The mean drift at 50 mmHg gain was 0.83 mmHg (range 1–6 mmHg). The gain measured by each Camino catheter in vitro prior to insertion at 0, 12.5, 25 and 50 mmHg underread by a mean

0.69 mmHg. When similarly checked after removal each Camino catheter underread by a mean 0.39 mmHg.

Ventriculitis developed after flushing the ventricular catheter in two patients. In two other patients dual monitoring was performed although the ventricular trace was damped and there was no free flow of CSF from the catheter.

In one patient the Camino catheter became dislodged during physiotherapy.

Discussion

Overall, Camino intraparenchymal pressure correlated well with fluid filled ventricular ICP, over a clinically relevant range of pressures, but overread by 2–3 mmHg. The Camino system was easy to use, with negligibe drift and stable calibration, offering a safe alternative to ventricular catheterisation, and remaining accurate up to 11 days after insertion. There was little difference in accuracy with different levels of ICP. Limits of agreement in individual catheters was good except for two, where a difference between mean ICP of more than 8 mmHg was found (D and K). This could not be explained by underreading of ICP by the ventricular catheter.

References

1. Altman DG, Bland JM (1983) Measurement in medicine: the analysis of method comparison studies. The Statistician 32:307–317
2. Ostrup RC, Luerssen TG, Marshall LF, Zornow MH (1987) Continuous monitoring of intracranial pressure with a miniturized fibre optic device. J Neurosurg 67:206–209
3. Piek J, Bock WJ (1990) Continuous monitoring of cerebral tissue pressure in neurosurgical practice-experiences with 100 patients. Intensive Care Medicine 16(3):184–188
4. Sundbarg G, Nordstrom C-H, Messeter K, Soderstrom S (1987) A comparison of intraparenchymatous and intraventricular pressure recording in clinical practice. J Neurosurg 67:841–845

Continuous Monitoring of Supratentorial Cerebral Tissue Pressure in Neurosurgical Routine. Experience with 125 Patients

J. PIEK and W.J. BOCK

Neurosurgical Clinic, Moorenstr. 5, Heinrich-Heine-University, W-4000 Düsseldorf, Germany

Introduction

Following the pioneering work of Lundberg [1] monitoring of ICP has become a routine investigation in most neurosurgical units. The ideal clinical method of ICP recording, however, has yet to be developed [2].

The advantages of the ventricular method, besides its proven reliability in thousands of patients, are that it provides a method for calibration *in vivo* and the ability to withdraw ventricular fluid for reduction of elevated ICP. The main disadvantages are transcerebral puncture and intracranial infections. In cases of narrow ventricles ICP recordings may be difficult to establish. Epidural transducers reduce infection rates but are expensive, have re-zeroing and drift problems and cannot be used in cases of open head injuries when the dura mater is destroyed [2].

Monitoring of cerebral tissue pressure (CTP) with a new type of transducer was introduced by our group in 1987 [3] with a present experience of 125 supratentorial recordings.

Material and Methods

An implantable, piezoresistive microtransducer located at the end of a 5 French–Catheter (Fig. 1; Table 1; SENSODYN, B. Braun AG, 3508 Melsungen, FRG) was used for CTP monitoring in all cases. To establish pressure recordings the tip of the catheter is placed approximately 1.5 cm into the brain tissue via a frontal burr-hole or into the surrounding tissue following open surgery with the exact procedure described elsewhere [3, 5].

Up to now we have used this method in 125 patients with various diseases (Table 2). Duration of monitoring (mean: 81.2 hours) as well as the pressures recorded (4 to 143 mmHg) varied widely depending on the clinical situation.

In 13 patients ventricular fluid pressure (VFP) and CTP were measured simultaneously. In 21 patients we performed parallel recordings of CTP to measure CTP gradients [4]. In 91 patients CTP recording was the only ICP device.

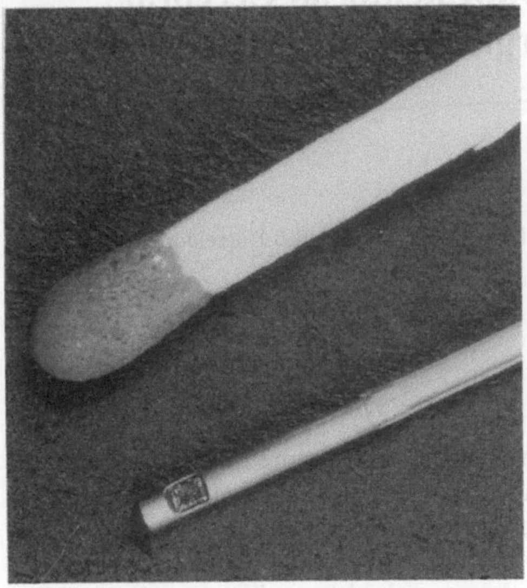

Fig. 1. Catheter (tip) used for CTP – monitoring

Table 1. Technical characteristics of the transducer

Total pressure range: −300 to +300 mm Hg
Max. pressure allowed: 4.000 mm Hg
Nonlinearity and hysteresis: max. 0.5% of end pressure
Temperature effect on zero point: max. 0.075 mm Hg/°C; operating temperature: 22 to 42°C
Zero point drift in water: max. 3 mm Hg after the first 16 hours; less than 1 mm Hg afterwards

Table 2. Clinical data: patient group and CTP recordings

Total: 125 patients (Sex: 68 male, 57 female; Age: 6–71 years)
Parallel recordings of CTP and VFP: 13 patients (SAH: 11 patients; Head Injury: 2 patients)
Intrahemispheric CTP gradients: 21 patients (Brain tumour: 19 patients; Head Injury: 1 patient; SAH: 1 patient)
CTP alone: 91 patients (Head Injury: 60 patients; SAH and IVH: 14 patients; ICH: 11 patients; Brain tumor: 6 patients)
Recording time: 8.25 to 448.2 hours (mean: 81.2 hours) Pressure range: 4–143 mm Hg

SAH, subarachnoid haemorrhage; IVH, spontaneous intraventricular haemorrhage; ICH, spontaneous intracerebral haematoma

Results

Establishing and Maintaining of Pressure Recordings

Pressure recordings were initially obtained in 122 patients (3 failures due to catheter defects following multiple re-sterilization). In 11 patients CTP recordings were lost during monitoring. The main causes of these failures were catheter destruction or dislocation (e.g. during CT transport). In simple burr-hole procedures no additional complications were observed until the end of the monitoring period. An initial drift of up to 4 mmHg during the first 24 hours is due to swelling of the silicone membrane which covers the transducer and can be avoided by placing the catheter tip into fluid for 30 min. before implantation and corrected by re-zeroing the system with the zero-point simulator. No drift problems were observed after this time.

In most cases where CTP was recorded following open surgery it took up to 3–4 hours before typical ICP waves were recorded. If epidural suction drains are used following open surgery, an exact closure of the dura is necessary, as negative CTP values may be recorded in these cases. For the same reason the catheter should be placed 3 cm into the surrounding brain tissue, if drainage of the operation cavity is used.

Parallel Recordings of VFP and CTP

CTP and VFP correlated closely with a CTP continuously 4–8 mmHg below VFP. This was the case in all pressure ranges. All typical ICP waves were recorded. Usually the pulse-wave shape is different in CTP and VFP. As VFP is transmitted by a fluid-filled system, the pulse-wave amplitude is higher due to the phenomenon of resonance. Compared with VFP, CTP reacted differently to therapeutical interventions. In cases of barbiturate injection VFP started to fall up to 2 minutes after CTP which usually decreased 5–15 seconds following injection. Mannitol infusions also reduced CTP first and VFP second.

Recordings of CTP Alone

In 91 cases CTP was recorded either via a frontal burr-hole after subarachnoid/intraventricular haemorrhages or to assist postoperative supervision following open surgery (brain tumours, poor-grade aneurysm surgery, spontaneous intracranial haematomas).

a) CTP After Closed Head Injury or Subarachnoid Haemorrhage. In these cases the catheter tip was placed via a frontal burr-hole 1.5 cm into the brain. The typical behaviour and different waves of elevated ICP were observed. Pupil dilatation was noted in 18 patients with CTP pressures ranging from 44 to 71 mmHg. In 14 of these patients the rise in CTP was caused by brain edema. Plateau waves were recorded in all of these cases and were subsequently treated with mannitol infusions and barbiturate coma. In one patient a steep rise in CTP without any pathological wave four hours after evacuation of a right temporal epidural haematoma was the first sign of a frontal extradural haematoma on the same side.

In 3 cases CTP was monitored ipsilaterally after large osteoclastic trauma flaps. Although high CTP values were recorded no plateau waves occurred. This can be explained by the pathogenesis of these waves.

b) CTP After Brain Tumour Operations. The typical CTP course following the operation of a brain tumour was a low CTP during the first postoperative day with a slight elevation up to 25 mmHg on day 2 and 3 and a reduction thereafter. B-waves were recorded in approximately half of these cases. Postoperative edema resulted in a rise of CTP which was accompanied by pathological waves. Postoperative haemorrhage in 5 patients resulted in a steep rise of ICP and was always noted during the first 8 postoperative hours.

Complications

No infection resulted from CTP recording although no prophylactic antibiotics were given. Bacteriological examinations of the catheter tip were routinely performed only in the first 30 patients. *Staphylococcus albus* was found in 4 cases and *Enterococcus species* in 1 case at the catheter tip. Only in the last

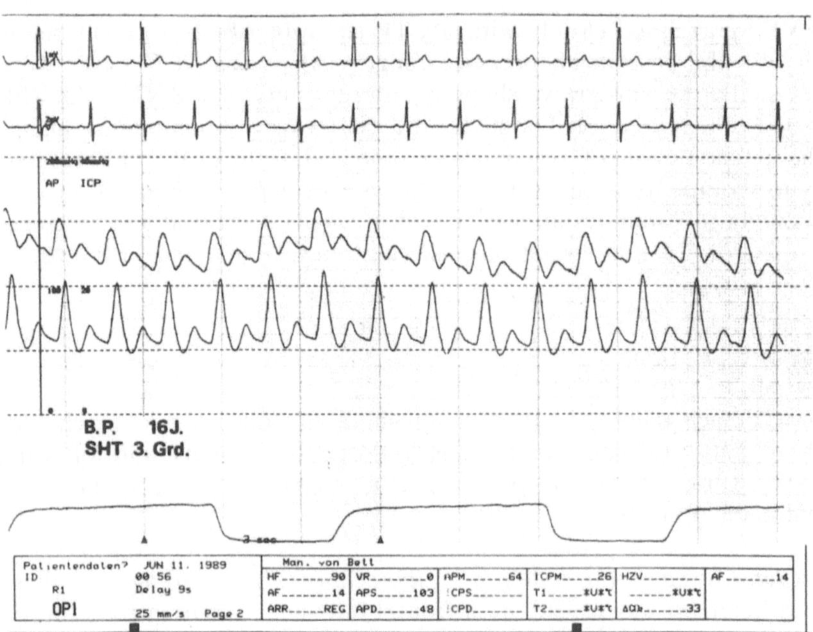

Fig. 2. Initial pressure curves of cerebral tissue pressure (ICP), blood-pressure (AP), and exspiratory CO_2

patient an antibiotic (Ampicillin) was administered. No additional intracranial bleedings were observed due to CTP recordings.

Costs

The initial costs are 1900,- DM for a catheter with one transducer, 400,- DM for the zero-point simulator and 250,- DM for the monitor adapter. Eight catheters were damaged due to mechanical lesions caused by implanting, removing, or cleaning the catheter. We used our catheters up to 14 times and had an average cost of 225,- DM per CTP recording.

Discussion

Up to now CTP monitoring as a new method of ICP control is used only in very few hospitals. Our results clearly show that it is a safe, harmless, and reliable method with low costs for control of ICP. In spite of new microtransducers some problems with conventional ICP recordings remain unsolved [2]. In cases of large craniectomies or open head injuries with the dura torn ipsilaterally epidural ICP monitoring is not possible. CTP recordings offer an alternative method in these cases.

After elective surgery ventricular catheters for VFP measurement often require an extra burr-hole with an additional risk for the patient. In severe head injuries ventricular puncture is often impossible. Infection rates may be as high as 5% [2]. Occlusion of the catheter by blood or brain tissue may occur in cases of elevated ICP. CTP recordings allow ICP monitoring in all of these cases. They have a lower infection rate and penetration of the catheter into the brain is less (CTP: 1.5 cm versus VFP: approx. 4 cm). On the other hand the main advantage of ventricular catheters is the possibility of ICP reduction by CSF drainage. From approximately 150 VFP recordings per year and our experiences with the present series, monitoring of CTP has the following indications:

a) postoperative ICP control following open surgery;
b) primarily narrow ventricles,
c) as an additional device together with a ventricular catheter via the same burr-hole, if obstruction of the ventricular cannula or ventricular collapse is expected,
d) in open head injuries with the dura torn or following large craniectomies.

References

1. Lundberg N (1960) Continuous recording and control of ventricular fluid pressure in neurosurgical practice. Acta Psychiat Scand [Suppl 149] 36:1–193
2. Miller JD (1989) Measuring ICP in patients – its value now and in the future? In: Hoff JT, Betz AL (eds) Intracranial Pressure VII. Springer, Berlin Heidelberg New York London Paris Tokyo Hong Kong, pp 5–15

3. Piek J, Kosub B, Küch F, et al. (1987) A practical technique for continuous monitoring of cerebral tissue pressure in neurosurgical patients. Acta Neurochir 87:144–149
4. Piek J, Plewe P, Bock WJ (1988) Intrahemispheric gradients of brain tissue pressure in patients with brain tumours. Acta Neurochir 93:129–132
5. Piek J, Bock WJ (1990) Continuous monitoring of cerebral tissue pressure in neurosurgical practice – experiences with 100 patients. Int Care Med 16:184–188

Continuous Monitoring of Cerebral Tissue Pressure After Elective Posterior Fossa Surgery

J. PIEK, G. ERN, and M. MESSING

Neurosurgical Clinic, Moorenstr. 5, Heinrich-Heine-University, W-4000 Düsseldorf, Germany

Introduction

If free communication exists between the supra- and the infratentorial space, the intracranial pressure is equally transmitted between these two compartments [1]. In cases of impaired communication ("compartment block"), however, supratentorial ICP may not reflect infratentorial pressure [4]. Direct ICP monitoring in the posterior fossa is indicated in these cases. Thus the aim of this pilot study was to determine the value of cerebral tissue pressure (CTP) monitoring after elective posterior fossa surgery.

Material and Methods

Infratentorial tissue pressure recordings were obtained from 18 patients (Table 1) undergoing surgery of various large (>6 cm diameter) space-occupying lesions.

An implantable, piezoresistive microtransducer located at the end of a 3 French-Catheter (SENSODYN, B. Braun AG, 3508 Melsungen, FRG) was used for CTP monitoring in all cases. To establish pressure recordings the tip of the catheter is placed approximately 1.5 cm into the surrounding cerebellar tissue or just left in the tumour cavity at the end of the operation (Fig. 1). The exact procedure and the technical data of the transducer have been described previously [2, 3].

Results

Recording data are given in Table 1. Postoperative CTP recordings were obtained in 16 cases. Of those, 12 patients had an uneventful postoperative course and showed no abnormalities on postoperative CT scans. CTP values in these patients remained below 20 mmHg and showed no abnormal pressure waves. The device was removed in all of these cases on the first or second postoperative day. Four patients developed postoperative complications (2 haemorrhages, 2 edemas). These were always followed by a rise in CTP above

Table 1. Clinical data: patient group and CTP recordings

Total: 18 patients
(Sex: 8 male, 10 female; Age: 26–71 years)

Diagnosis:
5 metastatic lesions
3 haemangioblastomas
3 ependymomas
2 meningiomas
1 acoustic schwannoma
1 medulloblastoma
2 spontaneous cerebellar haemorrhages
(all >6 cm in diameter)

Recording time: 16.75 to 204.75 hours (mean: 46.25 hours)
Pressure range: 0–121 (mean: 13.2) mm Hg

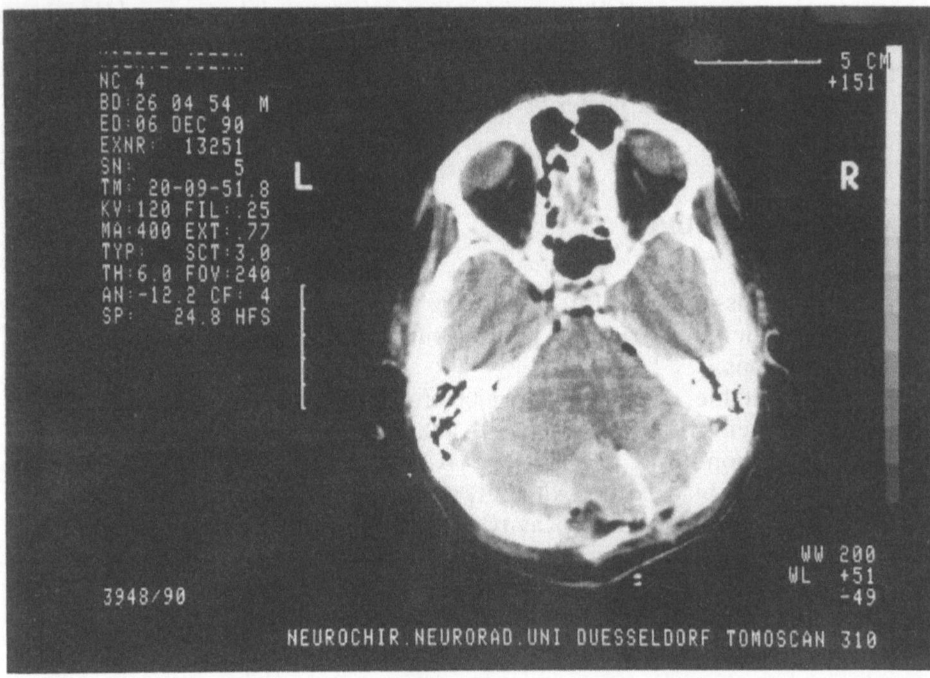

Fig. 1. Catheter (tip) in situ for CTP – monitoring

20 mmHg (mean) and subsequently treated by re-operation or conservative management. Three of these patients received an additional supratentorial ventricular catheter. ICP values showed typical signs of an impaired communication between the supra- and the infratentorial space with higher infratentorial pressures. Pressure differences up to 112 mmHg were observed in a patient who was clinically brain-stem dead with an "Alpha Coma".

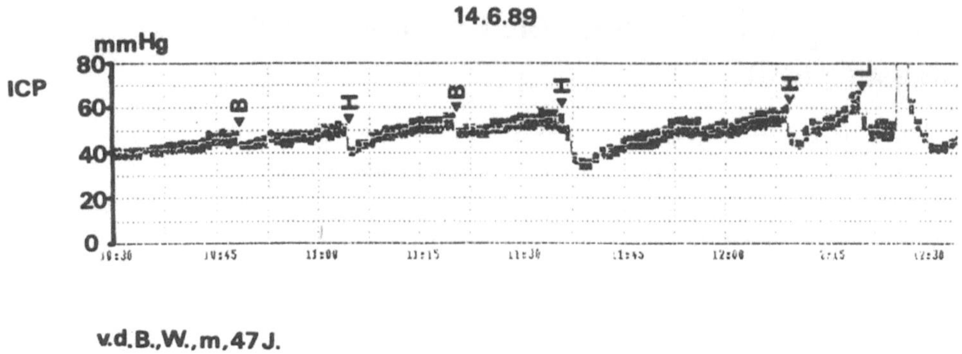

Fig. 2. Conservative management of raised infratentorial CTP by supratentorial CSF drainage (L), Hyperventilation (H), and barbiturate injection (B).

Brain stem auditory evoked potentials in all cases with impaired supa-/infratentorial CSF-communication revealed signs of inverse transtentorial herniation. In cases with infratentorial edema CTP recordings were able to guide conservative treatment (e.g. supratentorial CSF drainage, mannitol, barbiturates; Fig. 2). Medical treatment of elevated posterior fossa CTP, however, seemed to have less beneficial effects than in comparable cases with supratentorial elevated ICP.

No additional complication due to CTP monitoring was observed.

Conclusions

From our preliminary results we conclude that infratentorial monitoring of cerebral tissue pressure is a safe and reliable method which is especially indicated in cases of complicated infratentorial surgery.

References

1. Langfitt TW, Weinstein JD, Kassell NF, et al. (1964) Transmission of increased intracranial pressure. I. Within the craniospinal axis. J Neurosurg 21:989–997
2. Piek J, Kosub B, Küch F, et al. (1987) A practical technique for continuous monitoring of cerebral tissue pressure in neurosurgical patients. Acta Neurochir 87:144–149
3. Piek J, Bock WJ (1990) Continuous monitoring of cerebral tissue pressure in neurosurgical practice – experiences with 100 patients. Int Care Med 16:184–188
4. Rosenwasser RH, Kleiner LI, Krzeminski JP, et al. (1989) Intracranial pressure monitoring in the posterior fossa: a preliminary report. J Neurosurg 71:503–505

A Fiberoptic Device Suitable for Subdural Pressure Measurement

M. Yoshihara, A. Marmarou, J. Dunbar, D. Deyo, J. Weaver, N. Baldwin, M. Smith, and H.F. Young

Richard Roland Reynolds Neurosurgical Research Laboratories, Division of Neurosurgery, Medical College of Virginia, Richmond, VA, USA

Introduction

The benefit of ICP management has been clearly established in patients with severe brain injury. Elevated ICP above 20 mmHg should be avoided as it has been demonstrated that time above this critical level is correlated with poor outcome [1]. Although the monitoring of intracranial pressure by direct ventricular catheterization as introduced by Janny and Lundberg remains the gold standard, the recent introduction of fibre optic devices (FOD) for measurement of ICP has added a new dimension to ICP monitoring [2, 3]. Parenchymal recordings of ICP are now considered routine in many centers. However, the use of an FOD device in the subdural space and the relationship of subdural FOD pressure to tissue FOD and ventricular fluid pressure (VFP) pressure remains to be clarified. The objective of this study was to evaluate the capability of a highly flexible FOD device (Innerspace Inc. Irvine CA. USA) for measurement of subdural and tissue pressure in cats. A second objective was to determine the ability of parenchymal FOD's to reflect tissue pressure gradients in response to expansion of an epidural balloon and to determine whether these gradients are sustained.

Material and Methods

Eight adult cats weighing 2.4–3.2 kg were anesthetized with halothane (0.5–1.5%), mechanically ventilated and maintained normocapnic. The animals were positioned in a stereotactic frame and ventricular and cisternal fluid pressures and arterial blood pressure were monitored by fluid filled catheters connected to conventional gauges. The outer diameter of the new FOD measured 1.3 mm and was positioned in the subdural space through a burr hole 4 mm in diameter. The Innerspace FOD was compared to a Camino device for tissue pressure measurements and both were placed at 3 mm depth at symmetrical locations in the parietal white matter. A computer (Macintosh SE30) with specialized software recorded all pressures for at least 8 hours. Intermittent ICP elevation to 50 mmHg, using cisternal fluid injection at a rate of 0.35 ml/min, was performed five times during monitoring. Comparison of pressures was obtained from the average of these cycles. Abdominal compression, ventricular fluid injection (0.1 ml), hyper- and hypoventilation were also used to test the dynamics of the catheters under a variety of conditions.

In a parallel series of experiments using a similar preparation, the response of VFP, subdural pressure sensed by the Innerspace device (ISDP) and bilateral tissue pressure by Innerspace (ITP) and Camino (CTP) were studied in response to epidural balloon expansion study after intermittent ICP elevation. The epidural balloon was inserted in the right temporal area and inflated to 0.35 ml at a rate of 0.1 ml/min.

Results

Evaluation of Subdural FOD

The responses of subdural and tissue pressure catheters were similar to that of the ventricle during manipulations of fluid injection, abdominal compression, hyper- and hypoventilation. Typical examples of simultaneous recordings from all pressure monitors are shown in Fig. 1 recorded at a slow rate of speed. A high speed recording demonstrated the fidelity of the pulsatile pressure from each of the catheters.

Correlation of FOD Catheters with VFP

The Innerspace tissue, subdural and Camino tissue pressures were compared to VFP using linear regression. Each graph was derived from approximately 2000 data points of each pressure recording during the course of the experiment. Figure 2 demonstrates the typical graph of subdural pressure. The regressions indicate that the FOD catheters correlate well with VFP in both subdural and tissue placement (Table 1).

Epidural Balloon Expansion Study – Comparison of Tissue Pressures

The linear regression line of the right (balloon) side was always steeper, indicating the development of a tissue pressure gradient with the magnitude of gradient increasing with pressure.

Table 1. The average regression equation and correlation coefficient of all studies

	Regression equation	Correlation coefficient
Innerspace subdural pressure (ISDP)	VFP = 1.12 + 1.059 × ISDP	0.994 (sd = 0.007)
Innerspace tissue pressure (ITP)	VFP = 0.74 + 1.014 × ITP	0.995 (sd = 0.006)
Camino tissue pressure (CTP)	VFP = 1.84 + 0.952 × CTP	0.991 (sd = 0.005)

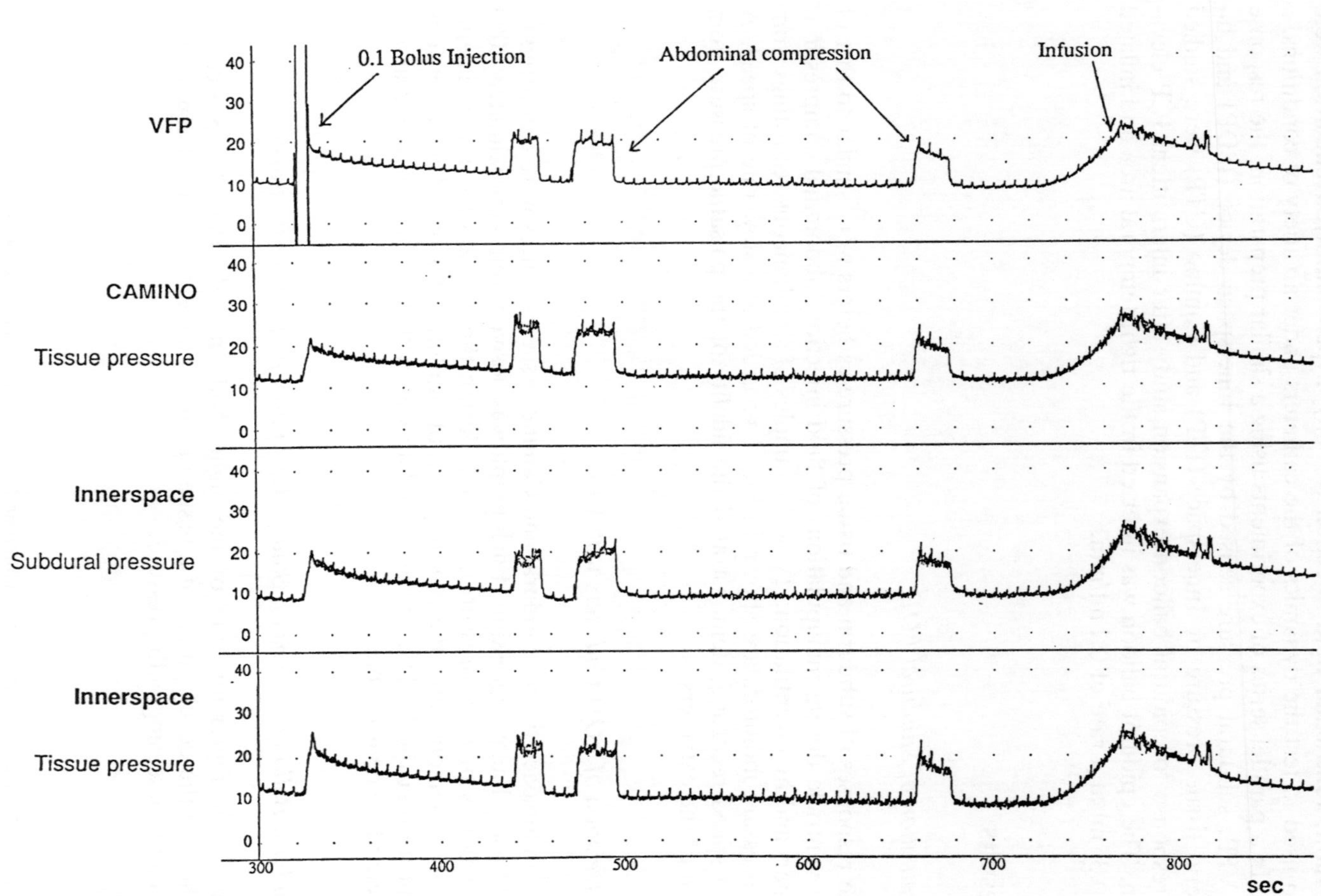

Fig. 1. Recording of various manipulations

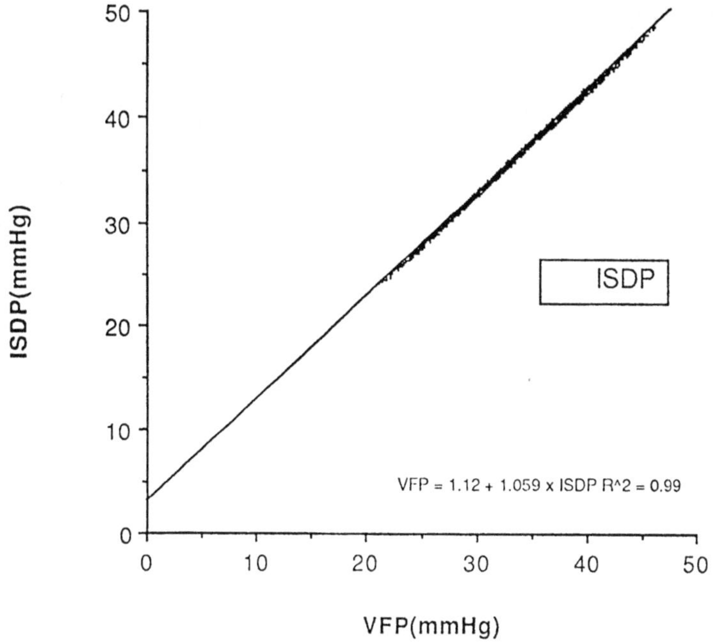

Fig. 2. VFP vs. ISDP (Innerspace subdural pressure)

Comparison of Subdural and Tissue Pressure Adjacent to Balloon

When the balloon was inflated, tissue pressure increased to 70 mmHg. The tissue pressure on the balloon side was slightly greater than the subdural pressure indicating the development of a maximum tissue-subdural gradient of 5 mmHg.

Comparison of VFP and Tissue Pressure in Hemisphere Opposite to Balloon

The VFP measured in the left ventricle was very close to that of the left tissue pressure catheter indicating that the tissue pressure tends to follow the local fluid compartment.

Dissipation of Tissue Pressure Gradients

When the balloon was inflated to increase VFP to 70 mmHg, a tissue pressure gradient developed between left and right hemispheres with pressure on the balloon side greater than in the contralateral hemisphere. The maximum tissue pressure gradient reached 7.0 mmHg at a corresponding VFP of 70 mmHg. This tissue pressure gradient gradually declined during a period of 30 minutes and stabilized at a fixed gradient of 2 mmHg at one hour.

Discussion

Ventricle fluid pressure is considered the average intracranial pressure and is regarded as the gold standard from which other devices are compared. However, the measurements of ICP at other sites not requiring tissue penetration have reduced the risk of complications. Subdural pressure measurement shares this advantage and is being used more widely. Heretofore, subdural measurement was restricted to fluid coupled devices. Our experimental study of the Innerspace catheter confirmed that tissue pressure and subdural pressure measured by this new device was identical to ventricle fluid pressure and Camino tissue pressure when elevated by cisternal infusion up to 50 mmHg. Moreover, the wave forms were in correspondence to those measured from the lateral ventricle. The balloon study showed the development of a brain tissue pressure gradient as pressure was increased. This gradient averaged approximately 10% of baseline pressure. However, other investigators have reported that tissue pressure ipsilateral and contralateral to an expanding epidural mass developed equal pressures. We suspect that a small gradient may be hidden by limitation of the recording method. In our studies, data were recorded and calibrated by computer which provided increased sensitivity and accuracy. This recording system allowed us to analyze ICP at higher sampling rates and subtract one pressure from the other easily to enhance the resolution of detecting small pressure gradients. These gradients were found to dissipate slowly within 30 minutes and small sustained gradients of 2 mmHg were observed at one hour. The observed reduction of pressure gradient over time is attributed to brain relaxation and accommodation of the expanding mass by other fluid compartments. We conclude that the new FOD is capable of providing an accurate recording of pressure and its unique flexibility allows placement in the subdural space, particularly in the lesion side where the pressure might be higher.

References

1. Alberico AM, Ward JD, Choi SC, Marmarou A, Young HF (1987) Outcome after severe head injury. J Neurosurg 67:648–656
2. Crutchfield JS, Narayan RK, Robertson CS, Michael LH (1990) Evaluation of a fiber optic intracranial pressure monitor. J Neurosurg 72:482–487
3. Chambers IR, Mendelow AD, Sinar E, Modha P (1990) A Clinical Evaluation of the Camino Subdural Screw and Ventricular Monitoring Kits. Neurosurgery 26:421–423

Anterior Fontanelle Pressure Monitoring in Infants

W.C.G. Overweg-Plandsoen[1], D.A. de Jong[3], M.C.B. Loonen[2], C.J.J. Avezaat[3], J.H.M. van Eijndhoven[4], and P.G.H. Mulder[5]

[1]Department of Pediatric Neurology, Academic Medical Center, Meibergdreef 9, 1105 AZ Amsterdam, The Netherlands
[2]Departments of Pediatric Neurology, [3]Neurosurgery and [4]Automation Informatics, Academic Hospital Dijkzigt, Dr Molewaterplein 40, 3015 GD Rotterdam, The Netherlands
[5]Department of Biostatistics, Erasmus University, Ee 2461a, P.O. Box 1738, 3000 DR Rotterdam, The Netherlands

Introduction

With the introduction of the lumbar puncture by Quincke [9], one century ago, the possibility of examining the cerebrospinal fluid (CSF) and of measuring the cerebrospinal fluid pressure (CSFP) was born. When continuous recording of intracranial pressure (ICP) became possible in clinical practice [4] a new dimension was given to research in the field of intracranial hypertension. In adult patients there are several indications for measuring ICP, e.g. in head-injury. The prognosis in these patients is poorer when ICP is higher [5]. In pediatric patients there are special indications for measuring ICP such as intraventricular haemorrhage in prematures and newborns, (posthaemorrhagic) hydrocephalus, bacterial meningitis, hypoxic-ischaemic encephalopathy and Reye's syndrome. Most techniques for monitoring ICP are invasive and many clinicians are reluctant to use those on younger children because of the infection risk and the technical problems, especially when longer monitoring periods are necessary. In children with an open fontanelle there is a natural access to the intracranial compartment; therefore, non-invasive anterior fontanelle pressure (AFP) monitoring seems an ideal method for measuring ICP. Up to today physicists and clinicians turned out to be geniuses in developing a large number of different devices for AFP monitoring. In reviewing all reports on non-invasive measuring devices it is clear that application and fixation methods are not standardized. Due to the different fixation procedures of the devices, application pressure tends to interfere with the actual pressure measurement. Few authors developed special holders for their measuring device, trying to overcome the problem of application pressure [2].

In the experimental neurological and neurosurgical department of the University Hospital of Rotterdam an implantable, stable, telemetric transducer with a fast dynamic response has been developed for epidural pressure (EDP) measurements in adult patients [1]. After developing a special light weight skull adaptor for this Rotterdam Teletransducer (RTT) it was possible to measure AFP reliably. Using the special skull adaptor and the soft, silicone fixation frame, the application pressure does not interfere with the actual ICP measurement since surplus of application pressure runs off to the skull [8]. With this fixation frame short term and long term (continuous) measurements were feasible. We tested this measuring device in a clinical setting. Normal

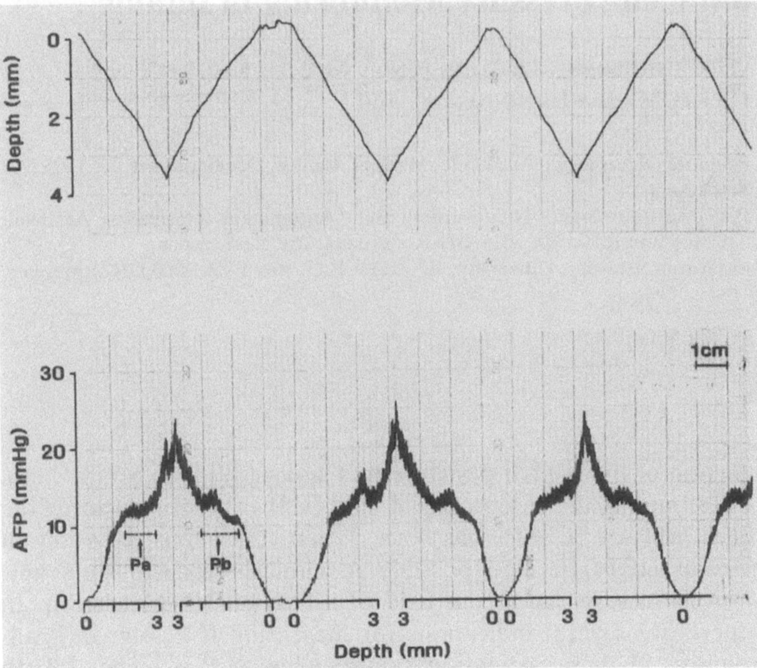

Fig. 1. Part of an AFP recording in an infant showing three consecutive pressure depth curves (PDC's). Pa = ascending plateau of the PDC, Pb = descending plateau of the PDC

values for AFP were gathered and AFP measurements were done in patients. The results of these investigations will be presented.

Material and Methods

AFP Recordings

For the recording of AFP we used the RTT in the special skull adaptor and fixation frame [6, 8]. Accurate depth positioning of the transducer is essential; this is done manually. The accurate depth of the RTT is determined by performing the pressure depth curve (PDC). The plateau in the PDC represents actual ICP. By repeatedly applying the RTT subsequent identical pressure recordings can be obtained (Fig. 1). These curves resemble the ones described by Schettini and Walsh [10] during epidural pressure measurements. The AFP value is calculated as the average of the ascending plateau (Pa) and the descending plateau (Pb). In each recording the AFP value was calculated as the average of the AFP values of the first three PDC's with clearly discernable plateau's.

Normal Babies

In 82 healthy newborns and infants normal values of AFP were established. These children were divided into two groups according to age (Group I: 30 newborns, 0–9 days, Group II: 52 infants, 30–330 days). The results are reported in a separate paper.

Patients

In 141 pediatric patients with various neurological and non-neurological diseases 253 AFP measurements were performed. The age of the patients ranged from 30 weeks gestational age to 24 months calender age.

Continuous Measurements

In 48 of the patients a total of 79 continuous (lasting for 30 minutes or more) AFP measurements were performed with a maximal duration of 39 hours. All recordings were analyzed for the calculation of the mean AFP value and the occurrence of specific wave forms such as A-waves or B-waves [4].

Pre- and Postoperative Measurements

In 23 patients with hydrocephalus a total number of 52 AFP measurements was performed before and after 26 shunting procedures to evaluate the effect of the operation on the level of ICP.

Comparitive Measurements

In 13 patients with neurological diseases 16 comparitive measurements were done between AFP and CSFP. The techniques were puncture of the fontanelle, the ventricle (during operation), the Rickham reservoir, or the lumbar space with a needle connected to either an open end or closed manometer.

Statistics

Data are represented as mean ± standard deviation (SD). For the statistical analysis the Kruskal-Wallis test, the Mann-Whitney U-test and the Wilcoxon test were used. A p-value <0.05 was considered to be significant.

Results

In the group of normal babies the mean AFP value in Group I was 8.9 ± 3.0 mmHg. In Group II mean AFP was 11.0 ± 1.9 mmHg. There was a

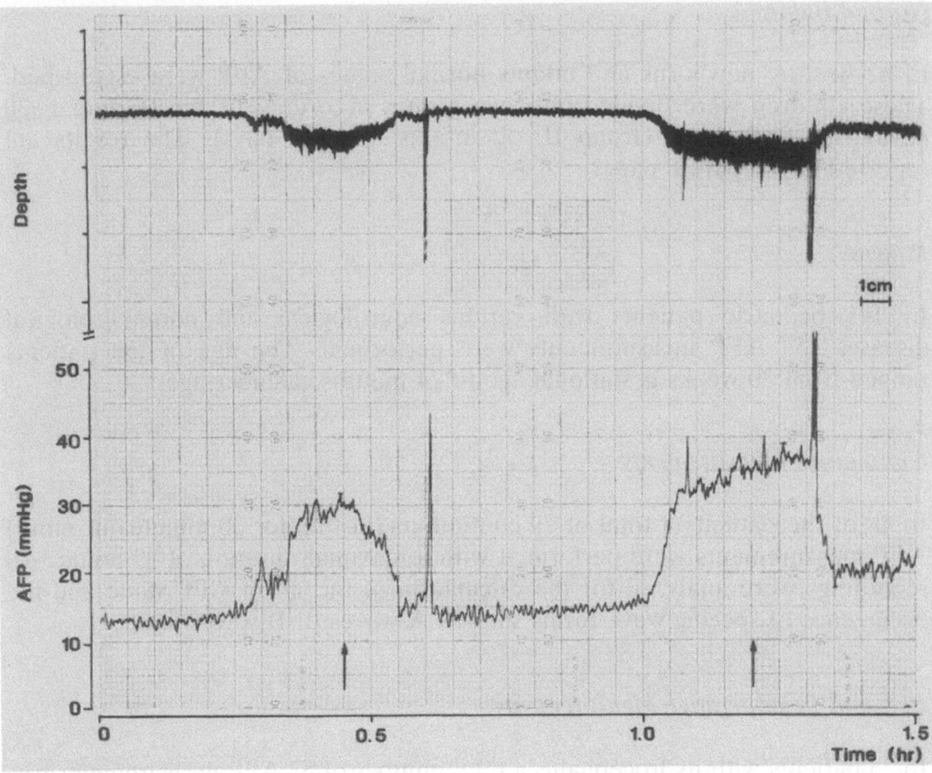

Fig. 2. Part of the continuous AFP recording in an infant with hydrocephalus showing two A-waves (arrows) occurring within one hour. The baseline pressures are 13.8 and 17.8 mmHg, the peak level pressures are 31.6 and 38.9 mmHg

statistically significant difference between the mean AFP value of Group I and Group II.

In the patient group all children with clinical signs of raised ICP and hydrocephalus established by ultrasound or CT scan of the brain had AFP values above 15 mmHg. In children with non-neurological diseases normal AFP levels were usually found [6]. In evaluating the continuous AFP recordings there was no significant difference between the visually estimated AFP level and the calculated AFP level (Wilcoxon $p = 0.2 = NS$). B-waves and A-waves were recorded in a number of patients e.g. in patients with hydrocephalus. An example of such a recording is shown in Fig. 2.

AFP monitoring was tested on 23 patients in whom 26 shunting operations or revisions were performed. The results of the 52 AFP measurements before and after operation are shown in Fig. 3. The average AFP level of the recordings before operation was 23.0 ± 7.9 mmHg and 12.7 ± 4.0 mmHg after operation. The difference was statistically significant (Wilcoxon $p < 0.01$).

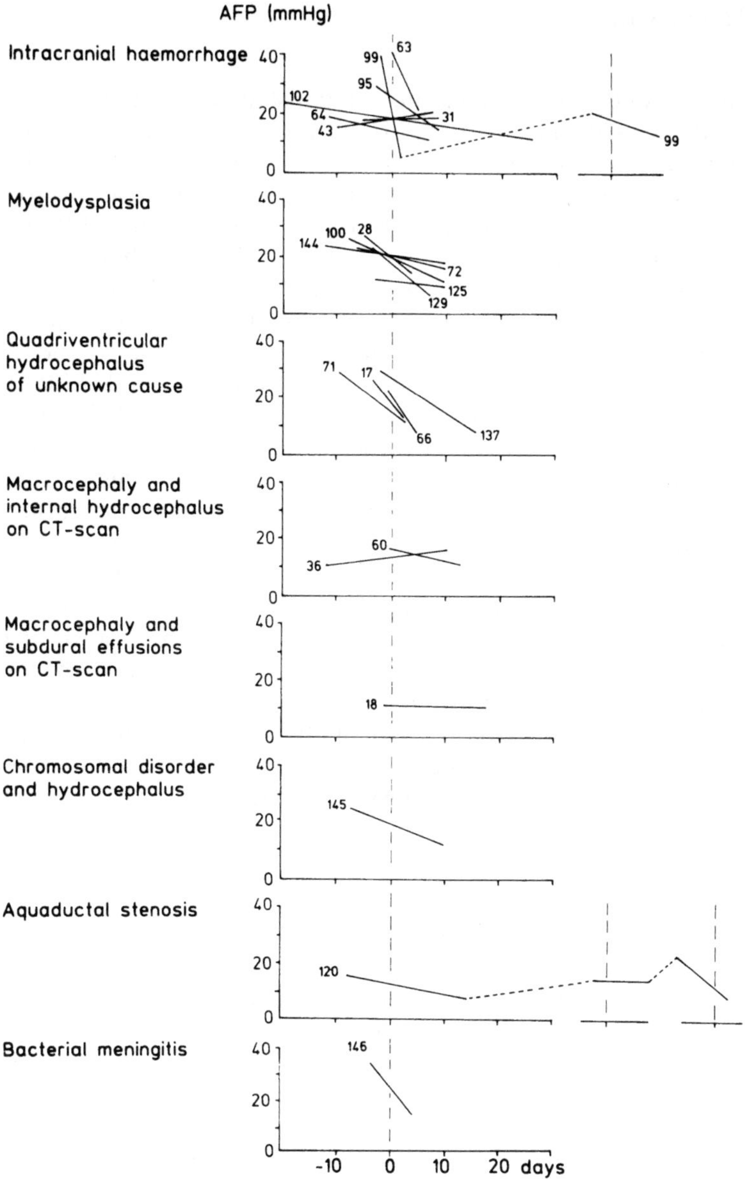

Fig. 3. Effect of a shunting or shunt revising operation on the level of ICP in 23 patients. Pre- and postoperative AFP values (mmHg) of 26 operations are represented according to the time of the pre- and postoperative measurements (days). The patients are identified by their number. The vertical broken lines represent the time of operation

In infants with low pressures (<10 mmHg) the difference between AFP and CSFP was less than one mmHg. If AFP was above 15 mmHg the difference between AFP and CSFP measured with an open end manometer was between 3.0 and 10.4 mmHg. The closed type comparitive measurements showed a good relationship of AFP and CSFP with a mean difference of 1.9 mmHg.

Discussion

In this study an age-pressure relationship was established [7]. This is in accordance with the literature. In all patients with clinical overt signs of raised ICP and hydrocephalus AFP values of more than 15 mmHg were found. In children with minor clinical signs of raised ICP, such as macrocephaly, elevated pressure levels were not always found. If continuous AFP measurements were performed it was sometimes possible to detect either an elevated AFP level during sleep or to detect A-waves and B-waves. The shape of the A-waves was different from the A-waves found in adult patients probably due to a greater expansibility of the skull. The amplitudes of both the A- and the B-waves could be easily determined. In a few patients an elevated AFP level was already detected before clinical signs of raised ICP appeared. In these cases AFP was indicative of developing hydrocephalus. The pre- and postoperative AFP measurements showed, as expected, a significant decrease of AFP after the shunt operation. Shunt dysfunction could be detected during follow-up measurements. Although the number of comparitive measurements was few, a good relationship between AFP and CSFP could be established. When an open end manometer was used and AFP was raised the difference in pressure levels was greater. This is easily understood, since in the range of higher pressures the compliance is lower and the craniospinal system is changing from the flat part to the steep part of the volume-pressure curve resulting in a greater change in pressure in non-isovolumetric measurement [3]. AFP monitoring, in combination with neurological examination and brain-imaging techniques, is a valuable dynamic tool to answer the question whether a child has to be shunted or not?

Conclusions

In children with an open fontanelle AFP monitoring is superior to invasive methods, however, only if proper attention is paid to the measuring device and to its application on the fontanelle. The ideal fixation method should overcome the influence of application forces in order not to interfere with the actual ICP measurement. With the RTT in the special skull adaptor and fixation frame the externally exerted pressure does not interfere with the pressure recording since surplus of application force runs off to the skull. With this reliable method we gathered normal values of AFP. These values were in accordance with the literature. In patients with signs of raised ICP elevated levels of AFP could be detected. The continuous measurements were all successful. A-waves and B-waves were monitored with this non-invasive method. Drain function could be checked. The few comparitive measurements with a closed manometer showed a good relationship between AFP and CSFP. In addition to clinical signs and ancillary examinations in patients with various neurological and non-neurological diseases, both short term and continuous measurement of ICP via the anterior fontanelle seem valuable parameters in deciding whether a child needs to be shunted or not.

References

1. Jong DA de, Maas AIR, Berfelo MW, Ouden AH den, Lange SA de (1982) The Rotterdam Teletransducer: A telemetric device for measuring epidural pressure. Biotelemetry Patient Monitg 9:154–165
2. Horbar JD, Yeager S, Philip AGS, Lucey JF (1980) Effect of application force on non-invasive measurement of intracranial pressure. Pediatrics 66:455–457
3. Löfgren J, Essen C von, Zwetnow NN (1973) The pressure-volume curve of the cerebrospinal fluid space in dogs. Acta Neurol Scand 49:557–574
4. Lundberg N (1960) Continuous recording and control of ventricular fluid pressure in neurosurgical practice. Acta Psych Neurol Scand 36, Suppl 149:1–193
5. Miller JD (1985) Intracranial pressure monitoring. Arch Neurol 42:1191–1193
6. Overweg-Plandsoen WCG (1990) Anterior Fontanelle Pressure Monitoring in Infants. Thesis, Erasmus University Rotterdam, pp 123
7. Philip AGS, Long JG, Donn SM (1981) Intracranial pressure. Sequential measurements in full-term and preterm infants. Am J Dis Chil 135:521–524
8. Plandsoen WCG, Jong DA de, Maas AIR, Stroink H, Eijndhoven JHM van (1986) The pressure depth curve in anterior fontanelle pressure monitoring. In: Miller JD, Teasdale GM, Rowan JO, Galbraith SL, Mendelow AD (eds) Intracranial pressure VI. Springer, Berlin Heidelberg New York Tokyo, pp 193–198
9. Quincke H (1891) Die Lumbalpunktion des Hydrocephalus. Berl Klin Wochenschr 28:929–933
10. Schettini A, Walsh EK (1974) Experimental identification of the subarachnoid and subpial compartments by intracranial pressure measurements. J Neurosurg 40:609–616

Anterior Fontanelle Pressure Values in Normal Young Children of Various Ages

W.C.G. Overweg-Plandsoen[1], D.A. de Jong[3], M.C.B. Loonen[2], P.W. Hanlo[4], and C.J.J. Avezaat[3]

[1] Department of Childneurology[1], Academic Medical Center, Meibergdreef 9, 1105 AZ Amsterdam, The Netherlands
[2] Departments of Childneurology and [3] Neurosurgery, Academic Hospital Dijkzigt, Dr Molewaterplein 40, 3015 GD Rotterdam, The Netherlands
[4] Department of Childneurology, University Hospital, Heidelberglaan 100, 3584 CX Utrecht, The Netherlands

Introduction

Every new measuring technique for use in human beings requires its own "normal values". For the purpose of establishing normal values of anterior fontanelle pressure (AFP) with the Rotterdam Teletransducer (RTT) [1] in the fontanelle-adaptor [7] we investigated a number of healthy infants of various ages. A positive relationship between intracranial pressure (ICP) and age was reported earlier [6, 9]. We wondered whether with this non-invasive method also an age/pressure relationship could be established.

The aims of the study were: (1) To record AFP in normal newborns and infants and to estimate its normal range. (2) To study the relation between AFP and age of newborns and infants.

Material and Methods

Eighty-two infants were studied, divided into two groups. *Group I* consisted of 30 newborn babies (12 males, 18 females) aged 0–9 days. These babies were born in the obstetrical ward of the University Hospital of Rotterdam. *Group II* consisted of 52 infants (28 males, 24 females) aged 30–330 days. These infants were measured in the child health clinic in the "Zevenkamp" district of Rotterdam.

AFP Recordings

AFP was recorded with the Rotterdam Teletransducer (RTT) in the special skull adaptor and fixation frame [7, 3, 4]. The application pressure does not interfere with the actual measured pressure since surplus of application force runs off to the skull [7, 3]. During each AFP recording a number of at least three pressure depth curves (PDC's) was performed. An example of such a PDC is shown elsewhere in this book [4].

Statistical Analysis

Data are presented as mean ± standard deviation (SD). Differences in AFP between the various age classes both in Group I and in Group II were assessed with the Kruskal-Wallis test, a non-parametric test. Differences in AFP between Group I and Group II were assessed with the Mann-Whitney U-test. A p-value <0.05 was considered to be significant.

Results

In Group I the mean value of AFP was 8.9 ± 3.0 mmHg. Figure 1 shows the AFP values, including the median and the range, for each age class. There was no statistical difference between the various age classes in group I ($p = 0.65$ = NS). In Group II the mean value of AFP was 11.0 ± 1.9 mmHg. Figure 2 shows the AFP values, including the median and the range, for each age class. There was no statistical difference between the age classes in group II ($p = 0.49$ = NS). There was a statistically significant difference between the mean AFP value of Group I and the mean AFP value of Group II ($p < 0.01$).

Discussion

It is necessary to distinguish between invasive and non-invasive methods. By means of invasive techniques for measuring ICP in preterm and term babies lower pressures were recorded than in older children [6]. Also with non-

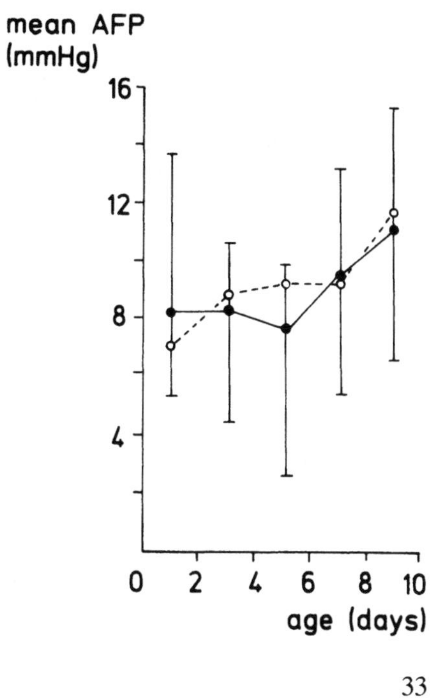

Fig. 1. Mean AFP values (mmHg) for each age class in Group I including the median and the range. AFP values are represented by closed circles, the median by open circles and the range by vertical bars

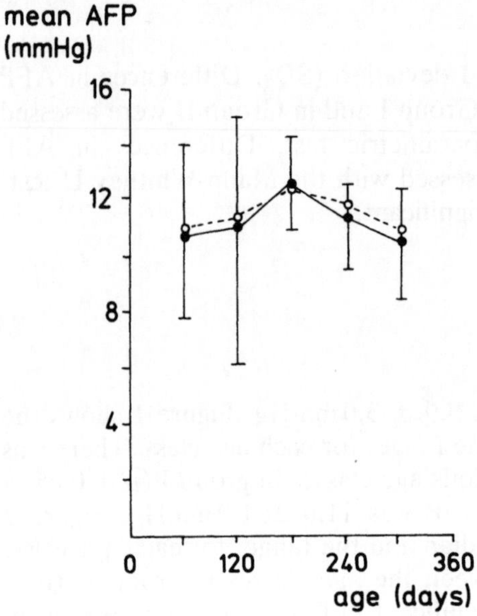

Fig. 2. Mean AFP values (mmHg) for each age class in Group II including the median and the range. AFP values are represented by closed circles, the median by open circles and the range by vertical bars

invasive techniques an age/pressure relationship was established [5, 8]. Why infants have lower ICP levels than adults is not exactly clear. Methods for measuring AFP vary, as do the fixation procedures. This could explain some of the differences in recorded AFP levels. Another explanation might be found in some of the parameters of the "steady state" condition (Pss = RoFi + Pd), implying equal CSF-formation and CSF absorption rates [2].

Further Research

Intracranial pressure values in prematures need attention. A frequently occurring problem in these patients is haemorrhage and (post-haemorrhagic) hydrocephalus. If normal pressure values are even lower than the values found in newborns then the "pathological values" are also at a lower level. Non-invasive ICP monitoring with the RTT offers the possibility to establish normal AFP values and to gain more insight into this interesting problem.

Conclusions

Normal AFP values recorded with the RTT are within the range of AFP values reported in the literature and obtained with other non-invasive methods. The difference in mean AFP values between newborns (Group I) and infants (Group II) is statistically significant and in accordance with age dependent AFP levels reported by others.

The mechanism of the lower ICP levels in young children is still not well understood.

References

1. Jong DA de, Maas AIR, Berfelo MW, Ouden AH den, Lange SA de (1982) The Rotterdam Teletransducer: A telemetric device for epidural pressure. Biotelemetry Patient Monitg 9:154–165
2. Marmarou A, Shulman K, LaMorgese J (1975) Compartmental analysis of compliance and outflow resistance of the cerebrospinal fluid system. J Neurosurg 43:523–534
3. Overweg-Plandsoen WCG (1990) Anterior fontanelle pressure monitoring in infants. Thesis, Erasmus University Rotterdam, pp 123
4. Overweg-Plandsoen WCG, Jong DA de, Loonen MCB, Avezaat CJJ, Eijndhoven JHM van, Mulder PGH (1991/2) Anterior Fontanelle Pressure monitoring in Infants. In: Avezaat CJJ, van Eijndhoven JHM, Maas AIR, Tans JThJ (eds) Intracranial Pressure VIII. Springer, Berlin Heidelberg New York Tokyo
5. Peabody JL, Schneider H, Huch R, Huch A (1981) A new device for non- invasive measurements of intracranial pressure (ICP) in newborns. J Perinat Med 9, suppl 1:125–128
6. Philip AGS, Long JG, Donn SM (1981) Intracranial pressure. Sequential measurements in full-term and preterm infants. Am J Dis Child 135:521–524
7. Plandsoen WCG, Jong DA de, Maas AIR, Stroink H, Avezaat CJJ (1987) Fontanelle Pressure monitoring with the Rotterdam Teletransducer; a reliable technique. Med Progr Technol 13:21–27
8. Vidyasagar D, Raju TNK (1977) A simple non-invasive technique of measuring intracranial pressure in the newborn. Pediatrics 59:957–961
9. Welch K (1980) The intracranial pressure in infants. J Neurosurg 52:693–699

A New Way to Monitor External Ventricular Drainage

G. BOULARD[1], P. RAVUSSIN[2], C. GROSS[3], and J. GUÉRIN[4]

[1] Neuro-Intensive Care Unit, Pellegrin Hospital, 33076 Bordeaux, France
[2] Anesthesiology Department, CHUV, 1011 Lausanne, Switzerland
[3] URA 1200 CNRS, University of Bordeaux II, 33076 Bordeaux, France
[4] Neurosurgery Department, Pellegrin Hospital, 33076 Bordeaux, France

Introduction

External ventricular drainage (EVD) is mainly used in the treatment of intracranial hypertension and when problems occur in the circulation or reabsorption of cerebrospinal fluid (CSF) [3]. EVD exposes the brain to infectious and mechanical complications [1]. Much has been said about infection caused by EVD. This is not the case for the mechanical problems which can seriously endanger the therapeutic efficiency of EVD and cause clinical aggravation. Mechanical complications occur due to an obstruction, especially if the CSF is hemorrhagic or rich in proteins. In some rare cases, this is caused by a kink in the drainage line. Finally, if the system is wrongly adjusted, it can cause limitations or exaggerations in the CSF drainage. Disconnection can also occur. Once the EVD is in place, monitoring is mandatory. Up to now, surveillance has basically required repeated checking of the level of liquid in the bag, and/or the presence of a drip. Clinical experience shows that this type of surveillance is difficult, giving rise to delayed diagnosis of an obstruction of EVD with worsening of the patient's neurological condition. The authors have thus put forward the hypothesis that a system based on continual weighing of the drained CSF should provide a useful and reliable means of monitoring EVD.

Equipment and Methods

With the approval of the Departmental Ethics Committee and the informed consent of a next of kin, 16 intubated and ventilated comatose patients (11 males, 5 females, age 40.9 ± 6 years (range 6–71 yrs)) were studied. Eleven of the cases were subarachnoid and/or ventricular hemorrhages and 5 cases hydrocephalus.

EVD was at all times performed using the Codman system (ventricular catheter 82-1705 and drainage bag 82-1688, Codman and Smurtleff, Randolph, Massachussetts, USA). The CSF bag was hung from the socle of an electronic Sartorius 1401 balance, characterized by a precision of 0.01 g (Sartorius, Göttingen, Germany). This balance had first to be zeroed on an empty bag. It was then connected via a digital/analogue converter (Sartorius 7287) to a low speed recorder (Siemens Kompensograph, Siemens, Erlangen, Germany)

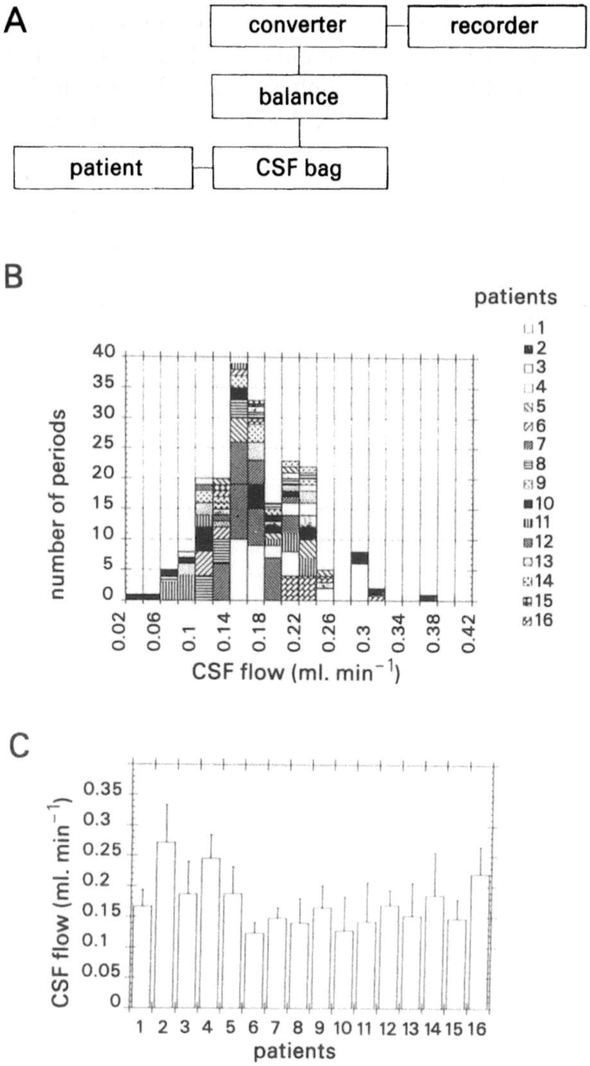

Fig. 1. A Schematic view of the installation. **B** Distribution of the 204 flows observed in the 16 patients. **C** Mean flow for each of the 16 patients (mean value ± SD)

(Fig. 1A) which graphically displays the CSF weight (4 cm = 100 g) as a function of time (3 cm = 1 hr) i.e. flow, in ml.min^{-1} if the specific gravity of the CSF is 1, which is usually the case as an approximation. Results are presented as means ± SD.

Results

The EVD monitoring was used for 4632 hours in 16 patients with a total of 204 recorded periods with a mean duration of 22.7 hours ±2.8 (range 14.6–39.5 hrs).

The mean number of recorded periods per patient was 12.7 ± 6.8 (range 2–25). For the 16 patients the lowest flow per period was 0.03 ml.min^{-1} (patient 10) and the highest was 0.37 ml.min^{-1} (patient 2) (Fig. 1B). Mean flow was then calculated for each patient taking all his recorded periods into account. The lowest mean flow per patient was 0.12 ± 0.02 ml.min^{-1} (patient 6) and the highest was 0.27 ± 0.06 ml.min^{-1} (patient 2) (Fig. 1C). For the 204 periods (4632 hrs), mean flow was 0.17 ± 0.05 ml.min^{-1}.

For each patient, CSF flow was stable during each recorded period. However, it could vary from one period to another i.e. from one day to another. To show this variability for each patient and between the patients, the

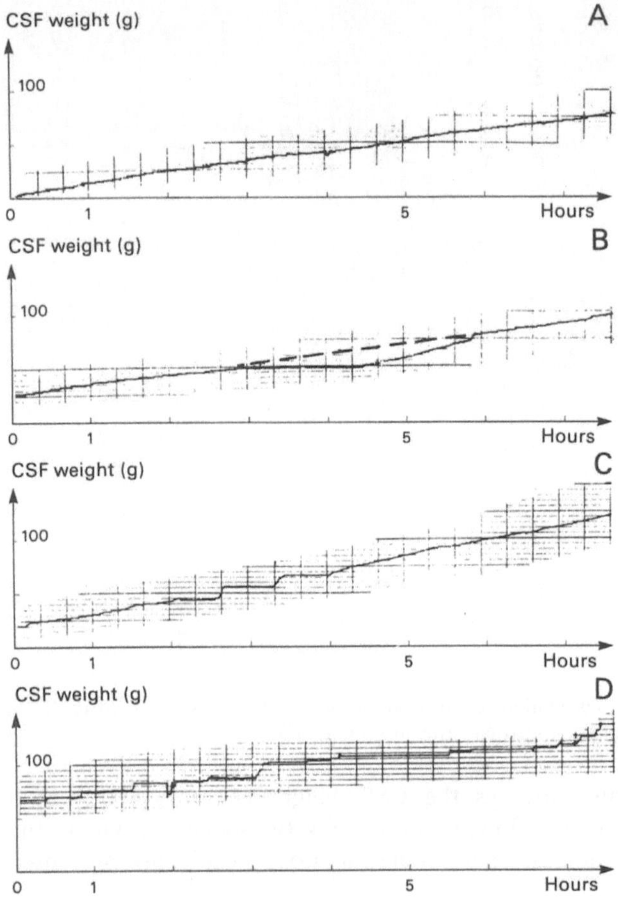

Fig. 2. A Continuous recording, normal graph. **B** Type 1 modification of the normal graph: stoppage in the drainage (plateau) followed by an increased CSF flow (increased slope) due to the rapid restitution of the exact amount of accumulated CSF. **C** Type 2 modification of the normal graph: the patient coughed twice; brief flush of CSF (increased slope) due to the increased CBV followed by a stoppage of the CSF flow (plateau) until the CSF secretion has compensated for the sudden ventricular loss. **D** Successive plateaus separated by short episodes of CSF flow due to nociceptive stimuli (increased slope)

flow of each recorded period was compared to the mean flow per patient. Thus each recorded period had a Δ which varied from 0 to 0.12 $ml.min^{-1}$ (patient 2). When averaging out these Δ for each patient, a mean Δ per patient was obtained ranging from 0.013 ± 0.01 $ml.min^{-1}$ (patient 7) to 0.06 ± 0.02 $ml.min^{-1}$ (patient 11). Mean Δ for the 16 patients was 0.034 ± 0.01 $ml.min^{-1}$ which corresponds to 19.5% of the mean CSF flow.

In 79.9% of the periods, the recorded curve appeared oblique with a stable CSF flow (Fig. 2A). On this oblique curve 2 types of occurences were noted: *Type 1 modification of the graph*: the oblique curve becomes horizontal (Fig. 2B). This phenomenon was observed 18 times and was due to an accidental stop in the ventricular drainage. Fifteen times, manipulation of the drainage tube was sufficient to solve the problem. On three occasions, a new EVD had to be inserted. Once the drainage was restored, CSF flow was higher than before, represented graphically by an increased slope of the oblique curve until the initial equilibrium was regained (Fig. 2B); *Type 2 modification of the graph*: a brief increase in the slope is followed by a plateau becoming progressively oblique again with the same slope (Fig. 2C). This sudden increase in the CSF flow occured when a nociceptive stimulus was applied to the patient or when he coughed and was followed by a pause of variable duration.

In 41 of the 204 periods (20.1%), observed in 3 patients, the curve was different. The recording shows a succession of plateaus separated by a brief increase in the slope (Fig. 2D). Only nociceptive stimuli and/or coughing created a CSF flow.

Discussion

By continuously recording the weight of the CSF bag during EVD, the CSF flow can be graphically visualized. It has to be pointed out that the observed flow is not equal to its rate of secretion, but rather to the difference between CSF secretion and reabsorption. In most of the cases studied, the observed CSF flow was stable in the same period, but it could vary from one period to another and from one patient to another by around 19.5%.

Type 1 modification of the graph, i.e. the normal ascending curve becomes a plateau, indicates that CSF drainage has suddenly stopped. Such a change of form of the graph immediately necessitates a search for the cause of the obstruction in the drainage, which can be a simple kink or a clot or pus, before the patient's neurological state deteriorates. Often simple adjustments may be sufficient to solve the problem. Rarely does a new drain have to be inserted.

Type 2 modification of the graph represents a brief CSF flush due to a sudden increase in the cerebral blood volume (CBV) caused by coughing and/or a rise in mean arterial pressure (MAP) in a patient with impaired autoregulation in whom nociceptive stimuli are applied [2].

The increases in CSF flow which occur in a mirror-like fashion in Type 1 and Type 2 modifications of the graph are easily explained. In the first case, CSF ventricular volume is increased due to drainage obstruction (plateau on the graph). Once the obstruction has been cleared, there is a rapid restitution

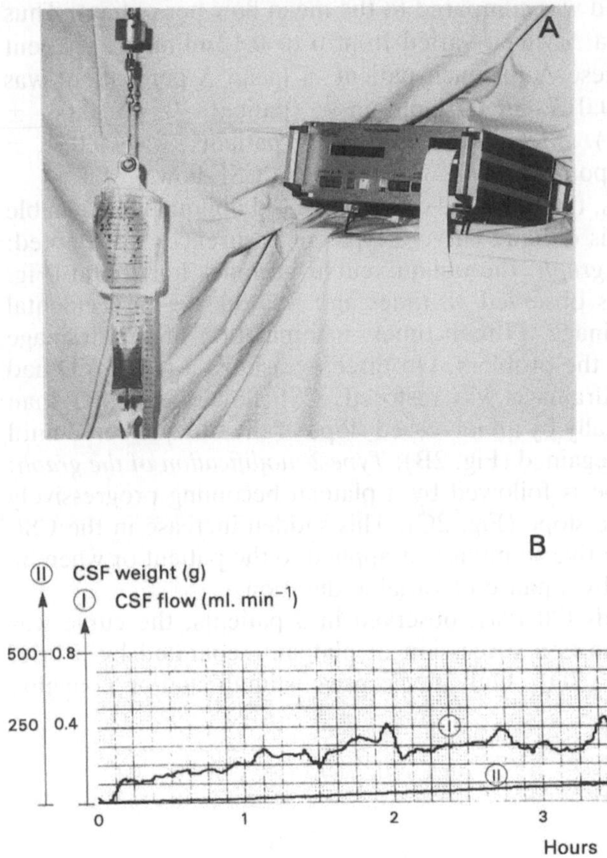

Fig. 3. **A** The compact device under investigation. **B** Example of the obtained recording – Curve I: CSF instantaneous flow, 4 cm = 0.8 ml.min^{-1} Curve II: Cumulated CSF weighing, 4 cm = 500 ml

of the exact amount of accumulated CSF (increased slope). Conversely, in the second case, following the Monro-Kellie hypothesis, the instantaneous rise in CBV, due to coughing or an increase in MAP, causes a brief CSF flush (increased slope) followed by a stoppage in the flow until the CSF secretion has compensated for this sudden ventricular loss (plateau).

The clinical situation, noted in only 3 patients (20.1% of the studied periods), where there was no slope on the graph but successive plateaus separated by brief CSF flushes due to nociceptive stimuli, evokes an efficient CSF absorption with a controllable ICP, and gives rise to the question of the clinical use of EVD. The answer must take into account the clinical and evolutive data of this kind of patient.

From the data and the experience gained from this study, a compact device was designed following the same principle of continuous weighing of the CSF, and manufactured by Sepame Inc., Chambray-les Tours, France. It works with a gauge extentiometer and is equipped with adjustable alarms of minimum and maximum flow, and a variable recuperation period also adjustable. The values are displayed as a continuous graph (monitoring function) and as a curve of instantaneous flow in $ml.min^{-1}$ which also appears as a digital display. This monitor is presently undergoing investigation.

Conclusion

The hypothesis that continuous weighing of the CSF bag of EVD could be a safe and accurate way to monitor the drainage system has been confirmed. This simple and non invasive device, by providing a visual display in $ml.min^{-1}$, ensures continuous monitoring of the CSF flow in real time. It helps to immediately detect a stoppage in the CSF flow, before any worsening of the patient's neurological condition. It indicates precisely when to look for the cause of the CSF flow interruption and to restore the initial situation. It can help to evaluate the utility of EVD in place. Futhermore, it could help to study CSF secretion and absorption in the framework of the disease but also their variations due to certain drugs, although the absorbed CSF fraction is not known in EVD.

References

1. Saunders RL, Lyons TA (1979) External ventricular drainage: a technical note. Critical Care Med 7:556–558
2. Shapiro HM (1975) Intracranial hypertension: therapeutic and anesthetic considerations. Anesthesiology 43:445–471
3. Shapiro HM, Drummond JC (1990) Neurological anesthesia and intracranial hypertension. In: Miller RD (ed) Anesthesia, 3rd edn. Churchill Livingstone, New York Edinburgh London Melbourne, pp 1747–1749

Post Traumatic Cerebrospinal Fluid Infections in the Traumatic Coma Data Bank: The Influence of the Type and Management of ICP Monitors

T.G. Luerssen[1], R.M. Chesnut[2], M. Van Berkum-Clark[2], L.F. Marshall[2], M.R. Klauber[2], B.A. Blunt[2], and the Traumatic Coma Data Bank Investigators

[1] Division of Neurosurgery, Indiana University Medical Center, Indianapolis, IN, USA
[2] Division of Neurosurgery, University of California San Diego Medical Center, San Diego, CA, USA

Introduction

Of the variety of complications associated with ICP monitoring, CSF infection is the most common. Multiple factors have been associated with an increased rate of infection, including increased age, prolonged duration of monitoring, concomitant use of steroids, multiple changes of monitors, and the presence of a concurrent infection [1, 6]. Although numerous studies have indicated that the ventricular catheter (VC) has the highest reported infection rate of all currently used ICP monitors, the advantages afforded by CSF drainage for the management of elevated ICP justify the use of VC assuming that the complication rate is acceptably low.

This study was undertaken to determine the influence of the type of ICP monitor on the occurrence of infection in head injured patients and to determine whether routine changing of the monitor had a beneficial effect in preventing an CSF infection.

Methods

The Traumatic Coma Data Bank was a four center North American study of severe head injury from 1984–1987. Epidemiologic, clinical, radiographic and outcome information were prospectively acquired on 1030 severely head injured patients. Part of the collected information included the type of ICP monitor, either ventricular catheter (VC), or subarachnoid bolt (SB), the management and duration of placement of each type of monitor, and any complications of the head injury or management. During the study, the centers also began using a fiber optic subarachnoid or intraparenchymal bolt system. Because the complication rate of subarachnoid bolt and the fiber optic system have been reported to be similarly low [3], these types of monitors were grouped together as SB.

CSF infection was defined as pleocytosis in the CSF and positive bacterial cultures obtained during the period of monitoring or immediately after the monitor was discontinued. Alterations in monitoring or replacement of monitors occurring as a consequence of infection were excluded from this analysis. The methods of survival analysis were applied for this study of infection [4]. The event "CSF infection" was treated in the same way as death would be in a survival or mortality study.

In order to test whether the patient's risk of infection actually increased with each successive change of monitor, the Cox proportional hazards model was used. This model provides estimates of risk as well as the degree of statistical significance (p-value). In addition to the number of times the monitor had been changed, the following other covariates were included: age, skull fracture, length of time monitored, removal of monitor without subsequent replacement, surgery for skull fracture or craniotomy for surgical mass.

Results

Seven hundred and eleven patients with closed head injury underwent ICP monitoring. Of these patients 500 (70%) were monitored for at least 48 hours and had complete infection data. The overall rate of CSF infection for these patients was 9.2% (46/500). 199 patients were monitored by SB alone and had an infection rate of 2.5% (5/199). Two hundred and eleven patients were monitored by VC and had an infection rate of 11.9% (25/211).

The effect of basilar skull fracture, depressed skull fracture requiring surgery, and craniotomy for surgical mass on the CSF infection rate for ICP monitors is shown in Table 1. The presence of a surgical procedure, a basilar skull fracture with CSF leak or a depressed fracture requiring operative elevation increased the likelihood of CSF infection, especially in the presence of a VC.

The Cox model results (Table 2) for patients with VC only show the importance of basilar skull fractures as a risk factor for infection. Depressed skull fracture with surgery (not shown in Table 2) showed a 2.8 fold excess risk comparable to basilar skull fracture, but was not statistically significant due to small numbers. Time on monitor showed a trend for increasing risk of infec-

Table 1. CSF infection rates for ICP monitors by type and mutually exclusive complicating factors

	None	Basilar skull FX only	Craniotomy only	Depressed skull FX with surgery
Ventricular catheter	7/93 (7.5%)	2/10 (20%)	8/68 (11.8%)	2/5 (40%)
Bolt	2/93 (2.2%)	2/23 (8.7%)	0/38 (0.0%)	0/8 (0.0%)
Difference[a]	p = 0.17	p = 0.57	p = 0.048	p = 0.13

[a] Fisher's Exact Test

Table 2. Cox proportional hazards model for the 211 patients monitored by ventricular catheter only

Variable	p Value	Excess risk
Basilar skull fracture	0.039	2.6
Time on monitor	0.099	12.7%/day
Basilar fracture and time interaction	0.099	
Replacement of monitors	0.98	

Table 3. Infection rate by duration of monitoring by ventricular catheter for cases with no replacements

	Duration of monitoring (hrs)		
	0–120	121–240	>240
Infection rate	7.6%	10.4%	22.2%
Number of patients	79	77	18

tion, which carried through to all groups. This increased risk was in addition to that due to other factors, for instance basilar skull fractures. Elective replacement of monitors (see below) is included in Table 2 to highlight its clear lack of significance and its neutral effect on infection.

The rate of CSF infection for VC increased for duration of monitoring (Table 3). It also appeared to increase with each replacement of the monitor, but this was shown to be an artifact of the correlation between the length of monitoring and the number of monitor changes; the infection in some instances preceded the replacement.

In has been suggested that prophylactically changing the VC will reduce the incidence of CSF infection [3, 5]. It was possible to analyze the effect of routinely changing the VC, because some centers in the TCDB adopted a policy of routinely changing VC every fifth day in order to prevent infection. For centers that routinely changed VC, the rate of CSF infection was 16/95 (16.8%). While the infection rate for those centers not routinely changing VC was 9/116 (7.8%). This difference showed borderline significance ($p = 0.054$) by Fisher's exact test.

Conclusions

Although multiple factors must account for the occurrence of CSF infection in head injured patients, this study of the influence of type and management of ICP monitors suggests the following conclusions:

1. The baseline CSF infection rate in the TCDB for patients with "uncomplicated" severe closed head injury who underwent at least 48 hours of ICP monitoring was just over 2%.

2. The contribution of subarachnoid or intraparenchymal bolts to additional CSF infection was essentially nil.
3. The overall rate of CSF infection for patients monitored by VC was 11.9%, but much lower (7.6%) for patients continuously monitored by VC for less than 5 days with no replacements.
4. The rate of CSF infection was increased for patients with basilar skull fractures, depressed skull fractures requiring operative elevation, and craniotomy for surgical mass lesions for those patients monitored by VC but not for those patients monitored by SB. A greater sample size is needed to substantiate an elevated risk of infection due to depressed skull fracture with surgery.
5. Prolonged use of VC increases the rate of CSF infection.
6. Routine prophylactic changes of VC apparently do not affect the rate of CSF infection.

Finally, the data suggest that ICP is best monitored by subarachnoid or parenchymal monitors unless CSF drainage is necessary for therapy. If a VC is necessary, the duration of use should be as brief as possible in order to minimize the occurrence of CSF infection.

Acknowledgements. This work was supported by the Traumatic Coma Data Bank (TCDB) under Contracts NO1-NS-3-2339, NO1-NS-3-2340, NO1-NS-3-2342, No1-NS-6-2305 from the National Insititute of Neurological Disorders and Stroke (NINDS). The TCDB Manual of Operations which includes the TCDB data forms is available from the National Technical Information Service (NTIS), U.S. Department of Commerce, 5285 Port Royal Road, Springfield, VA 22161 (NITS Accession No. PB87 228060/AS).

References

1. Clark WC, Muhlbauer MS, Lowrey R, Hartman M, Ray MW, Watridge CB (1989) Complications of intracranial pressure monitoring in trauma patients. Neurosurgery 25:20–24
2. Luerssen TG, Shields PF, Vos HR, Marshall LF (1989) Clinical experience with a fiber optic brain parenchymal pressure monitor. In: Hoff JT, Betz AL (eds) Intracranial Pressure VII. Springer, Berlin Heidelberg New York London Paris Tokyo Hong Kong, pp 35–37
3. Mayhall CG, Archer NH, Lamb VA, Spadora AC, Baggett JW, Ward JD, Narayan RK (1984) Ventriculostomy-related infections. N Engl J Med 310:553–559
4. Miller RG (1981) Survival analysis. John Wiley and Sons, New York
5. Narayan RK, Kishore PRS, Becker DP, Ward JD, Enas GG, Greenberg RP, Da Silva AD, Lipper MH, Choi SC, Mayhall CG, Lutz HA, Young HF (1982) Intracranial pressure: To monitor or not to monitor? J Neurosurg 56:650–659
6. Rosner MJ, Becker DP (1976) ICP monitoring: Complications and associated factors. Clin Neurosurg 23:494–519

Intracranial Distension in Neurosurgical Pathology

E. Sirovskiy

N.N. Burdenko Research Institute of Neurosurgery, Moscow, Russian Federation

Introduction

Since the classical studies on ICP by Cushing, the main methodological principle for most investigators is based on the *a priori* postulate that the pressure in the cranial cavity is evenly distributed. This starting point made it possible to characterize the overall ICP by the pressure in one compartment only: the epidural, subdural or the, most widely used, ventricular fluid pressure (VFP). During recent decades, two important facts have emerged. 1. The mechanical pressures of the intracranial constituents [brain tissue, cerebrospinal fluid (CSF), interstitial fluid (ISF)] are different in their absolute values [3, 4, 5, 6, 8]. 2. An uneven distribution of pressures between the various intracranial compartments has been demonstrated in neurosurgical pathology [2, 6, 7].

The aim of this study was to examine the difference between the mechanical pressures of CSF and ISF, as well as to assess the lack of correlation between these pressures in patients with different types of brain lesions.

Material and Methods

Comparitive measurements of VFP and ISFP were performed in 166 patients in the early post-operative period. Three groups of patients were studied. The first group consisted of 57 patients who were operated on because of basal, extracerebral tumours. The second group consisted of 64 patients after removal of a glioma, and the third group of 45 patients after removal of an infratentorial tumour.

The VFP was measured according to Lundberg's technique. Local ISFP was measured in the region adjacent to the removed tumour and/or in intact tissue by a special catheter with a double microperforated wall. This method proved to be more sensitive than the traditional wick-catheter [3].

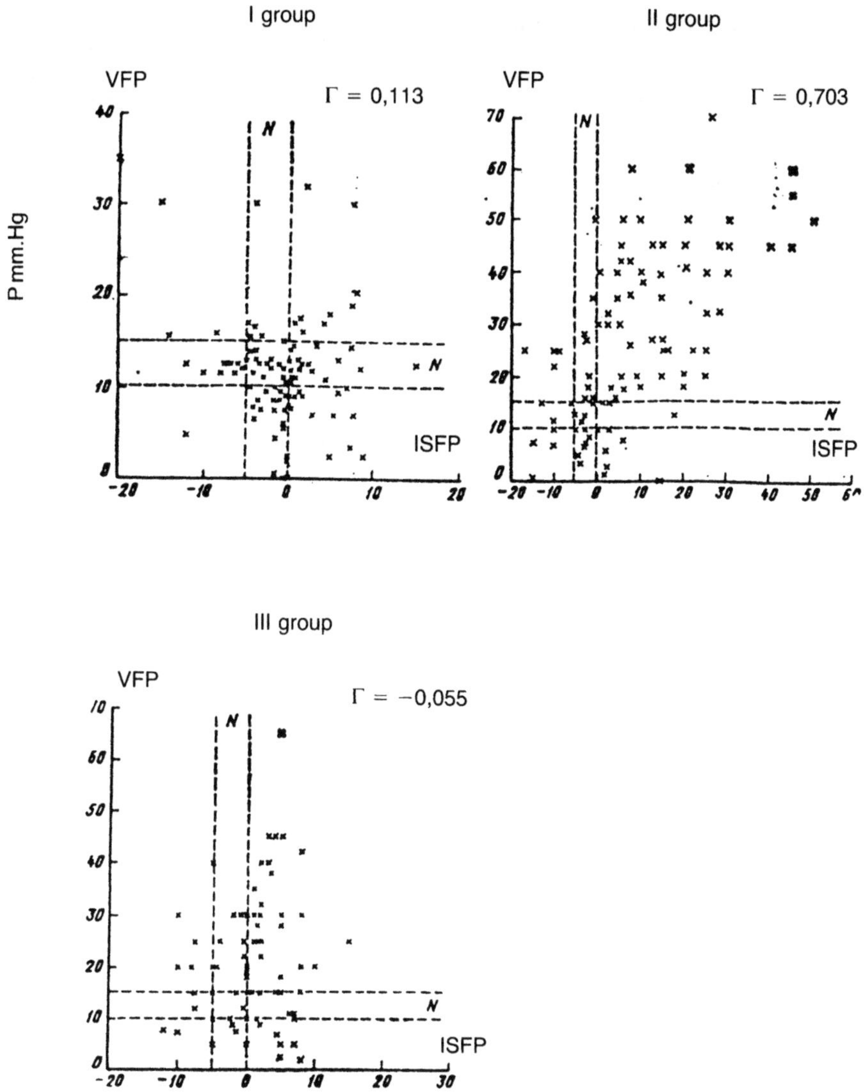

Fig. 1. Relationship between VFP and ISFP in the three patient groups: Group 1, basal-extracerebral tumours; Group 2, supratentorial, intracerebral gliomas; Group 3, infratentorial tumours

Results

The extreme and mean (±SD) values of the VFP and ISFP are shown in Table 1. In nearly all patients ISFP was significantly lower than VFP. The mean values of ISFP were almost the same in the patients of the three groups, slightly above or below the atmospheric pressure. Statistically significant mean ISFP differences were found between "normal" tissue and the perifocal zone of removed tumour (region of maximal edema). A significant correlation between

Table 1. VFP and ISFP after removal of basal, intracerebral and infratentorial tumours

P mmHg	VFP	ISFP	ISFP (edema reg.)
I. Basal-extracerebral	13.7 ± 2.9 (0–35)	−0.8 ± 1.5 (−20–16)	
II. Intracerebral gliomas	27.1 ± 12.4 (1–70)	−0.7 ± 2.1 (−18–45)	7.8 ± 5.6 (−5–60)
III. Infratentorial tumours	20.2 ± 3.5 (2–60)	1.1 ± 1.6 (−16–16)	

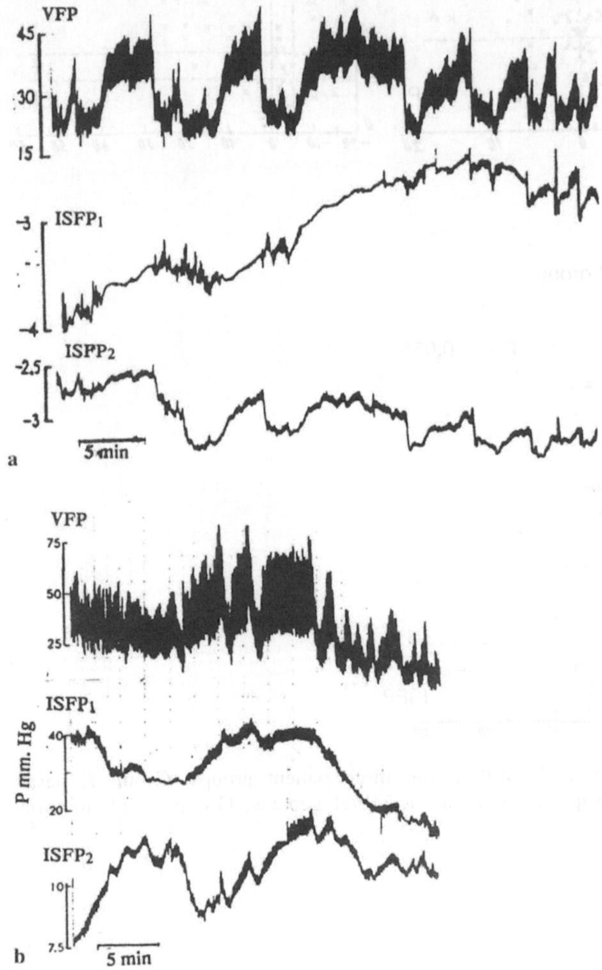

Fig. 2. a Patient C. (glioma of left parietal region): increased VFP with pressure waves and intracerebral normotension with "negative" ISFP both in perifocal region (ISFP1) and in intact tissue (ISFP2). **b** Patient H. (biopsy of corpus callosum tumour). Increased VFP and ISFP in perifocal region (ISFP1). The pressure gradient between perifocal region and intact tissue (ISFP2) decreased from 30 to 10 mmHg after spontaneous decrease of VFP

VFP and ISFP was only found in the glioma group. In the majority of cases, CSF normotension was not accompanied by a normal intracerebral pressure. Similarly, CSF hypo- and hypertension were not always associated with a low or high intracerebral pressure. Not seldom, a high VFP was accompanied by a normal, or even negative, ISFP. Even during pressure waves in the VFP recording, ISFP often remained constant (Fig. 2a).

The relationships between VFP and ISFP varied between the three groups. After removal of a basal tumour, both VFP and ISFP remained normal in 29%

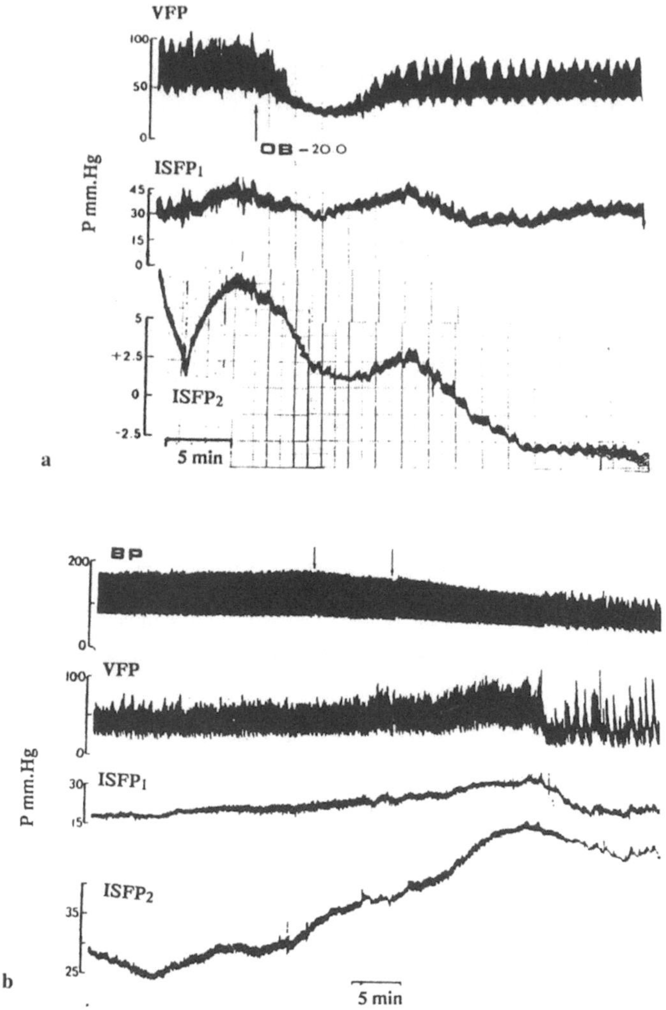

Fig. 3. a Patient W. (left fronto-parietal malignant glioma). Increased VFP, intracerebral hypertension in perifocal edema (ISFP1) and normotension in non-dominant hemisphere (ISFP2). (OB: oxybate sodium, i.v. anesthetic). **b** Patient A. (malignant glioma of thalamus). Diffuse brain edema. Increased VFP and ISFP1, both in perifocal region (ISFP2) and in intact tissue (ISFP1). The pressure gradient between these regions increased from 10 to 30 mmHg after lowering of blood pressure (arrows)

of the patients, whereas 60% of the patients demonstrated a lack of correlation between VFP and ISFP. After removal of an intracerebral glioma, only 7% of the patients demonstrated a normal VFP and ISFP, whereas in 53% of cases ISF hypertension was accompanied by a high VFP. After removal of an intratentorial tumour, only 10% of the patients had a normal VFP and ISFP. In the remaining percentage, the lack of correlation between VFP and ISFP was mainly caused by a combination of a high VFP and a normal ISFP.

All patients in whom an intracerebral tumour was removed, displayed an uneven distribution of ISFP. This was usually associated with brain edema, as

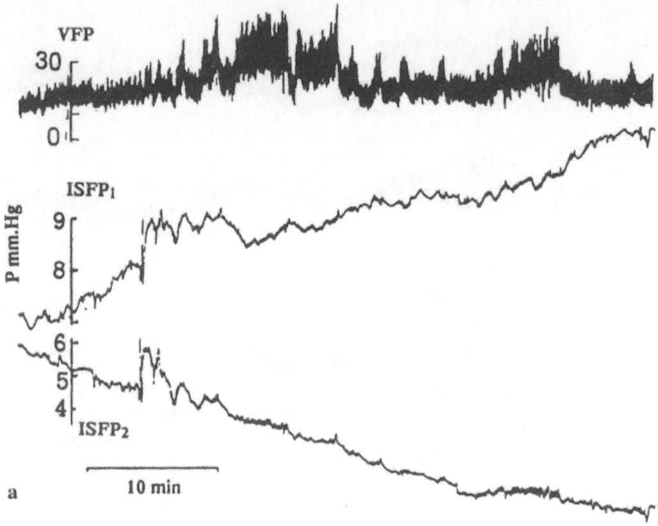

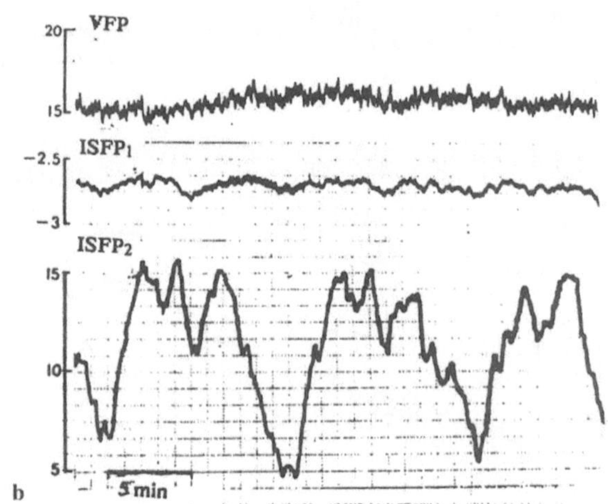

Fig. 4. **a** Patient K. (right occipital glioma). Increased VFP and contrasting dynamics of ISFP. The pressure gradient between perifocal region (ISFP1) and intact tissue (ISFP2) increased from 1 to 15 mmHg during one hour. **b** Patient Ar. (left parietal glioma and decompressive craniotomy). Normal VFP, normal intracerebral pressure with "negative" ISFP in non-dominant hemisphere and moderate intracerebral hypertension with pressure waves under decompression (ISFP2)

shown by CT-examination. In focal brain edema, ISFP was increased in the edematous region, whereas ISFP in the non-edematous tissue was normal (Fig. 3a). In diffuse edema, both VFP and ISFP were increased, in perifocal tissue as well as in "intact" tissue. The pressure gradients between these regions varied from 2 to 40 mmHg (Figs. 3a,b). ISFP in regions of maximal edema could reach considerable values and even exceeded VFP (Fig. 3b). Quite often the dynamics of ISFP in two regions of the brain could differ significantly (Figs. 2b, 4a,b).

In some cases the uneven distribution of intracerebral pressure can be explained by an inhomogeneous distribution of the cerebral circulation. This might be the reason of the opposite ISFP dynamics of the type shown in figure 4a. Another observation was made in a patient in whom a malignant glioma was removed, after which the bone flap was not replaced. The VFP was normal as was intracerebral pressure in intact tissue, whereas the pressure in the decompressed area was moderately increased showing quite different dynamics (Fig. 4b).

Discussion

These results show that the mechanical pressures of ISF and CSF are different as far as their absolute values are concerned. There is no direct hydrostatic connection between CSF and ISF. Physiological pressure gradients exist between the main intracranial components. Within each of these components, the pressure is evenly distributed. Under pathological conditions, the physiological equilibrium between these pressures is disturbed. In view of this uneven distribution of pressures, the term intracranial hypertension should be avoided. It would be more correct and precise to define this status as "intracranial distension". CSF, intracerebral and intracranial distensions should be considered separately. CSF distension is an uneven distribution of pressures within the CSF-containing spaces. Partial or complete obstruction of fluid pathways is the main cause of uneven pressure distribution in the CSF system. Thus, a pronounced supra-infratentorial CSFP gradient is the main factor for dislodging and wedging of the brainstem at the tentorial level. Intracerebral distension is an uneven distribution of pressure (tension) inside the brain. Additional volume is the primary cause of this condition. A tumour, haematoma or abscess compresses the surrounding tissues and the pressure in the perifocal zone is significantly higher than in distant areas. An uneven increase in the volume of tissue fluid, as in brain edema, is one of the leading causes of intracerebral distension. In this study, the ISFP gradient between edematous and "normal" tissue amounted to 20–40 mmHg. An uneven distribution of ISFP during edema has also been described in experimental studies [1, 3, 4].

Another cause for intracerebral distension may be the inhomogeneous distribution of the cerebral circulation, resulting from changes in vascular tone, e.g. vasoconstriction in one hemisphere and dilatation in the other. The dysbalance of the cerebral circulation causes an uneven transfer of blood pressure to the ISF giving rise to an uneven distribution of ISFP.

Intracranial distension is a disturbance of the physiological heterogeneity of pressure distribution between the intracranial components. This means a significant imbalance of tensions in the intracranial system, i.e. the co-existence of regions with normal, elevated and decreased pressure within the cranium.

References

1. Marmarou A, Takagi H, Shulman K (1980) Biomechanics of brain edema, and effects on local cerebral blood flow. In: Cervos-Navarro J, Ferozt R (eds). Advances in neurology. Brain edema. Raven Press, New York 28:345–358
2. Pick J, Bock WJ (1990) Continuous monitoring of cerebral tissue pressure in neurosurgical-practice. Experiences with 100 patients. Intensive Care Med 16:184–188
3. Poll W, Brock M, Markakis E, Winkelmuller W, Dietz H (1972) Brain tissue pressure. In: Brock M, Dietz H (eds). Intracranial pressure, Springer, Berlin Heidelberg New York, pp 188–194
4. Reulen HJ, Kreysch HG (1973) Measurement of brain Tissue Pressure in Cold Induced Cerebral Oedema. Acta Neurochir. 29:29–40
5. Schettini A, McKay L, Modell GH (1972) The response of brain surface pressure to hypercapnic hypoxia and hyperventilation. J Anaesthesiology 36:4–12
6. Sirovsky EB, Paltsev EI, Manevich AZ (1979) Clinico-experimental data on differences between intracerebral and CSF pressure and their biomechanical interpretation, Seara M. Neurochirurgica 3:261–268
7. Weaver D, Winn H, Jane J (1982) Differential intracranial pressure in patients with unilateral mass lesions. J Neurosurg 56:660–665
8. Weinstein JD, Langfitt TW, Bruno L, Zoren HA, Jackson JLF (1968) Experimental study of patterns of brain distortion and ischemia produced by intracranial mass. J Neurosurgery 28:513–521

On-Line Acquisition and Analysis of ICP and Physiologic Data in the Neurosurgical Intensive Care Unit

J.D. Crouch, C.F. Contant, Jr., and C.S. Robertson

Department of Neurosurgery, Baylor College of Medicine, Houston, TX, USA

Introduction

A real-time data acquisition and analysis system for use in the Neurosurgical Intensive Care Unit has been developed for research on ICP wave-shape changes and concurrent changes in physiologic variables. The system is an extension of the design of Bray and Sherwood [1]. The system has been designed to allow flexibility for research purposes, while providing a reliable system for real-time data collection.

Hardware

The acquisition and analysis system is based on a Compaq 386S-16 MHz computer with a Scientific Solutions 16 channel acquisition board. Analog signals representing physiologic data are collected through the acquisition board for data analysis and data storage.

The system obtains values for the following nine variables: Intracranial Pressure (ICP), Mean Arterial Pressure (MAP), Electrocardiogram (EKG), Jugular Venous Oxygen Saturation (SjvO2), peripheral Arterial Oxygen Saturation (SaO2), End-Tidal CO2 (ETCO2), Capnogram (CAPNO), Tissue Oxygen Saturation percent change (NIRO2), and Tissue Blood Volume percent change (NIRBV). Each parameter is represented as an analog voltage signal from its respective monitor.

The EKG, ICP, and MAP analog signals are taken directly from the hospital bedside monitor. ICP and MAP are collected through a special module that provides a voltage representation of the pressure wave forms. The ICP is measured via ventriculostomy or Camino catheter. The EKG signal is taken through the output provided for defibrillator synchronization. A Novametrix monitor (Model No. 1260/7000) measures SaO2 and ETCO2 and displays the capnograph and plethysmograph waveforms. A pulse oximeter finger probe allows measurement of the SaO2. A CO2 sensor connects to the patient-respirator airway circuit for measurement of the ETCO2. SjvO2 is obtained using the analog output port on the Oximetrix 3 SO2/CO Monitor with the Opticath fiber optic catheter placed in the jugular venous bulb.

NIRBV and NIRO2 are determined using technology developed by Dr. Britton Chance at the University of Pennsylvania. The instrument calculates oxygen saturation and blood volume of tissue beneath the probe. Presently, NIRBV and NIRO2 are relative values.

A junction box receives the analog signal from each component of the system. The signals are routed to the computer's acquisition board and to a data backup system. The backup system combines a Medical Systems Corporation A/D Recorder Adapter (Model No. PCM-8) and a VCR. The Recorder Adapter accepts up to 8 channels of analog or digital voltage signals and alters the signals for storage on VCR video tapes of up to 8 hours in duration. The video tapes are used as backup.

Software

The acquisition and analysis program is written in ASYST (Keithley ASYST, Rochester, NY). ASYST is a high level programming language using Forth-like commands. The language offers built-in commands for data acquisition, analysis, and graphics, including statistical computations and Fast Fourier Transforms (FFT). New commands can be formed based on ASYST commands or previous user-defined commands. The programs are compiled into a turnkey system requiring no programming experience use in the ICU. Menus provide access to various functions available in the program, and, if other input is necessary, the user is provided with self explanatory prompts.

Use of the system proceeds through several steps. Data specific to each patient are entered first. The system is then calibrated to the monitors. Each monitor has a specific routine for calibration, but a general calibration routine is to estimate the slope and intercept of the line relating the analog voltage to the true value. When calibration is complete a menu with several options is presented to the user. These options include reentering the patient information, entering a comment into the comment file, recalibrating the instruments, altering certain program parameters, acquiring data, or exiting the program. Two displays are available for viewing the information during data acquisition. The Wave Monitoring display provides values for all of the calculated variables as well as displaying the ICP waveform being analyzed. The Blood Flow Response display shows the predicted cerebral blood flow graphically. This display also includes values for all monitored parameters and values for several calculated parameters.

Data acquisition begins by continuously scanning the Capno channel until an end of expiration is detected. This event triggers the scanning of 9 channels at 200 Hz for 10 seconds with a 0.1 micro-second offset between each channel. Arrays of 2000 points are collected for ICP, EKG, MAP, and Capno. Arrays of 100 points are collected for SjvO2, SaO2, ETCO2, NIRBV, and NIRO2.

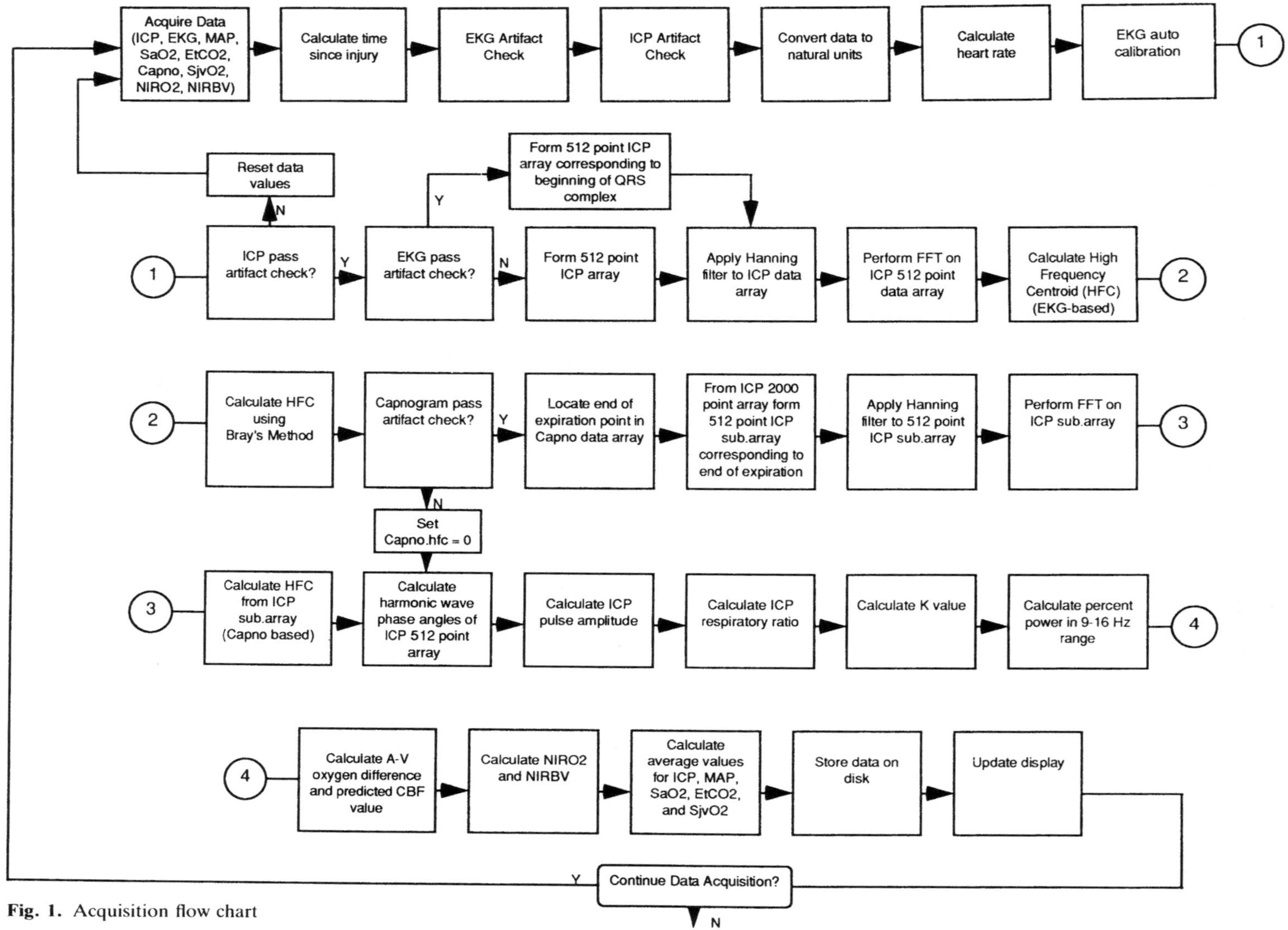

Fig. 1. Acquisition flow chart

Both arrays are collected simultaneously. At the end of collection of the arrays, the elapsed time since injury is calculated, the EKG and ICP are checked for artifacts, the data are converted to natural units, and the heart rate is calculated based on the EKG. The system then performs the analysis of the ICP wave shape and related calculations are performed. The Acquisition Flow Chart in Fig. 1 describes the order and restrictions of these calculations. At the completion of this processing all values are stored to disk, and the display is updated. Data are stored on files indexed by the patients last name. A file is created for user comments and an error file is created to store error messages generated by the program. The process repeats indefinitely unless the user interrupts data collection. When data collection ceases, the menu is displayed until further commands are issued.

Discussion

The intent of this project is to design a system that will collect data at the bedside and provide beneficial information regarding the patient's status. The system should not be obtrusive and should require minimal effort to extract the desired information. In its current form, the system adequately meets these requirements, but a more compact design is currently being developed. The design must provide physical space for new instruments until the system reaches the acquisition board's 16 channel capacity. Two channels of EEG signals are being incorporated into the program using a Neurowave Systems 2 monitor. This monitor provides a left- and right-channel EEG signal and calculates the percent change of total power and mean frequency of each channel. The acquisition system will acquire the raw amplified EEG signals and calculate the power in each of the alpha, beta, delta, and gamma frequency ranges. New routines based on the EEG will be written as needed.

A display that presents information which is unavailable from standard bedside monitors is the long range goal. As new information is learned from the data being collected, new parameters could be discovered and eventually displayed either graphically or numerically to indicate the status of the patient.

References

1. Bray RS, Sherwood AM, Halter JA, Robertson CS, Grossman RG (1986) Development of a clinical monitoring system by means of ICP waveform analysis. In: Miller JD, Teasdale GM, Rowan JO, Galbraith SL, Mendelow AD (eds) Intracranial Pressure VI. Springer, Berlin Heidelberg New York Tokyo, pp 260–264

Continuous Monitoring and Recording of Cerebral Perfusion Pressure

I.R. Chambers[1], A. Clark[1], P.J. Kane[2], D.A. Allcutt[2], and A.D. Mendelow[2]

[1] Regional Medical Physics Department and [2] Department of Neurosurgery, Newcastle General Hospital, Newcastle upon Tyne, UK

Introduction

The measurement of intracranial pressure (ICP) and arterial blood pressure (BP) by invasive techniques in severely head injured patients is routine in many neurosurgical Intensive Care Units. The cerebral perfusion pressure (CPP) can be calculated from these parameters such that:

CPP = Mean Arterial BP − Mean ICP

In areas of traumatised brain where normal regulation is disturbed the blood flow may become passively dependent on CPP. It has been suggested by Changaris et al. (2) that CPP may be an important determinant for outcome following head injury.

Whilst the calculation of CPP is a relatively trivial computation it can become an irksome task for the ICU nurse when repeated charting of a wide variety of physiological parameters is also needed. We have designed and constructed a module which performs this calculation automatically and displays the CPP value. Incorporated into the module is an RS232 digital communications interface which allows transmission of the ICP, BP and CPP data for recording on a PSION Organiser. This can subsequently be analysed.

CPP Module

The Simonsen and Weel 8000 modular monitoring system consists of a display monitor onto which a variety of modules can be attached for monitoring different physiological parameters (ECG, ICP, BP, respiration rate). In head injured patients, ICP and blood pressure are routinely monitored using invasive techniques (i.e. Camino subdural bolt and arterial cannulation). Two pressure modules are attached on to the top of the monitor to measure these parameters, connected electrically to each other by means of a bus system at the rear of the unit. We have designed and constructed a module which is connected between the monitor unit and the two pressure modules which calculates the CPP automatically. Each pressure module on the monitoring stack is of intelligent design and digitally calculates the systolic, diastolic and mean values of the pressure waveform. It displays this information on its

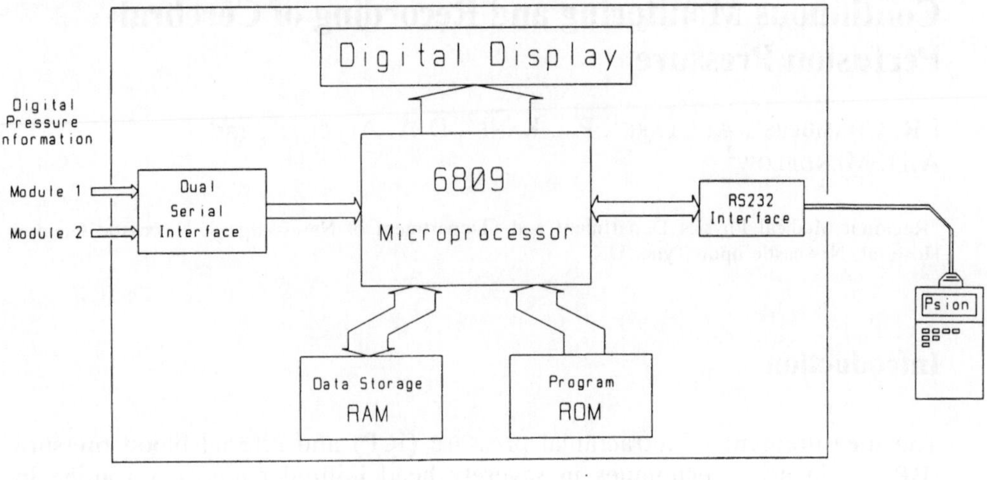

Fig. 1. Schematic construction of CPP module

front display and also makes the information available on the inter-module connector bus. Our CPP module extracts this information from each of the pressure modules and calculates the absolute difference between the two mean pressure values (the CPP) and displays this on the front of the unit.

At the heart of the module is a Motorola 6809 microprocessor, EPROM to store the program, a random access memory (RAM), LED digital display and parallel-to-serial and serial-to-parallel converters (Fig. 1). Serial pressure information is transmitted from each pressure module and transferred via the serial-to-parallel converters to the microprocessor. The microprocessor then calculates the absolute difference in the mean pressure values. The fact that an absolute calculation is performed means that it does not matter which module is used to measure ICP and which to measure blood pressure. The CPP module also incorporates a RS232 digital communications port which is capable of transmitting information to other devices. We have configured the module to average the values from both pressure modules over a two minute period and transmit this information from the serial communications port.

Recording

The RS232 output from the CPP module is connected to a PSION II Organiser model XP. This is a small hand held computer which has already been successfully used in the hospital environment [1, 3]. It is available in several versions of varying memory capacity and screen size and can be programmed using Organiser Programming Language which is similar to rudimentary versions of BASIC. The internal capacity of the Organiser can be substantially increased by the utilisation of its two internal expansion ports which can each accommodate a Rampack; these are 32 Kbyte random access memory (RAM) modules. This increase in internal memory is such that by sampling the ICP

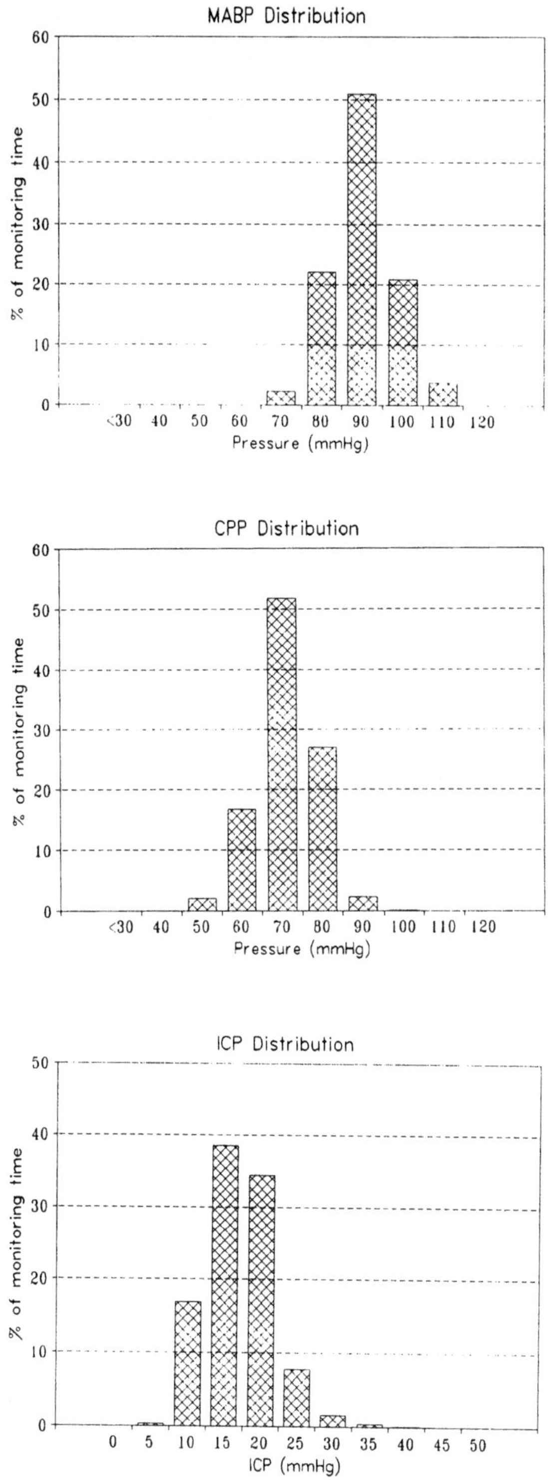

Fig. 2. Sample distributions of MABP, CPP and ICP

and blood pressure readings every two minutes up to five days of continuous monitoring can be undertaken before the memory capacity of the Organiser is reached. Once the monitoring period has been completed the data can be very easily transferred to a personal computer for analysis and display.

Output

Software programs have been developed to structure the output of the data. Graphs showing ICP, MABP and CPP are constructed for each twelve hour epoch of the monitoring period. Histograms are determined to show the distribution of the pressure readings (Fig. 2) and can be useful in describing their consistency or variability.

Discussion

Automation of the calculation of CPP and its display increases the awareness of Intensive Care staff regarding CPP. The digital display of ICP, BP and CPP at the bedside has been popular and encouraged the more frequent use of such monitoring. The immediate storage on a PSION Organiser reduces the need for bulky chart recorders and other hardware at the bedside. Also statistical analysis has been greatly facilitated in each patient. Whether easier access to immediate pressure measurements of this type and greater awareness of these parameters leads to improved outcomes for patients in ICU remains to be seen.

References

1. Chambers IR, Faulkner K, Marshall NW (1991) Recording dose-area product information using an electronic personal organiser. J Radiol Prot 11(2):137–138
2. Changaris DG, McGraw CP, Greenberg RA (1989) Optimal cerebral perfusion pressure in head injury. In: Hoff JT, Betz AL (eds). Intracranial pressure VII. Springer, Berlin Heidelberg New York London Paris Tokyo Hong Kong, pp 640–642
3. Hammond JE, Fawcett W (1989) The PSION II Organiser in ITU. Today's Anaesthetist 4:272–276

Attempts to Continuously Monitor Autoregulation and Compensatory Reserve in Severe Head Injuries

D.J. Price, M. Czosnyka, and M. Williamson

Pinderfields Hospital, Wakefield, UK, and Warsaw University of Technology, Warsaw, Poland

Introduction

Some neurosurgical units in Britain have been measuring ICP in patients with severe head injuries for the last 25 years and yet even now, in over half of the units, ICP monitoring has not been established as a routine component of intensive management.

The significance of just the mean ICP as an isolated piece of information at any moment of time is of limited value. Not only is it important to be able to visualise trends at the bedside, but it is necessary to explore the use of other parameters derived from the ICP signal to give information on autoregulation and compensatory reserve.

Methods – Signal Analysis

During the 1980s, a minicomputer was used for on-line averaging, trend display, distribution histogram generation and estimation of "elastivity". This "elastivity" was calculated from the amplitude of the cardiac pulse wave divided by the mean and presented as a mean of 600 values every 15 minutes [3]. The on-line generation of histograms of the distribution of ICP values were of no practical use and a simple continuously updated trend has proved to be of more value [4].

For a time, data was transmitted by modem to a mainframe computer some 12 miles from Wakefield enabling us to carry out on-line Fourier transformation to look at the sub-respiratory components of the signal but understandably this arrangement was not practical long-term [2].

More recent data acquisition and analysis software had been developed in Warsaw for implementation on a PC and arrangements were made to fully test this on 90 head injured patients in Wakefield. This Polish program written in the language C required a slower analogue-to-digital conversion rate of 18.1 Hz and is based on a unique fast Fourier transform [1] which is able to efficiently separate the cardiac from the respiratory wave-forms. It provides on-line means of amplitudes of the subrespiratory, respiratory, and cardiac components, of the heart rate, the regression value of the amplitude/ICP and the regression value of the heart rate/ICP. For those patients with on-line arterial pressure monitoring, it also displays perfusion pressure. Calculations are easily made on-line or retrospectively of the linear and non-linear relationships between any of these derived variables which are stored on the disc every 14 seconds over any selected time epoch.

Results of Evaluation

Software Calibration

During the first month, the software was rigorously tested with a signal generator. The frequency and power of the spectral analysis proved accurate. Adjustments were necessary to the frequency bandwidth of the pre-amplifiers to eliminate aliasing. A 20 Hz bandwidth upper cut-off proved optimal.

Between February 1989 and June 1991, 92 patients have been monitored using the software described. The software is intuitively easy to use and problems only arose when the hard disc on the computer developed intermittent faults. In an initial analysis of the first 25 patients who had both ICP and arterial pressure monitoring, the overall distributions of values recorded on the data-files are as described in Table 1.

Autoregulation and Compensatory Reserve

When the gradient of the cardiac pulse wave amplitude/mean had been studied during the earlier experience with signal analysis using the minicomputer,

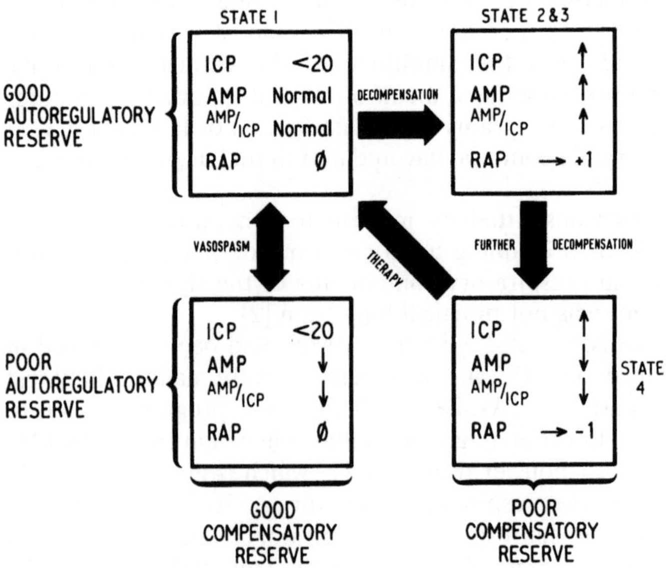

Fig. 1. A diagrammatic representation of the possible changes from one state to another

Table 1.

ICP	% Time	CPP	% Time
<20	66.7	>100	7.3
20–29	24.2	90–99	11.8
30–39	6.7	80–89	16.7
40–49	1.3	70–79	19.1
50–59	0.6	60–69	20.3
60–69	0.4	50–59	12.8
>70	0.1	40–49	8.1
		20–39	3.9

we had hoped that the "elastivity" might prove to be a useful short-term predictor of a rising ICP, but the relationship between a rise in elastivity and a subsequent rise in ICP did not appear very clear. We had failed to appreciate that the regression coefficient itself might contain information concerning autoregulation and compensatory reserve. The software developed in Warsaw provides a continuous assessment of the regression coefficient of the amplitude/pressure characteristic (RAP) and when head injuries were monitored, the significance of the RAP soon became apparent.

We then rationalised our interpretation of the RAP by arbitrarily defining four states:

1. Good autoregulatory reserve and good compensatory reserve.
2. Good autoregulatory reserve and reduced compensatory reserve.
3. Good autoregulatory reserve and severely reduced compensatory reserve.
4. Poor autoregulatory reserve and severely reduced compensatory reserve.

Figure 1 shows the relationship between the four states and also includes the combination of a poor autoregulation and good compensation which we had not recognised in this group of head injuries but which others have reported in patients with subarachnoid haemorrhage.

State 1: Mean ICP is less than 20 mmHg or the perfusion pressure is above 60 mmHg. The amplitude/ICP ratio is in the normal range between 0.15 and 0.4. And the RAP is around zero.

State 2: The ICP is between 15 and 25 mmHg. Or the CPP is greater than 60 mmHg. The amplitude/ICP ratio is above 0.3 or the RAP is rising above zero (0.2–0.5).

State 3: The ICP is between 25 and 40 mmHg. Or the CPP is between 50 and 60 mmHg. The amplitude/ICP ratio is above 0.4. Or the RAP is between 0.6 and 0.9.

State 4: The ICP is above 40 mmHg. Or the CPP is less than 50 mmHg. The amplitude/ICP ratio has fallen. Or the RAP has fallen below zero.

The four states are shown in Fig. 2 and there is an inference that the RAP and the amplitude/mean ratio rise prior to a rise in ICP and therefore discriminating between State 1 and State 2 on the flat portion of the PV curve. Eleven

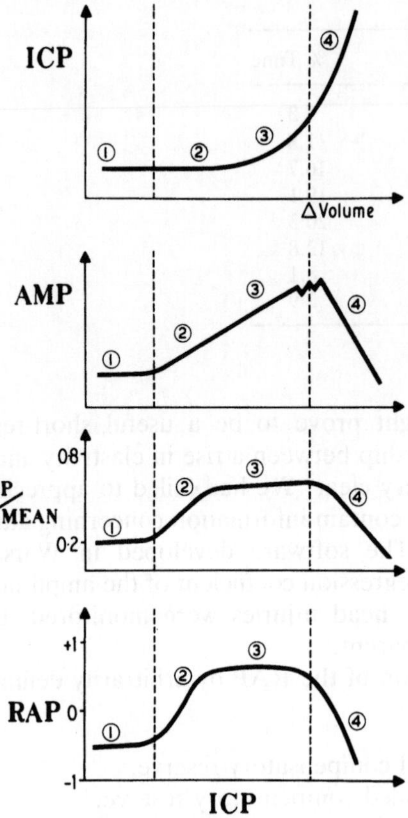

Fig. 2. Observed changes in amplitude, the amplitude/mean ratio and the regression coefficient of that relationship (RAP) in the four states

Table 2.

	% Time	Mean ICPmmHg	Mean CPPmmHg
State 1	65.7	18 ± 6	64 ± 14
State 2 & 3	30.6	24 ± 7	58 ± 13
State 4	3.7	37 ± 9	46 ± 16

patients from Wakefield were selected on the basis of having a wide range of ICP measurements. The relationship between the mean RAP and mean ICP is show in Fig. 3. The graph emphasises that at above an ICP of 60 mmHg, the RAP falls below zero indicating the transition between State 3 and State 4.

For a series of the first 25 head injured patients the proportion of time in each state is shown in Table 2.

The arterial line is often placed peripherally and this may therefore lead to some underestimation of the perfusion pressure and could account for the lower perfusion pressures.

Fig. 3. The data-files from 11 head injured patients were analysed by computer. The graph shows the relationship between ICP and RAP. Above an ICP of 60 mmHg, the RAP becomes negative

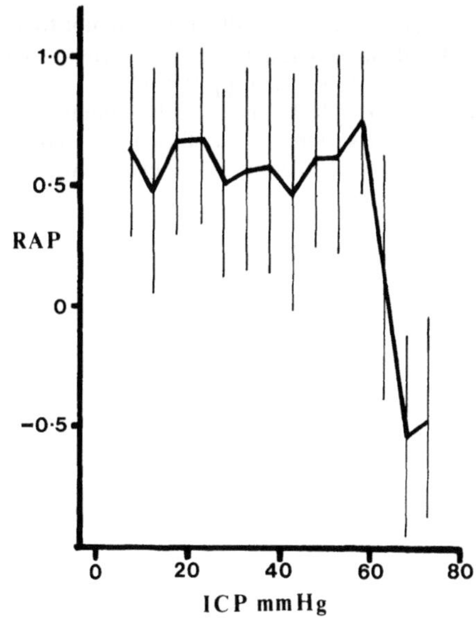

Although the logic of the selection of the state is quite simple, it has been incorporated into an expert system shell and the result displayed on a monitor as a line of colour – green, yellow, red or black. With further experience of this, we hope to improve the logical statements in the future and will then conduct a formal acceptability study to establish as to whether this system does improve understanding and management of raised intracranial pressure following head injury.

Conclusion

The generation of derived ICP variables on-line improves our understanding of a patient's progress and provides guidance about management. Too much information at the bedside can confuse the nursing staff and interpretation becomes necessary. A simple expert system integrated within the monitoring software may help solve the dilemma of the "information explosion" at the intensive care bedside.

References

1. Czosnyka M (1985) Determination of periodic or quasi-periodic signal parameters via interpolation of DFT. In: Luque A, Figueiras Vidal AR, Cappellini V (eds) Digital signal processing volume 2, Elsevier Science Publishers BV (North-Holland), pp 5–9
2. Price DJ, Dugdale RE, Mason J (1980) The control of ICP using three asynchronous control closed-loops. In: Shulman K, Marmarou A, Miller JD, Becker DP, Hochwald GM, Brock M (eds) Intracranial IV Springer, Berlin, Heidelberg, New York, pp 395–399

3. Price DJ, Mason J (1982) An attempt to automate the control of cerebral oedema. In: Go KG, Baethmann A (eds) Recent progress of the study and therapy of brain edema, Plenum Press, New York, London, pp 597–607
4. Price DJ (1987) The use of computers in neurosurgical intensive care. In: Jewkes DA (ed) Bailliere's Clinical Anaesthesiology – Anaesthesia for neurosurgery. Baillieres Tindall, London, Philadelphia, Toronto, Sydney, Tokyo, pp 533–556

Further Attempts to Anticipate Post-traumatic Intracranial Hypertension by On-line Analysis

M. WILLIAMSON, D.J. PRICE, and M. CZOSNYKA

Pinderfields Hospital, Wakefield, UK, and Warsaw University of Technology, Warsaw, Poland

Introduction

At every ICP symposium since 1972, attempts to monitor a patient's state of compensatory reserve have been presented [3, 5]. Despite considerable research into methodology with the increasingly more sophisticated computer processing, no widely accepted automated technique has yet emerged to identify significant changes in morphological characteristics of the ICP waveform. Unfortunately, the measurement of mean pressure only does not satisfactorily predict the future course of ICP in the head injured patient.

Methods

Earlier Waveform Analysis

Some 14 years ago, inspired by the pioneering work of Avezaat and his colleagues [1], an on-line ICP signal analysis using a minicomputer was introduced. Every 15 minutes a linear regression of 600 pairs of ICP mean and cardiac pulse wave amplitudes was calculated [4]. When the ICP was stable, the regression coefficient was too low for the calculated gradient to be useable. An estimated gradient "elastivity" was then derived by averaging the 600 amplitude/mean ratios and we accepted that this presumed a zero intercept. We had hopes that an increase in gradient would produce an increase in ICP within an hour with the intention of preventing such rises by prophylactic Mannitol administration. Unfortunately, no clear predictive correlation was found at that time and the gradient was useful only as a surrogate for elastance within the mathematical model which drove an automated closed-loop controller for the infusion of Mannitol [4].

More Recent Waveform Analysis

In a continuing search for an on-line method of estimating a patient's current position on the flat part of the pressure/volume curve, software developed in Poland using a unique Fourier Transform Algorithm implemented on an IBM

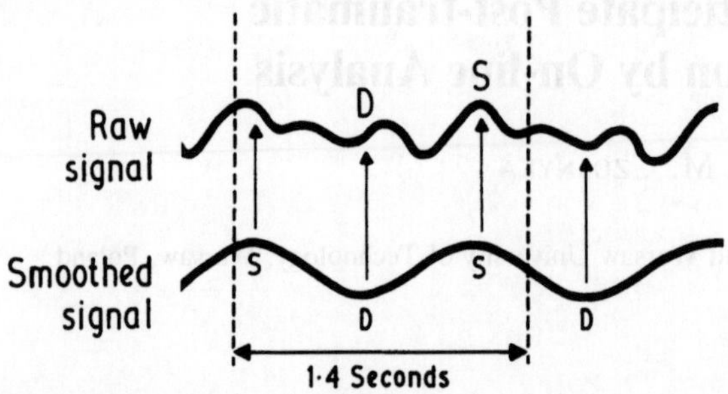

Fig. 1. Both the smoothed signal and the raw signal were analysed. The troughs and peaks were identified from the smoothed signal and the actual diastolic (*D*) and systolic (*S*) values were taken from the raw signal

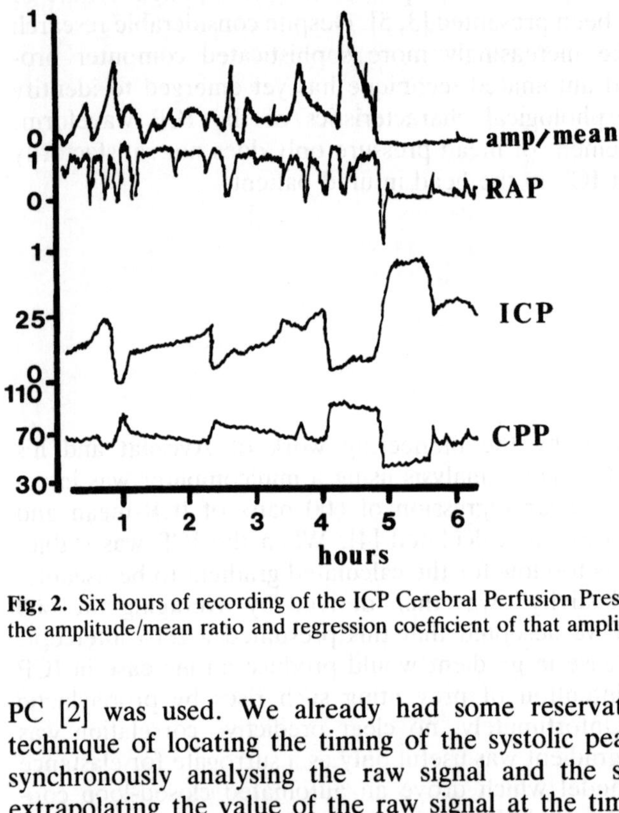

Fig. 2. Six hours of recording of the ICP Cerebral Perfusion Pressure (CPP) along with changes in the amplitude/mean ratio and regression coefficient of that amplitude/mean relationship (RAP)

PC [2] was used. We already had some reservations about the necessary technique of locating the timing of the systolic peak and diastolic trough by synchronously analysing the raw signal and the smoothed signal and then extrapolating the value of the raw signal at the times indicated by the peaks and troughs of the smoothed signal (Fig. 1).

After a period of validation, the Polish software was accepted in Wakefield with enthusiasm. The fast Fourier transform produced a very accurate measure of the cardiac and respiratory amplitudes and for the first time, it was possible to look at both the regression coefficient of the amplitude/mean relationship (RAP) and the gradient itself. The RAP trends are available as a continuous display on the screen on-line and software has recently been written in Wakefield to provide a display of the gradient trends off-line (Fig. 2).

We reviewed the recordings to find the following events.

1. A rise in ICP of at least 10 mmHg for at least 10 minutes.
2. A rise in the gradient of amplitude/mean of 0.3 or more over a period of no more than 30 minutes.
3. An increase of the mean RAP regression coefficient over a period of one hour of 0.3 or more.

We allowed a gap of up to one hour between an event relating to ICP and one relating to a change in the amplitude/mean relationship.

Results

The relative frequency of a rise in ICP of at least 10 mmHg preceeded by a rise in the amplitude/mean gradient of 0.3 or more over a 30 minute period is shown in Table 1. The statistical summary of this is as follows: Sensitivity = 48.4%, Specificity = 28.5%, Predictive value of positive result = 47.7%, Predictive value of negative result = 57.3%, % correct = 50.3%.

The relative incidence of a rise in ICP of at least 10 mmHg was preceeded by a regression coefficient of the amplitude/mean relationship (RAP) of 0.3 or more is shown in Table 2. The statistical summary of this is as follows: Sensitivity = 39.3%, Specificity = 98.4%, Predictive value of a positive result = 56.9%, Predictive value of a negative result = 96.8%, % correct = 98.5%.

Table 1.

32 Patients	No rise in ICP	Rise in ICP
No preceding rise in amp/mean ratio	59 (True−ve)	44 (False−ve)
Rise in amp/mean ratio	148 (False+ve)	135 (True+ve)

Table 2.

90 Patients	No rise in ICP	Rise in ICP
No preceding rise in RAP	3130 (True−ve)	102 (False−ve)
Rise in RAP	50 (False+ve)	66 (True+ve)

Conclusion

We conclude that the RAP (the regression coefficient of the amplitude/mean relationship) provides a better warning of impending intracranial hypertension than the gradient of that relationship. The gradient is less specific and the overall performance of correctness is half of that of the RAP. Although the sensitivity of the RAP is disappointingly low, the specificity is high. It is necessary to continue to search for the perfect predictor!

References

1. Avezaat CJJ, van Eijndhoven JHM, Wyper DJ (1979) Cerebrospinal fluid pulse pressure and intracranial volume-pressure relationships. J Neurol Neurosurg Psych 42:687–700
2. Czosnyka M (1985) Determination of periodic or quasi-periodic signal parameters via interpolation of DFT. In: Luque A, Figueiras Vidal AR, Cappellini V (eds) Digital signal processsing volume 2. Elsevier Science Publishers BV (North-Holland), pp 5–9
3. Janny P, Jouan JP, Janny L, Gourgano M, Gueitum (1972) A statistical approach to long-term monitoring of intracranial pressure. In: Brock M, Dietz H (eds) Intracranial pressure Springer, Berlin Heidelberg New York, pp 59–64
4. Price DJ, Mason J (1984) An attempt to automate control of cerebral edema. In: Go KG, Baethmann A (eds) Recent progress in the study and therapy of brain edema. Plenum Press, New York, London, pp 597–607
5. Szewczykowski J, Dytko P, Kunicki A et al. (1975) Determination of critical ICP levels in neurosurgical patients: A statistical approach. In: Lundberg N, Ponten U, Brock M (eds) Intracranial pressure II Springer, Berlin Heidelberg New York, pp 392–393

Mass Lesions

The Mechanism of Formation of Brain Tumor Cysts

K.G. Go, P.N.M. Lohle, I.T.H.J. Verhagen, A.W. Teelken, and E.H. Blaauw

Departments of Neurosurgery, Neurology, Electron Microscopy, University of Groningen, The Netherlands

Introduction

There are brain tumors which are associated with cysts. With respect to control of intracranial pressure, the occurrence of large cysts is of clinical significance, especially when removal of the tumor per sé is not possible, since evacuation of the cyst may readily achieve considerable increase of intracranial compliance. Yet the study of the mechanism of formation of tumor cysts, and of the conditions determining their prevalence and recurrence, has generally received little attention. Tumor cysts typically contain a protein-rich fluid. It is the protein that probably maintains cyst volume by retarding its resolution, as in the case of protein-rich vasogenic edema fluid. Conceivable origins of cyst fluid are necrosis or degeneration of tumor tissue versus vasogenic edema accompanying the tumor. If the cyst fluid originates from tumor tissue, it should predominantly contain cell proteins, whereas a vasogenic origin would imply a fluid constitution in which plasma proteins prevail.

Material and Methods

From 22 patients with cerebral gliomas (2 low-grade oligodendrogliomas, 4 low-grade and 11 high-grade astrocytomas, and 5 glioblastomas) cyst fluid and blood serum was obtained and subjected to cellulose acetate electrophoresis for the measurement of concentrations of the plasma protein fractions: albumin, IgA, IgC and IgM.

1. Dividing the sum of concentrations of plasma protein fractions in cyst fluid by the measured total protein concentration in cyst fluid provided the contribution (in %) of plasma proteins to cyst fluid.
2. The measured concentrations of plasma protein fractions were expressed by the ratio Q = serum concentration/cyst fluid concentration. These ratios were plotted against the molecular diameter of the protein to obtain a protein-gradient curve (Fig. 1) [1].

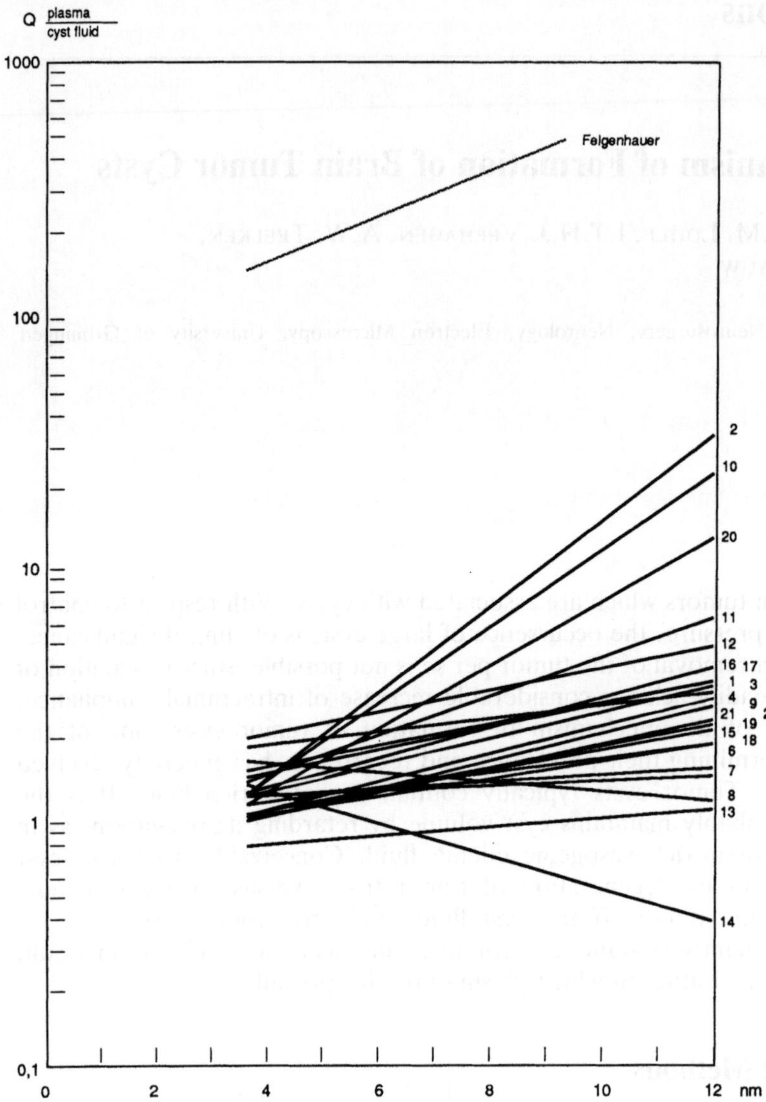

Fig. 1. Protein gradient curves, obtained by plotting the Q-values of cyst fluids (the numbers refer to the cases) against the molecular diameter (in nm) of the protein. The Felgenhauer curve denotes the normal gradient for CSF proteins; compared to this curve those of tumor cyst fluids are 50-fold lower (i.e. the protein concentrations are 50-fold higher)

Results and Discussion

Plasma proteins appeared to constitute 92.2 ± 5.2% of cyst fluid proteins. The Q-values indicated that the plasma protein fractions occurred in concentrations that are ~50-fold of those in normal CSF.

The prevalence of plasma proteins in cyst fluids clearly denotes their vasogenic origin, with intrinsic brain tissue proteins (e.g. resulting from

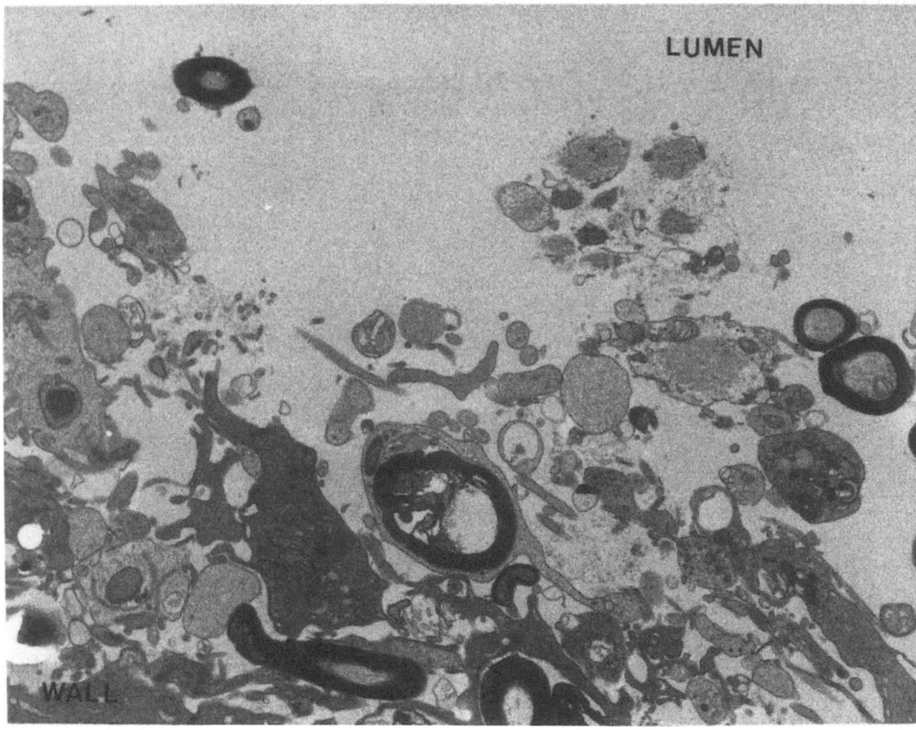

Fig. 2. Transmission electron micrograph of the wall of a gliomatous cyst. There is gradual transition of the edematous spongy tissue (lower half) into the cyst fluid (upper half)

necrosis) only constituting a minority. The vasogenic origin is in accordance with the Q-data indicating blood-brain barrier impairment, and with the frequent finding of contrast enhancement on the CT-scans. From a pathophysiological point of view, blood-brain barrier disruption is inherent with the occurrence of vasogenic brain edema [3], such as peritumoral edema. The presence of contrast-enhancement on CT or MRI-scans in the majority of gliomas denotes blood-brain barrier disruption. The ultrastructural basis for a defective blood-brain barrier may be found in the fenestrated type of endothelium often observed in the capillary walls of gliomas [2].

That cyst fluid may derive from peritumoral edema is, moreover, supported by the morphological findings. Next to areas showing a well-defined cell lining, which is apparently the result of expansion and compression, electron microscopy of cyst walls notably showed areas in which there was gradual transition of spongy edematous tissue to the debris of the cyst cavity (Fig. 2). It may be concluded that brain tumor cyst fluid, like peritumoral edema fluid, has a vasogenic origin in relation to blood-brain barrier disruption, and that it probably develops from peritumoral edema by gradual liquefaction of the edematous tissue.

References

1. Felgenhauer K, Schliep G, Rapic N (1976) Evaluation of the blood-CSF barrier by protein gradients and the humoral immune response within the central nervous system. J Neurol Sci 30:113–128
2. Hirano A, Matsui T (1975) Vascular structures in brain tumors. Human Pathol 6:611–621
3. Klatzo I (1967) Neuropathological aspects of brain edema. J Neuropathol Exp Neurol 26:1–14

Spontaneous Putaminal Haematoma. Does Post-operative ICU Management Improve Outcome?

W. POON, S. REHMAN, C. POON, and A.K.C. LI.

Neurosurgical Unit, Dept of Surgery, Prince of Wales Hospital, Chinese University of Hong Kong, Shatin, Hong Kong

Introduction

Surgical management of spontaneous intracerebral haemorrhage remains controversial because its mortality, in the region of 38%–61%, does not differ significantly whether treated conservatively or operatively [5, 6]. In the absence of any general agreement, surgical decision-making is at the level of each individual case, based upon the individual neurosurgeon's background of training and personal experience. The orthodox teaching of strongly considering surgical evacuation of lobar haematoma >30 ml, but never of thalamic haemorrhage, is recommended by modern textbooks of neurosurgery [2]. There is no concensus of opinion in spontaneous putaminal haematoma. Most recently published studies failed to demonstrate any benefit in the surgical group [1, 7, 8]. However, in a selected group of patients with putaminal haematoma, surgical evacuation has been shown to improve both mortality and morbidity [4].

We have focussed our study of intracranial pressure (ICP) and clinical outcome on a selected group of patients with putaminal haematoma treated by early surgical evacuation and intensive care (ICU) management.

Patients and Methods

In a 30-months-period between May 1988 and December 1990, nine patients with spontaneous putaminal haematoma entered the study of early surgical evacuation and post-operative ICU management. Selection criteria include [1] age 30–60 years; [2] Glasgow coma score 6–12/15; and [3] haematoma size >30 ml. The course of ICP and its response to treatment were followed. Management outcome was compared with an identical group of nine patients treated by a conventional policy in the 2 years preceding the study period (May 1986–April 1988) matched for age, coma score, site and size of the haematoma. These nine patients were closely observed and were treated conservatively unless clinical deterioration occurred, when surgical evacuation of the haematoma was carried out. ICP was not monitored. Post-operative ventilation was not routine and was only instituted if there was a respiratory indication.

Table 1. Demographic and clinical data of the two groups of patients

	N	Age (mean ± SE)	Coma (score)	Haematoma size (ml)
Early surgery + ICU (1988–90)	9	43 ± 3 yr	9 ± 1	54 ± 7 ml
Conventional (1986–1988)	9	40 ± 4 yr	10 ± 1	58 ± 8 ml

Table 2. Management outcome of the two groups of patients

	N	Good recovery	Moderate disability	Severe disability	Death
Early surgery + ICU (1988–90)	9	0	7	1	1
Conventional (1986–1988)					
• conservative	2	0	1	0	1
• surgery	7	0	1	2	4

DF = 2, chi-square = 5.78, p = 0.056

Results

A summary of the demographic and clinical data is listed in Table 1. One patient of the study group died from uncontrollable intracranial hypertension whereas 5 died in the conventional group (Table 2). Four patients in the study group had a post-operative ICP in the range of 30 mmHg (Fig. 1) and survived.

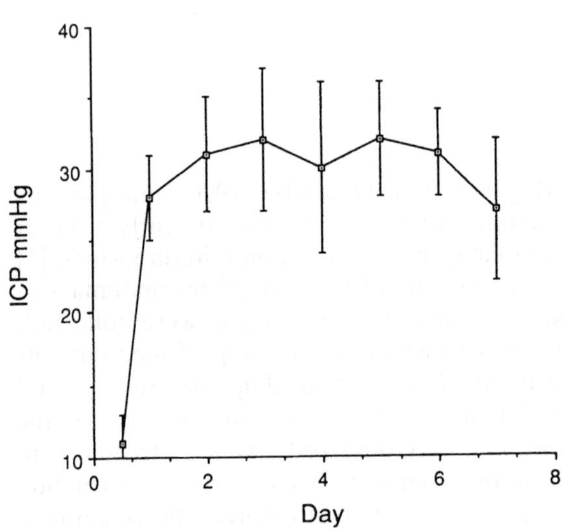

Fig. 1. ICP management in 4 patients in the study group was straightforward. They were routinely ventilated, requiring intermittent mannitol infusion

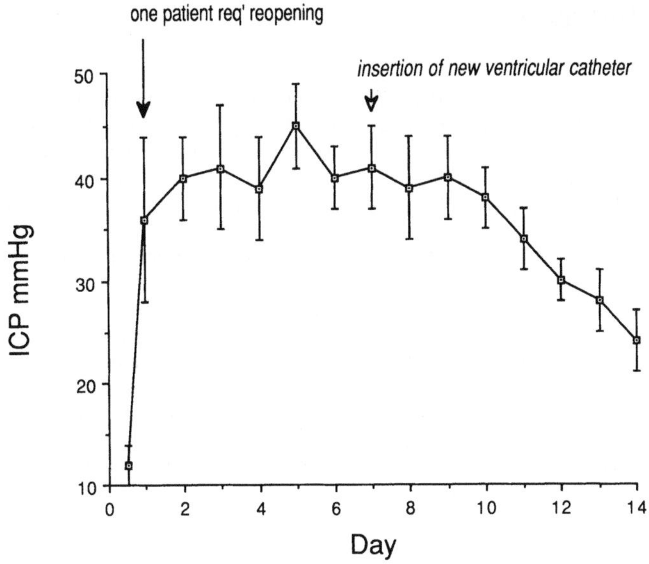

Fig. 2. ICP management in another 4 patients in the study group was difficult but manageable

In four others, the post-operative ICP in the first week was in the range of 40 mmHg: one patient required a re-opening for evacuation of a post-operative clot; they all required insertion of a second ventricular catheter in the contralateral frontal horn for prolonged monitoring in the second week; one patient developed meningitis and brain abscess at the operative site and was subsequently severely disabled (Fig. 2).

Discussion and Conclusion

Early surgery and routine post-operative ICU management of this selected group of patients with spontaneous putaminal haematoma clearly saves life in comparison with the conventional policy. However, even the good quality survivors failed to return to their previous employment and remained in the category of "moderate disability" at six months.

Zero mortality has been reported in spontaneous intracerebral haemorrhage treated by ICU management alone without surgery [3]. In spontaneous putaminal haematoma, a small group of patients with "rapidly progressive" symptoms and signs, surgical treatment was reported to be superior to conservative management [4]. The relative roles of surgery and ICU management in the reduction of mortality and morbidity in our patients therefore remain uncertain. A randomized trial comparing early surgery and ICU management vs. ICU management alone in this group of patients is needed.

References

1. Auer LM et al. (1989) Endoscopic surgery versus medical treatment for spontaneous intracerebral haematoma: a randomized study. J Neursurg 70:530–535
2. Castel JP, Kessel P (1990) Spontaneous intracerebral and infratentorial haemorrhage. In: Youmans JR (ed) Neurological Surgery, third edition, WB Saunders, 1890–1917
3. Duff TA et al. (1981) Nonsurgical management of spontaneous intracerebral haematoma. Neurosurgery 9:387–393
4. Fujitsu K et al. (1990) Indications for surgical treatment of putaminal haemorrhage. J Neurosurg 73:518–525
5. Juvela S et al. (1989) The treatment of spontaneous intracerebral haemorrhage, a prospective randomized trial of surgical and conservative treatment. J Neurosurg 70:755–758
6. McKissock W et al. (1961) Primary intracerebral haemorrhage, a controlled trial of surgical and conservative treatment in 180 unselected cases. Lancet 2:221–226
7. Waga S et al. (1983) Hypertensive putaminal haemorrhage, treatment and results. Is surgical treatment superior to conservative one? Stroke 14:480–485
8. Waga S et al. (1986) Hypertensive putaminal haemorrhage, analysis of 182 patients. Surg Neurol 26:159–166

Assessment of Brainstem Distortion Associated with Extraaxial Supratentorial Mass by Magnetic Resonance Imaging

S. Inao, H. Kuchiwaki, H. Kanaiwa, K. Sugita, S. Takada, A. Izawa, and M. Furuse

Department of Neurosurgery, Nagoya University, and Imaging Laboratory, Department of Radiology, Nakatsugawa Municipal General Hospital, Japan

Introduction

The characteristic findings on CT associated with transtentorial herniation have been studied [2], and the relationship between the lateral displacement of the brain and level of consciousness has also been reported [1]. However, quantitative measurement of brain distortion or the relationship between cerebral shift and brainstem displacement in patients with supratentorial space-occupying lesions did not receive much attention.

Using magnetic resonance imaging (MRI), we studied the types of brainstem distortions associated with cerebral hemisphere displacement secondary to a unilateral supratentorial mass. The horizontal and rotational movements of the hemisphere and brainstem were measured in the axial and coronal planes. The displacements were analysed and a mechanism for cerebral and brainstem injury is presented.

Material and Methods

Twenty-five cases of chronic subdural hematoma (age range 39–87 yrs, mean 66.4 ± 3.5) were studied with axial and coronal T1 weighted MR images. The hematoma thickness and the midline shift of the septum pellucidum, pineal body, intercollicular sulcus, interpeduncular fossa, and IVth ventricle were measured. The rotational movement at the septum, prepontine cistern, and intercollicular sulcus were also measured on axial or coronal images. The angles between the midline and the septum-pineal line and prepontine-IVth ventricle line were measured in the axial plane. The angles between the midline and septum-IIIrd ventricle line and the intercollicular sulcus-pontomedullary junction line were measured in the coronal plane.

Table 1. Hematoma thickness and midline shift

	Mean ± SD (mm)
Hematoma Thickness	21.7 ± 5.6
Axial Image	
Septum Pellucidum	8.1 ± 3.6
Pineal	6.3 ± 2.5
Intercollicular	2.9 ± 1.7
Interpeduncular	3.1 ± 1.8
IVth ventricle	0.7 ± 0.9
Coronal Image	
Septum Pellucidum	7.7 ± 2.9
Intercollicular	3.8 ± 1.5

Table 2. Rotational movement

	Mean ± SD (°)
Axial Image	
Septum – Pineal	5.7 ± 3.4
Prepontine – IV vent	5.2 ± 3.5
Coronal Image	
Septum – III vent	9.0 ± 3.3
IntC – Pontomedullary	5.7 ± 2.7

Results

Hematoma Thickness and Midline Shift

The average values of hematoma thickness and midline shift measured at multiple points are summarized in Table 1. The relationship between hematoma thickness and horizontal shift of the cerebrum (septum) and brainstem (interpeduncular fossa) is logarithmic and the best correlation is for the septum displacement ($r < 0.65$).

The horizontal shift of the cerebrum (septum) and the horizontal shift of the pineal and brainstem were also logarithmically correlated: pineal $r = 0.96$, interpeduncular $r = 0.73$, and intercollicular $r = 0.74$. In the early phase of an expanding supratentorial mass brainstem movement was not evident. The brainstem began to shift markedly with the concomitant cerebral shift, reaching a plateau despite further cerebral shift.

Rotational Movement

The average angles of the brain rotational movements are summarized in Table 2. In the axial plane, the rotation in the central cerebrum (septum-pineal line) and brainstem (prepontine-IVth ventricle) changed in a logarithmic manner.

Although the rotational movement of the brainstem changed by the same magnitude as the cerebrum, the axis of the rotation was different. The axis of cerebral rotation moves in direct response to the cerebral displacement, but the axis of pontine rotation was centered around the fixed position of the IVth ventricle.

In the coronal plane, the rotational movement of the cerebral hemisphere (septum-IIIrd ventricle) and the brainstem (intercollicular sulcus-pontomedullary junction) also changed logarithmically. The difference between the rotational movement of the cerebrum and the rotational movement of the brainstem develops as the hemispheric shift increases and finally results in midbrain kinking.

Discussion

The relationship between horizontal shift and rotational movement of the cerebrum and brainstem is logarithmic. The types of shift changed in the rostral-caudal direction. The cerebral hemisphere shifted and rotated in the axial plane, the midbrain shifted laterally with no rotation, and the pons shifted minimally in the axial plane but rotated moderately. The marked rotation of the cerebral hemisphere and the mild rotation of the brainstem result in marked midbrain kinking measured in the coronal plane. We propose that the major brainstem injury resulting from an expanding supratentorial mass is secondary to the combined shift and rotational movement at the midbrain rather than transtentorial herniation with brainstem compression. This occurs as a result of the differential movement of the hemisphere and brainstem and results in midbrain kinking. MRI has elucidated the types of brain displacements associated with a supratentorial mass.

References

1. Ropper AH (1986) Lateral displacement of the brain and level of consciousness in patients with an acute hemispheric mass. N Engl J Med 314:953–958
2. Storvring J (1977) Descending tentorial herniation; finding on computed tomography. Neuroradiology 14:101–105

Bilateral Intraparenchymal Pressure in Patients with Unilateral Supratentorial Mass Lesions

G. GAMBARDELLA, D. D'AVELLA, C. STAROPOLI, S. TOSCANO, and F. TOMASELLO

Institute of Neurological and Neurosurgical Sciences, Neurosurgical Clinic, University of Messina, Italy

Introduction

Limited information is available in the literature about the intracranial compartmental pressure relationships in patients harbouring unilateral supratentorial mass lesions. Moreover, studies that have examined this issue have yielded conflicting results [5, 6].

Weaver et al. [5] using subarachnoid bolts to measure ICP in four patients, reported higher pressures on the side of mass lesions. Conversely, more recently, Yano et al. [6] reported no difference in subarachnoid pressures with bifrontal catheters used in 15 patients. It has been suggested that the reported differences were a function of the device employed to monitor ICP [1, 6]. In the experimental setting, changes in ICP secondary to a unilateral mass lesion were identical in both supratentorial parenchymal compartments, when measured simultaneously by means of the fiberoptic device. Therefore, studies using the fiberoptic device in a clinical setting would be useful in resolving this issue [1, 4]. The purpose of this study was to determine concurrent comparative intracranial pressures by means of bilateral intraparenchymal fiberoptic device recording, in patients with unilateral supratentorial expanding masses.

Subjects and Methods

The subjects consisted of 6 patients, of both sexes, 12 to 80 years old, who showed differences in the pathological status between the right and left hemisphere caused by lesions such as cerebral contusions (3 cases), intraparenchymal hematomas (2 cases), and a brain tumor with marked peripheral edema (1 case). All patients had midline shift, and were not treated surgically. Each of the patients underwent simultaneous insertion of two intraparenchymal Camino fiberoptic devices into the frontal white matter of both sides. These ICPs were measured continuously for 36–96 hours.

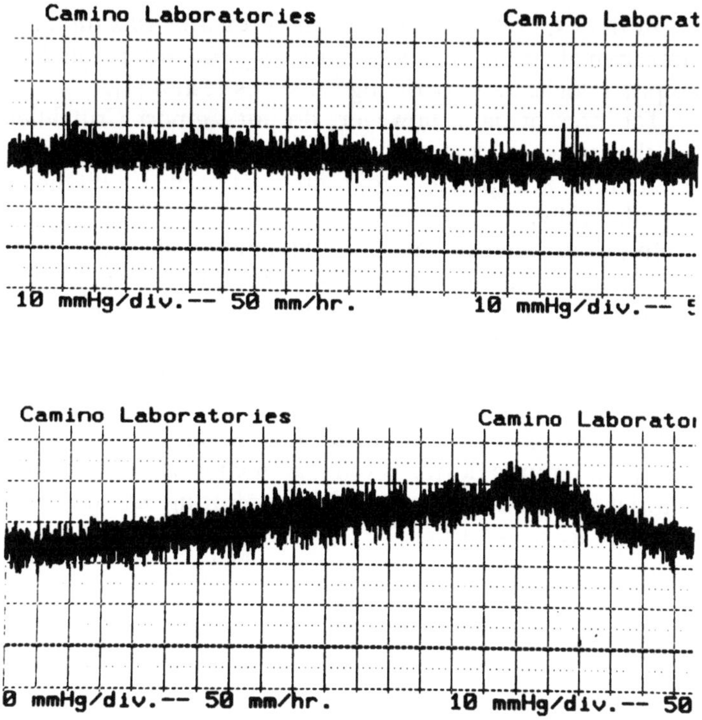

Fig. 1. ICP Tracings showing different pressure values between the two hemispheres during unilateral rapid volume increase

Results

In general, ICP tracings from the fiberoptic devices corresponded very closely to one another. In four cases, however, transient significant gradients of pressure between the right and left sides were observed, averaging 10–20 mmHg, and lasting no more than 1–2 hours (Fig. 1). These gradients were associated with the occurence of a rapid increase in volume of the mass lesion and the corresponding clinical deterioration.

CT scan studies showed in these patients an acute subdural hematoma, a delayed intracerebral hematoma, and two cases of acute worsening of the perilesional edema.

Discussion

Although based on a limited number of patients, these results corroborate and confirm previous clinical observations by Yano [6] and Marshall [6] that the supratentorial space can generally be considered as one compartment regardless of the differences in types and localization of chronic or slowly evolving unilateral intracranial lesions.

In the experimental setting, the pressures recorded in the subdural, intraparenchymal and intraventricular compartments paralleled each other in all of the physiological and pathological states tested [1].

The present data, however, do not support Crutchfield's observations [1] that the pressure changes between the brain parenchyma ipsilateral and contralateral to an expanding epidural mass occur simultaneously and at the same rate bilaterally.

In our experience, an abrupt volume increase in one hemisphere results in a significant increase in ipsilateral ICP. This unequal pressure distribution may last for 1–2 hours. When pressures equilibrate, differential pressures are no longer observed. Our clinical observations are in keeping with the concept of "local pressure", the pathomechanisms of which, involving CSF dynamics, regulation of CBF, or viscoelastic properties of the brain, have been extensively discussed [5]. In conclusion, intraparenchymatous pressure monitoring with the fiberoptic device is reliable in clinical practice. In patients with supratentorial unilateral lesions, ICP monitoring should include areas in close proximity to mass lesions.

References

1. Crutchfield JS, Narayan RK, Robertson CS, Michael LH (1990) Evaluation of a fiberoptic intracranial pressure monitor. J Neurosurg 72:482–487
2. Ostrup RC, Luerssen TG, Marshall LF, Zornow MH (1987) Continous monitoring of intracranial pressure with a miniaturized fiberoptic device. J Neurosurg 67:206–209
3. Robertson CS, Narayan RK, Contant CF, Grossman RG, Gokaslan ZL, Pahwa R, Caram P, Bray RS, Sherwood AM (1989) Clinical experience with a continous monitor of intracranial compliance. J Neurosurg 71:673–680
4. Sundbarg G, Nordstrom CH, Messeter K, Soderstrom S (1987) A comparison of intraparenchymatous and intraventricular pressure recording in clinical practice. J Neurosurg 67:841–845
5. Weaver DD, Winn HR, Jane JA (1982) Differential intracranial pressure in patients with unilateral mass lesion. J Neurosurg 56:660–665
6. Yano M, Ikeda Y, Kobayashi S, Otsuka T (1987) Intracranial pressure in head-injured patients with various intracranial lesions is identical throughout the supratentorial intracranial compartment. Neurosurgery 21, 5:688–692

Effects of Glycerol on Cerebral Blood Flow and Neural Function in Patients with Intracranial Space Occupying Lesions

H. KUYAMA, M. GOTOH, S. NISHINO, T. SHIRAKAWA, T. SAIJO, H. NIIMI, T. MUROTA, T. OHMOTO, and A. NISHIMOTO

Department of Neurological Surgery, Okayama University Medical School, 2-5-1 Shikata-cho, Okayama, Japan

Introduction

Hyperosmolar agents are often administered to obtain a rapid decrease in elevated intracranial pressure (ICP). Numerous workers have reported the effects of glycerol but little is known about its actions on cerebral circulation in the area of peritumoral edema and neural function. This study was undertaken to elucidate the effect of glycerol on regional cerebral blood flow (rCBF) and neural function in patients with intracranial space occupying lesions.

Clinical Material and Methods

A total of 26 patients were admitted to this study. Table 1 presents a clinical summary of patients. The patients were divided into two groups on the basis of the severity of cerebral edema which was estimated by computerized tomography (CT). Group 1 consisted of 11 patients. In 9 of 11 patients, the peritumoral hypodensity on CT was limited to a small area. The remaining two patients showed no peritumoral hypodensity area. In Group 2, CT showed extensive peritumoral hypodensity. All of these patients underwent rCBF measurements before glycerol administration and at 20 minutes after administration. rCBF was measured quantitatively using the inert gas washout technique with xenon-133 and single-photon emission computed tomography. The size of the region of interest (ROI) was 3 × 3 cm and the ROI was positioned adjacent to the tumor and in a symmetrically placed region in the contralateral hemisphere. All patients received 0.5 gm/kg of 10% glycerol within 30 minutes. Somatosensory evoked potentials (SEP) were recorded by median nerve stimulation in 8 patients with peritumoral edema located in the somatosensory cortical area on CT. Seven of eight patients belonged to Group 2 and the remaining one to Group 1.

Recording electrodes were placed at the C3/4 position of the international 10–20 system, using a frontal reference (Fpz). Visual evoked potentials (VEP) were recorded by transient hemi-field pattern-reversal stimulation in one patient of Group 2, who had a hypodensity area in the occipital lobe on CT. A midoccipital (MO) electrode was placed 5 cm above the external occipital protuberance. The left and right occipital electrodes were placed 5 cm to the

Table 1. Clinical summary of 26 patients. Case 21, 22, 25 and 26 showed the improvement of clinical symptoms following glycerol infusion.

Case no.		Age (yr)	Sex	Pathological diagnosis	Peritumoral edema	Percent increase in CBF following glycerol infusion Lesion side	Contralateral side
Group I							
1	Y.O.	63	F	malignant lymphoma	+	−15.4	−11.1
2	E.T.	61	F	tentorial meningioma	−	12.5	10.2
3	S.Y.	62	M	convexity meningioma	−	10.0	3.4
4	Y.K.	34	F	metastatic tumor	+	3.2	−9.8
5	K.H.	36	M	low grade astrocytoma	+	5.9	4.8
6	M.M.	70	M	high grade astrocytoma	+	14.3	13.6
7	M.T.	52	F	high grade astrocytoma	+	0.0	−2.6
8	M.U.	34	M	high grade astrocytoma	+	9.7	8.1
9	T.N.	29	M	low grade astrocytoma	+	2.4	−2.3
10	Y.S.	36	F	falx meningioma	+	2.6	0.0
11	K.A.	52	M	cavernous angioma	+	5.4	2.5
					mean ±S.D.	4.6±8.0	1.5±7.8
Group II							
12	F.H.	61	M	metastatic tumor	++	30.4	2.5
13	H.S.	44	M	metastatic tumor	++	36.8	8.8
14	H.S.	56	F	high grade astrocytoma	++	29.7	2.4
15	T.M.	41	M	high grade astrocytoma	++	30.4	20.7
16	S.T.	52	F	oligodendroglioma	++	17.6	26.8
17	S.N.	70	F	high grade astrocytoma	++	26.9	20.6
18	K.F.	60	F	metastatic tumor	++	21.4	5.0
19	S.H.	36	M	high grade astrocytoma	++	30.8	8.1
20	M.M.	51	F	metastatic tumor	++	−22.2	−26.0
21	S.U.	58	F	metastatic tumor	++	21.2	2.2
22	K.H.	60	M	malignant lymphoma	++	12.0	9.1
23	M.N.	67	F	metastatic tumor	++	17.9	19.4
24	T.M.	41	M	high grade astrocytoma	++	13.6	9.4
25	K.K.	66	F	metastatic tumor	++	19.2	2.4
26	T.Y.	43	M	metastatic tumor	++	20.0	10.7
					mean ±S.D.	20.4±13.8	8.1±12.3

− : none, + : mild, ++ : severe

left and right of the MO electrode respectively. Reference electrode was placed at the Fpz position. A black and white checkerboard was displayed on the same television screen, reversing at 1 Hz. During hemi-field stimulation the subject fixated on a red dot placed one degree of arc laterally from the stimulated hemi-field.

Results

Glycerol did not significantly alter systemic blood pressure in any cases. Resting rCBF in Group 1 was 37.0 ± 12.0 ml/100 g/min in the ROI adjacent to the tumor and 38.5 ± 10.1 ml/100 g/min in the contralateral side. In Group 2, rCBF on the lesion side was 29.1 ± 8.9 ml/100 g/min which was significantly

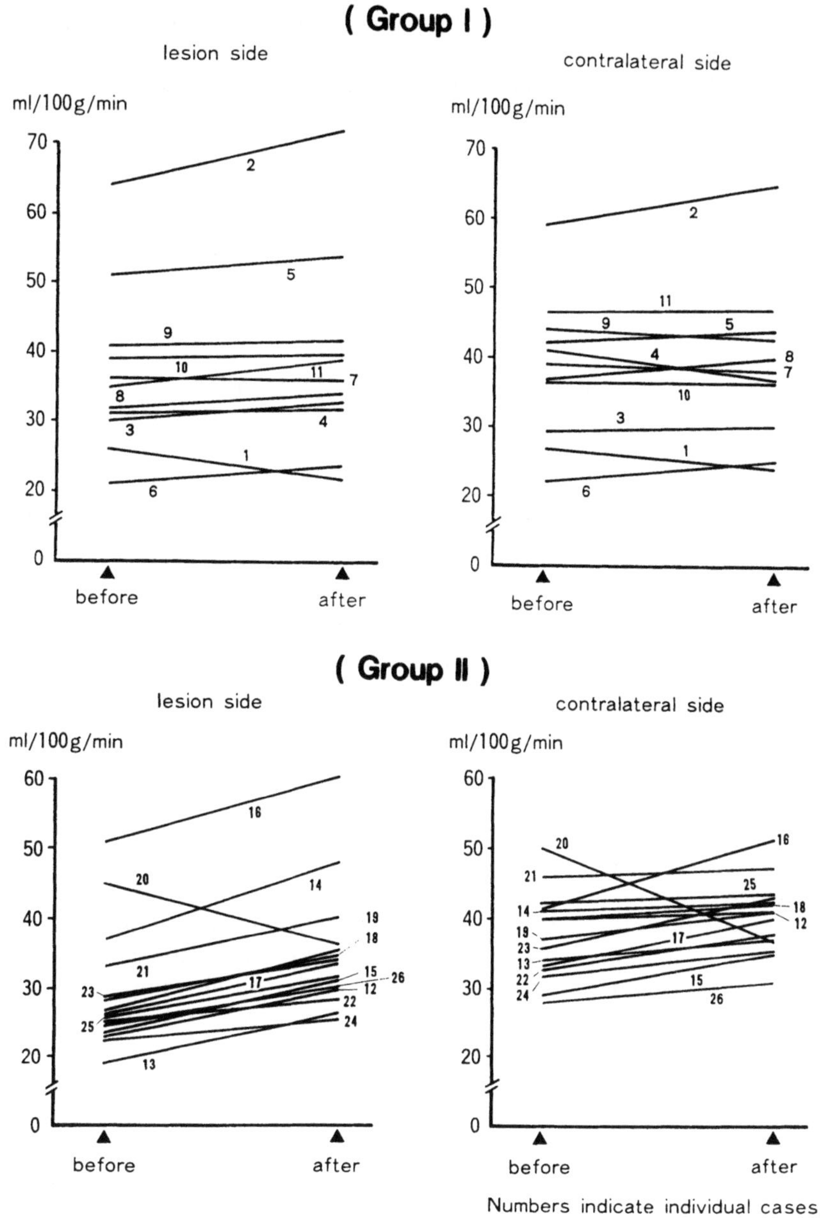

Fig. 1. Changes in rCBF before and after glycerol infusion in cases with mild cerebral edema (Group 1) and severe cerebral edema (Group 2)

decreased ($p < 0.01$) and rCBF in the contralateral side was 37.5 ± 6.1 ml/100 g/min (Fig. 1). After glycerol infusion, percent increase in rCBF in Group 1 was 4.6 ± 8.0 and 1.5 ± 7.8 on the lesion and contralateral sides respectively. In Group 2, percent increase in rCBF was 20.4 ± 13.8 on the lesion side, which was significantly increased compared to that of the contralateral side ($p < 0.05$)

(Table 1, Fig. 1). The later components of SEP (N33 and all other subsequent wave forms) were lost in 5 out of 8 patients and the latency of P24 was prolonged to 28.5 ± 2.1 msec in 6 patients. After glycerol infusion, prolonged P24 latency was shortened in 2 patients and the abolished later components recovered in 3 patients. The VEP showed a clear P100 peak and the peak latency tended to shorten in one case. Four of these 6 patients showed a rapid improvement of the clinical symptoms following glycerol infusion.

Discussion

Glycerol infusion can decrease ICP by dehydration of brain tissue. In this study, rCBF increased after glycerol infusion. The increase in rCBF was more marked in the affected areas in Group 2 patients who showed extensive peritumoral edema. This result suggests that glycerol can improve rCBF in the area of cerebral edema. Meyer et al. [3] reported that the improvement of CBF observed after glycerol infusion seemed to be due to the reduction of regional cerebral edema rather than to a decrease of overall intracranial pressure, because the CBF started to increase before the decrease in ICP. The other mechanisms of increasing rCBF are considered to be improved microcirculation produced by hemodilution [5] and increased deformability of red cells [2].

We employed SEP and VEP for assessment of electrophysiologic activity of the cortex and observed the improvement of evoked potentials in 6 patients. The late latency components of SEP relate to cortical integration processes [4] and pattern-reversal VEPs reflect the complex interaction of electrical field potentials within primary visual cortex and visual association areas [1]. Improvement of these evoked potentials following glycerol infusion probably may account for the amelioration of clinical symptoms. These results support the report on the improvement in the electroencephalogram and neurological function in patients with acute cerebral infarction after glycerol infusion [3]. The improvement of electrophysiologic activity following glycerol infusion is thought to be attributed to the improvement of cerebral metabolism [1] as well as cerebral circulation.

Conclusion

It is concluded from this clinical study that glycerol may increase rCBF in the area of peritumoral cerebral edema and improve the neural functions.

References

1. Celesia GG, Polcyn RD, Holden JE, Nickles RJ, Gatley JS, Koeppe RA (1982) Visual evoked potentials and positron emission tomographic mapping of regional cerebral blood flow and cerebral metabolism: Can the neuronal potential generators be visualized? Electroenceph Clin Neurophysiol 54:243–256

2. Hatashita S (1982) Protective effects of barbiturate, mannitol and glycerol on experimental global cerebral ischemia (Part 2). Neurol Med Chir (Tokyo) 22:972–981
3. Meyer JS, Fukuuchi Y, Shimazu K, Ohuchi T, Ericsson AD (1972) Effect of intravenous infusion of glycerol on hemispheric blood flow and metabolism in patients with acute cerebral infarction. Stroke 3:168–180
4. Pfurtscheller G, Schwarz G, Gravenstein N (1985) Clinical relevance of long-latency SEPs and VEPs during coma and emergence from coma. Electroenceph Clin Neurophysiol 62:88–98
5. Sasaki T, Matsuzaki T, Nakagawara J, Sato S, Kawai Y, Suematsu K (1983) Improvement of CBF by glycerol administration in hypertensive intracerebral hemorrhage. Brain Nerve 35:505–510

Peritumoral Edema and Regional Cerebral Blood Flow in Brain Tumors

S. TSUCHIDA, H. KUYAMA, S. ASARI, T. OHMOTO, and A. NISHIMOTO

Department of Neurological Surgery, Okayama University Medical School, 2-5-1 Shikata-cho, Okayama, Japan

Introduction

Brain tumor is often associated with peritumoral edema and the extent of the edema has been reported to be related to many factors especially meningiomas. The possible mechanisms for the production of severe edema surrounding meningioma include clinical evolution, tumor size, location, histological subtype, cellularity, vascularity, secretory-excretory activity, mechanical compression of a draining vein and disruption of the cortical layer between the tumor and the underlying white matter [1–5]. However, any of these factors are not sufficient to explain the production of peritumoral edema in brain tumors. In this study, peritumoral edema was analysed with special attention to the regional cerebral blood flow (rCBF).

Materials and Methods

rCBF was measured with the stable xenon-enhanced CT method in 21 cases of intracranial tumors (13 meningiomas, 5 gliomas, 3 metastatic brain tumors). The CBF studies were performed on a xenon-enhanced CT CBF system adapted to the 9800 CT scanner (General Electric Company). The patient inhaled a mixture of 33% stable xenon gas in 67% oxygen via a face mask for 5 minutes while the end-tidal xenon gas concentrations were recorded. CBF images were obtained at two levels including the tumor. The findings from these studies were compared with those obtained by CT scan and/or magnetic resonance imaging (MRI) studies, and the assessment of distribution patterns of intratumoral blood flow was made in association with peritumoral edema. The other factors such as histological subtype, tumor size, location, angiographical vascularity and clinical course were also evaluated. Peritumoral edema was graded as mild, moderate and severe on the basis of the extent of the edema on CT and MRI.

Results

Summarized data of the 21 cases are given in Tables 1 and 2. Intratumoral blood flow distribution patterns were classified into three types: central type

Table 1. Summary of gliomas and metastatic tumors

No.	Age	Sex	Tumor type	CE-CT	Location	Vascularization in angiogram	Length of clinical history	rCBF pattern of tumor on Xe-CT	Peritumoral edema
Gliomas									
1	54	M	Astrocytoma (grade 3)	Irregular Ring-enhanced	Thalamus	+++	1 M	Marginal	Mi
2	48	M	Astrocytoma (grade 3)	Irregular Cystic	Frontal	++	1.5 M	Marginal	Se
3	42	M	Astrocytoma (grade 3)	Ring-enhanced	Frontal	+	3.5 M	Marginal	Mo
4	50	M	Astrocytoma (grade 4)	Irregular Ring-enhanced	Temporal	+	4 M	Marginal	Mo
5	27	F	Astrocytoma (pleomorphic xantho-astrocytoma)	Cystic	Temporal	–	3 M	–	Mi
Metastatic tumors									
1	70	F	squamous	Homogeneously enhanced	Occipital	+	1.5 M	Marginal	Se
2	65	M	–	Homogeneously enhanced	Frontal	+	1 M	Marginal	Mo
3	53	M	–	Ring-enhanced	Corpus callosum	N	1 M	Marginal	Mo

+: poor, ++: moderate, +++: rich N: angiography was not performed
Mi: mild $\leqq$ 1 cm, 1 cm < Mo: moderate < 3 cm, 3 cm $\leqq$ Se: severe (maximum extension of peritumoral edema on CT or MRI)

Table 2. Summary of meningiomas

No.	Age	Sex	Tumor type	Size (cm)	Location	Vascularization in angiogram	Length of clinical history	rCBF pattern of tumor on Xe-CT	Peritumoral edema
1	49	F	Meningothelial	6.5	Tuberculum sellae	+++	29 Y	Central	Mi
2	60	F	Meningothelial	4.5	Convexity	+	2 M	Central	Mi
3	29	M	Meningothelial	4.5	Parasagittal	++	3 M	Central	Mi
4	39	F	Meningothelial	2.5	Sphenoid ridge (medial type)	+	1 M	Marginal	Mi
5	56	F	Vacuolated	4.5	Falx	++	2 M	Homogeneous	Mo
6	65	F	Angiomatous	3.0	Falx	+++	1 M	Homogeneous	Mo
7	62	M	Transitional	6.5	Convexity	++	5 Y	Marginal	Mo
8	76	M	Transitional	4.0	Convexity	+	3 M	Marginal	Mo
9	62	M	Meningothelial	4.5	Olfactory groove	+	1.5 M	Marginal	Se
10	58	M	Meningothelial	6.0	Falx	++	7 M	Marginal	Se
11	41	M	Meningothelial	3.0	Sphenoid ridge (lateral type)	++	8 M	Marginal	Se
12	41	F	Malignant	4.5	Occipital	–	1 M	Marginal	Se
13	69	F	Angiomatous	3.5	Convexity	++	2 M	Marginal	Se

+: poor, ++: moderate, +++: rich, Mi: mild $\leqq$ 1 cm, 1 cm < Mo: moderate < 3 cm, 3 cm $\leqq$ Se: severe

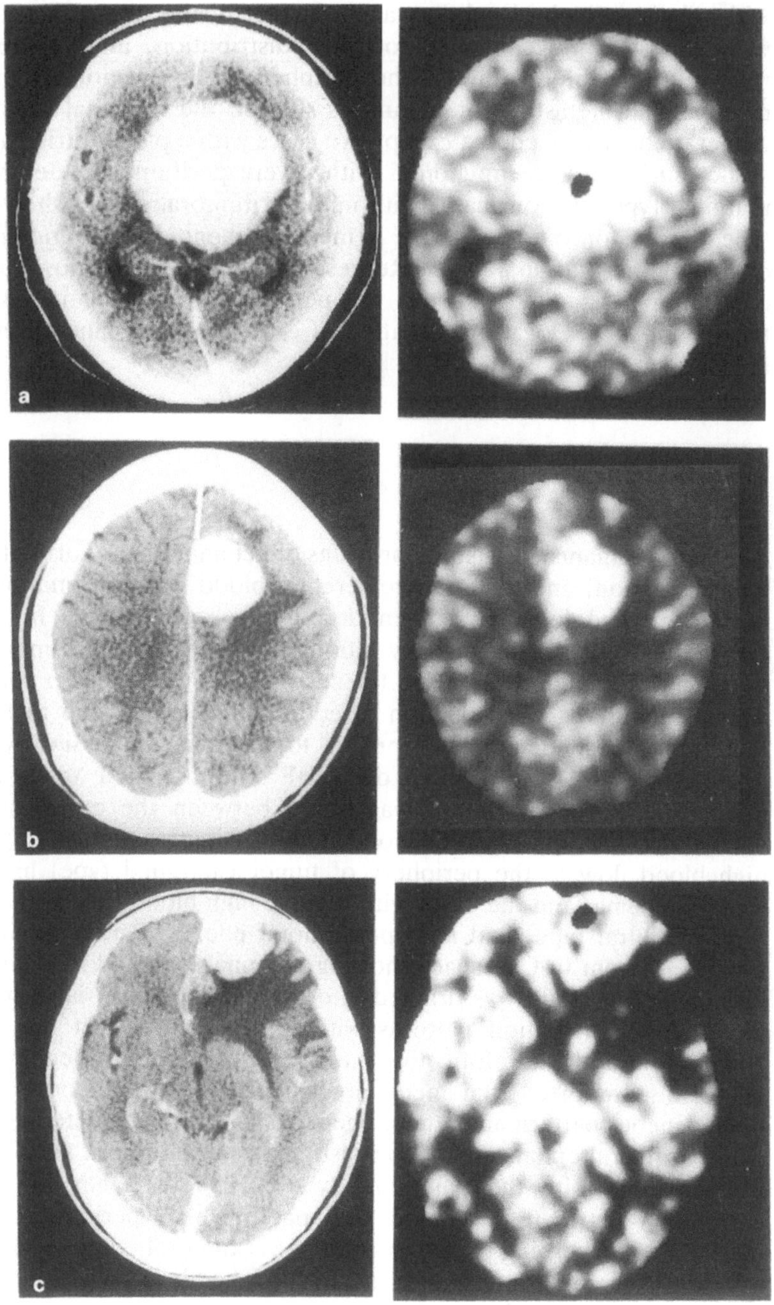

Fig. 1. **a** Central type (Case 1). Contrast enhanced CT shows a large meningioma with mild edema in the frontal region. rCBF image shows relatively high blood flow at the center of the tumor. Central small defect is due to calcification. **b** Homogeneous type (Case 6). Contrast enhanced CT shows a meningioma with moderate edema in the frontal region. rCBF image shows homogeneous blood flow distribution. **c** Marginal type (Case 13). Contrast enhanced CT shows olfactory groove meningioma with severe edema. rCBF image shows relatively high blood flow at the periphery of the tumor

with relatively high blood flow at the center of the tumor, homogeneous type with almost homogeneous blood flow distribution, and marginal type with relatively high blood flow at the periphery of the tumor. High grade astrocytomas and metastatic brain tumors showed the marginal type and revealed moderate or severe edema except two cases with a paraventricular tumor and a cystic tumor. Five meningiomas with severe peritumoral edema revealed the marginal type and four cases with mild peritumoral edema showed the central type except for one case with a medial sphenoid ridge meningioma which exhibited the marginal type. Representative cases are shown in Fig. 1. No correlation was found between the peritumoral edema and histological subtype, tumor size, location, duration of clinical history, and vascularization on angiogram.

Discussion

The xenon-enhanced CT study provides direct anatomical correlation, relatively high resolution, and quantitative cerebral blood flow information. The details of this methodology have been described elsewhere [8]. In brain tumors, edema fluid escapes from leaky blood vessels within the tumor, whereas the permeability of blood vessels in the surrounding white matter remains normal. This means that the production of edema fluid is confined to the tumor and that the leaked edema fluid spreads to the adjacent tissue by the pressure gradient [5, 6]. According to our CBF study using a xenon-enhanced CT method, a close correlation was found between the extent of peritumoral edema and the intratumoral blood flow distribution patterns: the cases with high blood flow at the periphery of tumor (marginal type) had severe peritumoral edema, and the cases with relative high blood flow at the center of the tumor (central type) had mild peritumoral edema. Paraventricular tumors or tumors adjacent to CSF space showing marginal type had mild edema probably because edema fluid was drained into the CSF space. It is suggested that the blood flow distribution patterns within the tumor affect the production of edema fluid and, therefore, the extension of peritumoral edema. Tatagiba et al. [7] also reported that meningiomas revealed two blood flow patterns: a homogeneous pattern and a heterogeneous pattern. The heterogeneous pattern with peripheral enhancement contrasting a central area of very low blood flow is compatible with the "marginal type". However, they did not state the correlation between the blood flow patterns and peritumoral edema. The mechanism concerning the production of peritumoral edema is speculated to be relevant to the hydromechanical factor [6]. The "leak" of the edema fluid from the tumor may be influenced by the balance between the production and the resolution of edema fluid.

References

1. Bradac GB, Ferszt R, Bender A, Schorner W (1986) Peritumoral edema in meningiomas. A radiological and histological study. Neuroradiology 28:304–312
2. Gilbert JJ, Paulseth JE, Coates RK, Malott D (1983) Cerebral edema associated with meningiomas. Neurosurgery 12:599–605
3. Go KG, Wilmink JT, Molenaar WM (1988) Peritumoral brain edema associated with meningiomas. Neurosurgery 23:175–179
4. Philippon J, Foncin JF, Grob R, Srour A, Poisson M, Pertuiset BF (1984) Cerebral edema associated with meningiomas: Possible role of a secretory-excretory phenomenon. Neurosurgery 14:295–301
5. Reulen HJ, Graber S, Huber P, Ito U (1988) Factors affecting the extension of peritumoural brain oedema. A CT-study. Acta Neurochir (Wien) 95:19–24
6. Stevens JM, Ruiz JS, Kendall BE (1983) Observations on peritumoural oedema in meningioma. Part 2: Mechanisms of oedema production. Neuroradiology 25:125–131
7. Tatagiba M, Mirzai S, Samii M (1991) Peritumoral blood flow in intratumoral meningiomas. Neurosurgery 26:400–404
8. Yonas H, Gur D, Latchaw R, Wolfson SK Jr (1987) Stable xenon CT/CBF imaging: Laboratory and clinical experience. Adv Tech Stand Neurosurg 15:1–37

Session II: Experimental Aspects

Chairmen: A. Baethmann and K.G. Go

Compression-induced Brain Edema: Regional Changes of Superoxide Free Radicals in the Development of Vasogenic Edema and Tissue Damage in Intracranial Hypertension

N. HAYASHI and T. TSUBOKAWA

Emergency Center and Department of Neurosurgery Nihon University, Tokyo, Japan

Introduction

Intracranial hypertension following severe head injury continues to remain a serious problem affecting morbidity and mortality. The major causes of such a seriously elevated intracranial pressure (ICP) are mainly either vascular engorgement (brain swelling) or brain edema. Engorgement occurs when there is a loss of normal regulation of vascular tone, and brain edema can occur due to an increased vascular permeability [7]. Recent studies have indicated that the oxygen derived free radicals may modify the changes of vascular tone, permeability and cell membrane damage in ischemic injury [1], resulting in brain edema and swelling. Despite this conceptual framework, previous studies have failed to elucidate the precise location, characteristics, and magnitude of free radical-induced alterations of the injured tissue. An accurate understanding of the regional changes in free radicals occurring in intracranial hypertension-injured tissue is important for investigating the mechanisms of brain edema and swelling in the central nervous system. One of the problems in such research is that free radicals are extremely labile and difficult to detect *in vivo*.

We recently developed a new technique for mapping the distribution of superoxide anion radicals, energy metabolism, tissue pH, Ca-Calmodulin (Ca-M) and vascular permeability in frozen tissue sections, simultaneously [4, 5]. In this paper, we report details of the localized changes in free radicals occurring in mass lesions induced by intracranial hypertension, and discuss the role of free radicals in the development of brain edema and metabolic changes.

Materials and Methods

Operative and Sampling Techniques

Forty-five male Sprague-Dawley rats weighing 250–350 g were fasted overnight but given free access to water. Anesthesia was initiated with 4.5% halothane in a mixture of 70% nitrogen and 30% oxygen, and was maintained with Nembutal (1.8 mg/kg, IV). The animals were placed in stereotaxic frames and were permitted to breath spontaneously. They were mounted on an Aquamatic K module heating pad (German Rupp Industries, Ont.). The body temperature was measured rectally and maintained at 37.0 ± 0.5°C.

Consistent long-lasting intracranial hypertension was produced by implantation of a piece of 3-mm diameter dual-hole silastic tubing into the left parietal epidural space. The levels of ICP were controlled through changes in the size of the silastic tubing in the epidural space. Blood gases analysis was performed before freezing to ensure that normoxic and normocapnic (arterial $PO_2 > 100$ mmHg; PCO_2, 35–40 mmHg) conditions prevailed. The brains were frozen *in situ* by pouring liquid nitrogen via a funnel onto the skull [9] and sliced to 15 μ in thickness on cryostats.

Experimental Protocol

The animals were divided into three groups according to the level of the ICP. The role of free radicals in the development of brain edema and damage to the energy metabolism was studied by simultaneous mapping of various pathophysiological changes such as of the tissue ATP, NADH, Ca-M, vascular permeability by extravasation of Evans Blue dye, and superoxide free radicals until 72 hr after epidural cerebral compression.

Group I (n = 15). After recording a stable baseline for the systemic arterial blood pressure and blood gases, a sham operation was performed. The localized distribution of superoxide anion free radicals in the normal brain tissue was then examined.

Group II (n = 10). Mild intracranial hypertension (lower than the cerebral mean capillary pressure) was produced by implantation of a 3-mm length of dual-hole silastic tubing. The regional changes in superoxide free radicals in the compressed brain tissue and the effects leading to damage of the vascular permeability, energy metabolism and Ca regulation as evaluated from the changes in Ca-M, were investigated at 24, 48 and 72 hr after cerebral compression.

Group III (n = 10). Moderate intracranial hypertension (higher than the cerebral mean capillary pressure) was produced by implantation of a 5-mm length of dual-hole silastic tubing. The intraparenchymal pathophysiology was examined in the same manner as in group II.

Technique for Mapping Superoxide Free Radicals

The distribution of superoxide anions in the CNS was determined by our new method based on the 380 nm chemiluminescence of 2-methyl-6-phenyl-3,7-dihydroimidazo[1,2a]pyrazin-3-one (CLA-phenyl, A5307, Tokyo Kasei Kogyo Co., Ltd., Tokyo, Japan), which reacts with superoxide anions [8]. The 15-μ sliced frozen tissue section was mounted on millipore filter paper (CA 250/0, Schleicher & Schuell Co., Germany) saturated with CLA-phenyl solution in

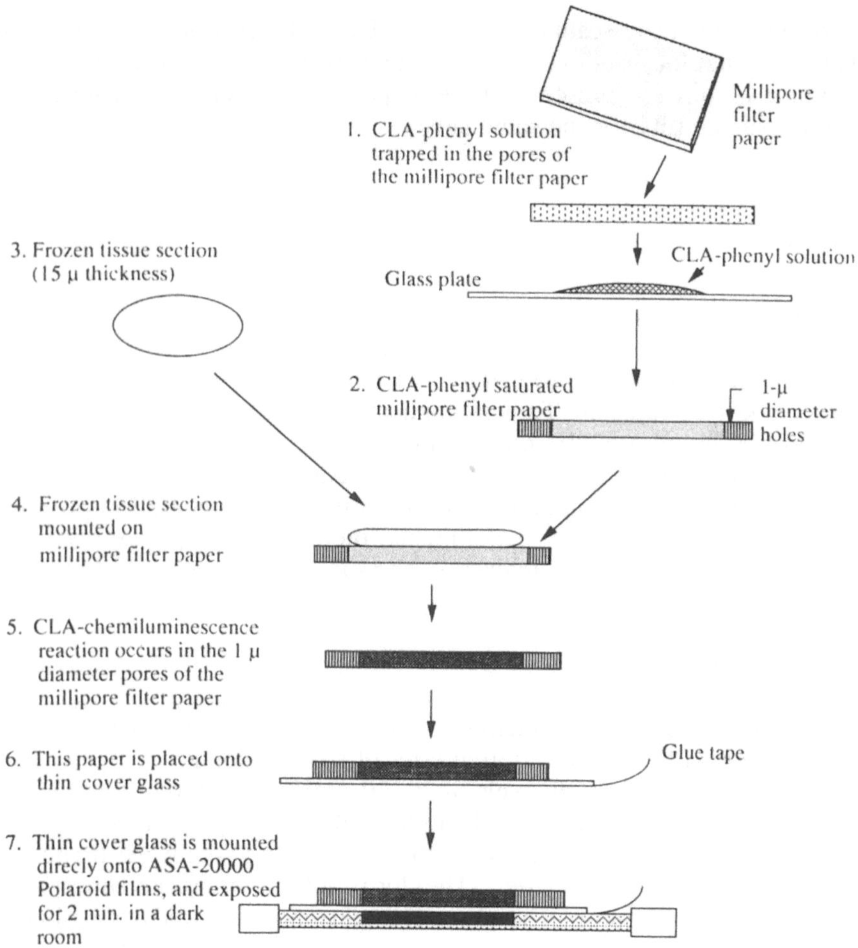

Fig. 1. Scheme of the procedure for mapping the superoxide free radical concentration in frozen tissue section employing a millipore hybrid paper technique. Frozen tissue sections (15μ) were mounted on millipore hybrid paper saturated previously with CLA-phenyl solution. The CLA-chemiluminescence reaction occurs in the 1μ diameter pores of the millipore hybrid paper. The photochemical reactions were recorded directly on ASA-20000 Polaroid films

the millipore holes. The frozen tissue section was first melted and then trapped in the filter pores at room temperature. Superoxide-CLA-phenyl photochemical reactions occurred immediately within the 1-μ diameter pores of the millipore filter paper. The paper was pasted onto a thin cover glass and then placed directly onto ASA-20000 Polaroid film in a dark room. The light emitted by the superoxide-CLA-phenyl photochemical reactions in the pores of the filter paper was recorded on the Polaroid film as a picture after exactly 2 min of exposure (Fig. 1). Next, the frozen tissue slices were prepared for mapping studies of the tissue ATP, Ca-M and extravasation of Evans Blue dye [4, 5]. The densities of superoxide anion radicals on the Polaroid films were determined by scanning with a SPCCA-II densitometer (Olympus Co., Tokyo). The localized changes in superoxide free radical density in the ischemic lesions are presented here as percent (%) changes from the normal brain tissue density for the same site.

Results

Normal Brain Tissue

Normal brain tissue showed very low intensity CLA-chemiluminescence by superoxide free radicals. Topical applications of ascorbic acid (0.25 mM) and superoxide dismutase (10 units) inhibited the CLA-chemiluminescence. In contrast, $FeCl_3$ (0.01 mM) saturated with oxygen activated the intensities. The current of the CLA-chemiluminescence on the films increased in proportion to the exposure time. In these experiments, therefore, pictures exposed for 2 min were used for quantitative analysis of the superoxide free radicals.

Intracranial Hypertension

Two different levels of intracranial hypertension were produced by epidural compression with the two different sizes of silastic tubing.

Group 1 revealed ICP levels of 20–30 mmHg ICP during the investigation period. Metabolic changes, such as loss of tissue ATP, increasing vascular permeability, and disturbances of the microcirculation were limited to the compressed brain tissue area. The localized increases in superoxide free radicals were severest at 24 hr after cerebral compression. The distribution was closely correlated with the changes in vascular permeability and loss of tissue ATP. No progressive pathological changes were noted, however, until 72 hr after compression. The increases of superoxide free radicals were limited to less than 1.2% of the normal values in this mild intracranial hypertension.

Group 2 revealed ICP levels of 30–45 mmHg during the investigation period. Severe localized changes in energy metabolism, loss of tissue ATP, activation of Ca-M binding, and increasing vascular permeability were observed heterogeneously in all the experimental animals throughout the observation period. Superoxide free radicals increased immediately and were strongly focused in the compressed brain tissue area at 24 hr after cerebral compression. These changes extended in the direction of the brain stem (stress concentration shift zone) and contralateral hemisphere heterogeneously throughout the white matter with changes in the blood brain barrier (BBB), Ca-M and loss of tissue ATP at 48 hours, as shown in Figs. 2 and 3. The distribution of free radicals had a wider extent than the area of extravasation of Evans Blue dye and loss of tissue ATP at any observation period. The changes in Ca-M binding, however, displayed a similar distribution to that of the increasing superoxide free radicals. The critical level of superoxide free radicals for producing vasogenic edema was 2.5 times higher than the normal values. Superoxide free

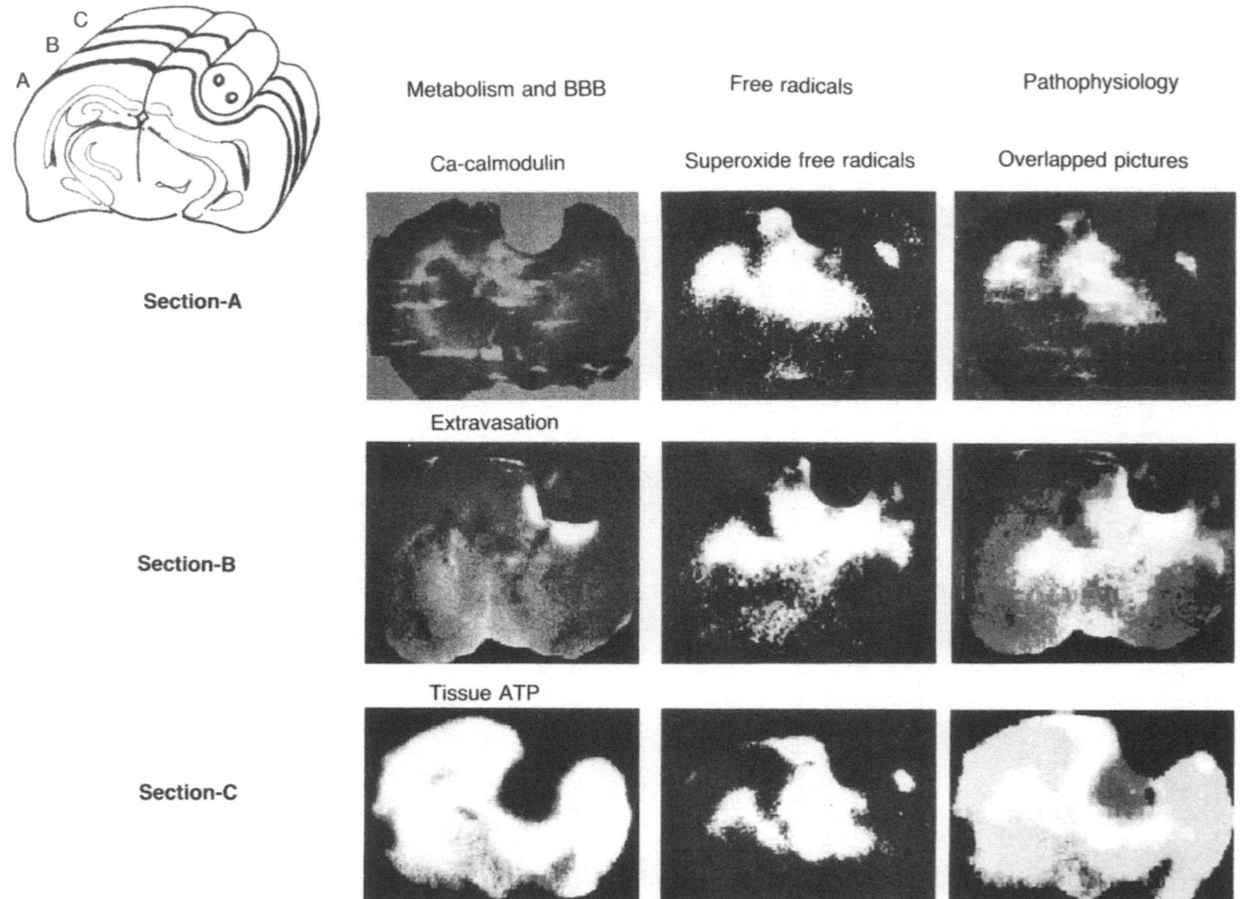

Fig. 2. Simultaneous topographic changes in metabolism (Ca-M binding and tissue ATP), extravasation of Evans Blue dye, superoxide free radicals and their relationships as indicated by the overlapped pictures in coronary transected brain slices at 48 hr after epidural compression in group 2. A great distribution of free radicals rather than extravasation and loss of tissue ATP was observed. Similar distributions of superoxide free radicals and Ca-M were, however, demonstrated in all the necrotic lesions

radicals were distributed more strongly and widely in the white matter than in the cortex at the extra-perifocal lesions (Fig. 2). Quantitative analysis of the superoxide free radicals, extravasation of Evans Blue dye and ATP crisis revealed no recovery at 72 hr after cerebral compression.

Discussion

Recent studies have demonstrated that oxygen free radicals involving superoxide anions, hydrogen peroxides, and hydroxy radicals, can facilitate damage to the endothelial and parenchymal cell membranes by disrupting their structure and functions. This process leads to puncture and damage to the enzymatic regulation of ion transport [1, 10]. Subsequently, vasogenic edema, cytotoxic edema and intravascular neutrophil aggregation [3] may cause the ischemic lesions to expand further. Good results for free radical scavengers against cerebral edema have therefore been proposed. Despite this conceptual framework, previous studies have failed to elucidate the precise location, characteristics, and magnitude of the free radical-induced alterations of ischemic lesions *in vivo*.

The present study has permitted detailed visualization of the localized changes in superoxide free radicals for the first time, and demonstrated specific quantitative distribution patterns of superoxide free radicals in relation to further expansion of the ischemic lesions, changes in vascular permeability and tissue ATP in compression-induced brain edema. In the present experiments, group 1 showed an increase in ICP to the level of the mathematically calibrated capillary pressure (25–35 mmHg). No localized mass effects in the brain tissue were observed at 72 hr after cerebral compression. Long-term localized brain tissue damage by mass effects was observed only in group 2. For the progression of serious localized vasogenic edema, the ICP needed to increase to a level at least higher than the capillary pressure.

In the compression-induced parenchymal lesions, the distribution of free radicals increased to a greater extent than the lesions of tissue ATP crisis and extravasation of Evans Blue dye (Fig. 2). The critical level of superoxide free radicals for producing the vasogenic edema was 2.5–3.2 times higher than the normal values. In the development of brain tissue damage in mass lesions, the occurrence of low perfusion ischemia, intravascular high pressure with venous stasis, and localized vascular compression and stretching by mechanical stress concentration were proposed as basic vascular changes of intraparenchymal pathophysiology. Vascular damage with vasogenic edema can thus occur more easily and severely, resulting in continuous serious brain edema as opposed to that encountered with traditional cerebral ischemic insults. Quantitative analysis of the superoxide free radical distribution, indeed, revealed much greater and severer changes in the compression-induced ischemic lesions than in the same size of necrotic lesions produced by four-vessel occlusion ischemic models in the rat.

As a possible mechanism for the secondary tissue damage occurring in the area around the lesion, progressive production of free radicals from the concomitant oxygen supply has been hypothesized. In the present experimental study, the large densities of superoxide free radicals rather than ATP crisis and changes in NADH in the lesions, supported this hypothesis and suggested that free radicals can directly cause secondary tissue damage in the areas surrounding ischemic lesions.

Previous studies have demonstrated various sources of superoxide anions in biological systems. These include the oxidization of ubisemiquinone radicals in the respiratory chain, prostaglandin synthesis, conversion from available nucleotides (NADPH), purine degradation with oxidization of xanthine oxidase, conversion of xanthine to urea, and activation of neutrophils [2, 6].

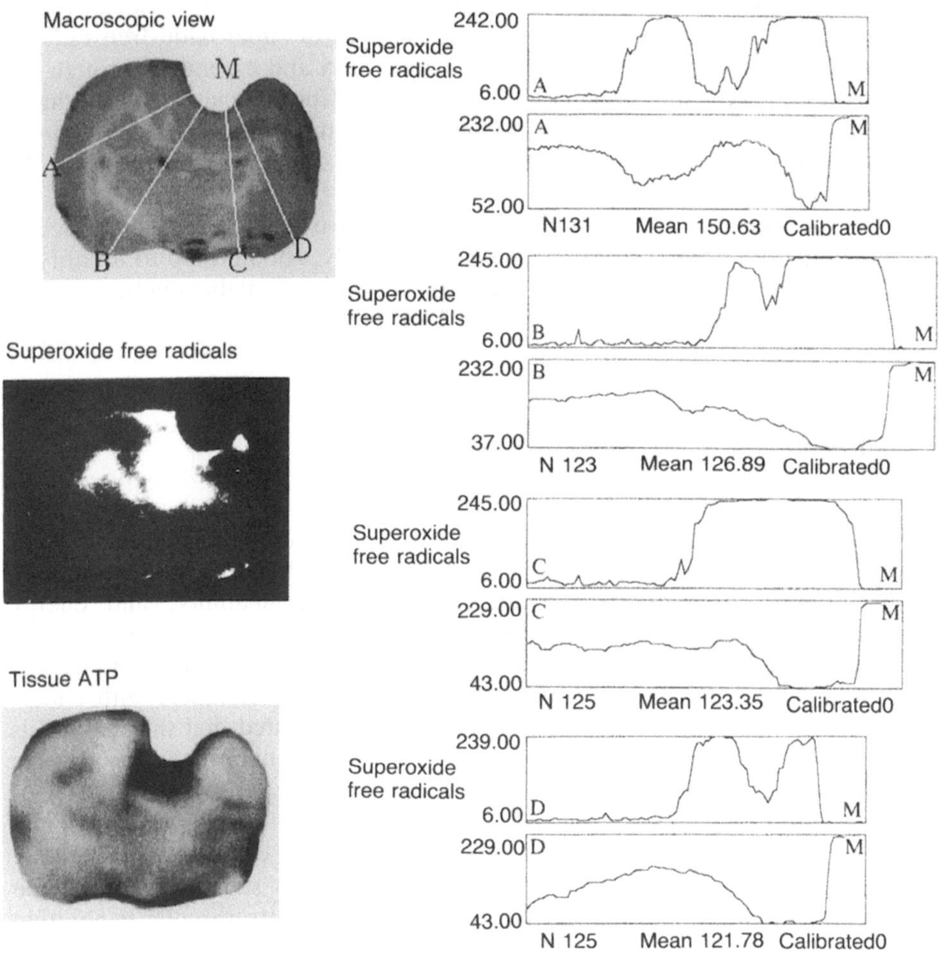

Fig. 3. Quantitative regional distribution of superoxide free radicals and tissue ATP in 48-hr compressed brain tissue. Changes of superoxide free radicals were observed severely in the center of the compressed area and extended towards the center of the brain stem through the stress concentration shift zone between lines MB and MC. However, outside of the stress concentration shift zone as demarcated by the lines MA and MD, free radicals were increased heterogeneously and extended into the white matter

The fact that a greater distribution of free radicals than tissue ATP crisis was observed in the necrotic tissue at 48 hr after compression, suggested that the sources of free radicals might be the activation of neutrophils (intravascular generating factors) and or synthesis of prostaglandin [6] rather than those of oxygen metabolic origin such as oxidization of ubisemiquinone, conversion from available nucleotides, and degradation of ATP to xanthine and conversion to urea. The similar distributions of the high densities of superoxide free radicals and Ca-M indicated that prostaglandin synthesis could represent the major cause of the free radical production in the compression-induced ischemic lesions.

Previous investigations have concentrated on mechanical pressure effects for the development of localized brain tissue damage as a major cause. In the present experiments, the effects involving changes of superoxide free radicals were observed in the center of the compressed area and extended through the stress concentration shift zone (Fig. 3). However, free radicals increased more easily in the white matter than in the gray matter, and extended heterogeneously outside of the stress concentration shift zone as demarcated by the lines MA and MD in figure 3.

The present new technique for mapping superoxide free radicals, vascular permeability and energy metabolism simultaneously, should help to identify in greater detail how free radicals are involved in the pathogenetic changes occurring in various ischemically injured CNS tissues.

Conclusion

To examine the role of free radicals in the regional pathogenesis of compression-induced intracranial hypertension, we developed a new technique for mapping superoxide free radicals, vascular permeability, and energy metabolism simultaneously. The distribution of superoxide anions in the CNS was based on the 380 nm chemiluminescence of 2-methyl-6-phenyl-3,7-dihydroimidazo[1,2a]pyrazin-3-one (CLA-phenyl) when it reacts with superoxide anions in frozen tissue sections. The results indicated that the ICP needs to increase to a level higher than the cerebral capillary pressure for the progression of serious localized vasogenic edema. The strong distribution of free radicals rather than vasogenic edema and tissue ATP crisis in all the necrotic lesions, suggested that free radicals can directly cause secondary tissue damage in the areas surrounding the mass lesions. As sources of these free radicals, arachidonic acid release and interventions by intravascular generating factors such as activation of neutrophils are strongly suggested rather than an ATP-related metabolic origin. The critical level of free radicals which caused vasogenic edema with tissue ATP crisis is 2.5 times higher than the normal value. Clear relationships between the production of superoxide free radicals, increased vascular permeability, and changes of energy metabolism in the necrotic tissue occurring in mass lesions were thus documented visually in our experiments.

References

1. Chan PH, Schmidley W, Fishman RA, Longer SM (1984) Brain injury, edema, and vascular permeability induced by oxygen-derived free radicals. Neurology 34:315–320
2. Fantone C, Ward PA (1985) Polymorphonuclear leucocyte mediated cell and tissue injury. Prog. Pathol 16:973–978
3. Fridovich I (1983) Superoxide free radical: an endogenous toxicant. Ann Rev Pharmacol Toxicol 23:239–257
4. Hayashi N (1990) Photochemical mapping technique for superoxide free radicals, vascular permeability, and metabolism in frozen tissue sections. Jap J Soc Laser Med 11:37–44
5. Hayashi N, Tsubokawa T, Green BA, Watson BD, Prado R (1990) A new mapping study of superoxide free radicals, vascular permeability and energy metabolism in central nervous system. Acta Neurochir (Suppl) 51:31–33
6. Kukreja RC, Kontos HA, Hess MH, Ellis EF (1986) PGH synthetase and lipoxygenase generate superoxide in the presence of NADH or NADPH. Cir. Res 59:612–619
7. Langfitt TW, Tannenbaum HM, Kassell NF (1966) The etiology of acute brain swelling. J Neurosurg 24:47–56
8. Nakano M, Sugioka K, Ushijima Y, Goto T (1986) Chemiluminescence probe with cypridin luciferin analog, 2-methyl-6-phenyl-3,7-dihydroimidazo[1,2a]pyrazin-3-one, for estimating the ability of human granulocytes to generate superoxide. Anal Biochem 159:363–369
9. Poten U, Ratcheson RA, Salford LG, Siesjo BK (1973) Optimal freezing conditions for cerebral metabolites in rats. J Neurochem 21:1127–1138
10. Wei EP, Christman CW, Kontos HA, Povlishock JT (1985) Effects of oxygen radicals on cerebral arterioles. Am J Physiol 248:H157–H162

The Effect of Lazaroid on Cerebral Elastance and Edema in a Cryogenic Injury Model

E. Arbit, G.R. DiResta, M. Wronski, J. Lee, and J.H. Galicich

Neurosurgery Service, Department of Surgery, and Department of Anesthesiology, Memorial Sloan-Kettering Cancer Center, New York, NY 10021, USA

Introduction

Lazaroid belongs to a novel group of compounds – aminosteroids (AS) which are potent inhibitors of central nervous system tissue lipid peroxidation, and are devoid of classical glucocorticoid and mineralocorticoid activities. Recent studies have shown that aminosteroids possess cerebral-protective properties and are efficacious in attenuating damage to the CNS imparted by trauma, ischemia, and vasospasm. The purpose of this study was to determine the effect of AS on (a) brain elastance, a measure of the protective volumetric buffering capacity of the brain, and (b) on cerebral perilesional edema. We used the cryogenic brain injury rat model, the constant rate and continuous infusion method to study brain elastance, and the gravitometric method to determine brain edema.

Methods

Male Sprague-Dawley rats (250–350 grams) were used in these experiments. The cryogenic lesion was created by a 2 mm. diameter cryo-probe, cooled to −65°C for 10 minutes placed on the dura mater through a craniotomy.

Edema Studies

Thirty rats were anesthetized with 2% halothane in oxygen for the duration of creating the cryogenic lesion. Twelve hours after lesion creation, animals were randomly divided into five treatment groups: (a) Lazaroid (5 mg/kg), (b) dexamethasone (20 mg/kg), (c) saline, (d) vehicle, and (e) sham. Drugs were administered through a cannula in the tail vein in equivolume of fluids except for the sham procedures. Six hours after treatment initiation the animals were decapitated and the brains removed. Brain edema was measured in four regions including the lesion, perilesional, and contralateral hemisphere. Specific gravity of the samples was determined and converted to percent water content. Group results were compared using independent t-tests ($p < 0.05$ was considered significant).

Elastance Studies

Eighteen rats were included in this study. After induction with 2% halothane the femoral artery vein and trachea were cannulated, and the animals were mounted in the stereotactic head frame. Anesthesia consisted of IV alpha-chloralose (45 mg/kg) initially, and maintenance with 15–20 mg/kg. Animals were paralyzed and artificially ventilated. Temperature, arterial pressure, heart rate, arterial blood gases were monitored and recorded. The cryogenic lesion was performed in the right occipital area. A Camino intracranial pressure probe was introduced through a left frontal burr hole, and inserted intra-parenchymally. Intracranial pressure was raised by a continuous infusion of petrolatum grease, infused at a constant rate through an epidural cannula. All the cranial openings were sealed at the end of the preparation. After surgical preparations were completed, the animals were divided into three groups; sham (n = 6), cryogenic lesion (n = 6), cryogenic lesion and lazaroid (5 mg/kg) (n = 6). Drug infusion began 10 mins. after lesion creation. Intracranial pressure increase was begun 15 min. after drug administration at a rate of 0.085 ml/min.

Results

1. Edema Studies

Effect of drug therapy on % water content following cryogenic injury

n = 6	Lazaroid	Dexamethasone	Vehicle	Saline	Control
mean	86.97	88.00	90.94	91.88	89.45
SD	1.32	1.32	1.68	1.86	2.44

Student's T-Test Statistics: Lazaroid & Dexamethasone statistically different ($p < 0.02$) from Saline and Vehicle.

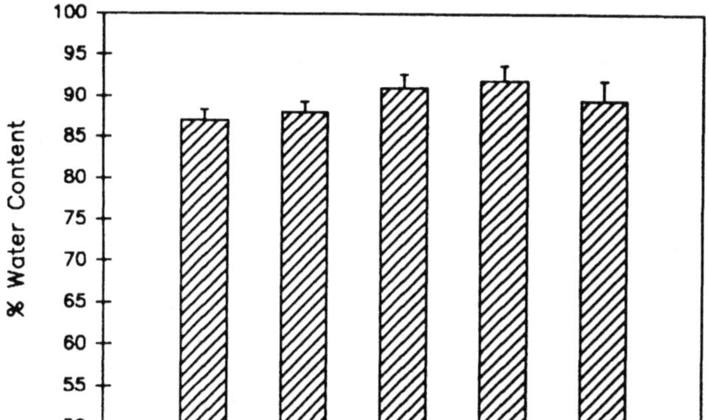

Fig. 1. The effect of manipulation on % water content following cryogenic lesion

2. *Elastance Studies*

Compliant Volume, G_0, in Control; Cryogenic Lesioned; and Lazaroid treated Cryogenic Lesioned Rats

	Control	Cryogenic Lesion	Cryogenic Lesion & Lazaroid
mean	0.0246	0.0024	0.0069
SD	0.0055	0.0031	0.0085
n	5	5	6

Student's T-Test Statistics: Cryogenic Lesion & Cryogenic lesion with Lazaroid statistically different ($p < 0.05$) from Control.

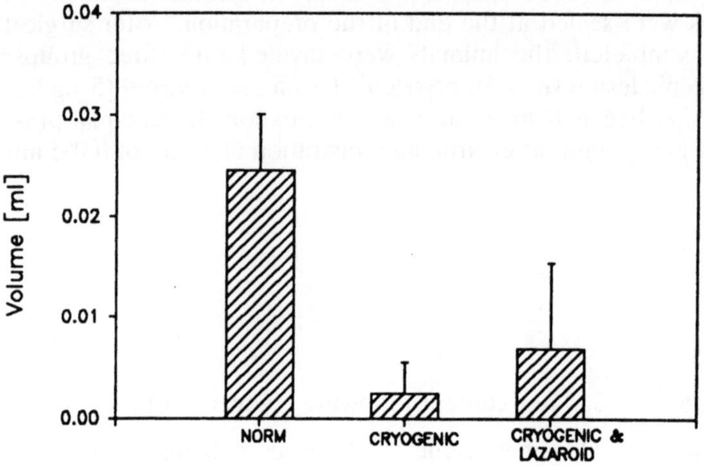

Fig. 2. Maximal volume (G_0) that may be added without intracranial pressure change

Discussion

Aminosteroids, a novel group of components, has an amino-group substituted on the 21 carbon of the steroid molecule. This substitution inactivates the corticosteroid receptor activity of the compound, thus making the drug devoid of the classical side effects of glucocorticosteroids. It has been shown that aminosteroids are potent iron catalized lipid peroxidation reaction inhibitors. The aminosteroids have demonstrated impressive *in vivo* CNS protection in models of trauma [3], subarachnoid hemorhage [4], ischemia [1, 5], spinal cord injury [2]. Recently a multicenter phase 2 prospective randomized clinical study has begun to assess the role of aminosteroids in head injury. The effect of aminosteroids on brain elastance as such have not been previously studied, although their effect to reduce intracranial pressure in models of subarachnoid hemorrhage have been reported [6]. This effect on intracranial pressure was attributed to decrease of vasogenic edema by way of reducing blood-brain barrier permeability. Reduction in ion shifts and brain edema has been similarly demonstrated in a model of regional ischemia [5].

In this experiment of cryogenic-induced injury we have demonstrated a reduction edema by the aminosteroid of the magnitude of 1.4% ($p < 0.05$). The reduction in edema was similar to the reduction achieved with dexamethasone and was significantly higher than the reduction achieved in saline or vehicle treated animals. The brain elastance, however, was not affected by the aminosteroids in this experimental model. Although one would expect a direct correlation between reduction of perilesional brain edema and increase in brain elastance, this has not been substantiated in this experiment. A posited mechanism to reconcile this observation is the concurrent increase in cerebral blood flow and volume known to occur under certain conditions with aminosteroids [2]. Enhancement of blood flow – hence an increase in intracranial blood volume – while beneficial to outcome under specific circumstances, may counterbalance the effect of reduction of edema as occurs in cryogenic injury, and in turn attenuate the intracranial pressure decrease and the increase in brain elastance.

In conclusion, the findings in these experiments reveal that aminosteroids are effective in reducing edema produced by cryogenic brain injury, yet have not altered the intracranial pressure-volume relationship. Cerebral elastance is a measure of the volumetric buffering capacity of the brain, and the fact that it has not been reduced by aminosteroids implies that the usage of Lazaroid is safe under specific conditions.

References

1. Hall ED, Pazara KE, Braughler JM (1988) 21 Aminosteroid lipid peroxidation inhibitor U74006F protects against cerebral ischemic in gerbils. Stroke 19:997–1002
2. Hall ED (1988) Effect of the 21 aminosteroid U74006F on posttraumatic spinal cord ischemic in cats. J Neurosurg 68:462–465
3. Hall ED, Yonkers PA, McCall JM, Barughler JM (1988) Effects of the 21 aminosteroid U74006F on experimental head injury in mice. J Neurosurg 68:456–461
4. Kanamaru K, Weir BKA, Findlay JM, et al. (1990) A dosage study of the effect of the 21 aminosteroid U74006F on chronic cerebral vasospasm in a primate model. Neurosurgery 27:29–38
5. Young W, Wojak JC, DeCrescito V (1988) 21 Aminosteroid reduces ion shifts and edema in the rat middle cerebral artery occlusion model of regional ischemia. Stroke 19:1013–1018
6. Zuccarello M, Anderson DK (1989) Protective effect of a 21 aminosteroid on the blood brain barrier following subarachnoid hemorrhage in rats. Stroke 20:367–371, 1989

Effects of Corticosteroid and Mannitol on the Early and Developed Stage of Vasogenic Brain Edema Evaluated by Proton Relaxation Behaviour

Y. HANDA, Y. NOGUCHI, H. ISHII, H. KOBAYASHI, H. KAWANO, T. KUBOTA, and M. HAYASHI

Department of Neurosurgery, Fukui Medical School, Matsuoka, Fukui 910-11, Japan

Introduction

It is recognized that development of vasogenic type of brain edema strongly affects the morbidity in patients with head injury, in whom development of brain edema elevates intracranial pressure resulting in brain herniation. In clinical situations, dexamethasone and mannitol are generally used to prevent the further development of brain edema, while the effects of these agents on brain edema are still controversial. In the present study, we investigated how these agents affect the progress or resolution of brain edema in its early and developed stage by evaluating the changes of proton relaxation behavior using NMR technique.

Materials and Methods

Thirty-six cats were used in this study. The animals were divided into three groups of twelve animals each: non-treated group (control group), dexamethasone-treated group (steroid group) and mannitol-treated group (mannitol group). Vasogenic edema was induced by the cold injury method in all animals. Under pentobarbital anesthesia, a rod of dry ice (5 cm diameter) was applied on the surface of the dura mater over the right parietal lobe for 30 seconds. Six animals in each group were sacrificed four hours after cold injury (early stage), and the other six were sacrificed 48 hours after injury (developed stage). The tissue samples were taken from the white matter beneath the cold lesion (WM1) and apart from the lesion (WM2), and corresponding regions in the contralateral hemisphere. After weighing, tissue samples were put into small tubes. For the measurements of proton relaxation rate, a 30 cm bore magnet operating at 2.0 T was employed. The small tube containing the tissue sample was placed in a double-turn coil of 1.6 cm diameter. The inversion recovery pulse sequence was used for the measurement of longitudinal relaxation rate ($R_1 = 1/T_1$). The Curr-Purcell-Meiboom-Gill sequence (16 spin echoes with echo time 25 ms) was employed to measure transverse relaxation rate ($R_2 = 1/T_2$). After the NMR study, the sample tubes were kept in the oven at 80°C for 2 days. The water content of tissue was calculated by the wet/dry weight method.

Table 1. Water content, relaxation rates and two-exponential transverse relaxation decay in edematous white matter in early and developed stages

	Early stage			Developed stage		
	Control group	Steroid group	Mannitol group	Control group	Steroid group	Mannitol group
Water content (%)	84.4 ± 1.3	82.8 ± 2.6	86.0 ± 2.6	88.9 ± 1.5	86.7 ± 2.8	83.5 ± 2.4[a]
R_1 (1/S)	0.97 ± 0.04	1.00 ± 0.03	0.91 ± 0.06	0.91 ± 0.05	0.94 ± 0.05	1.00 ± 0.04[a]
R_2 (1/S)	4.54 ± 0.63	5.95 ± 0.58[a]	4.53 ± 0.65	4.32 ± 0.82	6.20 ± 0.68	8.13 ± 0.78[a]
R_{2f} (1/S)	8.98 ± 0.71	10.20 ± 0.51	9.67 ± 0.65	8.50 ± 0.60	9.62 ± 0.53	10.12 ± 0.62
R_{2s} (1/S)	3.25 ± 0.36	4.10 ± 0.40[a]	3.76 ± 0.41	2.85 ± 0.31	3.98 ± 0.29[a]	3.28 ± 0.33[a]
%S (%)	22 ± 5	11 ± 4[a]	19 ± 6	38 ± 6	28 ± 5[a]	18 ± 5[b]

Values are mean ± SD. [a]$p < 0.05$ compared to the control group; [b]$P < 0.01$ compared to the control group; R_1, longitudinal relaxation rate; R_2, transverse relaxation rate (weighted average); R_{2f}, fast component of R_2; R_{2s}, slow component of R_2; %S, amount of signal contributing to R_{2s}.

In the steroid group, dexamethasone (2.5 mg/kg) was administered intraperitoneally 12 hours prior to the induction of injury, and an equivalent dose was administered every 12 hours. In the mannitol group, a solution of 20% mannitol (1.5 mg/kg) was infused intravenously for 60 minutes, and the infusion began 90 minutes before sacrifice.

Results

In the early stage, there were significant ($p < 0.05$) increases in water content and decreases in relaxation rates in the white matter of the injured hemisphere compared to the contralateral side in all three groups. While the water content and R_1 value in the edematous white matter showed no significant differences between three groups, a decrease in the weighted average of R_2 in the WM1 of the injured side was significantly ($p < 0.05$) smaller in the steroid group than in the other groups. The R_2 decay in the WM1 of the injured side showed two-components when two-exponential analysis was applied. The mean amount of signal contributing to the slow component of R_2 (R_{2s}) was significantly smaller in the steroid group than in the other groups (Table 1).

In the developed stage of brain edema, the increase in water content and decrease in relaxation rates (R_1 and R_2) in the mannitol group were significantly less than those in the control and steroid groups. The R_2 decay both in the WM1 and WM2 at the injured side showed two components in all the groups. The amount of signal contributing to R_{2s} was significantly ($p < 0.05$) smaller in the steroid group (28 ± 5%, mean ± SD) as well as in the mannitol group (18 ± 5%) compared to the control group (38 ± 6%) (Table 1).

Discussion

The present study revealed that the separation of R_2 into two components was observed from the early stage of vasogenic brain edema despite minimal changes in the water content and R_1 value. It has been reported that R_1 is mainly affected by an increase of free water in tissues, whereas R_2 is more easily affected by the slow molecular movements of water in tissues [1]. The R_{2s} refer to the extracellular fraction of water and the fast components to the intracellular fraction [2]. Exchange of water molecules between these two fractions can be observed in the edematous tissue by the NMR time scale, while it can not be observed in the normal state [1]. Hence, the amount of signal contributing to R_{2s} is thought to represent the impairment of the mobile movement of the water molecules between intra- and extracellular space as well as the amount of water in the extracellular space. Although dexamethasone could not alter the characteristics of vasogenic brain edema (extravasation of macromolecules) [5], it has been reported that its effect seems to be localized also at the cellular membranes or intracellular junctions [3]. Hence, the effect of dexamethasone on the R_{2s} in the acute stage may reflect its preventive effect on the movement of water into the extracellular space.

In the developed stage of brain edema, the R_2 decay showed an increase in signal contributing to slow components compared to the early stage. It is well recognized that water accumulates mainly in the extracellular space in the tissue of vasogenic edema at the developed stage [4]. In the present study, administration of mannitol demonstrated a significant reduction of the amount of signal contributing to R_{2s} accompanied with a decrease in water content. These results suggest that mannitol effectively withdraws the fluid accumulating in the extracelluar space at the developed stage of vasogenic edema.

References

1. Bakay L, Kurland RJ, Parrish RG, Lee JC, Peng RJ, Bartkowski HM (1975) Nuclear magnetic resonance studies in normal and edematous brain tissue. Exp Brain Res 23:241–248
2. Dea P, Chan SI, Dea FJ (1972) High-resolution proton magnetic resonance spectra of a rabbit sciatic nerve. Science 175:206–209
3. Herrman HD, Neuenfeldt D, Dittmann J, Palleske H (1972) The influence of dexamethasone on water content, electrolytes, blood-brain barrier and glucose metabolism in cold injury edema. In: Reulen HJ, Schürmann K (eds) Steroid and brain edema. Springer, Berlin Heiderberg New York, pp 77–85
4. Klatzo I (1967) Neuropathological aspects of brain edema. J Neuropathol Exp Neurol 26:1–14
5. Pappius HM (1972) Effects of steroid on cold injury edema. In: Reulen HJ, Schürmann K (eds) Steroid and brain edema. Springer, Berlin Heiderberg New York, pp 57–63

The Effect of Hypoxia, Hypercapnia, and Hypertension on Brain Edema

K. Ohashi, H. Kita, K. Shima, and H. Chigasaki

Department of Neurosurgery, National Defense Medical College, Saitama 3-2 Namiki, Tokorozawa city, Saitama, 359, Japan

Introduction

Many authors have reported that in various neurologic diseases, hypoxia can enhance edema development and cerebral damage. However, there are only a few reports on the mechanisms responsible for such deterioration. We studied the effect of hypoxia on brain tissue water content and electrical activity, and we also evaluated the influences of superimposed hypercapnia and hypertension on edema development.

Materials and Methods

This experiment included 3 groups as follows:

Group I:	hypoxia alone group, 350–400 g Sprague-Dawley rats (S.D. rat) maintained at PaO_2 35–40 mmHg, $PaCO_2$ 35–40 mmHg	(n = 15)
Group II:	hypoxia and hypercapnia group, 350–400 g S.D. rats maintained at PaO_2 35–40 mmHg, $PaCO_2$ 60–70 mmHg	(n = 22)
Group III:	hypoxia and hypertension group 300–350 g stroke-prone spontaneously hypertensive rats (SHR-SP) maintained at PaO_2 35–40 mmHg, $PaCO_2$ 35–40 mmHg	(n = 15)

After the induction of anesthesia with halothane, all rats were intubated and artificially ventilated. Anesthesia was maintained with a gas mixture containing 0.4% halothane. In all groups, the inspired oxygen content was gradually lowered and hypoxia was maintained at the above oxygen and carbon dioxide levels for one hour. In Group II, a small amount of carbon dioxide was added to the inspired gas mixture, and hypercapnic hypoxia was maintained at the above level.

During the experiment, evoked potentials [auditory brain stem response (ABR) and somatosensory evoked potentials (SEP)] and brain tissue pH were periodically recorded.

For the gravimetric study, animals were killed immediately, 1 day, and 2 days after the hypoxic insult respectively, and then the brains were removed. Brain tissue water content was determined by the gravimetric method described by Marmarou [1].

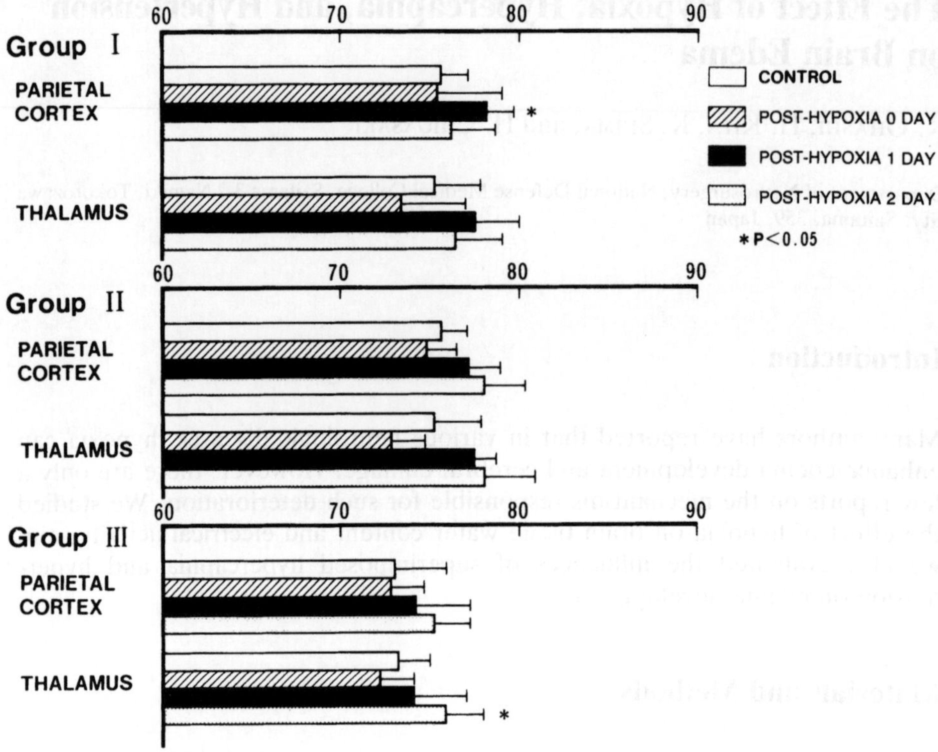

Fig. 1. Changes in brain tissue water content (%) after hypoxia in each group, showing a tendency to increase 1 day after hypoxic insult in Group I and on both 1st and 2nd days in Group II and Group III

Animals that were maintained at normocapnic normoxia under the same anesthesia served as controls.

Results

The mean arterial blood pressure (MABP) in Group III was significantly higher during the experiment. In all groups, the MABP showed a tendency to decrease during the hypoxic insult.

Figure 1 shows the change in brain tissue water content immediately, 1 day, and 2 days after the hypoxic insult in each group. In Group I, the brain tissue water content showed a tendency to increase only on the 1st day after the hypoxic insult. By contrast, in Group II and Group III, the brain tissue water content showed a tendency to increase both on the 1st and 2nd day after the insult.

The changes of evoked potentials are shown in Fig. 2. In Group I, interpeak latency of ABR or peak latency of SEP was significantly prolonged during the hypoxic insult. However, on the 1st and 2nd day, it returned to equal the

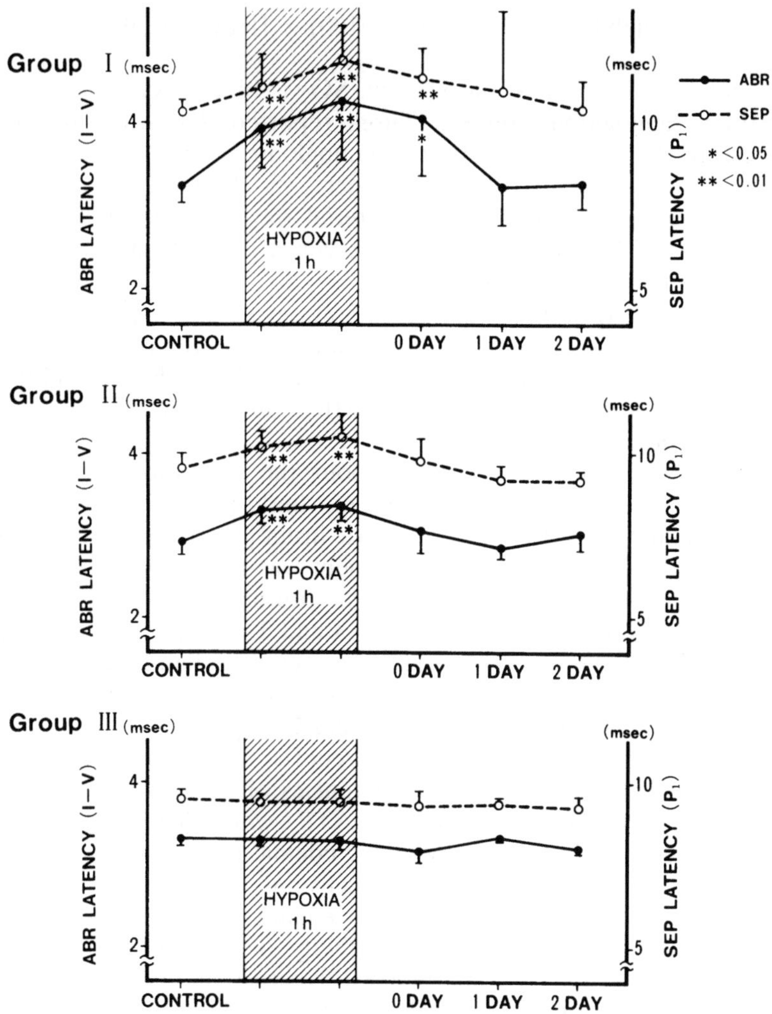

Fig. 2. Changes in each peak latency of ABR and SEP during and after hypoxia, showing significant prolongations during hypoxic insult in Group I and Group II, but no significant prolongation during the experiment in Group III

controls. In Group III, there was no significant prolongation found throughout the experiment.

The brain tissue pH/blood pH ratio in Group I decreased immediately after the insult of hypoxia and returned to the control level.

Discussion

Oxygen availability is an important factor that contributes to cerebral dysfunction and metabolic disorders. Siesjö presented the equation of oxygen availability as follows [5]:

$$O_2 \text{ availability} = CBF \times (SO_2/100) \times [Hb] \times 1.39$$

where CBF is cerebral blood flow, SO_2 is blood oxygen saturation (%), and [Hb] is hemoglobin content. Turek reported that when the arterial oxygen pressure (PaO_2) is 38 mmHg, the hemoglobin in rat blood is 50% saturated [7]. However, during hypoxia, CBF increases dramatically and increased CBF compensates for a decrease in arterial oxygen content [6]. Because of this increase in CBF during hypoxia, oxygen availability does not decrease unless PaO_2 decreases markedly [6].

Then the question arose as to how severe the hypoxia in our experiment was. McPherson reported that each wave of ABR or SEP was not suppressed unless brain tissue oxygen availability and $CMRO_2$ decreased [2]. According to his results, it is assumed that the $CMRO_2$ decreased during hypoxia in Group I and Group II.

There are also few studies about the formation of brain edema after hypoxia. In 1970, Norris et al. did not find any significant increase in specific gravity and Na^+ content after hypoxic insult [4]. In contrast to their results, the condition of hypoxia in our experiment was more severe. Because, in the rat, the PaO_2 at which hemoglobin is 50% saturated (P_{50}) is 38 mmHg [7] and CBF and $CMRO_2$ of the rat brain are 2–3 and 3–4 times greater than that of man [3], the metabolic rate of the rat brain is greater than that of larger animals and the resistance to severe hypoxia is quite low. Furthermore, hypotension was associated with hypoxia in Group I and Group II.

Based on our results and other reports, we can speculate as follows. First, in Group I, the prolonged peak latencies of each evoked potential suggest a decrease in $CMRO_2$ and cellular ATP, which leads to dysfunction of the Na^+-K^+ pump. Therefore, cytotoxic edema mainly developed on the 1st day, as a result of water movement into cells due to the pump dysfunction. Second, in Group II and Group III, vasogenic edema mainly developed after hypoxia as a result of an increase in permeability of capillaries or arterioles due to excessive dilatation by superimposed hypercapnia in Group II and continuous high hydrostatic pressure on dilated vessels in Group III.

Data of this study are insufficient to confirm the hypothesis as mentioned above. In the future, further detailed studies will be required.

Conclusions

This study suggests that brain edema develops within 2 days after a hypoxic insult and that superimposed hypercapnia or hypertension promotes such brain edema.

The prolonged latencies of each evoked potential in Group I and Group II may be due to associated hypotension during hypoxia.

According to our results, we speculate that cytotoxic edema is the main factor for edema development in Group I and vasogenic edema in Group II and Group III.

References

1. Marmarou A, Poll W, Shulman K, Bhagavan H (1978) A simple gravimetric technique for measurement of cerebral edema. J Neurosurg 49:530–537
2. McPherson RW, Eimerl D, Traystman RJ (1987) Interaction of hypoxia and hypercapnia on cerebral hemodynamics and brain electrical activity in dogs. Am J Physiol 253:H890–H897
3. Norberg K, Siesjö BK (1974) Quantitative measurement of blood flow and oxygen consumption in the rat brain. Acta Physiol Scand 91:154–164
4. Norris JW, Pappius HM (1970) Cerebral water and electrolytes. Effect of asphyxia, hypoxia, and hypercapnia. Arch Neurol 23:248–258
5. Siesjö BK (1978) Hypoxia. In: Siesjö BK (ed) Brain Energy Metabolism. Chichester, New York, Brisbane, Toronto, pp 398–452
6. Siesjö BK, Berntman L, Rehncrona S (1979) Effect of hypoxia on blood flow and metabolic flux in the brain. In: Fahn S et al. (eds) Advances in Neurology, vol 26. Raven Press, New York, pp 267–283
7. Turek Z, Kreuzer F, Hoofd LJC (1973) Advantage or disadvantage of a decrease of blood oxygen affinity for tissue oxygen supply at hypoxia. A theoretical study comparing man and rat. Pflügers Arch ges Physiol 342:185–97

Role of Stimulation of Medullary Reticular Formation on Centrally Released Arginine Vasopressin in Cold Induced Edema

T. Kuniyoshi, S. Nagao, M. Kagawa, T. Ogawa, Y. Honma, T. Ohmoto, T. Itano[1], and O. Hatase[1]

Departments of Neurological Surgery and Physiology[1], Kagawa Medical School, 1750-1, Ikenobe, Miki-Cho, Kita-Gun, Kagawa, 761-07, Japan

Introduction

We previously reported that in cold injured brain, stimulation of the medullary reticular formation (MORF) for 40 minutes results in a widespread significant increase in brain water content in white matter of the injured hemisphere by approximately 1.5 to 3 percent [3]. Recent studies indicate that centrally released arginine vasopressin (AVP) influences water permeability of the brain in both normal [1, 5] and pathological conditions [2, 6]. The present study was carried out to clarify the effect of stimulation of MORF on centrally released AVP by measuring AVP in the cerebrospinal fluid (CSF).

Materials and Methods

Animal Preparation

Experiments were conducted on 37 unselected cats. A burr hole, 10 mm in diameter, was made in the left frontoparietal bone. The cold injury was inflicted by applying a freezing probe of −50°C for one minute directly on the dura. Seventeen hours later, the animals were anesthetized and a tracheal cannula was inserted for ventilation with a respirator. Catheters were placed in both the femoral artery for measurement of blood pressure and the femoral vein. The ICP was continuously measured with a plate-type pressure transducer (Gaeltec, Dunvegan, UK) placed in the right parietal, epidural space.

Stimulation of Medullary Reticular Formation

Concentric circular electrodes connected to an electric stimulator were bilaterally inserted into the reticular formation of the medulla oblongata at P: 10.0, L: ±2.5, H: −9.0 via small holes in the posterior fossa in accordance with Snider and Niemer's atlas [8]. The site corresponded with the nucleus reticularis parvocellularis to gigantocellularis. Stimulus parameters were intensity 5 V, duration 1 msec, and pulse-repetition frequency 50 pulse/sec.

Stimulation was performed eight times with a duration of 10 minutes each at intervals of 2 to 5 minutes.

Animal Groups

The animals were divided into three groups. In group I (16 animals), electrical stimulation of MORF was carried out for 80 minutes in normal cats. In group II (11 animals), stimulation was started 17 hours after cold injury under the same conditions and carried out for 80 minutes. In group III (10 animals), angiotensin II was administered to elevate blood pressure to the same degree as during MORF stimulation 17 hours after cold injury.

CSF and Plasma AVP and Osmolality Analysis

In each group, CSF and blood samples were taken via the cisterna magna and femoral artery before, and during 40 and 80 minutes stimulation and induced hypertension, for measurement of AVP concentrations and plasma osmolalities. AVP concentrations in CSF and plasma were measured by radioimmunoassay (Amersham, UK) after extraction with Sep-pak C_{18}. Plasma osmolality was determined by the freezing point depression method (Model 5004, Precision Systems, USA). Student's t-test was used for statistical analysis.

Results

Changes in CSF, plasma AVP and plasma osmolality before, and during 40 and 80 minutes medullary stimulation and induced hypertension are presented in Table 1. Normal values of CSF and plasma AVP were 4.0 ± 2.2 and 9.9 ± 3.6 pg/ml respectively. Plasma AVP and osmolality did not show significant changes before and at the end of the experiments in all groups.

Table 1. Changes in cerebrospinal fluid (CSF) and plasma arginine vasopressin (AVP) concentrations and plasma osmolalities before, 40 and 80 minutes after medullary stimulation (Group I, II) and induced hypertension (Group III). Values are means ± S.D.

Time (min)	CSF AVP (pg/ml)			Plasma AVP (pg/ml)		Plasma Osmolality (mOsm/l)	
	0	40	80	0	80	0	80
Group I (n = 16)	4.0 ± 2.2	5.5 ± 0.9*	6.8 ± 3.2**	9.9 ± 3.6	11.0 ± 1.5	323.3 ± 8.1	323.5 ± 7.9
Group II (n = 11)	6.6 ± 3.4	12.0 ± 6.5*	14.4 ± 6.3***	19.9 ± 9.0	22.5 ± 9.1	313.6 ± 6.8	319.2 ± 8.5
Group III (n = 10)	2.9 ± 1.1	3.1 ± 1.4	2.6 ± 1.1	12.4 ± 4.9	14.6 ± 8.5	319.6 ± 9.8	321.0 ± 7.4

*, **, ***: values significantly different from prestimulation level by $P < 0.05$, $P < 0.01$, and $P < 0.005$.

There were no significant changes in CSF AVP by induced hypertension for 80 minutes (Group III). Stimulation of the medullary reticular formation resulted in significant and progressive increase in CSF AVP in normal and injured brain (Group I, II). The mean values of CSF AVP became approximately two times the pre-stimulation level after 80-minutes of stimulation in injured brain (Group II).

Discussion

Raichle et al. demonstrated that electrical stimulation of the locus ceruleus produced a prompt increase in brain water permeability and a reduction of cerebral blood flow [4]. They also reported that intraventricular administration of AVP resulted in a highly significant increase in brain water permeability [5]. With these results, Raichle et al. proposed a mechanism that stimulation of the central noradrenergic pathways activates secretion of centrally released AVP in the hypothalamus which has a significant effect on brain water permeability.

In normal brain, intraventricular administration of AVP (125 ng) brought about a 1–1.3% water accumulation [1]. Reeder et al. demonstrated that intraventricular AVP facilitates the production of vasogenic cold induced edema in cats [6].

Our previous report [3] showed that after 40 minutes of stimulation of the medullary reticular formation, widespread significant increase by approximately 1.5 to 3% in brain water content occurred in the white matter of the injured hemisphere. Stimulation of medullary reticular formation may exert some effects on brain water permeability by neurally modulated neuropeptides that act on the blood-brain barrier.

Our data clearly show that stimulation of the medullary reticular formation results in a significant increase in CSF AVP in both normal and cold-injured brain. The afferent projections to the anterior hypothalamus from the lower brain stem have been demonstrated by means of the horseradish peroxidase method [7]. These structures are in and near the site that is stimulated in this experiment. It is reasonable to assume that stimulation of the medullary reticular formation has some effects on production of central AVP via these pathways. When released with stimulation of the medullary reticular formation, AVP may act directly on the capillary bed to increase water permeability.

If our hypothesis is true, administration of an AVP receptor antagonist may be useful in the treatment of brain edema.

References

1. Doczi T, Szerdahelyi P, Gulya K, Kiss J (1982) Brain water accumulation after the central administration of vasopressin. Neurosurgery 11:402–407
2. Doczi T, Laszlo FA, Szerdahelyi P, Joo F (1984) Involvement of vasopressin in brain edema formation: Further evidence obtained from the Brattleboro diabetes insipidus rat with experimental subarachnoid hemorrhage. Neurosurgery 14:436–441

3. Nagao S, Ogawa T, Kuniyoshi T, Ohmoto T (1989) Effect of stimulation of the medullary reticular formation on vasogenic brain edema. Advances in Experimental Neurotrauma Res 1:35–40
4. Raichle ME, Eichling JO, Grubb RL, Hartman BK (1976) Central noradrenergic regulation of brain microcirculation. In: Pappius H, Feindel W (eds) Dynamics of Brain Edema. Springer-Verlag, New York, pp 11–17
5. Raichle ME, Grubb RL (1978) Regulation of brain water permeability by centrally-released vasopressin. Brain Res 143:191–194
6. Reeder RF, Nattie EE, North WG (1986) Effect of vasopressin on cold-induced brain edema in cats. J Neurosurgery 64:941–950
7. Sakumoto T, Tohyama M, Satoh K, Kimoto Y, Kinugasa T, Tanizawa O, Kurachi K, Shimizu N (1978) Afferent fiber connections from lower brain stem to hypothalamus studied by the horseradish peroxidase method with special reference to noradrenaline innervation. Exp Brain Res 31:81–94
8. Snider RS, Niemer WT (1961) Stereotaxic atlas of the cat brain, University of Chicago Press, Chicago

Amino-Acids Release in Cerebrospinal Fluid After Injury of Cat Brain with Cold Lesion

H. KUCHIWAKI, S. INAO, H. KANAIWA, T. HIRANO, and K. SUGITA

Department of Neurosurgery, Nagoya University School of Medicine, 65 Tsurumai-Cho, Showa-Ku, Nagoya, 466, Japan

Introduction

Excessive concentration of some amino-acids have recently been found to injure neurons in the central nervous system [2]. Similar injuries to the nervous system seem to occur in patients with head injury due to excessive release of amino-acids from the lesion in the brain into the extracellular space or the cerebrospinal fluid (CSF) space. We investigated the relationship between changes in electrical activity and in concentrations of amino-acids in the CSF during edema formation after a brain contusion. We constructed a model of a cat brain with a cold injury to clarify the relationship.

Materials and Methods

Twenty adult cats weighing 2.8 to 4.2 kg were anaesthetized with Ketamine hydochloride (30 mg/kg, i.m.), Chloralose (20 mg/kg, i.v.), and Urethane (80 mg/kg, i.v.). An intratracheal tube was inserted through a tracheostomy. The animals were immobilized with Pancuronium bromide (i.v.) and artificially ventilated. Expired CO_2 gas was monitored using a gas monitor (1H21A, Nec-SANEI Co.) and was maintained in the 4.8 to 5.1% range. Values of $PaCO_2$ were also checked. Arterial blood pressure (SAP) was measured in the abdominal aorta. Lactate Ringer's solution was continuously infused intravenously at a rate of 0.6 ml/min through a catheter in the vena cava inferior. Then the animals were placed on a stereotaxic operation table according to the "Animal Experimentation Guide, Nagoya University School of Medicine". A small unilateral craniectomy was performed over the motor area to make a cold lesion. Electroencephalogram (EEG) was recorded with monopolar leads (G1: lt. and rt. parietal region, G2: nasion) and was stored on a data recorder (R80 TEAC Co.). The power array of frequency spectrum was analyzed with a computer system (7T17, NEC-SANEI Co.). A suboccipital puncture was performed using a 27G needle for sampling 0.5 to 1.0 ml of CSF. Samplings for the control data were performed 30 min after the end of the experimental set-up. Thereafter, a lesion was made by touching the epidural surface for 30 sec with a metal bar (d = 7.7 mm) cooled in a dry ice and alcohol mixture. Sampling times were scheduled hourly for eight hours after the cold lesion had been made. Each individual animal was sampled for CSF and blood at three randomly selected times during the eight hours. Cerebrospinal fluid was slowly aspirated and rapidly stored at −80°C within a few minutes until the time for analysis. The serum of the samples from the arterial blood was rapidly extracted and stored in the same manner and schedule as CSF. Analysis of amino-acids was performed with liquid chromatography (JLC 300, Nihondenshi. Co.). Amino-acid concentrations at each experimental time were compared with control data by t-test ($p < 0.05$) to determine statistical significance.

Results

Constitution of Amino-Acids in Blood and CSF at Control State

Thirty-three kinds of amino-acids and related substances were examined. Of these, phosphethanolamine in CSF was found at higher levels than in blood. Concentration of glutamine and urea in CSF nearly equaled the concentration in blood. Control values were: alanine [Ala]: 47.6 (nmol/ml), tyrosine [Tyr]: 6.1, phenylalanine [Phe]: 11.2, Methionine [Met]: 2.7, and Glycine [Gly]: 3.4 in CSF. Glutamic acid and aspartic acid were not detected in CSF.

Changes in Concentration of Amino-Acids After a Cold Lesion Was Made

Concentrations of [Ala], [Tyr], [Phe], and [Met] were gradually and significantly increased as experimental time passed. These amino-acids also increased gradually in blood. In CSF glutamic acid increased for the initial four hours in more than one half of the animals. In contrast, in the later four hours glutamic acid decreased and was rarely detected. In the blood, glutamic acid concentration gradually decreased. Glycine in CSF increased insignificantly for the later four hours. Aspartic acid was detected more rarely in 10 to 16% of the animals throughout the experimental time. Other amino-acid concentrations did not change significantly. Changes in amino-acid concentrations in the blood were also not significant.

Changes in EEG Study

During the first four hours alpha waves extinguished and low voltage records were the general tendency. During this periods positive or negative spikes and sharp waves were more frequently observed than in the later four hours. After this period, high voltage sharp wave bursts less frequently appeared, but were observed with a long periodicity. From the sixth to the eighth hour low voltage slow waves mixed with high voltage slow waves became dominant in the EEG recordings. Spikes or sharp waves were rarely seen in this period.

Discussion

An acute change in EEG indicates local inactivity caused by injury to the brain. After the injury, most of the depressed activity of the brain function recovered. In this initial period the brain needs energy for it's recovery to the normal state.

There are controversial opinions with regard to increasing or decreasing blood flow in edematous brain. Our previous results showed that hyperemia shifted from the gray matter to the white matter, with a delay of two to three hours, in the edematous area of the same model as reported here [1]. In this area the blood brain barrier (BBB) was injured.

Spikes or sharp waves in the initial four hours seem to have a close relation to an increase in excitatory amino-acids and glutamic acid in CSF. During this period, a significant increase in Ala may also be of importance with regard to brain excitation and injury. The origin of amino-acids in CSF may be the blood by impairment of BBB in relation to the hyperemic area in the edema formation. In this early stage, the increase in the concentration of Gly and Ala is related to gamma-aminobutyric acid (GABA) activity.

In the second half of our experimental time, high voltage slow waves and the disappearance of fast components indicate progressive reduction in brain function. These findings are supported by increasing concentrations of amino-acids [Phe, Tyr] which are precursors of neurotransmitters. Increasing Met concentration in CSF indicates metabolic impairment in the production of biogenic amines involved by the edema front, although it does not accurately reflect the metabolism of the brain. These changes in amino-acid concentration suggest functional deterioration associated with an expanding edema area with ischemia in the later four hours [1].

In conclusion, amino-acid concentrations in CSF suggest a progression of the edema front by biomolecular aspects. An early increase in concentration of excitatory amino-acids may closely correlate with early epileptic discharges. Increasing concentrations of amino-acids, which are precursors of neurotransmitters, suggest biomolecular degradation in the brain parenchyma in the progression of the edema front.

References

1. Kuchiwaki H, Inao S, Nagasaka M, Andoh K, Hirano T, Sugita K (1990) The effects of cerebral hemodynamics on the progression of cold-induced oedema. Acta Neurochirurgica, Suppl 51:77–78
2. Olney JW, de Gubareff T, Labruyere J (1983) Seizure-related brain damage induced by cholinergic agents. Nature 301:520–522

Regional Tissue Compliance of Edematous Brain After Cryogenic Injury in Cats

T. Kuroiwa, I. Taniguchi[1], and R. Okeda

Department of Neuropathology, [1] Department of Auditory Disorders, Medical Research Institute, Tokyo Medical and Dental University, Yushiuma 1-5-45, Bunkyo-ku, Tokyo 113, Japan

Introduction

Brain edema is a major complication of several types of intracranial pathology such as ischemia, tumor and hemorrhage. Since the deleterious influence of brain edema is related primarily to a mass effect, basic knowledge of the mechanical properties of brain tissue is necessary in order to understand the process of edema-mediated tissue injury such as cerebral herniation and demyelination. In the present investigation, we measured regional differences in the tissue compliance of edematous as well as normal brain tissue in cats subjected to cryogenic injury. We observed that an increase in regional tissue compliance was closely associated with an increase in the tissue water content.

Materials and Methods

Eight adult cats of either sex, each weighing between 2.7 and 4.0 kg, were used. Anesthesia was induced by intramuscular injection of ketamine (30 mg/kg) and maintained by additional injections during surgical preparation. Catheters were inserted into the femoral artery and vein for monitoring of arterial blood pressure (ABP), and injection of tracers and drugs. A cold lesion was made by application of a metal plate cooled with a mixture of dry ice and acetone to the exposed suprasylvian gyrus for 1 min [2, 3]. The cranial window was then closed with dental wax, and 2% Evans blue solution (EB), 2 ml/kg, was injected as a tracer for assessment of edema fluid distribution. Each animal was sacrificed 4 h after cold lesioning, then the brain was removed rapidly and cut in the coronal plane through the center of the lesion to obtain rostral and caudal blocks, 5 mm thick, for measurement of specific gravity and regional compliance. Samples, each about 2 mm in diameter, were dissected from the areas showing EB staining, and from the normal unstained area in the white matter of the rostral coronal block, and submerged in a kerosene-bromobenzene gradient column for determination of specific gravity. Regional tissue compliance was measured in the caudal block in the areas corresponding to sites of specific gravity measurement by an indentation method. For the measurement, a compression probe attached to a strain gauge was inserted to a predetermined depth (about 400 μm) into the region of interest at a constant

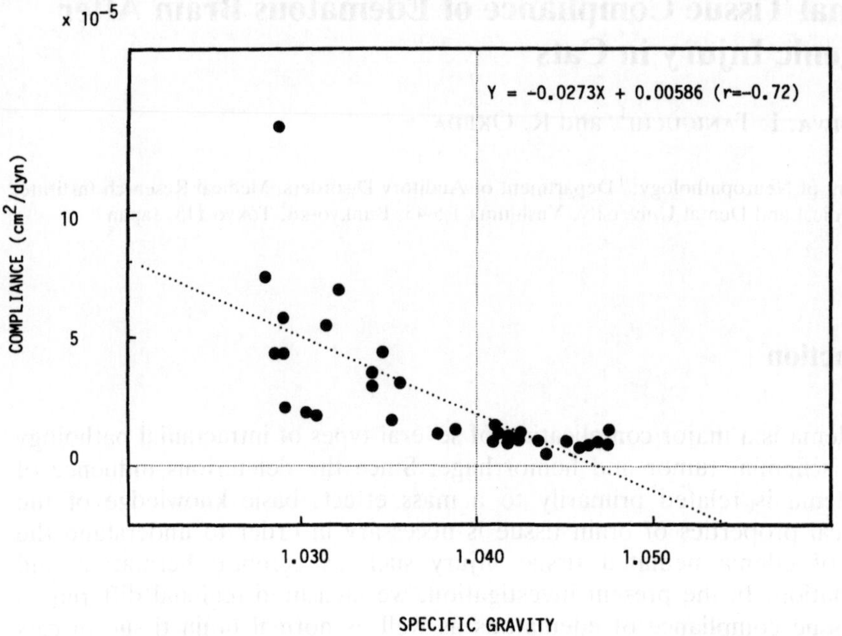

Fig. 1. Correlation between the specific gravity and regional tissue compliance in the white matter 4 h after cryogenic injury in cats. Note a significant correlation between the two parameters

speed (about 25 μm/s), the pressure-depth response was recorded by an X-Y recorder, and tissue compliance was calculated according to the method described by Walsh et al. [5]. The caudal block was immersion-fixed in buffered formalin, and prepared for histological examination with luxol fast blue staining. Four control animals were operated on as described above, but were not given cold lesions, and then similarly examined.

Results

ABP and blood gas values remained within the normal range during the experiment, and showed no significant differences between the experimental and control groups. The coronal plane of the brain from cats sacrificed 4 h after cold-lesioning showed spreading of EB staining into the white matter of the injured gyrus, centrum semiovale toward the lateral ventricle and also to the white matter of the adjacent gyri. Specific gravity measurement showed that the spread of edema fluid was confined to the area of EB staining, i.e. the area containing extravasated serum protein.

The specific gravity of the normal white matter was 1.0439 ± 0.0024 (mean ± SD), corresponding to a tissue compliance of $1.001 \times 10^{-4} \pm 0.264 \times 10^{-4}$ cm²/dyne. In the edematous area, tissue compliance increased in parallel with the decrease in specific gravity, i.e. the increase in water content [2, 3, 4].

The correlation of the two parameters was statistically significant ($p < 0.05$), and the regression coefficient was 0.72. The average specific gravity measured in the edematous area was 1.0322 ± 0.0035, corresponding to a tissue compliance of $4.027 \times 10^{-4} \pm 2.74 \times 10^{-4} cm^2/dyne$. Histologically, widening of the inter-fiber space was observed in the edematous white matter showing macroscopic EB staining.

Discussion

The mechanical properties of brain tissue have been measured in both human and animal brain. Fallenstein et al. [1] measured the dynamic elastic modulus of the human brain obtained at autopsy using a dynamic mechanical apparatus. Walsh et al. [5] measured the properties of brain tissue using a pressure-displacement transducer system applied to the brain of normal mongrel dogs. However, to our knowledge, regional differences in the tissue compliance of the brain in relation to a neuropathological process have never been measured.

The present findings can be summarized as follows:

1. Both tissue specific gravity and regional tissue compliance are uniform in the normal white matter.
2. Regional tissue compliance increases in close association with a decrease in tissue specific gravity, i.e. an increase of tissue water content.
3. Widening of the inter-fiber space due to accumulation of edema fluid seems to increase the regional tissue compliance.

The observed increase in regional tissue compliance may have a causative role in the development of edema-mediated tissue injury. Demyelination is a common tissue injury mediated by brain edema, especially around intracranial mass lesions. From the above findings we speculate that edema increases the tissue compliance of the white matter around a mass lesion, making the tissue vulnerable to mechanical stress, and ultimately resulting in demyelination of the white matter.

References

1. Fallenstein G, Hulce VD, Melvin JW (1969) Dynamic mechanical properties of human brain tissue. ASME paper No. 69-BHF-6:2–8
2. Klatzo I, Chui E, Fujiwara K, Spatz M (1980) Resolution of vasogenic brain edema. In: Cervos-Navarro J, Ferszt R (eds) Advances in Neurology, vol 28. Raven Press, New York, pp 359–373
3. Kuroiwa T, Yokofujita J, Kaneko H, Okeda R (1990) Accumulation of oedema fluid in deep white matter after cerebral cold injury. Acta Neurochir, Suppl 51:84–86
4. Marmarou A, Tanaka K, Shulman K (1982) An improved gravimetric measure of cerebral edema. J Neurosurg 56:246–253
5. Walsh EK, Schettini A (1976) Elastic behavior of brain tissue in vivo. Am J Physiol 230(4): 1058–1062

Microautoradiographic Examination of Edema Fluid Distribution in the Cat Brain After Cryogenic Injury

T. KUROIWA[1], J. YOKOFUJITA[2], H. KANENO[3], and R. OKEDA[1]

[1] Department of Neuropathology, [2] Department of Cell Regulation, Medical Research Institute, Tokyo Medical and Dental University, Yushima 1-5-45, Bunkyo-ku, Tokyo 113, Japan
[3] Unique Medical Co. Ltd., Tokyo, Japan

Introduction

We recently reported that maximal accumulation of edema fluid after cold-lesioning was not observed in the white matter of the injured gyrus but in the deeper white matter under the gyrus [3]. However, this result was equivocal, since the observed accumulation of the tracer for edema fluid, ^{125}I-labeled albumin, may have merely reflected the change in the vascular space due to the cold injury. The purpose of the present study was (i) to examine micro-autoradiographically the distribution of ^{125}I-labeled albumin in the edematous area to clarify whether the increase was, in fact, due to increased extravascular accumulation, and (ii) to elucidate histologically the structural characteristics of the deep white matter showing maximal accumulation of edema fluid in cold-lesion edema.

Materials and Methods

Cold lesions were made on the suprasylvian gyrus of cats under ketamine anesthesia, while monitoring blood pressure and blood gases [1]. ^{125}I-labeled serum albumin dissolved in 2% Evans blue solution was infused continuously for 6 h after the cold-lesioning according to the method of Patlak and Pettigrew [2, 5] so as to keep the serum specific activity constant. Each animal was sacrificed at 6 h after cold injury. The brain was then removed and cut coronally through the lesion. A coronal block was frozen and cut for macro-autoradiography. The degree and extent of edema was assessed from the quantitative image of the tissue albumin, assuming a close correlation with the content of edema fluid in the early stage of vasogenic brain edema [2]. Micro-autoradiography was carried out to examine the histological distribution of the tracer according to the method of Mizuhira et al. [4].

Results

Physiological parameters were stable during the experiment. The accumulation of edema fluid assessed by measurement of tissue albumin content was not maximal in the white matter of the lesioned cortex, but in the deeper white

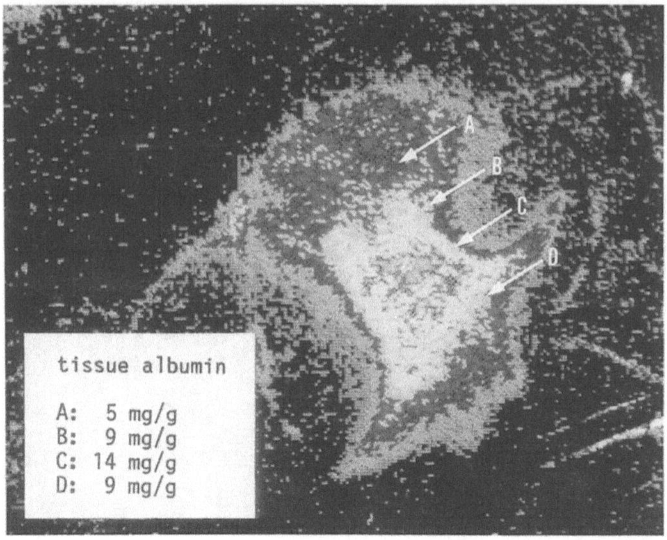

Fig. 1. Distribution of edema fluid in the white matter after cold-lesioning assessed in terms of tissue albumin (mg/g.brain). Note that the greatest accumulation occurs in the deeper white matter

matter of the centrum semiovale (Fig. 1). Micro-autoradiographic examination showed that the ^{125}I-albumin was localized in the intravascular space in the non-edematous white matter (Fig. 2a). In the area showing maximal accumulation of edema fluid in the deeper white matter, marked accumulation of ^{125}I-albumin was observed predominantly in the extravascular space (Fig. 2c). The amount of intravascular tracer in this area was not increased, but rather reduced in comparison with the control white matter and mildly edematous white matter (Fig. 2b). Thus, accumulation of ^{125}I-albumin in the deep white matter is not due to the increased vascular space, but to the increase in tissue albumin reflecting the accumulation of edema fluid. Histological examination revealed that the area showing maximal accumulation of edema fluid in the white matter had the following characteristics; (a) no close association with the surrounding gray matter, (b) presence of crossing and interweaving fiber bundles (Fig. 2e,f).

Conclusions

(1) The maximal accumulation of the tracer for edema fluid was observed in the deeper white matter under the subcortical white matter after cortical cold-lesioning. (2) Micro-autoradiography showed that the maximal accumulation corresponded to the maximal extravascular accumulation of the tracer. (3) The observed heterogeneity of edema fluid accumulation may be explained by regional differences in the structural characteristics of white matter such as the arrangement of fibers. (4) Preferential accumulation of edema fluid in the deep

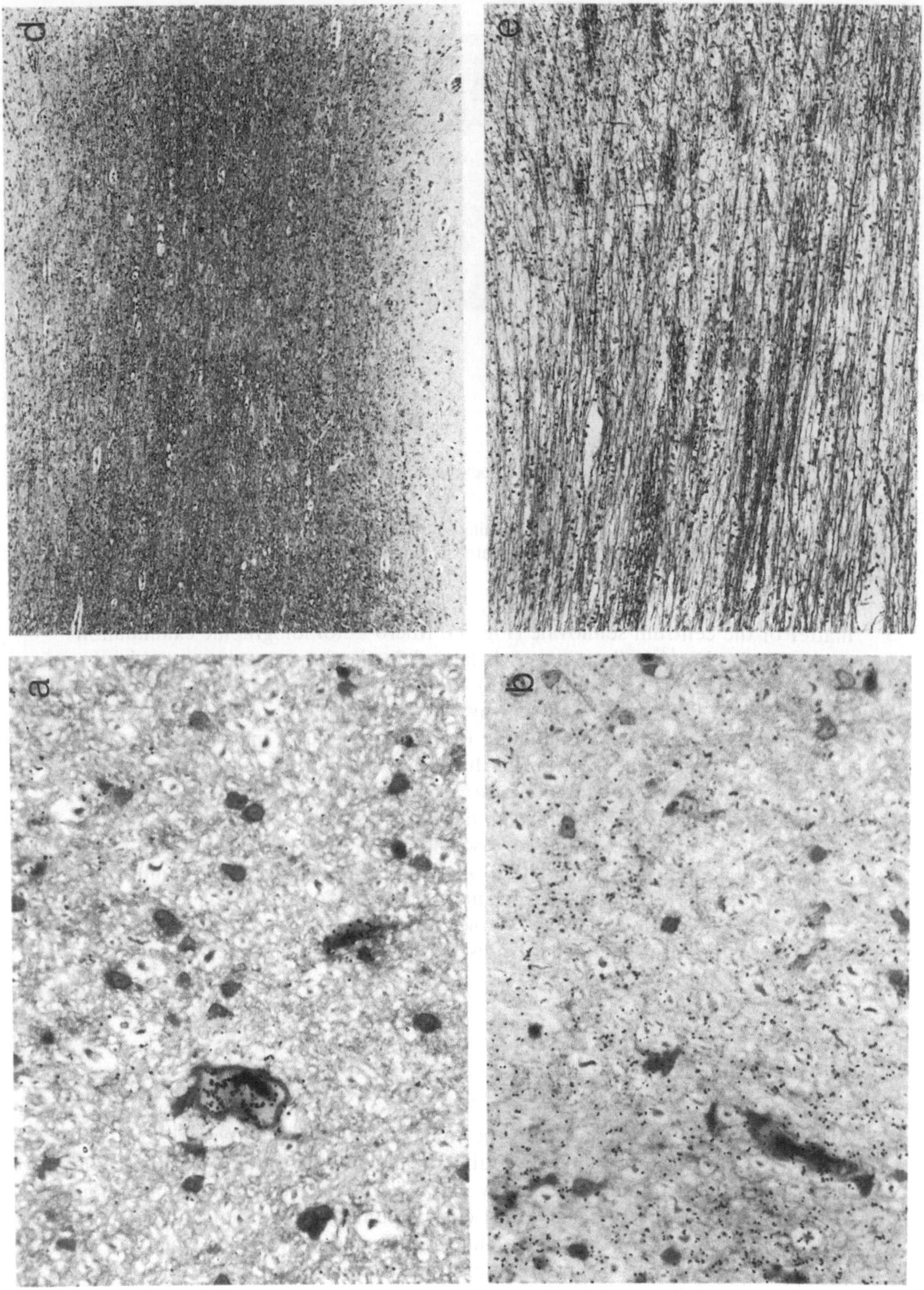
d
e
a
b

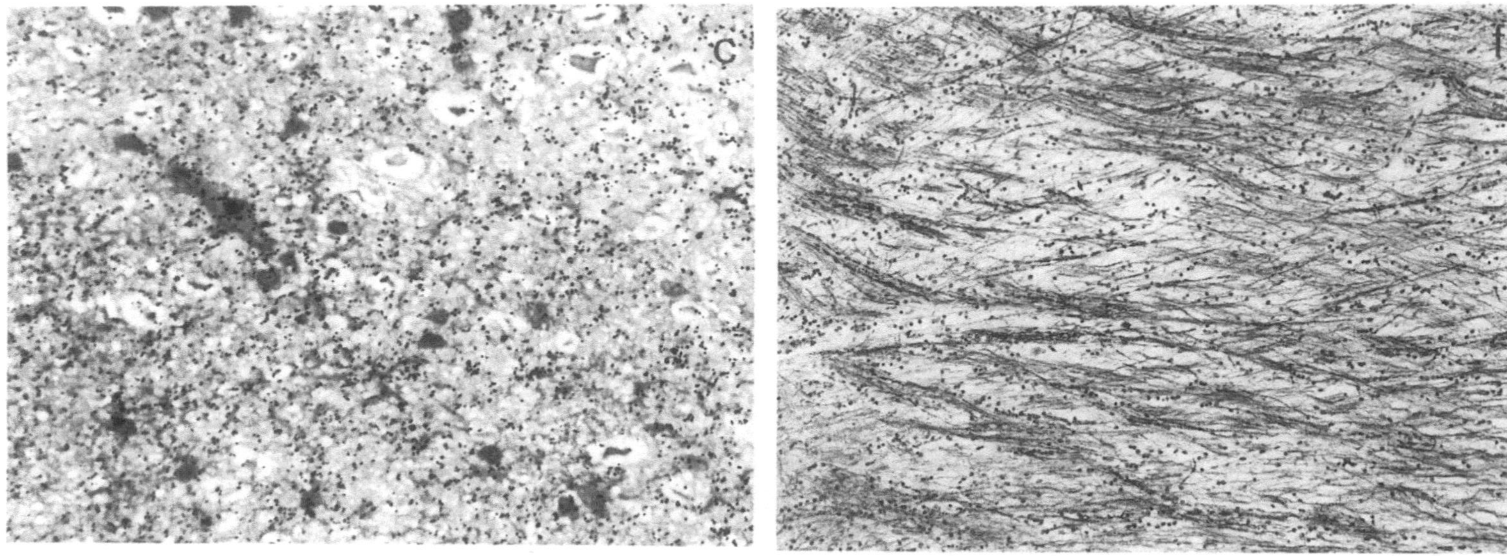

Fig. 2. Micro-autoradiogram of control white matter (**a**), and mildly and severely edematous white matter (**b,c**). Histology corresponding to the above three locations (**d,e,f**). Note the extravascular accumulation of the tracer in the edematous white matter. The white matter showing greatest accumulation of edema fluid is characterized by interweaving fibers and enlargement of the interfiber space

white matter in vasogenic edema may play a pathogenic role in certain diseases such as subcortical encephalopathy, where edema and demyelination are observed frequently in the deep white matter.

References

1. Klatzo I, Chui E, Fujiwara K, Spatz M (1980) Resolution of vasogenic brain oedema. In: Cervos-Navarro, J, Ferszt R (eds) Advances in neurology vol 28: Brain oedema: Pathology, diagnosis and therapy. Raven Press, New York, pp 359–373
2. Kuroiwa T, Cahn R, Juhler M, Gopping G, Campbell G, Klatzo I (1985) Role of extracellular proteins in the dynamics of vasogenic edema. Acta Neuropathol (Berl) 66:3–11
3. Kuroiwa T, Yokofujita J, Kaneko H, Okeda R (1990) Accumulation of edema fluid in deep white matter after cerebral cold injury. J Neurochir, Suppl 51:84–86
4. Mizuhira V, Yokofujita J, Suzuki H, Sugiura Y (1986) Demonstration of membrane-bound receptors by means of autoradiography. Acta Histochem Cytochem 687–700
5. Patlak C, Pettigrew K (1976) A method to obtain infusion schedules for prescribed blood concentration time courses, J Appl Physiol 40:458–463

Gray Matter Edema Following Subarachnoid Hemorrhage

H. Nihei[1], S. Manaka[1], M. Hirakawa[1], J. Sashida[1], and N. Fuke[2]

[1]Department of Neurosurgery and [2]Intensive Care Center, University of Teikyo Ichihara Hospital, 3426-3, Anegasaki, Ichihara Chiba, 299-01, Japan

Introduction

The treatment of subarachnoid hemorrhage patients has been improved in the last ten years. However, there still remains a very difficult problem to save those who are suffering from severe subarachnoid hemorrhage. One of the causes of death in those patients is increased intracranial pressure due to diffuse brain swelling. We have investigated the brain swelling after subarachnoid hemorrhage using a magnetic resonance imaging scan (MRI).

Clinical Material

Four severe subarachnoid hemorrhage patients were brought to our hospital last year. Three of them were, so-called, dead on arrival (DOA), and resuscitated immediately after their arrival. The last patient was comatose (Glasgow Coma Scale 5), and circulatory function was well preserved. MRI and CT scan were performed, and diagnosed by a radiologist. Intracranial pressure was monitored via a ventricular catheter in three cases.

Results

Intracranial pressure was extremely high in all patients. The initial CT scan showed diffuse subarachnoid hemorrhage with or without ventricular hemorrhage, and there was no significant brain swelling. However, cerebral hemispheres became severely swollen on the sequential CT scans, and the density of both cerebral hemispheres was decreased so that the difference between white matter and gray matter became difficult to see (Fig. 1a,b). In contrast, the anatomical structure was quite well differentiated on MRI. T1-weighed images showed diffuse cerebral swelling, and the intensity of the basal ganglia was high in two cases (Fig. 1c). The contrast between gray matter and white matter became more remarkable on T2-weighed images, because gray matter, including thalamus, putamen and insular cortex, appeared to be more intense and thicker in comparison with a T2-weighed image of normal brain (Fig. 1d).

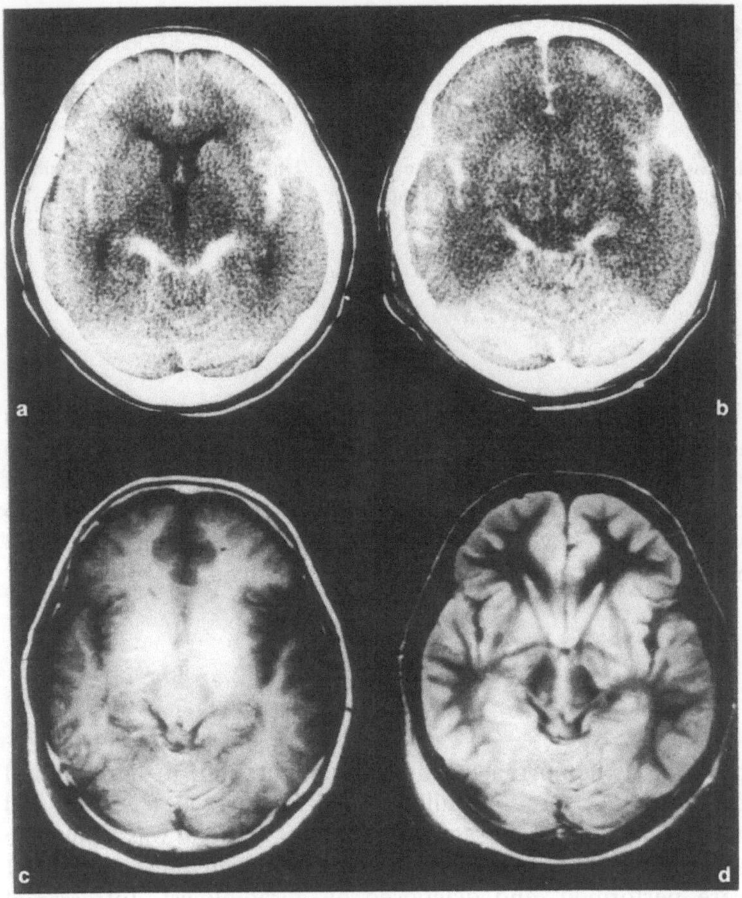

Fig. 1a–d. A patient with severe subarachnoid hemorrhage whose circulation was preserved. CT scan on day 0 (**a**), and day 6 (**b**). T1-weighed (**c**), and T2-weighed (**d**) image of MRI scan on day 3

There was no significant increase in white matter intensity. Because MRI is not a suitable instrument for quantitative analysis compared with X-ray CT, it might be difficult to interpret these findings. However, we concluded that edema occurs mainly in gray matter following severe subarachnoid hemorrhage.

Discussion

Brain edema is well described on T2-weighed images of MRI, and white matter is involved more readily than gray matter in brain tumor or intracerebral hemorrhage. In ischemic situations, both white and gray matter are involved. Our four cases of severe subarachnoid hemorrhage showed intense and thick gray matter on MRI, but no increase of intensity in white matter. This indicates that diffuse cerebral swelling after subarachnoid hemorrhage is different from commonly encountered brain edema in patients with tumor, intracerebral hemorrhage or infarction. We interpreted these MRI findings as gray matter edema, but there might be two speculations about the pathomechanism of gray matter edema: true edema, and petechial hemorrhage.

It has been reported that subarachnoid clot causes breakdown of blood-brain barrier resulting in brain edema [1]. The authors suggested that certain vasoactive products derived from subarachnoid clot cause endothelial damage and increase permeability. Another report stresses the significance of increased intracranial pressure after subarachnoid hemorrhage in breaking down the blood-brain barrier [4]. Both hypotheses are not persuasive enough to explain why only gray matter is involved rather than white matter.

We have experienced a case of post-cardio-pulmonary resuscitation and noticed that the MRI findings were very similar to those of severe subarachnoid hemorrhage. We propose the hypothesis that this gray matter edema is caused by reperfusion following cerebral ischemia of a certain period. Three cases were DOA, and underwent cardio-pulmonary resuscitation. The fourth was not a DOA case, but it has been reported that intracranial pressure increases until it becomes nearly equal to systemic arterial pressure when an aneurysm ruptures [2]. This suggests that there was also an ischemic period after severe subarachnoid hemorrhage. It is well known that gray matter, especially hippocampus, basal ganglia, and layer 3, 5 and 6 of neocortex, is more vulnerable to ischemia than other brain tissue [3]. The gray matter seems to be injured more severely during global transient ischemia than other parts of the brain. When the cerebral circulation is restored, brain edema may occur in the more severely injured parts, i.e. gray matter. It is impossible to determine whether this is true edema or petechial hemorrhage, and a further pathological study is anticipated.

Conclusion

The nature of diffuse brain swelling after severe subarachnoid hemorrhage might be gray matter edema judging from MRI findings. We speculate that gray matter edema occurs when cerebral blood flow is restored after a certain period of cerebral ischemia as a result of the tissue vulnerability to ischemia.

References

1. Doczi T (1985) The pathogenetic and prognostic significance of blood-brain barrier damage at the acute stage of aneurysmal subarachnoid hemorrhage. Clinical and experimental studies. Acta Neurochir 77:110–132
2. Dorsch N, Branston NM, Symon L, Jakubowski J (1989) Intracranial pressure change following primate subarachnoid hemorrhage. Neurological Research 11:201–205

3. Plum F (1983) What causes infarction in ischemic brain? The Robert Wartenberg Lecture. Neurology (NY) 33:222–233
4. Sasaki T, Kassell NF, Yamashita M, Fujiwara S, Zuccarello M (1985) Barrier disruption in the major cerebral arteries following experimental subarachnoid hemorrhage. J Neurosurg 63: 433–440

Effects of Leukotriene C_4 and Acivicin on the Blood-Brain Barrier Permeability of Ischemic Rat Brains: Proof of Existence of Enzymatic Barrier

T. Baba, K.L. Black, K. Ikezaki, and D.P. Becker

The Brain Research Institute and Division of Neurosurgery, UCLA Medical Center, CA, USA

Introduction

We previously demonstrated that leukotriene C_4 (LTC_4) infused into the carotid artery ipsilateral to an experimental glial tumor increased the unidirectional transfer constant for permeability, Ki, two-fold within the tumor while no effect on permeability was seen in the normal brain [2]. Normal brain capillaries are rich in γ-glutamyl transpeptidase (γ-GTP), an enzyme which inactivates LTC_4. In contrast, γ-GTP was absent in tumor capillaries. We suggested that normal brain capillaries may resist the vasogenic effects of LTC_4, and hypothesized that this could relate to the ability of γ-GTP to act as an "enzymatic barrier" and inactivate leukotrienes in normal brain capillaries. We further speculated that leukotrienes could be important mediators of capillary permeability in pathological conditions where the ability of brain capillaries to inactivate LTC_4 is impaired. To support this hypothesis, we already showed the ability of intracarotid infusions of LTC_4 to selectively open the blood-brain barrier (BBB) in the ischemic tissue of the middle cerebral artery (MCA)-occluded rats [1]. Here, we further present the effects of leukotrienes on BBB permeability in ischemic tissue with or without acivicin, inhibitor of γ-GTP.

Materials and Methods

The right MCA of female Wistar rats, weighing 110 to 190 g, were occluded by the technique of Tamura et al. [5].

For intracarotid infusion experiments, rats were divided into two groups, acivicin pretreated group and non-pretreated group. Three hours prior to the sacrifice, rats of pretreated group were given intraperitoneal injection of acivicin (5 mg/1 ml saline). Twenty-four hours, or 72 hours after right MCA occlusion, rats were anesthetized and a catheter was inserted retrograde through the right external carotid artery to the right common carotid artery bifurcation ipsilateral to the MCA occlusion. Both femoral arteries and one femoral vein were also cannulated. Body temperature was maintained at 37°C, and arterial blood gases, blood pressure, and hematocrit were monitored. LTC_4 (0.8 ml) at a concentration of 5 μg/ml or 0.8 ml of vehicle (2.5% ethanol in PBS, pH 7.1) was infused into the right carotid artery using a constant infusion pump at a rate of 53.3 μl/min for 15 min. Five minutes after the start of the intracarotid infusion, 100 μCi/kg of ^{14}C-aminoisobutyric acid (AIB) was injected as an intravenous bolus. Femoral arterial blood was withdrawn at a constant rate immediately after injection of ^{14}C-AIB for determination of serum radioactivity. Fifteen minutes after the start of intracarotid infusion, animals were sacrificed. Standard techniques were employed for autoradiography. Sections were stained with hematoxylin and eosin to correlate areas of histologically verified ischemia with autoradiograms. Quantitative analysis was performed using a computer-assisted digital image analyzer [6]. Ki was calculated using the method of Blasberg et al. [3] and expressed in μl/g/min. ANOVA analysis and unpaired student t test were applied to the mean values.

Gamma-GTP histochemistry was performed for 5 rats of each subgroup, acivicin pretreated and non-pretreated [4].

Results

The pH, $PaCO_2$ and PaO_2 were 7.408 ± 0.037, 33.5 ± 5.1 mmHg, 96.7 ± 15.7 mmHg, respectively (mean ± SD). The mean arterial blood pressure and hematocrit were 124.4 ± 12.8 mmHg and 35.0 ± 4.9%, respectively. Size of ischemic core was measured in the section in which the infarcted area is maximum. There was no significant difference among subgroups.

Table 1 shows a summary of the results, 24 hours after MCA occlusion. Without pretreatment of acivicin, intracarotid infusion of LTC_4 ($n = 7$) failed to increase Ki within ischemic tissue when compared to vehicle alone ($n = 7$). With pretreatment of acivicin, however, intracarotid infusion of LTC_4 ($n = 7$) resulted in more than two fold increase of Ki within both the ischemic core and tissue adjacent to the ischemic core when compared to vehicle alone without acivicin ($n = 7$) (17.2 ± 16.3 vs. 8.2 ± 6.6, $p < 0.05$, and 11.8 ± 8.1 vs. 4.6 ± 1.9, $p < 0.01$, respectively). With pretreatment of acivicin, even intracarotid infusion of vehicle ($n = 7$) produced a tendency of increase of Ki within the ischemic core (14.3 ± 6.1 vs. 8.2 ± 6.6) and a significant increase of Ki within the tissue adjacent to the ischemic core (9.1 ± 5.2 vs. 4.6 ± 1.9, $p < 0.05$). There was no significant change in BBB permeability within the extratumoral normal tissue.

Table 2 shows a summary of the results, 72 hours after MCA occlusion. Without pretreatment of acivicin, intracarotid infusion of LTC_4 ($n = 7$) resulted in more than two fold increase of Ki within both the ischemic core and tissue adjacent to the ischemic core when compared to vehicle alone ($n = 7$) (15.5 ± 6.0 vs. 8.4 ± 3.6, $p < 0.05$, and 8.8 ± 4.0 vs. 4.5 ± 2.2, $p < 0.05$,

Table 1. Effect of LTC_4 on Ki (μl/g/min; mean ± SD) of rat brains with or without pretreatment of acivicin, 24 hrs after MCA occlusion

	vehicle i.c.a.	LTC_4 i.c.a.
A. Ischemic tissue		
1. Ischemic core		
acivicin(−)	8.2 ± 6.6	8.7 ± 5.8
acivicin(+)	14.3 ± 6.12	17.2 ± 16.3*
2. Tissue adjacent to ischemic core		
acivicin(−)	4.6 ± 1.9	3.9 ± 2.7
acivicin(+)	9.1 ± 5.2*	11.8 ± 8.1**
B. Extratumoral ipsilateral hemisphere		
1. Frontal cortex		
acivicin(−)	1.2 ± 1.6	1.1 ± 1.3
acivicin(+)	1.2 ± 1.5	1.6 ± 1.6
2. Basal ganglia		
acivicin(−)	1.2 ± 1.6	3.0 ± 3.3
acivicin(+)	2.6 ± 4.9	3.1 ± 2.1
C. Contralateral hemisphere		
1. Frontal cortex		
acivicin(−)	1.7 ± 1.9	2.2 ± 2.4
acivicin(+)	1.2 ± 1.5	2.8 ± 2.0
2. Basal ganglia		
acivicin(−)	1.2 ± 1.6	1.1 ± 1.3
acivicin(+)	1.2 ± 1.5	1.6 ± 1.6

i.c.a.: intracarotid administration; * significantly different from control group at $p < 0.05$; ** significantly different from control group at $p < 0.01$

respectively). LTC_4 (n = 7) with pretreatment of acivicin also produced more than two fold increase of Ki within both the ischemic core and tissue adjacent to the ischemic core (17.2 ± 5.7 vs. 8.4 ± 3.6, $p < 0.01$, and 9.6 ± 3.5 vs. 4.5 ± 2.2, $p < 0.01$, respectively), but intracarotid infusion of vehicle with pretreatment of acivicin (n = 7) did not produce significant increase of Ki within the ischemic tissue. There was no significant change in BBB permeability within extratumoral normal tissue.

Gamma-GTP activity in capillaries was seen in normal rat brains without pretreatment of acivicin (n = 5). With pretreatment of acivicin, however, it almost completely disappeared in all examined rat brains (n = 5).

Discussion

We previously demonstrated that the BBB could be selectively opened by intracarotid infusion of LTC_4 in ischemic tissue, 48 to 72 hours after MCA, but it could not be opened in ischemic tissue, 24 hours after MCA occlusion

Table 2. Effect of LTC_4 on Ki ($\mu l/g/min$; mean ± SD) of rat brains with or without pretreatment of acivicin, 72 hrs after MCA occlusion

	vehicle i.c.a.	LTC_4 i.c.a.
A. Ischemic tissue		
1. Ischemic core		
acivicin(−)	8.4 ± 3.6	15.5 ± 6.0*
acivicin(+)	10.7 ± 3.5	17.2 ± 5.7**
2. Tissue adjacent to ischemic core		
acivicin(−)	4.5 ± 2.2	8.8 ± 4.0*
acivicin(+)	4.7 ± 2.3	9.6 ± 3.5**
B. Extratumoral ipsilateral hemisphere		
1. Frontal cortex		
acivicin(−)	1.7 ± 1.6	2.2 ± 2.0
acivicin(+)	1.8 ± 1.1	2.7 ± 0.9
2. Basal ganglia		
acivicin(−)	3.6 ± 4.9	2.0 ± 2.0
acivicin(+)	1.8 ± 1.1	3.6 ± 4.9
C. Contralateral hemisphere		
1. Frontal cortex		
acivicin(−)	2.2 ± 2.1	3.1 ± 1.8
acivicin(+)	1.8 ± 1.1	2.4 ± 1.4
2. Basal ganglia		
acivicin(−)	1.7 ± 1.6	2.0 ± 2.0
acivicin(+)	1.8 ± 1.1	2.4 ± 1.4

i.c.a.: intracarotid administration; * significantly different from control group at $p < 0.05$; ** significantly different from control group at $p < 0.01$

[1]. We suggested that this is due to the difference in amount of γ-GTP of capillaries; i.e. almost all γ-GTP activity in capillaries is lost in ischemic tissue, 72 hours after MCA occlusion, while a moderate amount of γ-GTP activity in capillaries still remains in ischemic tissue, 24 hours after MCA occlusion [1]. In this study, we demonstrated that the BBB could be selectively opened by intracarotid infusion of LTC_4 in ischemic tissue, even 24 hours after MCA occlusion, with pretreatment of acivicin, inhibitor of γ-GTP. These results indicate that our hypothesis that normal brain capillaries might use γ-GTP as an enzymatic barrier to inactivate LTC_4 is right.

In this study, BBB within the ischemic tissue of the acivicin-pretreated rats could be selectively opened not only by intracarotid infusion of LTC_4, but also by intracarotid infusion of vehicle. This is supposed to be because endogenous LTC_4, after 24 hours after MCA occlusion, was enough to increase the BBB permeability in the brain where activity of γ-GTP was inhibited by acivicin. It is also suspected that the result that acivicin alone failed to increase the BBB permeability in the ischemic tissue, 72 hours after MCA, is due to decreased endogenous LTC_4.

Conclusion

Seventy-two hours after MCA occlusion, LTC_4 infused into the carotid artery ipsilateral to the MCA occlusion selectively increased Ki within ischemic brain tissue. No effect on BBB permeability was seen within non-ischemic brain tissue or in ischemic tissue after only 24 hours post MCA occlusion. These findings show that normal brain capillaries resist the vasogenic effects of LTC_4 while LTC_4 increases permeability in capillaries of ischemic tissue. With pretreatment of acivicin, inhibitor of γ-GTP, intracarotid infusion of LTC_4 increased Ki in ischemic tissue even at 24 hours after infarction, when γ-GTP is still supposed to exist in capillaries. We speculate that γ-GTP may act as an "enzymatic barrier" and inactivates leukotrienes in normal brain capillaries.

References

1. Baba T, Black KL, Ikezaki K, Chen K, Becker DP (1991) Intracarotid infusion of leukotriene C_4 selectively increased blood-brain barrier permeability after focal ischemia. J Cerebr Blood Flow Metabol (in press)
2. Black KL, King WA, Ikezaki K (1990) Selective opening of the blood-tumor barrier by intracarotid infusion of leukotriene C_4. J Neurosurg 72:912–916
3. Blasberg RG, Patlak CS, Jehle JW, Fenstermacher JD (1978) An autoradiographic technique to measure the permeability of normal and abnormal brain capillaries. Neurology 28:363
4. Gardell SJ, Tate SS (1980) Affinity labeling of g-glutamyl transpeptidase by glutamine antagonists. Effects of the g-glutamyl tranfer and proteinase activities. FEBS Letters 122:171–174
5. Tamura A, Graham DI, McCulloch J, Teasdale GM (1981) Focal cerebral ischemia in the rats: 1. Description of technique and early neuropathological consequences following middle cerebral artery occlusion. J Cerebr Blood Flow Metabol 1:53–60
6. Toga AW, Santori EM, Samaie M (1986) Regional distribution of flunitrazepam binding constants: visualizing Kd and Bmax by digital image analysis. J Neurosci 6:2747–2756

Temporary Blood Brain Barrier Damage and Continued Edema Formation in Experimental Closed Head Injury in the Rat*

W.A. VAN DEN BRINK[1], B.O. SANTOS[1], A. MARMAROU[1], and C.J.J. AVEZAAT[2]

[1] Division of Neurosurgery, Medical College of Virginia, Richmond, VA, USA
[2] Department of Neurosurgery, Erasmus University Rotterdam, The Netherlands

Introduction

The disruption of the blood brain barrier (BBB) and development of brain edema concomitant with traumatic brain injury has been well established [5, 7]. In experimental studies, at least two factors contribute to this disruption immediately upon impact; the mechanical deformation of tissue and cerebral vessels and the hypertensive surge that accompanies the injury. This hypertensive surge is seen with experimental fluid percussion injury [1]. In fact, hypertension alone is sufficient to cause BBB disruption and models of pharmacologic induced hypertension mimicking the surge observed with experimental models have produced similar defects in the barrier [8]. The objective of this study was to determine if a similar hypertensive surge and BBB disruption occurred with impact-acceleration to the closed calvarium as has been observed with direct dural impact. This would help clarify the role that hypertension plays in the degree of barrier disruption in mechanical trauma under conditions more allied to the clinical experience.

Materials and Methods

In this report, the BBB was studied using iodine −125 radio active labelled bovine albumin as a tracer of a blood borne high molecular weight substance to show a general BBB-dysfunction [2]. The edema analysis was performed using micro gravimetrical techniques [6] to quantify regional edema formation. Studies at 4, 15, and 24 hours after trauma provided temporal information of total brain water content.

Trauma Model

The Closed Head Injury (CHI) model in the rat was produced by weight drop (450 gm – 2.0 meter) on the intact and partially restrained skull. The skull was

* This study was funded by NIH grant 2P0INS12587 and NIDRR HI33B80029. Further support was obtained from: the Richard Roland Reynolds Research Laboratories and the Sophia Foundation for Medical Research from the Netherlands.

protected from fracture by cementing a small stainless steel disc in the midline between bregma and lambda.

Animal Preparation

Rats were maintained under anaesthesia using Isoflurane in a 1–2% concentration in an oxygen : nitrous oxide mixture (33% : 66%). In studies of the BBB 30 μCi I^{125} Radio labelled Bovine Serum Albumin was injected in the left femoral vein. The albumin was allowed to circulate for 30 minutes. Just prior to the injury a control blood sample was obtained. Either 4, 15 or 24 hours after injury the animal was intraperitoneal injected with pentobarbital. Animals were sacrificed with 2 ml KCl intra cardiac (edema studies) or perfused with saline (BBB studies). The brain was removed and frosted to facilitate standardized cutting. Water contents of survivors of severe CHI were obtained using micrograviметrical techniques [6]. For BBB studies the radioactivity of each segment was counted in a gamma counter and a Cumulative Permeability Index (CPI) was calculated as follows:

$$\mathrm{CPI} = \frac{\text{background corrected brain counts per minute/brain weight}}{\text{background corrected blood counts per minute/blood weight}} [2].$$

Results

Of 47 animals tested, three animals suffered skull fracture and were discarded from analysis. The overall mortality in the remaining 44 closed head injured animals equaled 41%. This mortality (450 gm – 2 meter) was indicative of severe trauma.

Hypertension at Impact

A slight increase in blood pressure was observed directly after impact. This brief rise of BP reached 124 mmHg from a baseline of 107 mmHg and returned to baseline within 3 seconds. Thereafter, sustained hypotension was observed for 10 minutes.

Blood Brain Barrier Studies

In all slices, the CPI for I-125 albumin was consistently higher in injured animals than in sham operated animals demonstrating BBB disruption. Table 1 displays the CPI-values after 4 and 15 hours for both sham and traumatized animals. The highest levels in the supratentorial compartment were found in the brain slices just under the helmet, the area where most of the skull and brain deformation was expected. After 15 hours, the increase in CPI was much smaller than early after trauma.

Table 1. CPI at 4 and 15 hours after injury (mean ± sem). In each group there were 5 animals. The CPI increase after trauma is less after 15 hours, indicating an early sealing of the blood brain barrier.

CPI	4 hr injury	sham	15 hr injury	sham
slice 1	2.36 (0.22)	1.59 (0.20)	2.01 (0.18)	1.39 (0.61)
slice 2	2.90 (0.43)	1.34 (0.16)	1.42 (0.20)	0.88 (0.21)
slice 3	3.42 (0.73)	1.50 (0.25)	1.53 (0.14)	0.77 (0.16)
slice 4	4.47 (0.84)	1.50 (0.35)	1.81 (0.26)	0.73 (0.13)
slice 5	7.04 (1.32)	1.66 (0.29)	2.21 (0.35)	0.99 (0.15)
stem	10.34 (2.23)	1.89 (0.34)	2.96 (0.39)	1.37 (0.28)
cer	14.50 (5.52)	1.48 (0.34)	2.44 (0.29)	1.21 (0.22)

Table 2. Brain water contents after 4, 15 and 24 hours. Over time there is a gradual increase in traumatic brain edema

% Water	4 hr injury	sham	15 hr injury	sham	24 hr injury	sham
slice 1	78.90 (0.10)	78.74 (0.09)	79.96 (0.13)	79.54 (0.14)	78.67 (0.07)	77.85 (0.09)
slice 2	79.21 (0.08)	78.92 (0.06)	80.27 (0.08)	79.95 (0.05)	79.06 (0.08)	78.77 (0.07)
slice 3	79.00 (0.07)	79.08 (0.07)	80.39 (0.09)	80.06 (0.06)	79.07 (0.08)	78.67 (0.08)
slice 4	79.16 (0.08)	79.02 (0.06)	80.37 (0.08)	80.02 (0.05)	79.14 (0.11)	78.64 (0.08)
slice 5	79.60 (0.11)	79.27 (0.12)	80.74 (0.08)	80.53 (0.08)	79.50 (0.10)	79.01 (0.11)

Edema Studies

Edema was clearly evident in CHI by 4 hours post trauma. The brain water content was higher in the traumatized animals compared to sham controls (Table 2). Over time the water content increased, and after 24 hours all brain slices of traumatized rats contained significantly more water. The distribution of water content after 4, 15, and 24 hours for traumatized and sham operated animals (Table 2) showed a gradual increase over time.

Discussion and Conclusion

Early qualitative studies on the dysfunction of the BBB have determined that an arterial pressure surge, in absence of craniocerebral trauma, compromises the barrier [3]. In these studies, the pharmacologic pressure surge was matched to that observed with fluid percussion. However, it appears from our experiments that a dramatic pressure surge is not associated with CHI. Our studies show that CHI is typically followed by a prolonged period of hypotension after a preceding short transient period of mildly increased arterial pressure [9]. This would suggest that CHI might produce less BBB disruption and edema than that observed with direct dural impact. Increased CPI's after CHI indicate trauma induced barrier dysfunction. We observed that the CPI after 4 hours is considerably higher than after 15 hours. Following this initial stage, no further accumulation of radioactive albumin in the brain parenchyma was found. However, during this period, it is likely that clearance mechanisms are operative and a portion of the protein that was extravasated initially was cleared into CSF. We suspect on the basis of these observations that barrier opening ceases at some time point within 4 hours after trauma. However, this study shows the gradual increase of brain water content over time. Thus, mechanisms other than vascular permeability attribute to the continuously increasing edema. Based on these data it is likely that the initial edema after CHI is of a vascular origin. As time progresses, other secondary mechanisms, such as oncotic forces may develop after introduction of blood borne high molecular weight substances in the brain parenchyma. The slow clearance of these relatively large molecules can further attribute to edema formation [4].

We conclude that CHI, as expected, produces BBB disruption. Unlike percussion to the exposed dura, this BBB disruption occurs in the absence of a dramatic arterial pressure surge. Thereafter, edema formation continues despite the sealing of the BBB within 4 hours.

References

1. Dixon CE, Lighthall JW, Anderson TE (1988) Physiologic, histopathologic, and cineradiographic characterization of a new fluid percussion model of experimental brain injury in the rat. J Neurotrauma 5:99–104
2. Ellis EF, Chao J, Heizer ML (1989) Brain kininogen following experimental brain injury: evidence for a secondary event. J Neurosurg 71:437–442
3. Haggendal E, Johansson B (1972) On the pathophysiology of the increased cerebrovascular permeability in acute arterial hypertension in cats. Acta Neurol Scand 48:265–270
4. Kuroiwa T, Shibutani M, Tajima T, Hirasawa H, Okeda R (1990) Hydrostatic pressure versus osmotic pressure in the development of vasogenic brain edema induced by cold injury. In: Long D (ed) Advances in Neurology, Raven Press, New York, pp 11–19
5. Marmarou A, Shima K (1990) Comparative studies of edema produced by fluid percussion injury with lateral and central modes of injury in cats. In: Long D (ed) Advances in Neurology, Raven Press, Ltd., New York, pp 233–236
6. Marmarou A, Tanaka K, Shulman K (1982) An improved gravimetric measure of cerebral edema. J Neurosurg 56:246–253
7. McIntosh TK, Soares H, Thomas M, Cloherty K (1990) Development of regional cerebral oedema after lateral fluid-percussion brain injury in the rat. Acta Neurochir, Suppl 51:263–264
8. Zhang XM, Ellis EF (1990) Superoxide dismutase reduces permeability and edema induced by hypertension in rats. Am J Physiol (In Press)
9. van den Brink WA, Marmarou A, Avezaat CJJ (1990) Brain oedema in experimental closed head injury in the rat. Acta Neurochir, Suppl 51:261–262

Breakdown of the Blood-Brain Barrier to Horseradish Peroxidase After Experimental Post-Traumatic Hypoxic Brain Injury

H. Tanno, L. Pitts, and L.J. Noble

Department of Neurosurgery, San Francisco General Hospital and the University of California at San Francisco, San Francisco, CA 94110, USA

Introduction

Clinical studies have clearly demonstrated that severe head injury is frequently accompanied by hypoxic insult and that there is a close association between post-traumatic hypoxic brain injury (PTHI) and poor neurologic outcome. We therefore developed a rat model of PTHI combining a fluid percussion injury and hypoxic insult [3].

Vasogenic edema is a consequence of breakdown of the blood-brain barrier (BBB) and is characterized by permeability to both water and plasma proteins. In previous studies we assessed water content in the brain after PTHI by measuring specific gravity and by using magnetic resonance imaging. These studies demonstrated an increase in water content in the brain after PTHI [3].

In the present study we focused on alterations in permeability of the BBB to the protein horseradish peroxidase (HRP) and evaluated the pattern and time course of breakdown of the BBB after PTHI.

Materials and Methods

Adult male Sprague-Dawley rats (350–400 g) were prepared for fluid percussion brain injury as previously described [3]. Briefly, each animal was anesthetized with 4% chloral hydrate (8 ml/kg b.w., i.p.). A catheter was inserted into the femoral artery to monitor blood pressure and analyze blood gases. Each animal was subjected to a lateral fluid percussion injury (4.8–5.2 atm.) for 20 msec and exposed to hypoxic conditions (10% O_2) for 45 min. immediately after injury. Animals were allowed to breathe spontaneously throughout the procedure.

Horseradish peroxidase (HRP, M.W. 40,000; Sigma, Type VI; 75 mg/kg b.w.) was given i.v. either prior to impact (Study 1) or 10 min. prior to sacrifice (Study 2). Since HRP may stimulate histamine release, diphenhydramine-hydrochloride (Benedryl), a histamine antagonist, was given 10 min. before the administration of HRP. In Study 1 rats were examined at 1 h (n = 4), 3 h (n = 3), and 6 h (n = 5) and in Study 2 at 1 h (n = 4), 3 h (n = 5), 6 h (n = 7), and 24 h (n = 5).

Animals were sacrificed by intracardiac perfusion with fixative. Each brain was removed and 100 μm sections were cut on a vibratome. The protein was

Fig. 1. Study 1. Localization of HRP at 1 hour after injury. *Arrow*: impact site; *shading*: distribution of HRP; *closed circles*: hematoma in external capsule

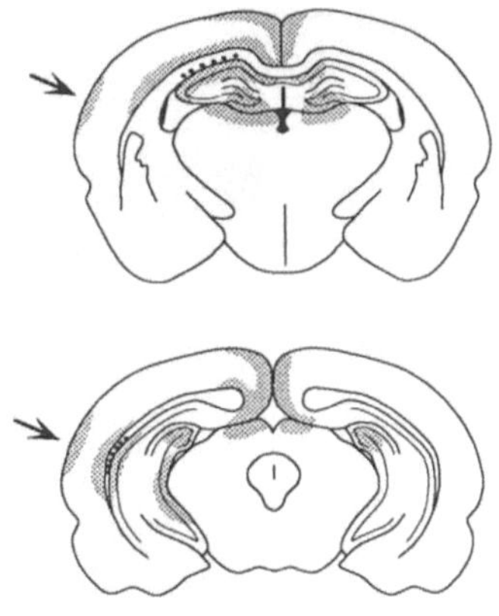

visualized in brain sections at the light microscopic level using diaminobenzidine as the chromogen in the presence of hydrogen peroxide.

Results

After PTHI a moderate amount of parenchymal hemorrhage was present in the ipsilateral external capsule. Small hematomas were infrequently found, in the hippocampus (CA3) and/or superior colliculus ipsilaterally. There were no hematomas in the cortex, including the impact site (Fig. 1).

In Study 1 breakdown of the BBB to HRP and sites of extravascular accumulation of this protein were evaluated. Prominent leakage of HRP occurred in multiple sites in the ipsilateral cortex, hippocampus, thalamus, and midbrain at 1 h after impact. A diffuse pattern of staining appeared localized to the extracellular space (Fig. 1, 2A). In addition HRP was identified within neuronal cell bodies and their processes (Fig. 2B). The contralateral hemisphere exhibited minimal extravasation in the cortex and hippocampus as compared to the ipsilateral hemisphere. There was no difference in this staining pattern at 1, 3, and 6 h.

In Study 2 the time course for abnormal permeability to HRP was evaluated at 1 to 24 h after PTHI (Fig. 3). Up to 6 h after impact, leakage of HRP occurred in various regions of the cortex including the paramedian cortex, impact site, and deep cortical layers. At 24 h after impact, the BBB appeared to be re-established at most cortical sites. The impact site, however, remained permeable.

Discussion

Our study elucidated the pattern and time course of abnormal permeability of the BBB to the protein HRP in the acute stage after PTHI. Protein leakage was not restricted to the impact site but was distributed in various brain regions

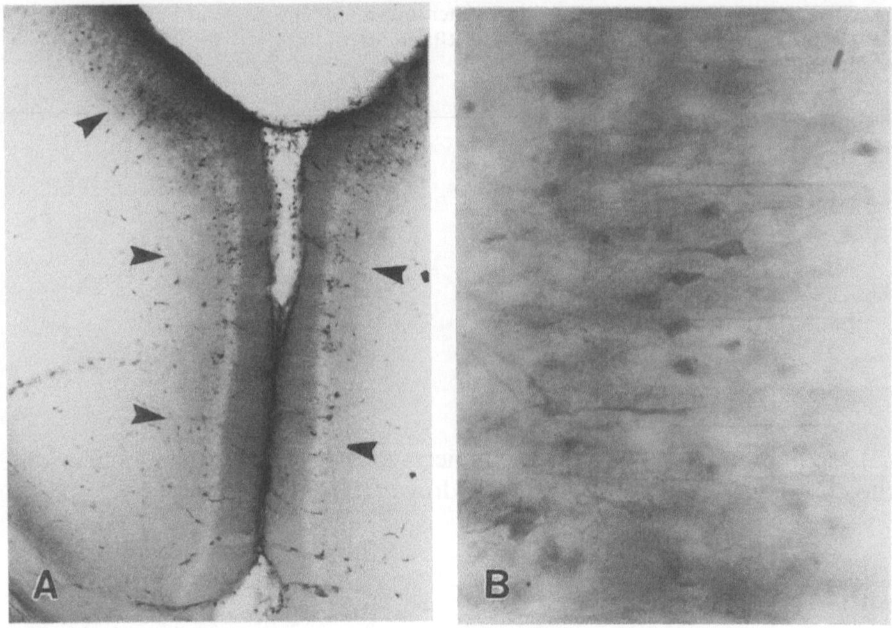

Fig. 2. A Paramedian cortex exhibits diffuse staining (arrowheads). **B** Higher magnification reveals intraneuronal staining

in the ipsilateral and contralateral hemispheres. This widespread leakage is similar to the distribution of increased tissue water content after PTHI [3]. Thus, vasogenic edema, which is characterized by permeability to both water and plasma proteins, is a prominent pathologic event after PTHI.

The pathological consequences of this widespread vasogenic edema are not well understood. Increased brain water content can lead to compression and/or elevation of intracranial pressure. In addition abnormal permeability to plasma components such as biogenic amines, calcium, and/or glutamate may alter the microenvironment and contribute to secondary tissue destruction.

The mechanisms of vasogenic edema after brain trauma are not yet well defined. Vasogenic edema is closely correlated with directly traumatized (hemorrhagic) blood vessels. However, vascular thrombosis quickly prevents further edema formation from this source [5]. The widespread and prolonged leakage of HRP in the present study may be due to vasoactive plasma components that have crossed the BBB (bradykinins, histamine, excitatory amino acids), as well as substances that may be released or activated from membrane phospholipids of injured cells (arachadonic acid, prostaglandins, and free radicals; [1, 6]).

There are at least 3 potential routes for the passage of proteins across the BBB: diffusion across either damaged plasma membranes or through opened tight junctions and transport across the cell in membrane-bound vesicles. Ultrastructural studies support the hypothesis that transendothelial vesicular

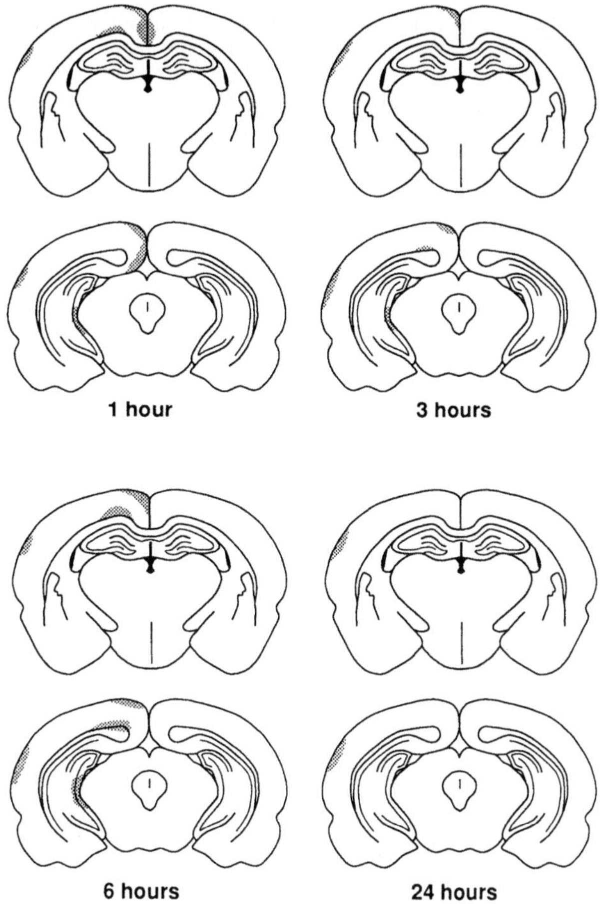

Fig. 3. Study 2. Time course for abnormal permeability to HRP. *Shading*: distribution of HRP

transport is the primary mechanism for protein permeability after brain injury [4].

In the present study, we observed a diffuse staining of HRP in neurons. Whether this neuronal inundation reflects irreversible cell injury or a transient neuronal response remains unclear [2]. We plan to examine this neuronal response in more detail in future studies.

References

1. Chan PH, Schmidley JW, Fishman RA, Longar SM (1984) Brain injury, edema, and vascular permeability changes induced by oxygen-derived free radicals. Neurol 34:315–320
2. Brightman MW, Klatzo I, Olsson Y, Reese TS (1970) The blood-brain barrier to protein tracer under normal and pathological conditions. J Neurol Sci 10:215–239

3. Ishige N, Pitts LH, Berry I, Carlson S, Nishimura MC, Moseley ME, Weinstein PR (1987) The effect of hypoxia on traumatic head injury in rats: alterations in neurologic function, brain edema, and cerebral blood flow. J Cereb Blood Flow Metab 7:759–767
4. Povlishock JT, Becker DP, Sullivan HG, Millar JD (1978) Vascular permeability alterations to horseradish peroxidase in experimental brain injury. Brain Research 153:223–239
5. Tornheim PA (1985) Traumatic edema in head injury. In: Becker DP, Povlishock JT (eds). Central nervous system trauma status report 1985. National Institute of Neurological and Communicative Disorders and Stroke. William Byrd Press, Richmond, VA, pp 431–442
6. Wahl M, Unterberg A, Baethmann A, Schilling L (1988) Mediators of blood-brain barrier dysfunction and formation of vasogenic brain edema. J Cereb Blood Flow Metab 8:621–634

Delayed Opening of the Blood-Brain Barrier in Direct Infusion Edema Model

H. Sakamoto, J. Katsuyama, S. Nishimura, and A. Hakuba

Department of Neurosurgery, Osaka City University Medical School, Osaka, Japan

Introduction

Marmarou et al. developed a unique model for studying brain edema by infusing a relatively large amount of fluid into the white matter [2]. Such intraparenchymal infusion did not induce local breakdown of the blood-brain barrier (BBB): the BBB was found intact at 0 hour, 72 hours and at 7 days after the infusion [1]. Therefore, this model could be considered suitable for investigations on the resolution process of brain edema in terms of no new edema fluid supplied from the blood vessels. A recent study using this model showed that the fluid infused into the brain migrated, in an extremely short period after infusion, to the ventricular system and also to the cortical surface [4]. Such a fast movement of fluid along the intraparenchymal vessels may change their permeability in a short time after the infusion. In the present study we reinvestigated the effect of intraparenchymal infusion on the BBB within 24 hours after the infusion.

Methods

Adult cats were anesthetized with halothane and nitrous oxide under mechanical ventilation. The mean blood pressure was kept under 140 mmHg. Intracranial pressure (ICP) was continuously monitored through a 25-gauge needle inserted into the lateral ventricle. Infusion edema was produced by direct infusion of the fluid through a 25-gauge needle into the centrum semiovale [2]. Animals of the bilateral infusion group were infused symmetrically into the left and right centrum semiovale with 0.25 ml of autoserum and 0.25 ml of protein-free mock cerebrospinal fluid (CSF), respectively, at the same time. The infusion required 136 minutes and the animals were sacrificed at 0 minute (n = 2), 30 minutes (n = 4), 3 hours (n = 4), and at 24 hours after the completion of the infusion (n = 4). In the delayed infusion group, mock CSF was at first infused into the centrum semiovale on one side, followed by a second infusion of the same amount of mock CSF into a symmetrical site on the other side. The volume of the infusate was 0.25 ml (n = 2), 0.125 ml (n = 4) and 0.03 ml (n = 4). The second infusion was made in a fashion identical to the first one, except that the time interval between the first and second infusion

Table 1. Evans blue staining in relation to time after infusion

	0 min (n = 2)		30 min (n = 4)		3 hrs (n = 4)		24 hrs (n = 4)	
	serum	CSF	serum	CSF	serum	CSF	serum	CSF
number of	0	0	0	0	5	1	4	1
slices stained	0	0	1	0	4	3	1	0
			3	0	5	3	3	0
			0	0	4	3	0	0

was 3 hours. The animals of this group were killed within 1 minute after the completion of the second infusion. Evans blue (2 ml/Kg), an indicator of BBB opening, was administered intravenously 30 minutes prior to the sacrifice in all animals. Upon the conclusion of the experiment the brain was quickly removed and sectioned coronally at 2 mm thickness. The blue staining of the brain slices by Evans blue was observed macroscopically and also the water content was measured by a gravimetric method [3]. Samples for measuring the water content were obtained from the center of the white matter in each coronary slice.

Results

In the bilateral infusion group, staining by Evans blue was consistently observed in both serum- and CSF-infusion sites 3 hours after the completion of the infusion (Table 1). The area of dark staining corresponded to the infusion site, and light staining was seen in the white matter up to the subcortical area, often to the overlying cortex, and down to the head of the caudate nucleus. The area of the staining in the serum-infused hemisphere was significantly larger than that in the CSF-infused hemisphere. No staining was found in the animals sacrificed 0 minutes after the completion of the infusion. Only faint staining was seen in the animals sacrificed 24 hours after the infusion. The delayed infusion group showed that the first infusion of smaller amounts of fluid induced a BBB opening 3 hours after the infusion, though no staining was found at the second infusion side of the hemisphere where the infusion was finished at the time of sacrifice (Table 2). In this group, infusing a less amount of fluid reduced the area stained by Evans blue, which was restricted to the center of the infusion site.

Table 2. Evans blue staining in relation to volume of infusate

	0.25 ml (n = 3)		0.125 ml (n = 3)		0.03 ml (n = 3)	
	first	second	first	second	first	second
number of	4	0	2	0	1	0
slices stained	3	0	2	0	2	0
	3	0	1	0	2	0

The water content of the white matter infused with 0.25 ml of serum showed no significant change at 0 hour, 3 hours and 24 hours after the completion of the infusion. Animals infused with 0.03 ml at each side showed no significant change in ICP before and after the infusion. Other groups of animals infused with a larger amount of fluid, either serum or mock CSF, showed that ICP increased significantly after the infusion.

Summary

The present study showed a delayed opening of the BBB in the infusion edema model. The bilateral infusion group showed that the infusion, either of autoserum or of protein-free mock CSF, into the white matter consistently developed a BBB opening 3 hours after completion of the infusion. BBB opening was observed at the infusion site of the white matter and its adjacent area which often included the overlying gray matter. It is very unlikely that BBB opening observed in the present study resulted from a needle injury: in the delayed infusion group, the second infusion showed no BBB opening in that hemisphere, though the first infusion carried out in an identical fashion induced BBB opening on the ipsilateral side in the same animal. It is unlikely that significant advancement of the edema occurred and that the BBB opening lasted long. There was no significant increase in water content at 3 hours or 24 hours after serum infusion, and the area and intensity of the BBB opening diminished at 24 hours after the infusion. The opening of the BBB produced by serum infusion was found to be over a significantly larger area than that produced by mock CSF. Infusing protein-free and iso-osmolar mock CSF, in amounts as small as 0.03 ml, induced delayed BBB opening. These results indicate that chemical compounds contained in the infusate influenced the BBB opening and that a mechanical distension of the extracellular space could break the BBB.

We conclude that the infusion edema model can be used for investigations on the water content without significant error and that a delayed opening of the BBB should be considered in this model.

References

1. Hirano A, Marmarou A, Nakamura T, Inoue A (1985) The fine structural study of brain response to intracerebral infusion of serum in the cat. In: Inaba Y, Klatzo I, Spatz M (eds) Brain edema. Springer, Berlin Heidelberg New York Tokyo, pp 32–39
2. Marmarou A, Tanaka K, Shulman K (1982) The brain response to infusion edema: Dynamics of fluid resolution. In: Hartmann A, Brock M (eds) Treatment of cerebral edema. Springer, Berlin Heidelberg New York, pp 11–18
3. Marmarou A, Tanaka K, Shulman K (1982) An improved gravimetric measure of cerebral edema. J Neurosurg 56:246–253
4. Ohata K, Marmarou A, Povlishock JT (1990) An immunocytochemical study of protein clearance in brain infusion edema. Acta Neuropathol 81:162–177

Effect of Osmotic Opening of Blood-Brain Barrier on the Learning of Rats

T. NAGASHIMA[1], M. YAMAGUCHI[2], I. KINOSHITA[2], H. SUZUKI[1], S. CHAKARABORTTY[1], and N. TAMAKI[1]

[1] Department of Neurosurgery, Kobe University School of Medicine, and
[2] School of Allied Medical Sciences, Kobe University, Japan

Introduction

Osmotic opening of the blood brain barrier (BBB) has been used in the chemotherapy of brain tumors [2]. However, the potential risk of the procedure is still controversial [4, 5]. The purpose of the present study is to determine the effect of osmotic opening of BBB on learning of rats.

Materials and Methods

Osmotic Opening of Blood-Brain Barrier

Adult Wister rats of both sexes, each weighing 250–300 gm, were anesthetized with Pentobarbital sodium (50 mg/kg, i.p.). A catheter (PE-50 polyethylene tube) filled with heparinized saline was introduced into the right external carotid artery for retrograde infusion. A 1.4-M Mannitol solution, which was prefilterd with a 0.45 μm filter, was infused at a constant rate of 0.083 ml/sec for 30 seconds in 10 rats. As a control, the same infusion with normal saline was performed in 5 rats. The perfusate was kept at 37°C during the whole procedure in order not to produce microcrystals. Carotid artery pressure was continuously monitored.

In 5 rats, 2 ml of 1% Evans blue (EB) solution was injected intravenously just after the Mannitol infusion to confirm the opening of BBB. One hour after the injection of the EB solution, the brain was removed and the hemispheres were separately homogenized in 50% trichloracetic acid. The EB content was measured by a fluorescence spectometer [6]. EB content of the plasma was similarly measured as well as the ratio of tissue to plasma Evans blue.

Active Avoidance Learning

Twenty-four hours after the infusion, the animals were tested on the avoidance learning. A box (12 × 58 × 24 cm) was divided into two compartments: an open room without top roof and a dark room with a floor of aluminium grid which was programmed to load a scrambled alternative current of 200 volt exactly 5 seconds after the initiation of the learning procedure. A swinging door between the two compartments was programmed to be unlocked at the initiation of lighting of a signal lamp on the dark room wall. When unlocked, the rats should push the door open to run out of the dark room.

The electric shock of 200 volt was given continuously from the aluminium floor exactly 5 seconds after the lighting of the small lamp. After several trials, the rats learned to escape from the electric shock. When a series of 5 escapes without receiving the electric shock was obtained, the avoidance from shock was considered to be learned. The minimal numbers of trials up to the successful learning were counted.

The Mannitol infused rats, the normal saline infused rats, and no insult rats were tested on avoidance learning. Statistical significance was evaluated by unpaired t-test.

Results

Immediately after the infusion of Mannitol, transient hypotension and respiratory suppression were observed in all animals (Fig. 1). Some showed prolonged hypotension. Infusion of normal saline did not affect blood pressure and respiration. The rats recovered from the Mannitol infusion and showed no gross neurological abnormality.

Infusion of 1.4-M Mannitol increased EB content of the Mannitol infused brains 10 times higher than that of the control brains, which confirms the successful opening of BBB.

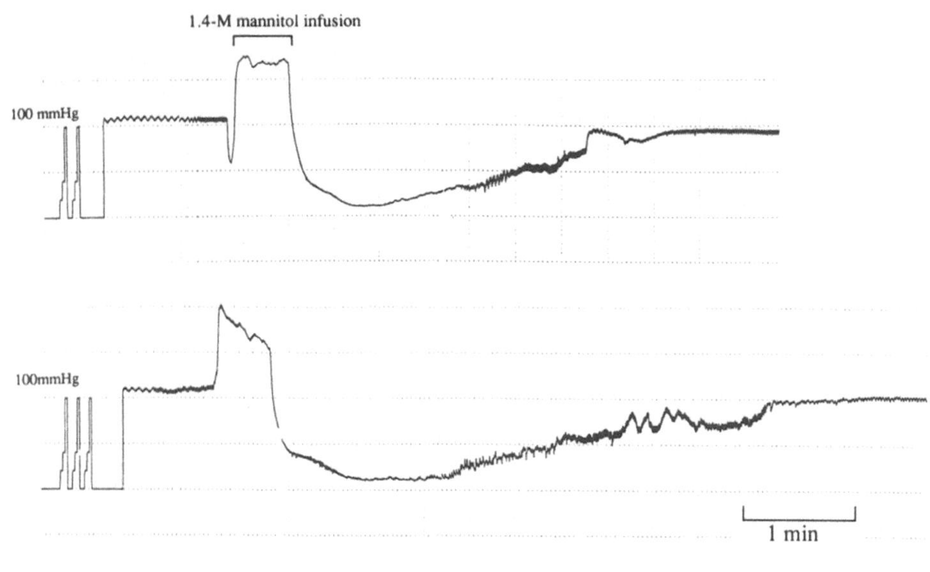

Fig. 1. Arterial pressure recording during and after Mannitol perfusion. The recording shows transient profound hypotension

Table 1. Minimal trial numbers for active avoidance learning

Group	Minimal trial number
No insult	9.14 ± 1.30 (14)
Saline infusion	4.80 ± 1.48 (5)
Mannitol infusion	6.50 ± 2.12 (10)

Values: number of trials, as mean ± S.E.M.
( ): number of animals

The active avoidance learning test showed no statistical difference between the mean trial numbers of the three groups (Table 1).

Discussion

Rapoport reported that gross neurological and behavioral abnormality and histological evidence of brain damage were not produced by osmotic opening of BBB [3]. Clinical application of this method to chemotherapy of malignant brain tumor revealed an increased incidence of seizures in 15–20% and transient exacerbation of preexisting neurological deficits [2]. Suzuki and his colleagues reported ischemic neuronal death of delayed onset in the CA-1 region of the hippocampus, in the cerebellum, and in the thalamus [5].

Although the potential risk was pointed out [5], the carefully conducted osmotic opening of blood-brain barrier with 1.4-M Mannitol did not disturb the active avoidance learning of Wister rats.

Post-infusion hypotension did not cause neurological deficit or learning disability. However, the prolonged hypotension may cause ischemic neuronal death of late onset in the CA-1 of the hippocampus and cerebellum which are selectively vulnerable to ischemia [1].

References

1. Kirino T (1982) Delayed neuronal death in the gerbil hippocampus following ischemia. Brain Res 239:57–69
2. Neuwelt EA, Frenkel EP, Diehl JT (1980) Reversible osmotic blood-brain barrier disruption in humans: Implications for the chemopthrapy of malignant brain tumors. Neurosurgery 7:44–52
3. Rapoport SI, Fredericks WR, Ohno K, Pittigrew KD (1980) Quantitative aspect of reversible osmotic opening of the blood-brain barrier. Am J Physiol 238:R421–431
4. Rapoport SI: Microinfarction (1991) Osmotic BBB opening or microcrystals in perfusate? Letter to the editor, J Neurosurg 74:685
5. Suzuki M, Iwasaki Y, Yamamoto T, Konno H, Kudo H (1988) Sequelae of the osmotic blood-brain barrier opening in rats. J Neurosurg 69:421–428
6. Uyama O, Okamura N, Yanase M, Narita M, Kawabata K, Sugita M (1988) Quantitative evaluation of vascular permeability in the gerbil brain after transient ischemia using evans blue fluorescence. J of Cerebral Blood Flow and Metabolism 8:282–284

Ischemia

Improved Recovery With 21-Aminosteroid (U74006F) Pretreatment After Incomplete Cerebral Ischemia

Y. Maruki, R.C. Koehler, J.R. Kirsch, and R.J. Traystman

Department of Anesthesiology and Critical Care Medicine, The Johns Hopkins Medical Institutions, Baltimore, MD 21205, USA

Introduction

Incomplete cerebral ischemia resulting from intracranial hypertension causes intracellular acidosis. One potential mechanism of acidosis-induced injury during ischemia and reperfusion is augmentation of oxygen radical-mediated lipid peroxidation [4].

The 21-aminosteroids are a class of agents that inhibit lipid peroxidation, but have little glucocorticoid activity [1]. The 21-aminosteroid, tirilazad (U74006F), ameliorates delayed hypoperfusion and somatosensory evoked potential deficit after brief global ischemia [2] and ameliorates edema in border zones during focal ischemia [5]. We tested whether pretreatment with tirilazad improves recovery of brain pH, metabolism and evoked potentials after global incomplete ischemia produced by intracranial hypertension.

Methods

Dogs were anesthetized with intravenous fentanyl (50 μg/kg) and low dose pentobarbital (10 mg/kg plus 3 mg/kg/hr). They were mechanically ventilated and catheterized for measurement of cerebral blood flow by the radiolabeled microsphere technique. Cerebral O_2 consumption was calculated using sagittal sinus blood samples. Foreleg stimulation was used to generate somatosensory evoked potentials.

The dog was placed in a 1.9 Tesla magnet to obtain phosphorus magnetic resonance spectra. Relative changes in cerebral ATP, phosphocreatine and inorganic phosphate were measured, and intracellular pH was calculated from the chemical shift of inorganic phosphate. Incomplete cerebral ischemia was produced by infusion of warmed artificial cerebrospinal fluid into the lateral ventricle. Intracranial pressure was regulated to be within 10–15 mmHg of mean arterial pressure for a duration of 30 minutes. This procedure produces stable reductions in blood flow during the ischemia period [3]. A three hour period of reperfusion followed ischemia. Two groups of eight dogs were studied: vehicle group (citrate buffered saline; pH = 3) and tirilazad group (1 mg/kg pretreatment plus 0.18 mg/kg/hr).

Results

During ischemia, cerebral blood flow decreased from 30 ± 3 to 6 ± 1 ml/min/100 g (±SE) in both groups. During reperfusion, hyperemia was equivalent in both groups followed by recovery to baseline levels without significant hypoperfusion. Cerebral O_2 consumption decreased from 3.3 ± 0.3 to 0.6 ± 0.2 ml O_2/min/100 g during ischemia and recovered to baseline during reperfusion in both groups. Likewise, ATP decreased to 20% of baseline levels and rapidly recovered to baseline by 12 minutes of reperfusion. Blood glucose was 72 ± 11 mg/dl in the vehicle group and 96 ± 10 mg/dl in the tirilazad group. Brain temperature was 37°–38°C.

Intracellular pH decreased from 7.09 ± 0.03 to 6.09 ± 0.07 in the vehicle group, and from 7.04 ± 0.03 to 5.98 ± 0.08 in the tirilazad group. During reperfusion, pH recovered to near baseline levels, but the rate of pH recovery was significantly faster with tirilazad (15 ± 3 minutes) than with vehicle (31 ± 5 minutes). Recovery of somatosensory evoked potential amplitude was significantly greater with tirilazad (49 ± 5% of baseline amplitude) than with vehicle (32 ± 6%). Fractional water content of cortical grey matter measured at 3 hours of reperfusion was significantly less with tirilazad (0.819 ± 0.003) than with vehicle (0.831 ± 0.002).

Conclusion

The results indicate that treatment with tirilazad prior to 30 minutes of global incomplete cerebral ischemia results in some improvement in recovery of somatosensory evoked potential amplitude and attenuation of cerebral edema. The ischemic insult was equivalent in terms of the reduction in blood flow, O_2 consumption, ATP and intracellular pH. Moreover, metabolic recovery in terms of ATP and O_2 consumption is rapid and complete in this model. The major metabolic parameter that showed any improvement was the rate of recovery of intracellular pH. Doubling of the pH recovery rate may reflect improved membrane function resulting in more efficient antiporter extrusion of protons, or it may reflect decreased lactic acid production as a result of improved mitochondrial function during the early minutes of reperfusion. The decrease in cerebral edema at 3 hours of reperfusion supports either interpretation. If the drug's mechanism of action is inhibition of lipid peroxidation, then the more rapid brain pH recovery with tirilazad suggests that lipid peroxidation occurs in the early minutes of reperfusion. Moreover, the more rapid pH recovery itself may limit further lipid peroxidation related to acidosis [4].

Acknowledgement. Supported by a grant of the National Institutes of Health (NS 20020).

References

1. Braughler JM, Pregenzer JF, Chase RL, Jacobsen EJ, McCall JM (1987) Novel 21-aminosubstituted steroids as potent inhibitors of iron-dependent lipid peroxidation. J Biol Chem 262:10438–10440
2. Hall ED, Yonkers PA (1988) Attenuation of postischemic cerebral hypoperfusion by the 21-aminosteroid U74006F. Stroke 19:340–344
3. Hurn PD, Koehler RC, Norris SE, Blizzard KK, Traystman RJ (1991) Dependence of cerebral energy phosphate and evoked potential recovery on end-ischemic pH. Am J Physiol 260: H532–H541
4. Rehncrona S, Hauge HN, Siesjö BK (1989) Enhancement of iron-catalyzed free radical formation by acidosis in brain homogenates: difference in effect by lactic acid and CO_2. J Cereb Blood Flow Metab 9:65–70
5. Young W, Wojak JC, DeCrescito V (1988) 21-aminosteroid reduces ion shifts and edema in the rat middle cerebral artery occlusion model of regional ischemia. Stroke 19:1013–1019

Effects of Respiratory Depression on Cytoprotective Effect of the Competitive NMDA Antagonist, D-CPPene

C.K. Park, J. McCulloch, J.K. Kang, and C.R. Choi

Department of Neurosurgery, Catholic University Medical College, Seoul, 138-040, Korea

Introduction

Numerous experimental data suggest that the excitatory amino acid neurotransmitter glutamate is involved in the pathophysiology of ischaemic neuronal injury [8] as well as traumatic brain injury [3], and that the glutamate subtype receptor, N-methyl-D-aspartate (NMDA) antagonists have cytoprotective effect against ischaemic neuronal damage [6]. Since secondary ischaemia is one of the major contributing factors in the pathology of traumatic injury of the brain and patients with head injury can arrive at a hospital at a time before the development of secondary ischaemia, it can be a promising therapeutic area for NMDA antagonists. However, many patients with severe head injury suffer from respiratory problems such as apnea, atelectasis and aspiration in acute stage, while in animal experiment an optimal physiological state has been emphasized. The objective of this study was to examine the effect of systemic acidosis induced by respiratory depression under halothane anesthesia upon the extent of ischaemic brain damage as well as upon the cytoprotective efficacy of the competitive NMDA receptor antagonist, (E)-4-(3-phosphonoprop-2-enyl)-piperazine-2-carboxylic acid(D-CPPene) in the middle cerebral artery occlusion (MCAO) model of rats.

Materials and Methods

Twenty-four adult male Sprague-Dawly rats (300–390 g) were anesthetized with a nitrous oxide mixture containing 1.0 to 1.5% halothane. Self-respiration was maintained during the time required for surgery (around 30 min). Anesthesia was discontinued immediately following MCAO. The right femoral artery and vein were catheterised for monitoring of blood pressure and blood sampling and administration of the drug. The arterial catheter was removed 5 min after MCAO, but the venous catheter was kept with a swivel system throughout the experiment. The animals were maintained normothermic by external heating. All animals underwent left MCAO via a subtemporal approach [6]. The animals were divided into four groups and each group had six rats. Two groups (groups 3 and 4) received D-CPPene (4.5 mg/kg IV) 15 min before MCAO and maintenance doses (3 mg/kg/hr IV) as a treated group. Two other MCAO groups (1 and 2) received only saline as a control group. Respiratory acidosis was induced in group 2 and 4 and in the other two groups (1 and 3) normo- to mild hyper-capnia was maintained. Arterial gases and pH (178 pH/blood gas analyser, Corning, USA) were measured at two points, one before the administration of the drug and the other just following MCAO. The results of pH measured at the second time more clearly differentiated the groups.

Immediately after sacrifice the brain was removed and frozen at −10°C for 10 min. The forebrain was cut into 1 mm-thick coronal slices by a rat brain slicer, which were processed with the tetrazolium chloride (TTC) emulsion technique [1]. The areas of ischaemic damage were measured with a planimeter and integrated to determine the volumes as previously described [5]. All data are expressed as means ± SD. Two-way ANOVA and Student's t test were used to analyse the data.

Results

The respiratory depression groups (2 and 4) showed mild acidosis and hyper- capnia at MCAO (pH: 7.284 ± 0.037; $PaCO_2$: 62.05 ± 7.49), whereas the other two groups (1 and 3) showed only mild hypercapnia (pH: 7.370 ± 0.014; $PaCO_2$: 51.27 ± 2.96). Bolus infusion of the drug decreased transiently the baseline MABP by 3–6%. The decreased MABP recovered within 1 min. The values for the physiological variables except for the respiratory ones were similar in the 4 groups throughout the surgical period.

Changes of Infarct Volume

In the treated groups (3 and 4) D-CPPene reduced the mean ischaemic volume by 60% and 30% in the hemisphere, by 73% and 32% in the cortex, and by 16% and 34% in the caudate nucleus repectively, compared with the MCAO control groups (1 and 2). In the control groups, the group with acidosis showed larger ischaemic damage than the group with normal pH, but the difference was minimal and not statistically significant. Statistical analysis of the volumes of ischaemic damage with two-way ANOVA revealed that the differences between the control and the treated groups were significant not only in the hemisphere ($p < 0.001$) and the cortex ($p < 0.001$), but also in the caudate nucleus ($p < 0.001$). The differences between the two different pH groups were not significant in the hemisphere, the cortex or the caudate nucleus (Fig. 1).

Discussion

The acidosis accompanying cerebral ischaemia has been viewed as deleterious to neurons [9]. However, it was recently reported that moderate acidosis (pH 6.6) abolishes NMDA receptor-activated currents in hippocampal neurons in

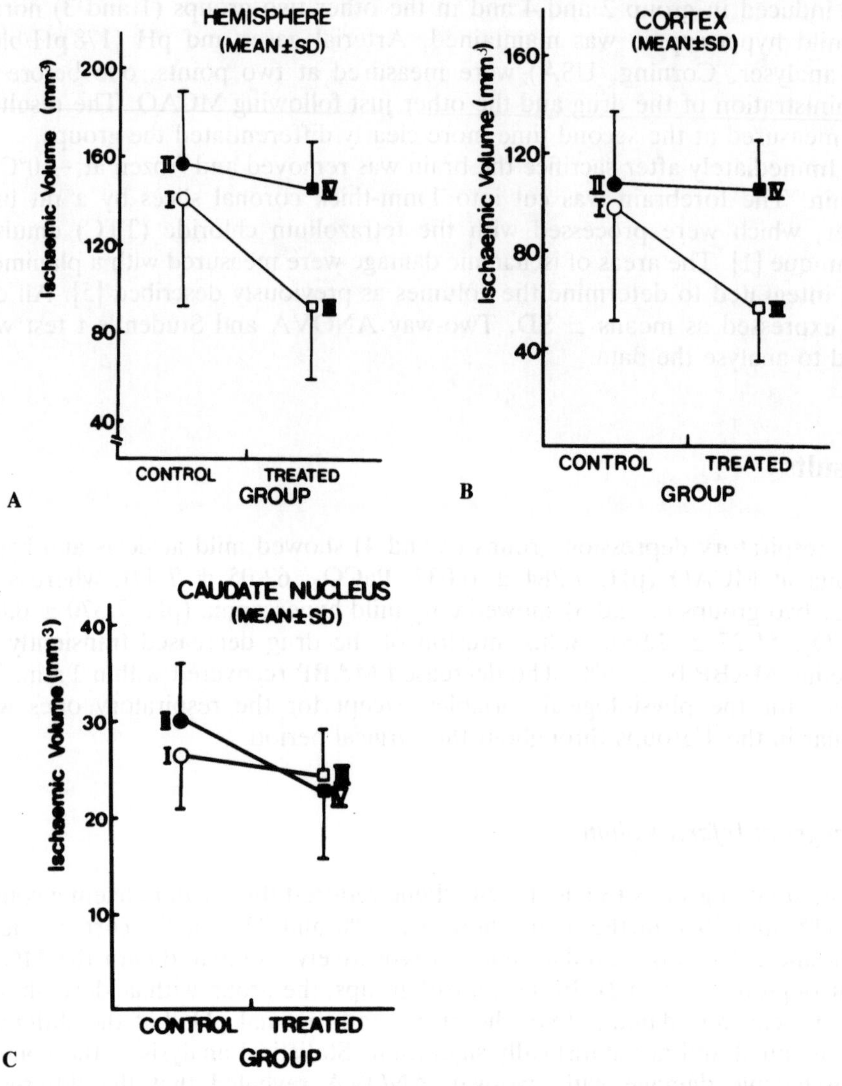

Fig. 1A–C. Changes of ischaemic volume assessed by two-way ANOVA to compare two different factors simulataneously. Factor 1: control (circle) versus treated (square); Factor 2: normal pH (open symbol) versus acidosis (closed symbol). For factor 1 there is a significant difference ($p < 0.001$) between hemisphere (**A**), cortex (**B**) and caudate nucleus (**C**), but for factor 2, the difference between hemisphere, cortex and caudate nucleus is not significant

vitro [4] and can be protective against ischaemic brain injury [2]. Considering these reports from a therapeutic standpoint, there are two points that have to be elucidated. The first one is whether the reduced NMDA receptor activation by acidosis exerts any influence upon the anti-ischaemic effects of NMDA antagonist. The other one is whether the cytoprotective effect of systemic acidosis can be observed in vivo. This study shows that despite induced respiratory acidosis, the competitive NMDA receptor antagonist D-CPPene achieved cytoprotective effects in focal cerebral ischaemia in rats, even though the efficacy of its anti-ischaemic effects was much less in acidosis than in normal pH state. On the contrary, we have shown in the same experimental model [7] as in the present one, that such a short duration (less than 30 min) of respiratory acidosis significantly attenuated the cytoprotective effects of NMDA ion channel blocker. In both experiments there was no significant difference between the MCAO control groups in normal pH and in acidosis, although the control groups in acidosis showed rather large ischaemic damage. Taking these studies in concert, it is clear that the anti-ischaemic effects of NMDA antagonists, particularly NMDA ion channel blockers, come under the negative influence of systemic acidosis, which reduces NMDA receptor activation [2, 4]. It appears that mild systemic acidosis (7.20 < pH < 7.35) of short duration (less than 30 min) does not have any significant effect upon the extent of ischaemic damage in focal cerebral ischaemia in the rat.

Acknowledgements. This research was supported in part by the Catholic Medical Center, Seoul, Korea. The present address of Professor J. McCulloch is Wellcome Surgical Institute, University of Glasgow, Glasgow, United Kingdom.

References

1. Burt JT, Kapp JP, Smith RR (1987) Hyperbaric oxygen and cerebral infarction in the gerbil. Surg Neurol 28:265–268
2. Giffard RG, Monyer H, Christine CW, Choi DW (1990) Acidosis reduces NMDA receptor activation, glutamate neurotoxicity, and oxygen-glucose deprivation neuronal injury in cortical cultures. Brain Res 506:339–342
3. McIntosh TK, Vink R, Soares H, Simon R (1989) N-methyl-D-aspartate (NMDA) receptor antagonists in the treatment of experimental brain injury: P magnetic resonance spectroscopy and behavioral studies. In: Hoff JT, Bez AL (eds) Intracranial pressure VII. Springer, Berlin Heidelberg New York London Paris Tokyo Hong Kong, pp 581–583
4. Morad M, Ditcher M, Tang CM (1988) The NMDA activated current in hippocampal neurons is highly sensitive to [H+]. Soc Neurosci Abstr 14:791
5. Osborne KA, Shigeno T, Ford I, McCulloch J, Teasdale GM, Graham DI (1987) Quantitative assessment of early brain damage in a rat model of focal cerebral ischaemia. J Neurol Neurosurg Psychiatry 50:402–410
6. Park CK, Nehls DG, Graham DI, Teasdale GM, McCulloch J (1988) The glutamate antagonist MK-801 reduces focal ischemic brain damage in the rat. Ann Neurol 24:543–551
7. Park CK, McCulloch J, McBurney RN, Kang JK, Choi CR (1991) Respiratory depression attenuates the anti-ischaemic effects of the NMDA ion channel blocker, CNS 1102. J Cereb Blood Flow Metab 11 (Suppl) (in press)
8. Rothman SM, Olney JW (1987) Excitotoxcity and the NMDA receptor. Trens Neurol Sci 10:299–302
9. Siesjö BK (1981) Cell damage in the brain: A speculative synthesis. J Cereb Blood Flow Metab 1:155–185

Electrical Impedance, ICP and Histology in Rats with Sagittal Sinus Occlusion

A. RÜTHER[1], K. FRERICHS[1], L. SCHÜRER[1], O. KEMPSKI[2], and A. BAETHMANN[1]

[1] Institute for Surgical Research, Ludwig-Maximilians-University, 8000 München 70, Germany
[2] Institute for Neurosurgical Pathophysiology, Johannes Gutenberg-University, 6500 Mainz, Germany

Introduction

The diversity of clinical symptoms developing after thrombosis of the cerebral superior sagittal sinus is not well understood [2, 4]. This is largely related to our ignorance of the underlying pathophysiology. An improvement in the pathophysiological understanding can be expected by experimental studies. Although animal models are available for that purpose they are, however, in short supply. A few years ago, our laboratory in collaboration with the department of neurology at the University of Munich made another attempt to establish a reproducible experimental model for the induction of thrombosis of the superior sagittal sinus in rats. In the present studies this model has been used to evaluate ischemic cell swelling, intracranial pressure and extension of venous infarction within the first 24 hours after induction of thrombosis.

Methods and Materials

Male wistar rats of ca. 300 g body weight were used for the study. Anaesthesia was induced and maintained by intraperitoneal injection of chloralhydrate (36 mg/100 g body weight and 12 mg/100 g body weight per hour). The body temperature was kept constant at 37°C. Catheters were inserted into the right jugular vein and into the tail artery in order to obtain central venous pressure and the mean arterial pressure. After stereotactical immobilization of the animal, the skull was exposed and two windows were prepared rostral and caudal of the bregma. An operating microscope was used. Electrodes were inserted into the left ventricle and the right temporal lobe of the brain in order to obtain the electrical cerebral impedance. The electrode in the left ventricle moreover served as cannula for the measurement of the intracranial pressure. After a control phase of 35 minutes the sinus was ligated 3 mm frontal and 4 mm caudal to the bregma. Then 100 μl thrombotic material (PTT-agent: kaolin-cephalin suspension; Boehringer Mannheim Inc.) was slowly injected into the sinus within 5 minutes. Thirty-five minutes later the induced thrombus was visualized and its extension documented by fluorescence microangiography performed by intravenous injection of Na^+-fluorescein (0.1 ml of 2% solution per 100 g body weight). Then the electrodes and catheters were pulled out, the removed bone flap of the skull repositioned and the skin closed with a running suture. Three hours and 24 hours later the animals were sacrificed and perfused with 2% paraformaldehyde. The whole brain was removed and coronal sections were stained according to Nissl. The venous infarct volume was quantitatively determined [7] in brain tissue blocks cut at three mm frontal and four mm caudal from the bregma. Volume assessment was made by computer based image analysis. Thereby the total volume of infarction was expressed as volume fraction of the whole brain tissue block, which was cut and studied.

The animals with registration of the intracranial pressure were not studied by fluorescence and histological analysis.

As a control, animals with craniectomy and sinus ligature alone were used.

Results

Extension of Thrombosis

In all experimental animals ($n = 54$) fluorescence observation proved the successful induction of thrombosis. Two different spontaneous groups could be distinguished: Either the thrombus was confined to the superior sagittal sinus alone (group 1, $n = 19$, 35.2%) or it involved one or more bridging veins (group 2, $n = 35$, 64.8%). Eleven animals of group 2 (group 2b, 20.4%) died within 24 hours.

Systemic Parameters

The mean arterial pressure of all groups fell to 50% of control immediately after thrombosis induction and reached the normal value again five minutes later. Afterwards the mean arterial pressure remained constant in all groups. There was no change in central venous pressure in all groups.

Electrical Cerebral Impedance

The cerebral impedance of controls and group 1 remained stable and showed no change during the whole examination. The impedance of groups 2 and 2b increased after thrombosis induction up to 20% over control and remained elevated. The difference was highly significant versus group 1 and control ($p < 0.01$) from 5 minutes after thrombosis induction to the end of examination. Groups 2 and 2b did not differ.

Intracranial Pressure

Before thrombosis induction all animals with intracranial pressure cannulas ($n = 7$) had similar pressure values (Table 1), which corresponds to the

Table 1. ICP-course in sinus vein thrombosis of animals with increasing impedance (n = 4) and animals without increasing impedance (n = 3) after thrombosis induction

No changes of impedance		Increasing impedance
Control	1 hr after thrombosis induction	1 hr after thrombosis induction
5.2 mmHg	4.7 mmHg	12.8 mmHg
not significant	not significant	$p < 0.05$

literature [8]. One hour after thrombosis induction four animals had an elevation of intracranial pressure paralleled by a raised impedance. The other three animals had an unchanged impedance and intracranial pressure. The difference between both groups was significant ($p < 0.05$, Table 1).

Volume of Necrosis

Three hours after thrombosis induction in group 2 the necrosis volume was significantly ($p < 0.05$) larger than in group 1, and reached on average 15% of the total volume of the investigated tissue block after 24 hours. The necrosis volume of group 1 remained unchanged ($p < 0.01$ vs. group 2). The subgroup of animals which did not survive the whole observation period, was perfusion fixed earlier, as soon as their impending death became visible. In this group spread of thrombosis appeared to be even more extensive than in the other group which survived 24 hours.

Discussion

The model of sinus vein thrombosis used in this study combines long-term survival of the animals [3, 5] with successful, reproducible thrombosis induction. The thrombogenic material (PTT-agent) employed contains the surface-active agent kaolin and the phospholipid cephalin. Both activate coagulation, resulting in a red fibrinous thrombus [6] similar to thrombosis caused by lesion of blood vessels. Moreover, the venous system of the rat is similar to the cerebrovenous system of man [9, 1]. Taken together, this experimental model is suitable for the investigation of the pathophysiology of sinus vein thrombosis. The present study has demonstrated that ligation of the sagittal sinus and injection of thrombogenic material causes thrombosis of the sinus alone in one-third of the animals while thrombosis of the sinus and ascending cortical veins occurs in two-thirds. In a subgroup with thrombosis spreading into the ascending cortical veins survival was less than 24 hours.

The electrical impedance change was related to the extent of thrombosis formation. A marked increase of impedance was found only when thrombosis involved both the sinus and the ascending cortical veins. Alteration of the electrical tissue impedance is, as Van Harreveld has demonstrated [10], a parameter reflecting corresponding alterations of the size of the extracellular compartment. Hence, ischemic cell swelling from uptake of extracellular fluid causes shrinking of the extracellular compartment and, consequently rise in electrical impedance. Therefore, the increase of electrical impedance in the group with spread of thrombosis into the bridging veins infers marked ischemic cell swelling, while in the group with thrombosis of the sinus only no cell swelling was detected. The findings of the ICP study are in agreement with the above results. Only animals with an increased impedance after thrombosis induction showed an increase in intracranial pressure.

Finally, the histological investigations three hours and 24 hours after thrombosis induction underline a relationship between the extension of thrombosis and the resulting structural damage. Venous infarction was limited to the group of animals with thrombosis of the sinus together with that of the ascending cortical veins.

The current findings lead to the conclusion that ischemic cell swelling, intracranial pressure rise, and ischemic tissue damage are closely related with the spread of sinus thrombosis into the cortical ascending veins. In other words, the pathophysiological consequences of sinus thrombosis relate closely with the extent of the venous flow obstruction. Taken together, the present experimental model appears useful not only to explore pathophysiological mechanisms of sinus vein thrombosis but also novel methods of treatment.

References

1. Bar T, Scheck T (1983) The vascular system of the rat cerebral cortex: basic pattern of leptomeningeal vessels and numerical densities of neocortical arteries and veins. In: Auer LM, Loew F (eds) The cerebral veins. Springer, Wien, pp 65–71
2. Bousser M-G, Chiras J, Bories J, Castaigne P (1985) Cerebral venous thrombosis – A case review of 38 cases. Stroke 16:199–213
3. Deckert M, Frerichs K, Mehraein P, Kempski O, Baethmann A (1990) A new experimental model of sinus vein thrombosis. In: Einhäupl KM, Kempski O, Baethmann A (eds) Cerebral sinus thrombosis: Experimental and clinical aspects, Plenum Press, New York, pp 39–42
4. Einhäupl K (1986) Klinik und Pathophysiologie von blanden Hirnvenen- und Sinusthrombosen. Thesis, Ludwig-Maximilians-University, Munich
5. Frerichs K, Deckert M, Kempski O, Einhäupl KM, Baethmann A (1990) Brain function, pathophysiology and heparin therapy in experimental sinus vein thrombosis. In: Einhäupl KM, Kempski O, Baethmann A (eds) Cerebral sinus thrombosis: Experimental and clinical aspects, Plenum Press, New York, pp 53–58
6. Frerichs K (1990) Die Pathophysiologie zerebraler Sinus- und Hirnvenenthrombosen – Eine experimentelle Untersuchung-. Thesis, Ludwig-Maximilians-University, Munich
7. Uylings H, Van Eden C, Hofman M (1986) Morphometry of size/volume variables and comparison of their bivariate relations in the nervous system under different conditions. J Neurosc Methods 18:19–37
8. Kingman TA, Mendelow AD, Graham DI, Teasdale GM (1988) Experimental intracerebral mass: Description of model, intracranial pressure changes and neuropathology. J Neuropathol Exp Neurol 47:128–137
9. Schumacher M (1984) Microangiographic study of the normal anatomy of the cerebral venous system in rats. Neuroradiology 26:137–140
10. Van Harreveld A, Murphy T, Nobel KW (1963) Specific impedance of rabbit's cortical tissue. Am J Physiol 205:203–207

Experimental Study on Cerebral Venous Circulatory Disturbance

T. Saijo, M. Gotoh, S. Nishino, T. Shirakawa, H. Niimi, T. Murota, H. Kuyama, T. Ohmoto, and A. Nishimoto

Department of Neurological Surgery, Okayama University Medical School 2-5-1 Shikata-cho, Okayama, Japan

Introduction

It is well known that the disturbance of cerebral venous circulation, such as resulting from dural sinus thrombosis or occlusion of large cerebral veins or dural sinus during surgery, often leads to brain swelling which causes neurological deficits. However, the pathophysiology of venous circulatory disturbance is poorly understood because of difficulties in making standardized experimental models. In this study, the authors have developed a new experimental model and studied the pathophysiology of cerebral venous circulatory disturbance using this model.

Experiment I (Studies on the anatomy of the venous system of cats)

Method

Five adult cats were anesthetized by ketamine hydrochrolide, and 300 ml of saline and 40 ml of 5% glutaraldehyde were injected into the carotid arteries to fix the brain. Subsequently, the polymer consisting of 20 g of methacryl resin (Mercox) mixed with 1 g of sclerosing agent was injected bilaterally into the internal and external jugular veins. After polymerization, the brain was dissolved in 20% potassium hydroxide and a mold of the cerebral veins was obtained.

Results

The cerebral venous system was composed of the superficial venous system and deep venous system. The superficial venous system had two draining pathways. One of these draining pathways is from the superior sagittal sinus (SSS) to the internal jugular veins via the transverse sinuses. The other pathway is from the SSS to the external jugular veins via diploic veins (Fig. 1A,B).

Experiment II (Studies on the pathophysiology of cerebral venous circulatory disturbance)

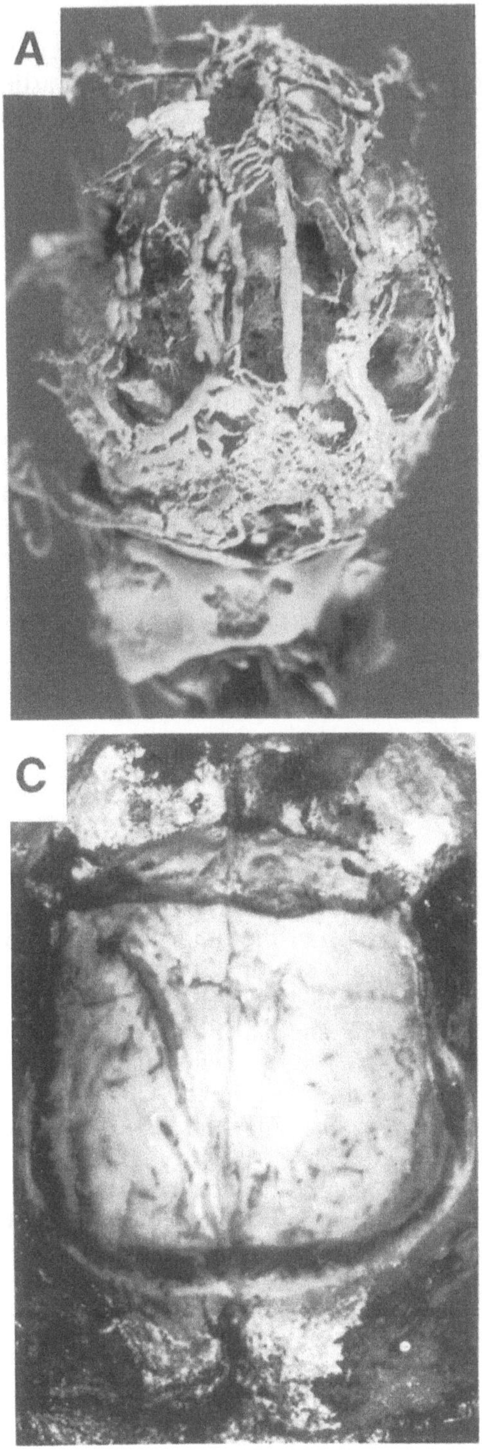

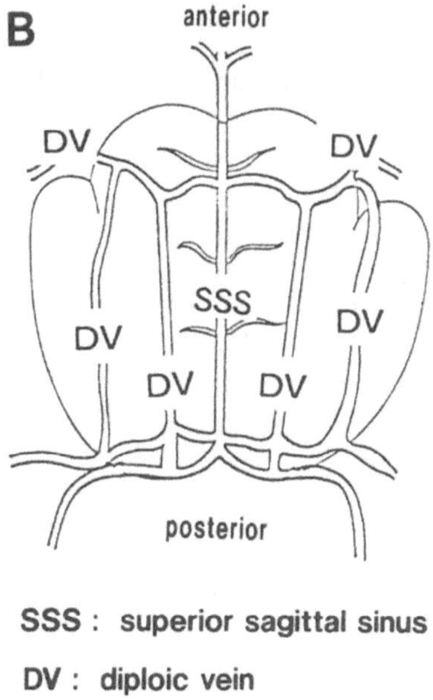

Fig. 1. **A** A mold of cerebral veins. **B** Scheme of cerebral venous system. **C** A groove around the cranium for exposing diploic veins

Method

Thirty adult cats were anesthetized by ketamine hydrochloride and artificially ventilated under relaxation with panchronium bromide. The parieto-temporal bone was exposed bilaterally. Two small burr holes were made in the anterior end of the SSS and near the confluens. The outer table of the skull was drilled away to make a groove in width of 3–5 mm around the cranium to expose diploic veins as shown in Fig. 1C. The SSS was occluded by coagulation through the burr holes, and diploic veins were occluded by packing bone wax into the groove. These cats were divided into three groups on the basis of the occlusion sites as follows: Group I: SSS occlusion, Group II: diploic veins occlusion, Group III: occlusion of both SSS and diploic veins.

Six hours after the occlusion, a vessel mold was obtained in each group by the same method as in Experiment I. ICP and cerebral blood volume (CBV) were continuously monitored. CBV was measured by the photoelectric method using a tissue spectrum analysis instrument (Sumitomo Denki, TS-200). Local cerebral blood flow (l-CBF) was measured by the hydrogen clearance method [1]. Somatosensory evoked potentials (SEP) were also recorded. Cerebral water content was calculated by the specific gravimetric technique [5] 6 hours after the occlusion. Evans blue was injected intravenously 5 hours after the occlusion in Group III to evaluate blood-brain barrier permeability. Histological examinations were also performed after the experiment.

Results

The polymer was injected into cortical veins via diploic veins and the external jugular veins in Group I (Fig. 2A), and via the transverse sinuses and the internal jugular veins in Group II (Fig. 2B). On the other hand, no mold of polymer was seen in the superficial cortical veins in Group III; however, a mold of the deep veins was obtained (Fig. 2C).

There were no significant changes in ICP and l-CBF in Group I and II. In Group III, however, ICP increased and l-CBF decreased significantly 2 hours after the occlusion. ICP increased to 19.9 ± 8.8 mmHg and l-CBF decreased to 19.6 ± 4.7 ml/100g/min 6 hours after the occlusion (Fig. 3A,B). N1 latency of SEP was significantly prolonged 6 hours after the occlusion.

The cerebral water content showed a significant increase in group III but no significant change in Group I and II compared with the control (Fig. 4B).

In Group III, CBV demonstrated an abrupt increase immediately after the occlusion and, with a further increase thereafter, CBV was $24.4 \pm 10.0\%$ at 10 minutes after the occlusion. However, a uniform tendency was not seen afterwards (Fig. 4A). Evans blue was not extravasated in Group III.

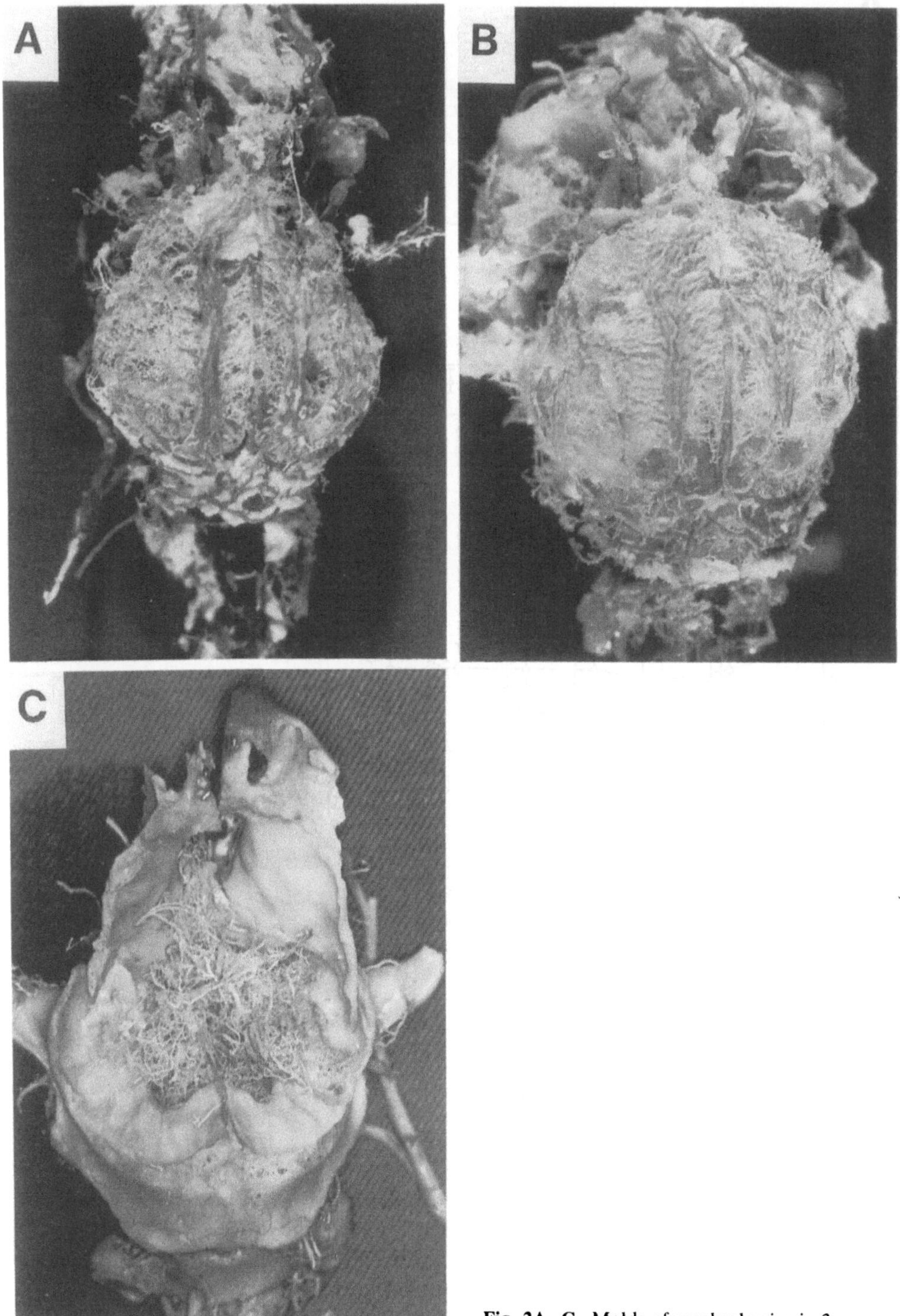

Fig. 2A–C. Molds of cerebral veins in 3 groups
A Group I, **B** Group II, **C** Group III

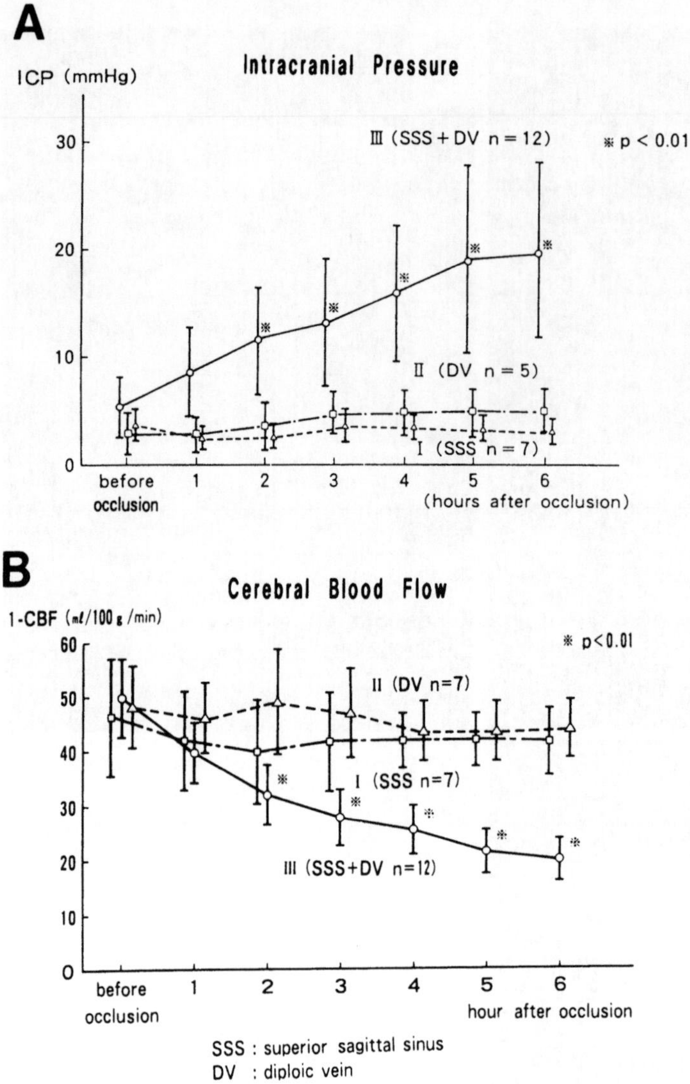

Fig. 3. Changes in ICP (**A**) and l-CBF (**B**) following the venous occlusion in 3 groups

Discussion

Several experimental studies have been performed to clarify the pathophysiology of cerebral venous system disturbance, and different results have been obtained. The reasons for these differences include the different animals used and various methods of venous occlusion as well as individual variations of cerebral venous system. Fujita et al. [3] reported an experimental model of venous occlusion by embolization in dogs. He emphasized that cortical veins play an important role as a collateral channel in sinus occlusion, because

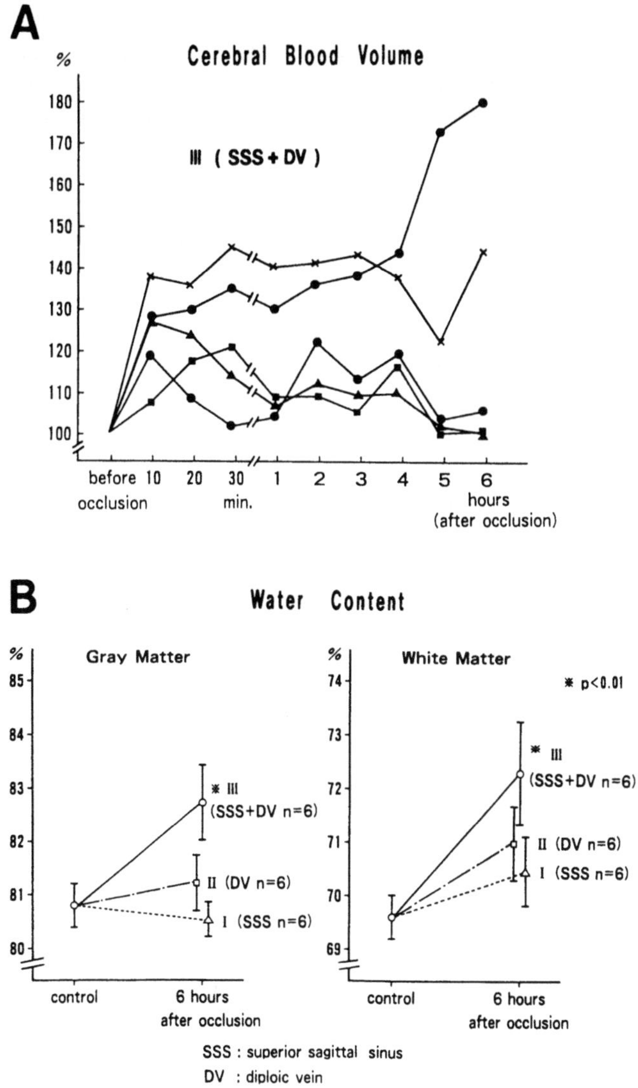

Fig. 4. Changes in CBV (**A**) and water content (**B**) following the venous occlusion in 3 groups

marked venous congestion is caused by cortical vein occlusion and not by sinus occlusion. On the other hand, Kyoi et al. [4] observed massive brain swelling with subarachnoid hemorrhage and intracerebral hemorrhage only by clipping the SSS in cats.

Our preliminary study demonstrated that the SSS drained into the external jugular vein via diploic veins and to the internal jugular veins via the transverse sinuses. The internal jugular system could be occluded by coagulation of the SSS at its anterior end and near the confluens. However, the SSS coagulated at both ends of the sinus still has interconnecting collaterals with diploic veins which drain into the external jugular veins. Therefore, only SSS occlusion appeared to be inadequate in producing venous circulatory disturbance. The external jugular system could be occluded by packing bone wax into the groove, which was made around the extensively exposed skull. This method facilitates the obstruction of the widely distributed diploic veins in the skull and the production of an adequate congestion of cerebral venous channels without the danger of brain damage.

The CBF after venous occlusion decreased due to an elevation of venous pressure rather than to an increase in ICP, because ICP did not increase enough to decrease CBF. Although the venous pressure was not measured in this study, it was reported in a previous study in dogs [8] that CBF decreased significantly when cerebral perfusion pressure decreased to values below 60 mmHg with an elevation in jugular venous pressure. Six hours after the occlusion, l-CBF value was below 20 ml/100 g/min and N1 latency was significantly prolonged. This neural suppression has to be attributed to the reduction of l-CBF, because the flow threshold for synaptic transmission failure is below 20 ml/100 g/min [2].

This experiment demonstrated no extravasation of Evans blue, and electromicroscopic observation showed the preservation of tight junctions [6]. We confirmed that external decompression for the brain swelling in this model increased the transmural pressure gradient through cerebral capillaries and enhanced cerebral edema [6]. From these results the brain edema in this model seems to be hydrostatic edema. Cytotoxic edema may also be responsible for the cerebral edema in this model, as l-CBF was reduced to the flow threshold for the development of cytotoxic edema [7].

Summary

We developed a new experimental model of cerebral venous circulatory disturbance. This model will be useful in the study of dural sinus occlusion. It was confirmed that the increase of CBV and cerebral water content after the venous occlusion led to an intracranial hypertension and to a decrease in CBF, thus resulting in a neural dysfunction. The cerebral edema in this model seemed to be mainly hydrostatic edema but cytotoxic edema may also play a role.

References

1. Aukland K, Bower BF, Berlinger RN (1964) Measurement of local blood flow with hydrogen gas. Circ Res 14:164–187
2. Branston NM, Symon L, Crockard HA, Pasztor E (1974) Relationship between the cortical evoked potential and local cortical blood flow following acute middle cerebral artery occlusion in the baboon. Exp Neurol 45:195–208
3. Fujita K, Kajima N, Tamaki N, Matsumoto S (1986) Changes in regional cerebral blood flow in intracranial venous hypertension. Neurol Med Chir (Tokyo) 26:111–115

4. Kyoi K, Tsujimoto S, Sakaki T, Yokoyama K, Morimoto T, Utsumi S (1988) Experimental studies on cerebral hemodynamics in venous circulatory disturbance; Reversibility of cerebral blood circulation and sinus occlusion. J Nara Med Ass 39:414–420
5. Marmarou A, Tanaka K, Shulman K (1982) An improved gravimetric measure of cerebral edema. J Neurosurg 56:246–253
6. Nishino S, Gotoh M, Shirakawa T, Saijo T, Niimi N, Murota T, Kuyama H, Ohmoto T, Nishimoto A. Effect of external decompression on cerebral venous system occlusion. In: Avezaat CJJ, van Eijndhoven JHM, Maas AIR, Tans JThJ (eds) Intracranial pressure VIII. Springer, Berlin, Heidelberg, New York, Tokyo, pp 186–190
7. Symon L, Branston NM, Chikovani O (1979) Ischemic brain edema following middle cerebral artery occlusion in baboons: Relationship between regional cerebral water content and blood flow at 1 to 2 hours. Stroke 10:184–191
8. Wargner EM, Traystman RJ (1983) Effect of cerebral venous and cerebrospinal fluid pressure on cerebral blood flow. Auer LM, Loew F (eds) The Cerebral Veins, Springer, Wien New York, pp 223–230

Measuring the Degree of Ischemic Change by $AVDO_2$ and EEG

A. Yabuki[1], H. Mishina[2], M. Maeda[2], S. Takagi[1], K. Sato[3], and S. Ishii[3]

[1] Department of Neurosurgery, Hiroo Metropolitan City Hospital 2-34-10 Ebisu, Shibuya-ku, Tokyo, Japan
[2] Department of Neurosurgery, Juntendo Izu Nagaoka Hospital, Shizuoka, Japan
[3] Department of Neurosurgery, Juntendo University school of Medicine, 2-1-1 Hongo, Bunkyo-ku, Tokyo, Japan

Introduction

Brain ischemia in the early phase of severe head trauma, will give rise to many adverse secondary changes such as cerebral edema, infarct, and swelling. The present study aims to measure the severity of this early ischemia using $AVDO_2$ and EEG, and to select the most suitable mode of treatment.

Material and Method

Clinical Cases

Twenty-six severely head injured patients were divided into three groups. Group 1 with controllable ICP and good recovery according to the Glasgow Outcome Scale. Group 2 with delayed swelling and uncontrollable ICP but with some brain function for at least 24 hours. Group 3 with acute swelling and brain dead within 24 hours. $AVDO_2$, mean ABP, and mean ICP were continuously measured, starting within 1 hour of surgical decompression either by removal of clot or ventricular drainage. It was continued for 24 hours.

Experiment. Fifty-four cats were anesthetized, paralyzed and ventilated. Brain compression was produced by inflating a right frontal epidural rubber balloon to the point of global ischemia lasting for 60 sec, 5 min, and 15 min. Seven cats with 60 seconds ischemia having no or transient brain swelling were named "0 minutes no swelling group". Out of cats which showed post ischemic fatal brain swelling following a "silent" interval of at least 10 hours, ten were grouped in the "5 minutes ischemia delayed swelling group" and ten in the "15 minutes delayed swelling group". The time course of $AVDO_2$, CBF (by hydrogen clearance method), and EEG fast wave component (isolated by fast fourier transfer) was observed and compared.

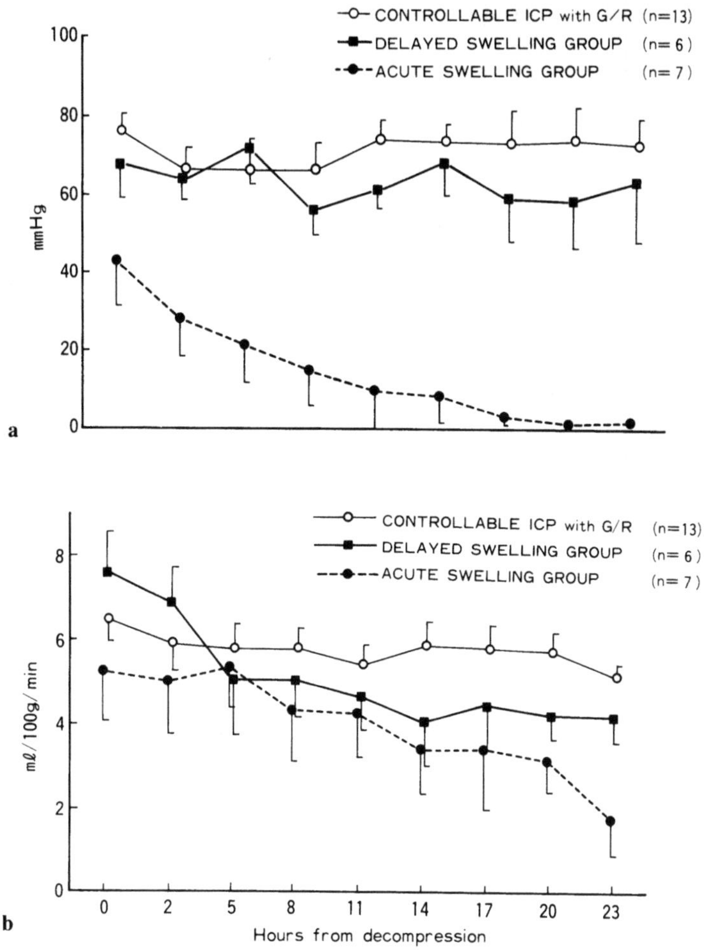

Fig. 1. **a** Time course of CPP. **b** Time course of $AVDO_2$ in three clinical groups

Results

Clinical Cases

As shown in Fig. 1A, there was no difference in CPP between group 1 and 2 for the first 24 hours. On the other hand, group 3 showed remarkably low values just after the surgical decompression that decreased rapidly. $AVDO_2$ (Fig. 1B), was very stable in group 1. In group 3, it started with values slightly smaller than in group 1 and rapidly declined thereafter. $AVDO_2$ of group 2 was greater than of the other two groups, and declined within 24 hours to become lower than in group 1.

Experiment. CBF rapidly increased following decompression (Fig. 2A). The rate of increase was smallest in group 3. There was a marked reduction of CBF following this hyperemia (postischemic delayed hypoperfusion). Recovery of

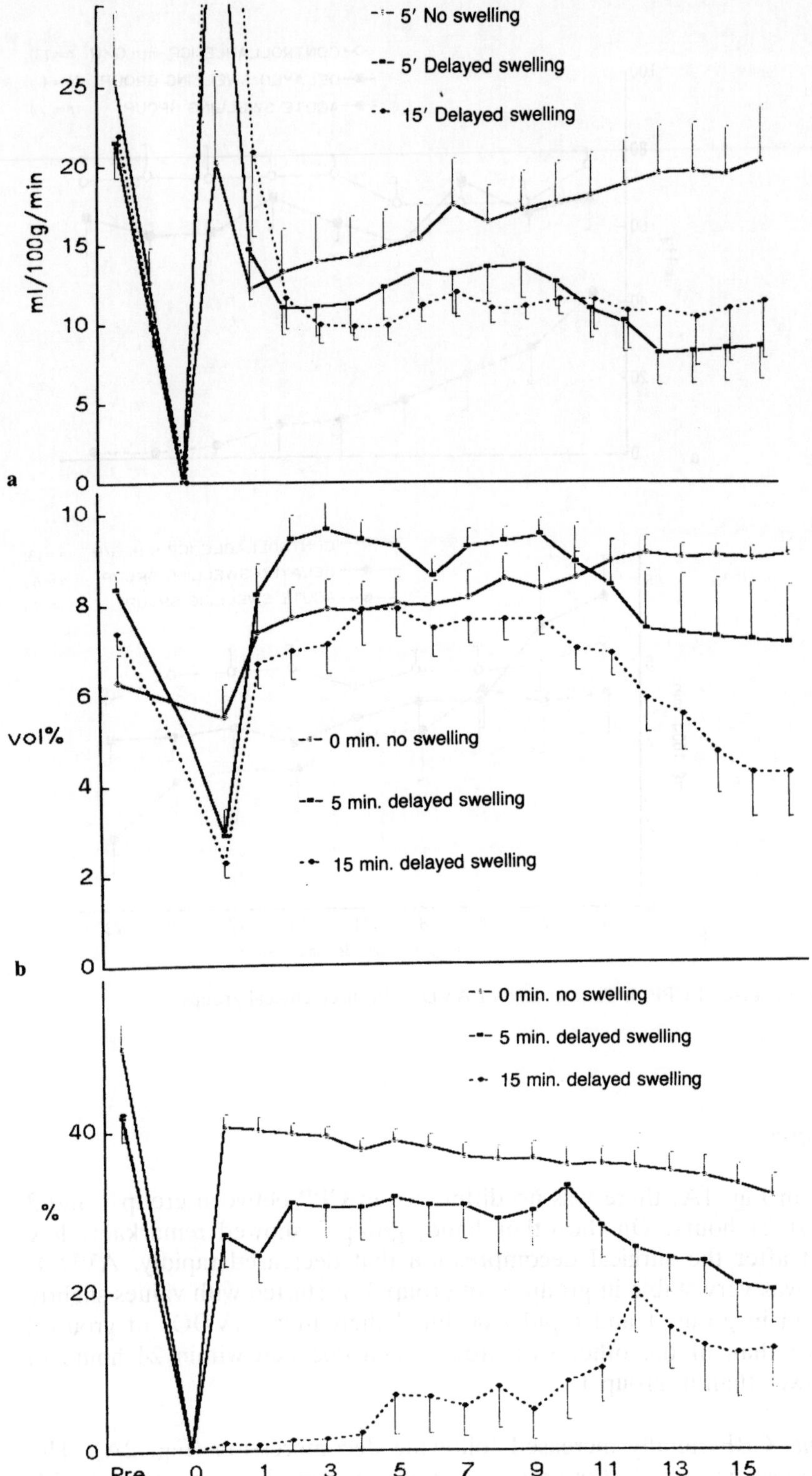
5′ No swelling
5′ Delayed swelling
15′ Delayed swelling
ml/100g/min
25
20
15
10
5
0
a
10
8
6
vol%
4
2
0
0 min. no swelling
5 min. delayed swelling
15 min. delayed swelling
b
0 min. no swelling
5 min. delayed swelling
15 min. delayed swelling
40
%
20
0
Pre
0
1
3
5
7
9
11
13
15
c
Hrs.from deflation

CBF was remarkable in the 0 min no swelling group, as compared to the other two groups. $AVDO_2$ of this group, as shown in figure 2B, only moderately declined during the period of post-decompression hyperemia and was stable after a rapid recovery. In the 15 min delayed swelling group, $AVDO_2$ never exceeded the pre-compression values, and a rapid decline was seen after 9 hours. $AVDO_2$ exceeded the pre-compression level in group 2, and also in the other two groups for several hours. Again, a sharp decline was seen 8 hours after deflation. Recovery of the fast wave component of the EEG, as seen in figure 2C, was paradoxical to the duration of ischemia.

Discussion

Although $AVDO_2$ is the ratio of $CMRO_2$ to CBF, and the time course of its value seems to be a good landmark for tracing the process of ischemia, interpretation of its value requires great caution, because either of two parameters can be responsible for the change in $AVDO_2$. We think that this problem can be overcome by simultanously recording the ratio of the EEG fast wave component and using it as a substitute for $CMRO_2$. From the result of the experimental study, the rapid decline of $AVDO_2$ with extremely poor EEG recovery in the 15 min ischemia delayed swelling group can be interpreted as catastrophic metabolic failure resulting from the most severe form of ischemia, where no kind of treatment will be useful. High $AVDO_2$ with moderate recovery of EEG during the early post-decompression period in group 0 and 5 min ischemia group is probably due to the reduction of CBF mismatching the recovering $CMRO_2$, causing relative ischemia, leading to secondary metabolic failure manifested by decline of both $AVDO_2$ and EEG. This group will require most vigorous efforts to increase CBF, to decrease the oxygen demand, and to avoid secondary ischemic insults such as the formation of oxygen free radicals. The treatment should be by hyperosmolar agents, metabolic depressants like barbiturates, and SOD. This should be started early, even without ICP elevation. Finally, stable values of $AVDO_2$ with rapid recovery of EEG in the 0 min no swelling group is a sign of good metabolic recovery and good CBF recovery, requiring only little supportive therapy by hyperosmolar agents. There was a striking similarity in the behavior of the $AVDO_2$ between clinical and experimental cases, the clinical controllable ICP group being compatible with the experimental 0 min no swelling group, the delayed swelling group with the 5 min ischemia delayed swelling group, and the acute swelling group with the 15 min ischemia delayed swelling group. Therefore, we conclude that our method using $AVDO_2$ and EEG to measure the degree of post traumatic brain ischemia is suitable for the use in patients.

Fig. 2. a Time course of CBF. **b** Time course of $AVDO_2$. **c** Time course of EEG fast wave component

Local Cerebral Blood Flow, Glucose Content and Glucose Utilization in Focal Cerebral Ischemia in Spontaneously Hypertensive Stroke-Prone Rats

H. KITA, K. SHIMA, M. IWATA, and H. CHIGASAKI

Department of Neurosurgery, National Defense Medical College, 3-2 Namiki, Tokorozawa, Saitama 359, Japan

Introduction

Previous studies of local glucose utilization (lCGU) in the acute phase of focal ischemia showed that there is an increase in lCGU in the border zone of the infarct. These findings were obtained in normotensive animals and in models of stroke. We attempted to demonstrate correlations between post-ischemic metabolic changes and neuronal damage in the acute stage of focal ischemia in spontaneously hypertensive stroke-prone rats (SHRSP).

Materials and Methods

Thirty-seven male SHRSP were obtained from Shin Nihon Dobutsu Co., Ltd. and, at the age of 12–14 weeks, anesthetized with halothane, intubated and normoventilated. The right middle cerebral artery (MCA) was occluded distal to the striate branches and 0.7–1 mm dorsal to the hinal fissure via a transtemporal approach [1]. Systemic blood pressure, rectal temperature, hematocrit and arterial blood gases were monitored. Four hours following occlusion of the MCA, local cerebral blood flow (lCBF), local cerebral glucose content (lCGC) and lCGU were measured, using quantitative autoradiographic techniques.

LCBF was measured using ^{14}C-iodoantipyrine (IAP). After confirming that the physiological state of each animal was acceptable, 100 μCi/kg of IAP was intravenously infused for 30 sec and arterial blood samples were taken every 5 sec to assess the ^{14}C activity. At 30 sec the rat was decapitated. The brains were rapidly removed and frozen. Twenty μm sections were cut, dried over a hot plate and exposed to Kodak SB-5 film for 7 days together with calibrated ^{14}C-methylmethacrylate standards. Adjacent sections were collected and stained with hematoxylin and eosin for histological identification of individual structures and the infarct area. The density of the autoradiograms was measured using a densitometer. Optical densities were converted to radioactivities by means of a standard curve. LCBF was calculated using the tissue-blood partition coefficient of 0.8 and the equation of Sakurada et al. [4].

LCGC was measured using 3-0-^{14}C-methylglucose (MG). Two hundred μCi/kg of MG was given and was allowed to circulate for 15 min. In these experiments, the final plasma concentrations of MG and glucose were measured [2]. Autoradiographs were prepared in the same manner as for lCBF. LCGC and the lumped constant were calculated from the MG content, as described by Nedergaard et al. [2, 3]. LCGU was measured using ^{14}C-2-deoxyglucose (2-DG). The animals were given an intravenous injection of 100 μCi/kg of 2-DG. Timed blood samples were taken for analysis of ^{14}C activity and glucose concentrations, and the animals were decapitated 45 min after the injection of 2-DG. Autoradiographs were prepared in the same manner as for lCBF, and lCGU was calculated according to Sokoloff et al. [5]. The lumped constant, determined from corresponding MG autoradiograms, was used as described by Nedergaard et al. [3].

Results

Physiological parameters did not differ among the groups studied. Location of the infarct was limited to the ipsilateral cerebral cortex, but some portions of the external capsule and most of the lateral striatum showed mild ischemic changes. The average infarct size was 8.3 ± 0.9 (mean ± SD) %. LCBF, LCGC and lCGU were markedly depressed in the ischemic core. A significant reduction in the lCBF in most of the cerebral hemisphere was observed in the MCA occluded group compared with the sham control. LCBF showed a widespread and marked decrease in the MCA occluded hemisphere surrouding the ischemic core, thalamus and medial portion of striatum, but the lateral

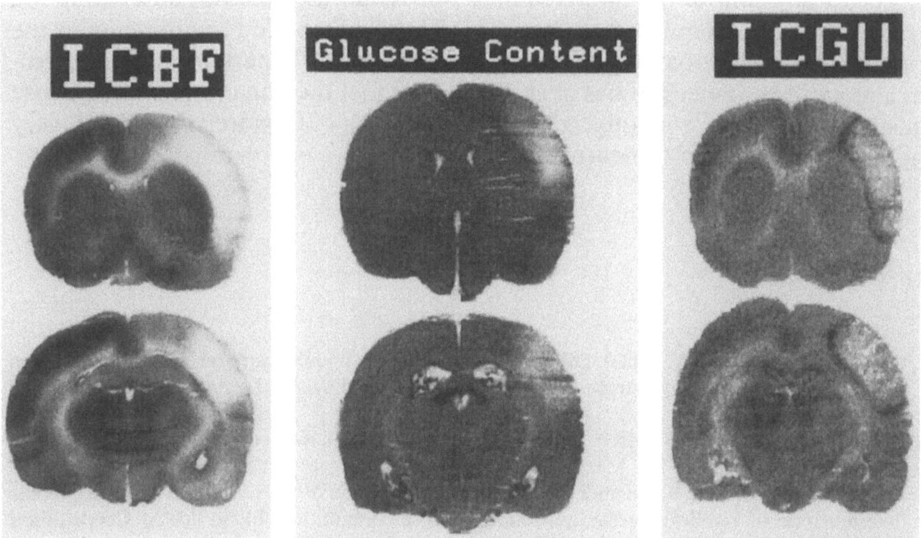

Fig. 1. Brain sections showing changes in local cerebral blood flow (lCBF), local cerebral glucose content and local glucose utilization (lCGU) after occlusion of right middle cerebral artery in the rat

segment of the striatum showed an increase of 136%, compared to the findings on the contralateral side. LCGC showed little regional variation, but increased to 138% in the border zone of ischemia and the lumped constant of this zone was reduced to 86% compared to the contralateral hemisphere. The ischemic rim represented a 155% increase when compared to the contralateral hemisphere. The area of increased glucose content was wider than that for the accumulation of 2-DG. LCGU in the contralateral hemisphere showed no significant difference between sham control and MCA occluded groups. The MCA occluded hemisphere surrounding the ischemic core, thalamus and lateral segment of the striatum showed significant decreases in lCGU.

Discussion

We used the SHRSP rat, a model of focal ischemia in the presence of hypertension. The distal MCA occlusion results in focal ischemia limited to the cortex in SHRSP, but not in normotensive rats. We found a widespread correlation between the decreased 2-DG accumulation and low CBF, perfusion-metabolic coupling, in the ipsilateral hemisphere surrounding the ischemic area and thalamus. A hyperemic border zone was evident in the lateral segment of the striatum, the medial border of the infarcted area. The glucose content increased in the border zone and the lumped constant was reduced. Therefore, the increased 2-DG accumulation represented a pronounced increase in glucose utilization. The zone of increased glucose content was wider than that for 2-DG accumulation. Other investigators found that MG accumulation in the cortex adjacent to the infarcted area was reduced or did not differ from the level in the nonischemic hemisphere [3]. Thus, metabolic requirements in the border areas are probably greater in the presence of hypertension and microcirculatory disturbances. It has been speculated that the enhancement of glucose consumption reflects anaerobic glycolysis as a result of impaired oxygen delivery and is a manifestation of neuronal repair [6].

References

1. Coyle P, Jokelainen PT (1983) Differential outcome to middle cerebral artery occlusion in spontaneously hypertensive stroke-prone rats (SHRSP) and Wister Kyoto (WKY) rats. Stroke 14:605–610
2. Gjedde A, Diemer NH (1983) Autoradiographic determination of regional brain glucose content. J Cereb Blood Flow Metab 3:303–310
3. Nedergaard M, Gjedde A, Diemer NH (1986) Focal ischemia of the ratbrain: Autoradiographic determination of cerebral glucose utilization, glucose content, and blood flow, J Cereb Blood Flow Metab 6:414–424
4. Sakurada O, Kennedy C, Jehle J, Brown JD, Sokoloff L (1978) Measurement of local cerebral blood flow with [14C]iodoantipyrine. Am J Physiol 234:H59–H66
5. Sokoloff L, Reivich M, Kennedy C, Des Rosiers MH, Patlak CS, Pettigrew KD, Sakurada O, Shinohara M (1977) The [14C]deoxyglucose method for measurement of local cerebral glucose

uitilization: Theory, procedure, and normal values in the conscious and anesthetized albino rat. J Neurochem 28:897–916
6. Welsh FA, Greenberg JH, Jones SC, Ginsgerg MD, Reivich M (1980) Correlation between glucose utilization and metabolic levels during focal ischemia in cat brain. Stroke 11:79–84

Effect of External Decompression on Cerebral Venous System Occlusion

S. Nishino, M. Gotoh, T. Shirakawa, T. Saijo, H. Niimi, T. Murota, H. Kuyama, T. Ohmoto, and A. Nishimoto

Department of Neurologiucal Surgery, Okayama University Medical School, 2-5-1 Shikata-cho, Okayama, Japan

Introduction

Decompressive craniectomy (external decompression) is available for patients with uncontrollable intracranial hypertension. However, some authors have reported that external decompression has no beneficial effects due to edema enhancement [1]. We have developed a new experimental model of cerebral venous system occlusion [8]. The venous occlusion in this model led to intracranial hypertension. In this study, we investigated the effect of decompressive craniectomy on the cerebral circulation and cerebral edema in this model.

Materials and Methods

Adult mongrel cats (weight 3–5 kg) were intubated under general anesthesia with ketamine hydrochloride (40 mg/kg, i.m.). The animals were immobilized with pancronium bromide (2 mg/kg, i.v.) and artificially ventilated. After fixation of the head in a stereotactic frame, the scalp was incised in the midline and the bilateral temporal muscles were reflected laterally for exposing the skull. A groove was made around the skull to expose the diploic veins. The diploic veins were occluded by packing bone wax into the groove and the superior sagittal sinus (SSS) was coagulated at the anterior end and near the confluens. The left convexity cranium was removed and the dura was opened for external decompression. Local cerebral blood flow (l-CBF) was measured using the H_2 clearance method before and every one hour after venous occlusion in the bilateral ectosylvian cortex. Cerebral water contents of bilateral cortical gray matter and white matter were measured by specific gravimetric method [6]. Evans blue (EB) was administered intravenously 5 hours after venous occlusion. Six hours after venous occlusion, the animals were sacrificed, and the brains were removed, fixed and examined with light and electron microscope.

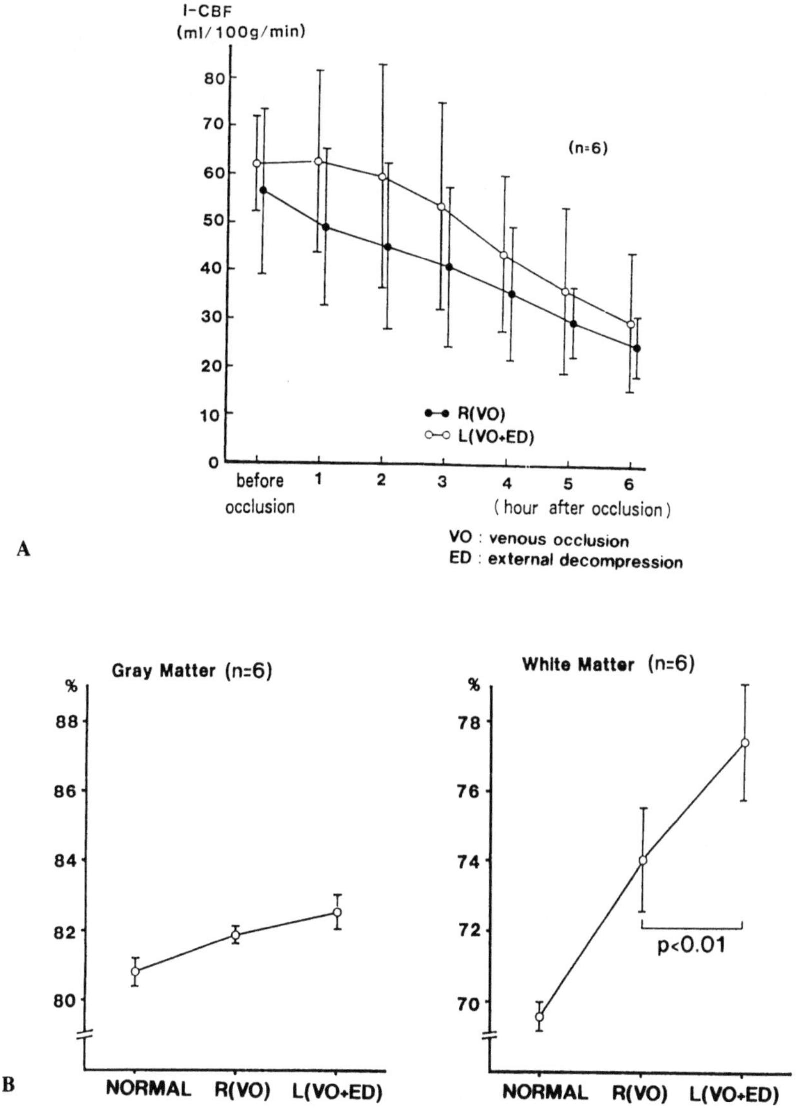

Fig. 1. A Sequential changes of l-CBF before and after venous occlusion. **B** The changes of cerebral water content in bilateral cortical gray matter and subcortical white matter

Results

l-CBF at 2 hours after venous occlusion and external decompression was 45.4 ml/100 g/min on the non-decompressed (right) side and 60.2 ml/100 g/min on the decompressed (left) side. However, l-CBF decreased below 30 ml/100 g/min at the end of the experiment on both sides (Fig. 1A). Cerebral water content increased in the decompressed side at 6 hours after venous occlusion and external decompression, particularly (+3.3%) in the white matter (Fig.

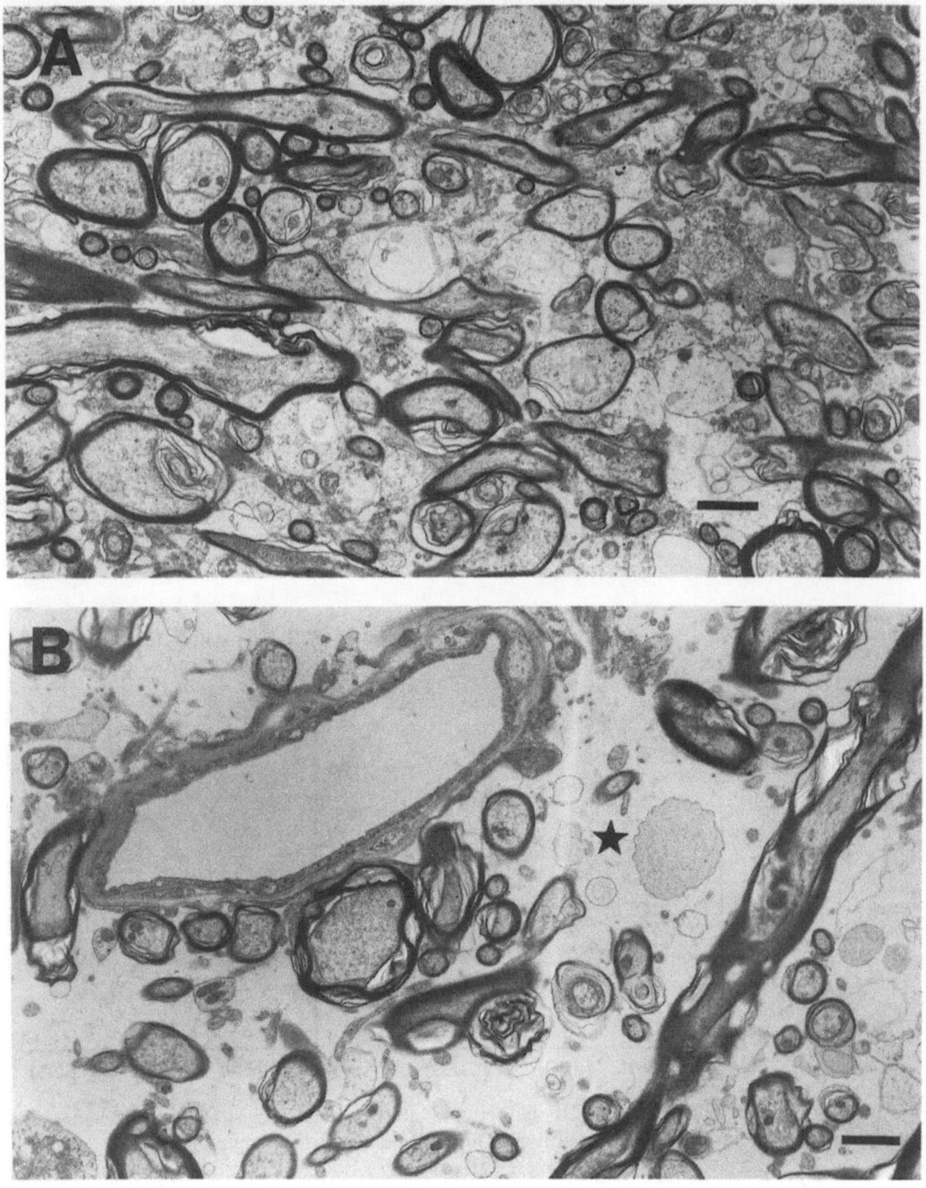

Fig. 2. Electron micrograph **A** Taken from the white matter in normal control. **B** Taken from the white matter in decompressed side 6 hours after venous occlusion, showing enlarged extracellular space (*asterisk*) which separated neuropiles

1B). In half of the animals, EB extravasated in the left hemisphere under the craniectomy, extending into the underlying subcortical white matter [2]. Histological investigation with light microscopy revealed an unclear border between cortical gray matter and white matter, and rarefaction in the decompressed hemisphere. Electron micrograph showed an enlarged extracellular space which separated neuropiles in the white matter on the decompressed side (Fig. 2A,B) [4]. But a blood-brain barrier (BBB) destruction, such as the disruption of the tight junctions, was not demonstrated morphologically 6 hours after venous occlusion.

Discussion

We have developed a new experimental model of venous system occlusion, and reported the change in the cerebral circulation and cerebral water content [8]. In our previous report, cerebral venous occlusion led to intracranial hypertension which was produced by the increase of cerebral blood volume and enhanced by cerebral edema. We suggested that the type of cerebral edema in this model may be classified as hydrostatic.

Sato et al. concluded that the main cause of cerebral edema in sagittal sinus occlusion was BBB dysfunction [9]. Koike et al. reported the effect of combined craniectomy and arterial hypertension, and they demonstrated an important role of hydrostatic pressure gradients between blood vessels and surrounding extracellular space [3, 5, 7].

In this study, we employed external decompression as the method of enhancement of the transmural pressure gradient over the cerebral capillary wall. The results suggest that this increase of transmural pressure gradient by external decompression enhances cerebral edema in experimental cerebral venous system occlusion.

References

1. Cooper PR, Hagler H, Clark WK, Barnett P (1979) Enhancement of experimental cerebral edema after decompressive craniectomy: Implications for the management of severe head injuries. Neurosurgery 4:296–300
2. Fujita K, Kojima N, Tamaki N, Matsumoto S (1984) Brain edema in intracranial venous hypertension. In: Inaba Y, Klatzo I, Spatz M (eds) Brain edema (Proceedings of the sixth international symposium). Springer, Berlin Heidelberg New York Tokyo, pp 228–234
3. Hatashita S, Koike J, Sonokawa T, Ishii S (1985) Cerebral edema associated with craniectomy and arterial hypertension. Stroke 16:661–668
4. Klatzo I (1967) Presidential Address. Neuropathological aspects of brain edema. J Neuropathol Exp Neurol 26:1–14
5. Koike J (1983) Permeability change of cerebral vessels in acute hypertension and external decompression. Neurol Med Chir (Tokyo) 23:325–335
6. Marmarou A, Poll W, Schulman K, Bhargavan H (1978) A simple gravimetric technique for measurement of cerebral edema. J Neurosurg 49:530–537
7. Reulen HJ, Graham BS, Spatz M, Klatzo I (1973) Role of pressure gradients and bulk flow in dynamics of vasogenic brain edema. J Neurosurg 46:24–35

8. Saijo T (in press) Experimental study on cerebral venous circuratory disturbance. Okayama Igakkai Zasshi
9. Sato S, Toya S, Ohtani M, Kawase T (1984) The effect of sagittal sinus occlusion on blood-brain barrier permeability and cerebral blood flow in the dog. In: Inaba Y, Klatzo I, Spatz M (eds) Brain edema (Proceedings of the sixth international symposium). Springer, Berlin Heidelberg New York Tokyo, pp 235–239

Epidural Pressure and Cerebral Perfusion Pressure in Cerebral Infarction with Massive Brain Swelling

T. SHIMA, Y. OKADA, M. NISHIDA, S. OKITA, and A. YOSHIDA

Departments of Neurosurgery and Critical Care Medicine, Chugoku Rousai Hospital, 1-5-1 Hiro-Tagaya, Kure City, 737-01, Japan

Introduction

Massive brain swelling has been noted following extensive cerebral infarction [3]. Experimentally, we have reported a rapid increase in epidural pressure (EDP) after the embolic occlusion of MCA in dogs [4]. However, few reports can be found concerning the ICP changes in clinical cases [6, 7]. The authors measured the changes in EDP and cerebral perfusion pressure (CPP) in serious cerebral infarction. Furthermore, the effects of treatment were investigated.

Clinical Material and Methods

This study included seven patients who manifested a large hemispheric low-density area on computed tomogram (CT) following the sudden onset of hemiparesis (Table 1). In each patient, ICP was measured by epidural transducer (Ladd/Steritek), and systemic arterial blood pressure (SABP) was monitored at the level of the external auditory meatus. CPP was obtained by subtracting the mean EDP from the mean SABP. In addition to conventional therapies for intracranial hypertension (hyper-ventilation, osmotic agents and steroids), external decompression was carried out in six patients, and barbiturate therapy was performed in five. The clinical outcomes were evaluated by the Glasgow outcome scale at three months after the onset.

Results

The changes in the mean EDP and CPP are shown in Fig. 1. The EDP had its peak value at the third to eighth day after the onset. Although EDP showed an abrupt increase before the development of uncal syndrome, no significant correlation could be found between the maximum values of EDP and the outcomes. On the other hand, a good correlation was seen between the mean CPP and the outcomes; namely, a CPP less than 40 mmHg indicated a fatal condition, 40–60 mmHg CPP corresponded to vegetative or a severely disabled state, and CPP persistently over 60 mmHg related closely with an independent daily life.

Table 1. Profiles of patients

Case No.	Age (yrs)	Sex	Admission GCS[a]	Distribution of LDA on CT	Cardiac disorders
1	58	M	14	Rt) MCA distribution	Congestive heart failure
2	58	M	15	Rt) MCA distribution	Atrial septal defect
3	69	M	15	Rt) MCA distribution	Congestive heart failure
4	47	F	15	Rt) MCA ~ PCA distribution	Atrial fibrillation
5	72	F	7	Lt) MCA distribution	Atrial fibrillation
6	43	F	11	Lt) MCA distribution	–
7	51	M	14	Rt) MCA distribution	Old myocardial infarction

[a] GCS, Glasgow coma scale score, LDA: low density area

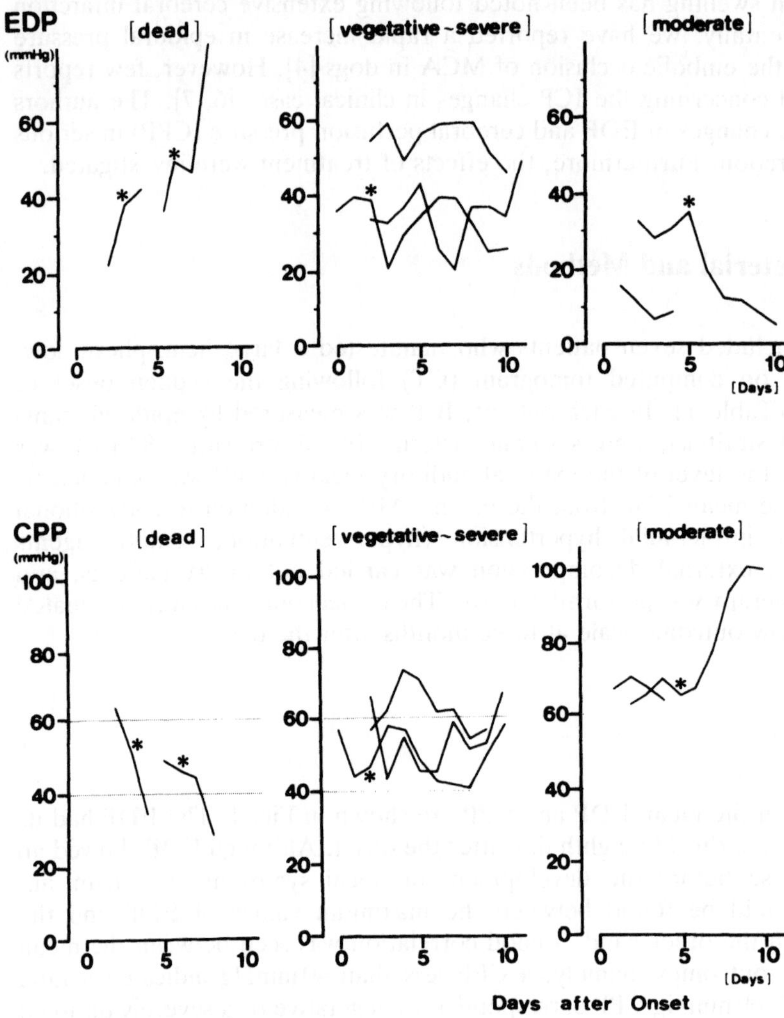

Fig. 1. The changes of epidural pressure (EDP) and cerebral perfusion pressure (CPP) in the seven patients. * the onset of uncal syndrome

Table 2. Effects of Therapies

Case No	Effects of Craniectomy on		Effects of Barbiturates on		Prognosis (GOS)
	EDP	Brain Edema*	EDP	CPP	
1	decreased	increased	decreased	unchanged	moderate
2	–	–	–	–	moderate
3	decreased	increased	decreased	decreased	severe
4	decreased	increased	decreased	decreased	vegetative
5	unchanged	increased	–	–	vegetative
6	decreased	increased	decreased	decreased	dead
7	decreased	increased	unchanged	decreased	dead

* Diagnosed by follow-up CT, GOS: Glasgow outcome scale, moderate: moderate disability, severe: severe disability, vegetative: persistent vegetative state

The effects of external decompression and barbiturate therapy are summarized in Table 2. While external decompression was effective in reducing EDP, it aggravated brain edema producing massive brain bulging at the craniectomy site on follow-up CT. Barbiturate therapy was also effective in reducing EDP in four of the patients, although CPP was reduced at the same time in three patients.

Discussion

Our results suggest that not only the reduction in EDP, but also the maintenance of CPP was of the utmost importance in the management of patients with serious cerebral infarction. Although an optimum CPP for adequate cerebral circulation could not be determined by the present study, a CPP of 60 mmHg was considered to be a critical level.

Patients with cerebral infarction are known to have a high incidence of serious cardiac disorders. Therefore, therapeutic management for brain swelling should be determined by its influence on cardiac function in addition to its effects on ICP and CPP.

In our six patients, external decompression was carried out to prevent fatal brain swelling. Controversy still exists regarding the effects of external decompression, because of its aggravation of brain edema [1, 2, 5]. However, in our opinion, external decompression would be indicated in patients whose ICPs are extremely high and whose cardiac function cannot tolerate a large amount of osmotic agents. External decompression was able to reduce ICP without suppressing cardiac function except for the perioperative period.

In our study, barbiturate therapy was effective in reducing EDP, but a simultaneous decrease in CPP was observed. Therefore, barbiturate therapy must be adopted with great caution in patients with serious cerebral infarction.

In summary, the therapeutic management of patients with serious cerebral infarction should be selected by considering both ICP and CPP as well as cardiac function.

References

1. Delashaw JB, Broaddus WC, Kassell NF et al. (1990) Treatment of right hemispheric cerebral infarction by hemicraniectomy. Stroke 21:874–881
2. Hatashita S, Koike J, Sonokawa T, Ishii S (1985) Cerebral edema associated with craniectomy and arterial hypertension. Stroke 16:661–668
3. Ng LKY, Nimmannitya J (1970) Massive cerebral infarction with severe brain swelling. Stroke 1:158–163
4. Okada Y, Shima T, Yamamoto M et al. (1983) Regional cerebral blood flow, sensory evoked potentials, and intracranial pressure in dogs with MCA occlusion by embolization or trapping. J Neurosurg 58:500–507
5. Rengachary SS, Batnitzky S, Morantz RA et al. (1981) Hemicraniectomy for acute massive cerebral infarction. Neurosurgery 8:321–328
6. Ropper AH, Shafran B (1984) Brain edema after stroke. Clinical syndrome and intracranial pressure. Arch Neurol 41:26–29
7. Young PH, Smith KR, Dunn RC (1982) Surgical decompression after cerebral hemispheric stroke. South Med J 75:473–474

Effects of Prostacyclin Analog (OP-2507) on Experimental Focal Cerebral Ischemia

H. Kobayashi, M. Hayashi, H. Ide, Y. Handa, M. Kabuto, and H. Aradachi

Department of Neurosurgery, Fukui Medical School, Matsuoka, Fukui, Japan

Introduction

Prostacyclin produced in endothelial cells has vasodilating and antiplatelet activities. The effects of prostacyclin have been reported in experimental ischemic studies and in patients with ischemic stroke [3, 5]. Prostacyclin is too unstable to serve as a drug. The purpose of this study was to evaluate the effects of a stable prostacyclin analog, OP-2507 (15-cis-(4-n-propylcyclohexyl)-16,17,18,19,20-pentanor-9-deoxy-6,9alpha-nitrilo-prostaglandin F1 methylester), on acute focal cerebral ischemia in cats.

Materials and Methods

The experiments were carried out using 21 adult cats of either sex weighing between 3.5 to 5.0 kg. The animals were anesthetized with alpha-chloralose (50 mg/kg, i.v.), intubated and connected to a respirator. Ventilation was adjusted to maintain normocapnia. Arterial blood pressure and arterial blood gases were monitored. Normal body temperature was maintained using a heating blanket and Ringer's lactate was infused intravenously at a rate of 0.25 ml/min to counteract fluid losses. The animal was placed in a stereotaxic frame and the left middle cerebral artery (MCA) was exposed by a transorbital approach [4]. The area was then covered with gelfoam until the remainder of the surgical preparation had been completed.

Laser-Doppler flowmetry was used to measure changes in cerebral blood flow, blood velocity and blood volume in the cortical area [1]. We used a commercially available Laser-Doppler flowmeter monitor (BPM 403A, TSI Inc., St. Paul, MN) equipped with a small caliber probe (P-433, TSI Inc.). A burrhole of 3 mm in diameter was made over the anterior ectosylvian gyrus on the left side. The probe head that we used is 0.84 mm in diameter and was fixed 1 mm above the surface of the anterior ectosylvian gyrus. Infrared light from a laser diode (wavelength of 780 nm, intensity of 1.6 mW) is delivered to and detected from a tissue area of approximately 1 mm^3 by a flexible fiber optic. The light is scattered by both stationary tissue and moving red cells. Scattering by a moving red blood cell results in a Doppler frequency shift, whereas light scattered by stationary cells remains unshifted. Analysis of the backscattered light yields the frequency of the Doppler shift, which is proportional to the red cell velocity. The fraction of the backscattered light that is Doppler shifted is proportional to the total volume of moving blood cells in the tissue sample. An index of red cell flow is then derived from the multiplication of the mean Doppler shift by the fraction of light that is Doppler shifted.

Animals were divided into three groups. In group 1 (n = 5), intact animals received a bolus injection of OP-2507 (10^4 ng/kg). Group 2 cats (n = 8) received continuous infusion of OP-2507 (50 ng/kg/min) intravenously for 3 hours just after the MCA occlusion. Group 3 cats (n = 8) received continuous infusion of the vehicle as a control. A novel stable prostacyclin analog, OP-2507, was supplied by ONO Pharmaceutical Co. Ltd. (Osaka, Japan).

The % water content of the brain tissue was determined after 3-hour-measurement in group 1, 2 and 3 [2]. In each animal cortical samples were carefully obtained from bilateral anterior ectosylvian gyrus apart from the probe head. Values are reported as mean ± SEM. Statistical significance was assessed by analysis of variance.

Results

The intravenous bolus injection of OP-2507 at 10^4 ng/kg produced 26% decrease in blood pressure. About 10 minutes were required for return of the arterial pressure to baseline levels. The systemic arterial blood pressure remained stable throughout the experiment with no significant difference between the OP-2507 group and the vehicle-treated control group. The regional cerebral blood flow (CBF) was 88 ± 5 ml/100 g/min. CBF fell to about 20% immediately after the middle cerebral artery occlusion. There was no sig-

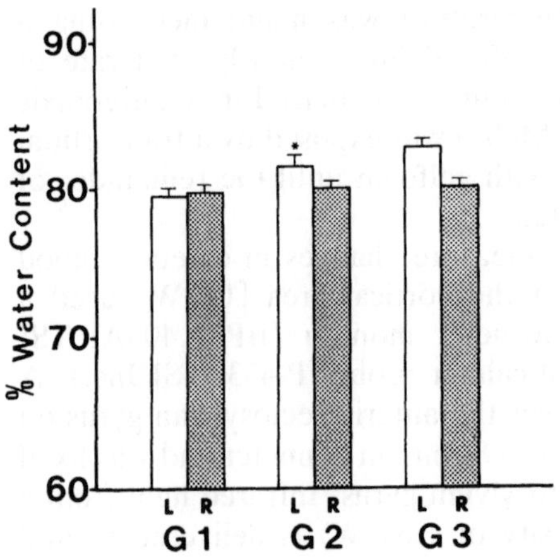

Fig. 1. Effect of a novel prostacyclin analog, OP-2507, on the water content of the cerebral cortex. *G1*, group 1 (n = 5) or intact animals. *G2*, group 2 (n = 8) or OP-2507 treated group, *G3*, group 3 (n = 8) or vehicle control, *L*, left hemisphere, *R*, right hemisphere. *Asterisk* indicates a significant difference from the vehicle control ($p < 0.05$)

nificant difference in CBF between group 2 and 3. Figure 1 shows % water content of the cerebral cortex in 3 groups. There was a significant increase in water content of the cortex of the left hemisphere in group 2 and 3 compared with the contralateral intact hemisphere. The water content in the cortex of the left hemisphere was 81.4 ± 0.4% in group 2 and 82.7 ± 0.4% in group 3. These results indicate that OP-2507 has a preventive effect on cerebral edema induced by middle cerebral artery occlusion ($p < 0.05$).

Conclusions

Effects of a novel prostacyclin analog, OP-2507, are reported on focal cerebral ischemia induced by left middle cerebral ischemia in cats. A continuous intravenous infusion of OP-2507 (50 ng/kg/min) just after the left MCA occlusion did not increase regional CBF on the left side, but showed a preventive effect on postischemic brain edema. Prostacyclin has been reported to produce vasodilatation, improvement of the microcirculation by antiplatelet aggregation and a membrane-stabilization effect. OP-2507, a stable prostacyclin analog, has promising effects on ischemic cerebral disease.

References

1. Dirnagl U, Kaplan B, Jacewicz M, Pulsinelli W (1989) Continuous measurement of cerebral cortical blood flow by Laser-Doppler flowmetry in a rat stroke model. J Cereb Blood Flow Metab 9:589–596
2. Elliott KAC, Jasper H (1949) Measurement of experimentally induced brain swelling and shrinkage. Am J Physiol 157:122–129
3. Gryglewski RJ, Nowak S, Kostka-Trabka E, Kusmiderski J, Dembinska-Kiec A, Bieron K, Basista M, Blaszczyk B (1983) Treatment of ischemic stroke with prostacyclin. Stroke 14: 197–202
4. Kobayashi H, Hayashi M, Kawano, Handa Y, Kabuto M, Ide H (1990) Phosphorus-31 magnetic resonance spectroscopy of cerebral ischemia in cats. Neurosurgery 27:240–246
5. Nikolov R, Nikolova M, Miyares C, Milanova D (1982) Antihypoxic effect of prostacyclin. Meth Find Exp Clin Pharmacol 4:211–219

Intracranial Pressures and Fever in the Rat, Rabbit and Cat*

T.J. MALKINSON, W.L. VEALE, and K.E. COOPER

Faculty of Medicine, University of Calgary, Calgary Alberta, Canada T2N 4N1

Introduction

Fever, characterized by a core body temperature rising above the usual range of normal is often associated with disease. The most frequent cause of fever is infection from bacteria (and their toxins) and viruses. Experimentally, Prostaglandin E_1 (PGE_1) when delivered into specific brain loci and bacterial endotoxin when administered intravenously both elicit fever in the rat, rabbit, and cat. The resulting febrile response gives rise to a characteristic sequence of physiological changes which occur in four phases: prodrome, chill, flush, and defervesence.

Little is known about the effects of fever on cerebral pressure dynamics. Clinical reports describe the occurrence of increased intracranial pressure with some bacterial or viral infections and with meningitis. Our investigations focused first on the validation of our pressure measurement technology and subsequently on the effects of experimentally induced fever upon cranial pressures in four animal models. In this discussion intracranial pressure (ICP) will refer to pressures continuously recorded from the subarachnoid space utilizing the subarachnoid bolt, and lateral cerebral ventricular pressure (LCVP) will refer to pressures continuously recorded from within a lateral cerebral ventricle (LCV) measured by direct cannulation of that ventricle.

Validation of the ICP and LCVP Transduction Systems

Adult male Wistar rats and New Zealand White rabbits were anesthetized to a surgical level with sodium pentobarbitone and positioned in a stereotaxic frame. Following standard surgical techniques either a subarachnoid bolt was

* This work is supported by the Medical Research Council of Canada. All animal experiments were conducted in accordance with the American Physiological Societies "Guiding Principles for Research Involving Animals"

positioned to measure ICP, or a LCV was cannulated to measure LCVP. A catheter connection was made to a high sensitivity pressure transducer and waveforms were continuously recorded.

Bolus volume-pressure and infusion volume-pressure relationships were determined. Pharmacological agents such as osmotic diuretics, adrenergics, vasodilators, peptides, and antihypertensives were administered to groups of rats and rabbits. The ICP and LCVP response to these interventions were all appropriate and dose-dependent [1]. These results proved the ability of our pressure transduction system to meet essential features for cranial pressure monitoring devices [4].

Effect of PGE_1 Fever Upon ICP and LCVP in the Urethane Anesthetized Rat

In these series of experiments we first assessed the ability of the urethane anesthetized (1.5 gm/kg) adult male Wistar rat to develop a fever. We found that when basal body temperature was maintained within the range (36.8–37.4°C), PGE_1 when delivered into a LCV or into the anterior hypothalamic/preoptic area (AH/POA) resulted in a dose-dependent rise in colonic body temperature which was similar in time of onset, magnitude, and duration to that observed in conscious animals [2].

Using this anesthetized animal model for fever we next continuously measured ICP or LCVP in groups of ten animals before and after the administration of PGE_1 at two concentrations into the LCV or AH/POA [2]. Following delivery of PGE_1 a significant ($p < 0.05$) rapid dose-dependent increase in ICP or LCVP and colonic body temperature occurred (Table 1-A). Pulsation pressure amplitude also increased. Shortly prior to the peak of body temperature pressures started to return to normal levels. Physiological systems measured in other groups of animals revealed a dose-dependent increase in heart rate, oxygen consumption, arterial and central venous blood pressure. Shivering, and skin vasoconstriction and vasodilatation occurred at appropriate phases of the fever. $PaCO_2$ fell significantly during the latter stages of the rise in body temperature, no change occurred in PaO_2 and there was a small but insignificant increase in blood pH. Experiments in which the animal was externally heated to simulate a PGE_1 fever resulted in no change in cranial pressures.

These results demonstrate that the urethane anesthetized rat responds with a significant increase in ICP and LCVP during the rising "chill" phase of a PGE_1 induced fever.

Effect of PGE_1 Fever Upon LCVP in the Conscious Rat

In these series of experiments groups of ten Wistar rats were surgically prepared with a telemetric intraperitoneal body temperature transducer and re-

Table 1. Maximum changes in body temperature (°C) and ICP or LCVP (mm saline) with administration of control artificial cerebrospinal fluid (aCSF) or control intravenous saline and doses of various pyrogenic agents. Values represent the mean ± standard error of the mean from groups of ten rats or groups of six rabbits or cats. Significance from control experiments utilized single factor Analysis of Variance

A. Effect of PGE$_1$ fever upon ICP and LCVP in the urethane anesthetized rat						
PGE$_1$ into the LCV						
	Temperature			ICP		
aCSF	0.05	(0.07)		−2.10	(3.60)	
100 ng	0.70	(0.17)	< 0.01	21.90	(2.60)	< 0.001
400 ng	1.68	(0.07)	< 0.001	41.20	(5.10)	< 0.001
	Temperature			LCVP		
aCSF	0.01	(0.14)		3.86	(3.58)	
100 ng	0.77	(0.09)	< 0.001	30.89	(5.87)	< 0.01
400 ng	1.56	(0.12)	< 0.001	51.91	(4.54)	< 0.001
PGE$_1$ into the AH/POA						
	Temperature			ICP		
aCSF	−0.03	(0.09)		3.15	(3.36)	
10 ng	0.76	(0.15)	< 0.01	13.64	(3.75)	< 0.01
40 ng	1.33	(0.18)	< 0.01	37.92	(6.04)	< 0.001
	Temperature			LCVP		
aCSF	−0.09	(0.12)		−4.39	(3.63)	
10 ng	0.91	(0.11)	< 0.001	16.70	(1.62)	< 0.001
40 ng	1.28	(0.13)	< 0.001	42.67	(5.97)	< 0.001
B. Effect of PGE$_1$ fever upon LCVP in the conscious rat						
PGE$_1$ into the LCV						
	Temperature			LCVP		
aCSF	−0.17	(0.15)		2.10	(10.99)	
100 ng	1.10	(0.18)	< 0.001	47.40	(11.16)	< 0.05
800 ng	2.05	(0.11)	< 0.001	91.70	(12.07)	< 0.001
C. Effect of intravenous bacterial endotoxin fever upon ICP and LCVP in the conscious rabbit						
	Temperature			ICP		
Saline	0.25	(0.07)		3.20	(1.78)	
0.025 μg/kg	1.84	(0.11)	< 0.05	14.30	(3.01)	< 0.05
	Temperature			LCVP		
Saline	0.07	(0.08)		−9.31	(8.67)	
0.0075 μg/kg	1.02	(0.12)	< 0.05	19.86	(4.77)	< 0.05
D. Effect of intravenous bacterial endotoxin fever upon LCVP in the conscious cat						
	Temperature			LCVP		
Saline	0.24	(0.09)		−4.33	(11.22)	
0.02 μg/kg	1.56	(0.13)	< 0.05	36.83	(4.11)	< 0.05

entrant tubes were stereotaxically positioned above each LCV. After recovery from surgery LCVP was continuously measured by a catheter lowered through the guide tube until its tip entered the LCV. PGE$_1$ was delivered at two concentrations into the contralateral LCV [3].

We found that as was the case with the urethane anesthetized rat LCVP and intraperitoneal body temperature increased significantly ($p < 0.05$) in a dose-dependent manner during the rising "chill" phase of the fever (Table 1-B) and then returned to normal levels. Experiments in other groups of animals demonstrated that during the "chill" phase of the fever a dose-dependent increase in heart rate, oxygen consumption, arterial and central venous blood pressure occurred. Vigorous shivering resulted in bursts of increased LCVP.

These data from the conscious rat support the hypothesis that an increase in LCVP occurs during the "chill" phase of a PGE_1 induced fever.

Effect of Endotoxin Fever Upon ICP and LCVP in the Conscious Rabbit

In these series of experiments groups of six adult male New Zealand White rabbits each were surgically prepared with either a subarachnoid bolt or a re-entrant tube to allow for the later measurement of ICP or LCVP. After full recovery from surgery the cranial pressure and rectal body temperature were monitored [5]. The pyrogenic agent was intravenous bacterial pyrogen extracted from *Salmonella abortus equi*.

We found that as was the case with the rats a significant increase in ICP or LCVP and colonic body temperature occurred during the rising "chill" phase of the fever (Table 1-C). In complementary experiments heart rate, arterial and central venous blood pressure also increased at this time. A fall in $PaCO_2$, no change in PaO_2, and a slight rise in blood pH occurred. These data from the conscious rabbit using a different pyrogenic agent (endotoxin) support the hypothesis of intracranial hypertension during fever.

Effect of Endotoxin Fever Upon LCVP in the Conscious Cat

In these series of experiments LCVP was measured from one group of six conscious cats [5]. The pyrogenic agent was intravenous endotoxin extracted from *Salmonella abortus equi*. As was the case with the rat and rabbit these animals also responded with increased LCVP during the "chill" phase of the endotoxin fever (Table 1-D).

Conclusion

Our results on the effects of two different pyrogenic agents administered by several different methods to three animal species all resulted in a significant dose-dependent increase in intracranial pressure as measured by means of the subarachnoid bolt and lateral cerebral ventricular pressure as measured by direct cannulation of a lateral cerebral ventricle during the rising "chill" phase of the resultant fever. Pressures started returning to normal levels slightly prior to the peak of the temperature. These changes are likely the result of the physiological changes which we have shown to occur during the fever. In particular the increase in central venous pressure in conjunction with increased arterial pressure, heart rate, and shivering during the rising phase of body temperature are major contributors to the intracranial hypertensive response.

References

1. Malkinson TJ, Cooper KE, Veale WL (1985) Induced changes in intracranial pressure in the anesthetized rat and rabbit. Brain Research Bulletin 15:321–328
2. Malkinson TJ, Cooper KE, Veale WL (1988) Physiological changes during thermoregulation and fever in urethan-anesthetized rats. Am J Physiology 255:R73–R81
3. Malkinson TJ, Cooper KE, Veale WL (1990) Cerebrospinal fluid pressure in conscious rats during Prostaglandin E_1 fever. Am J Physiology 258:R783–R787
4. Malkinson TJ, Veale WL, Cooper KE (1984) Essential features of intracranial pressure monitoring devices. Proceedings International Congress on Medical Instrumentation. Vereniging van Ziekenhuiselektronici 1:18–19
5. Malkinson TJ, Veale WL, Cooper KE (1985) Fever and intracranial pressures. Brain Research Bulletin 15:315–319

Influences of Total Body Hyperthermia by Extracorporeal Circulation on Intracranial Hemodynamics in Dogs

H. Katsumura, K. Hosotani, M. Kabuto, Y. Handa, H. Kobayashi, T. Kubota, and M. Hayashi

Department of Neurosurgery, Fukui Medical School, Matsuoka, Fukui 910-11, Japan

Introduction

There has been great interest in utilization of hyperthermia in patients with malignant neoplasms. Clinical applications of hyperthermia are classified into two categories; localized hyperthermia and total body hyperthermia (TBH). TBH has been utilized in patients with advanced and wide-spread malignancies. Although it has been reported that TBH is well tolerated in patients as long as the body temperature dose not exceed 41.8°C [4], few studies have been carried out to investigate the influences of TBH on the intracranial hemodynamics. In the present study, using an experimental model of TBH in dogs, we studied the effects of hyperthermia on the intracranial pressure (ICP), cerebral blood flow (CBF) and the autoregulation of CBF.

Materials and Methods

Twenty-one dogs were anesthetized with intravenous administration of sodium thiopental (10 mg/kg/hr). The animals were paralyzed with an intravenous injection of pancronium bromide. The animals were intubated and artificially ventilated with room air, and the tidal volume was controlled to maintain $PaCO_2$ between 38 and 39 mmHg. TBH was induced by using an extracorporeal circuit incorporating a heat exchanger [3]. Rectal temperature was raised to 41.5°C and maintained between 41.5 and 42.0°C for two hours (hyperthermic period), and was lowered to normothermia by cooling. The ICP was recorded continuously by using an epidural pressure sensor. Regional CBF in the parietal lobe was measured by a hydrogen clearance technique before hyperthermia, during the hyperthermic period and after cooling. In order to evaluate the cerebral autoregulation, the changes in both ICP and CBF were studied during either drug-induced hypertension and hypotension, before hyperthermia, during the hyperthermic period, and after cooling.

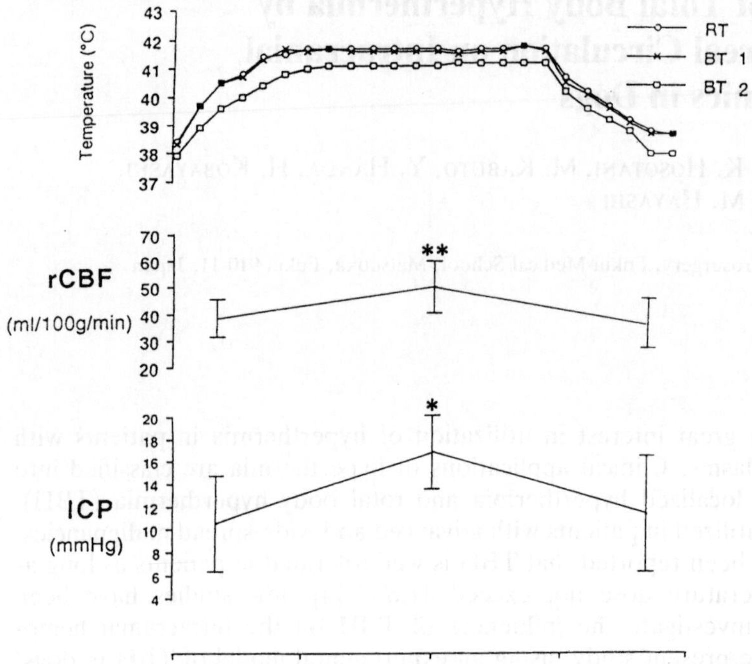

Fig. 1. The changes of temperature, regional cerebral blood flow (rCBF) and intracranial pressure (ICP) during total body hyperthermia. The values are mean ± SD. *$p < 0.05$ compared to the control value. **$p < 0.01$ compared to the control value. RT, rectal temperature; BT 1, brain temperature at the depth of 15 mm under the brain surface. BT 2, brain temperature at the depth of 5 mm under the brain surface

Results

The value of ICP was 10.3 ± 4.2 mmHg (mean ± SD) before hyperthermia, and increased significantly ($p < 0.05$) to 16.8 ± 3.4 mmHg during the hyperthermic period. After cooling, the mean ICP decreased to 10.7 ± 5.2 mmHg. The mean CBF during hyperthermia (49.1 ± 9.8 ml/100 g/min) showed a significant ($p < 0.05$) increase compared to the control value before hyperthermia (38.1 ± 8.2) and the value after cooling (36.8 ± 8.2) (Fig. 1). During the hyperthermic period, the mean ICP and CBF changed in parallel with the increase or decrease in mean arterial blood pressure (ABP), indicating the impairment of cerebral autoregulation. In contrast, the mean ICP and mean CBF was fairly constant, in spite of alterations in mean ABP, before treatment of hyperthermia and after cooling (Fig. 2).

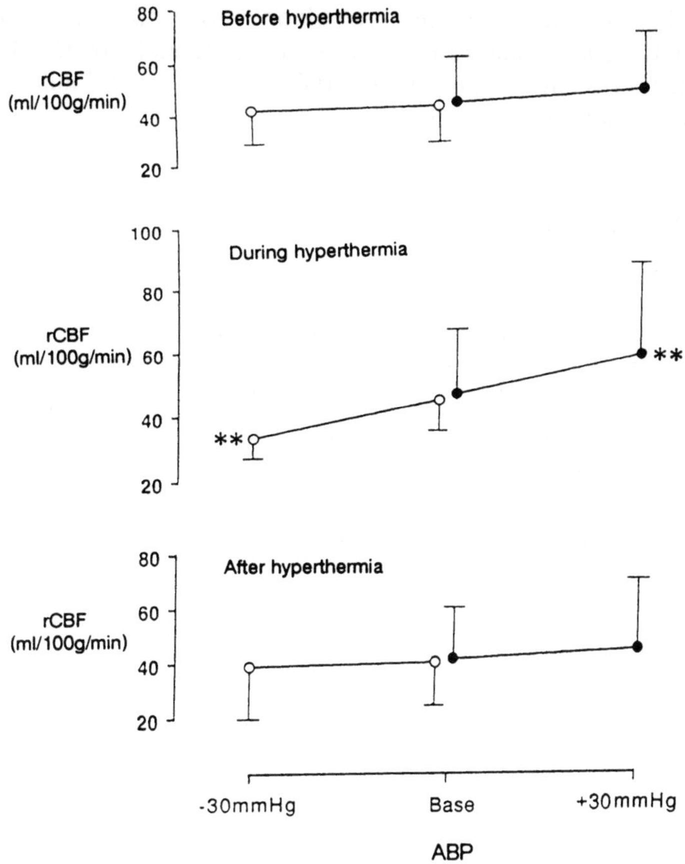

Fig. 2. The effect of induced hypotension and hypertension on the regional cerebral blood flow (rCBF) before hyperthermia, during hyperthermia and after hyperthermia. The values represent mean ± SD. $^{**}p < 0.01$ compared to the baseline value

Discussion

These results indicate that during hyperthermia CBF autoregulation is impaired and ICP is elevated. It has been reported that ICP does not increase during TBH for two hours when rectal temperature is less than 42.5°C [5], whereas the present study demonstrates a slight increase in ICP when hyperthermia is produced in normal dogs. The fact that TBH causes vasodilatation of cerebral blood vessels [2] may explain the elevation in ICP. Furthermore, dilated blood vessels cannot dilate further to maintain CBF when cerebral perfusion pressure is reduced. This may explain why autoregulation is impaired when cerebral perfusion pressure is decreased. It is well recognized that hyperthermia affects the enzymes or membranes of nerve cells [1]. Hence, it is suspected that the impairment of the upper limit of autoregulation with hypertension may be affected by the functional impairment of the sympathetic nervous system, which constricts the cerebral blood vessels following a marked elevation of ABP. The present results indicate the potential risk of TBH for the intracranial hemodynamics implying an impairment of cerebral autoregulation as well as a significant elevation of ICP.

References

1. Carlsson C, Hagerdal M, Siesjö K (1975) The effect of hyperthermia upon oxygen consumption and upon organic phosphates, glycolytic metabolites, citric acid cycle intermediates and associated amino acid in rat cerebral cortex. J Neurochem 26:1001–1006
2. Meyer JS, Handa J (1967) Cerebral blood flow and metabolism. Minnesota Med 50:37–44
3. Parks LC, Minaberry D, Smith DP, Neely WA (1979) Treatment of far-advanced bronchogenic carcinoma by extracorporeally induced systemic hyperthermia. J Thorac Cardiovasc Surg 78:883–892
4. Pettigrew RT, Galt JM, Ludgate CW, Horn DB, Smith AN (1974) Circulatory and biochemical effects of whole body hyperthermia. Br J Surg 61:727–730
5. Rhoon GC, Zee J (1983) Cerebral temperature and epidural pressure during whole body hyperthermia in dogs. Res Exp Med 183:47–54

Control of ICP by The Medullary Reticular Formation

M. Maeda, M. Miyazaki, and S. Ishii

Department of Neurosurgery and Casualty Center, Juntendo University School of Medicine, Izunagaoka Hospital, Shizuoka-ken, 410-22, Japan

Introduction

Spontaneous episodic elevation of intracranial pressure (ICP), named "plateau wave" by Lundberg [4], often occurs in patients with increased ICP caused by brain tumor, hydrocephalus and other conditions. There are two possible causes for the development of plateau waves: persistent intracranial hypertension and cerebral vasomotor reaction [2]. Plateau waves are associated with increased cerebral blood volume (CBV) [9] due to dilatation of the cerebral blood vessels, and apparently result from intact autoregulation responding to changes in cerebral perfusion pressure (CPP) [7, 10]. Previously, we investigated the function of noradrenergic cell groups, especially the dorsal noradrenergic system (locus coeruleus complex, LC), and the cholinoceptive pontine area (CPA) [3] in the generation of plateau waves in ICP-VI [5] and VII [6]. This study investigated the function of the ventral noradrenergic system [1] (medullary reticular formation, MRF) in the control of ICP and neuronal organizations between the CPA and MRF.

Materials and Methods

Twenty chloralose-anesthetized cats with or without Kaolin-induced hydrocephalus were used for the experiments. The animals were immobilized by pancuronium bromide and artificially ventilated. The ICP was continuously monitored by a Camino fiber optic transducer inserted into the white matter of the right occipital lobe. The systemic arterial blood pressure (BP) and end-tidal CO_2 concentration ($ETCO_2$) were measured continuously. The first experiments recorded single unit spikes continuously during ICP variations using tungsten-microelectrodes in the medullary reticular formation [8] (N.R. parvocellularis and gigantocellularis (P10 level in the Atlas of the Cat Brain, Snider and Niemer). The frequency of successive discharges was measured

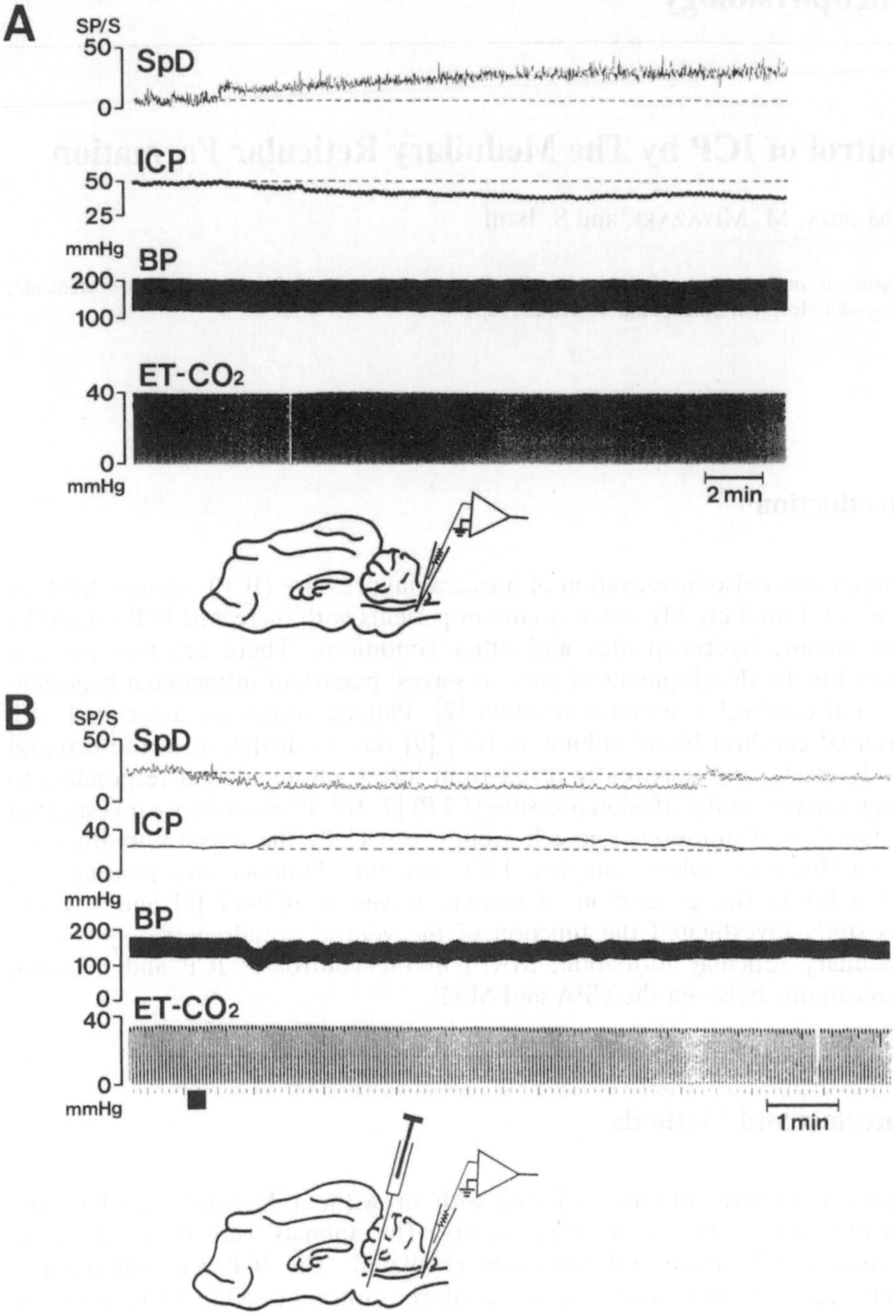

Fig. 1A,B. Discharge patterns of medullary reticular formation (MRF) neurons during ICP changes. Simultaneous recording of unit spike discharge (SpD), intracranial pressure (ICP), systemic blood pressure (BP) and end-tidal CO_2 concentration ($ETCO_2$). The frequency of successive discharges was measured during one second periods. Filled square in **B** indicates Ach microinjection into the cholinoceptive pontine area (CPA)

during 500 msec to 1 sec periods. In the second series of experiments injection needles were inserted for microinjection of glutamate or Ach into the CPA (ventromedial to the LC) and the MRF. In the third series, the medial part of the cerebellum (anterior and posterior vermis) was removed, and single spikes from MRF-neurons were recorded extracellularly using glass-micropipettes containing Ringer solution. The neurons were identified using the reference point at the end of the experiment. The bipolar stimulating electrodes were placed bilaterally in the CPA.

Results

Needle-insertion into the MRF evoked increased ICP resembling plateau waves, associated with slightly increased BP. Glutamate microinjection into the MRF produced a persistent decrease of ICP associated with a marked increase in BP.

Tonic MRF-neuron discharge increased before onset and during ICP decrease. The BP and $ETCO_2$ concentration changed little (Fig. 1A). Ach microinjection into the CPA caused consistent increases in ICP (see also [3]) associated with slightly decreased BP. The MRF-neurons spike activities associated with ICP increase are shown in Fig. 1B. Tonic MRF-neuron discharges were gradually suppressed about 30 seconds before onset of plateau wave like ICP-variations and were sharply suppressed during the plateau phase. Recovery began 10 to 30 seconds before the ICP decrease (Fig. 1B). Spike activity in some MRF-neuron was unchanged during ICP-variations caused by Ach microinjection into the CPA.

Extracellular unit recording showed that electrical CPA stimulation evoked predominantly inhibition in the MRF neurons. Spontaneous MRF-neuron spikes (Fig. 2Ba) were inhibited following ipsilateral (Fig. 2Bb) or contralateral (Fig. 2Bc) CPA stimulation. Early slight excitation followed by inhibition also occurred (Fig. 2C). Figure 2D shows the location and pattern of the MRF neurons studied by CPA stimulation. MRF or LC stimulation caused antidromic neuron behavior, showing that some CPA-neurons have axons in both the MRF and the LC [5] causing neuronal inhibition.

Some MRF-neurons demonstrated no suppression or promotion of spike activities during increased ICP caused by Ach microinjection into the CPA (Fig. 3C). Electrical CPA stimulation did not inhibit spontaneous spikes in these MRF-neurons (Fig. 3Ac). In contrast, spike activities were clearly suppressed before the ICP increase in MRF-neurons (Fig. 3B) inhibited by electrical CPA stimulation (Fig. 3Ab).

Discussion

Cerebral blood vessels have at least two types of adrenergic innervation: from the cervical sympathetic plexus affecting the extracerebral arteries and the cerebral arterioles, and from the medulla oblongata, pons, and midbrain (the

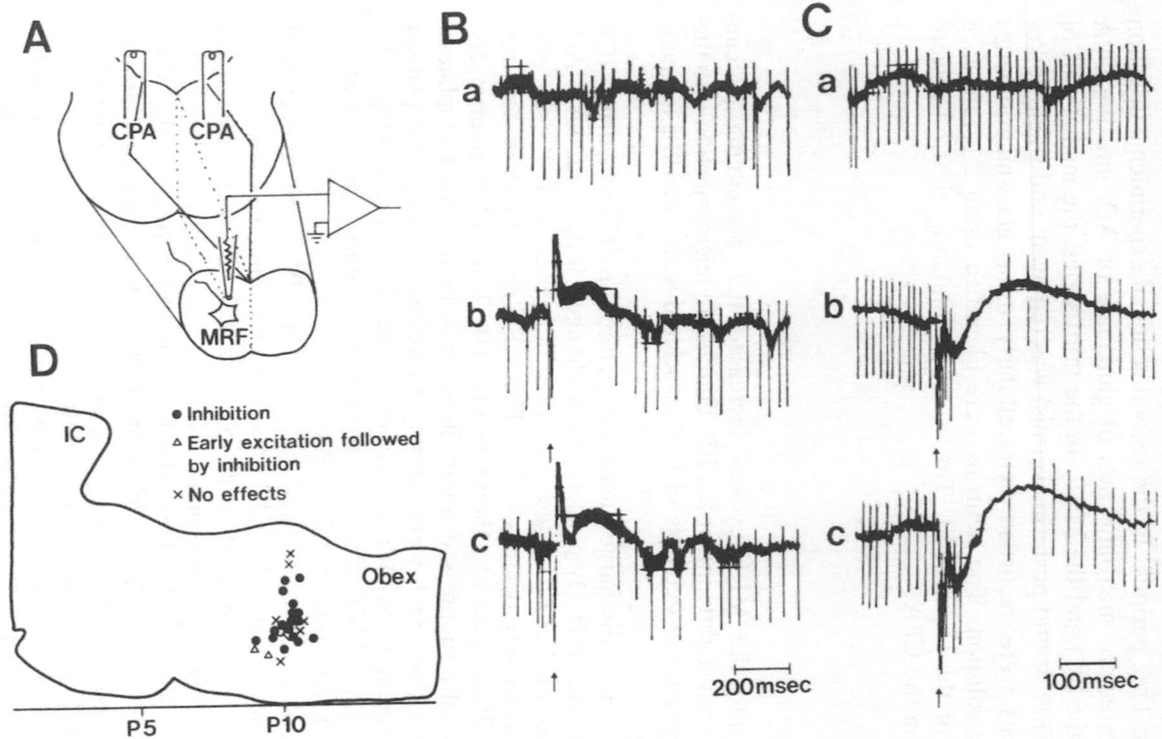

Fig. 2A–D. Effects of CPA stimulation on MRF neuronal activities **A** experimental arrangement, **B** and **C** two individual MRF neurons. Spontaneous discharges (**Ba**) are inhibited by electrical micro-stimulation of ipsilateral (**Bb**) or contralateral (**Bc**) CPA. Early excitation followed by inhibition (**Cb** and **Cc**) are also induced. Downward reflection in each trace represents negativity. **D** location and pattern of MRF-neurons studied by stimulation of CPA

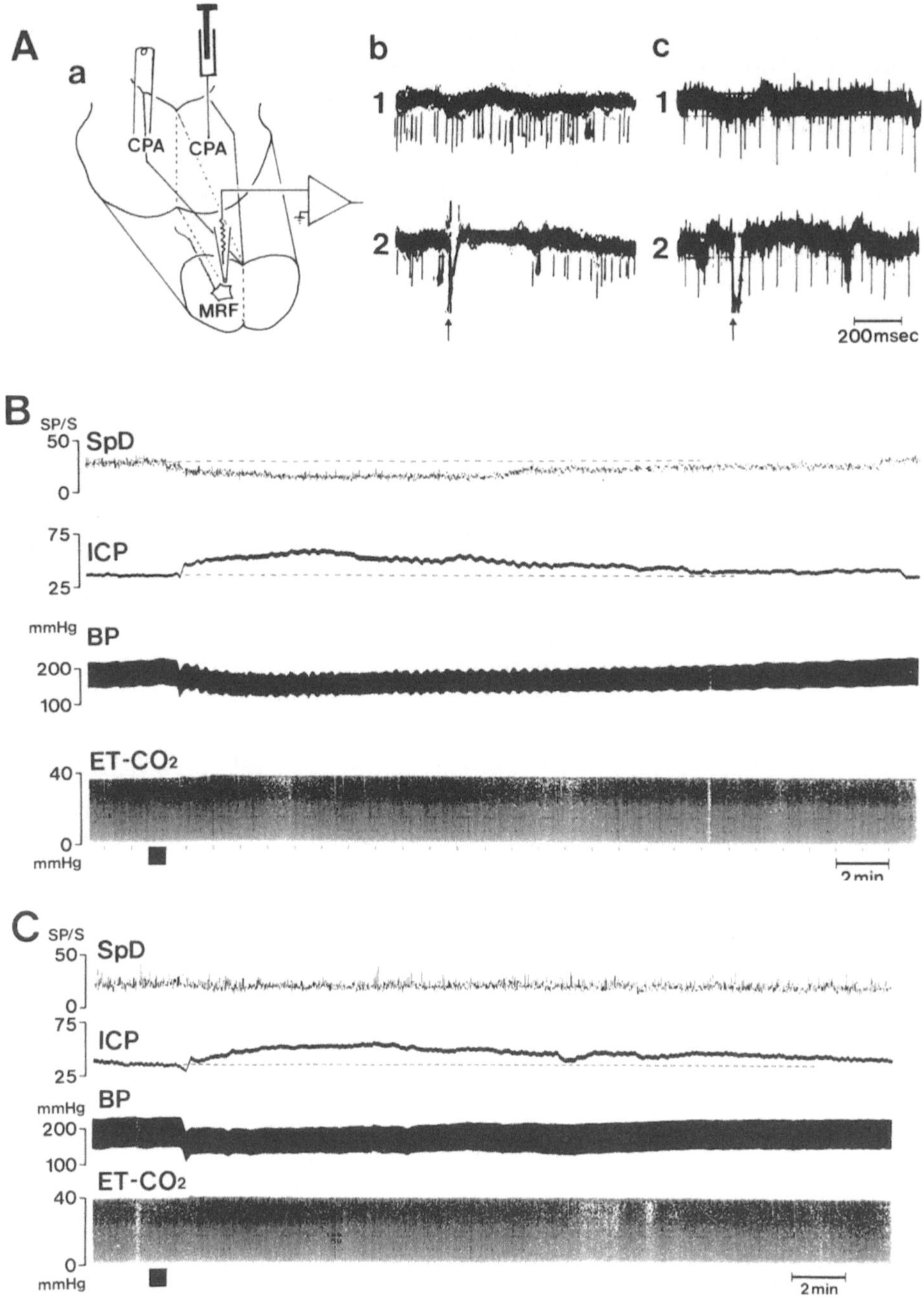

Fig. 3A–C. Discharge patterns of MRF-neurons during ICP changes. **Aa** experimental arrangement, **b,c** two individual MRF neurons. Spontaneous discharges (upper traces, 1) and after electrical CPA stimulation (lower traces, 2). **B** and **C** Simultaneous recording of spikes (SpD) of MRF neurons, ICP, BP and $ETCO_2$. The MRF-neuron in **B** or **C** is the same in **Ab** or **Ac**, respectively. Successive discharge frequency measured in each 1 second. Filled square in **B** and **C** indicates Ach microinjection into the CPA locus coeruleus complex) directly affecting the intramedullary arteriole walls. Thus, the central noradrenergic system may be analogous to the peripheral sympathetic system, with the special function of regulating brain vascular tone.

Previously, we found that spontaneous LC-neuron activity was clearly suppressed during plateau wave, CPA-neuron spikes were synchronized with the plateau waves, and a mutual inhibition mechanism of the LC and CPA neurons is important in plateau wave generation [5, 6]. This study showed that small lesions in the MRF evoked ICP changes resembling a plateau wave. In contrast, activation of MRF-neurons by glutamate microinjection produced a decrease in ICP. Spontaneous activities of MRF-neurons inhibited by the CPA were suppressed during increased ICP induced by Ach microinjection into the CPA. However, the MRF-neurons not inhibited by the CPA demonstrated little change. Therefore, the MRF- and LC-neurons had similar firing patterns during ICP changes.

Plateau waves may result from an increase in CBV [2–6, 8, 9]. Ach-induced ICP changes in the present study have resulted from increased CBV in response to reduced cerebral vasoconstrictor tone. Our previous [6] and present studies show that the CPA neurons suppress both the LC and MRF-neurons which make up the central noradrenergic system. Activation of the CPA neurons should suppress activity in the central noradrenergic system. The increase in CBV then occurs in response to dilatation of cerebral vessels. These results suggest that activity within the CPA, LC and MRF contributes to ICP changes and is the endogenous neuronal origin of plateau waves occurring in some conditions such as disturbed CSF absorption (Kaolin-induced hydrocephalus).

Acknowledgements. This work was supported in part by a grant awarded to Prof. M. Maeda (No. 03670690) from the Japanese Ministry of Education, Science and Culture.

References

1. Coyle JT, Snyder SH (1981) Catecholamines. In: Siegel GJ, Albers RW, Agranoff BW, Katzman R (eds) Basic Neurochemistry. Little, Brown and Company Boston, pp 205–217
2. Hayashi M, Ishii H, Handa Y, Kobayashi H, Kawano H, Kabuto M (1987) Role of the medulla oblongata in plateau-wave development in dogs. J. Neurosurg 67:97–101
3. Katayama Y, Nakamura T, Bedser DP, Hayes RL (1984) Intracranial pressure variations associated with activation of the cholinoceptive pontine inhibitory area in the unanesthetized drug-free cat. J. Neurosurg 61:713–724
4. Lundberg N (1960) Continuous recording and control of ventricular fluid pressure in neurosurgical practice. Acta Psychiatr Scand (Suppl 149) 36:1–193
5. Maeda M, Takahashi K, Miyazaki M, Ishii S (1986) The role of the central monoamine system and the cholinoceptive pontine area on the oscillation of ICP "pressure waves". In: Miller JD, Teasdale GM, Rowan JO, Galbraith SL, Mendelow AD (eds) Intracranial pressure VI. Springer, Berlin Heidelberg New York Tokyo, pp 151–155
6. Maeda M, Miyazaki M, Ishii S (1989) The role of the mutual interaction between the locus coeruleus complex and the cholinoceptive pontine area in the plateau wave. In: Hoff JT, Betz AL (eds) Intracranial pressure VII. Springer, Berlin Heidelberg New York London Paris Tokyo Hong Kong, pp 228–231

7. Matsuda M, Handa H (1989) Failure in aborting plateau waves by a temporary increase in cerebral perfusion pressure. In: Hoff JT, Betz AL (eds) Intracranial pressure VII. Springer, Berlin Heidelberg New York London Paris Tokyo Hong Kong, pp 245–247
8. Nagao S, Nishiura T, Kuyama H, Suga M, Murota T (1987) Effect of stimulation of the medullary reticular formation on cerebral vasomotor tonus and intracranial pressure. J. Neurosurg 66:548–554.
9. Risberg J, Lundberg N, Ingvar DH (1969) Regional cerebral blood volume during acute transient rises of the intracranial pressure (plateau waves). J. Neurosurg 31:303–310
10. Rosner MJ, Becker DP (1984) Origin and evolution of plateau waves, experimental observations and a theoretical model. J. Neurosurg 60:312–324

Analysis of Pyramidal Tract Function in Experimental Intracranial Hypertension by Magnetic Stimulation

N. Kawai, S. Nagao, M. Fujisawa, K. Fujita, T. Ito, and T. Ohmoto

Department of Neurological Surgery, Kagawa Medical School 1750-1, Ikenobe, Miki-Cho, Kita-Gun, Kagawa, 761-07, Japan

Introduction

Recent studies have demonstrated the usefulness of the motor evoked responses (MERs) recorded from spinal cord and muscle after electrical stimulation of the motor cortex for evaluating the function of the central motor pathways in humans [9] and animals [7]. In 1985, Barker et al. reported a new method of MERs recording by time-varied magnetic stimulation of the motor cortex. Their clinical studies [2] demonstrated the usefulness of magnetic stimulation for evaluating the motor function. However, there have been few studies concerning MERs recording by magnetic stimulation in experimental animals. In the present study, we first examined the physiological characteristics of the spinal MERs following the transcranial magnetic stimulation in cats. And next, we evaluated the electrophysiological changes in the central motor pathways by transcranial magnetic stimulation in experimental intracranial hypertension.

Materials and Methods

Twenty-four adult mongrel cats, weighing 3–5 kg each, were used. All cats were anesthetized with ketamine hydrochloride (10 mg/kg/hr), intubated and ventilated with room air using a respirator. The femoral artery and vein were cannulated for recording the arterial blood pressure and fluid infusion respectively. Blood gases were maintained within normal ranges. The rectal temperature was maintained at 37–38°C with a heating pad.

Stimulation and MERs Recording

The device used for magnetic stimulation consisted of capacitors (capacitor voltage 300–900 V) and a flat circular stimulation coil. A large current (3000–9000 A) was passed through the coil by the discharge of the capacitors. The time-varied magnetic field with a peak of 2.2 tesla around the coil induced an electric current within the conducting tissues of the brain and excited the neural tissues. The coil used in the present study had an outer diameter of 85 mm and was positioned tangentially just above the vertex. A laminectomy was performed at the L1–L2 level. Spinal MERs were recorded with a flexible, bipolar wire electrode at the posterolateral epidural space. In 6 animals, another laminectomy was performed at T10 level and spinal MERs were recorded for calculating the conduction velocities. Muscle MERs were recorded with a needle electrode inserted into the left gastrocnemius muscle. Sixteen signals from the spinal MERs were averaged by a signal processor (Neuropack 2, Nihon-Khoden, Japan) at a band pass of 100–3000 Hz.

Tract Ablation

In an attempt to identify the motor evoked response elicited from the sensorimotor cortex and travelling in the pyramidal tract, lesions were performed at various levels of the pyramidal tract. In three cats, bilateral craniotomies were performed and sensorimotor cortices (anterior and posterior sigmoid gyri) were exposed. The bilateral sensorimotor cortices were coagulated and ablated. Microsurgical transection of the bilateral pyramis at the brain stem by transclival approach was performed in another three cats. The spinal MERs were recorded before and after the lesions under the same conditions. At the end of the experiment, the animals were sacrificed by an intravenous KCl injection and the lesions were confirmed.

Experimental Intracranial Hypertension

The experiment was designed to investigate the effect of intracranial hypertension on the motor evoked responses by transcranial magnetic stimulation. A small rubber balloon was inserted into the right temporoparietal epidural space. Intracranial pressure (ICP) was measured at the right parietal epidural space with a plate-type pressure transducer (Gaeltec, type ICT/B, UK). The intracranial pressure was continuously increased by balloon inflation with saline at a rate of 0.01 ml/min. The MERs from the spinal cord and muscle were recorded at increased ICP, at approximately 10 mmHg intervals. The ICP was likewise increased until the muscle MER disappeared. Then the balloon content was evacuated and the recoveries of spinal and muscle MERs were observed in the following 3 hours.

Results

Spinal MERs Wave Form

Spinal MERs (MERs-S) were obtained in all 24 animals. The MERs-S were considerably affected by the stimulation conditions. However, stable waves appeared when the stimulus intensity was above 500 V, and the amplitude of those waves tended to increase when the stimulus intensity was increased. Representative MERs-S recorded from L1 epidural electrode by transcranial magnetic stimulation consisted of four negative peaks (N1 through N4) and following small, multiphasic waves. The peak latencies of the four waves were 2.56 ± 0.18, 3.19 ± 0.19, 4.06 ± 0.25 and 4.99 ± 0.37 msec respectively (mean ± S.D.). The peak amplitudes of the four waves at the stimulus intensity of 600 V were 19.76 ± 11.00, 18.42 ± 8.33, 25.69 ± 10.24 and 13.12 ± 5.52 μV respectively (mean ± SD).

Spinal MERs Conduction Velocities

The conduction velocities of each wave were calculated as follows in 6 cats. Δx represented the distance from T10 to L1 electrode and Δt represented the differences between negative peak latencies.

$$\text{C.V.} = \Delta x/\Delta t\,(\text{m/sec.}) \quad (\Delta t: \Delta t_1 \sim \Delta t_4)$$

The conduction velocities of each wave were estimated 115.4 ± 16.2, 97.2 ± 15.8, 88.9 ± 7.2 and 70.6 ± 8.4 m/sec respectively.

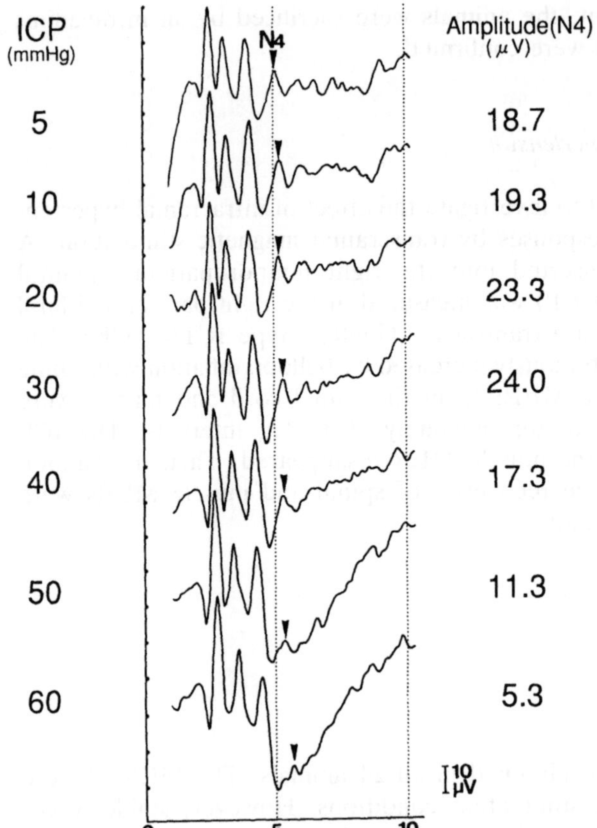

Fig. 1. Representative changes in MERs-S during increased ICP. According to an increase in ICP, the latency and amplitude of N4 component were progressively prolonged and suppressed

Tract Ablation Studies

In 3 cats in which the bilateral sensorimotor cortices were coagulated and ablated, N4 of spinal MERs decreased in amplitude and disappeared. After pyramidotomy in another 3 cats, the N4 of spinal MERs also diminished, whereas N1 to N3 remained unaffected.

These results indicated that the N4 component elicited by transcranial magnetic stimulation originated from the pyramidal tract. On the other hand, it was considered that N1 to N3 components originated and travelled in non-pyramidal tracts.

Changes in Pyramidal Tract Response in Intracranial Hypertension

The ICP was gradually increased by continuous balloon inflation. After two hours of inflation, the ICP reached approximately 60 mmHg. The blood pressure was stable during the experiment, but in some animals, the typical pressure response occurred above 70 mmHg.

Recordings of serial MERs-S during increased ICP were satisfactory in 12 animals. Representative changes in MERs-S during increased ICP are shown in Fig. 1. According to an increase in ICP, the latency and amplitude of the N4 component were progressively prolonged and suppressed. At 60 and 70 mmHg, the N4 component disappeared in 4 and 3 animals respectively. However, the amplitudes of N1 to N3 were well preserved until moderately high ICP. Changes in amplitude of the N4 component in increased ICP are shown in Fig. 2A. The ordinates are relative amplitude as percentage of the control. Some facilitation in the amplitude was observed transiently at 10 to 20 mmHg. The amplitude of N4 was significantly suppressed above 40 mmHg and it almost disappeared above 70 mmHg. Changes in latency of the N4 component at increased ICP are shown in Fig. 2B. The control value of the latency in these 12 animals was 5.11 ± 0.49 msec. The latency of the N4 component was significantly prolonged above 50 mmHg (latency: 5.60 ± 0.50 msec).

Muscle MERs (MERs-M) were obtained as a compound muscle action potential from the left gastrocnemius muscle. The MERs-M were also suppressed at increased ICP and became flat when the mean ICP reached approximately 65 mmHg. After that the balloon content was evacuated and the mean balloon volume was 1.65 ml.

After balloon deflation, the MERs-M reappeared within 30 min. The MERs-S (N4) and MERs-M gradually recovered in amplitude following three hours.

Discussion

Spinal MERs in Cats

These results show that transcranial magnetic stimulation as well as transcranial and direct motor cortex electrical stimulation [7] could easily produce descend-

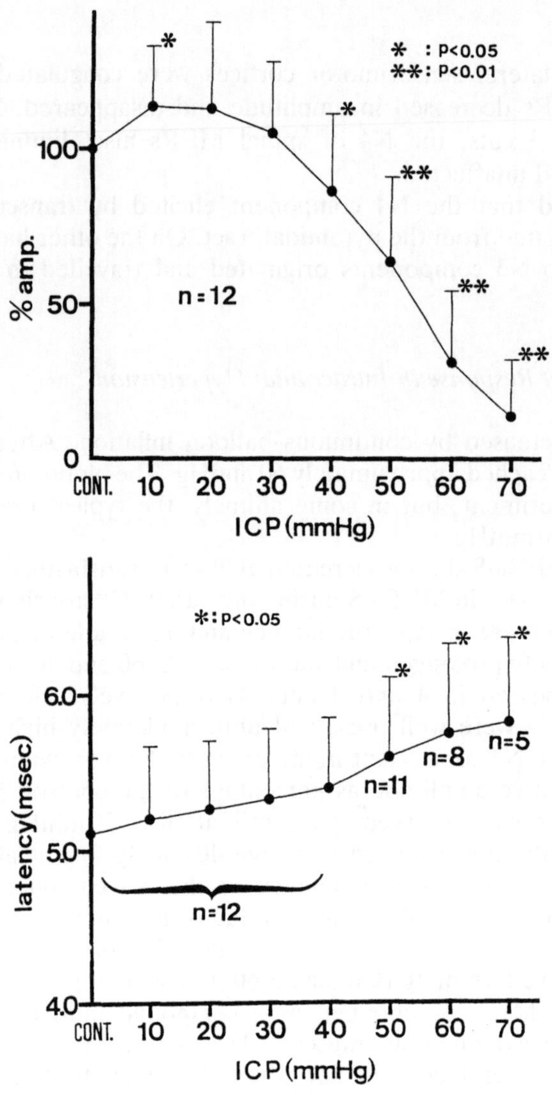

Fig. 2. Changes in amplitude (**A**) and latency (**B**) of N4 component in increased ICP. The amplitude and latency of N4 component were significantly suppressed and prolonged above 40 and 50 mmHg respectively

ing evoked potentials that were recorded from the spinal cord in the experimental animals.

The spinal MERs we obtained consist of four negative peaks (N1–N4) [5]. The peak latencies of N1 and N2 in the lumbar spinal cord (<3.2 msec) are much shorter than that reported for corticospinal tract activation in the classic neurophysiological experiments (4.0–4.5 msec). The conduction velocities calculated for the N1 to N3 peak are greater than 90 m/sec and, therefore, inconsistent with the corticospinal tract activation. The conduction velocities of

N1 to N3 correspond to the cerebellar evoked potentials (CEPs) including the rubrospinal, reticulospinal, vestibulospinal and fastigiospinal tracts [8]. It is considered that delivery of the wide spread magnetic stimulation current in experimental animals that have smaller brain volume may directly excite a number of neural elements at a significant distance from the stimulation site.

On the other hand, the N4 component of the spinal MERs has a conduction velocity of 70 m/sec which is consistent with corticospinal tract activation. The fact that the N4 component of the spinal MERs disappeared by sensorimotor cortex ablation and pyramidotomy suggests that the wave may originate from the sensorimotor cortex and travel in the corticospinal (pyramidal) tract.

In general, we conclude that the N4 component of the spinal MERs represents pyramidal tract activation whereas the N1 to N3 components represent nonpyramidal tract responses.

Pyramidal Tract Response in Increased ICP

This is a first report of changes in MERs following transcranial magnetic stimulation in a supratentorial pathophysiological condition using experimental animals.

Our results indicate that an increase in ICP highly correlated with suppression of the amplitude of the pyramidal tract response (N4) following transcranial magnetic stimulation. The amplitude of the pyramidal tract response transiently increased to approximately 120% of the control value at an ICP of 10 to 20 mmHg, so called "augmentation", and then gradually decreased. A significant decrease occurred at 40 mmHg, suggesting a significant electrophysiological suppression of the pyramidal tract [10].

The amplitude of the muscle MERs also correlated with an increase in the ICP and became flat at an ICP of 65 mmHg with a marked suppression of the amplitude of the pyramidal tract response (N4). At the stage of complete suppression of the muscle MERs, the mean balloon volume was approximately 1.65 ml which was equivalent to 8% of cat brain volume.

The latency of the pyramidal tract response (N4), which represents neural conductance of the pyramidal tract, was significantly prolonged at an ICP of 50 mmHg. But the latency shift was relatively small compared to the amplitude change, suggesting a good tolerance of the conduction system in myelinated axons [6] during supratentorial compression ischemia.

In many studies of pyramidal tract responses [3], multiple descending volleys (an initial descending D-wave and subsequent descending I waves) are reported. D-waves are thought to result from direct excitation of pyramidal neurons and I-waves are the results of indirect activation of the pyramidal cells through cortical interneurons. It is hypothesized that the direct motor cortex stimulation can elicit the D- and I-waves, but the transcranial magnetic stimulation may activate pyramidal neurons transsynaptically and produce only I-waves in the pyramidal tract [4]. During increased ICP by balloon expansion, compression ischemia occurs at the sensorimotor cortex and results in the prolongation of the synaptic delay for transsynaptic activation of the pyramidal neurons.

These findings suggest that compression ischemia of the sensorimotor cortex results in suppression of the number of neural activations and prolongation of transsynaptic activation of the pyramidal neurons following transcranial magnetic stimulation.

In conclusion, magnetic stimulation is considered to be an effective tool for evaluating the electrophysiological changes in the pyramidal tract at increased ICP, though detailed characteristics of the recorded signals should be taken into consideration.

References

1. Barker AT, Jalinous R, Freeston IL (1985) Non-invasive magnetic stimulation of human motor cortex. Lancet 1:1106–1107
2. Barker AT, et al. (1987) Magnetic stimulation of the human brain and peripheral nervous system: An introduction and the results of an initial clinical evaluation. Neurosurgery 20:100–109
3. Day BL, et al. (1987a) Motor cortex stimulation in intact man: 2. Multiple descending volleys. Brain 110:1191–1209
4. Day BL, et al. (1987b) Different site of action of electrical and magnetic stimulation of the human brain. Neurosci Lett 75:101–106
5. Fujiki M, Isono M, Hori S (1990) Spinal and muscle motor evoked potentials following magnetic stimulation in cats. Neuro Med Chir (Tokyo) 30:234–241
6. Konrad PE, et al. (1987) Motor evoked potentials in the dog: Effects of global ischemia on spinal cord and peripheral nerve signals. Neurosurgery 20:117–124
7. Levy WJ, McCaffrey M, York DH, Tanzer F (1984) Motor evoked potentials from transcranial stimulation of the motor cortex in cats. Neurosurgery 15:214–227
8. Levy WJ, McCaffrey M, Goldman D, York DH (1986) Non-pyramidal motor activation produced by stimulation of the cerebellum, direct or transcranial: A cerebellar evoked potential. Neurosurgery 19:163–176
9. Levy WJ (1987) Clinical experience with motor and cerebellar evoked potential monitoring. Neurosurgery 20:169–182
10. Nagao, S, Roccaforte P, Moody R (1981) Effect of brain compression on pyramidal tract response in cat. Exp Neurology 73:107–117

Neurophysiological Evidence of Preservation of Brain Stem Function in Experimental Closed Head Injury in the Rat*

W.A. van den Brink[1], W. Slomka[1], A. Marmarou[1], and C.J.J. Avezaat[2]

[1] Division of Neurosurgery, Medical College of Virginia, Richmond, VA, USA
[2] Department of Neurosurgery, Erasmus University, Rotterdam, The Netherlands

Introduction

The use of animal models of head injury have contributed substantially to the understanding of the pathophysiology, neuropathology, and underlying mechanisms of traumatic brain injury. Despite this progress, a reproducible model of severe closed head injury (CHI) without substantial brain stem damage was not yet available. This fact has been emphasized by Shima and Marmarou [5]. In the cat model of fluid percussion, using brain stem auditory evoked potentials (BAEP), these workers found a severe impairment of the neurophysiological function of the brain stem. Similar findings were observed in the rat model of FPI [1]. In contrast, our studies of CHI, using a simple weight drop model, shows a markedly different response from the fluid percussion injury (FPI) model. The CHI model is characterized by impact, which causes the compression and acceleration of the partially restrained skull. This mechanism is similar to many high velocity impact injuries seen in humans. However, it is unclear if similar brain stem disturbances seen in FPI would occur in closed head injury. The objective of this study was to investigate the functional integrity of the brain stem in response to CHI. This was accomplished utilizing BAEP's. Somatosensory evoked potentials (SSEP) were used to evaluate the cervical and cortical neuronal function. These neurophysiological methods are well described for evaluating the sensory tracts, and interposed synapses, which, from periphery to central nervous system, traverse a major part of the brain stem and spinal cord.

Materials and Methods

Surgical Preparation

Adult male Sprague Dawley rats weighing 342 ± 40 grams (mean ± sd) were kept under surgical anaesthesia with either alpha-chloralose, or halothane.

* This study was funded by NIH grant 2P0INS12587 and NIDRR HI33B80029. Further support was obtained from: the Richard Roland Reynolds Research Laboratories and the Sophia Foundation for Medical Research from the Netherlands.

Throughout the experiment a heating lamp was used to maintain the core body temperature to 38°C. The scalp and periosteum were reflected and the skull was carefully dried using a cold air source. A stainless steel disc measuring 10 mm in diameter and 3 mm thick was secured between lambda and bregma using dental acrylic. Four platinum needles (Grass), at the left and right mastoid (A1, A2), over the frontal sinus (Fpz), in the occipito-cervical muscles (Cz), and one skull screw over the right sensory cortex (C4) were placed and secured. The protocols were approved by the Institutional Animal Care and Use Committee, Medical College of Virginia, Richmond, Virginia.

Trauma Model

The CHI model in the rat produces trauma by weight drop on the intact skull. Limited movement and thus impact, compression and acceleration are provided by supporting the skull with foam. High levels of impact needed to cause severe brain damage generally causes the skull to fracture. However, the stainless steel disk has been shown to protect the skull while transmitting the force and acceleration of the impact. Both the foam bedding and the rat were positioned under a 2.20 meter long vertically placed plexiglass tubing. The helmet was aligned exactly under the center, and perpendicular to the opening of the tubing. The CHI was delivered to the animals by dropping a segmented brass cylinder of 450 gram through the tubing on the rat's "helmet". Care was taken that there was no obstruction of the air outflow caused by the falling weight. The weight was dropped from a height of either 1 or 2 meter. These levels will be referred to as "mild" or "severe" injury. Rebounding is prevented by quickly removing the foam bed with the rat sideways after the first contact.

Evoked Potentials

Needle electrodes at both mastoids, the vertex, nasal bone and an epidural screw electrode over the right sensory cortex (A1, A2, Cz, FPz and C4 respectively) were placed to record evoked potentials before trauma and at regular interval for 4 hours after trauma. BAEP's, elicited by 85 dB square wave click stimuli to the right ear, were recorded from Cz and A1 referred to A2. SSEP's, elicited by 5mA square wave current pulses delivered to both forepaws, were recorded from C4 referred to FPz.

Protocol

The rats were subjected to either mild or severe CHI; each group was accompanied by a sham control group. Double recordings of BAEP were acquired at 0, 5, 15, 30 minutes, and at each hour after trauma. SSEP's were recorded before trauma, every minute for the first 15 minutes after trauma, and every hour after trauma up to 4 hours. At the conclusion of the experiment the

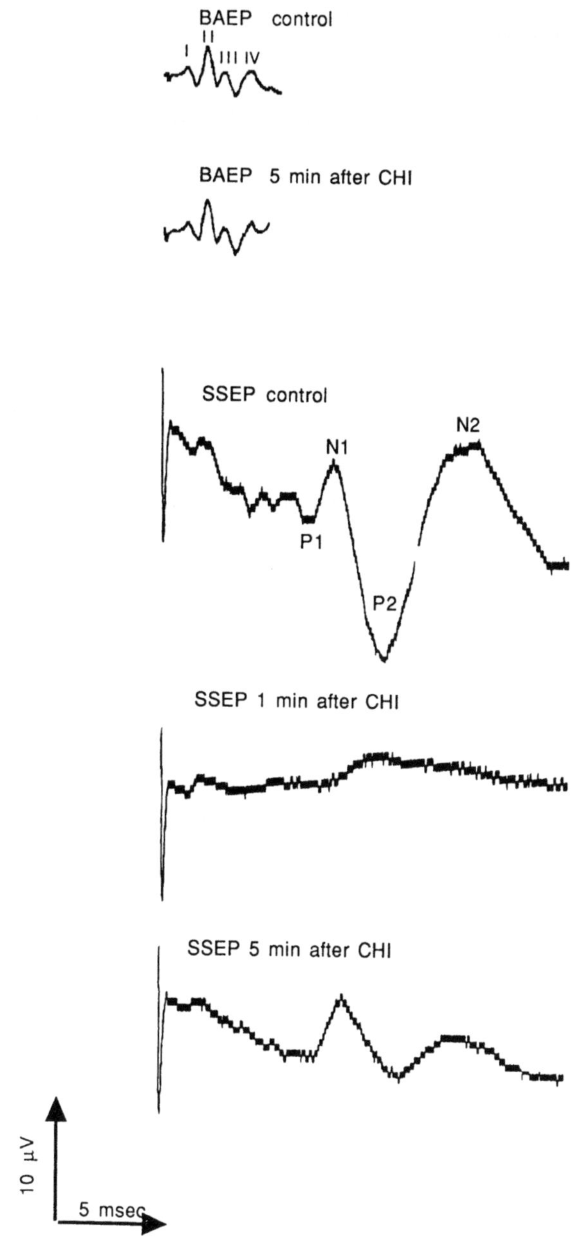

Fig. 1. Example of a BAEP and SSEP before and shortly after injury, positive peaks are labelled with roman numerals in the BAEP, in SSEP peaks are labelled conform their polarity and order of appearance

animal was sacrificed by systemic administration of 2 cc of saturated KCl. Statistics: Latency and amplitude parameters were analyzed using the student T-test. When appropriate a Bonferroni T-test was performed. P values of less than 0.05 were considered significant.

Results

Of 45 rats tested, two rats in the entire series of CHI were excluded because of skull fracture. Both were injured at the 450 gram 2 meter level. A third rat had a dura tear due to screw placement. Data from these three experiments were neglected. All rats in the mildly injured group survived, while the overall mortality in the severely injured group was 37%.

Brain Stem Auditory Evoked Potentials

There was no difference in the BAEP's as compared with the BAEP's obtained at baseline or from sham animals in animals subjected to mild trauma. Typical examples of the rat BAEP and SSEP before and just following severe CHI are shown in Fig. 1. The latencies and amplitudes of normal evoked potentials, obtained before trauma are shown in Table 1. After trauma wave form morphology remained intact and no peaks disappeared. In contrast, severe trauma caused a relative instability, but no disappearance, of the fourth wave. The fourth in the rat is considered to be generated in the inferior colliculus. The fourth wave and the I-IV interval as an indicator of global brain stem integrity did not show a prolongation in latencies nor a decrease in amplitudes in both mildly and severely injured animals.

Somatosensory Evoked Potentials

Mild injury caused a transient deterioration of near field wavelets for approximately 6 minutes. However, after severe injury all near field SSEP's were abolished. This was followed by a gradual recovery. Analysis of the waves consisted of the counting of the number of waves visible, averaging wave latencies and amplitudes. The wavelets with the short latencies tend to recover earlier than the long latency-peaks. Of the peaks that could be identified and had a latency within normal range, that is shorter than the mean +2 times the standard deviation, more than 50% P1 peaks were within normal range after

Table 1. Normal values of latencies and amplitudes of evoked potentials in the rat

Control values of normal rat BAEP's (mean ± sem)				
A1–A2	wave I	wave II	wave III	wave IV
latencies	1.14 (±0.01)	2.08 (±0.01)	2.77 (±0.02)	3.89 (±0.03)
amplitudes	0.86 (±0.04)	1.67 (±0.05)	1.56 (±0.05)	0.40 (±0.08)
Control values of normal rat SSEP's (mean ± sem)				
C4-FPz	P1	N1	P2	N2
latencies	6.89 (±0.08)	8.49 (±0.07)	10.66 (±0.10)	14.11 (±1.16)
amplitudes	6.78 (±0.34)	2.86 (±0.26)	14.30 (±1.31)	5.87 (±0.65)

2 min; followed by N1, >50% after 6 min; P2, >50% after 10 min; and N2, >50% after one hour. The three far field components did not show a post traumatic latency prolongation. Peak amplitudes remained severely affected after the initial abolition. Significant amplitude decrease of peaks N1 and N2 was present up to 30 minutes, for P2 up to 15 minutes.

Discussion

These studies show that a mechanical injury to the closed calvarium, sufficient in magnitude to be lethal in 50% of animals, does not produce brain stem damage in survivors. Indeed, the BAEP's remained unaffected in all animals surviving the initial trauma. Preservation of peaks and latencies provide strong evidence that brain stem function is not severely compromised. In contrast, evidence for supratentorial damage was found in the effect of injury on cortical generated SSEP waves. Mild injury caused cortical dysfunction of short duration with rapid and complete recovery. After severe injury only partial recovery of cortical function was seen; latencies were abnormal for at least 1 hour, and amplitudes did not return to baseline values during the 4 hour experimental period. Impact acceleration models often are associated with persistent severe damage to the cervical cord [3]. In this model the preservation of the three far field components and the rapid return of the early near field potential P1 indicate an absence of permanent damage to the cervical cord. It is well known that in the clinical situation brain stem injury is an indicator of the severity of brain injury, and predictive of bad outcome. Solitary injury to the brain stem is a rare entity [2]. This clinical experience is consistent with the experimental findings of Ommaya who observed that the distribution of damaging strains, as induced by inertial loading, would decrease in magnitude from the surface to the center of the brain [4]. With direct dural impact, these forces are sufficient in magnitude to cause structural damage. However, in the closed calvarium, as might be expected, the distortion of tissue is minimized.

Conclusion

In this study neurophysiological parameters were used to evaluate the function of neural pathways in the cervical cord, brain stem and cortical areas after mild and severe experimental CHI. The neurophysiological brain stem parameters after CHI survivors remain unaffected. The SSEP's suggest sustained dysfunction at cortical level, while the cervical cord potentials remain intact. We consider this new simple model to be of value in future trauma research.

References

1. Dixon CE, Lyeth BG, Povlishock JT, et al. (1987) A fluid percussion model of experimental brain injury in the rat. J Neurosurg 67:110–119
2. Marshall LF, Gautille T, Klauber MR, et al. (1991) The outcome of severe head injury. J Neurosurg 75 (Suppl): S28–S36
3. Nilsson B, Ponten U, Voigt G (1977) Experimental head injury in the rat. Part 1: Mechanics, pathophysiology, and morphology in an impact acceleration trauma model. J Neurosurg 47:241–251
4. Ommaya AK, Gennarelli TA (1974) Cerebral concussion and traumatic unconsciousness correlation of experimental and clinical observations on blunt head injuries. Brain 97:633–654
5. Shima K, Marmarou A (1991) Evaluation of brain stem dysfunction following severe fluid percussion head injury to the cat. J Neurosurg 74:270–277

Panel 1
Methodology and Experimental Aspects

Moderator: A. Baethmann

Members: K.G. Go, L. Pitts, R.J. Traystman, A. Wachi, and N. Zwetnow

BAETHMANN: The panel discussions form a new experimental part of the ICP symposium. We hope to discuss the work presented and hope that you will retain the main messages and be happy with the results and final conclusions; if you're not happy after our discussions, at least those who are sitting here you can blame, but don't blame the organizers. We have a huge ground to cover. I would like to present to you briefly which issues presented today in the oral session and in the poster sessions we found particularly important, although we admit that we may be ignorant and are leaving out other equally important subjects.

The first issue raised was that of brain tissue or parenchymal pressure versus ICP measured in the brain fluid compartments, such as the ventricular system or the subarachnoid space. In some papers, tissue pressures lower than ventricular fluid pressure had been found and even negative tissue pressures. This is of great clinical significance since, in clinical practice, more and more fiberoptic devices are being used, which are measuring occasionally, or by purpose, tissue pressures. What are we measuring if we are measuring tissue pressure?

MILLER commented that when fluid filled systems are used to measure tissue pressure, one tends to get negative values. The investigators using these systems advise to fill the system with a fluid which is 20 mosm higher than the serum, to infuse the system in order to keep the pressure stable, or to put a wick into the system. On the other hand, the tissue pressures obtained with closed systems seem to correlate quite well with the ICP. It was hypothesized that it is in the damaged areas of the brain, as in the study by Sirowski, where the most discordant measurements are obtained. This has to do with the osmotic pressure in these areas which is interfering with the hydrostatic pressure measurement. Presumably, the high protein content of the tissue fluid will tend to withdraw fluid from the catheter system and give a false, too low tissue pressure measurement.

According to the experience of BROCK, clotting is another factor that may lead to negative tissue pressures. When the system is filled with protein or with blood, the clotting process appears to produce negative pressures, because there seems to be a reduction in volume of the whole mass within the system.

PIEK performed brain tissue pressure measurements in 145 patients, in 20 in the posterior fossa, with a direct pressure transducer. The only situation in which he could observe negative pressures, was in the postoperative period when the dura had not been tightly closed and a negative epidural suction had been put in. These negative pressures were only present for a short period of time. He agreed with Miller that negative pressures are due to a technical failure if fluid filled systems are used.

ANDEWEG commented on the subject of osmotic versus hydrostatic pressures. The difference is that a hydrostatic pressure is active with or without a membrane present, whereas the osmotic pressure is only active when there is a semi-permeable membrane in between. So, when you put a catheter into whatever tissue, you will not get an osmotic action.

MARMAROU requested the panel to consider the importance of tissue pressure at least as a clinical monitoring tool. As we put more and more catheters into tissue, to what degree do they represent the ventricular fluid pressure which we are used to treat and which we use for calculation of cerebral perfusion pressure?

D'AVELLA had placed two fiberoptic devices bifrontally and had recorded intraparenchymal ICP in the presence of a unilateral, supratentorial expanding mass. With this technique transient pressure gradients could be observed lasting one or two hours.

NARAYAN had also used fiberoptic transducers to measure tissue pressure both ipsilateral and contralateral to an expanding epidural balloon and had observed a very little, if any, difference in pressure between the ventricular and parenchymal pressure, both ipsilateral and contralateral to the mass. He was of the opinion that these minimal pressure gradients were artifactual, but even if they were real, that, from a clinical point of view, they were without consequences. He had used these fiberoptic devices to measure pressures in clinical patients, simultaneously in parenchyma and in the ventricle, and had found only minimal differences.

TRAYSTMAN commented that in the brain, in terms of perfusion, we normally think of an inflow pressure, an outflow pressure and some surrounding pressure, which last pressure is usually considered to be ICP or CSF pressure. But now we have to think of another pressure, that pressure being intraparenchymal pressure, which may be equivalent to, higher than or lower than ICP, which some people might consider the back pressure to flow. Therefore, the issue of parenchymal pressure and how it compares with ICP, if it does at all, is very important. For if it doesn't, then all of our notions in terms of cerebral perfusion pressure and what controls that perfusion pressure may have to be re-thought of.

BROCK: I'm sorry, I think this discussion is late by 20 years. As long as a patient with an epidural hematoma develops a widening pupil, there is no way to deny intracranial pressure gradients. There is no way by which you can get mass displacement but by pressure gradients. The importance of tissue pressure is tissue perfusion pressure. If you consider that the arterial pressure at the level of the tissue is only 30 to 40 mmHg at the moment the vessels penetrate the pia mater and if you consider an ICP of 10 mmHg, then you have a tissue perfusion pressure of 30 mmHg only, which is normal. Now, if you increase ICP at the diseased area by 10 mmHg, it is nothing. Well, it is nothing if you take ICP, but if you take tissue pressure it is ⅓ of the available pressure head.

CHESNUT reported that he had put in well over 300 Camino catheters, some bilaterally, some in conjunction with ventricular catheters and he had certainly observed gradients both between the ventricular catheter and an ipsilateral intraparenchymal transducer, and interhemispherically between Camino's. He thought that the basic problem was what should be treated. The golden standard is the ventricular pressure, because we haven't been able to measure reliably the parenchymal pressure. We are all interested in the neurons themselves and the closer we get to the neurons, the more interesting the pressure becomes. The idea that we have marked gradients in the brain that may be related to changes in the tissue elastance is something that needs to be considered.

The second issue concerned the relevance of various experimental models of head injury to the clinical situation

BAETHMANN discussed the various experimental models of head injury. All models serve some specific purpose to analyse aspects of severe head injury, but there is no model in the laboratory which really represents all the qualitative and quantitative aspects of what is going on in severe head injured patients. This is a point we should never forget.

VAN DEN BRINK agreed that every model serves its own purpose. He claimed that his new model of closed head injury in the rat, without concomitant brainstem damage, comes very close to the common closed head injury seen in patients in which there is no skull fracture and also no mass lesion afterwards.

PITTS discussed the cold injury model. This model is often characterized as a vasogenic edema model and yet there is a great deal of necrosis and interstitial or intracellular edema. So, it is a very mixed model and the question is what it means in terms of human disease. It is probably a useful model for studying the flow of edema fluid, but it hardly relates to human head injury or any other specific human pathology. In fact very few patients in San Francisco actually freeze their brain.

MARMAROU pointed out that there is not yet a reliable model of contusion available. The best model we had ten years ago was the acceleration impact model of Gennarelli. Since this model cannot be used anymore, we have to resort to fluid percussion, closed head injury or cryogenic injury, which last model gives us the opportunity to study the dynamics of edema from a source that continues at least for a certain period of time. We have learned from fluid percussion that we must stay below a three atmosphere hit level, which gives us a predominant brainstem component and masks many of the supratentorial events. With closed head injury, we know that we have a hypertension immediately following impact that does not approach the level seen in fluid percussion. So, each model has its specific characteristics and certainly cryogenic injury does have its advantages to study the edema.

Bullock and co-workers looked with a number of different endpoints at patients with contusions to map the amount of breakdown at the blood brain barrier using gadolineum in MRI and pertechnetate in SPECT. The consensus of these studies has been to show that there is relatively little blood brain barrier change in the observed early phase, that is within about the first four days. The blood brain barrier change is largely secondary in the majority of the patients. The peak time for the biggest barrier lesion is after about the 7th day, which also accords with the phase of deterioration in patients with space-occupying contusions.

Pitts remarked that in focal ischemia or stroke in humans, the blood brain barrier defect starts showing up 18–24 hours after the lesion and suggested that the focal cold injury model is closer to a middle cerebral artery occlusion than it is to head injury. In reply to a question by Maas, Bullock mentioned that his studies were done in patients with contusions, specifically selected on CT and that they were mostly at the awake end of the spectrum. He referred to post mortem data from Graham confirming that the main barrier leak was later rather than very early.

Kojiva had compared the protein content of edema after ischemia and after cold lesion. He had found that the protein content was very similar between the two different types of edema from which he concluded that post ischemic edema had very similar features to cold injury edema.

The third issue raised concerned the significance of brain edema in severe head injury under clinical circumstances. Baethmann referred to some studies done in Richmond, on the fluid percussion model indicating that there was no increase in the brain water content.

Miller commented that they had been looking at the early rise in ICP immediately after the fluid percussion injury. At the period when the ICP was extremely high, in the first few minutes after the injury, there was no evidence of an increase in brain water content. However, taking the time dimension into account, it was clear that after more than 24 hours, brain water was increasing. The issue is a very important one, because if the ICU doctor is faced with a patient with raised ICP, the question is whether the predominant cause of the increased pressure is vascular, in which case there is one logic of treatment or nonvascular, in which case we may want to use different sorts of treatment.

A brief comment was made on the role of early MRI in head injury compared to early CT. On T2 weighted MR abnormal areas can be seen which may be assumed to indicate an increased water content. Early MRI may become a quantifiable measure of injury, more than early CT does.

Marmarou had discovered a controversy among the poster sessions with regard to the head elevation of patients, whether we should maintain our patients flat or we should elevate their heads at 30–35 degrees. The Rosner data, published in the Journal of Neurosurgery, indicate that maintaining patients flat optimizes cerebral perfusion pressure. On the other hand, work from Richmond and Houston indicates that there is no change in perfusion pressure with elevation of patients, but that there is a statistically marked reduction in ICP.

Session III: Cerebrovascular Dynamics I

Chairmen: G.M. Teasdale and J.P. Muizelaar

Effect of Increased ICP and Decreased Cerebral Perfusion Pressure on Brain Tissue and Cerebrospinal Fluid Oxygen Tension

A.I.R. MAAS, W. FLECKENSTEIN, D.A. DE JONG, and M. WOLF

Departments of Neurosurgery and Experimental Surgery, University Hospital Rotterdam, Rotterdam, The Netherlands

Introduction

Ischaemia is the central mechanism leading to secondary brain damage in patients with severe head injury. It would therefore seem appropriate to monitor cerebral oxygenation. Recent studies have focussed on continuous monitoring of oxygen saturation in cerebral venous blood by means of jugular oxymetry [2, 3, 7, 8, 9]. With this method the cerebral extraction of oxygen can be measured, but no direct information on the tissue oxygen content is available. We have investigated the possibilities of continuous monitoring of brain tissue and cerebrospinal fluid (CSF) oxygen tension (pO_2) as parameter for cerebral oxygenation. In previous studies we investigated the effect of changes in arterial pO_2 and pCO_2 on CSF oxygen tension [4, 5, 6].

Fast CSF-pO_2 changes were observed in response to changes in arterial pO_2; hyperventilation was shown to induce a marked decrease in CSF-pO_2. In the present studies we also focussed attention on brain tissue pO_2 and investigated the effect of raised ICP and decreased cerebral perfusion pressure (CPP) on brain tissue and CSF-pO_2.

Material and Methods

The studies were performed in ten dogs, all anaesthetised and artificially ventilated. Anaesthesia was maintained with fentanyl and N_2O. The animals were paralysed (pancuronium) for artificial ventilation. Arterial pO_2 and pCO_2 were kept within narrow limites, mean values 110 and 38 mmHg respectively. Catheters were inserted for continuous monitoring of arterial blood pressure, rectal temperature, brain temperature, ventricular fluid pressure, ventricular and brain tissue pO_2. CSF-pO_2 was measured with a sterilisable, polarographic needle probe (low sensitive "Licox" probe type, GMS mbH, Kiel FRG); brain tissue pO_2 was measured with a flexible polarographic micro-catheter (Shiley). The pO_2 probe's current values were measured at intervals of four seconds and stored electronically (device Licox, manufactured by GMS mbH, Kiel Mielkendorf, FRG). Raised ICP was induced by cisternal infusion of Ringer's Lactate. ICP was raised stepwise by increments of 10 mmHg, each sustained for 15 minutes. A problem resulted from increasing arterial blood pressure secondary to raised ICP. This "Cushing response" could not adequately be prevented by pharmacologic agents, and it was necessary to induce artificial pericardiac tamponade. With this technique the "Cushing response" was effectively prevented in six animals.

Results

In the experiments in which ICP was raised without preventing secondary increase in the blood pressure, no effect was seen on brain tissue pO_2 or CSF-pO_2 (Table 1). In these experiments CPP did not decrease. In the experiments in which the blood pressure was controlled with pericardiac tamponade, and reflectory increase of CPP was effectively prevented, a decrease of both brain tissue pO_2 and CSF-pO_2 was noted (Table 2, Fig. 1). Although there was a slight decrease in brain tissue pO_2 when reducing CPP from 120 to 100 mmHg, a sharper decrease was noted below CPP of 80 mmHg. Interestingly enough the brain temperature, measured simultaneously with the brain tissue pO_2 so as to be able to correct for temperature differences, decreased suddenly when CPP fell below 40 mmHg. In some of the experiments the CPP was reduced to values of zero or below (ICP $\geqslant$ mean arterial blood pressure). Brain tissue pO_2 in the absence of cerebral perfusion remained at 7 ± 1.6 mmHg and CSF-pO_2 at 1.4 ± 1 mmHg. During the reperfusion phase a discrepancy occurred between brain tissue and CSF-pO_2: CSF-pO_2 was rapidly restored to normal or even

Table 1. Brain tissue pO_2 and CSF-pO_2 at increased ICP, but normal CPP

	ICP	CPP	MABP	PaO_2	$PaCO_2$	Br.T. pO_2	VCSF pO_2
Without BP control	11.3 ± 3.8	102 ± 22	113 ± 25	112 ± 6	39 ± 5	28 ± 7	65 ± 12
	38 ± 3	108 ± 21	122 ± 17	114 ± 8	35 ± 5	28 ± 9	63 ± 15
	57 ± 3	110 ± 19	168 ± 18	112 ± 13	38 ± 5	29 ± 10	59 ± 13

Table 2. Brain tissue pO_2 and CSF-pO_2 at decreased CPP

	ICP	CPP	MABP	PaO_2	$PaCO_2$	Br.T. pO_2	VCSF pO_2
With BP control	12 ± 5	122 ± 10	134 ± 8	111 ± 11	39 ± 7	31 ± 11	60 ± 7
	39 ± 2	61 ± 2	100 ± 2	105 ± 6	40 ± 8	22 ± 8	45 ± 9
	51 ± 4	51 ± 2	102 ± 3	106 ± 8	41 ± 5	19 ± 8	39 ± 10
	59 ± 1	40 ± 2	99 ± 2	104 ± 7	43 ± 4	15 ± 7	34 ± 10
	65 ± 5	29 ± 2	94 ± 4	102 ± 11	45 ± 8	12 ± 6	25 ± 13

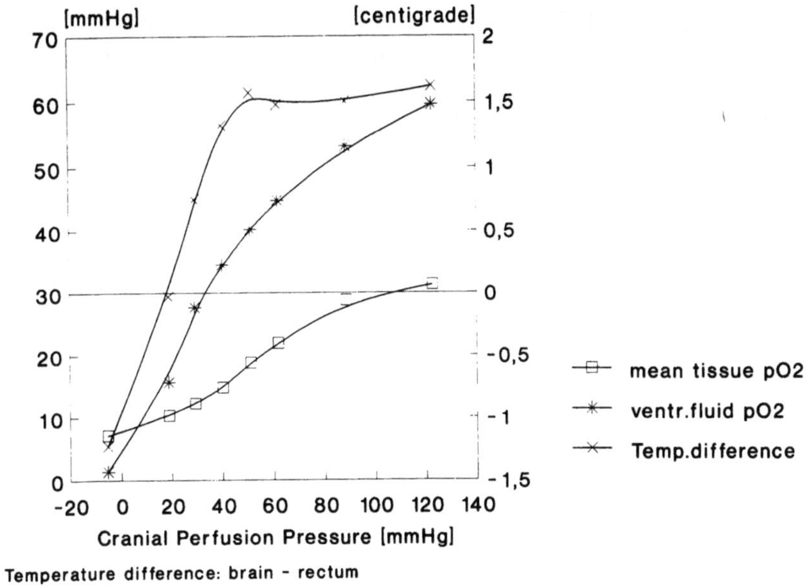

Fig. 1. Effect of decreased cerebral perfusion pressure on brain tissue pO_2, CSF-pO_2 and brain temperature. Values averaged from 6 dogs

above normal levels, but brain tissue pO_2 remained low or even decreased further.

Discussion

The experiments previously reported on monitoring of brain tissue pO_2 and CSF-pO_2 and the results of the present studies show that both parameters are influenced by changes in arterial pO_2, arterial pCO_2 and cerebral perfusion pressure. As both hyperventilation and reduced CPP decrease cerebral blood flow, it seems probable that the noted decrease in brain tissue pO_2 and CSF-pO_2 due to lowering CPP reflects decreasing cerebral blood flow. The results of the experiments reported in this study indicate that a CPP of approximately 80 mmHg appears to be critical for brain tissue- and CSF-pO_2. Below this level brain tissue and CSF-pO_2 decrease by 3 and 6 mmHg respectively per 10 mm decrease in CPP. In the CPP range of 40–60 mmHg a sharper decline is noted, indicating developing ischaemia. Chan et al. [1] have reported a critical CPP level of 70 mmHg in patients with severe head injury. Our results would sustain his conclusion that critical levels of CPP may well be higher than previously reported. Moreover, it may be that the critical level of CPP is different between individual patients. Monitoring brain tissue pO_2 could potentially ascertain the critical CPP level in individual patients.

When monitoring cerebral oxygenation we need to consider the effects of oxygen offer and oxygen demand. Oxygen offer is determined by arterial pO_2, and cerebral blood flow. The oxygen demand is determined by the rate of cerebral metabolism. The fact that brain tissue pO_2 does not decrease to zero in the absence of cerebral perfusion probably reflects the absence of oxygen demand from the brain tissue in this situation.

It is our opinion that both brain tissue pO_2 and CSF-pO_2 monitoring may be of great clinical value as the parameters reflect the net effect of oxygen offer and demand. When considering clinical application, the question is whether brain tissue pO_2 or CSF-pO_2 monitoring should be adopted. For practical and theoretical reasons it would seem more appropriate to monitor brain tissue pO_2. First of all, it may be difficult in patients with raised ICP and mass lesions to insert a catheter into the ventricle; secondly, a changing position of the catheter in the ventricular CSF, caused by increasing or decreasing mass shift may influence the result of the measurements; thirdly, in brain tissue pO_2 monitoring measurements are obtained from the brain tissue itself in contrast to CSF-pO_2 measurements, thus reflecting the net effect of oxygen offer and demand at tissue level. The most important reason, however, is the discrepancy noted between brain tissue and CSF-pO_2 during the reperfusion fase after very low CPP values. This discrepancy is probably caused by restoration of perfusion of the larger capillaries of the choroid plexus, whilst brain tissue reperfusion does not occur due to irreversible ischaemic damage.

In the experiments performed a sharp fall of brain temperature was noted at CPP levels below 40 mmHg. This probably reflects the development of severe ischaemia. Combined monitoring of brain tissue pO_2 and brain temperature would seem to be indicated. We should hope that brain tissue pO_2 monitoring could indicate the critical perfusion pressure in individual patients below which a relative risk of ischaemia is present. Brain temperature monitoring would show the absolute critical level of CPP for development of brain ischemia.

References

1. Chan KH, Dearden NM, Miller JD (1993) Multi modality monitoring of Intracranial Pressure therapy after Severe Brain Injury. In: Avezaat CJJ, van Eijndhoven JHM, Maas AIR, Tans JThJ (eds) Intracranial Pressure VIII, Springer, Berlin Heidelberg New York London Paris Tokyo Hong Kong Barcelona
2. Cruz J, Miner ME, Allen SJ, Alves WM, Gennarelli TA (1993) Relationship Between Cerebral Oxygenation and Perfusion Pressure in Acute Brain Injury. In: Avezaat CJJ, van Eijndhoven JHM, Maas AIR, Tans JThJ (eds) Intracranial Pressure VIII, Springer, Berlin Heidelberg New York London Paris Tokyo Hong Kong Barcelona
3. Dearden NM (1991) Jugular Bulb Venous Oxygen Saturation Monitoring in the Management of Severe Head Injury. Current Opinion in Anaesthesiology 4:279–286
4. Fleckenstein W, Maas AIR (1989) Continous recordings of oxygen pressure in the cerebrospinal fluid of cat, dog and men. Funktions Analyse biologischer Systeme. J. Grote and E. Witzleb Eds. Gustav Fischer Verlag Stuttgart-New York 19:211–224
5. Fleckenstein W, Maas AIR, Nollert G, de Jong DA (1990) Oxygen pressure in cerebrospinal fluid. 1: Dynamics of oxygen transfer at normal, increased and decreased oxygen offer. 2: Effects of hypocapnia and hypercapnia. In: AM Ehrly, W Fleckenstein, J Hauss, R Huch (eds) Clinical oxygen pressure measurements II, Blackwell Ueberreuter Wissenschaft Berlin: 368–395

6. Maas AIR, de Jong DA, Fleckenstein WA (1989) CSF oxygen tension and ICP. In: Hoff JT, Betz AL (eds) Intracranial pressure VII, Springer, Berlin Heidelberg New York London Paris Tokyo Hong Kong, pp 434–436
7. Midgley S, Dearden NM, Miller JD (1993) CPP and SJO_2 with ICP Reduction Therapy after Severe Head Injury. In: Avezaat CJJ, van Eijndhoven JHM, Maas AIR, Tans JThJ (eds) Intracranial pressure VIII, Springer, Berlin Heidelberg New York London Paris Tokyo Hong Kong Barcelona
8. Obrist WD, Langfitt ThW, Jaggi JL, Cruz J, Gennarelli ThA (1984) Cerebral blood flow and metabolism in comatose patients with acute head injury. Relationship to intracranial hypertension, J Neurosurg 61:241–253
9. Robertson CS, Narayan RK, Gokaslan ZL, Pahwa R, Grossman RG, Caram P, Allen E (1989) Cerebral arteriovenous oxygen difference as an estimate of cerebral blood flow in comatose patients, J Neurosurg 70:222–230

The Effect of Hypoxia on Intracranial Pressure and Cerebral Blood Flow

J.B. North[1], P.L. Reilly[1], D. Gorman[3], C. Grant[1], and G.L. Ludbrook[2]

[1] Departments of Neurosurgery, and [2] Anaesthesia, Royal Adelaide Hospital, North Terrace, Adelaide, South Australia 5000, Australia
[3] Royal New Zealand Naval Hospital, Naval Base, Auckland, New Zealand

Introduction

The cerebrovascular response to oxygen has been well described previously by McDowall and others [3, 5]. These studies were primarily directed towards observing changes in cerebral blood flow (CBF), rather than intracranial pressure (ICP). ICP was often not recorded, or if it was, a fluid filled catheter or cisternal needle and external transducer were used. In view of advances in ICP methodology in the form of catheter tip transducers, we decided to reinvestigate the ICP and CBF responses to hypoxia using this technique. We were also interested in the relationship between ICP and CBF.

In addition, a variety of anaesthetic agents have been used in previous studies, many of which are well known to significantly alter cerebro-vascular reflexes. Synthetic opioids have been shown to minimally affect these reflexes and therefore we chose to use alfentanil as an anaesthetic agent in this study [6, 9].

Methods

Eight New Zealand White rabbits were induced with halothane, anaesthetised with alfentanil, paralysed with gallamine and ventilated via a tacheostomy. The animal was then placed in a stereotaxic frame in the sphinx position. ICP was measured continuously using a Camino transducer placed in the subdural space via a frontal burrhole [8].

CBF was measured at intervals using the hydrogen clearance method [1]. Platinum electrodes 0.2 mm in diameter were inserted via burr holes into the right and left cerebral cortex, to a depth of 1 mm. Arterial blood was sampled from the femoral artery and blood gas analysis was performed by a micro technique using a Corning blood gas analyser.

Cortical somatosensory evoked potentials were recorded from an extradural electrode in the left somato-sensory area after a stimulus was applied to the right forepaw. We measured the first negative (N_1) and the second positive (P_2) wave voltages, and recorded the P_2–N_1 voltage [2].

After establishing control values for ICP and CBF on room air, hypoxia was produced in a stepwise manner by increasing the level of nitrogen in the inspired air of the breathing circuit. The PaO_2 was then reduced to about 60 mmHg, and CBF was measured. Preliminary work had shown that there were no ICP or CBF changes in the PaO_2 range of 60 to 100 mmHg. From 60 mmHg, further reductions in PaO_2 were made, each of about 10 mmHg, down to PaO_2 of 20 to 30 mmHg. Three CBF measurements were performed at each of these levels. Arterial PCO_2 levels were maintained within the range ±3 mmHg.

We analysed ICP and CBF data by plotting those values against PaO_2, fitting a polynomial regression curve to these data points.

Results

Figure 1 shows the pooled data showing the change in mean ICP as PaO_2 was lowered. There was no change in ICP until about 50 mmHg PaO_2. Below that level, we observed a progressive increase in ICP. There was a 1.5 mmHg increase in ICP when PaO_2 dropped to 35 mmHg, and a 2 mmHg increase at PaO_2 levels of 25 mmHg. The ICP data in figure 1 refers to the peak ICP value

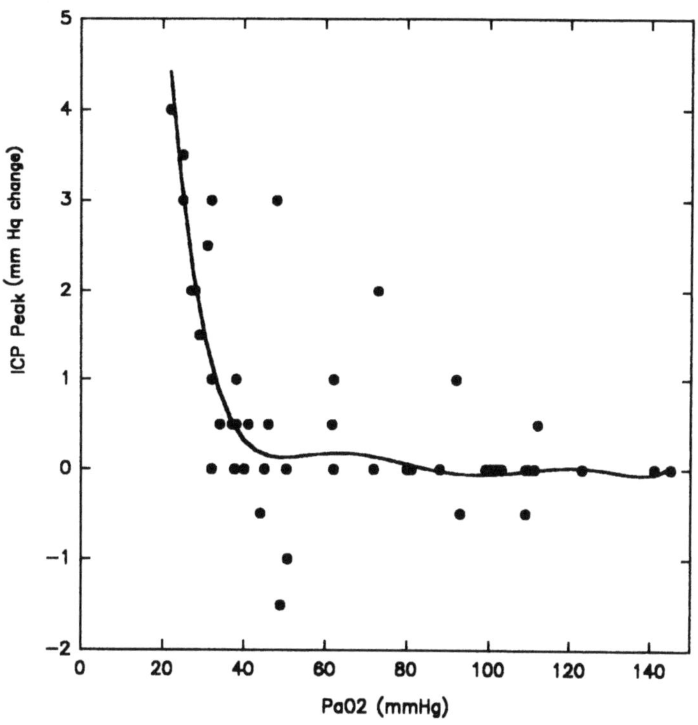

Fig. 1. The relationship between PaO_2 and mean ICP, measured in mmHg at a peak

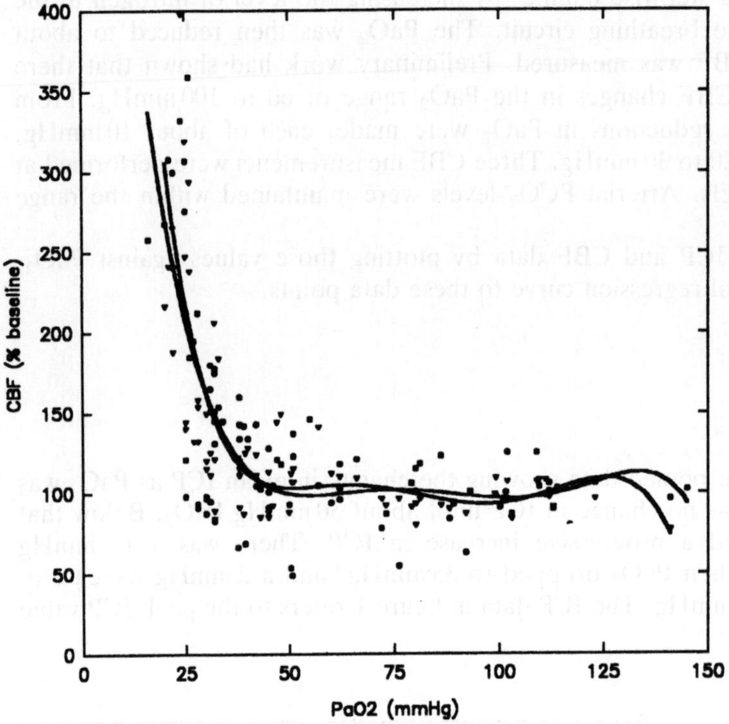

Fig. 2. The relationship between PaO_2 and right and left cortical CBF

observed after each decrement in PaO_2. We observed that this rise was not sustained, and tended to return towards the previous level.

Figure 2 shows CBF measurements plotted against PaO_2. No change was observed from normoxia down to a PaO_2 of 50 mmHg. Below that, CBF increased progressively, with a 150% increase from baseline at a PaO_2 of 30 mmHg and a 200% increase at a PaO_2 of 25 mmHg. There was no difference between right and left hemisphere flows. Cerebral perfusion pressure remained constant. Systemic arterial pressure only fell when a PaO_2 of 20 mmHg was reached and this heralded a terminal event; this data was excluded. The ICP rise was transient and fell after 5 minutes of each new condition of hypoxia. Figure 3 shows ICP and CBF data at PaO_2 levels between 20 and 30 mmHg. The degree of hypoxia is constant during the times indicated on the y axis. For the first 5 minutes, ICP and CBF rose at the same rate. Following that time, ICP falls towards baseline, whereas CBF remains relatively constant. This divergence between ICP and CBF after 5 min is an apparent trend and does not reach statistical significance. However, it was a consistent finding.

Cortical somatosensory evoked responses remained unchanged throughout most levels of hypoxia (Fig. 4). In some of the animals, the evoked responses suddenly dropped at very low levels of PaO_2, but this was usually a terminal event.

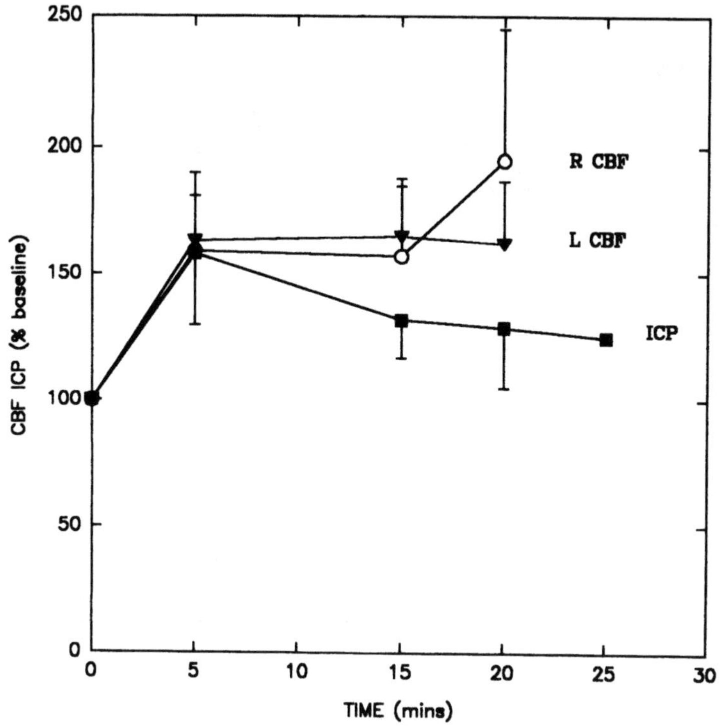

Fig. 3. The relationship between mean ICP and CBF (% baseline) during periods of constant hypoxia. Mean data from runs at PaO_2 20–22 mmHg (+SEM)

Discussion

We have confirmed that ICP rises in response to hypoxia in animals. This response begins at PaO_2 levels of 50 mmHg and rises steeply below that. We found an almost identical rise in cortical CBF as measured by the hydrogen clearance method. Thus we have confirmed the relationship described by McDowall and others with regard to CBF and hypoxia, adding ICP data to these CBF findings.

The close similarity between the ICP and CBF response to hypoxia may confirm that initially at least, ICP passively follows the vasodilatation seen in hypoxia. We observed similar rates of change in both ICP and CBF when hypoxia was first produced. Likewise, both ICP and CBF began to rise at comparable levels of PaO_2. The exact mechanism by which this occurs seems unclear to us but a direct effect of oxygen on vessel walls and lactacidosis have both been suggested.

The fall of mean ICP after 5 minutes of hypoxia in the presence of relatively constant CBF may indicate that a compensating mechanism is acting. Krasney has suggested that the primary CBF response to hypoxia does not adapt [4].

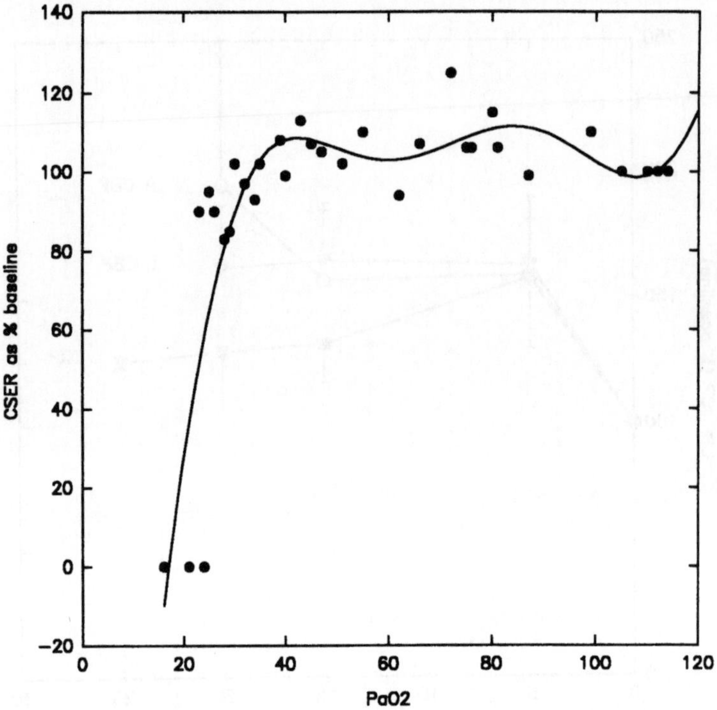

Fig. 4. The relationship between PaO_2 (mmHg) and cortical somatosensory evoked responses (% baseline)

Presumably the pressure/volume status of our animals was intact and this compensation may have occurred through the known avenue of CSF displacement out of the cranium [7].

Our experience was that the animals tolerated severe degrees of hypoxia for periods of several hours. Previous experience in rabbits and other animals indicates a poorer tolerance of hypoxia. Perhaps our use of alfentanil as an anaesthetic agent may be a partial explanation of this tendency.

Conclusions

1. In an animal series to investigate ICP responses to hypoxia, we concluded that ICP and cortical CBF were unchanged until a PaO_2 of 50 mmHg was reached and then they both rose in a similar manner. This may mean that there is a common mechanism causing each to change, perhaps simply through changes in cerebral blood volume.
2. We observed a trend where ICP fell from a peak after 5 minutes of hypoxia, with persisting elevation of CBF.
3. In this model, cerebral function as measured by cortical evoked responses was preserved down to PaO_2 20 mmHg.

References

1. Aukland K, Bower FB, Berliner RW (1964) Measurement of local blood flow with hydrogen gas. Circ Res 14:164–187
2. Iragui-Madoz VJ, Wiederholt WC (1977) Far-field somatosensory evoked potentials in the cat. Electroencephalogr Clin Neurophysiol 43:646–657
3. Jones MD, Traystman RJ, Simmons MA, Molten RA (1981) Effects of changes in arterial O_2 content on cerebral blood flow in the lamb. Am J Physiol 240:H209–215
4. Krasney JA, Jensen JB, Lassen NA (1990) Cerebral Blood Flow Does Not Adapt to Sustained Hypoxia. J Cereb Blood Flow Metab 10:759–764
5. McDowall DG (1966) Interrelationships between blood oxygen tensions and cerebral blood flow. In: Payne JP, Hill DW (eds) A Symposium on Oxygen measurements in Blood and Tissues. Churchill, London, pp 205–219
6. Milde LN, Milde JH, Gallagher WJ (1989) Cerebral effects of fentanyl in dogs. Brit J Anaesth 63:710–715
7. Miller JD (1985) Head Injury And Brain Ischaemia- Implications For Therapy. Brit J Anaesth 57:120–130
8. Ostrup RC, Luerssen TG, Marshall LF, Zornow MH (1987) Continuous monitoring of intracranial pressure with a minaturized fiberoptic device. J Neurosurg 67:206–209
9. Sebel PS, Bovil JG, Van Der Haven A (1982) Cardiovascular effects of alfentanil anaesthesia. Brit J Anaesth 54:1185–1189

Intracranial Hypotension: A Feline Model and Effects on Cerebral Blood Flow

S. Pomeranz[1], L. Beni[1], J. Gomori[2], and M. Shalit[1]

[1] Departments of Neurosurgery and [2] Radiology, Hadassah University Hospital, Ein Karem, Jerusalem 91120, Israel

Introduction

Intracranial hypotension is a frequently noted phenomenon in the clinical neurosurgical setting [1, 3, 4, 5, 9]. A typical picture of severe headaches, nausea, general malaise, and occasionally, decreased consciousness are the well-known nonspecific hallmarks of this syndrome [1]. A variety of situations such as traumatic cerebrospinal fluid (CSF) leak, lumbar puncture or continuous CSF drainage, craniotomy, intra- and extracranial drainage systems, overdrained hydrocephalus, and spontaneous intracranial hypotension have been described as causative [3, 4, 5, 9].

Though the clinical spectrum of intracranial hypotension is well known, its pathophysiology is obscure. Singular animal models of this pathology have been described [2], and no clear physiological correlates have been demonstrated. In 1953 Shenkin [8] proposed decreased cerebral blood flow (averaging 34 cc/100 g/min) as the cause of impaired consciousness in three patients following the evacuation of subdural hematomas with a relatively low intracranial pressure of +30 mm water. This explanation has not been accepted in the relevant literature. We know of no systematic study describing basic physiological changes secondary to intracranial hypotension and no study that has attempted to understand the mediators of the symptoms in this entity. The purpose of this study was to develop an animal model of intracranial hypotension to study the cause of the symptomatology of intracranial hypotension.

A preliminary study (unpublished results) in our laboratory in four cats, draining CSF from the cisterna magna to attain a negative lateral ventricular pressure of up to −10 torr for up to four hours with a stable normal arterial blood pressure, did not result in any change in the thalamic, caudate nucleus, or cerebral cortical blood flows as measured by the H_2 clearance technique [10]. This study was similar in method and degree of maximal intraventricular hypotension to that by Blanks et al. [2] in rabbits. The purpose of the present study was to produce a greater degree of intracranial hypotension than in the previous studies and to observe the accompanying cerebral blood flows.

Materials and Methods

Eleven mongrel cats weighing 2.5–3.0 kg underwent injection of a sterile suspension of 150 mg kaolin in normal saline into the cisterna magna. Computerized tomography was performed 45–70 days following the injection to demonstrate that the maximal width of the lateral ventricles was at least 0.4 of the width of the brain at that level. The cats were anesthesized with intraperitoneal pentobarbitone 30 mg/kg. An inguinal artery and vein were catheterized and a tracheostomy was placed. The rectal temperature was continuously measured and maintained between 37.5–38.5°C by a heating pad under the cat. The electrocardiogram, arterial pressure, and end-tidal pCO_2 were constantly monitored. The cats were paralyzed with 0.2 mg intravenous pancuronium as needed and mechanically ventilated to maintain an arterial pCO_2 of 38–42 torr. In a stereotactic frame, according to stereotactic coordinates, 1 mm diameter holes were drilled in the skull. A plastic cannula, 1 mm outer diameter, was inserted into each of the lateral ventricles. 0.3 mm diameter epoxy coated platinum electrodes, with the distal 1 mm exposed, were inserted 1.5 mm deep into the anterior and posterior cerebral cortex, and into the thalamus and caudate nucleus, all on the right side. All the holes in the calvarium were sealed, and the catheters and electrodes fixed with acrylic adhesive. Intracranial hypotension was created by connecting the left ventricular catheter to saline-filled tubing and draining by gravity. The hypotension was regulated by adjusting the height of the free end of the tubing while monitoring the right ventricular pressure.

The regional cerebral blood flows were measured by the H_2 clearance method [10] following several seconds of breathing a 75% H_2:25% O_2 mixture. At the end of the experiment the cat was killed by administering pentobarbitone and air intravenously. The brain was fixed in formalin and coronally sectioned to ascertain catheter and electrode placement.

Statistical comparison of the cerebral blood flows and arterial blood pressures was done utilizing the T-test.

Results

The initial lateral ventricular mean pressure in these cats was 4.8 ± 2.5 (standard deviation) torr. In two cats the intraventricular pressure was decreased by drainage to −80 torr. This pressure was maintained for 9 and 12 minutes, when the CSF stopped draining from the left ventricle and the right ventricular pressure rapidly rose in both cats to 3 and 6 torr, and could not be reduced by attempted additional CSF drainage. Four cats had intraventricular pressure reduction to −35 torr, which could be maintained for an average of 28 minutes (range 14–39 minutes), when the CSF ceased to drain and the contralateral ventricular pressure rose to an average of 4 torr. Seven cats had CSF drainage to bring the contralateral ventricular pressure to −15 torr. Of these cats, two had a rise to pressure to 2 and 4 torr after 165 and

215 minutes respectively. The other five cats maintained this intracranial hypotension until the end of the experiment, for at least four hours. Multiple simultaneous pressure measurements of both lateral ventricles while CSF drainage was momentarily stopped, showed interventricular differences no greater than 2 torr in all of the cats.

Following at least two baseline measurements, the cerebral blood flows were measured once for the cats with intracranial hypotension of −80 and −35 torr, 3 and 10 minutes respectively, after reaching the target pressures. The cats with intracranial pressure of −15 torr underwent blood flow measurements every approximately 35 minutes. The resulting cerebral blood flows are presented in Table 1. There were no significant changes in cerebral blood flow at any of the electrode sites for any of the intracranial pressure groups or for the combination of the groups between the baseline values and the flows during intracranial hypotension. The mean arterial pressure average for all of the cats before CSF drainage was 118 ± 13 torr and during drainage 113 ± 13 torr, an average decrease of 4%. The mean CSF volume drained per cat was 3.5 cc.

Examination of the formalin-fixed brains of the cats showed that the ventricular catheters had been in place in all of them and that all of the cats whose pressure rose when the CSF ceased to drain had collapse of the ventricles. Those cats that continued to drain CSF and maintain intracranial hypotension to the end of the experiment had moderately dilated ventricles, with the drained ventricle invariably smaller than its contralateral counterpart.

Discussion

Intracranial hypotension is an important clinical entity due to the spectrum of circumstances within which it arises and the possible dire consequences, including loss of consciousness and death. An experimental model with values

Table 1. Combined regional cerebral blood flows (CBF) of 11 hydrocephalic cats before and during intracranial hypotension of −15 to −80 torr (see text for durations)

Region of CBF	Stage of CSF drainage	Mean CBF cc/100 gr/min	% Change in CBF	p-Value
Anterior cerebral cortex	baseline	29.6 ± 9.6	−8	0.57
	during	27.1 ± 8.2		
Thalamus	baseline	15.1 ± 5.5	+8	0.60
	during	16.3 ± 3.7		
Caudate nucleus	baseline	14.3 ± 4.5	+10	0.46
	during	15.8 ± 4.0		
Posterior cerebral cortex	baseline	23.8 ± 4.9	+5	0.75
	during	25.1 ± 6.6		

of intracranial hypotension of -20 cm H_2O as measured by Foltz [5] in symptomatic shunted hydrocephalic patients has not been described. The most appropriate animal model was described by Foltz himself in rabbits [2], with acute CSF drainage from the cisterna magna to attain a lateral ventricular pressure of 15 cm H_2O *less than the initial pressure*. In an attempt to emulate Foltz's model we obtained intracranial hypotension of -24 torr (-31 cm H_2O) for a few minutes and up to -10 torr during several hours in cats. These results are similar to those of Foltz, even with extreme negative cisterna magna values of -90 torr. This transtentorial pressure gradient is apparently due to the same known mechanism of such a gradient in increased ICP. This gradient limits the degree of intracranial hypotension that can be created in this model.

The kaolin-induced hydrocephalic model presented here produced a greater degree of hydrocephalus and substantially lower initial ventricular pressures than more acute preparations following kaolin administration (our unpublished results). This suggests a pressure "compensation" by the brain parenchyma and perhaps intracranial venous space contraction. This balance allows a consistent drainage of CSF from a lateral ventricle to maintain intracranial hypotension of up to -15 torr for several hours.

A criticism could be made of this model, that it is secondary to the artificial induction of hydrocephalus with kaolin, and thereby may give a distorted picture of intracranial hypotension pathophysiology. It is accepted that the mechanism of hydrocephalus induction by kaolin is absorptive at the arachnoid villi and does not directly affect the cerebral parenchyma itself [6]. Moreover, many of the patients with symptomatic intracranial hypotension are hydrocephalic.

According to classical neurophysiology, the cerebral perfusion pressure (CPP) equals the mean arterial pressure (MAP) less the intracranial pressure (ICP) (assuming the sagittal sinus pressure (SSP) to be normally minimal and therefore negligible). Cerebral vascular autoregulation is the maintenance of a stable cerebral blood flow (CBF) in spite of changes in the CPP due to changes in the MAP, ICP, or SSP. To the best of our knowledge, this is the first report of autoregulation with increased CPP due to decreased ICP. It implies that cerebral vasoconstriction occurs secondary to the increased CPP (according to the classical definition) that is the result of a prominently negative ICP. Traystman et al. [7] have demonstrated, at least for positive ICPs, that the higher of the ICP or SSP determines the back pressure for cerebral perfusion and that the lower value of the two is not a factor in determining the CPP. Their work implies that this holds true for negative ICPs, and that the CPP and CBF would not be expected to change as a result of the ICP becoming increasingly negative. Our findings support the observations and conclusions of Traystman. It is possible though, that the negative ICP is at least partially transmitted to the cerebral venous space through the vessel walls and thereby increases the CPP. This could be a regional phenomenon within the brain and not necessarily a global intracranial effect, depending on vein wall compliance and venous backflow secondary to the intravascular pressure gradients.

We conclude that cerebral blood flow is unchanged with prominently negative ICP and therefore the symptomatology of negative ICP is not due to a change in the cerebral blood flow. The significance of unchanged cerebral blood flow during overt intracranial hypotension is yet to be determined. The model presented should be useful in further investigating the pathophysiology of negative ICP and the cause of its symptoms.

References

1. Bell WE, Joynt RJ, Sahs AL (1960) Low spinal fluid pressure syndromes. Neurology (Minneap) 10:512–521
2. Blanks JP, McPherson D, Foltz EL (1985) Acute negative intracranial pressure effects on the auditory evoked response in rabbits. Neurosurgery 17:877–882
3. Chorobski J (1950) Postoperative Intracranial Hypotension. J. Neurol Neurosurg and Psychiat 13:280
4. Dana C (1917) Puncture headache. JAMA 68:1017
5. Foltz EL, Blanks JP (1988) Symptomatic low intracranial pressure in shunted hydrocephalus. J Neurosurg 68:401–408
6. Ingraham FD, Alexander E, Matson DD (1947) Experimental Hydrocephalus. J Neurosurgery 4:164–176
7. McPherson RW, Koehler RC, Traystman RJ (1988) Effect of jugular venous pressure on cerebral autoregulation in dogs. Am J Physiol 255:H1516–H1524
8. Shenkin H (1953) The cerebral circulation in postoperative intracranial hypotension. J Neurosurg 10:48–51
9. Shenkin H, Finnenson B (1958) Clinical significance of low cerebral spinal fluid pressure. Neurology 8:157
10. Young W (1980) H_2 Clearance measurement of blood flow: a review of technique and polarographic principles. Stroke 11:552–564

Change of Cerebral Electrophysiological Activity, Regional Cerebral Blood Flow and Regional Cerebral Blood Volume in Acute Intracranial Hypertension

T. KOJIMA, K. IWAT, and K. TAMAI

Department of Neurological Surgery, Aichi Medical University, Aichi-ken Japan

Introduction

The intracranial volume is composed of three components, i.e. cerebral parenchyma, cerebrospinal fluid and blood. In case of the presence of space-occupying lesions such as cerebral hemorrhage, brain tumor, etc., it is thought that intracranial pressure (ICP) is determined by these three components.

In recent years, the measurement of time-courses of cerebral blood flow (CBF) and cerebral blood volume (CBV) in vivo has become possible, leading to subsequent measurement of the change in cerebral blood circulation to cope with intracranial hypertension. In the present study, we made consecutive measurements of ICP, CBF and CBV in the epidural balloon expansion model and we examined the cerebral blood circulatory dynamics in acute intracranial hypertension.

Material and Methods

Adult male cats, weighing 2–3 kg, were used. The cats were anaesthetized with i.v. injection of ketamine hydrochloride (5–10 mg), tracheostomized, immobilized with pancuronium bromide (0.005 mg/kg/min), and kept on controlled ventilation. The systemic arterial pressure was measured in the femoral artery. After minor craniotomy, intracranial hypertension was produced by expansion of an epidural balloon and ICP was measured by the Camino device. Regional cerebral blood flow (r-CBF) was measured by a heat clearance type tissue blood flowmeter embedded in the subdural space. Regional cerebral blood volume (r-CBV) was measured by a measuring probe put on the cerebral surface, using a reflection spectrophotometer (Biomedical Science Co., Ltd.).

In experiment A, the epidural balloon was inflated with physiological saline using a continuous infusion pump and anisocoria was caused for 15 minutes. Changes in BP, ICP, r-CBF, r-CBV and EEG were measured for 2 hours after decompression of the balloon.

In experiment B, pressurization was repeated until mydriasis appeared and the EEG became flat; changes were recorded after decompression.

Results

Before the start of the experiments, BP, ICP, r-CBF and r-CBV were 97.8 ± 16.9 mmHg, 63 ± 4.5 mmHg, 49.1 ± 7.4 ml/100g/min and control 100%, respectively.

Experiment A. As ICP began to rise, r-CBF increased and when ICP became above 20 and 30 mmHg, r-CBF and r-CBV started to decrease. Anisocoria appeared when the ICP rose above 45 mmHg. Decompression 15 minutes later led to an abrupt decrease in ICP and transient increases in r-CBF and r-CBV, after which both r-CBF and r-CBV recovered to control values (Fig. 1).

Experiment B. At ICP > 80–100 mmHg, r-CBF fell to 15.3 ± 2.2 ml/100g/min, mydriasis occurred and the EEG became flat. More pressurization and subsequent 30 min-decompression led to a decrease in ICP and subsequent re-increase. r-CBF and r-CBV increased temporarily, but with a further increase in ICP, r-CBF became oligemic and r-CBV showed no difference from the control value. No recovery of the EEG was noted (Fig. 2).

Discussion

r-CBV was measured by means of reflection spectrophotometry in which cerebral tissue is illuminated with white light and analysis of the Hb absorption spectrum is made from the difference between absorption at 569 mm not

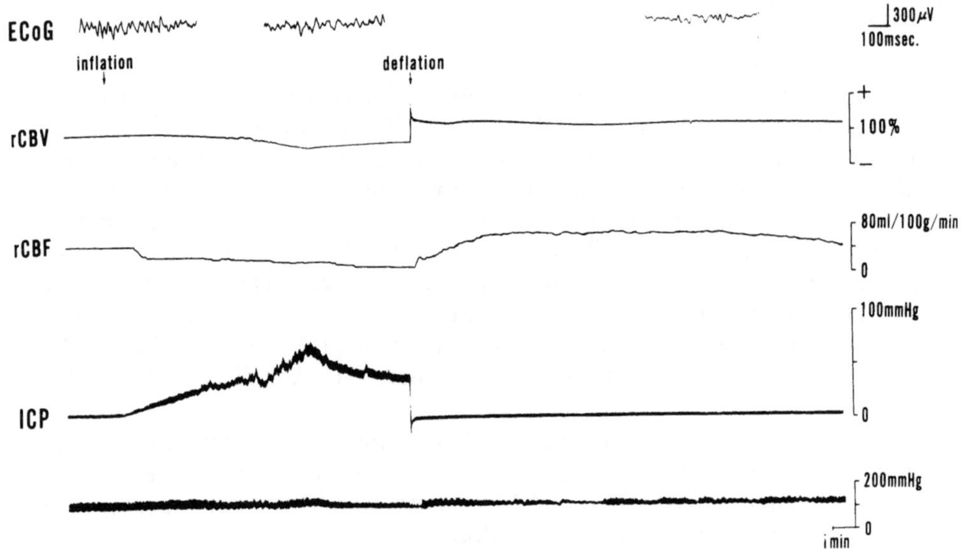

Fig. 1. Polygraphic illustration of ICP, BP, r-CBF, r-CBV and ECoG in cat (A)

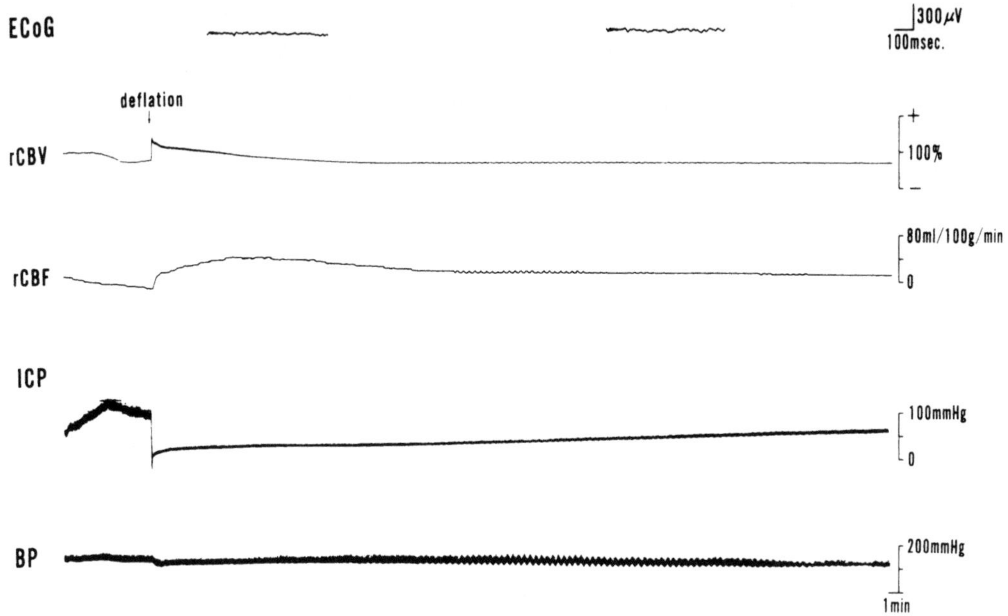

Fig. 2. Polygraphic illustration of ICP, BP, r-CBF, r-CBV and ECoG in cat (B)

influenced by oxidation and reduction and absorption at 650 mm not influenced by Hb. However, the measurement is not quantitative and yields relative changes.

With an increase in ICP, CBF initially remained unchanged and CBV increased, and with further increase in ICP, both CBF and CBV decreased. The first increase in CBV is thought to be caused by the relaxation of the resistance vessels under the influence of small vein blood flow disturbance at the cerebral surface, but with further increase in ICP, mechanical vessel compression rather than venous reflux disturbance is thought to cause a decrease in CBF and CBV. This requires further study of the venous side of the cerebral vascular bed.

In experiment A, transient increases in CBF and CBV were observed after decompression, but no new increase in ICP was observed. In experiment B, however, ICP increased again after balloon deflation, but CBF and CBV did not increase above their control values.

This suggests that intracranial hypertension after decompression can not be explained by high perfusion hyperemia.

References

1. Kuhl DE, Alavi A, Hoffman EJ, Phelps ME, Zimmerman RA, Obrist WD, Bruce DA, Greenberg JH, Uzzel B (1980) Local cerebral blood volume in head injured patients. J Neurosurg 52:309–320

2. Langfitt TW, Weinstein JD, Sklar HS, Zaren HA, Kassel NF (1968) Contribution of intracranial blood volume to three forms of experimental brain swelling. John Hopkins Med J 122:261–270
3. Lowell HM, Bloor BM (1971) The effect of increased intracranial pressure on cerebrovascular hemodynamics. J Neurosurg 34:760–769

Local Cerebral Blood Flow Mapping Before and After Removal of Acute Subdural Hematoma in the Rat

Y. Kuroda, K. Kusumoto, G.M. Teasdale, and R. Bullock

Department of Neurosurgery, Institute of Neurological Sciences, Southern General Hospital, Glasgow G51 4TF, Scotland
Wellcome Surgical Institute, Garscube Estate, Bearsden Road, Glasgow, G61 1QH, Scotland

Introduction

High intracranial pressure (ICP) and hemispheric swelling occurs post-operatively in about 60–70% of patients with acute subdural hematomas (SDH) [5], and this may present great difficulty for the neurosurgeon. The cause for this swelling remains unknown. In order to study this process, we have used a model of acute subdural hematoma in the rat, to compare local cerebral blood flow (LCBF), and ischemic tissue volume before and after removal of the hematoma. We have also measured the change in hemispheric volume, by making a comparison between the ipsilateral and the contralateral hemisphere, four hours after inducing the hematoma.

Materials and Methods

Six adult Sprague-Dawley rats were anesthetised and mechanically ventilated to maintain $Paco_2$ between 35–41 mmHg. Femoral arteries and veins were cannulated bilaterally. Mean arterial blood pressure, blood gases, and rectal temperature were measured throughout, and maintained within the physiological range.

To produce the hematoma, a scalp incision was made, and a 3 mm burr hole was drilled 2 mm to the left side of the sagittal suture and 1 mm posterior to the coronal suture. A blunt "J" shaped 23 gauge needle was inserted subdurally and cemented to the skull. Four hundred ul non-heparinised autologous blood was then injected over 7 minutes [4]. Three hours after induction of the SDH, a craniotomy measuring 15 mm × 8 mm was performed with a dental drill and the hematoma was removed using the operating microscope and the scalp closed.

Double Label Autoradiographic Measurement of LCBF

^{99m}Tc labelled d,l-hexamethyl propylene amine oxime (HMPAO) was used to measure LCBF with the hematoma in situ, two hours after induction of the SDH [2].

LCBF was measured one hour after removal of the hematoma, using ^{14}C-iodoantipyrene (IAP) by the method of Sakurada [7]. After the 30 second IAP infusion, the anaesthetised animals were decapitated, the brains were removed and frozen (−42°C). Coronal sections were cut, mounted on glass cover slips, and immediately incubated for four hours against ^{3}H sensitive x-ray film together with pre-calibrated standards, to obtain the [^{99m}Tc] HMPAO autoradiogram. The sections were then removed from the film, and left to stand for three days to allow all remaining Technetium radioactivity to decay. The same brain sections were then incubated for two weeks against Kodak GRL film to obtain the IAP autoradiogram.

The tissue concentrations of ^{99m}Tc-HMPAO were measured by densitometry and normalised to the contralateral (right) caudate nucleus. Lassen's correction (alpha = 2) was applied [2]. LCBF after removal of hematoma was calculated from the tissue ^{14}C-IAP concentration, using the equation of Sakurada [7] and normalised to the contralateral caudate nucleus.

To measure hemispheric and ischemic volume, eight brain sections at predetermined stereotaxic planes were examined [6]. The area of ischemia at each section was measured using an image analysing computer and the volume obtained by integrating the areas. The ischemic threshold for IAP was taken to be $25\,ml \cdot 100g^{-1}1^{1} \cdot min^{-1}$, corresponding to half the optical density of white matter, on the HMPAO film.

Results

Figure 1 demonstrates the patterns of LCBF change before and after removal of the subdural hematoma. The zone of profound ischemia enlarged significantly after removal of the hematoma. The ischemic volume with the hematoma in situ (HMPAO) was $98 \pm 25\,mm^3$ ($19 \pm 5\%$ of hemisphere volume). After hematoma removal (IAP) this increased to $144 \pm 17\,mm^3$ ($26 \pm 3\%$ of hemisphere volume) ($p < 0.01$ paired t-test). Reperfusion after hematoma removal was not observed within the previously ischemic cortex. Hyperaemia (over $230\,ml \cdot 100\,g^{-1} \cdot min^{-1}$) was, however, seen in some animals in the thalamus after hematoma removal. Enlargement of the ischemic area was associated with a 60% decrease in LCBF in the peri-ischemic region, after hematoma removal ($p < 0.05$ paired t-test). The ipsilateral hemispheric volume ($552 \pm 10\,mm^3$) was significantly increased in comparison with the contralateral side ($494 \pm 10\,mm^3$). ($p < 0.01$ unpaired t-test)

Discussion

This study has shown that even though the hematoma was removed surgically three hours after its induction, the volume of the cortical ischemic zone enlarged significantly.

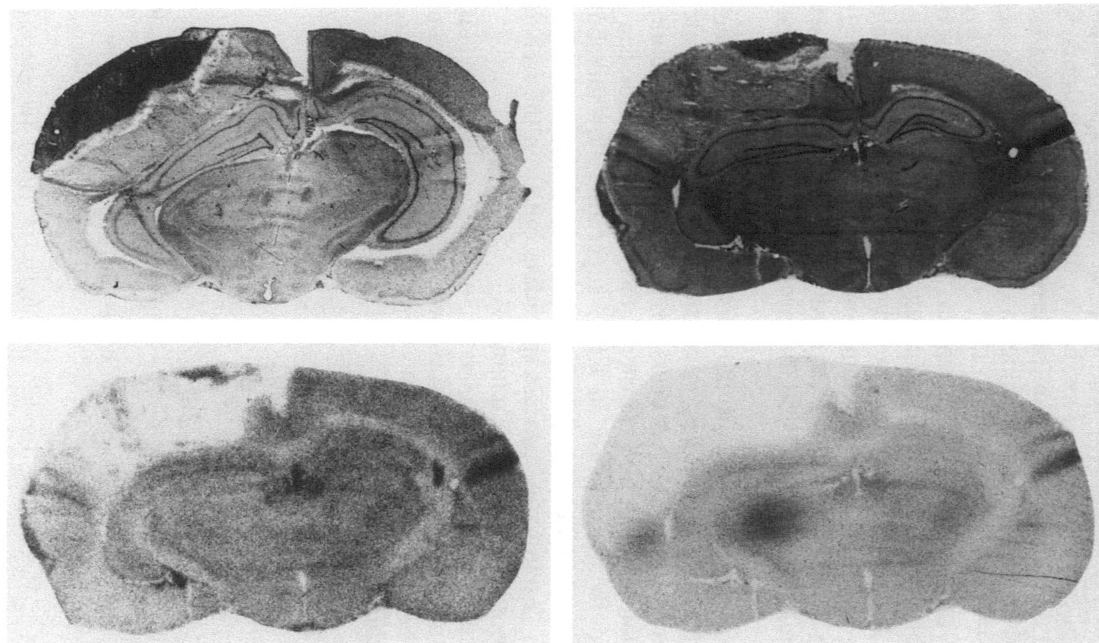

Fig. 1. **a** H + E stained histological section (×10) through the hippocampal region, three and a half hours after subdural hematoma. Note the zone of underlying ischemia damage. (From a previous study). **b** H + E stained section (×10) 1 hour after hematoma removal. **c** ^{99m}Tc-HMPAO CBF autoradiogram from the same section as top right. Note the zone of ischemia corresponding to the area of histological damage and pallor of staining. **d** ^{14}C-IAP CBF autoradiogram from the same section as top right. Note enlargement of the ischemic zone (CBF $< 25\,ml \cdot 100\,g^{-1} \cdot min^{-1}$) and patchy hyperaemia (CBF $= 240\,ml \cdot 100\,g^{-1} \cdot min^{-1}$)

After hematoma removal, the brain was swollen, with slight herniation into the craniotomy defect, similar to appearances at surgery in some patients. Ipsilateral hemisphere volume at four hours after the hematoma was significantly increased compared to the contralateral side, but this was largely due to enlargement of the ischemic zone, which was edematous, as judged by pallor of staining on H + E sections. In two of the six animals, patches of hyperaemia were seen in the thalamus and basal ganglia, which may be a less important contributing factor to the hemisphere swelling.

In other studies with this model, we have shown that ICP is elevated to >100 mmHg five minutes after hematoma induction, and remains 2–3 times above normal up to four hours [3]. Cerebral perfusion pressure is well preserved after the initial surge of ICP, so that prolonged global ischemia does not occur.

The progressive enlargement of the zone of focal ischemia seen in this model, despite hematoma removal, is consistent with our previous studies, which indicate an "excitotoxic" process in the peri-ischemic zone, characterised by glutamate release, and transient glucose hypermetabolism [1]. This is unaccompanied by an increase in CBF, suggesting flow-metabolism uncoupling. These data invite the speculation that ischaemic damage may be propagated by an "excitotoxic" process spreading out from the ischemic core, which is *uninfluenced* by hematoma removal.

We further speculate that a vasospastic process, induced by the clotted subdural blood, may initiate focal cortical ischemia under the hematoma, and that this process persists after hematoma removal. Further studies are needed to more fully evaluate these events.

References

1. Bullock R, Butcher S, Chen M-H, Kendall L, McCulloch J (1991) Extracellular glutamate concentration correlates with the extent of blood flow reduction after subdural hematoma in the rat. J Neurosurg (In press)
2. Bullock R, Patterson J, Park C, McCulloch J, Wyper D (1991) Estimation of ^{99m}Tc HMPAO cerebral blood flow mapping in cerebral ischemia: A double label autoradiographic study. Stroke (In press)
3. Kuroda Y, Strebel S, McCulloch J, Teasdale GM, Bullock R (1993) The effects of NMDA antagonists on intracranial pressure in a model of acute subdural haematoma in the rat. In: Avezaat CJJ, van Eijndhoven JHM, Maas AIR, Tans JThJ (eds) Intracranial pressure VIII. Springer, Berlin Heidelberg New York London Paris Tokyo Hong Kong Barcelona
4. Miller JD, Bullock R, Graham DI, Chen MH, Teasdale GM (1990) Ischemic brain damage in a model of acute subdural hematoma. Neurosurgery 27:433–439
5. Miller JD, Butterworth JF, Gudeman SK, et al. (1981) Further experience in the management of severe head injury. J Neurosurg 54:289–299
6. Osborne KA, Shigeno T, Balarsky AM, Ford I, McCulloch J, Teasdale GM, Graham DI (1987) Quantitative assessment of early brain damage in a rat model of focal cerebral ischemia. J Neurol Neurosurg Psychiatry 50:402–410
7. Sakurada O, Kennedy C, Jehle J, Brown JD, Carbin GL, Sokoloff L (1978) Measurement of local cerebral blood flow with iodo[^{14}C]antipyrine. Am J Physiol 234:H59–H66

The Effects of NMDA Antagonists on Intracranial Pressure in a Model of Acute Subdural Haematoma in the Rat

Y. Kuroda, S. Strebel, J McCulloch, G.M. Teasdale, and R. Bullock

Department of Neurosurgery, Institute of Neurological Sciences, and Wellcome Surgical Institute, University of Glasgow, Glasgow, G12 8QQ, Scotland

Introduction

NMDA antagonists have demonstrated neuroprotective efficacy in reducing focal cerebral ischaemic damage in many laboratory studies [1, 4, 6]. Patients with high intracranial pressure (ICP) due to head injury, stroke and subarachnoid haemorrhage are likely to be among the first candidates for these drugs, yet their effects on ICP are unknown.

In this study, we have used a rat model of acute subdural haematoma (SDH), which produces high ICP [5], to evaluate the effect of neuroprotective doses of the competitive NMDA antagonist D-CPP-ene and the noncompetitive NMDA antagonist MK801 upon ICP and cerebral perfusion pressure (CPP). We have compared their effects to those seen in a positive control group (20% mannitol) and a negative control group (0.9% saline).

Materials and Methods

Thirty adult male Sprague-Dawley rats weighing 310–520 g were divided into four treatment groups: (six animals in each group): (1) physiological saline 1 ml/kg; (2) 20% mannitol 1 g/kg; (3) D-CPP-ene 4.5 mg/kg; and (4) MK801 0.5 mg/kg. The drugs were given as a slow (5 minute) intravenous bolus.

Under 2% isoflurane and 70% nitrous oxide anaesthesia, tracheostomy was performed, unilateral femoral artery and vein were cannulated and mechanical ventilation was commenced. Blood gases and rectal temperature were maintained within the physiological range, using a heating pad, and by adjusting the ventilator. The animals' head was immobilised in a stereotaxic frame. For the induction of the subdural haematoma, a "J"-shaped needle was inserted into the subdural space over the left parietal cortex, and cemented into position, thus sealing the burr hole [5]. ICP was measured continuously using a zero calibrated fiberoptic implanted device through a burr hole over the right parietal cortex. (Camino Laboratories, San Diego, California) [7]. After completion of surgery, the isoflurane concentration was decreased to 1%. The haematoma was induced by injecting 350 ul non-heparinised autologous venous blood into the subdural space. Twenty-five minutes after induction of the subdural haematoma, the drugs were infused intravenously. Mean arterial blood pressure (MABP), ICP, and cerebral perfusion pressure (CPP: MABP-ICP) were measured for four hours. $PaCO_2$ was carefully controlled throughout the procedure and did not vary by more than 5 mmHg (38–43 mmHg).

Statistical differences were tested by a one-way analysis of variance and the Bonferroni method. To test the overall effect of the drugs upon ICP, MABP, and CPP the mean values for eight time points over 210 minutes were obtained for each animal, giving 48 observations per group (Table 2). Significance was assumed at $p < 0.05$. All values were expressed as mean ± SEM.

Results

The peak ICP increased to 125 ± 7 mmHg five minutes after induction of haematoma, for all animals. It decreased to 22 ± 2 mmHg by 25 minutes after the haematoma, the time point at which the drug infusions were commenced. CPP was maintained over 50 mmHg except during the induction of haematoma (Fig. 1). Prior to drug infusion, there were no significant differences in the haemodynamic parameters between the four groups (Table 1).

Table 2 shows the haemodynamic parameters after the drugs were given. For the mannitol treated group, MABP (13%) and CPP (14%) were significantly higher than the saline group. None of the NMDA antagonists increased

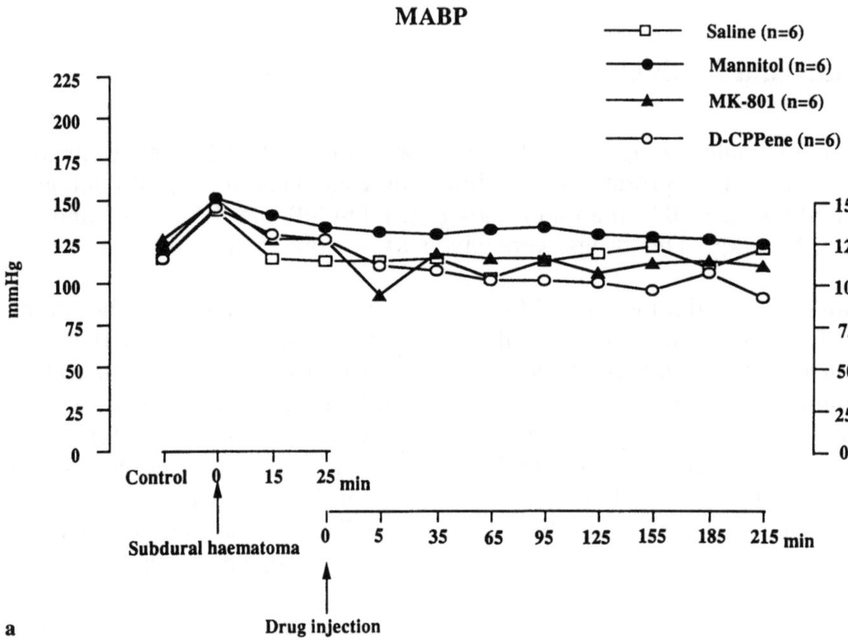

a

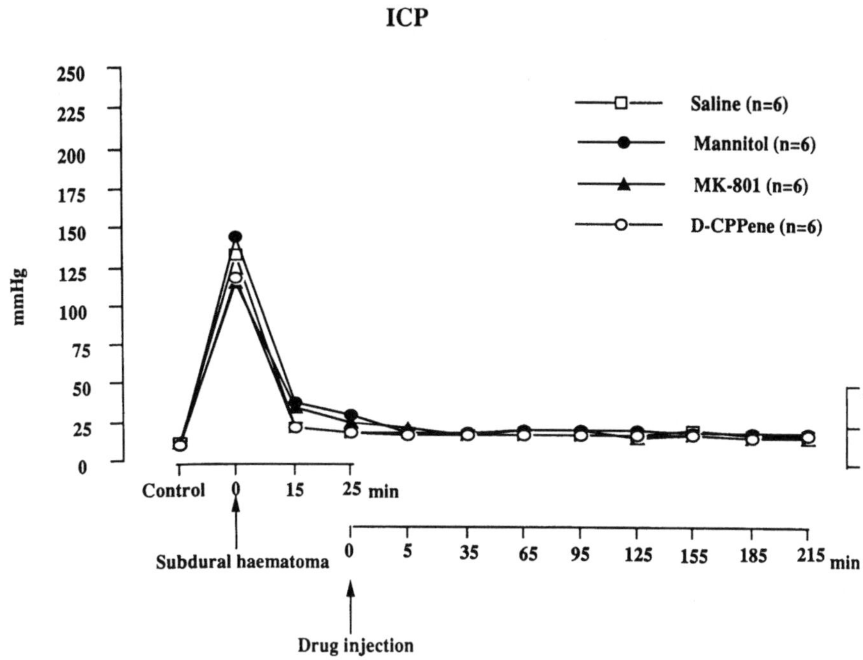

b

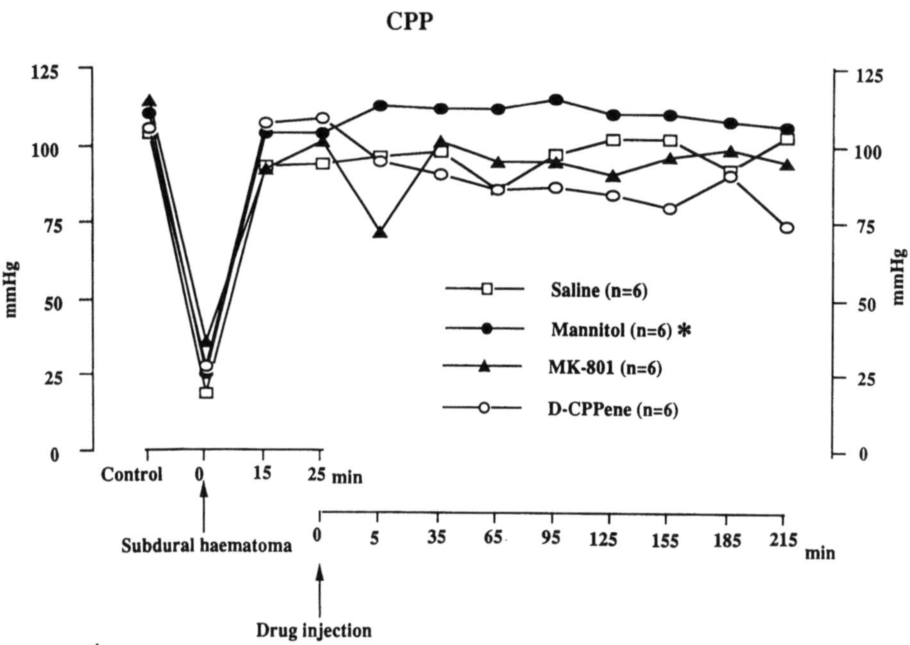

c * Only Mannitol Significantly Improved Cerebral Perfusion Pressure.

Fig. 1 a–c. MABP, ICP and CPP after subdural haematoma: effect of mannitol and NMDA antagonists

Table 1. MABP, ICP and CPP before drug injection

	Saline (n = 6)	Mannitol (n = 6)	MK801 (n = 6)	D-CPP-ene (n = 6)
MABP (mmHg)	113 ± 12	134 ± 12	126 ± 7	127 ± 8
ICP (mmHg)	18 ± 2	30 ± 6	25 ± 8	18 ± 2
CPP (mmHg)	94 ± 12	104 ± 12	101 ± 3	109 ± 8

Values are mean ± SEM.
There are no significant differences between the five groups.

Table 2. MABP, ICP and CPP after drug injection

	Saline (n = 48)	Mannitol (n = 48)	MK801 (n = 48)	D-CPP-ene (n = 48)
MABP (mmHg)	114 ± 3	129 ± 4**	110 ± 3	102 ± 4*
ICP (mmHg)	17 ± 1	19 ± 2	17 ± 2	16 ± 1
CPP (mmHg)	97 ± 3	111 ± 4*	93 ± 3	86 ± 4

Values are mean ± SEM.
,: Significantly different from Saline group (* $p < 0.056$, ** $p < 0.01$)

ICP, or significantly decreased CPP. Although MK801 decreased MABP (26%) and CPP (29%) transiently, five minutes after injection, there was no ICP change. D-CPP-ene slightly decreased MABP (by 11%) but ICP and CPP were not significantly reduced, in comparison to the saline treated controls.

Discussion

Both competitive and non-competitive NMDA antagonists cause activation and increased metabolism in parts of the limbic system so that an increase in regional CBF, and possibly ICP, might occur. However, these results indicate that neuroprotective doses of NMDA antagonists do not cause an increase in ICP or jeopardise CPP. The increased MABP and CPP seen after mannitol treatment may be due to its early volume expansion effect. Mannitol acutely decreased the ICP from 30 to 18 mmHg. The combined result of these two effects produced an increase in CPP. This accords with clinical experience. The transient decrease in MABP induced by MK801 is probably a function of anaesthesia. In the conscious animal, MK801 produces a transient elevation of MABP [2, 3] by its centrally mediated sympathomimetic effects, via blockade of the NMDA receptor [3]. Although MABP also decreased after D-CPP-ene injection in this study, CPP was adequately maintained.

This data suggests that NMDA antagonists are unlikely to cause an increase in ICP or a decrease in CPP, especially when $PaCO_2$ is controlled and anaesthesia or sedation is concomitantly used.

References

1. Chen MH, Bullock R, Graham DI, Fret P, Lowe D, McCulloch J (1991) Evaluation of a competitive NMDA antagonist (D-CPP-ene) in feline focal cerebral ischaemia. Ann Neurol. 29:(in press)
2. Kurumaji A, Nehls DG, Park CK, McCulloch J (1989) Effects of NMDA antagonists, MK801 and CPP, upon local cerebral glucose use. Brain Res 496:268–284
3. Lewis SJ, Barres C, Jacob HJ, Ohta H, Brody M (1989) Cardiovascular effects of the N-methyl-D-aspartate receptor antagonist MK801 in conscious rats. Hypertension 13:759–765
4. Meldrum B (1990) Protection against ischaemic neuronal damage by drugs acting on excitatory neurotransmission. Cerebrovasc Brain Metab Rev 2:27–57
5. Miller J, Bullock R, Graham DI, Chen MH, Teasdale GM (1990) Ischaemic brain damage in a model of acute subdural haematoma. Neurosurgery 27:433–439
6. Simon R, Shiraishi K (1990) N-methyl-D-aspartate antagonist reduces stroke size and regional glucose metabolism. Ann Neurol 27:606–611
7. Verlooy J, Selosse P, Reempts JV, Haseldonckx M, Borgers M (1990) Fiberoptic intracranial pressure monitoring in rats. J Neurosci Methods 31:1–6

Intracranial Pressure and Phosphorus-31 Magnetic Resonance Spectroscopy in Cats

H. Kobayashi, H. Ide, M. Kabuto, Y. Handa, H. Kawano, and M. Hayashi

Department of Neurosurgery, Fukui Medical School, Matsuoka, Fukui, Japan

Introduction

Cerebral metabolic alterations in an experimental study have been reported by many investigators. Recent advances in magnetic resonance spectroscopy (MRS) allow a non-invasive study of brain metabolism in vivo [1]. In this study, changes of intracranial pressure and P-31 MRS were observed after inflation and deflation of an epidural balloon in the cat.

Materials and Methods

Twenty adult cats were anaesthetized, intubated, and ventilated with a respirator. Arterial blood pressure (BP), intracranial pressure (ICP) and arterial blood gases were monitored. A latex rubber balloon was placed epidurally over the right frontal cortex through a burrhole. The P-31 MR spectra were recorded at 35.288MHz on a spectrometer (2.0 Tesla) constructed in the Phospho-Energetics, Inc. A radiofrequency surface coil (20 mm in diameter) was placed on the right parietal bone, apart from the balloon over the frontal lobe on the same side. The peak of phosphocreatine (Pcr) was assigned a chemical shift of zero. The tissue levels of Pcr, inorganic phosphate (Pi) and ATP were estimated from the areas under individual peaks. The intracellular pH was calculated from the chemical shift difference between Pi and Pcr in P-31 spectra [2].

Animals were randomly divided into four groups. In group 1 animals, the balloon was inflated with 1 ml of water at a speed of 1 ml/sec. Then, the balloon was deflated after obtaining a spectrum, or 4 minutes later. P-31 MRS, physiological parameters and the size of the pupils were observed for one hour. The balloons in group 2, 3 and 4 were inflated with 2, 3 and 4 ml of water at a speed of 1 ml/sec, respectively. The balloons were deflated 4 minutes after the inflation. The blood pressure in animals with herniation was kept stable during the study as much as possible with an intravenous drip injection of dopamine hydrochloride in Ringer's lactate. After the 1 hour measurement, animals were killed with pentobarbital sodium. The brains were carefully removed, grossly examined, weighed and fixed with 10% formalin for pathological study.

The data presented are expressed as mean value ± SEM and statistical significance was assessed by analysis of variance.

Results

The baseline values of arterial blood pressure and blood gases showed no significant change among 4 groups. The inflation of the epidural balloon produced an increase in mean ICP of 36 ± 3 mmHg in group 1, 60 ± 3 mmHg in group 2, 92 ± 3 mmHg in group 3 and 130 ± 6 mmHg in group 4. Three of 5 animals in group 3 showed ipsilateral oculomotor palsy when the epidural balloon was inflated and the other 2 animals in group 3 had bilateral dilated pupils. They recovered from the palsy during the 1 hour measurement after the balloon deflation. A rise in BP occurred when the epidural balloon was inflated in group 2 and 3, and the BP returned to the previous level after the deflation of the balloon. In group 4, all the animals showed bilateral oculomotor palsies and a drop in BP. The BP was restored with an intravenous drip injection of dopamine hydrochloride. But the bilateral oculomotor palsies lasted during the one hour measurement. After the deflation of the balloon, the ICP in each group rapidly returned to the baseline value and remained there in group 1 (13 ± 1 mmHg) and group 2 (14 ± 2 mmHg). The ICP in both group 3 and 4 gradually increased again to 21 ± 2 mmHg ($p < 0.01$) and 25 ± 3 mmHg ($p < 0.01$) in 1 hour, respectively.

There were several peaks in the spectrum of the normal brain: β ATP, α ATP, γ ATP, Pcr, Phosphodiester (PDE), Pi and phospho-monoester (PME). Figure 1 shows sequential changes of P-31 MRS in group 1. The inflation of the epidural balloon produced peaks of Pcr, ATP, PDE and PME decrease in the second spectrum and the peaks gradually recovered to the baseline levels with the passage of time. Spectra in group 2, 3 and 4 did not

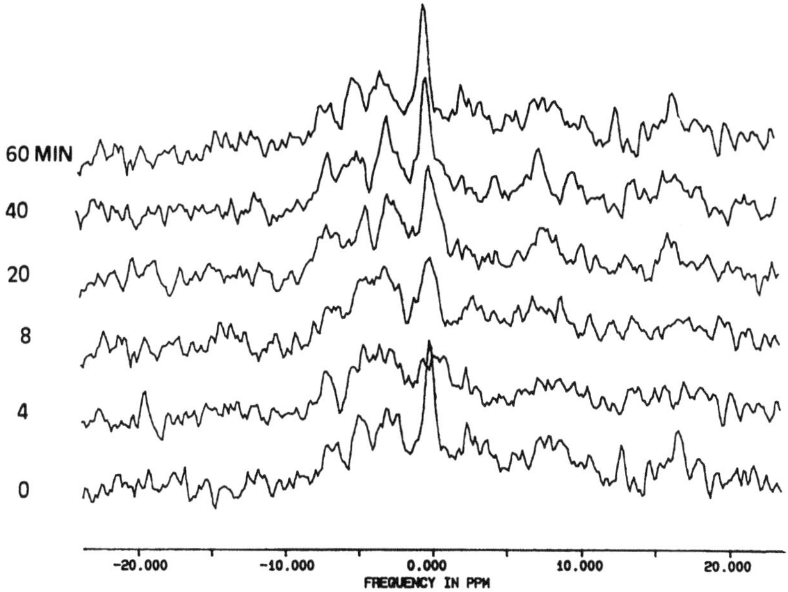

Fig. 1. Sequential changes of P-31 magnetic resonance spectroscopy in group 1

recover completely during the one-hour-observation. The mean pH of the normal brain was 7.20 ± 0.01. The mean pH during the balloon inflation decreased to 6.94 ± 0.02 in group 1, 6.82 ± 0.09 in group 2, 6.77 ± 0.07 in group 3 and 6.66 ± 0.06 in group 4. The mean pH increased to the normal value in group 1, 7.10 ± 0.02 ($p < 0.01$) in group 2, 7.11 ± 0.02 ($p < 0.01$) in group 3 and 7.05 ± 0.02 ($p < 0.001$) in group 4 during the course of the one hour measurement after the balloon deflation. Pcr decreased to 83.3 ± 2.9% in group 1, 66.7 ± 4.0% in group 2, 51.8 ± 2.5% in group 3 and 44.3 ± 4.0% in group 4 by the balloon inflation and recovered to 95.9 ± 1.3% in group 1, 88.0 ± 2.4% ($p < 0.05$) in group 2, 78.6 ± 5.8% ($p < 0.05$) in group 3 and 64.8 ± 2.2% in group 4 ($p < 0.001$) during the one hour measurement after the balloon deflation. The changes in β ATP values were more moderate than the changes in Pcr values. ATP decreased to 79.0 ± 1.6% in group 1, 75.8 ± 2.7% in group 2, 76.8 ± 1.7% in group 3 and 59.4 ± 1.9% in group 4 by the balloon inflation and recovered to 98.0 ± 3.7% in group 1, 87,7 ± 4.5% in group 2, 87.5 ± 1.4% ($p < 0.05$) in group 3 and 74.2 ± 6.5% ($p < 0.05$) in group 4, during the one hour measurement after the balloon deflation. The mean weight of the cat brains was 40.5 ± 1.0 g and there was no significant difference in the weight among the groups. Autopsy revealed the normal configuration without a shift of the midline in group 1 and 2. The shift of the midline with brain swelling and petechial hemorrhages in the pontomesencephalic zone of the brain stem were observed in group 3 and 4.

Conclusions

The inflation of the epidural balloon suddenly decreased phosphocreatine (Pcr), ATP, phosphodiester (PDE) and phosphomonoester (PME), and these gradually recovered after deflation of the epidural balloon. Acidosis progressed by the cerebral compression for 4 minutes and it gradually recovered during the time course. The degree of the recovery was volume related. This study demonstrates that P-31 MRS can provide non-invasive, serial, in vivo measurements of critical, high energy phosphate metabolites and intracellular pH after inflation and deflation of an epidural balloon in cats.

References

1. Kobayashi H, Hayashi M, Kawano H, Handa Y, Kabuto M, Ide H (1990) Phosphorus-31 magnetic resonance spectroscopy of cerebral ischemia in cats. Neurosurgery 27:240–246
2. Petroff OAC, Pricard JW, Behar KL, Alger JR, den Hollander JA, Shulman RG (1985) Cerebral intracellular pH by ^{31}P nuclear magnetic resonance spectroscopy. Neurology 35:781–788

Biomechanical Regulation of Cerebral Blood Flow

C. ANILE[1], A. RINALDI[1], A. MANGIOLA[1], P. AMANTE[1], P. PALMA[1], G. MAIRA[1], F. DELLA CORTE[2], R. CALIMICI[2], and A. FERRARESI[3]

[1] Institutes of Neurosurgery, [2] Anaesthesiology, and [3] Physiology, Catholic University, Largo Gemelli 8, 00168 Rome, Italy

Introduction

It is generally accepted that myogenic, metabolic and neurogenic regulation mechanisms exist for the cerebral blood flow (CBF). Recently, a hydraulic control acting at the predural level has been suggested by Chopp et al. [2] These mechanisms, however, do not take into consideration the problem represented by the peculiar feature of the brain (an incompressible organ) within the skull and dura mater (a rigid box and a stiff envelope), perfused by a pulsatile blood flow through a vascular tree with elastic walls. On the basis of this consideration we think that the progressive CBF reduction up to cerebral circulatory arrest following severe intracranial hypertension is probably due to an unbalance between cerebral blood volume variations during each cardiac cycle and the compensatory systems, primarily the venous vascular bed.

Material and Methods

To investigate these phenomena we carried out an experimental study on a model of intracranial hypertension induced by intraventricular mock CSF infusion in two different animal species (lamb and pig). Arterial blood pressure, venous CBF velocity (at the sagittal sinus level), ventricular fluid pressure, and electrocortical activity (ECoA) were simultaneously recorded.

Results

Six experiments were performed on four pigs and four experiments on three lambs. The following phenomena were noted:

1. Sagittal sinus blood flow velocity (SSBFV) remains constant, showing a pulsatile morphology synchronous with the cardiac cycle (Fig. 1), until the cerebral perfusion pressure (CPP) decreases to approximately 25–30 mmHg (Fig. 2). At lower CPP values the SSBFV progressively decreases reaching zero value while the CPP is still positive.

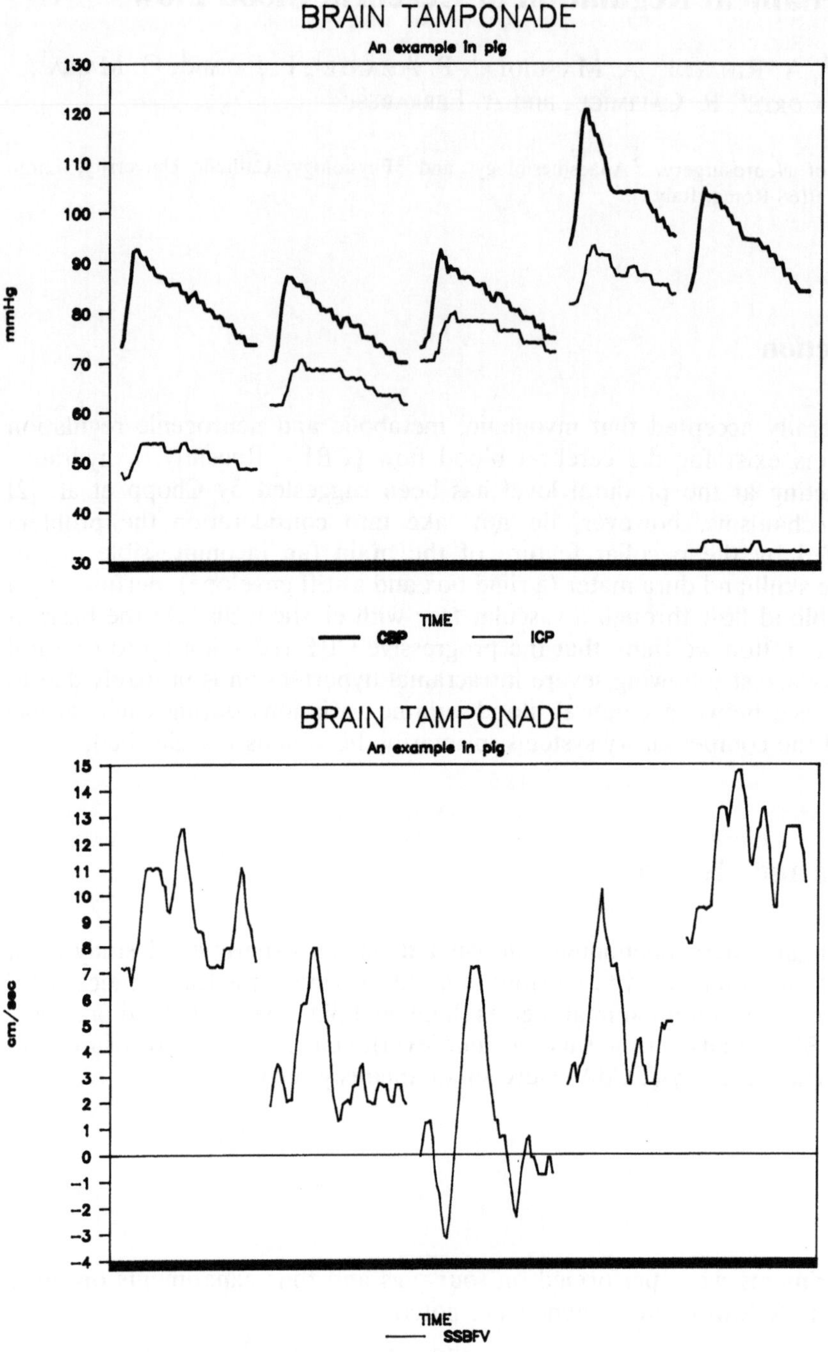

Fig. 1. Brain tamponade, example in pig. ICP, carotid blood pressure (CBP) (**a**) and sagittal sinus blood flow velocity (SSBFV) (**b**) synchronously recorded during a trial of intracranial hypertension produced by intraventricular mock CSF infusion

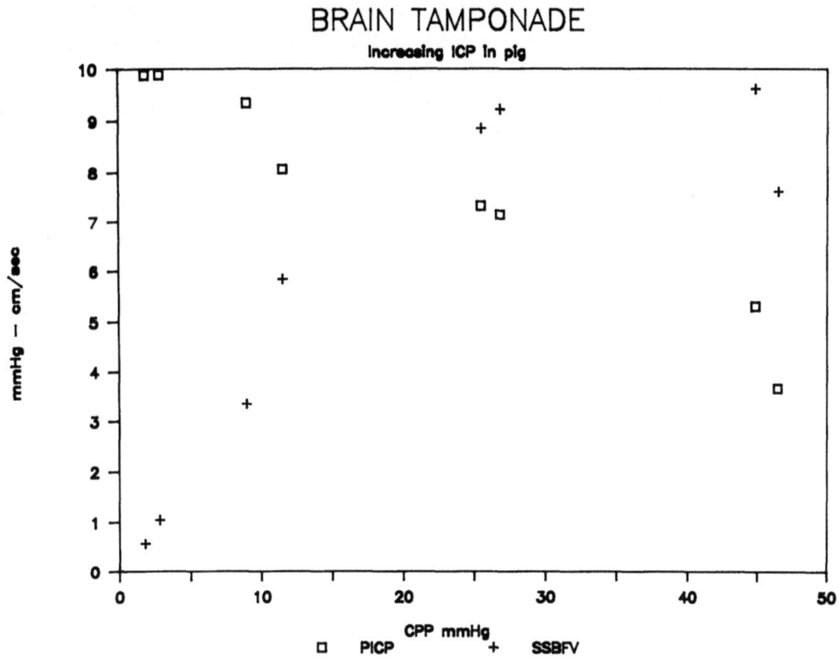

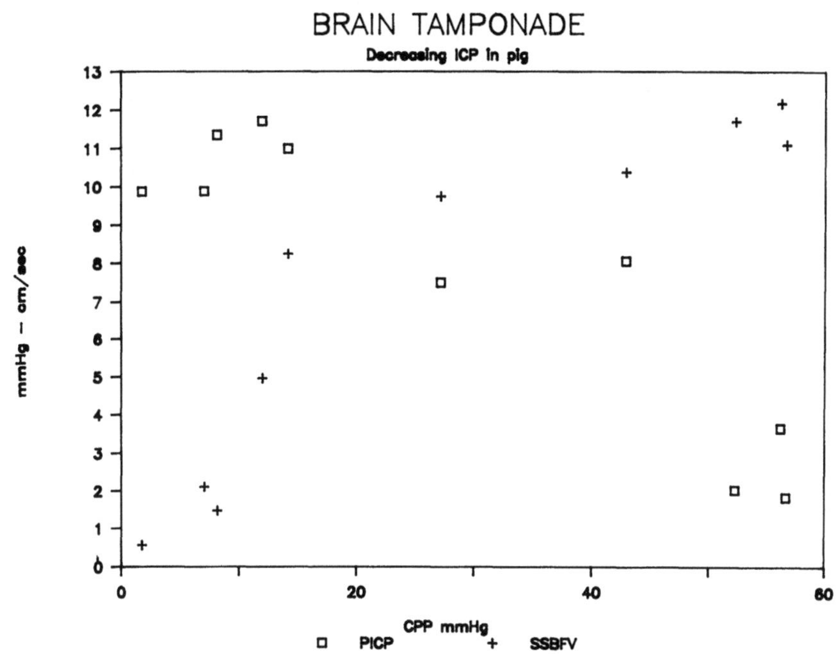

Fig. 2. Correlations between cerebral perfusion pressure (CPP), amplitude of pulse intracranial pressure (PICP) and mean value of sagittal sinus blood flow velocity (SSBFV) during a trial of intracranial hypertension produced by intraventricular mock CSF infusion. The top figure (**a**) shows the ascending phase of intracranial hypertension; the bottom figure (**b**) shows the results obtained in the descending phase after stop of infusion

2. The point at which the SSBFV approaches zero is marked by the appearance of a "reverberating wave" at the sagittal sinus level (Fig. 1) mimicking the phenomenon already described by others [3, 4] in humans. This phenomenon has also been noted by us [1] at the extracranial level of the internal carotid artery in a previous experimental model in rabbits [1].
3. In our experiments, the intracranial elastance, as determined by the slope of the amplitude of the pulse ICP (PICP) versus the CPP, does not show the steeper increase described by others [5]. Moreover, mainly in the decreasing phase of intracranial hypertension after the stop of the infusion, when fluid buffering factors are probably less active, the intracranial elastance shows a tendency to decrease (Fig. 2).
4. The ECoA disappears a few seconds after the SSBFV zero value is reached.
5. A reversal of the initial cerebral hemodynamic conditions follows immediately after the stop of intraventricular CSF mock infusion.
6. The recovery of ECoA, however, is always delayed, mostly depending on the duration of cerebral circulatory arrest.

Discussion

Our results, especially those concerning the observation of a pulsatile morphology of the SSBFV and the appearance of a "reverberating wave" at venous outflow level, suggest a different interpretation of the well known "brain tamponade" phenomenon. We may need to reconsider both the mechanisms underlying CSF regulation and the significance of intracranial elastance. In a closed system, such as the intracranial system, the possibility to maintain adequate flow is determined by control of the internal volume. Our study shows that this control is obtained by means of a simple hydraulic mechanism which links inflow and outflow volume changes at Starling resistor level.

References

1. Anile C, Rinaldi A, Roselli R, Visocchi M, Ferraresi A, Serricchio M, Dal Lago A, Bradariolo S, Calimici R, Della Corte F, Maira G (1989) An experimental model of "brain tamponade". Preliminary observations on ICP dynamics, carotid blood flow velocitimetry and EEG activity. In: Hoff JT, Betz AL (eds) Intracranial pressure VII. Springer, Berlin Heidelberg New York London Paris Tokyo Hong Kong, pp 941–943
2. Chopp M, Portnoy HD, Branch C (1983) Hydraulic model of the cerebrovascular bed: An aid to understanding the volume-pressure test. Neurosurgery 13:5–11
3. Hassler W, Steinmetz H, Pirschel J (1989) Transcranial Doppler study of intracranial circulatory arrest. J Neurosurg 71:195–201
4. Lindegaard K-F, Grip A, Nornes (1980) Precerebral haemodynamics in brain tamponade. Neurochirurgia 23:133–142
5. Van Eijndhoven JHM, Avezaat CJJ (1986) Cerebrospinal fluid pulse pressure and the pulsatile variation in cerebral blood volume: an experimental study in dogs. Neurosurgery 19:507–522

Cerebral Blood Flow Restoration After Decompressive Craniectomy in Cold Induced Brain Edema

A. Rinaldi[1], A. Mangiola[1], C. Anile[1], G. Maira[1], P. Amante[1], P. Palma[1], and A. Ferraresi[2]

[1] Institutes of Neurosurgery and [2] Physiology, Catholic University, Rome, Italy

Introduction

In neurosurgical practice different viewpoints have been expressed about the value of decompressive craniectomy as a last resource to control untreatable ICP elevations [2]. In an experimental model of cold induced brain injury we examined the effects of an appropriately tailored cranio-dural opening on whole brain perfusion and on local fluid dynamics. An edematous lesion induced by cold injury produces a critical mass effect and compromises the volume buffering capacity of the intracranial system. This produces an increase in the cerebrovascular resistance (CVR) thereby generating a vicious circle which can enhance edema formation. It is supposed that cranio-dural removal, opening the intracranial system to the atmosphere and reducing ICP, could facilitate the cerebral venous outflow from the skull, thereby decreasing the CVR and disrupting the vicious circle linking primary and secondary pathological events.

Material and Methods

The experiments were carried out on 10 albino rabbits of 3–4 kg weight, under conditions of assisted ventilation and general anaesthesia (Ketamine, Tubocurarine). Rabbits were selected as both the anatomy and function of the carotid-vertebral system and the anastomotic circle at the base of the skull is analogous to that of the human being [3]. The following parameters were simultaneously recorded:

- ICP by a 18G needle inserted stereotactically into the left lateral ventricle
- carotid blood pressure (CBP) by a catheter in the left common carotid artery
- internal carotid artery blood flow velocity (ICABFV) by means of a continuous wave 8 MHz Doppler probe firmly placed on the right common carotid artery after ligation of the external branch.

After positioning the animal in the stereotactic frame the experimental protocol started with surgical removal of a right parietal rectangular shaped (1.5 × 1.0 cm) cranio-dural flap and reconstruction of the dura by a thin silastic layer sealed to the external boundaries of the residual skull defect to prevent CSF leakage and to allow brain displacement without damage. In 3 control animals this initial step was followed by the recording procedure lasting for 3 hours, without any other manipulation. In the remaining 7 rabbits the bone flap was then rigidly replaced and sealed with acrylic cement; thereafter a cold lesion in the same right parietal region was induced through the replaced bone by topical application of liquid nitrogen (−180°C) for the duration of 1 min utilizing an appropriately sized tube sealed to the skull. The lesion was followed by a 4 hours period of observation. In 4 animals, when high values of ICP were reached (>50 mmHg), usually within 2 hours of the lesion, the bone flap was again removed and the recording procedure continued to complete the 4 hours of observation as in the non-craniectomized animals. Histologic staining with Evan's blue was utilized to check fluid extravasation.

Results

Non-Craniectomized Cold Lesioned Animals

After the lesion, while CBP remained relatively stable, ICP showed a progressive increase in about 2–3 hours up to 40–60 mmHg. This rise was concomitant with a reduction in the diastolic ICABFV and an increase in the ratio between systolic and diastolic values, which reached and even passed zero flow velocity, thus indicating a remarkable increment in CVR.

Craniectomized Cold Lesioned Animals

In this group of animals the first 2 hours of the experiment showed the same findings as those in the control group; the bone removal was immediately followed by a dramatic decrease of ICP to basal levels with simultaneous restoration of ICABFV towards normal values, indicating a decrease in CVR (Fig. 1). No difference in the Evan's blue distribution was noticed between the two groups of animals.

Discussion and Conclusions

These preliminary results suggest the possibility that a decompressive craniectomy, if carried out timely and in a proper way, can be an efficacious therapeutic tool to mechanically disrupt the events' cascade which links the primary to secondary brain damage following a cold induced lesion. The opening of the intracranial system to the atmosphere, bypassing the action of the Starling resistor [1], primarily relieves the effects of increased ICP on the venous outflow resistance and rebalances the cerebral blood inflow-outflow regulation. As a consequence of this an arterio-venous gradient is restored. At the same

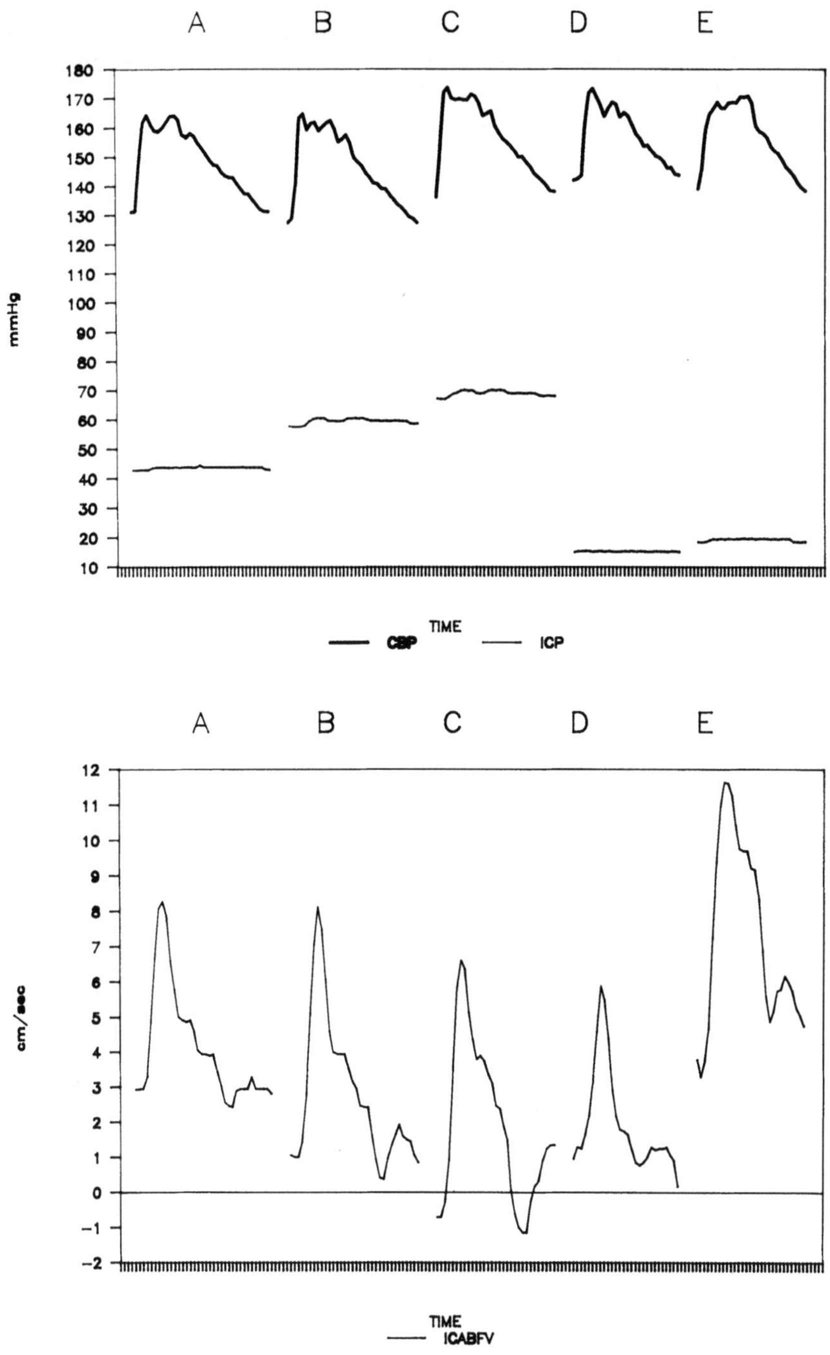

Fig. 1. Intracranial pressure (ICP), carotid blood pressure (CBP) and internal carotid artery blood flow velocity (ICABFV) synchronously recorded after cold lesion in a craniectomized animal. Craniectomy was carried out immediately after C and before D

time the transmural pressure at the capillary bed is reduced following the decrease in CSF and/or venous pressure. These phenomena facilitate the flow through the vessels and improve the fluid dynamics by reducing the formation and increasing the absorption of brain edema.

Acknowledgements. We are grateful to Mrs. Anna Capuano and Mr. Pietro Santini for their precious technical support.

References

1. Chopp M, Portnoy HD, Branch C (1983) Hydraulic model of the cerebrovascular bed: An aid to understanding the volume-pressure test. Neurosurgery 13:5–11
2. Clark K, Nash TM, Hutchison GC (1986) The failure of circumferential craniotomy in acute traumatic cerebral swelling. J Neurosurg 29:367–371
3. Meyer FB, Anderson RE, Sundt TM, Yaksh TL (1986) Intracellular brain pH, indicator tissue perfusion, EEG and histology in severe and moderate focal cortical ischemia in the rabbit. J Cereb Blood Flow Metab 6:71–78

The Metabolic Protection of Hypoxia by Etomidate Evaluated by Magnetic Resonance Spectroscopy*

K. Yoshida,[1] A. Marmarou[1], and M. Furuse[2]

[1] Division of Neurosurgery, Medical College of Virginia, USA
[2] Nakatsugawa Municipal General Hospital, Japan

Introduction

Prolonged hypoxia leads to increase of the rate of anaerobic glycolysis and hence the accumulation of lactate. There is a progressive fall in intracellular pH of brain and energy disturbances. The objective of this study was, using magnetic resonance spectroscopy, to determine if Etomidate could ameliorate brain metabolic derangements resulting from the hypoxic energy crisis.

Materials and Methods

Fourteen cats were anesthetized with intravenous methohexical sodium (1–2 mg/kg) and maintained with isoflurane (1.75%), nitrous oxide (70%) and oxygen during the surgical procedure. They were intubated and mechanically ventilated. Catheters were placed in the femoral artery for pressure monitoring and blood sample withdrawal and in the femoral vein for drug infusion. A small craniectomy (5 × 15 mm) was made above the sagittal sinus 1.5 cm posterior to the bregma and a polyethylene catheter was placed in the superior sagittal sinus to obtain cerebro-venous blood. Two burr holes were made in the frontal bone, and teflon-coated platinum electrodes were inserted in the gray matters for measurement of CBF. A 24 G teflon catheter (Jelco) was placed in the cisterna magna for ICP measurement. One 10 mm diameter circular ^{31}P magnetic resonance spectroscopy (MRS) surface coil was cemented on the right frontoparietal region. After surgical preparation, the animals were randomized to one of two groups; (1) etomidate treatment group (n = 7), (2) no treatment group (n = 7). In the etomidate treatment group, isoflurane was stopped and Etomidate administered intravenously after completion of the surgical preparation. Initially, a bolus dose (2.5 mg/kg) was given, followed by a continuous (0.25 mg/kg/min) maintenance dose administered intravenously. In the untreated group, isoflurane was kept within the range from 1.0 to 1.5%

* This work was supported in part by grants NS 12587 and NS 19235 from the National Institutes of Health. Additional facilities and support were provided by the Richard Roland Reynolds Neurosurgical Research Laboratories.

during the entire experiment. After control measurements, spontaneous ventilation was stopped by using muscle paralysis with intravenous pancronium bromide (1 mg/kg). After ventilation was stopped for 90 seconds, hypoventilation was begun approximately half of the initial rate of 10 to 15 breaths/min but no lower than 4 breaths/min to keep the value of PaO_2 35 ± 5 mmHg. In both groups, blood samples were taken at 30, 60, 90, and 120 minutes and CBF, CMRO2, CMRG1, and CMRLac were measured at 30 and 90 minutes after the onset of hypoventilation. The brain tissue pH, ATP, PCr, and Pi levels were measured between CBF measurements. At the end of the experiment, the animals were sacrificed by KCl injection and the brains removed for measurement of water content using gravimetric techniques.

Results

Control ICP values were 10.5 ± 2.3 and 5.8 ± 2.2 mmHg, and in 10 minutes after hypoventilation ICP values reached peak values of 33.8 ± 2.8 and 25.2 ± 2.6 mmHg, $p < 0.05$ in untreated and treated groups respectively. The ICP values in the untreated group were always higher than in the treated group (Table 1).

CMRGlu and CMRLac increased significantly in the untreated group during hypoxia, indicating increased anaerobic cerebral metabolism. An index of oxidative metabolic stores, the PCr/Pi ratio, markedly decreased during hypoxia and the PCr/Pi ratio remained suppressed for 2 hours after resuscitation and return to normal ventilation. In contrast, CMRGlu and CMRLac remained unchanged in animals treated with Etomidate while the PCr/Pi ratio decreased only slightly during hypoventilation.

Discussion

Etomidate, an intravenous anesthetic induction agent, is a non-barbiturate hypnotic without analgesic properties that has less cardiovascular and respiratory depressant actions than sodium thiopental [2]. It has been believed that hypoxia leads to increase of the rate of anaerobic glycolysis and hence the

Table 1. Intracranial pressure during hypoxia

	Control	Peak value	30 (min)	60	90	120
No treatment	10.5	33.75[a]	26.5	19.8	12.5	13.0
	2.3	2.8	2.1	1.4	1.4	1.1
Etomidate	5.8	25.2	24.0	18.8	11.0	10.6
	2.2	2.6	3.1	2.5	2.9	2.9

All data are mean ± SEM (mmHg)
[a] $p < 0.05$ vs. treated group

accumulation of lactate [5, 6]. The lower rate of lactate accumulation in the Etomidate treated group indicates a concomitant reduction in anaerobic metabolism in brain tissue. Hypoxia caused a marked depletion of this ratio and a reduction in brain pH without changes in ATP. And even during normal ventilation, the ratio did not completely return to normal. However, with Etomidate treatment cerebral oxidative metabolites were preserved during hypoxia. Etomidate, given by continuous infusion in the cat, provides the advantages of systematic hemodynamic stability [4], decreased cerebral metabolism, and decreased cerebral blood flow, resulting in decreased ICP without the reduction of cerebral perfusion pressure [3, 4, 1]. In conclusion, Etomidate has a possible role in brain protection because of its ability to decrease cerebral metabolism, thereby decreasing oxygen demand at a time when oxygen supply is decreased. Further, Etomidate can preserve brain function by prolonging tolerance of the brain to ischemia when the possibility of hypoxia or ischemia can be anticipated. These results suggest that Etomidate could be very useful especially in the management of critically ill or head-injury patients when it is desirable to decrease cerebral metabolism and intracranial pressure without interfering with vital functions.

References

1. Dearden NM, Mcdowell DG (1985) Comparison of etomidate and althesin in the reduction of increased intracranial pressure after head injury. Br J Anaesth 57:361–368
2. Giese JL, Stanley TH (1983) Etomidate: A new intravenous anesthetic induction agent. Pharmacotherapy 3:251–258
3. Gilsanz FJ, Sola G, Mateos LT, Hernandez C (1986) Effects of etomidate, sodium pentothal and lidocaine on cerebral elastance. ICP 6:736–739
4. Moss E, Powell D, Gibson RM, Mcdowall DG (1979) Effect of etomidate on intracranial pressure and cerebral perfusion pressure. Br J Anaesth 51:347–352
5. Norberg K, Siesjo BK (1975) Cerebral metabolism in hypoxic hypoxia 1. Pattern of activation of glycolysis: A re-evaluation. Brain Res 86:31–44
6. Siesjo BK, Nilsson L (1971) The influence of arterial hypoxemia upon labile phosphates and upon extracellular and intracellular lactate and pyruvate concentration in the rat brain. Scand J Clin Lab Invest 27:83–96

Effect of Torasemide – A New Cl^--Transport Inhibitor on Glial Swelling by Lactacidosis and Glutamate

F. Staub[1], J. Peters[1], O. Kempski[2], G.-H. Schneider[3], L. Schürer[1], and A. Baethmann[1]

[1] Institute for Surgical Research, Ludwig-Maximilians-University, 8000 München 70, Germany
[2] Institute for Neurosurgical Pathophysiology, Johannes Gutenberg-University, 6500 Mainz, Germany
[3] Department of Neurosurgery, Free University, 1000 Berlin 65, Germany

Introduction

Cytotoxic brain edema, i.e. swelling of glial- and nerve cells is a common result of cerebral ischemia, brain trauma, metabolic disorders, and develops secondarily in vasogenic edema. During ischemia and severe head injury, brain tissue homeostasis is severely changed, and many parameters are simultaneously affected. To dissect and isolate the causal mechanisms leading to swelling of nerve- and glial cells, our laboratory has established an in vitro model [4, 5]. Thereby pathomechanisms can be studied in isolation without interference of epiphenomena taking place in damaged brain tissue under circumstances of cerebral ischemia or trauma. In previous studies the role of acidosis in cell swelling has been analyzed by using C6 glioma cells or astrocytes obtained from primary culture [5, 8]. Cell swelling was found at a pH of 6.8 and below, i.e. at a level of acidosis which occurs in ischemia or trauma [7] of the brain. Another aspect is related with glutamate. The excitatory neurotransmitter is released in large amounts in ischemic or traumatized brain tissue [1] and likely to be involved in cell swelling [9].

Methods for the treatment of cell swelling or permanent cellular injury in the brain, which is specifically aiming at the underlying pathophysiological processes are in short supply. The purpose of the present study was to investigate the therapeutic effect of a potent diuretic, torasemide [1-isopropyl-3-((4-(3-methylphenylamino)pyrid-3-yl)-sulfonyl)urea] on swelling of C6 glioma cells induced by lactacidosis or by glutamate in vitro. Torasemide is structurally related to furosemide. It is a blocker of the $Na^+/K^+/Cl^-$ cotransporter and of Cl^- channels in the thick ascending limb of the loop of Henle [10]. In clinical trials torasemide was a more effective diuretic than furosemide and was well tolerated.

Materials and Methods

The currently used experimental model has been previously described in detail [4, 5]. In brief, C6 glioma cells originate from a chemically induced glial tumor in rats. The cells have similar properties as astrocytes isolated from brain tissue [6]. The cells were cultivated as monolayers in Petri dishes using Dulbecco's modified minimal essential medium with 25 mM bicarbonate. The medium was supplemented with 10% fetal calf serum and 100 IU/ml penicillin G and 50 μg/ml streptomycin. The cells were grown in a humidified atmosphere of 5% CO_2 and 95% room air at 37°C. For the experiments, C6 glioma cells were harvested with 0.05% trypsin-0.02% ethylenediaminetetraacetate (EDTA) in phosphate-buffered saline and washed twice thereafter. After resuspension in serum-free medium the glial cells were transferred into a plexiglas incubation chamber supplied with electrodes to control pH, temperature, and pO_2. A gas-permeable silicon rubber tube in the chamber provided the single cell suspension with a mixture of O_2, CO_2, and N_2. Sedimentation of the cells was prevented by a magnetic stirrer. The cell volume of glial cells was determined by flow cytometry using an advanced coulter system with hydrodynamic focusing. This method allows to recognize alterations in cell size of <1%.

The experiments were performed after a 60 minute control period used for measurements of normal cell volume, cell density of the suspension, and medium osmolality. The mean of the cell volume taken from 3 serial measurements obtained during the last 15 min of the control period was utilized as control value. Acidosis was induced by addition of isotonic lactic acid titrating the pH of the medium from 7.4 down to 6.2, or 5.0. The cell volume was monitored for 60 min during lactacidosis. In another set of experiments the C6 glioma suspension was added with 1 mM glutamate after a control period, the cell volume was monitored then for 120 min. Parallel experiments were performed in the presence of 1 mM torasemide (Boehringer Mannheim, Mannheim, FRG) administered 15 min before induction of acidosis, or elevation of the glutamate concentration in the medium, respectively.

Results and Discussion

As in previous experiments, lactacidosis led to a reproducible volume increase of C6 glial cells [8]. At pH 6.2 cell volume increased within 1 minute to 108.5 ± 0.3% of control followed by further gradual swelling during 30 minutes (Table 1). After 60 minutes the cell volume had reached 117.9 ± 0.7% at this level of acidosis. By addition of 1 mM torasemide the swelling of C6 glioma cells at pH 6.2 was significantly reduced during the whole observation period (Table 1, $p < 0.01$). The increase in cell size by acidosis was only half of what was found without torasemide. Lactacidosis of pH 5.0 led to a more intensive cell swelling. At pH 5.0, the initial increase in cell size amounted to 115.7 ± 0.8% of control during the first minute. Cell swelling continued for about 40 minutes reaching 146.9 ± 2.3% after 60 minutes. The swelling response at this level of acidosis was also significantly inhibited in the presence of torasemide. Addition of the agent attenuated the increase in cell volume from acidosis by 7–10%. As mentioned above, torasemide is a blocker of the $Na^+/K^+/Cl^-$ cotransport as well of Cl^--channels in the thick ascending limb of the loop of Henle of rabbit nephrons [10]. According to previous findings on

Table 1. Swelling of C6 glioma cells in percent from lactacidosis of pH 6.2 with (B) or without (A) addition of torasemide. The increase of the cell volume is given in percent of the normal cell size obtained during the final 15 minutes of the control period. Four experiments were performed per group. Torasemide was significantly inhibiting cell swelling during the entire observation period ($p < 0.01$)

Time [Min]	Control			Lactacidosis pH 6.2					
	−15	−10	−5	1	5	10	20	40	60
A Volume [%]	100.27	100.14	99.59	108.50	111.64	113.37	115.91	116.68	117.87
SEM	0.33	0.16	0.43	0.29	0.75	0.75	1.70	2.15	0.70
B Volume [%]	101.11	100.21	98.68	104.05[a]	104.32[a]	106.48[a]	108.11[a]	109.78[a]	113.08[a]
SEM	0.52	0.46	0.44	0.54	0.78	1.43	0.81	1.17	0.69

[a] $p < 0.01$

Table 2. Volume response of C6 glioma cells by addition of 1 mM glutamate to the cell suspension. The data of four control experiments (A) are shown together with four experiments performed in the presence of torasemide (B). The diuretic agent had no effect on the continuing volume increased by glutamate

Time [Min]	Control			+1 mM Glutamate					
	−15	−10	−5	1	10	30	60	90	120
A Volume [%]	100.37	99.26	100.4	100.45	101.90	104.19	107.01	109.66	111.28
SEM	0.22	0.43	0.29	0.14	1.06	0.42	0.75	1.30	0.46
B Volume [%]	100.88	100.16	98.96	99.65	100.64	103.42	107.38	111.15	112.35
SEM	0.35	0.52	0.65	0.53	0.53	1.22	0.67	0.98	0.52

acidosis induced swelling of glial cells activation of the Na^+/H^+- and the Cl^-/HCO_3^- antiporters is proposed as a central mechanism of acidosis induced glial swelling. These mechanisms are sensitive to amilorid or SITS [5]. Accordingly, addition of acid to the suspension medium buffered by bicarbonate causes formation of CO_2, which diffuses into the cell, resulting in an intracellular acidosis by hydration of CO_2 to H_2CO_3 and subsequent dissociation. The resulting H^+ and bicarbonate ions are exchanged against extracellular Na^+ and Cl^- ions by activation of the antiporters mentioned above. Accumulation of Na^+ and Cl^- in the cell is the final step of glial swelling from osmotic reasons. The inhibition of swelling of C6 glial cells by torasemide from acidosis might, therefore, be attributed to an interference with activation of anion exchange mechanisms caused by the intracellular acidosis (cf. above). This contention is supported by observations on inhibition of SITS- or DIDS-sensitive anion carriers by pharmacological agents which are structurally related to torasemide [3].

Addition of 1 mM glutamate to the C6 glioma cell suspension led to a quasi linear increase in cell size, irrespective whether torasemide was administered or not (Table 2). Exposure of the cells to glutamate resulted in an increase in volume to 107.0 ± 0.8% of control after 60 min. In the presence of torasemide, cell swelling from glutamate approached also 107.4 ± 0.7%. After 120 min, cell volume approached a value of 111.3 ± 0.5% under control conditions whereas 112.4 ± 0.5% when torasemide was administered (Table 2). Swelling of the glial cells by an increased glutamate concentration in the medium is considered to result from active accumulation of the amino acid by the cells [2]. Accumulation of glutamate by the glial cells can be interpreted as clearance function of the extracellular compartment as a requirement of a normal activity of nerve cells. Since uptake of glutamate into the glial cells occurs against a steep extra-/intracellular concentration gradient, energy is required which is provided by the concurrent influx of Na^+-ions along their electrochemical gradient [2]. Accumulation of both Na^+-ions and glutamate in the cells raises the osmotic concentration as a basis for the influx of water resulting in cell swelling. The current findings indicate that torasemide does not interfere with the uptake of glutamate into the C6 glioma cells. Taken together, the present findings demonstrate therapeutical properties of torasemide in the swelling of C6 glioma cells from lactacidosis, whereas the agent appears to be ineffective against cell swelling induced by glutamate. The findings are encouraging for further studies on the therapeutical potential of torasemide under *in vivo* conditions, for instance to reduce brain edema from trauma or ischemia.

Acknowledgements. The excellent technical assistance of Ingrid Kölbl and Ulrike Goerke is gratefully acknowledged. The current project was supported by grants provided by the Deutsche Forschungsgemeinschaft: Ba 452/6-7.

References

1. Baethmann A, Maier-Hauff K, Schürer L, Lange M, Guggenbichler C, Vogt W, Jacob K, Kempski O (1989) Release of glutamate and of free fatty acids in vasogenic brain edema. J Neurosurg 70:578–591
2. Barbour B, Brew H, Attwell D (1988) Electrogenic glutamate uptake in glial cells is activated by intracellular potassium. Nature 335:433–435
3. Brazy PC, Gunn RB (1976) Furosemide inhibition of chloride transport in human red blood cells. J Gen Physiol 68:583–599
4. Kempski O, Chaussy L, Gross U, Zimmer M, Baethmann A (1983) Volume regulation and metabolism of suspended C6 glioma cells: An in vitro model to study cytotoxic brain edema. Brain Res 279:217–228
5. Kempski O, Staub F, Jansen M, Schödel F, Baethmann A (1988) Glial swelling during extracellular acidosis in vitro. Stroke 19:385–392
6. Pfeiffer SE, Betschart B, Cook J, Mancini P, Morris R (1977) Glial cell lines. In: Fedoroff S, Hertz L (eds) Cell, Tissue, and Organ Culture in Neurobiology. Academic Press, New York, pp 287–346
7. Siemkowicz E, Hansen AJ (1981) Brain extracellular ion composition and EEG activity following 10 minutes ischemia in normo- and hyperglycemic rats. Stroke 12:236–240
8. Staub F, Baethmann A, Peters J, Weigt H, Kempski O (1990) Effects of lactacidosis on glial cell volume and viability. J Cereb Blood Flow Metab 10:866–876
9. Van Harreveld A, Fifkova E (1971) Light- and electron-microscopic changes in central nervous tissue after electrophoretic injection of glutamate. Exp Mol Pathol 15:61–81
10. Wittner M, Di Stefano A, Schlatter E, Delarge J, Greger R (1986) Torasemide inhibits NaCl reabsorption in the thick ascending limb of the loop of Henle. Pflügers Arch 407:611–614

The Effects of Vasopressin on Intracranial Pressure and Cerebrovascular Dynamics in the Rat*

L.K. SALADIN[1], J.E. BRUNI[2], and E.R. CARDOSO[3]

[1] Physical Therapy Education Department, College of Health Related Professionals, Medical University of South Carolina, Charleston, SC, USA
[2] Departments of Anatomy and [3] Surgery, Section of Neurosurgery, The University of Manitoba, Winnipeg, Manitoba, Canada

Introduction

Vasopressin (AVP) in the cerebrospinal fluid (CSF) has been implicated in the control of intracranial pressure (ICP). Evidence suggests that central AVP has a separate origin and exerts different effects than AVP in the peripheral circulation. Increased concentrations are present in the CSF of patients with a variety of neurological disorders associated with elevated ICP [2, 6] and a positive relationship exists between ICP and AVP levels in the CSF [5].

Equivocal results, however, have been obtained from experimental studies which have attempted to determine the relationship between changes in ICP and AVP. Central administration of AVP has both increased [4, 7] decreased [3] and produced no change [1] in ICP.

This study was undertaken to determine the effect of intracerebroventricular (ICV) vs intravenous (IV) administration of AVP on ICP and arterial blood pressure (BP) in rats.

Materials and Methods

Sprague-Dawley rats (250–350 g BW) were anesthetized with ketamine (90 mg/kg) – xylazine (10 mg/kg) at a dose of 0.23 ml/100 g BW and artificially ventilated following tracheotomy and administration of tubocurarine (5 mg/kg). The tail artery was cannulated to record arterial BP; ICP was recorded from the cisterna magna and IV and ICV injections were made via cannulae placed in the femoral vein and frontal horn of the lateral ventricle, respectively. Core body temperature was maintained at 36.5–37.5°C with a thermal blanket. Cerebral blood flow/volume was monitored by laser-Doppler flowmetry of the pial-cortical microvascular circulation.

* The authors acknowledge with gratitude the technical assistance provided by Mr. P. Perumal and R. Strachan. We also thank the St. Boniface General Hospital Research Foundation and the Spina Bifida Association of Canada for funding this investigation.

Following surgery, if arterial PaO_2 was >70 mmHg and $PaCO_2$ ranged from 30–40 mmHg, a 30 min baseline recording of BP and ICP was taken. At the end of this time, 14 rats were given a single ICV injection of 0.125 or 0.5 μg synthetic AVP (Sigma) in 1 μl of 0.9% saline and 4 sham controls received an equivalent volume of vehicle alone. For comparison, 12 others received a single IV injection of 0.004 or 0.125 μg AVP in 0.05 ml saline and 3 controls were given saline only. All injections were followed by a 40 min post-injection recording period. All data were acquired directly to computer.

Results

The mean ICP and BP during the pre-injection period was 3.9 ± 0.8 mmHg and 79.4 ± 7.9 mmHg (X ± SD), respectively. Average arterial blood gas values during the control period were $PaCO_2$, 35.3 ± 2.9 mmHg; PaO_2, 76.2 ± 11.4 mmHg and pH = 7.4 ± 0.04. Average blood gas values at the end of the post-injection period were $PaCO_2$, 36.5 ± 3.6 mmHg; PaO_2, 72.8 ± 7.3 mmHg and pH = 7.35 ± 0.04.

ICV injections of 0.125 or 0.5 μg AVP significantly ($p < 0.05$) reduced ICP. ICP decreased within minutes of injection and attained a mean maximum decrease of about 6% or 0.2 mmHg 4–6 min after injection and remained significantly decreased. ICV administration of an equivalent volume of vehicle alone produced no significant changes in ICP.

ICV administration of both doses of AVP also produced a concomitant decrease of cerebral blood volume (CBV) that reached a maximum of 11–14% within 4–12 min and was sustained for the duration of the experiment.

In contrast, administration of 0.004 and 0.125 μg of AVP IV produced significant ($p < 0.05$) and sustained increases in ICP that reached mean maxima of 6.5–17% (0.3–1.0 mmHg) within 2–12 min of injection. IV administration of 0.05 ml of 0.9% NaCl only produced no significant changes in ICP.

BP and ICP exhibited a negative linear relationship following ICV administration of AVP. BP increased significantly ($p < 0.05$) from 5–44% (4–34 mmHg) within 4–6 min following ICV injection of 0.125 and 0.5 μg of AVP, remained elevated but never exceeded 103–113 mmHg.

IV administration of either 0.004 or 0.125 μg of AVP resulted in significant ($p < 0.05$) but transient increases in arterial BP. A mean maximum increase of 34–100% was attained within 1–2 min of injection but returned to baseline by 9–18 min. The largest increases did not exceeded 124 mmHg with the former dose but ranged from 156–171 mmHg with the latter.

Conclusions

Consistent with reports in the literature, our results show that single ICV injections of AVP reduce ICP in rats; this contrasts with reports of increased or unchanged ICP following continuous ICV infusion of AVP.

IV administration of AVP significantly but transiently increased ICP. The larger dose (0.125 μg) also increased BP beyond the upper autoregulatory limit of 150–170 mmHg in the rat. The concomitant increase in ICP, therefore, was likely BP induced. This does not appear to be the case with the lower dose (0.004 μg) of AVP, however.

The opposite ICP responses elicited by AVP administered via the two different routes suggest that the reduction in ICP following ICV injection is likely due to a direct central effect rather than spill-over into the systemic circulation. The differences in BP responses also support this conclusion.

ICV administration of AVP appears to reduce cerebral blood volume suggesting that the ICP response may be due to cerebral vasoconstriction. AVP receptors (V_1) are present in cerebral microvessels and they also appear to be innervated by AVP containing nerve fibers. Whether the reduction in ICP reflects an effect of AVP on the cerebral vessels or on central neural loci, like the locus coeruleus, which may modulate the noradrenergic system and thereby influence both the cardiovascular system and the cerebrovasculature remains speculative at this time. Other mechanism(s), however, such as increased CSF absorption, increased ependymal and capillary permeability also cannot be precluded at this time.

References

1. Barbella YR, Keil LC, Wurpel JND, Severs WB (1983) Cerebrospinal fluid pressure during cerebroventricular infusion of angiotensin and vasopressin. Exp Neurol 82:325–334
2. Mather HM, Ang V, Jenkins JS (1981) Vasopressin in plasma and CSF of patients with subarachnoid hemorrhage. J Neurol Neurosurg Psych 44:216–219
3. Noto T, Nakajima T, Saji Y, Nagawa Y (1978) Effect of vasopressin on intracranial pressure of rabbit. Endocrinol Japon 25:591–596
4. Seckl JR, Lightman SL (1987) Intracerebroventricular arginine vasopressin causes intracranial pressure to rise in conscious goats. Brain Res 423:279–285
5. Sorensen PS, Gjerris F, Hammer M (1984) Cerebrospinal fluid vasopressin and increased intracranial pressure. Ann Neurol 15:435–440
6. Sorensen PS (1986) Studies of vasopressin in the human cerebrospinal fluid. Acta Neurol Scand 74:81–102
7. Sorensen PS, Gyring JA (1990) Intracerebroventricular infusion but not bolus injection of vasopressin increases the cerebrospinal fluid pressure in awake rabbits. Neurological Res 12:83–88

Cerebral Aerobic Index and Oxygen/Glucose Ratio in Acute Brain Injury

J. Cruz[1], W.M. Alves[1], T.A. Gennarelli[1], S.J. Allen[3], and M.E. Miner[2]

[1] Division of Neurosurgery and Head Injury Center, University of Pennsylvania, 3400 Spruce St., Philadelphia, PA 19104, USA
[2] Division of Neurologic Surgery, Ohio State University, Columbus, OH 43210, USA
[3] Department of Anesthesiology, University of Texas, Houston, TX 77030, USA

Introduction

We have previously found a strong association between global cerebral luxury perfusion (hyperemia) and intracranial hypertension, in severe acute brain trauma [7]. In the same work, we found an excellent inverse relationship between mean regional cerebral blood flow (CBF) values and the arterio-jugular oxygen content difference ($AJDO_2$), so that decreased $AJDO_2$ values were consistent with global cerebral hyperperfusion relative to oxygen consumption ($CMRO_2$), and vice versa. We therefore adopted and proposed clinical monitoring of the arteriojugular oxygen difference for both intermittent and continuous assessment [1–5]. The present work was aimed at investigating the relationship between global cerebral glucose and oxygen extraction in severe acute brain trauma, as a means of assessing a possible etiological basis for cerebral anaerobic metabolism, and its association with cerebral luxury perfusion and related intracranial hypertension.

Clinical Material and Methods

Ten adults with severe acute closed brain trauma were prospectively evaluated during an average period of 2.5 days. The Glasgow Coma Scale [8] scores were in the range of 4 to 7, and the admission computerized tomography (CT) scans of the head disclosed predominantly diffuse brain swelling. The intracranial pressure (ICP) and the systemic arterial pressure (SAP) were continuously monitored. The cerebral perfusion pressure (CPP) was monitored as the difference between mean SAP and ICP. Intermittent monitoring at approximately four-hour intervals was carried out for the arterial PCO_2 ($PaCO_2$), arterio-jugular bulb oxygen content difference ($AJDO_2$), and glucose concentration difference (AJDGL). Blood samples were of approximately 1 ml each. In each study, the mean AJDGL values were calculated from an average of 8.7 arterial and jugular determinations of the glucose concentration in whole blood. The average standard deviation of the AJDGL determinations corresponded to only 12.9% of the mean AJDGL values. Observations were carried out during the course of therapeutic sedation, muscle paralysis, and optimized hyperventilation (based on the $AJDO_2$), for ICP control below 20 mmHg. All patients received intravenous 5% glucose in 0.45% saline solution (average infusion rate of 100 ml/hr) during the study period. Fasting for over 48 hours prior to trauma and a premorbid history of diabetes mellitus were ruled out by the next of kin. After the study period, follow-up head CT scans showed no evidence of cerebral infarction.

The relationship between cerebral oxygen and glucose extraction was assessed in terms of the oxygen/glucose ratio (OGR), and the aerobic index (AI), where $AJDO_2$ and AJDGL are expressed in mMol/dl. The OGR and the AI were calculated according to the following equations: $OGR = [(AJDO_2/22.4)/(AJDGL/180)]$, and $AI = [(AJDO_2/22.4)/(6 * AJDGL/180)]$, where $AJDO_2$ is in vol% and AJDGL is in mg%. Stoichiometrically, the normal OGR is 6. The normal AI range was estimated from reported norms for the $AJDO_2$ and AJDGL [6], from which we assessed raw data and calculated the AI values. The normal AI range was estimated as 0.64 to 1.24 (0.94 ± 0.30, mean ± 2 SD). The normal ranges for $AJDO_2$ and AJDGL are 4.9 to 8.5 vol% and 7 to 12.2 mg% (respectively, 6.7 ± 1.8 vol% and 9.6 ± 2.6 mg%, means ± 2 SD), at a mean $PaCO_2$ of 39.5 mmHg.

Correlations among the variables under study were assessed by Pearson's correlation coefficient. Differences among separate groups of observations were assessed by one-way analysis of variance. Simultaneously assessed physiological parameters will be presented as means ± SD, for 4 groups of observations: Group 1 – where the AI was below the normal range (anaerobic oxygen/glucose uncoupling); Group 2a – where the AI was on the low side of the normal range, but the OGR was decreased in the range of 4 to 5 ("impending" anaerobic uncoupling); Group 2b – where the AI and the OGR were higher than in group 2a, but within the normal range; and Group 3 – where the AI was above the normal range, with corresponding increased OGR values (nonanaerobic uncoupling). Data from Groups 2a and 2b were also combined in a single Group 2. Since all observations were carried out during hyperventilation, the $AJDO_2$ values were presumably increased (due to hypocapnic CBF decreases). Thus, in order to estimate the natural occurrence of cerebral luxury perfusion, the measured $AJDO_2$ values were subsequently corrected for normocapnia ($PaCO_2$ of 40 mmHg), by adopting a 3% change in $AJDO_2$ per unit change in $PaCO_2$ [7]. No corrections were applied for the AJDGL, as no correction factors are known from simultaneous studies of corrected CBF and AJDGL.

Results

A total of 102 studies were performed in the 10 patients. In these studies, the arterial glucose concentration was 119 ± 34 mg%, the arterial pH was 7.49 ± 0.05, the hemoglobin content was 11.5 ± 1.5 gm/dl, and the rectal temperature was 37.6 ± 0.9 degrees Celsius. Nine of the studies, in 5 of the 10 patients, had an AI below 0.64 (Group 1); 75 in the 10 patients had an AI from 0.64 to 1.24 (Group 2), and 18 in 6 patients had an AI above 1.24 (Group 3). Of the 75 observations in Group 2, 27 in 8 of the patients had an OGR in the range of 4 to 5 (Group 2a). Adding up observations from Groups 1 and 2a, the rate of anaerobic oxygen/glucose uncoupling was of 35.2%, in 80% of the patients. Tables 1 and 2 present data on 7 simultaneously assessed variables, respectively for Groups 1, 2, and 3, and Groups 1, 2a, and 2b. The $AJDO_2$ values in the two Tables are uncorrected for normocapnia.

In Groups 1, 2, and 3 (Table 1), significant ICP differences were found, higher ICP values being found in Group 1. Also significant were the $AJDO_2$ differences, lower values found in Group 1, in a trend opposite to that of the AJDGL (lower values found in Group 3), which differences were also significant. The AI and OGR differences were also statistically significant. The $PaCO_2$ differences were not statistically significant, although a trend was found for lower $PaCO_2$ levels to be required for control of higher ICP values. When Group 3 was excluded (Table 2), the same overall significant changes were found, as in Table 1; that is, a tendency was found for Group 2a to behave as that of "impending" anaerobiosis, which associated with higher ICP and lower $AJDO_2$ values than in Group 2b.

In the 102 studies, there was an inverse correlation between AI and ICP ($r = -0.41$, $p < 0.0001$), and positive correlation between AI and uncorrected $AJDO_2$ ($r = 0.33$, $p = 0.0006$). The OGR correlated with these variables in the same way as did the AI, as expected. There was a modest inverse cor-

Table 1. Physiological variables in 10 patients (Groups 1, 2, and 3)

Variable	Group 1	Group 2	Group 3	p value
ICP (mmHg)	20 ± 4.7	15 ± 4.5	12 ± 3.2	0.0001
CPP (mmHg)	83 ± 16	78 ± 12	85 ± 11	0.08 (NS)
$PaCO_2$ (mmHg)	22.3 ± 6.5	24.9 ± 4.2	26.6 ± 4.5	0.07 (NS)
$AJDO_2$ (vol %)	4.8 ± 1.4	6.16 ± 1.22	6.66 ± 1.63	0.003
AJDGL (mg %)	10.9 ± 2.8	9.1 ± 2.17	6.22 ± 1.65	<0.0001
AI	0.58 ± 0.04	0.92 ± 0.17	1.45 ± 0.17	<0.0001
OGR	3.5 ± 0.29	5.56 ± 1.04	8.72 ± 1.03	<0.0001

Values are means ± standard deviation. NS = not statistically significant.

Table 2. Physiological variables in 10 patients (Groups 1, 2a, and 2b)

Variable	Group 1	Group 2a	Group 2b	p value
ICP (mmHg)	20 ± 4.7	17 ± 3.8	14 ± 4.6	0.0005
CPP (mmHg)	83 ± 16	76 ± 12	80 ± 11	0.19 (NS)
$PaCO_2$ (mmHg)	22.3 ± 6.5	24.3 ± 3.9	25.3 ± 4.4	0.17 (NS)
$AJDO_2$ (vol %)	4.8 ± 1.4	5.78 ± 1.1	6.38 ± 1.2	0.001
AJDGL (mg %)	10.9 ± 2.8	10.5 ± 2.2	8.34 ± 1.6	<0.0001
AI	0.58 ± 0.04	0.74 ± 0.05	1.03 ± 0.12	<0.0001
OGR	3.5 ± 0.29	4.45 ± 0.35	6.19 ± 0.73	<0.0001

Values are means ± standard deviation. NS = not statistically significant.

relation between ICP and uncorrected $AJDO_2$ ($r = -0.21$, $p = 0.02$). The latter was much stronger when the $AJDO_2$ values were corrected for normocapnia ($r = -0.53$, $p < 0.0001$), which better disclosed the association between cerebral luxury perfusion and intracranial hypertension.

The uncorrected $AJDO_2$ values were below 4.9 vol% (luxury perfusion) 16 times (15.7%), in 6 of the 10 patients; from 4.9 to 8.5 vol% (normalized $CMRO_2$/CBF ratio) 79 times (77.4%), in the 10 patients; and above 8.5 vol% (oligemic hypoxia) 7 times (6.9%), in 5 of the patients. These early seven observations, however, did not associate with AI and OGR values from Groups 1 or 2a. Thus, by-and-large, the predominantly normalized $AJDO_2$ values reflected adequate (optimized) hypocapnia for ICP control. When corrected for normocapnia, 94 of the 102 $AJDO_2$ values (92.2%), in the 10 patients, were below 4.9 vol%. The remaining 8 values (7.8%), in 3 of the patients, were in the normal range. None of the corrected $AJDO_2$ values was abnormally increased. The corrected $AJDO_2$ values were significantly different for Groups 1, 2a, 2b, and 3 (respectively, 2.23 ± 1.07, 3.03 ± 0.85, 3.53 ± 0.91, and 3.92 ± 1.22 vol% – $p = 0.0001$). These findings revealed that observations in which the OGR was ≤ 5 tended to present with the most pronounced degrees of cerebral luxury perfusion.

Discussion

Our present findings indicated a close association among increased ICP, decreased AI (and OGR), and decreased $AJDO_2$ values. The significant association between elevated ICP and decreased $AJDO_2$ was previously reported by our group of investigators [7]. However, an etiological basis for the existence of posttraumatic cerebral luxury perfusion (and associated intracranial hypertension) has not been, to our knowledge, previously confirmed. Nor has the above described triple association been reported, which offers a possible etiological relationship between cerebral anaerobiosis and luxury perfusion. Perhaps most important, the above findings disclosed an anaerobic uncoupling between cerebral glucose and oxygen extraction, a logical explanation for cerebral lactate production. Even though cerebral lactate production has been reported in acute brain trauma, in studies where cerebral ischemia was assessed, a primarily metabolic etiological source for lactate production has not been previously addressed. It is particularly interesting that an association between cerebrospinal fluid lactic acidosis and cerebral luxury perfusion has been reported in acute brain trauma [9], however without an etiological background for the existence of the lactacidosis-hyperemia relationship. We believe our present findings may provide further insight into the pathophysiology of posttraumatic cerebral luxury perfusion, and plan to further study the relationships among $AJDO_2$, AJDGL, and the arteriojugular lactate difference. This would eventually allow us to establish "threshold" values for low OGR (and AI), at which cerebral lactate production would ensue. We would then attempt to investigate possible therapies to intervene upon the anaerobic uncoupling; that is, therapies that might allow us to actually increase low OGR (and AI) values, and presumably minimize cerebral lactate production. Such a therapeutic approach, to our knowledge not yet proposed, would basically aim at *selectively* decreasing cerebral glucose extraction *relative* to oxygen extraction, its reciprocal, or both.

Our findings also indicated that AJDGL measurements alone may provide misleading information regarding the status of the global cerebral oxygen metabolism – flow relationship. In fact, in Groups 1 and 3, the AJDGL would, if measured alone, mistakenly suggest adequate or decreased CBF, and increased CBF (relative to metabolic demand), respectively; that is, in Group 1 the AJDGL was normal to high, while in Group 3 it was abnormally decreased. However, in Group 1, the uncorrected $AJDO_2$ was normal to low (consistent with adequate or increased CBF to metabolic demand), and in Group 3 it was normal (consistent with adequate CBF to metabolic demand). Thus, in this group of patients, cerebral glucose extraction may periodically behave relatively independently of oxygen extraction. Fortunately, the most significant AJDGL abnormality (an abnormal decrease, in Group 3) is not expected to result in the formation of deleterious products to brain function, as is the case when the OGR is decreased (Groups 1 and 2a), and lactate production is expected to ensue.

Acknowledgements. This work was supported in part by Grants R49/CCR303687-02 from the Center for Environmental Health and Injury Control of the Centers for Disease Control, and NS-08803-19 from the National Institute of Neurological Disorders and Stroke.

References

1. Cruz J, Allen SJ, Miner ME (1985) Hypoxic insults in acute brain injury. Crit Care Med 13:284
2. Cruz J, Miner ME (1986) Modulating cerebral oxygen delivery and extraction in acute traumatic coma. In: Miner ME, Wagner KA (eds) Neurotrauma. Treatment, Rehabilitation, and Related Issues, ed. 1. Butterworths, Boston, pp 55–72
3. Cruz J (1988) Continuous versus serial global cerebral hemometabolic monitoring: applications in acute brain trauma. Acta Neurochir 42 (Suppl):35–39
4. Cruz J, Miner ME, Allen SJ, Alves WM, Gennarelli TA (1990) Continuous monitoring of cerebral oxygenation in acute brain injury: injection of mannitol during hyperventilation. J Neurosurg 73:725–730
5. Cruz J, Miner ME, Allen SJ, Alves WM, Gennarelli TA (1991) Continuous monitoring of cerebral oxygenation in acute brain injury: assessment of cerebral hemodynamic reserve. Neurosurgery 29, no 5:743–749
6. Gibbs EL, Lennox WG, Nims LF, Gibbs FA (1942) Arterial and cerebral venous blood. Arterial-venous differences in man. J Biol Chem 144:325–332
7. Obrist WD, Langfitt TW, Jaggi JL, Cruz J, Gennarelli TA (1984) Cerebral blood flow and metabolism in comatose patients with acute head injury. Relationship to intracranial hypertension. J Neurosurg 61:241–253
8. Teasdale G, Jennett B (1974) Assessment of coma and impaired consciousness. A practical scale. Lancet 2:81–84
9. Zupping R (1970) Cerebral acid-base and gas metabolism in brain injury. J Neurosurg 33:498–505

Combined Monitoring of ICP and Cerebrovenous Oxygen Saturation to Estimate Cerebral Blood Flow

A. UNTERBERG, A. VON HELDEN, G.-H. SCHNEIDER, and W. LANKSCH

Department of Neurosurgery, Universitätsklinikum Rudolf Virchow, Free University of Berlin, 1000 Berlin 65, Germany

Introduction

In comatose patients, monitoring of intracranial pressure has become a routine procedure. To prevent secondary cerebral ischemia, representing a major secondary insult to the traumatized brain [2, 4], it would be of the utmost importance to monitor cerebral blood flow, in addition. Measurement of cerebral blood flow in these patients is difficult to perform and limited to stochastic determinations. Recently, it has been demonstrated that the cerebral arteriovenous oxygen difference can be used to estimate cerebral blood flow [5, 6]. Moreover, it has become possible to continuously monitor cerebrovenous oxygen saturation by a fiberoptic catheter system [1, 3]. Such a system (Oximetrix 3) was used to continuously measure oxygen saturation in the jugular bulb of comatose patients to estimate cerebral blood flow and identify cerebral ischemia.

Methods

In 22 comatose patients due to severe head injury (n = 9), subarachnoid hemorrhage (n = 7) and intracerebral hemorrhage (n = 6), intracranial pressure (ICP) and cerebrovenous oxygen saturation (CVOS) were continuously monitored for 1–10 days. A 4 F double-lumen fiberoptical catheter (Opticath, Abbott) was placed in the jugular bulb under X-ray-screening. The spectroscopically measured oxygen saturation was calibrated after insertion and twice daily thereafter. The catheter was furthermore used to withdraw cerebrovenous blood to determine pH, pO_2, pCO_2, glucose and lactate. An additional arterial line made it possible to determine the arteriovenous difference of oxygen saturation and lactate concentration ($AVDSO_2$, AVDL) [7].

Results and Discussion

The oximetric catheter yielded reliable values of the cerebrovenous oxygen saturation during the entire monitoring period (up to 10 days) as checked by

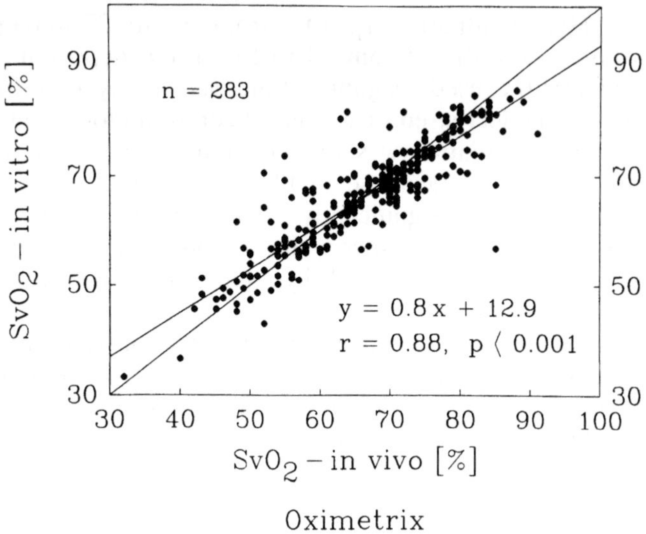

Fig. 1. Comparison of cerebrovenous oxygen saturation as determined by direct oximetry (in-vitro) and by fiberoptical measurements (Oximetry, in-vivo)

Table 1. Cerebrovenous oxygen saturation (CVOS) and arteriovenous difference of lactate (AVDL) in patients with "normal", and compromised cerebral blood flow

CPP	>50 mmHg	<50 mmHg
CVOS	69–90% (70 ± 4%)	<55%
AVDL	<3 mg/dl	>3 mg/dl
CBF	adequate	inadequate

CPP = cerebral perfusion pressure
CVOS = cerebro-venous oxygen saturation
AVDL = arterio-venous difference of lactate
CBF = cerebral blood flow

blood-gas analyses and direct oximetry. Oxygen saturation determined by direct oximetry in-vitro was found to correlate excellently with the fiberoptic measurements in-vivo (Fig. 1).

Within 12 hours there was a 4 ± 3% drift of the catheter measurements which was corrected by regular recalibration. There were no complications which might have been attributed to the jugular catheter, like thrombosis or infection.

The patterns of patients with supposedly normal, or decreased cerebral blood flow in respect to cerebral perfusion pressure, cerebro-venous oxygen saturation and lactate production are given in Table 1. In patients with compromised cerebral blood flow, CVOS fell below 55% and AVDL increased above 3 mg/dl.

In non-ischemic patients, CO_2-response and pressure autoregulation were tested.

Hyperventilation (pCO_2: from 34 to 27 mmHg) caused a decrease in oxygen saturation (from 70 to 58%) and hypoventilation (pCO_2: from 31 to 41 mmHg) caused a significant increase in oxygen saturation (from 65 to 76%), indicating decreased or enhanced cerebral blood flow, respectively.

Autoregulation was studied by infusion of etilefrin or urapidil, producing an increase or decrease in blood pressure, respectively. These manoeuvres usually did not significantly affect cerebral venous oxygen saturation. Only some patients with severe head injury showed an increase or decrease in CVOS due to hyper- of hypotension, respectively, indicating a disturbed autoregulation.

Further studies concerning the effect of head elevation on ICP and CVOS revealed that in patients with a moderately decreased intracranial compliance, head elevation reduced intracranial pressure, but did not significantly affect cerebrovenous oxygen saturation.

Conclusions

Continuous monitoring of cerebrovenous oxygen saturation in the jugular bulb supplemented by determination of the arteriovenous difference of lactate enables one to estimate cerebral blood flow. Thereby, it is possible to identify secondary ischemia, to test pressure autoregulation, and to analyze the effects of various therapeutic regimens on CBF.

It is hoped that this new monitoring modality will be a useful tool in the management of comatose patients.

Acknowledgements. The technical and secretarial assistance of J. Kopetzki and A. Riede is highly appreciated.

References

1. Andrews PJD, Piper IR, Dearden NM, Miller JD (1990) Secondary insults during intrahospital transport of head injured patients. Lancet 335:327–330
2. Baethmann A, Go KG, Unterberg A (eds) (1986) Mechanisms of Secondary Brain Damage. Plenum Press, New York
3. Cruz J, Miner ME, Allen SJ, Alves WM, Gennarelli TA (1990) Continuous monitoring of cerebral oxygenation in acute brain injury: injection of mannitol during hyperventilation. J Neurosurg 73:725–730
4. Miller JD, Sweet RC, Narayan R, Becker DP (1978) Early insults in the injured brain. JAMA 240:439–442
5. Robertson C, Narayan RK, Gokaslan ZL, Pahwa R, Grossman RG, Caram P, Allen E (1989) Cerebral arteriovenous oxygen difference as an estimate of cerebral blood flow in comatose patients. J Neurosurg 70:222–230
6. Sutton LN, McLaughlin AC, Dante S, Kotapka M, Sinwell T, Mills E (1990) Cerebral venous oxygen content as a measure of brain energy metabolism with increased intracranial pressure and hyperventilation. J Neurosurg 73:927–932
7. Unterberg A, Gethmann J, von Helden A, Schneider GH, Lanksch W: Treatment of "cerebral vasospasm" with hypervolemia and hypertension, in: Advances of Neurosurgery (in press)

Functional Exploration of the Internal Jugular Veins

N. Stocchetti, A. Paparella, T. Serioli, A. Vezzani, P. Zuccoli, and A. Marmarou

Ist Dept. Anesthesia & Intensive Care – Hospital of Parma, Via Abbeveratoia, 14, 43100 Parma, Italy
Div. Neurosurgery – Medical College of Virginia, Box 508 MCV Station 23298, Richmond, VA, USA

Introduction

The determination of clearance of metabolites and oxygen in the brain is based on the assumption that a reliable sample of mixed venous blood can be drawn from the internal jugular vein (IJ) [1, 6, 7, 9]. In the current literature many measurements ($AVDO_2$, $CMRO_2$, etc.) are reported based on IJ samples drawn from either side of the neck. We compared oxygen saturation in both IJs in head injured patients to establish similarities or discrepancies in the two veins.

Clinical Material and Methods

From February 1990 to April 1991, 20 head injured patients who were admitted to our Intensive Care Unit in coma (GCS $\leqslant$ 8 between admission and up to 6 hours post-trauma) were studied. These patients underwent standard treatment protocol. This included continuous monitoring of arterial pressure, central venous pressure and intracranial pressure (ICP) through ventricular catheters (13 cases) or subdural catheters (7 cases). All the patients were ventilated to maintain a $PaO_2 \geqslant 100\,mmHg$ and a $PaCO_2$ ranging from 30 to 35 mmHg. If standard measures failed to keep ICP less than 20 mmHg (CSF withdrawal, mannitol and sedation), lower levels of $PaCO_2$ were reached. The hemoglobin concentration was kept above 10 g% using red cell transfusions if necessary. Both internal jugular veins were cannulated according to the technique reported by Goetting [4]. In 10 cases 14 G introducers were used and in the remainder of cases 20 G catheters were placed (Leader Cath 115, Vygon France). The catheter position was verified by X-ray in two projections, antero-posterior and lateral. The lateral film was obtained in a position slightly less than perpendicular to the neck to allow visualization of both catheters. The correct placement of the catheters was indicated by the projection of the catheter tips into the superior jugular bulb. Through the introducer catheters, a 16 G silicon catheter (15 cm) (Viacath 730-7 Becton Dickinson France) was inserted upstream in 5 patients, reaching approximately the sigmoid sinus. An additional X-ray was obtained at this time to confirm the proper position of the catheter. At this point simultaneous samples were withdrawn from the catheters in equivalent position of the two IJs. After this maneuver a new 20 G catheter replaced the long one. In 5 patients a fiberoptic catheter (Oximetrix Abbot Critical Care System) was inserted through the introducer to obtain a continuous recording of the hemoglobin saturation. Both in the case of the silicon catheters and the Oximetrix catheters the introducer sheath was withdrawn as soon as a correct placement of the inside catheter was reached. Blood samples were taken simultaneously from the two IJs and immediately processed using a Co-Oximeter (Instrumentation Laboratory 482 Co-Oximeter).

During the first phase of this investigation we checked the precision and accuracy of the measurements, by processing the same sample with two Co-Oximeters and repeating the analysis of the same sample 3 times. The variability of the measures was approximately 1%. When fiberoptic catheters were used, we performed an *in vivo* calibration every 12 hr and accepted the recorded data only if the light intensity signal was in the recommended range.

The statistical analysis was performed using a "summary measures method" [5] with confidence limits calculation in order to analyze the maximum differences between the two IJs. A regression model was also fit in order to evaluate the contribution of some clinical factors to the degree of variability between the two IJs. Since the maximum difference in mean Hb saturation was exponentially distributed we used a log transformation. A forward selection procedure was performed in order to identify simultaneously influential variables.

Results

Twenty patients, 12 male and 8 female, with a mean age of 45.6 years (SD 20.4) were studied. The data about the patients are reported in Table 1. Eight patients showed differences in the hemoglobin saturation greater than 10% at some point during the investigation. Five more patients had differences ranging from 6 to 10%. The average of the differences in the two IJs for each patient is also reported in Table 1. The mean value of this data is 3.9 with a standard deviation of 4.1. Eight patients had the higher hemoglobin saturation in the right IJ, and 11 had the higher values in the left. One patient had no differences between the two sides. Each patient was classified into two groups according to CT scan results, patients with unilateral lesions (14 cases) and patients with bilateral lesions (6 cases). Eight patients had right hemisphere lesions, and 3 of these had differences between the two IJs greater than 5%. The side with the higher hemoglobin saturation was the left in all three cases. Six patients had left hemisphere lesions and 5 of them developed a difference between the two IJs greater than 5%. Three of these patients had the higher hemoglobin saturation in the right IJ. Among the six patients with bilateral lesions, we detected a difference between the two IJs greater than 10% in two cases, and between 6 and 10% in two more patients.

Table 1. Summary of data on the patient severity and the values of Oxygen Hemoglobin saturation in the left and right Internal Jugular veins

Pt. number	Sex	Age	CTScan	GCS	Right IJ Mean Hb Sat	Left IJ Mean Hb Sat	Difference in Mean Hb Sat	Max Difference in Mean Hb Sat
1	F	55	Diffuse Injury	4	72.5	70	2.5	4
2	M	81	Subdural H.	5	65	67.5	2.5	3
3	M	25	Subdural H.	6	73.5	77	3.5	4
4	F	76	Subdural H.	6	48	64.1	16.1	37
5	M	24	Diffuse Injury	7	63.4	64.4	1	2
6	M	60	Epidural H.	6	63.1	72	9.5	17
7	M	25	Subdural H.	6	78.7	78.7	0	2
8	M	24	Subdural H.	4	68.7	61.3	7.4	13
9	M	50	Contusions	7	69.5	64.6	4.8	11
10	F	53	Contusions	7	69.6	68.6	1	2
11	F	39	Subdural H.	4	69.5	70.7	1.1	7
12	F	77	Subdural H.	6	59.6	61.8	2.2	13
13	F	72	Subdural H.	7	69.4	71	1.5	7
14	M	18	Contusions	5	74.1	72.5	1.6	8
15	M	53	Subdural H.	8	60.2	70.2	10	19
16	F	34	Subdural H.	8	76.2	75.5	.7	10
17	M	21	Contusions	5	67	63	4	8
18	F	50	Diffuse Injury	7	64.5	69.5	5	20
19	M	53	Diffuse Injury	4	70.7	71	.2	5
20	M	21	Contusions	8	61.7	59.2	2.5	28

The time course of the Hb saturation is dependent on the relationships between flow and tissue needs and is therefore variable. Nevertheless, a consistent pattern in the difference between the two sides was measured in most of the cases.

In an attempt to identify the causes of such a variability, we explored both IJ veins at different levels in five patients starting from the jugular superior bulb and going up to the sigmoid sinus. In each IJ the hemoglobin saturation was higher at the jugular bulb than at the sigmoid sinus, by an average of 3% higher. The relationships between the two IJs were consistent: when the values showed some difference in the samples from the jugular bulb, the same difference was detected in the samples withdrawn from the sinus. These data suggest that the source of variability is upstream to the sigmoid sinus.

In the subset of patients monitored using fiberoptic catheters we observed a pattern of Hemoglobin saturation in good agreement with the data obtained through repeated blood samples in 3 cases. In two patients the side with the lower saturation at some point of the recording had the same saturation, or higher, than the contralateral.

The 95% confidence limits for the percentage of the patients with difference higher than 10 were 19–64%; at the same level of confidence the limits for the percentage of patients with difference higher than 5 were 41–85%. The per cent of variability explained by some clinical factors was assessed in many steps; when the mean value of the differences was entered it showed a significant p value ($p = 0.0009$). In the following steps the outcome, sex, age and

CT scan diagnosis were entered in the model, both combined and as single factors. The variables explained only a small fraction of the maximum difference, without any significant level of p. We concluded that, based on this sample, none of the clinical data examined could explain the variability of the Hb saturation measured in the two IJs.

Discussion

According to the literature we can estimate that roughly 1/3 of blood flow present in each IJ is flowing from the contralateral hemisphere [8], so the mixing of the blood is only partial. Therefore, we expect some difference in the hemoglobin saturation when the relationships between the oxygen supply and the oxygen consumption are not constant among different regions of the brain. In comatose head injured patients it has been shown [6] that 65% of cases have significant hemispheral and/or regional CBF differences. It is common clinical practice to calculate the $AVDO_2$ based on blood sampled from one IJ, and it is therefore of interest to establish whether we can estimate the true oxygen content from one IJ or whether we have to consider relevant differences between the two sides.

The proportion of patients with relevant discrepancies between the two IJs is higher than suspected, because we detected 8 of 20 patients with a difference greater than 10 points of Hb saturation. Looking at the confidence intervals we can estimate that a proportion varying from 19 to 64% of the patients can have such a difference, and that a higher proportion (41–85%) can have a difference between 6 and 10% in the Hb saturation. In other words, in a wide proportion of the patients this difference could change the $AVDO_2$ calculation as much as more than 30%, causing inaccurate estimates of parameters related to the $AVDO_2$.

It seems reasonable to expect wider differences in unilateral lesions, but this finding was not present in our study population, since 4 patients had relevant differences despite having a bilateral lesion present. Since the source of variability is upstream to the sigmoid sinus we hypothesize that some patients have venous return from the brain that is not mixed before entering the IJs and these regional differences in flow and/or metabolism are reflected in the different oxygen content. A search of the literature confirmed that a few data exist in this field of investigation [2, 3, 8] and some differences between the two IJs were detected in previous research [8].

At this point, the reliability of the data we obtained from a single IJ catheter should be carefully examined. It has been suggested that the IJ catheter should be placed on the side of most severe injury or on the right side in case of diffuse lesion [7] but our data do not support the concept of a "good" side for the cerebral venous hemoglobin saturation.

We conclude that, since blood can carry varying concentrations of metabolites and oxygen in the left IJ compared to the right, many measures based on oxygen content of the IJ should be reconsidered.

References

1. Cruz J, Miner ME, Allen SJ, Alves WM, Gennarelli TA (1990) Continuous monitoring of cerebral oxygenation in acute brain injury: injection of mannitol during hyperventilation. J Neurosurg 73:725–730
2. Gibbs EL, Lennox WG, Nims LF, Gibbs FA (1942) Arterial and cerebral venous blood. Arterial-venous differences in man. J Biol Chem 144:325–332
3. Gibbs EL, Lennox WG, Gibbs FA (1945) Bilateral internal jugular blood. Comparison of A-V differences, oxygen-dextrose ratios and respiratory quotients. Am J Psychiatry 102:184–190
4. Goetting MG, Preston G (1990) Jugular bulb catheterization: experience with 123 patients. Crit Care Med 18, 11:1220–1223
5. Matthews JNS, Altman DG, Campbell MJ, Royston P (1990) Analysis of serial measurements in medical research. Br Med J 300:230–235
6. Obrist WD, Langfitt TW, Jaggi JL, Cruz J, Gennarelli TA (1984) Cerebral blood flow and metabolism in comatose head injury. J Neurosurg 61:241–253
7. Robertson CS, Narayan RK, Gokaslan ZL, Pahwa R, Grossmann RG, Caram P, Allen E (1989) Cerebral arteriovenous oxygen difference as an estimate of cerebral blood flow in comatose patients. J Neurosurg 70:222–230
8. Shenkin HA, Harmel MH, Kety SS (1948) Dynamic anatomy of the cerebral circulation. Arch Neurol Psychiatry 60:240–252
9. Sutton LN, McLaughlin AC, Dante S, Kotapka M, Sinwell T, Mills E (1990) Cerebral venous oxygen content as a measure of brain energy metabolism with increased intracranial pressure and hyperventilation. J Neurosurg 73:927–932

Blood Pressure and ICP Dynamics in Severe Head Injury: Relation With CBF Autoregulation

G.J. Bouma, J.P. Muizelaar, K. Bandoh, and A. Marmarou

Division of Neurosurgery, Medical College of Virginia, Virginia Commonwealth University, Richmond, VA, USA

Introduction

There is controversy about the optimal blood pressure management in severely head-injured patients. Traditionally, high arterial blood pressure has been thought to break down the blood-brain barrier and cause cerebral edema, and therefore, antihypertensive therapy has been advocated [6]. However, when CBF is reduced, as is frequently the case in the first 24 hours, this procedure carries the risk of provoking cerebral ischemia by decreasing CPP, especially since $AVDO_2$ is usually still high in this period [2]. Thus, maintaining adequate CPP may be more important than control of ICP per se. It has also been suggested that maintaining slightly elevated CPP, if necessary even by pharmacologically induced arterial hypertension, would prevent ICP "plateau" waves or even reduce ICP by autoregulatory vasoconstriction [9].

Several factors should be taken into account when manipulating arterial blood pressure after severe head injury. First, the status of autoregulation (which may or may not be intact after severe head injury) will determine the effect on cerebral hemodynamics. However, it is important to determine whether increased CBF resulting from induced hypertension also leads to improved cerebral metabolism as measured by $CMRO_2$, or whether the increased CBF is merely "luxury perfusion". Second, the way in which changes in arterial blood pressure will affect ICP and brain stiffness, measured either as compliance, elastance, or pressure-volume index (PVI), is also dependent on the status of autoregulation [7]. However, these relationships are complex, and experimental data have been compounded by effects of anaesthesia [1, 3, 4].

In the present study, we have evaluated the responses of CBF, $CMRO_2$, ICP, and PVI to induced changes in blood pressure during tests of autoregulation in severely head-injured patients. Thus, we were able to examine the above relationships separately for both intact and defective autoregulation.

Clinical Materials and Methods

Forty-seven comatose severely head-injured patients (GCS ≤ 8) were studied. All patients were ventilated mechanically and paralyzed with pancuronium bromide, in order to achieve optimal control of pCO_2, and prevent movement artifacts. ICP was measured with an intraventricular catheter and mean arterial blood pressure (MABP) was monitored from an intra-arterial catheter. PVI was determined by intraventricular bolus injection or withdrawal as described by Marmarou [5]. Measurement of CBF was performed by the ^{133}Xe i.v. injection technique using a Novo 10-a apparatus. Autoregulation was tested by i.v. infusion of phenylephrine or trimethaphan camsylate (Arfonad) to respectively raise of decrease MABP by 25–30%. Autoregulation was defined intact if $\Delta\%CPP/\Delta\%CVR \leqslant 2$ [8]. Arterial blood gases were obtained during each CBF measurement. Small differences in pCO_2 between pre- and postdrug measurements were corrected for by assuming a 3% change in CBF per torr change in pCO_2. $AVDO_2$ was determined twice during each CBF measurement, by oximetry of simultaneously obtained arterial and jugular venous blood samples, and $CMRO_2$ was calculated by multiplying CBF and $AVDO_2$.

Results

A total of 58 autoregulation tests were performed. Autoregulation was found to be intact 40 times (69%) and defective 18 times (31%). The mean and S.D. of the measured parameters for both intact and defective autoregulation are shown in Table 1. When autoregulation was intact, increased blood pressure did not change ICP significantly, but lowering blood pressure resulted in a steep increase in ICP. With defective autoregulation, however, ICP varied directly with MABP ($p < 0.01$, paired t-test). The changes in CBF resulting from blood pressure manipulations in patients with impaired autoregulation did not significantly alter $CMRO_2$. The changes in brain compliance as indicated by PVI are shown in Fig. 1. There was a weak, yet significant ($p < 0.05$, paired t-test) positive correlation between CPP and PVI when autoregulation was preserved, but with defective autoregulation PVI was inversely related to CPP ($p < 0.01$).

Table 1.

Autoregulation		Hypotension	Hypertension
Intact	MABP	120 ± 13 → 91 ± 10	93 ± 11 → 119 ± 11
	ICP	20 ± 3 → 30 ± 2*	20 ± 6 → 20 ± 8
(n = 40)	PVI	22 ± 5 → 22 ± 6	19 ± 6 → 21 ± 7
	CBF	38 ± 6 → 35 ± 4	35 ± 10 → 37 ± 11
	$CMRO_2$	1.01 ± 0.29 → 0.99 ± 0.41	1.71 ± 0.62 → 1.60 ± 0.52
Defective	MABP	112 ± 19 → 90 ± 17	99 ± 12 → 126 ± 9
	ICP	16 ± 5 → 11 ± 7*	16 ± 7 → 20 ± 9*
(n = 18)	PVI	21 ± 9 → 24 ± 2**	22 ± 5 → 18 ± 4**
	CBF	79 ± 38 → 37 ± 10	34 ± 6 → 50 ± 14
	$CMRO_2$	2.07 ± 0.29 → 1.86 ± 0.49	1.32 ± 0.39 → 1.50 ± 0.65

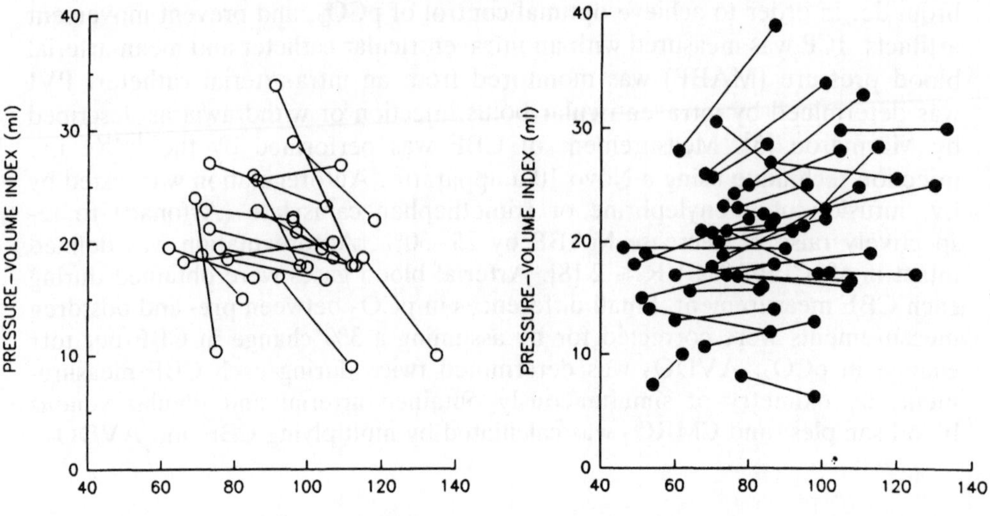

Fig. 1a,b. Pressure-volume Index (ml) versus cerebral perfusion pressure (mmHg) during blood pressure manipulations: negative correlation with defective Autoregulation ($p < 0.01$) and positive correlation with intact Autoregulation ($p < 0.05$). **a** autoregulation defective, **b** autoregulation intact

Discussion

The PVI is a measure of brain compliance and is thought to be a reflection of the vascular component of the intracranial contents [5]. As changes in CPP affect cerebrovascular status, dependent on autoregulation, they will also affect ICP and PVI. Contrary to earlier reports, where PVI did not change with CPP alterations within the limits of autoregulation [1, 4], Gray and Rosner [3] found that within the limits of autoregulation PVI and CPP were positively correlated. However, this relationship was hardly present in animals anesthetized with pentobarbital, which, presumably because of its own vasoconstricting effect, blunted the vascular responses to CPP changes, and obscured the relationship between PVI and CPP [3]. In the present study in patients without anaesthesia there was only a weak positive correlation between PVI an CPP with intact autoregulation, suggesting that vasoconstriction and subsequently reduced CBV had some effect on PVI, but that this effect is counteracted by increased transmural pressure. The increase in transmural pressure may be attenuated by thickening of the vessel wall due to vasoconstriction, but the degree of this effect probably differs from patient to patient, which may explain the variability in the results shown in Fig. 1B. The inverse correlation that we found between CPP and PVI with defective autoregulation is in agreement with earlier data. In these cases, higher transmural pressure across the vessel wall in not offset by arteriolar vasoconstriction, and transmitted to the distal parts of the cerebral microcirculation, leading to forced vascular expansion and high CBV with decreased compressibility of the venous part of the cerebrovascular bed. Conversely, reduced CPP causes vessel collapse and lower CBV, which makes the brain more "slack".

Based on the present data, a few comments with regard to blood pressure management in severe head injury can be made. First, a fall in blood pressure is always detrimental: with impaired autoregulation it may invoke the risk of cerebral ischemia, while with intact autoregulation it may lead to dangerous increases in ICP and brain stiffness, due to compensatory vasodilation. On the other hand, artificially raising blood pressure if necessary to maintain CPP, would only seem prudent when autoregulation is known to be intact. In these cases induced hypertension has little effect on ICP and PVI, and may thus be regarded safe. With defective autoregulation, however, this maneuver caused a significant deterioration of the biomechanical status of the brain. The increased CBF in most of these cases was not accompanied by an increase in $CMRO_2$, and could thus be considered "luxury perfusion". It should be emphasized, however, that when CBF is below ischemic levels at baseline, induced hypertension may be beneficial and lead to improved $CMRO_2$ [2].

References

1. Avezaat CJJ, van Eijndhoven JHM, Wyper DJ (1980) Effects of hypercapnia and arterial hypotension and hypertension on cerebrospinal fluid pulse pressure and intracranial volume-pressure relationships. J Neurol Neurosurg Psychiatry 43:222–234
2. Bouma GJ, Muizelaar JP, Choi SC, Newlon PG, Young HF (1991) Cerebral circulation and metabolism after severe traumatic brain injury: The elusive role of ischemia. J Neurosurg (In Press)
3. Gray WJ, Rosner MJ (1987) Pressure-volume index as a function of cerebral perfusion pressure. Part 1: The effects of cerebral perfusion changes and anaesthesia. J Neurosurg 67:369–376
4. Leech P, Miller JD (1974) Intracranial pressure-volume relationships during experimental brain compression in primates. 2. Effect of induced changes in systemic arterial pressure and cerebral blood flow. J Neurol Neurosurg Psychiatry 37:1009–1104
5. Marmarou A, Maset AL, Ward JD, Choi SC, Brooks D, Lutz HA, Moulton RJ, Muizelaar JP, DeSalles AAF, Young HF (1987) Contribution of CSF and vascular factors to elevation of ICP in severely head-injured patients. J Neurosurg 66:883–890
6. Marshall WJS, Jackson JLF, Langfitt TW (1969) Brain swelling caused by trauma and arterial hypertension. Arch Neurol 21:545–553
7. Muizelaar JP, Marmarou A, Wachi A (1989) ICP and PVI with blood pressure alterations and relation with CBF autoregulation. In: Hoff JT, Betz AL (eds) Intracranial Pressure VII. Springer, Berlin Heidelberg New York London Paris Tokyo Hong Kong, pp 825–828
8. Muizelaar JP, Ward JD, Marmarou A, Newlon PG, Wachi A (1989) Cerebral blood flow and metabolism in severely head-injured children. Part II: Autoregulation. J Neurosurg 71:72–76
9. Rosner MJ, Daughton S (1990) Cerebral perfusion pressure management in head injury. J Trauma 30:933–941

Reversibility of Cerebral Circulatory Arrest (CCA) Following Severe Intracranial Hypertension

D.G. Iacopino, G. Gambardella, C. Todaro, F. Salpietro, C. Alafaci, and F. Tomasello

Neurosurgical Clinic, University of Messina, Italy

Introduction

Severe increase of Intracranial Pressure (ICP) leads to a decrease of Cerebral Perfusion Pressure (CPP). The last step of these events is Cerebral Tamponade. It is general accepted that the absence of Cerebral Blood Flow (CBF) confirms brain death [2]. Transcranial Doppler (TCD) ultrasonography permits a non-invasive, bedside, real-time evaluation of the intracranial hemodynamics [1]. Changes in blood velocity in consequence of intracranial hypertension have been described [3], but as yet standard criteria have not been universally accepted. We report our experience using TCD in severe intracranial hypertension with particular attention to the possibility of reversibility of CCA.

Materials and Methods

We studied 54 patients who suffered severe intracranial hypertension from different neurosurgical diseases (Table 1), monitored by:

- ICP by intraparenchymal fiberoptic catheter (Camino).
- Flow velocity of the middle cerebral artery (MCA) by TCD (TC2-64EME).
- Arterial blood pressure (ABP).

Results

Cerebral tamponade occurred when ICP values reached systolic ABP values and CCP was O. At the same time TCD pattern was characterized by small systolic spikes and absence of diastolic flow.

Out of 54 patients, 10 had 24 critical episodes of CCA (Table 2). During the crisis, we performed all the common intensive therapeutic measures, including intravenous infusion of Mannitol 20%. In 14 cases there was a decrease of ICP and CCP was temporarily restored. In all these cases TCD pattern turned from a "small systolic spikes" picture to a pattern similar to the status quo ante the crisis. At last, all 10 patients died.

Table 1. 54 Patients

Head Injuries (HI)	28
Cerebral Hemorrhages (HM)	14
Brain Tumors (BT)	12

Table 2.

n	Sex	Pat	n of CCA	Reversible
1	M	HI	2	1
2	F	HM	3	2
3	M	HI	3	2
4	M	HM	3	2
5	M	BT	3	2
6	M	HI	1	0
7	M	HI	3	2
8	M	HM	1	0
9	F	BT	3	2
10	F	BT	3	2

Discussion

We could monitor the early changes of TCD pattern when CPP fell near to zero. In 10 patients there were 24 critical episodes of CCA, 14 of which were reversible and CPP was partially restored after rapid infusion of mannitol 20%. This was confirmed by a restoration of a positive diastolic flow in the TCD pattern. In the past, recovery has been reported despite reverse flow in the common carotid artery [4]. Recently, Powers [6] has described a case in which a post-operative TCD evaluation revealed an early reverberating flow. The neurological status of the patient improved to final recovery in the following days, with a normalization of the TCD pattern.

Precise time limitations for cerebral death after cessation of intracranial circulation have not been experimentally determined [5]. Pribam [7] found that in some patients, removal of ventricular fluid reduced ICP and allowed vessel filling, leading to recovery in certain patients.

In conclusion, although TCD ultrasonography holds great promise for the non-invasive monitoring of cerebral hemodynamics in intracranial hypertension, further clinical experience with this method is necessary before the impact of this new technology can be fully assessed.

References

1. Aaslid R, Lindegaard K-F (1986) Cerebral hemodynamics. In: Aaslid R (ed) Transcranial Doppler sonography. Springer, New York, Wien, pp 60–85

2. Brock M, Schurmann K, Hadjidimos A (1969) Cerebral blood flow and cerebral death. Preliminary report. Acta Neurochir. 20:195–209
3. Hassler W, Steinmetz H, Gawlowski J (1988) Transcranial Doppler ultrasonography in raised intracranial pressure and intracranial circulatory arrest. J. Neurosurg 68:745–751
4. Lewis RR, Padayachee TS, Beasley MG, Keen H, Gosling RG (1983) Investigation of brain death with doppler shift ultrasound. J. R. Soc Med 76:308–310
5. Neely WA, Youmans JR (1963) Anoxia of canine brain without damage. JAMA 183:1085–1087
6. Powers AD, Graeber MC, Smith RR (1989) Transcranial Doppler ultrasonography in the determination of brain death. Neurosurgery 24:884–889
7. Pribam HFW (1961) Angiographic appearences in acute intracranial hypertension. Neurology 11:10–21

ICP and Flow Dynamics After Subarachnoid Hemorrhage

T. HASHIMOTO, N. NAKAMURA, S. ABE, Y. HASEGAWA, and K. NAKAZAWA

Department of Neurosurgery, Jikei University School of Medicine, 3-25-8, Nishishinbashi, Minatoku, Tokyo 105, Japan

Introduction

The cerebral hemodynamics after subarachnoid hemorrhage (SAH) are very complicated due to vasospasm and increased ICP. The flow velocity in the circle of Willis can be observed non-invasively by transcranial Doppler (TCD) [1, 2]. Laser Doppler flowmetry now makes it possible to continuously measure microvascular flow (MVF) after surgery [3, 4]. In our department, flow velocity of the middle cerebral artery (MCA) and MVF have been measured in 50 patients after surgery using transcranial Doppler and Laser Doppler. Also ICP and cardiovascular parameters have been monitored simultaneously.

The aim of this study was to correlate the flow of MCA measured by transcranial Doppler and MVF measured by Laser Doppler, and to investigate the relationship between flow velocity, MVF and ICP.

Materials and Methods

In 50 patients undergoing early aneurysm surgery the flow velocity in the MCA was measured by TCD; MVF, blood volume and flow velocity of the brain cortex were measured by Laser Doppler. A flat probe of TCD was placed at the temporal region for continuous monitoring, and the low profile sensor of the Laser Doppler was placed on the surface of the cortex during surgery. ICP was measured by an epidural sensor. A Swan-Ganz catheter was introduced via the jugular vein. Blood pressure, pulmonary arterial pressure, pulmonary arterial wedge pressure, cardiac output and central venous pressure were measured simultaneously. These parameters were monitored for 2 weeks continuously.

Results

Continuous ICP monitoring demonstrated B waves on several occasions. Figure 1 shows the relation between B waves and flow velocity measured by TCD. The systemic arterial pressure and flow velocity fluctuated in response to

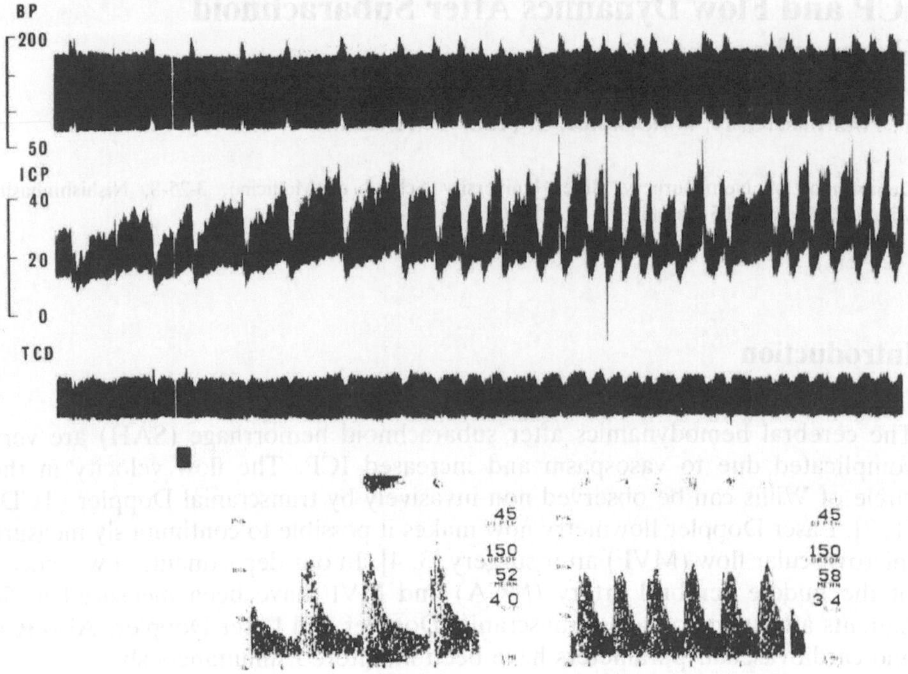

Fig. 1. Flow velocity in MCA measured by TCD fluctuates with ICP and decreases during pressure waves

the B waves. TCD showed particular flow patterns, indicating lower values of mean flow and a higher S/D ratio at the peak of a B wave and vice versa at the bottom of a B wave.

MVF, blood volume and flow velocity of cerebral cortex, measured by Laser Doppler also indicated undulations in response to ICP changes. The observed changes were comparable to those observed in the transcranial Doppler studies, showing a decrease in mean velocity at the ascending slope of the pressure wave and an increase in mean velocity at the descending slope. Systemic blood pressure, pulmonary arterial pressure and central venous pressure also showed fluctuations during the pressure waves (Fig. 2). Figure 3 demonstrates changes in MVF and velocity during a plateau wave observed in a patient with an aneurysm of the anterior communicating artery. MVF and flow velocity of the cortex were reduced during the plateau wave. Blood volume of the cortex showed a slight increase before the plateau wave. A decrease in mean flow velocity and an increase in S/D ratio was shown during the plateau wave. The flow pattern showed an increase in mean velocity and a decrease in S/D ratio when the plateau wave disappeared.

In some patients with sėvere SAH CSF flow was disturbed. This led to a gradual increase in ICP and a decrease in mean flow velocity measured by TCD, the S/D ratio becoming higher in proportion to the increased ICP.

In some selected cases the effect of Glycerol and Mannitol was evaluated on ICP, flow velocity and MVF. ICP gradually decreased after Glycerol

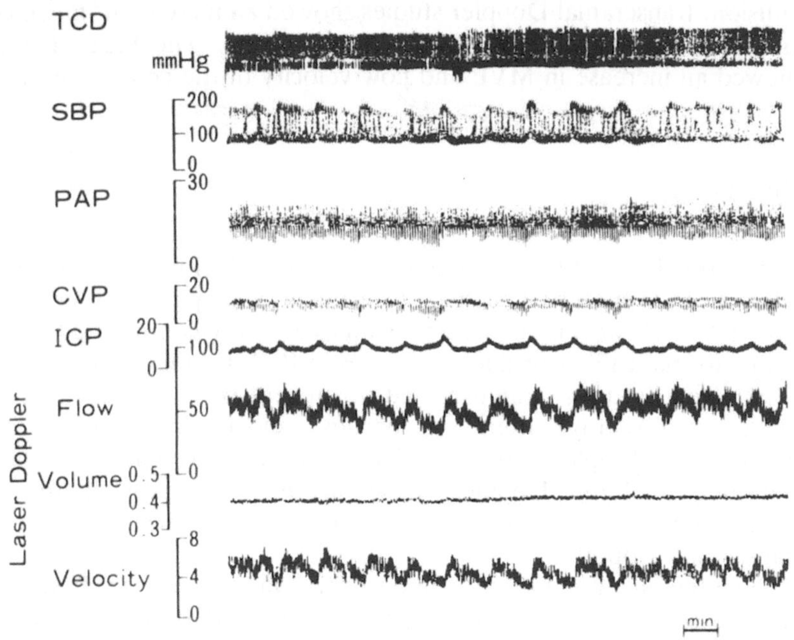

Fig. 2. Mean flow velocity in MCA measured by transcranial Doppler and MVF measured by Laser Doppler decrease at the peak of a pressure wave

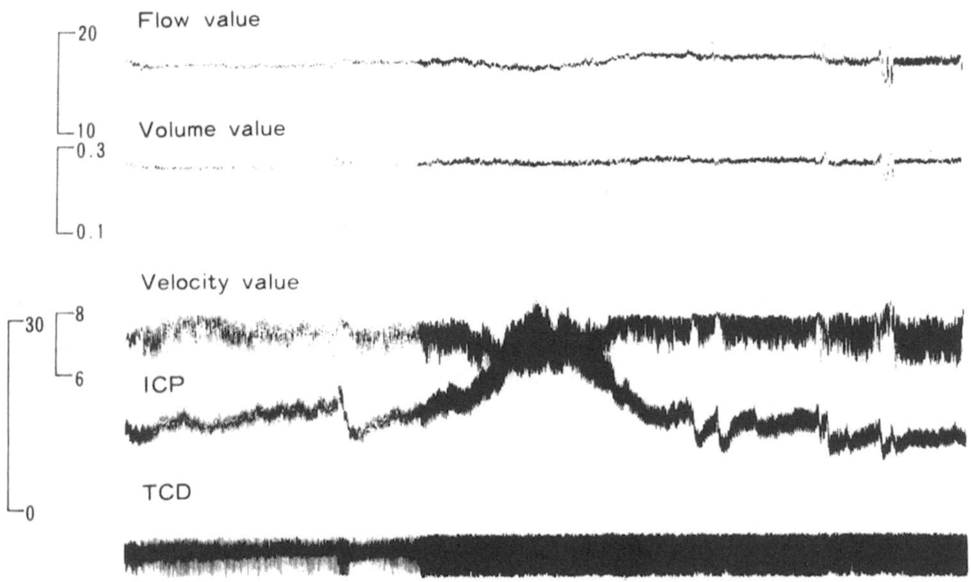

Fig. 3. Microvascular flow and flow velocity obtained by Laser Doppler decrease during a plateau wave

infusion; transcranial Doppler studies showed an increase of mean flow velocity and a decrease of the S/D ratio after infusion. The Laser Doppler studies showed an increase in MVF and flow velocity of the cerebral cortex.

Discussion

TCD provides real-time evaluation of flow velocity from the basal cerebral arteries. TCD may be beneficial to estimate vasospasm and cerebral ischemia after SAH. However, the hemodynamics are very complicated due to changes in the arterial caliber or due to changes in ICP. Furthermore, flow velocity can be affected by drugs administrated to prevent cerebral ischemia. Our studies suggest that relative alterations of flow velocity in the MCA obtained by transcranial Doppler resemble changes of microvascular flow and velocity measured by Laser Doppler. However, it was impossible to evaluate the critical reduction of MVF by absolute values of mean flow velocity using transcranial Doppler.

Continuous monitoring demonstrated fluctuations in flow velocity and microvascular flow in response to changes in ICP. During pressure waves changes in the transcranial Doppler studies and Laser Doppler studies were noted, suggesting that these methods may be used to evaluate the existence of pressure waves. An effect of both Glycerol and Mannitol infusion was shown during the flow studies. Our results suggest that continuous monitoring of flow velocity by transcranial Doppler and microvascular flow by Laser Doppler may be valuable to assess the hemodynamics in patients with SAH in addition to ICP recording.

References

1. Harders AG, Gilsbach JM (1987) The time course of blood velocity changes to vasospasm in the circle of Willis measured by transcranial Doppler ultrasound. J. Neurosurugery 66:718–728
2. Hashimoto T, Nakamura N, Kanki T, Abe S (1989) Monitoring of hemodynamics in subarachnoid hemorrhage using transcranial Doppler. Advances in Neurosurg. 17:337–343
3. Hashimoto T, Nakamura N, Kanki T, Abe S, Akachi K (1991) Monitoring of hemodynamics in subarachnoid hemorrhage with transcranial Doppler and Laser Doppler. Arteres et veines 10:29–34
4. Hashimoto T, Nakamura N, Abe S, Akachi K, Matsumoto M, Boku M (1990) Continuous monitoring of hemodynamics in subarachnoid hemorrhage using transcranial Doppler and Laser Doppler. In: Sano K, Takakura K, Kassell NF, Sasaki T (eds) Cerebral Vasospasm, University of Tokyo Press, pp 21–23

Session IV: Cerebrovascular Dynamics II

Chairmen: J.T. Hoff and C.J.J. Avezaat

Evaluation of Closed Head Injury Patients Using Transcranial Doppler Monitoring

D.W. NEWELL, R. AASLID, R. STOOSS, and H.J. REULEN

Department of Neurological Surgery, (DWN, RA) University of Washington Seattle, WA, USA
Department of Neurosurgery, (RA, RS, HJR) University of Bern, Bern, Switzerland

Introduction

Continuous recording of basal cerebral artery velocities using transcranial Doppler may provide a more practical alternative to CBF methods for the assessment of cerebrovascular responses in patients with head injury and other neurological conditions requiring ICP management. A method is described where continuous recordings of blood flow velocity (BFV), arterial blood pressure (ABP), intracranial pressure (ICP), and end tidal CO_2 (Et CO_2) are obtained by portable equipment which can easily be taken to the ICU. This unit can then be used to test blood flow response to CO_2 changes, autoregulation, response to barbiturates and response to mannitol therapy. By obtaining information on the effectiveness of these responses in head injury patients, it may be feasible to use this information to guide therapy.

Clinical Material and Methods

The feasibility of TCD monitoring was evaluated in 22 patients with a diagnosis of closed head injury Age range was 16–69 with a mean of 36. Average Glasgow coma score (GCS) was 6. These patients had continuous ABP, ICP, and Et CO_2 monitoring and were artificially ventilated during their initial hospital course.

Middle cerebral velocity (MCV) signals were located through a transtemporal window, using probes fixed with an elastic headband during the recording sessions. Analog signals from the 4 different modalities were then stored digitally by computer and a custom software program was used to analyze the results.

Reactivity to CO_2 was tested by inducing step changes in arterial CO_2 concentration by temporarily disconnecting the patient from the ventilator and hand ventilating, for at least 2 minutes. The values from stable recording periods from before and after the manipulation were then averaged, and the percentage response (blood flow velocity change per mm CO_2 change) was calculated.

Autoregulation was tested according to the method of Aaslid et al. by inflating leg cuffs around both thighs to a suprasystolic blood pressure for a period of 2 minutes and then rapidly deflating them, inducing a systemic blood pressure drop. The relative change in CBF (evaluated by the change in mean MCA velocity) was observed following the sudden blood pressure decrease and recovery. Relative changes in velocity in comparison to relative ABP changes were examined relative to their control values immediately following the BP drop. The rate of regulation (RoR), was defined as the change in calculated cerebrovascular resistance/the change in time, divided by the change in ABP. In a previous study of a group of healthy volunteers at normocapnia, the normal value for RoR was found to be 20 ± 3 [1].

Response to mannitol was tested by giving 4 mg/kg of 20% mannitol intravenously over 5 minutes. Continuous recording of all parameters was then performed for at least 20 minutes following the end of the infusion. Change in blood flow velocity was then calculated as the maximum percentage change that occurred following the infusion. This usually occurred 10 minutes after the mannitol was given.

Response to barbiturate was assessed by rapidly infusing a loading dose (5 mg/kg) of thiopentone according to the method of Cold et al., and observing the response in blood flow velocity, ABP, and ICP. Relative blood flow change was determined from the percent change in blood flow velocity following the infusion.

Results

CO_2 Testing

Middle cerebral artery velocity response to CO_2 was tested in 20 patients. The results obtained showed reactivities between 0 and 4.63% change/mmHg. The results of CO_2 reactivity within 48 hours of admission for both hemispheres were combined and compared to Glasgow outcome score at 1 month in 15 patients. CO_2 reactivity was higher in patients who made a good recovery or had a moderate disability (2.25%/mm $CO_2 \pm 0.87$) than those who died, were severely disabled, or were in a persistant vegetative state (1.51%/mm $CO_2 \pm 0.25$), but the difference was not statistically significant ($0.1 > p > 0.05$).

Autoregulation

The rate of regulation, which was calculated from the change in cerebrovascular resistance induced by sudden transient decreases in blood pressure, varied from 0 to 29.4 in the 118 studies performed. The results indicated that in this group of patients the autoregulation response was not either absent or present but could be impaired to varying degrees. In selected patients there were marked differences between the hemispheres. There was no correlation of RoR to admission GCS or outcome at 1 month.

Mannitol Response

Following mannitol infusion most patients had an increase in middle cerebral artery velocity. The greatest increase occurred ten minutes following the end of the infusion. The degree of increase in MCV was greatest in those patients with the most impaired autoregulation and least in patients with intact autoregulation but the number of patients with completely intact autoregulation was small. Regression analysis showed an inverse correlation between RoR and MCV increase following mannitol infusion ($r = -0.59$).

Barbiturate Response

Following barbiturate administration the typical response which was seen was a transient drop in blood pressure followed by a return to pre-infusion or near pre-infusion values in some patients, and a more persistant blood pressure drop in others. Patients judged to have a favorable response to barbiturates had a decreased blood flow velocity and a decreased ICP, without a significant drop, or in some cases an improvement, in perfusion pressure. Patients who were judged to have an unfavorable response had either a minimal change in blood flow velocity and ICP or a significant drop in cerebral perfusion pressure.

Discussion

Recording of blood flow velocities in the basal cerebral arteries does not give an absolute value for CBF; however, the velocity change is directly proportional to the changes in blood flow provided the diameter of the conducting artery remains constant [1, 2]. This has been demonstrated by Lindegaard et al. [7] in humans by observing spontaneous blood flow changes during carotid endarterectomy while simultaneously recording MCV using Doppler ultrasound and carotid blood flow using an electromagnetic flowmeter. These results indicate that under these circumstances basal artery diameter must not vary to any significant degree because the majority of the velocity changes are directly reflecting changes in flow. To gain an index of the effectiveness of autoregulation or CO_2 responsiveness in patients, knowledge of the absolute blood flow is not necessary [3, 4, 5, 8]. More valuable is a continuous measure of relative changes in blood flow under changing conditions of ICP, ABP, or CO_2. Recent experimental evidence has supported the validity of the TCD method for determining autoregulation [2, 6]. More research is needed to determine the relationship between CBF and MCA velocity in response to different medications.

References

1. Aaslid R, Lindegaard KF, Sorteberg W, Nornes H (1989) Cerebral autoregulation dynamics in humans. Stroke 20(1):45–52
2. Aaslid R, Newell DW, Stooss R, Sorteberg W, Lindegaard KF, Nornes H (1991) Assessment of cerebral autoregulation dynamics from simultaneous arterial and venous transcranial Doppler recordings in humans. Stroke (in press)
3. Cold, GE (1989) Measurements of CO_2 reactivity and barbiturate reactivity in patients with severe head injury. Acta Neurochir (Wien) 98:153–163
4. Cold GE, Jensen FT, et al. (1977) The cerebrovascular CO_2 reactivity during the acute phase of brain injury. Acta Anaesth. Scand 21:222–231
5. Enevoldsen EM, Jensen FT (1978) Autoregulation and CO_2 responses of cerebral blood flow in patients with acute severe head injury. J Neurosurg 48:689–703
6. Kontos HA (1989) Validity of cerebral arterial blood flow calculations from velocity measurements. Stroke 20(1):1–3
7. Lindegaard KF, Lundar T, Wiberg J, et al. (1987) Variations in middle cerebral artery blood flow investigated with noninvasive transcranial blood velocity measurements. Stroke 18:1025–1030
8. Muizelaar JP, Lutz III HA, et al. (1984) Effect of mannitol on ICP and CBF and correlation with pressure autoregulation in severely head-injured patients. J Neurosurg 61:700–706

The Significance of Increased Transcranial Doppler Flow Velocity After Severe Brain Injury

K.H. Chan, N.M. Dearden, and J.D. Miller

Department of Clinical Neurosciences, University of Edinburgh, Scotland, EH4 2XU

Introduction

Transcranial doppler (TCD) allows repeated or continuous non-invasive measurement of blood flow velocity in major intracranial vessels [1]. Flow velocity is proportional to cerebral blood flow (CBF) and inversely related to cross-sectional area of the insonated vessel. Increased blood flow velocity may therefore occur in association with elevated CBF or reduced vessel diameter. Both situations are known to occur following brain injury [6, 7]. The present study aims to examine the relationship between increased blood flow velocity and subsequent development of ischaemic neurological complications following severe brain injury.

Methods

Fifty patients with severe head injury defined as post-resuscitation admission Glasgow Coma Score of less than or equal to eight points with no eye opening, who survived for more than 24 hours after admission were studied. They were managed according to a standard regime that included artificial ventilation under muscle paralysis and sedation with continuous infusion of pancuronium and phenoperidine respectively, to a $PaO_2 > 13\,kPa$ and $PaCO_2$ between 3.5 and 4.5 kPa. Blood pressure, arterial oxygen saturation (SaO_2), end-tidal carbon dioxide concentration and body temperature were recorded continuously. Forty-one patients had intracranial pressure (ICP) monitoring. Twenty-two of these patients also had unilateral continuous monitoring of jugular bulb venous oxygen saturation (SJO_2) using the Oximetrics 3 system (Abbott Laboratories, Chicago, USA), on the side of predominant venous drainage [2]. The arterial-jugular venous oxygen content difference ($AVDO_2$) was calculated by multiplying the difference between SaO_2 and SJO_2 by the daily haemoglobin concentration and 1.39, divided by 100. Global cerebral hyperaemia was defined as $AJDO_2$ of less than 4 ml/dl. Treatment was initiated when ICP exceeded 25 mmHg or CPP fell below 60 mmHg.

Transcranial Doppler (Medasonics, California, USA) insonation of at least both middle cerebral arteries (MCA) was performed within 24 hours of admission according to the method described by Aaslid (1). The depth of insonation giving the highest timed-mean flow velocity (MFV) was chosen for recording. Subsequent daily measurements used the same window and depth previously employed. Continuous recordings of MCA velocity were obtained during periods of changing CPP by mounting the ultrasound probe in a head band. Velocity measurements were taken at the points of maximum and subsequent minimum CPP before treatment was instigated.

Average MFV from the MCA of 20 normal subjects was 60 ± 7 (± standard deviations) cm/second. In brain injured patients, MFV was considered abnormally elevated if it exceeded 100 cm/second.

Computerised tomography (CT) was performed on admission and repeated serially as clinically indicated. Intracranial pathology was classified into focal (haematoma and/or unilateral contusion or swelling) and diffuse. The amount of subarachnoid blood was estimated from CT according to the criteria of Fisher (4). Follow-up CT was obtained at three months in all survivors. Cerebral infarction was diagnosed from clinical, CT and post-mortem data. CT was used to classify infarction into contusion-related (at or around the site of previous contusion or hematoma) and noncontusion-related (NCI). NCI was identified as a hypodense area on CT with distinct margins restricted to an arterial territory, and persisting after the acute phase of injury based on CT or post-mortem examination. Statistical analysis was by either Chi Square with Yates' correction or Fisher's exact test.

Results

MFV exceeded 100 cm/second in 17 patients following severe brain injury (34%). The median time of onset of increased velocity was day 2 (range: 1–4) with a median duration of four days (range: 1–7). There was no significant relationship between the presence of subarachnoid blood on CT and increased MFV.

Increased Blood Flow Velocity and CPP and SJO_2

Raised MFV was observed in 17 of 41 patients with CPP measurements. MFV exceeded 100 cm/second only when CPP was above 60 mmHg ($p < 0.0001$).

Fourteen of 22 patients undergoing continuous SJO_2 monitoring developed elevated MFV. Raised MFV was associated with global cerebral hyperaemia on six occasions. The remaining eight cases had normal $AVDO_2$ (4–9 ml/dl). Diffuse injury was present in four of the six hyperaemic patients and two of the eight nonhyperaemic cases ($p = 0.12$). Bilateral increase in MFV was observed in all six hyperaemic patients. Six of eight nonhyperaemic cases had unilateral increase in MFV velocity ($p = 0.018$).

Increased Blood Flow Velocity and Noncontusion Related Infarction

Noncontusion related infarcts (NCI) developed in only four patients with increased MFV. Patients with NCI had unilateral increased MFV in the territory of the relevant cerebral artery ($p = 0.0011$). Contusion related infarcts were noted in four patients with increased MFV and eight cases without raised MFV. There was no relationship between increased MFV and development of contusion related infarct ($p > 0.05$).

Three of the four patients with NCI had SJO_2 monitoring and all were nonhyperaemic. Of the patients with increased MFV associated with hyperaemia, none developed NCI ($p > 0.05$).

CPP elevation therapy was required in 7 of 17 patients with increased MFV. All four patients who had elevated MFV and subsequently developed NCI had received treatment to restore a reduced CPP ($p = 0.03$). Only patients with NCI had both an unilateral increase in MFV of the relevant cerebral vessel and subsequently required treatment for a CPP below 60 mmHg ($p = 0.008$).

Discussion

Although TCD allows detection of elevated MFV, it was not possible to determine whether increased MFV represented raised cerebral blood flow (CBF) or narrowing of the insonated vessel. Data from patients with continuous CPP and SJO_2 monitoring partly address this issue.

Increased velocity was never observed when CPP fell below 60 mmHg. After cerebral trauma, CBF often falls below a critical limit of CPP [6]. Studies after subarachnoid haemorrhage (SAH) confirm that increased MFV cannot be demonstrated when CBF is low despite angiographic evidence of spasm [8].

Following severe head injury, CBF may be coupled to reduced metabolism with normal $AVDO_2$ or uncoupled with a normal (relative hyperaemia) or increased CBF (absolute hyperaemia) associated with low $AVDO_2$ [7]. Increased CBF has been associated with raised MFV [5]. After head injury, absolute global hyperaemia should therefore be associated with low $AVDO_2$ and increased MFV of all insonated vessels. Our observation of significant association between bilateral increases in MFV and hyperaemia may indicate that these patients have raised CBF and would be consistent with the observation that NCI was not seen in these patients.

Unilateral increases in MFV were usually associated with normal $AVDO_2$. After severe head injury, normal $AVDO_2$ indicates coupled reduction of CBF and metabolism although focal ischaemia cannot be excluded [7]. Angiographic evidence from patients suffering SAH demonstrates that vasospasm is accompanied by an increase in MFV [5]. Since reduced CBF without change in vessel calibre is associated with reduced MFV [5], the presence of unilateral increase in MFV, associated with normal $AVDO_2$, probably indicates reduction in diameter of the lumen of the insonated vessel. Significant reduction of flow would be expected to lead to infarction. In patients with $AVDO_2$ monitoring, NCI developed only in the three patients with normal $AVDO_2$ and unilateral increased MFV who also had subsequent compromise of CPP.

Absence of association between the amount of SAH and development of increased MFV contrasts with studies of spontaneous SAH [5]. Increased MFV occurred earlier, had shorter duration and never exceeded 200 cm/second, compared to SAH where higher MFV (>250 cm/second) is associated with an increased risk of neurological complications [5]. Development of infarction after head injury appears to occur at a lower MFV than SAH but in association with compromised CPP. Our findings are in accord with experimental observations that the combination of vasospasm and reduced CPP is associated with a much greater reduction in CBF when compared to the effect of either mechanism alone [3].

Aggressive management of severe brain injury by employing sedative and relaxant drugs obviates our ability to assess neurological status directly. TCD enables identification of increased MFV but, without comparative studies of CBF and angiography, the cause of increased MFV must remain speculative. This study emphasises the value of CPP measurement when interpreting MFV after severe head injury and shows that elevation of MFV significantly increases the risk of NCI especially if this is unilateral and CPP becomes compromised. We therefore suggest that daily measurement of TCD should be performed as an integral part of the monitoring of severely brain injured patients.

Conclusions

1. Demonstration of increased flow velocity is dependent upon an adequate CPP.
2. The combination of reduced CPP and unilateral elevated flow velocity is associated with an increased risk of infarction.
3. Increased velocity in nonhyperaemic patients probably indicates vasospasm.

References

1. Aaslid R, Huber P, Nornes H (1984) Evaluation of cerebrovascular spasm with transcranial doppler ultrasound. J Neurosurg 60:37–41
2. Andrews PJD, Dearden NM, Miller JD (1991) Jugular bulb cannulation; description of a technique and validation of a new continuous monitor. Br J Anesth (In press)
3. Farrar JK (1975) Chronic cerebral arterial spasm. The role of intracranial pressure. J Neurosurg 43:408–417
4. Fisher CM, Kistler JP, Davis JM (1980) Relation of cerebral vasospasm to subarachnoid hemorrhage visualized by computerized tomography scanning. Neurosurgery 6:1–9
5. Harders AG (1986) Neurosurgical applications of transcranial doppler sonography. New York: Springer-Verlag
6. Miller JD (1985) Head injury and brain ischemia. Implications for therapy. Br J Anaesth 57:120–129
7. Obrist WD, Langfitt TW, Jaggi JL, Cruz J, Gennarelli T (1984) Cerebral blood flow and metabolism in comatose patients with acute head injury. Relationship to intracranial hypertension. J Neurosurg 61:241–253
8. Sekhar LN, Wechsler LR, Yonas H, Luyckx K, Obrist W (1988) Value of transcranial doppler examination in the diagnosis of cerebral vasospasm after subarachnoid hemorrhage. Neurosurg 22:813–821
9. Sorteberg W, Lindegaard KF, Rootwelt A, Dahl D, Russell R, Nyberg-Hansen R, Nornes H (1989) Blood velocity and regional blood flow in defined cerebral artery systems. Acta Neurochir (Wien) 97:47–52

A Study of Alterations of Cerebral Circulation Following Head Injury Using Transcranial Doppler Sonography

H.M. Mehdorn[1,2] and C.H. Hoffmann[2]

[1] Department of Neurosurgery, University of Kiel, Weimarer Str. 8, 2300 Kiel 1, Germany
[2] Department of Neurosurgery, University of Essen, Hufelandstr. 55, 4300 Essen 1, Germany

Introduction

Transcranial Doppler sonography (TCD) has been recently applied to the non-invasive evaluation of patients with cerebrovascular disease, particularly following subarachnoid hemorrhage [1, 2], and head injury (3–6, 8–10). A previous study from our group [4, 8] as well as others had shown that TCD is helpful in single patients since it allows non-invasive repeat studies of intracranial blood flow velocities, particularly in patients who have sustained a major head injury and are at risk of intracranial circulatory arrest. In this group of patients, it allows the determination of a typical flow pattern of oscillating flow velocities or pure systolic peaks, which is equivalent to intracranial circulatory arrest. Since the first study was not able to determine a close correlation (better than $r = 0.6$) between intracranial pressure and TCD results such as pulsatility index [4], a second, prospective study was performed in 128 head trauma patients (age range from 7 to 75 years). In this study different types of head injury were considered separately with the intention to additionally distinguish between different mechanisms by which the trauma influences intracranial hemodynamics.

Material

Among 128 patients included in this study, 41 patients presented with open head injury, and 82 patients were admitted following a closed head injury. Five patients were admitted to determine intracranial circulatory arrest following severe head injury, prior to organ explant. Seventy-six patients showed signs of intracerebral hemorrhage or contusion, 37 had evidence of traumatic subarachnoid hemorrhage, 32 presented with acute subdural hematoma, and 17 presented with an epidural hematoma. Clinical status upon admission was determined using the Glasgow Coma Scale (GCS), outcome up to 6 months after discharge was evaluated using the Glasgow Outcome scale (GOS). A total of 732 complete TCD studies were performed (average 5.7 studies per patient) during an average stay in the ICU of 11, 9 days (maximum 77 days). As many arteries as possible were studied by the same investigator. The investigations were performed using a TC 2-64 manufactured by EME. The flow velocity values presented here represent the mean blood flow velocities for the middle cerebral artery at an insonation depth of 60 mm. If indicated on the basis of clinical judgement and on CT findings, intracranial pressure (ICP) was measured epidurally by using the Spiegelberg system. Blood pressure was kept within normal limits and blood gas analyses were performed regularly and artificial ventilation was set up in order to keep pCO_2 in the lower range. No trial of CO_2 reactivity was performed in these patients in order to test this part of cerebral autoregulation because it was thought too risky in patients with raised intracranial pressure.

Results

Sixty-three patients were initially in GCS 3–6, 30 patients in GCS 7–11, and 35 patients in GCS 12–15. Final outcome was evaluated by reviewing the charts, by follow-up visits, phone calls to the referring physicians or to the relatives. Thirty-seven patients had died (GOS = 1), 7 patients were in grade 2, 23 patients in grade 3, 27 patients in grade 4, and 34 patients were in grade 5.

Mean blood flow velocities (BFV) increased within the first week after trauma. As with all BFV values, the standard deviation is rather remarkable (up to ±0.63%). While initial BFV average values recorded within the first 24 hours after injury were 47.2 cm/sec, they rose to values around 72 cm/sec at the end of the first week. They rose further up to values of 84 cm/sec at the end of the second week, and declined within the next 2 weeks to normal values. At the same time, the pulsatility index (PI) decreased more rapidly from initial mean values of 1.64 to values as low as 0.154, although it needs to be mentioned that 5 patients who were admitted with the diagnosis of brain death and showed high initial PI values were not available for further studies. Within the first 4 weeks following brain trauma, a slight rise in mean PI values back to normal could be observed.

With regard to the initial clinical status, in 35 patients admitted with GCS 12–15, initial mean BFV was within normal limits, showed a rapid increase within the first few days following admission up to mean values around 90 cm/sec and returned to normal values within three weeks following trauma; on the other hand, in patients admitted with GCS 3–6, flow velocities rose slightly slower but to higher peaks (up to over 100 cm/sec) and they remained higher for a longer period of time.

Considering the type and location of lesion, no obvious difference was observed between mean BFV in patients with extra- or intra-axial lesions. The highest flow velocities were measured in patients who had undergone surgery for epidural hematomas, while the lowest flow velocities were measured in patients with subdural hematomas. While flow velocities were initially slightly higher in patients with extra-axial lesions, they remained slightly higher over time in patients with intra-axial lesions. Patients whose CT scans were suggestive of pure subarachnoid hemorrhage of traumatic origin did not exhibit higher BVF than the other patients with similar clinical grading.

In order to improve the correlation between PI and ICP, paired values of 139 measurements of ICP and PI were plotted (Fig. 1). In addition, the cerebral perfusion pressure (CPP) was calculated from arterial blood pressures and ICP and plotted against the PI (Fig. 2), distinguishing between patients who survived and those who were dead at time of examination or died within the next 6 hours. The figures show that the simple correlation between ICP and PI even with this high number of paired values is still low; a polynome of fifth order reaches a correlation coefficient of 0.768. Patients who present with pulsatility index below 3 have ICP values below 40 mmHg and cerebral perfusion pressure values calculated above 50 mmHg. A correlation between CPP and PI, however, was not found. Patients with ICP values below 40 mmHg resp. CPP values above 60 mmHg survived with one exception.

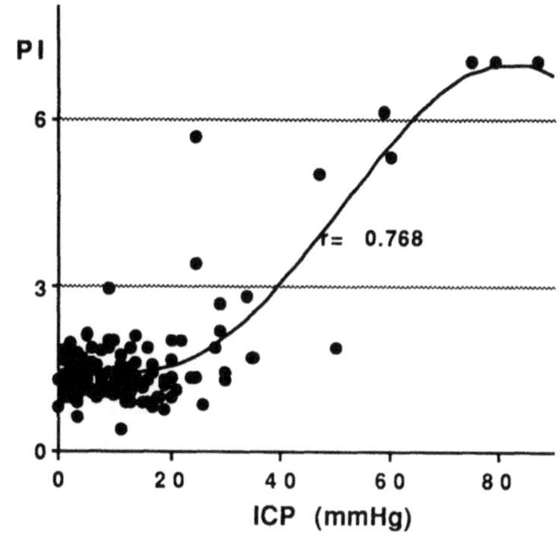

Fig. 1. Intracranial pressure and pulsatility index: Correlation coefficient for a polynome of fifth order: 0.768

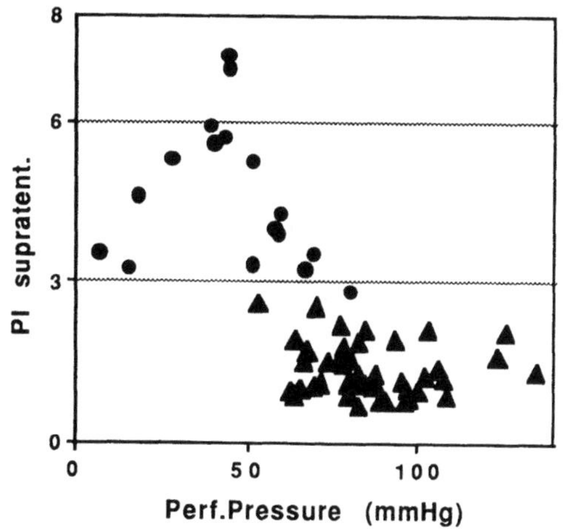

Fig. 2. Cerebral perfusion pressure and pulsatility index. The dots represent the patients dying within 6 hours while the triangles represent surviving patients

Discussion

The major finding from this study is the fact that brain trauma which leads to treatment in a neurosurgical ICU is nearly always associated with a rise of blood flow velocities and in the whole study population, mean blood flow velocities (mBFV) rose by an average of 78% when comparing the mBFV in the middle cerebral artery obtained within 24 hours following injury to the maximum mBVF. Previous studies on smaller number of patients had either obtained similar results [3, 6, 10] or reported the contrary [9]. However, there was no close correlation between the time pattern of flow velocities and clinical outcome. This is in contrast to previous suggestions, e.g. from experience in SAH, that TCD is able to detect patients who are at risk to suffer from ischemic damage due to vasospasm [1, 2]. Although it has been suggested that vasospasm may play an important role in the development of brain damage following brain trauma [7], this study has been unable to confirm this assumption for the different lesions and clinical outcomes. This disappointing result may be due to the great variability of flow velocities in the study population, which is a general problem in TCD findings. In particular it may partly be due to the great age variation, since pCO_2 values have been surveyed and kept in the lower range in order to treat or prevent rise of ICP. This great variability prevents from drawing general conclusions from mBVF values e.g. as they relate to different kinds of brain trauma such as intra- or extra-axial lesions, but still allows to use the results of this study in individual patients. At present, it further remains open for debate whether this rise of mBFV equals vasospasm or is a response of the cerebral circulation to the metabolic demand of the brain tissue following brain injury.

A more consistent finding has been previously reported [4, 8] that patients who had an PI value over 3 had a high probability to dy within the next 24 hours. This study showed that the probability of death within the next 6 hours was 94% when the PI value above 3. This is true despite the fact that, even when using a higher number of patients and simultaneous measurements of PI and ICP, the correlation between these values only rose to 0.768 for a polynomial regression of the fifth order. Still, the PI values below 3 were always associated with ICP values below 40 mmHg, so this suggests that PI is a good indicator for ICP-monitoring, in addition to clinical judgement.

Furthermore, Fig. 2 has shown that all patients died in whom a cerebral perfusion pressure below 50 mmHg had been calculated from blood pressure and ICP values. This is in good correlation with previous experience. On the other hand, among the 17 patients who died subsequently, there were also 8 patients with CPP values above 50 mmHg. This suggests that PI values are sharper prognostic indicators than CPP values.

References

1. Aaslid R (1986) Transcranial Doppler Sonography. Springer, Berlin Heidelberg New York
2. Aaslid R, Huber P, Nornes H (1984) Evaluation of cerebrovascular spasm with transcranial Doppler sonography. J Neurosurg 60:37–41

3. Compton JS, Teddy PJ (1987) Cerebral arterial vasospasm following severe head injury: a transcranial Doppler study. Br J Neurosurg 1:435–439
4. Feldges A, Mehdorn HM (1990) Zum Einsatz der transkraniellen Dopplersonographie auf einer neurochirurgischen Intensivstation. Wiener Med Wschr 140:567–570
5. Gomez CR, Backer RJ, Bucholz RD (1990) Transcranial Doppler ultrasound following closed head injury: vasospasm or vasoparalysis? Surg Neurol 35:30–35
6. Grolimund P, Weber M, Seiler RW, Reulen HP (1988) Time course of cerebral vasospasm after severe head injury. Lancet 1, 2:1173
7. MacPherson P, Graham DI (1978) Correlation between angiographic findings and the ischemia of head injuries. J Neurol Neurosurg Psychiatr 41:122–127
8. Mehdorn HM, Feldges A, Hoffmann B, Löhr E (1989) Comparative evaluation of angiography and transcranial Doppler sonography in the determination of intracranial circulatory arrest. Adv Neurosurg 17:299–303
9. Shigemori M, Moriyama T, Harada K, Kikuchi N, Tokutomi T, Kuramoto S (1990) Intracranial haemodynamics in diffuse and focal brain injuries. Evaluation with transcranial Doppler (TCD) ultrasound. Acta Neurochir 107:5–10
10. Weber M, Grolimund P, Seiler RW (1990) Evaluation of posttraumatic cerebral blood flow velocities by transcranial Doppler ultrasonography. Neurosurgery 27:106–112

Impaired Carbon Dioxide Reactivity Predicts Poor Outcome in Severe Head Injury: A Transcranial Doppler Study

D.G. Grosset, S. Strebel, J. Straiton, J.D. Miller, G.M. Teasdale, and R. Bullock

Institute of Neurological Sciences, Southern General Hospital, Govan Road, Glasgow G51 4TF, UK

Introduction

Regional cerebral blood flow is often reduced over the first few days after severe head injury, but it may also be increased. In some studies hyperaemia has been reported in over half the cases studied, so that regional CBF measurements have not been useful as an indicator of prognosis [1, 6, 7]. By contrast, impaired CO_2 responsiveness correlates well with the severity of the initial injury [1, 3], and with poor outcome [1]. Earlier methods of assessing CO_2 responsiveness, such as intraarterial 133Xe CBF measurement [2, 3, 7] were invasive, expensive, time-consuming and inaccurate. Less invasive techniques, such as intravenous or inhalational 133Xe CBF [7], and the thermal diffusion technique [8], allow measurements bilaterally and at greater frequency, but remain technically difficult and are not easily repeatable.

Transcranial Doppler sonography (TCD) is an easily repeatable, non-invasive technique for measuring cerebral artery flow velocities, and has been used to assess CO_2 responsiveness in subarachnoid haemorrhage and for the evaluation of collateral capacity in extracranial carotid disease. Flow velocities are often increased following severe head injury; hyperaemia can be distinguished from cerebral vasospasm by calculating a ratio of middle cerebral artery to internal carotid artery velocity, the Aaslid index [9].

The aim of the present pilot study was to measure the acute TCD velocity response in the middle cerebral artery to lowered $PaCO_2$, and to correlate this with computed tomography findings and functional outcome.

Materials and Methods

Ten patients (9 males, 1 female) with severe head injury, aged 9–31, mean 19 years, were studied. All patients were artificially ventilated, and sedated with propofol, morphine, or midazolam. Measurement of flow velocities in the middle cerebral arteries (MCA) and in the upper cervical portions of the internal carotid arteries was made using standard transtemporal and submandibular approaches, by transcranial Doppler sonography using an EME TC2-64B with 2 MHz probe (Überlingen, Germany). MCA velocity was measured before and after a period of acute hypocapnia, induced by increasing the ventilation rate for between 2 and 10 minutes. CO_2 responsiveness was calculated as a percentage change, according to the formula: (change in flow velocity/initial flow velocity * 100%) divided by change in $PaCO_2$, giving a % change in velocity per mmHg CO_2; and as an absolute change, according to the formula: (initial flow velocity – final flow velocity) divided by change in $PaCO_2$, giving a velocity change per mmHg CO_2.

A mean "whole brain" CO_2 response was calculated as a mean of responses from the right and left middle cerebral arteries. Results from individual hemispheres were also considered separately.

Intracranial pressure was monitored continuously by ventricular catheter or the Camino intraparenchymal system (Camino Laboratories, San Diego, USA). The Aaslid index was calculated as the mean MCA velocity divided by the ipsilateral mean ICA velocity. The Aaslid index was interpreted by comparison to a previously defined level of 3.0, above which significant vasospasm is considered to be present [9]. Outcome was assessed by the Glasgow outcome scale (GOS) at 2–4 months following injury. A poor outcome was scored if there was severe disability, vegetative survival, or death.

Results

A summary of clinical features, CT results, ICP, and CO_2 responses in the 10 patients is given in Table 1. The mean CO_2 level before hyperventilation was 31 mmHg (range 26–34 mmHg). The mean fall in $PaCO_2$ following hyperventilation was 6.0 mmHg (range 2.8–10.8 mmHg). Both the percentage change and the absolute change in flow velocity following CO_2 reduction were significantly lower in patients with poor outcome than in patients with good outcome. The mean hemisphere CO_2 response (i.e. mean of right and left hemispheres) was 1.0% per mmHg CO_2 (range 0.2–2.0%) in 5 patients with poor outcome, and 3.8% per mmHg CO_2 (range 2.2–6.6%) in patients with good outcome ($p = 0.01$, Mann-Whitney). Individual hemisphere CO_2 responses are shown in Figure 1. Corresponding results for absolute change were 0.92 cm/sec/mmHg CO_2 (range 0–2.3) in patients with poor outcome, and 4.0 cm/sec/mmHg CO_2 (range 1.2–7.5) in patients with good outcome ($p = 0.04$, Mann-Whitney). CO_2 responses were particularly impaired in hemispheres with severe damage on computed tomography (contusion/intracranial haematoma) (See Table 1). In 4 patients with poor outcome (cases 3–6), there was no fall in middle cerebral artery velocity in response to lowered CO_2; moreover in 3 of these patients there was a paradoxical increase (cases 4–6, with negative velocity change shown in Table 1), although a CO_2 response was obtained from the contralateral hemisphere (Table 1).

The Aaslid index recorded from right and left hemispheres immediately before starting CO_2 reactivity testing is shown in Table 1. The index tended to be lower in patients with good outcome (mean 2.1, range 1.0–2.8) than in

Table 1.

Patient number	Sex	Age	CT finding	ICP Before hyperventilation	ICP After hyperventilation	Patient number	CPP	% fall in MCAV per mmHg CO_2 R side	% fall in MCAV per mmHg CO_2 L side	Outcome	Aaslid index[a] R side	Aaslid index[a] L side
1	m	31	L frontotemporal contusion	22.0	13.0	1	88.0	2.9	1.9	good	2.0	2.4
2	f	13	R parietal, L frontal contusions (small)	20.5	11.5	2	82.5	4.9	8.3	good	1.0	2.1
3	m	9	R internal capsule ICH	21.5	17.5	3	57.5	0.0	1.0	poor	3.0	2.6
4	m	23	Bilateral multiple ICH	14.5	8.5	4	90.5	1.6	−1.1	poor	1.6	2.1
5	m	26	R subfrontal contusion	10.5	9.0	5	74.5	−0.7	4.8	poor	1.2	1.9
6	m	20	L basal ganglia ICH	39.0	14.5	6	69.0	6.7	−2.8	poor	3.8	3.5
7	m	18	L frontal ICH R frontal EDH	22.0	18.0	7	76.0	4.5	3.2	good	2.3	2.1
8	m	21	R SDH and ICH	10.0	8.0	8	78.0	5.0	3.3	good	2.1	2.8
9	m	14	Diffuse bilateral oedema	19.0	10.0	9	61.0	2.2	2.2	good	2.3	1.6
10	m	27	R SDH	28.0	24.0	10	99.0	0.2	0.2	poor	4.0	3.5

SDH: subdural haematoma, EDH: extradural haematoma, ICH: intracerebral haematoma; CPP = cerebral perfusion pressure; MCAV = middle cerebral artery velocity

[a] Aaslid index = MCA/ICA velocity; a value >3 indicates "vasospasm"

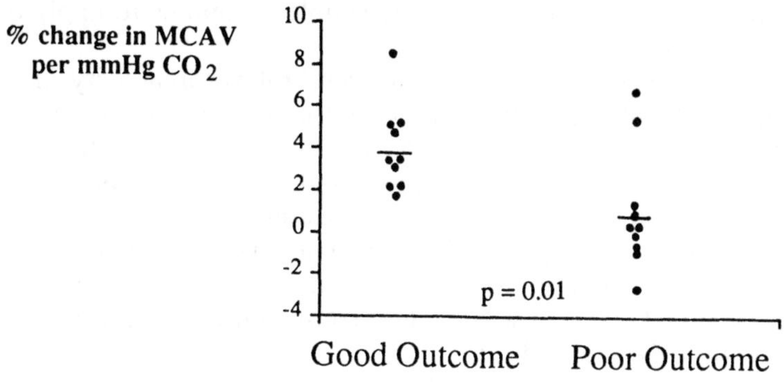

Fig. 1. Change in middle cerebral artery velocity (MCAV), expressed as a percentage change per mmHg CO_2, in 20 hemispheres of 5 patients with good outcome and 5 patients with poor outcome. Mean change was 3.8% per mmHg CO_2 in patients with good outcome, and 1.0% per mmHg CO_2 in patients with poor outcome

patients with poor outcome (mean 2.7, range 1.2–4.0), although the difference was not significant. Values of 3.0 and above, indicating significant vasospasm, were recorded in 5 cerebral hemispheres in 3 patients, all of whom had poor outcome, and in 4 of these cases there was impaired response to reduced CO_2. CT appearances in these 3 patients were suggestive of a high velocity (diffuse axonal injury) type of injury.

Intracranial pressure tended to be lower in patients with good outcome (mean 18.7 cm, range 10–22) than in patients with poor outcome (mean 22.7 cm, range 10.5–39), but the difference was not significant. The mean fall in ICP induced by hyperventilation was 1.93 cm/mmHgCO_2 (range 0.35–11.1) in patients with poor outcome, which was not significantly different from patients with good outcome (mean 1.02 cm/mmHgCO_2, range 0.36–2.71).

Discussion

Dynamic testing of the responsiveness of the cerebral circulation to physiological stimuli is useful after severe head injury for 3 reasons:

1. Patients with reduced or absent vasoreactivity to changes in $PaCO_2$ or systemic blood pressure have a poor outcome.
2. Measures to control high ICP, such as hyperventilation, or mild hypertension, depend on an intact autoregulatory response.
3. Putatively neuroprotective drugs, such as calcium antagonists and NMDA antagonists, are being evaluated for use in acutely head injured patients. These drugs may be hypotensive, and they may themselves impair vasoreactivity. These effects may therefore be detrimental, if vasoreactivity is already damaged.

We have chosen to test the CO_2 response in this study because data from animal studies indicate that CO_2 reactivity is the most robust of the 3 vasoregulatory responses (to MABP, PaO_2, $PaCO_2$), and because a change in

$PaCO_2$ is the least invasive and simplest stimulus to apply in the head injured patient [4].

In previous studies, testing cerebral vasoreactivity after head injury has been difficult. Usually, the responses of hemisphere or regional CBF to a change in $PaCO_2$ or MABP has been used, but the methods have been invasive, cumbersome, complex, and of limited reproducibility. In this pilot study, we have shown that TCD testing of CO_2 reactivity is a simple, easily repeatable technique, which correlates with outcome, and appears to be independently determined in each hemisphere to some extent. This accords with regional CO_2 response data derived by Marion et al. using the tomographic CT Xenon CBF method [5].

We have also evaluated the Doppler Aaslid index in this study. An Aaslid index of over 3 indicates vasospasm in patients with subarachnoid haemorrhage, and the index has also been applied in head injury [9]. We have found a high Aaslid index to be more common in patients with poor outcome. Although a raised Aaslid index has been described in patients with large intracerebral haematomas and/or heavy cisternal blood load, there was no correlation between Doppler vasospasm and outcome in this serial study [9]. We have found that some middle cerebral arteries with a high Aaslid index retain their CO_2 responsiveness. Interpretation of vasospasm on the basis of Doppler readings may thus be more difficult in patients with head injury than in subarachnoid haemorrhage, perhaps due to coexistence of hyperaemia and vasospasm.

Further studies are needed to validate our measurement of CO_2 reactivity using TCD, and to test the hypothesis that reduced CO_2 reactivity implies that pressure autoregulation and the hypoxic response are also reduced or lost. Such studies would then allow CO_2 response testing to become a useful bedside technique to improve the safety of head injury management.

References

1. Cold GE, Taagehoj FT, Malmros R (1977) The cerebrovascular CO_2 reactivity during the acute phase of brain injury. Acta Anaesth Scand 21:222–231
2. Cold GE, Christensen MS, Schmidt K (1981) Effect of two levels of induced hypocapnia on cerebral autoregulation in the acute phase of head injury coma. Acta Anaesth Scand 25:397–401
3. Enevoldsen EM, Jensen FT (1978) Autoregulation and CO_2 responses of cerebral blood flow in patients with acute head injury. J Neurosurg 48:689–703
4. Lewelt W, Jenkins LW, Miller JD (1982) Effects of experimental fluid-percussion injury of the brain on cerebrovascular reactivity to hypoxia and to hypercapnia. J Neurosurg 56:332–337
5. Marion D, Darby J, Yonas H (1991) Acute regional cerebral blood flow changes caused by head injury. J Neurosurg 74:407–411
6. Muizelaar JP, Marmarou A, DeSalles AAF, Ward JD, Zimmerman RS, Li Z, Choi CS, Young HF (1989) Cerebral blood flow and metabolism in severely head-injured children. Part 1: Relationship with GCS score, outcome, ICP, and PVI. J Neurosurg 71:63–71
7. Obrist WD, Langfitt TW, Jaggi JL, Cruz J, Gennarelli TA (1984) Cerebral blood flow and metabolism in comatose patients with acute head injury. J Neurosurg 61:241–253
8. Tenjin H, Yamaki T, Nakagawa Y, Kuboyama T, Ebisu T, Kobori N, Ueda S, Mizukawa N (1990) Impairment of CO_2 reactivity in severe head injury patients: an investigation using the thermal diffusion method. Acta Neurochir 104:121–125
9. Weber M, Grolimund P, Seiler RW (1990) Evaluation of posttraumatic cerebral blood flow velocities by transcranial Doppler ultrasonography. Neurosurg 27:106–112

Cerebrovascular Reactivity Assessed by Changes in ICP and Transcranial Doppler

K. BANDOH, C.B. ZERATE, M. YOSHIHARA, and A. MARMAROU

Division of Neurosurgery, Medical Collage of Virginia, Richmond, VA, USA

Introduction

The ability to control ICP following traumatic head injury depends in part on cerebrovascular reactivity (CVR). By definition, cerebrovascular reactivity is defined as the change in blood flow (CBF) per torr change in PCO2. With regard to ICP control, it is the concomitant reduction in blood volume achieved in response to hyperventilation which remains a potent therapeutic tool in the patient with raised intracranial pressure. However, with traumatic injury, vascular reactivity may be reduced thus compromising the volume compensatory response for ICP reduction as well as altering dynamics of cerebral blood flow. Thus, a quantitative measure of cerebrovascular reactivity is important to help determine the underlying mechanisms leading to metabolic crisis and pressure/volume instability following severe head injury.

A new and simple method for cerebrovascular responsivity assessment which does not require measurement of CBF was recently introduced [1] and was based upon changes in ICP per torr change PCO2, induced by either hyperventilation or hypoventilation. (See Methods). However, this technique is based upon the important assumption that the global response of ICP is an accurate reflection of the degree of vessel caliber change.

One objective of this study was to confirm that ICP responsivity is directly related to vascular change by comparing ICP responses with transcranial doppler (TCD) assessments of vascular dynamics [2]. A second objective was to determine if either technique was of sufficient sensitivity to detect altered cerebrovascular responsiveness following severe head injury.

Methods

Sixty studies were performed on 19 patients with severe head injury admitted to the Medical College of Virginia and stabilized in the Neuroscience Intensive Care Unit. Intracranial pressure was measured by ventricular catheter. We defined four indices for assessment of pressure responsivity of the vessels in response to PCO2 (Table 1) [1]. For example, the "*P*ressure *R*eactivity *C*oefficient to hype*R*ventilation" (PRCR) characterized the global response to hypocapnia. This index was determined by first noting the ICP level and endotidal PCO2 (PeCO2) and then modifying the ventilation setting to lower

Table 1.

PRCR	=	Change in ICP per torr reduction of PCO2* (ICPb-ICPr)/(PCO2b-PCO2r)
PRCO	=	Change in ICP per torr increase of PCO2 (ICPb-ICPo)/(PCO2b-PCO2o)
BVRR	=	Change in CBV per torr reduction of PCO2 PVI*Log(ICPb/ICPr)/(PCO2b-PCO2r)
BVRO	=	Change in CBV per torr increase of PCO2 PVI*Log(ICPo/ICPb)/(PCO2o-PCO2b)
VRCR	=	Change in MCAv per torr reduction of PCO2 (MCAvb-MCAvr)/(PCO2b-PCO2r)
VRCO	=	Change in MCAv per torr increase of PCO2 (MCAvb-MCAvo)/(PCO2b-PCO2o)

PRCR, PRCO, *P*ressure *R*eactivity in Hype*R* or Hyp*O*ventilation; BVRR, BVRO, *B*lood *V*olume *R*esponse in Hype*R* or Hyp*O*ventilation; VRCR or VRCO, MCAv Reactivity in HypeR or HypOventilation.
(ICPb, PCO2b, MCAvb) = Baseline values of each parameter, (ICPr, PCO2r, MCAvr) = Values of each parameter to Hyperventilaiton, (ICPo, PCO2o, MCAvo) = Values of each parameter to Hypoventilation.

PCO2 by 2–3 torr. When ICP stabilized at a new level, the change in ICP per torr change in PeCO2 defined the PRCR. Calculation of other pressure indices are described in Table 1.

Measurement of left and right MCA velocities were obtained using the TC2-64 transcranial doppler instrument by Eden Medical Electronics Inc. Lake Constance, West Germany [2]. Insonation was obtained consistently through the temporal cranial window. The MCA measures were obtained synchronously with baseline ICP and were repeated after steady state was achieved. The responsivity indices were calculated in a similar manner and were defined as the change in MCA velocity per unit torr change in PeCO2 [1].

Both ICP and MCA velocity responsivity measures were determined daily and were coupled with measures of pressure volume index (PVI) which measured the brain compliance.

Results

The ICP and PVI were maintained at moderate levels for the duration of the study period (ICP = 17.7 ± 7.1 to 20.7 ± 8.0, PVI = 18.5 ± 6.4 to 21.0 ± 6.6). The treat threshold of ICP at MCV equals 20 mmHg and was maintained by CSF drainage, Mannitol, mild to aggressive hyperventilation and barbiturates, administered in that order as needed. It is important to note that the average PCO2 of these patients during the first 5 days post injury ranged from 28.9 ± 6.11 to 31.4 ± 4.7 (SD). Thus, moderate hyperventilation was required for ICP control.

The MCA velocities measured within 24 hours post injury averaged 61.14 ± 12.10, 58.00 ± 19.02 (SD), in left side and right side, respectively, and were only slightly elevated above normal levels. However, as time progressed, both left and right MCA velocities increased to significantly elevated values at 3 (Rt MCAv = 77.2 ± 24.1, Lt MCAv = 81.7 ± 41.4, $p < 0.05$) and 4 days (Rt MCAv = 78.2 ± 21.8, Lt MCAv = 84.3 ± 23.9, $p < 0.01$) post injury. Three patients reached levels greater than 120 cm/sec on the third day and approached the range of velocities equated with "vasospasm".

The pressure reduction achieved per torr hyperventilation (PRCR) averaged 0.66 ± 0.92 (SD) within 24 hours post injury and this level, which describes the ability of the vessels to constrict, was sustained throughout the five day period. In contrast, the ICP response to raised $PeCO_2$, termed PRCO, was greater by more than two fold. Thus, the ability of the vessels to dilate was greater than the degree of vasoconstriction produced by the same change in $PeCO_2$.

In contrast to the relatively flat profile of the ICP indices (PRCR, PRCO) over time, the right MCA responsivity measures show a gradual increase which peaks at day 4 post injury. This would suggest a slight improvement in vascular reactivity as time progresses post injury. The response to hyperventilation (VRCR) is less than the velocity change to increased $PeCO_2$ (VRCO). This follows the same pattern as the ICP reactivity measures.

Using the right MCA velocity change as a standard for monitoring vascular reactivity, agreement between ICP and MCA changes to hypocapnia is 81%. For ICP and MCA responses to hypercapnia, the agreement is slightly less (76%). When MCA response includes either left or right MCA, then simultaneous ICP responses are in 100% agreement. This includes response to increased and decreased $PeCO_2$. Thus, pressure and vascular responsiveness by doppler may be in error if only right MCA velocity changes are used.

Highest values of PRCO correlated with better outcome (Table 2). The reduction in PRCO associated with patients who died relative to PRCO of the

Table 2.

	PRCR	BVRR	Rt VRCR	Lt VRCR	PRCO	BVRO	Rt VRCO	Lt VRCO
G/MD								
AVE	0.73*	0.33*	0.58	1.14	1.67*	0.61*	1.02	0.33
SD	0.80	0.26	2.81	1.45	1.01	0.21	6.26	7.09
N	7	7	7	5	8	8	8	4
SD/V								
AVE	0.96	0.58*	1.96	3.33	1.40	0.75	4.89	3.67
SD	0.93	0.24	0.73	1.89	1.44	0.46	5.00	0.47
N	3	3	3	2	3	3	3	2
DEAD								
AVE	−0.20	−0.03	0.51	0.82	0.86	0.31	1.00	0.78
SD	0.48	0.21	0.78	1.90	0.58	0.13	2.00	1.35
N	5	4	4	3	4	4	3	3

Dead cases due to Systemic Complications were excluded. * $p < 0.05$: Compared with Dead Group (t-test).

G/MD patients was significant ($p < 0.015$). In contrast, no pattern could be distinguished with PRCR index. And also no pattern of MCA velocity responsivity changes related to outcome could be distinguished with exception of the consistently lower values of both left and right MCA in patients who died.

Discussion

This study shows that changes in blood velocity as assessed by transcranial doppler correlate well with the global ICP indices of cerebrovascular responsivity. A 100% agreement between ICP change and MCA velocity change was achieved. It should be noted that both left and right MCA's should be insonated to indicate presence of vascular responsiveness. Restricting the measurement to the right MCA would result in error.

In 4 patients, ICP was unresponsive to hyperventilation. However, in two of these patients, concomitant changes in MCA velocity were noted. Thus changes in MCA velocity in response to the PCO_2 stimulus can occur without a measurable change in ICP. Consequently, by strict definition, absence of ICP reactivity to PCO_2 stimulus cannot be interpreted as total absence of vascular reactivity. It suggests that resistive changes can occur in the peripheral arterial segments sufficient to effect blood velocity but not cause a sufficient volume reduction to reduce ICP.

The pressure indices reveal that the resting diameters of the vessels are altered following traumatic injury. The observation that PRCO is greater than PRCR indicates that the ability of the cerebral vessels to constrict is limited. This might be explained either by a reduction in vessel responsivity or reflect a persistent vasoconstriction resulting from the sustained hyperventilation applied to control ICP. The fact that PCO_2 levels in this patient group were only in the 30 torr range would suggest an impairment in the ability of the cerebral vessels to constrict.

Conclusion

1. Concomitant changes in doppler MCA velocities with ICP changes confirm the use of the simple ICP indices as measures of vascular responsivity.
2. In absence of ICP monitoring, transcranial doppler can be used as an alternate, less invasive method for establishing presence of vascular responsiveness. However, the magnitude of MCA velocity change may reflect low volume segments of the arterial vasculature and not correlate directly with ICP indices of responsivity.
3. By these ICP measures, the ability of the vessels to constrict further is impaired for at least 5 days following head injury.
4. Reduced responsivity to both vasoconstriction and vasodilation is associated with poor outcome.

References

1. Marmarou A, Wachi A (1989) Blood Volume Responsivity to ICP Change in Head Injured Patients. In: Hoff JT, Betz AL (eds) Intracranial pressure VLL. Springer, Berlin Heidelberg New York London Paris Tokyo Hong Kong, pp 688–690
2. Aaslid R, Markwalder TM, Nornes H (1982) Noninvasive Transcranial Doppler Ultrasound recording of flow velocity in basal cerebral arteries. J Neurosurg 57:769–774

Relationship Between Cerebral Perfusion Pressure and Pulsatility Index of Transcranial Doppler Sonogram

A. Yoshida, T. Shima, Y. Okada, M. Nishida, and H. Kurino

Departments of Critical Care Medicine and Neurosurgery, Chugoku Rousai Hospital, 1-5-1, Hiro-Tagaya, Kure City 737-01, Japan

Introduction

Transcranial Doppler (TCD) sonography, a non-invasive ultrasonic method introduced by Aaslid et al. [1], has made it possible to evaluate the hemodynamics in basal cerebral arteries through the intact cranium. Characteristic changes of TCD sonogram, the reduction of the diastolic component and the augmentation of the pulsatility amplitude in flow velocity wave forms have been reported in patients with intracranial hypertension [4, 5, 6].

To define the validity of TCD as a simple screening test for early identification of intracranial hypertension in emergency patients, we investigated the relationship between the cerebral perfusion pressure (CPP) and the pulsatility index on TCD sonogram.

Clinical Material and Methods

This study included 41 emergency patients with a diagnosis of closed head injury [17], hypertensive intracerebral hemorrhage [14] and ruptured aneurysms [10]. Their age ranged from 16 to 75 years (mean 54 years) and their Glasgow coma scale scores on admission were 5 to 14. Patients with systolic blood pressure below 80 mmHg, or with angiographically verified cerebral vasospasm were excluded from this study.

ICP was measured by an epidural pressure transducer (Ladd/Steritek) placed in the frontal epidural space.

Systemic arterial pressure (SABP) was continuously recorded through a catheter in the radial artery, and the transducer was calibrated at the level of the external auditory meatus. Cerebral perfusion pressure (CPP) was defined as the difference between the SABP and the epidural pressure (EDP). In this study, we obtained three types of CPP by the following calculations; systolic CPP (CPPs) = systolic SABP − mean EDP, mean CPP (CPPm) = mean SABP − mean EDP, and diastolic CPP (CPPd) = diastolic SABP − mean EDP.

Transcranial Doppler study was performed using a 2-MHz pulsed Doppler device (EME TC 2-64), and the middle cerebral arteries (MCA) were insonated on the side of the EDP measurement. The pulsatility indices (PI) of Gosling were calculated from the Doppler sonogram according to the following equation.:

$$PI = \frac{\text{peak systolic velocity} - \text{end diastolic velocity}}{\text{mean velocity}}$$

To minimize the influence of arterial carbon-dioxide tension ($PaCO_2$), hematocrit, and heart rate upon TCD sonogram, these variables were kept in the range of 35–40 mmHg, 30–40%, and 50–100 beats/min, respectively, during the TCD examinations.

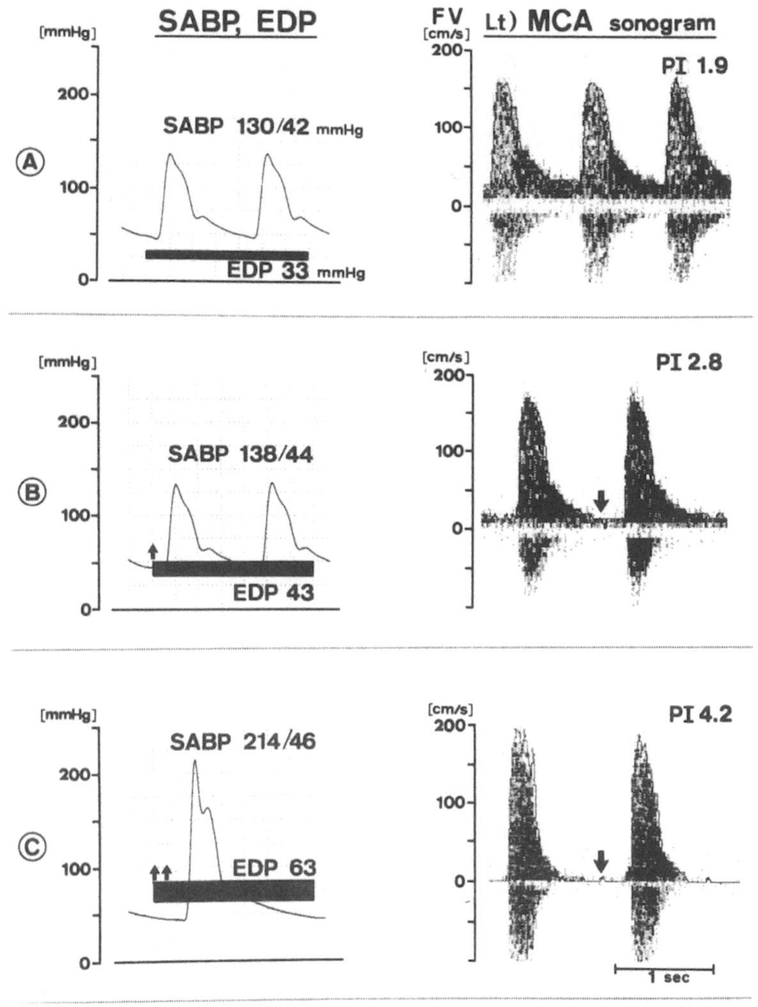

Fig. 1A–F. Changes in EDP, SABP and TCD sonogram of the left middle cerebral artery (MCA) in a patient with an acute subdural hematoma

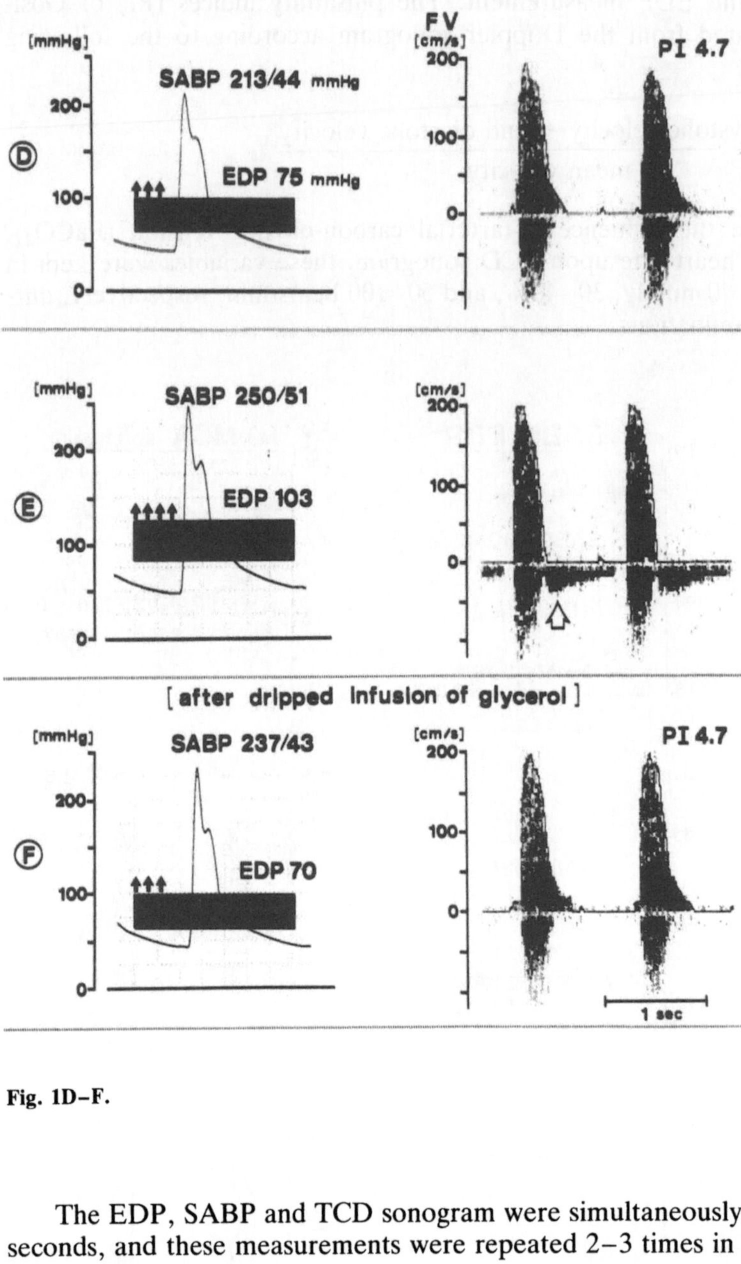

Fig. 1D–F.

The EDP, SABP and TCD sonogram were simultaneously recorded for 12 seconds, and these measurements were repeated 2–3 times in each patient.

Illustrative Case Report

Figure 1 shows the typical changes in the MCA sonogram corresponding to the elevation of the EDP in a patient suffering from an acute subdural hematoma.

An increase in EDP reduced the diastolic flow component of the MCA sonogram causing an increase in PI (Fig. 1A–B). When EDP increased above the diastolic SABP, no flow could be detected by TCD during diastole (large arrow in Fig. 1C–D), and an augmentation of PI could be observed. Further increase in EDP delivered a biphasic flow pattern with a reversed flow in the diastole (white arrow in Fig. 1E). This biphasic flow pattern vanished after the administration of glycerol (Fig. 1F).

These results suggest that the TCD flow pattern in the diastole is closely correlated with changes in EDP.

Results

In our 75 measurements, the PI increased with the progressive increase in EDP and the concomitant reduction in CPP.

Figure 2 shows the relationship between the PI and three calculated cerebral perfusion pressures; CPPs, CPPd, and CPPm. Of these three variables, the CPPd and CPPm demonstrated a significant correlation with the PI ($r = 0.871$ and 0.836, respectively). No significant correlation was observed between PI and CPPs ($r = 0.351$).

Moreover, no diastolic flow components could be detected by TCD whenever the EDP exceeded the diastolic SABP (open circles in Fig. 2B).

During a moderate decrease in CPP (CPPd above 40 mmHg, CPPm above 60 mmHg), no significant change in the PI could be observed.

Discussion

The present study demonstrated a good correlation between the CPPm and PI and, in particular, between the CPPd and PI.

The reason why CPPd had an excellent correlation with PI might be as follows.

As suggested by our case (Fig. 1), when the EDP was elevated, the systolic SABP was increased but the diastolic SABP remained unchanged. This means that the CPPs and CPPm increase parallel to the increase in EDP, but that the CPPd is inversely related to the EDP.

Although the present study suggests that a non-invasive estimation of ICP is possible through the measurement of PI and SABP, particularly diastolic SABP, there are some problems with regard to this method.

First, PI may be influenced by several factors such as heart rate, the wave form of systemic arterial pressure, arterial partial pressure of CO_2, etc. [2, 3]. These variables were kept in a normal range in our patients. However, in emergency patients with serious intracranial lesions, they would be hard to control because of the concomitant disturbances in circulation and/or respiration.

Secondly, the detection of a moderate intracranial hypertension by the analysis of PI was difficult, since the CPPd value of 40 mmHg was suggested to be a critical level to increase the PI in our study (Fig. 2B).

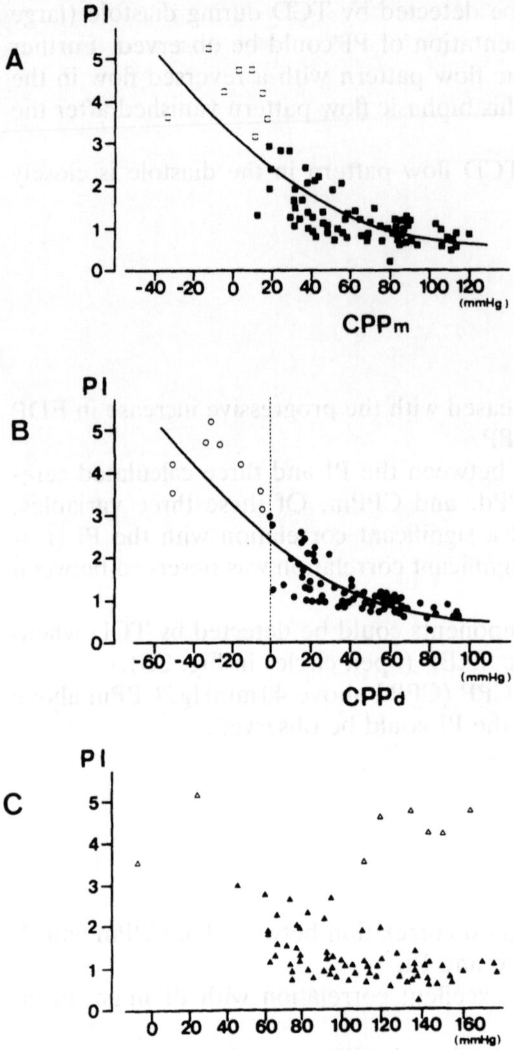

Fig. 2. A The relationship between the mean CPP (CPPm) and PI ($Y = 3.21 - 0.045\ X + 0.00019\ X^2$, $r = 0.836$, $p < 0.001$). Open squares: diastolic no flow pattern. **B** The relationship between the diastolic CPP (CPPd) and PI ($Y = 2.34 - 0.034\ X + 0.00015\ X^2$, $r = 0.871$, $p < 0.001$). Open circles: diastolic no flow pattern. **C** The relationship between the systolic CPP (CPPs) and PI. No significant correlation was observed ($r = 0.351$). Open triangles: diastolic no flow pattern

Regardless of such problems, the simultaneous measurement of the PI on TCD sonogram and the diastolic SABP was considered to be extremely useful in the non-invasive assessment of intracranial hypertension in emergency patients.

References

1. Aaslid R, Markwalder TM, Nornes H (1982) Noninvasive transcranial Doppler recording of flow velocity in basal cerebral arteries. J Neurosurg 57:769–774
2. Aaslid R, Lindegaard KF, Nornes H (1986) Estimation of cerebral perfusion pressure from arterial blood pressure and transcranial Doppler recordings. In: Miller JD, Teasdale GM, Rowan JO, Galbraith SL, Mendelow AD (eds) Intracranial pressure VI. Springer, Berlin Heidelberg New York Tokyo, pp 226–229
3. Giulioni M, Ursino M, Alvisi C (1988) Correlations among intracranial pulsatility, intracranial hemodynamics, and transcranial Doppler wave form: Literature review and hypothesis for future studies. Neurosurgery 22:807–812
4. Hassler W, Steinmetz H, Gawlowski J (1988) Transcranial Doppler ultrasonography in raised intracranial pressure and intracranial circulatory arrest. J Neurosurg 68:745–751
5. Klingelhöfer J, Conrad B, Benecke R, Sander D, Markakis E (1988) Evaluation of intracranial pressure from transcranial Doppler studies in cerebral disease. J Neurol 235:159–162
6. Saunders FW, Cledgett P (1988) Intracranial blood velocity in head injury. – A transcranial ultrasound Doppler study. Surg Neurol 29:401–409

Estimation of Cerebral Perfusion Pressure from Transcranial Doppler Sonography in Comatose Patients

T. Shiogai, Y. Tomita, M. Hara, K. Takeuchi, and I. Saito

Department of Neurosurgery, Kyorin University School of Medicine, 6-20-2 Shinkawa, Mitaka, Tokyo 181, Japan

Introduction

Transcranial Doppler sonography (TCD) can noninvasively assess the intracranial pressure (ICP) – volume relationship during intracranial hypertension. Non-invasive estimations of cerebral perfusion pressure (CPP) [1] and ICP [5] have been attempted without conclusive results. The aim of this study was to establish a method of noninvasively estimating CPP and ICP in comatose patients by multiple regression analysis of TCD and other physiological parameters.

Patients and Methods

A computer-controlled continuous, multimodal neuromonitoring system, consisting of TCD, ICP, systemic arterial blood pressure (BP), endtidal CO_2 partial pressure (PCO_2), and electrophysiological modalities (Fig. 1), was applied in 40 comatose patients with intracranial lesions. Supratentorial ICP was monitored with epidural (Gaeltec Ltd., Scotland) or intraparenchymal (intraventricular) probes (Camino Lab., USA). TCD was monitored with a 2-MHz flat probe (FP-2/TC2-64B, EME, FRG) on the middle cerebral artery (MCA).

Thirteen of the 40 cases were selected for the quality and continuity of acquired data. Patients' mean age was 53 (range, 16–72). Brain damage was caused by head injury (5 focal and 1 diffuse) in 6 cases, and stroke (3 subarachnoid and 2 intracerebral hemorrhages; 2 cerebral infarction) in 7 cases. A total 494 data (9–65 data per patient) were selected for calculation during 2–13 hours. Peak systolic velocity (VS), end-diastolic velocity (VD), mean velocity (VM), pulsatility index (PI = VS-VD/VM), and resistance index (RI = VS-VD/VS) derived from TCD waveform analysis, and PCO_2, hematocrit (HT), and BP were considered for selection of independent variables in multiple regression analysis.

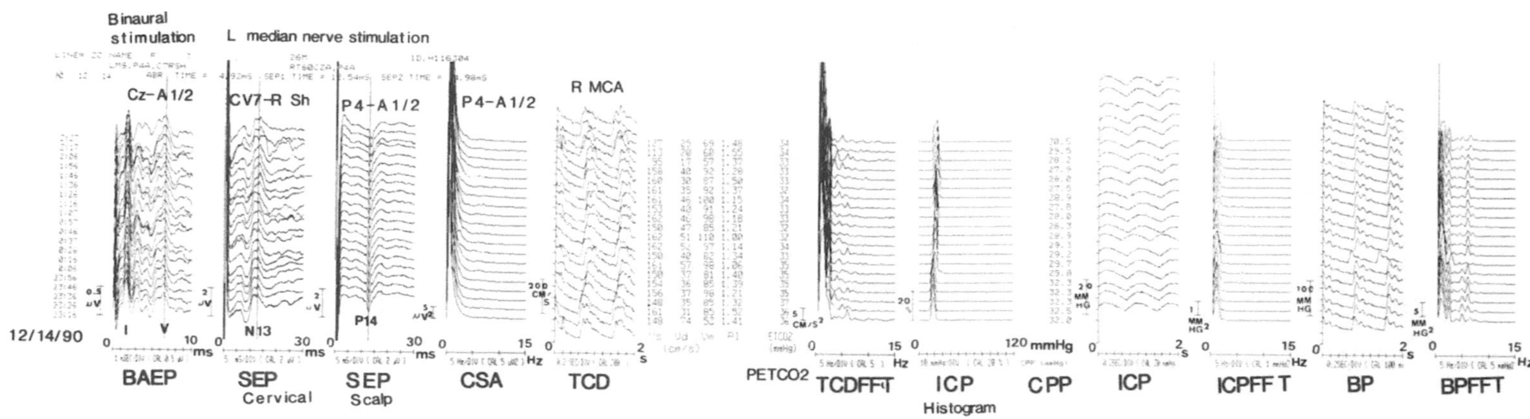

Fig. 1. Continuous, multimodal neuromonitoring of a 26-year-old comatose patient with right acute subdural hematoma. Left to right: Brainstem auditory evoked potentials (BAEP), somatosensory evoked potentials (SEP), compressed spectral arrays (CSA), TCD flow velocity waveforms in right MCA, TCD waveforms parameters (VS, VD, VM and PI), end-tidal PCO_2 ($PETCO_2$), Fourier analysis of TCD waveforms (TCDFFT), ICP histogram, CPP, and original and Fourier analysis of ICP and BP waveforms (ICPFFT and BPFFT). On-line data were analysed and presented every 10 minutes and stored in two floppy discs for later off-line analysis

Results

Simple Correlations Between Variables and CPP and ICP

Among the simple correlation coefficients (r) between variables derived from TCD and other physiological parameters, and CPP and ICP: BP (0.83), RI (−0.60) and VD (0.46) for CPP, and BP (0.42), PCO_2 (−0.36) and PI (−0.34) for ICP had high coefficient values in comparison with other variables. These results were significant at $p < 0.0001$ (paired t-test).

In the regression curve between CPP and VD (RI), there was a breaking point at about 40 mmHg CPP. Below this CPP level, zero VD (RI = 1) was observed in some cases.

Multiple Regression Analysis for Estimation of CPP and ICP

To avoid multi-collinearity [4] in the determination of independent variables for multiple regression analysis, five variables (1 velocity, 1 index, and 3 physiological parameters) were selected. There was a high rate of correlations among velocity parameters (VS, VD, and VM; $r > 0.9$, $p < 0.0001$) and indices of pulsatility (RI and VD, $r = -0.76$; PI and RI, $r = 0.66$: $p < 0.0001$).

If VD, PI, BP, PCO_2 and HT were selected, multiple correlation coefficients (r) for estimation of CPP and ICP were 0.86 and 0.50, respectively. To cancel the effects of other variables, partial correlation coefficients (r) were calculated; BP (0.82), PCO_2 (0.21), VD (0.11) and Pi (0.08) for CPP; PCO_2 (0.36), BP (0.25), VD (0.19), and PI (0.14) for ICP. These results were significant at $p < 0.0001$ (F test).

The multiple regression equations were calculated as: CPP = 0.84 BP (mmHg) + 0.86 PCO_2 (mmHg) + 0.09 VD (cm/s) + 0.93 PI − 41.5 and ICP = 41.5 − 0.86 PCO_2 (mmHg) + 0.16 BP (mmHg) − 0.09 VD (cm/s) − 0.93 PI. A scatter diagram of the relationship between measured and predicted values of CPP is shown in Fig. 2.

Discussion

Flow Velocity Pulsatility and Autoregulation During Intracranial Hypertension

Increased pulsatility of flow velocity waveforms during intracranial hypertension mainly results from decrease in diastolic flow velocity (approaching zero, finally changing to reverse flow) with severe reduction of CPP (approaching zero, finally becoming intracranial circulatory arrest) [3]. Precise relationships between flow velocity parameters and CPP or ICP have not been established. In our study, however, simple correlation analysis indicated the closest relation between RI and CPP. This close correlation has also been observed clinically

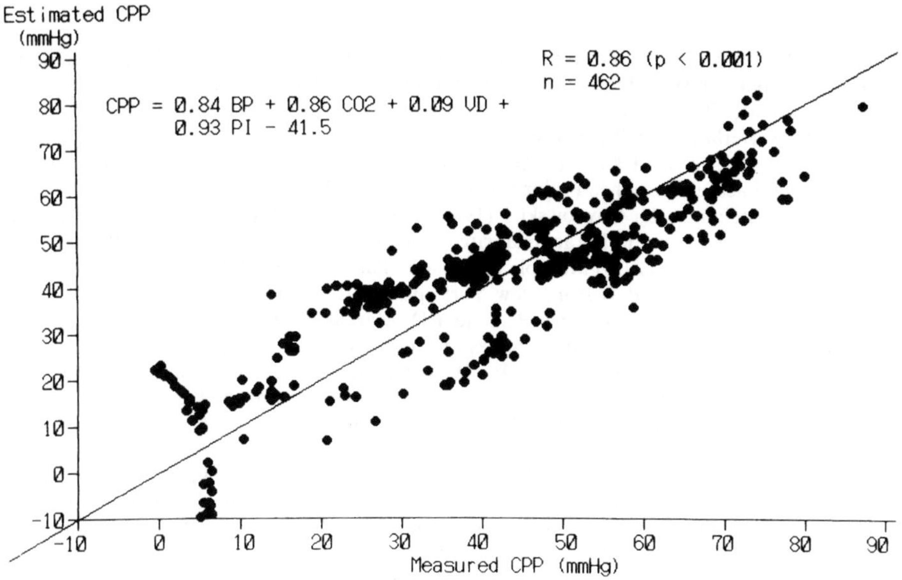

Fig. 2. Scatter diagram of relationship between measured and predicted values of CPP

[5] and experimentally [8]. These findings indicate highly disturbed autoregulation in comatose patients and experimental animals.

It is well known, on the other hand, that there is a breaking point between CPP and cerebral blood flow (CBF) at 40 mmHg CPP [7]. A similar breaking point was identified in our study of the relationship between CPP and VD (RI). A lower autoregulatory limit of 40–45 mmHg CPP was also speculated clinically [6]. Below this CPP level, zero VD and diastolic reverse flow appeared in some cases. Zero VD also appeared experimentally below 27 ± 11 mmHg CPP during hydrostatic pressure loading [8]. Clinically, this critical point may not always be stable due to the effect of other physiological and morphological factors, such as $PaCO_2$ change or intracranial mass lesions. Zero VD, however, highly indicates disturbed autoregulation and a grave prognosis for patients with severe brain damage [9].

Estimation of CPP Based on TCD and Physiological Parameters

Estimation of CPP by Fourier analysis of TCD and BP waveforms has been attempted [1]. In our study of comatose patients, BP and PCO_2 greatly contributed to estimation of CPP. The dissociation of autoregulation and CO_2 response of CBF in cases of severe head injury has been pointed out [2]. Precise CPP estimation based not only on TCD parameters and BP but also on PCO_2 is therefore necessary in the case of comatose patients with critical brain damage.

References

1. Aaslid R, Lundar T, Lindegaard K-F, Nornes H (1986) Estimation of cerebral perfusion pressure from arterial blood pressure and transcranial Doppler recordings. In: Miller JD, Teasdale GM, Rowan JO, Galbraith SL, Mendelow AD (eds) Intracranial Pressure Vl, Springer, V Berlin, Heidelberg New York Tokyo, pp 226–229
2. Enevoldsen EM, Jensen FT (1978) Autoregulation and CO_2 responses of cerebral blood flow in patients with acute severe head injury. J Neurosurg 48:689–703
3. Hassler W, Steinmctz H, Gawlowski J (1988) Transcranial Doppler ultrasonography in raised intracranial pressure and in intracranial circulatory arrest. J Neurosurgery 68:745–751
4. Hays WL, Winkler RL (1970) Multiple regression. Statistics: probability, inference and decision. Vol II. Holt Rinehart and Wiston, New York, pp 59–91
5. Kligelhoefer J, Conrad B, Benecke R, Sander D, Markakis E (1988) Evaluation of intracranial pressure from transcranial Doppler studies in cerebral disease. J Neurol 235:159–162
6. Lundar T, Lindegaard K-F, Nornes H (1990) Continuous recording of the middle cerebral artery blood velocity in clinical neurosurgery. Acta Neurochir (Wien) 102:85–90
7. Miller JD, Stanek A, Langfitt TW (1973) Cerebral blood flow regulation during experimental brain compression. J Neurosurg 39:186–196
8. Nakatani S, Ozaki K, Hara K, Mogami H (1989) Intracranial volume and pressure load tolerance evaluated by continuous measurement of Doppler flow velocity on intracranial vessel in cats. In: Hoff JT, Betz AL (eds) Intracranial Pressure VII. Springer, Berlin Heidelberg, New York London Paris Tokyo Hong Kong, pp 109–112
9. Shiogai T, Sato E, Tokitsu M, Hara M, Takeuchi K (1990) Transcranial Doppler monitoring in severe brain damage: relationship between intracranial haemodynamics, brain dysfunction and outcome. Neurol Res 12:205–213

Changes in Cerebral Blood Flow During ICP Monitoring

T. Cafiero[1], B. Gallicchio[2], G. Gargiulo[1], P. Mastronardi[1], B. Mazzarella[1], and L. Stella[2]

[1] I. Cattedra di Anestesiologia e Rianimazione, [2] Istituto di Neurochirurgia, II. Facoltà di Medicina e Chirurgia di Napoli, Naples, Italy

Introduction

The possibility of evaluating the cerebral blood flow by using the pulsed transcranial doppler (TCD) is a reliable and noninvasive technique [1]. This method can provide information on the ICP-cerebral hemodynamics relationship [2]. The aim of this study is to compare the changes in CBF during ICP monitoring in heterogeneous conditions.

Methods

Fifteen patients (11 males and 4 females), aging from 35 to 67 years, undergoing ICP monitoring for diagnostic or therapeutic purposes were studied. ICP and CBF were simultaneously monitored as follows: (a) for a 12 hours period in 6 patients suffering from severe head injury; (b) during bolus fluid injection test in 6 patients (5 with spontaneous subarachnoid or intracerebral hemorrhage and 1 with hydrocephalus); (c) during propofol 2.5 mg/kg single bolus administration in 3 patients with hydrocephalus. ICP monitoring was connected with a polygraph (Honeywell) with ICP zero reference at midcranial level. CBF was measured in the MCA at depths of 50–55 mm by TCD (TC 264 EME 2 MHZ). The parameters studied were S/D (range 2.1 – 2.4), mean velocity in MCA (Vmca) (range 62 ± 10 cm/sec) and pulsatility index (PI) (range 0.7 – 0.9). Statistical analysis was performed using the Student's t test. $P < 0.05$ was considered to be significant.

Results

Regarding the patients with head injury the results are shown in Table 1. Also during the infusion tests a good correlation between ICP changes and the hemodynamic parameters was noted. In one case especially, ICP increased significantly from a baseline value of 20 mmHg to 38 mmHg with a concomitant increase of S/D to a value of 3.8 and a decrease of Vmca to a value of 35 cm/sec. In patients who received propofol for sedation the results are shown in Table 2.

Table 1. ICP, PI and Vmca values during monitoring in patients with head injury (6 cases)

Time (hours)	1	2	3	4	5	6	7	8	9	10	11	12
ICP	24 ± 3	22 ± 4	26 ± 5	25 ± 2	25 ± 2	18 ± 3*	25 ± 5	26 ± 1	20 ± 1	24 ± 3	24 ± 2	26 ± 3
Vmca	50 ± 5	48 ± 3	55 ± 3	56 ± 4	50 ± 1	80 ± 4*	59 ± 3	50 ± 2	56 ± 3	50 ± 6	50 ± 5	45 ± 3
PI	2.0	1.8	1.8	1.3	1.8	0.8*	1.3	2.5	1.3	1.5	1.8	2.0

* = p 0.05

Table 2. ICP, Vmca and MAP changes during single bolus injection of propofol (2.5 mg.kg. −1)

Time	B	1	2	5
ICP	21.2 ± 2.3	15.2 ± 2.5*	12.2 ± 1.8*	15.9 ± 4.1*
Vmca	60 ± 5	40 ± 6*	45 ± 5*	70 ± 5
MAP	90.5 ± 5.6	75.5 ± 2.8*	78.3 ± 3.5*	85.5 ± 5.2

Time: B = basal; 1, 2, and 5 minutes after propofol administration.
* = p 0.05

Discussion

In all cases we found a good correlation between PI and ICP and inversely between Vmca and ICP. The use of TCD together with ICP monitoring is a valid method of great importance for assessing the efficacy of CBF autoregulation. It has been demonstrated that Vmca monitoring is a useful index of the cerebral hemodynamics. In patients who received propofol for sedation, ICP decreased significantly as demonstrated also in other studies [3]. Also Vmca decreased significantly at 1 and 2 minutes after propofol administration. Furthermore, we found MAP reduction at the same time. In this case, a direct correlation between ICP and Vmca was demonstrated because both ICP and Vmca decreased. This is probably due to the action of propofol on the peripheral vascular resistance which can influence the behaviour of the CBF. Another interesting factor to be considered is the concomitant reduction of S/D (about 20%). We can hypothesize that the S/D reduction depends on the decrease in cerebral vascular resistances during propofol injection. Although other investigations are necessary, we can conclude that TCD is a reliable noninvasive method in monitoring the cerebral perfusion state.

References

1. Bishop CCR, Powell S, Rutt D, Browse NL (1986) Transcranial Doppler measurement of middle cerebral artery blood flow velocity: A validation study. Stroke 17:913–915
2. Lundar T, Lindegaard KF, Aaslid R, Nornes H (1988) In: Hoff JT, Betz AL (eds) Intracranial Pressure VII. Springer, Berlin Heidelberg New York London Paris Tokyo Hong Kong
3. Parma A, Massei R, et al. (1988) Influence of single bolus of propofol on ICP and CBF velocity. In: Hoff JT, Betz AL (eds) Intracranial Pressure VII. Springer, Berlin Heidelberg New York London Paris Tokyo Hong Kong

Non-Invasive Monitoring of Intracranial Pressure Gradients by Means of Transcranial Doppler

E.R. Cardoso and J.A. Kupchak

Cerebral Hydrodynamics Laboratory and Department of Nursing Education and Research, Health Sciences Centre, Winnipeg, Canada

Introduction

The effects of diffuse elevations of ICP on TCD have been extensively investigated. Diffuse elevation of ICP lowers cerebral perfusion pressure, affecting mostly the diastolic TCD mean velocity in the major intracranial arteries, thus increasing the pulsatility index (PI) [3]. We investigated the possibility to identify side-to-side gradients of intracranial pressure (ICP) by means of transcranial Doppler (TCD) ultrasonography in patients with subacute and chronic subdural hematomas.

Materials and Methods

Patient Population

Eleven patients harbouring a subdural hematoma underwent pre- and post-operative TCD examinations of the internal carotid and middle cerebral arteries, bilaterally. Patients were included in the study if they harboured a single symptomatic subacute or chronic subdural hematoma, with attributable focal neurological findings and no steroid pre-treatment.

TCD Measurements

The TCD examinations through a model TC 2-64B EME TCD, coupled with a 2 MHz. PW probe were performed just prior to and 24 hours after surgical evacuation of the subdural hematoma. Values of mean velocity and pulsatility index (PI) obtained from the internal carotid and middle cerebral arteries at depth settings of 65, 60, 55, and 50 mm from the temporal ultrasonic window were averaged and compared to the contra-lateral counterpart by means of paired Student t-test. The hematomas were evacuated by means of burr hole drainage under local anesthesia. The subdural pressure was measured before hematoma evacuation in 8 cases. Blood pressure, Glasgow coma score (GCS) and arterial PCO_2 were recorded at the time of TCD readings. Surgical evacuation of hematomas was carried out through a single burr hole, on awake patients. Subdural pressure was measured prior to drainage, and a drain was left in the subdural space for post-operative pressure measurements.

Results

Eleven patients, including 10 males and 1 female had a mean age of 67.7 years, varying from 39 to 86 years. The pre-operative mean GCS was 12. The focal neurological deficits disappeared in all patients after surgery.

Lateralized intracranial mass produced side-to-side differences of mean TCD velocity and PI. Pre-operative TCD mean velocities were consistently lower on the side of the subdural hematoma in all but one patient. The mean side-to-side difference was 15.64 + 3.01 m.sec-1 ($P < 0.0005$). The mean TCD value on the side of the subdural hematoma was 34.18 + 2.22 m.sec-1, going up to 47.9 + 3.2 m.sec-1 ($P < 0.002$) following removal of the subdural hematoma (Table 1).

Pre-operative PI measurements also showed significant side-to-side differences, being significantly greater on the side of the hematoma by a mean side-to-side difference of 0.23 + 0.04 ($P < 0.0025$). These differences disappeared following evacuation of the hematoma. The mean pre-operative ipsi-lateral PI value of 1.33 + 0.01 went down to 1.08 + 0.01 ($P < 0.01$).

The mean pre-operative subdural pressure was 13.19 + 2.93 cm H_2O and correlated well with side-to-side differences of mean PI ($r = 0.85$).

Discussion

TCD is a recently developed, non-invasive technique of measurement of blood velocity in the major intra-cranial arteries [1]. It has shown to be useful in the investigation of critical elevations of the ICP, to the point of affecting cerebral perfusion pressure [3]. Here the diastolic portion of the velocity wave is

Table 1.

	Pre-OP		Post-OP	
	Ipsilateral	Contralateral	Ipsilateral	Contralateral
Mean Velocity (m/sec)	34.18 ± 2.22	49.2 ± 1.2*	47.9 ± 3.2	49.0 ± 3.0†
PI	1.33 ± 0.01	1.11 ± 0.05**	1.08 ± 0.01	1.05 ± 0.06†
ΔV (m/sec)	15.64 ± 3.01		2.55 ± 2.9	
ΔPI	0.23 ± 0.04		0.06 ± 0.1	

* $p < 0.0005$
** $p < 0.0025$
† NSD

predominantly affected leading to progressive alteration of the configuration of the TCD spectra as the ICP rises [3].

Our results suggest the possibility to use TCD for non-invasive monitoring of ICP gradients generated by mass lesions. We postulate that the side-to-side TCD differences are caused by intracranial pressure gradients generated by the subdural mass lesion, as it creates pressure gradients within the cerebral tissue [2, 4, 5]. Raised tissue pressure subsequently lowers intravascular blood flow velocity. Thus, we believe that the asymmetry of TCD readings was caused by the raised interstitial pressure underlying the subdural hematoma.

Our results showed a better correlation of subdural pressures with PI than with mean TCD velocities, suggesting that PI values might be more useful than mean TCD velocities to detect ICP gradients.

Acknowledgements. Project funded by the Grand Lodge of Free Masons of Manitoba, the Head Injury Association of Manitoba and the Children's Hospital Association.

References

1. Aaslid R, Markwalder T, Nornes H (1982) Non-invasive transcranial doppler ultrasound recording of flow velocity in basal cerebral arteries. J Neurosurg 57:769–774
2. Abe T, Black PM, Foley L (1984) Changes in parenchymal and ventricular pressure with experimental epidural compression. Surg Neurol 22:477–480
3. Hassler W, Steinmetz H, Gawlowski J (1988) Transcranial Doppler ultrasonography in raised intracranial pressure and in intracranial circulatory arrest. J Neurosurg 68:745–751
4. Penn RD, Bacus JW (1984) The brain as a sponge: a computed tomographic look at Hakim's hypothesis. Neurosurg 14:670–675
5. Weaver DD, Winn HR, Jane JA (1982) Differential intracranial pressure in patients with unilateral mass lesions. J Neurosurg 56:660–665

Wave Form Analysis

Comparison of Methods for ICP Waveform Analysis with Intracranial Hypertension in Head-Injured Patients

C.S. Robertson, C.F. Contant, R.K. Narayan, and R.G. Grossman

Baylor College of Medicine, One Baylor Plaza Houston, TX 77030, 713-798-4696 USA

Introduction

Continuous monitoring of intracranial pressure (ICP) permits early identification and treatment of intracranial hypertension. However, measurement of the mean ICP does not provide information about the cause of the intracranial hypertension, which can include mass lesions, cerebral edema, hyperemia, and/or hydrocephalus. A number of experimental and preliminary clinical studies have suggested that changes in the shape of the ICP waveform could suggest the underlying pathophysiological mechanism of an elevated ICP [3, 4, 5, 6]. This additional information would permit treatment of the elevated ICP to be directed more specifically at the underlying cause.

The purpose of this study was to determine if one or more of 8 parameters describing changes in the shape of the ICP waveform could distinguish between an ICP increase due to hyperemia and an ICP increase due to increasing cerebral edema or mass effect.

Methods

Seventy-eight adult patients admitted to the Neurosurgical intensive care unit at Ben Taub General Hospital between July 15, 1989 and December 31, 1990 with a Glasgow Coma Score (GCS) $\leq$8 due to severe head trauma had continuous monitoring of ICP and of 8 parameters quantitating changes in the shape of the ICP waveform. ICP was monitored by a ventriculostomy in 64 of these patients, by a subdural catheter in 3 patients, and by a Camino fiberoptic ICP monitor placed in the brain parenchyma in the remaining 11 patients. Forty-seven of the patients also had simultaneous monitoring of jugular venous oxygen saturation ($SjvO_2$). Arterial oxygen saturation (SaO_2), end-tidal CO_2 ($ETCO_2$), and mean arterial blood pressure (MAP) were collected in all patients.

Two types of ICP increases were identified and studied using the 8 parameters which are described below:

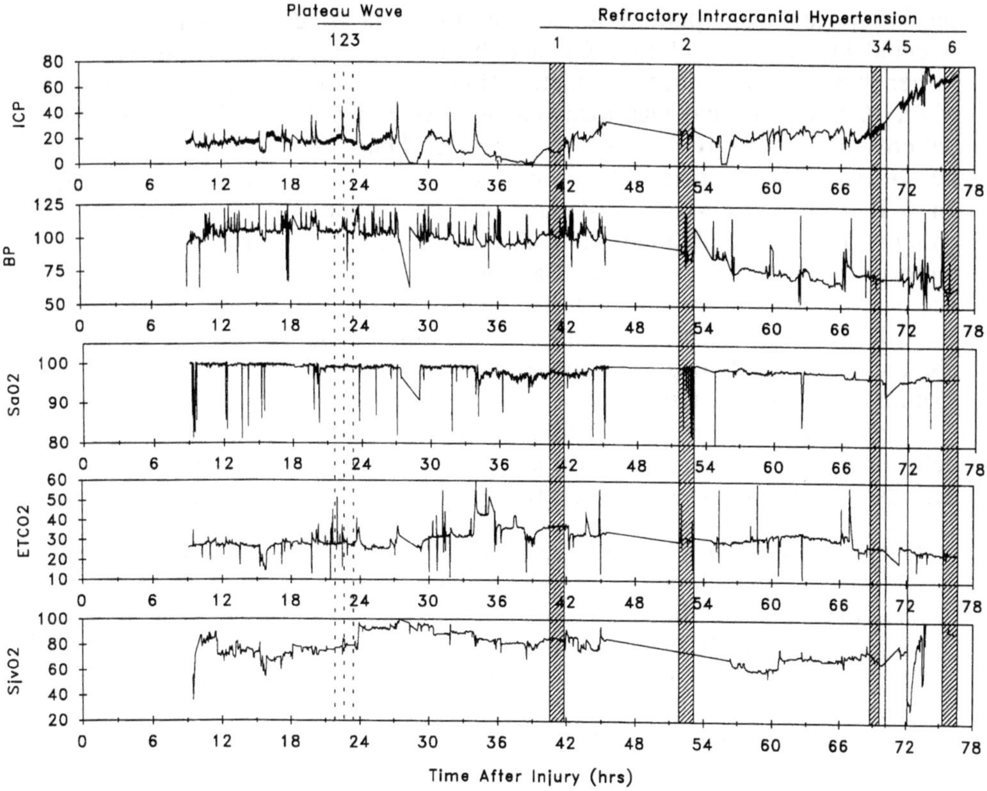

Fig. 1. Example of the time periods selected for analysis. This patient was admitted with a diffuse brain injury. For the first 24 hours the ICP required no treatment although several transient increases in the ICP occurred. One of these ICP spikes (at hour 22) was selected for examination as a plateau wave. At hour 28, a CT scan was repeated and showed multiple contusions that were not present on the initial CT scan. Over the next 48 hours, the ICP became increasingly refractory to treatment, and the patient eventually died with increased ICP. The time periods that were selected for analysis as the ICP became refractory are indicated

Plateau Waves

ICP increases characterized by an abrupt increase in ICP to at least 25 mmHg and to at least 50% greater than the previous hour's mean ICP were identified in 43 of the 78 patients. The sudden rapid and transient nature of the ICP increase suggested a vascular origin. Most often the ICP increase was precipitated by coughing, suctioning, or some other type of stimulation. Occasionally there was no obvious external precipitating event. As illustrated in Fig. 1, a 10–60 minutes time period prior to the ICP increase, at the peak of the ICP increase, and after the ICP increase were identified for study.

Refractory Intracranial Hypertension

Refractory intracranial hypertension developed in 11 patients who died of increased ICP. Because the time course of the progressing intracranial hypertension varied from patient to patient, the data used for comparison were selected by the level of the ICP and by the development of clinical events rather than by time course parameters (Fig. 1). A baseline set of data at a time when ICP was normal was available in 8 of the patients. The remaining 3 patients never had ICP values <20 mmHg. Data as the ICP increased but before clinical signs of herniation and before CBF dropped were obtained, at an ICP of 20–30 mmHg in 10 patients, and at an ICP > 30 mmHg in 10 patients. Data were obtained in all 11 patients at the time that clinical signs of tentorial herniation developed. Data were obtained in 6 patients as $SjvO_2$ decreased, indicating a fall in CBF. The drop in CBF usually followed the clinical signs of brainstem compression, often by hours. Finally data were obtained after CBF was very low or absent (cerebral perfusion pressure < 15 mmHg) in all 11 patients.

Eight ICP waveform descriptors derived from either the height of the ICP pulse or from a Fourier transform analysis were studied at the identified time periods. The 4 parameters derived from the height of the ICP wave included:

1. The *pulse amplitude* (PA) was defined as the systolic ICP minus the diastolic ICP. This is the simplest method for expressing the amplitude of the ICP waveform, and has been the single most widely used method in reported clinical studies of ICP waveform analysis [1, 7, 9].
2. The *pulse amplitude-ICP ratio* (PAICP ratio) was calculated from the PA divided by the ICP.
3. The *pulse-respiratory ratio* (PR ratio) was obtained from the PA divided by the amplitude of the respiratory variation in the ICP, as described by Dearden and Miller [4]. Hyperemia, or vascular dilatation, would increase primarily the PA, while cerebral edema or an expanding mass lesion would increase both the PA and the respiratory variation in the ICP. Therefore an increased PR ratio (>1.5) indicates intracranial hypertension due to vascular engorgement, which would be more likely to respond to treatment with barbiturates, while a decreased PR ratio (<0.8) indicates intracranial hypertension due to a condition which would be more likely to respond to mannitol.
4. *Slope* was defined as the maximal upgoing slope.
   The 4 parameters obtained from the Fourier transform analysis of the ICP wave included:
5. The *amplitude of the fundamental wave* (FW), and *second through fifth harmonics* (HW2–HW5) of the heart rate were calculated.
6. The *relative power contained in the fundamental wave* (%FW) and *in the second through fifth harmonics* (%HW2–%HW5) were calculated.
7. The distortion factor, or *k ratio*, was calculated by the formula:

$$\text{k ratio} = \frac{\sqrt{(HW2)^2 + (HW3)^2 + (HW4)^2 + (HW5)^2}}{FW}$$

as described by Takizawa et al. [8]. As the ICP waveform becomes rounded in appearance, losing the individual component waves, it's appearance approaches that of a pure sine wave, which has no harmonics. The k ratio of the ICP power density spectrum is an index that represents the extent to which the ICP waveform is distorted or different from a pure sine wave. The value of the k ratio is zero if it is a pure sine wave. The k ratio of a normal-appearing ICP waveform is usually 1–2.

8. The *high frequency centroid* (HFC) was calculated as the power-weighted mean frequency within a 4 to 15 Hz frequency band, as described by Bray et al. [2]. The HFC had an inverse relationship to the PVI in these studies. A HFC of 6.5–7.0 Hz was normal, and a HFC of 9.0 Hz corresponded with a reduction in PVI to approximately 13 ml.

Results

The data is summarized in Table 1. The baseline ICP was similar in the 2 groups of patients, as were the remainder of the physiological parameters. Of the waveform descriptors, only the HFC was significantly different in the patients who developed refractory intracranial hypertension, averaging 8.3 ± 0.2 Hz, compared to 7.7 ± 0.1 Hz in the plateau wave group.

Consistent changes in the physiological parameters occurred during the ICP increases identified as plateau waves. MAP, $ETCO_2$, and $SjvO_2$ increased with the ICP. The cerebral perfusion pressure (CPP) was unchanged. The ICP waveform parameters described an increase in the pulse height and rounding of the ICP waveform as the ICP increased. PA, FW, HW2–HW5, %FW, and the HFC all increased. The k ratio decreased.

Characteristic physiological changes were also observed during intracranial hypertension prior to the development of clinical neurological changes. BP and HR tended to decrease, although the differences were not significant. $SjvO_2$ and $ETCO_2$ were unchanged as the ICP increased. The ICP waveform parameters quantitated primarily an increase in pulse height as the ICP became refractory. The PA, FW, and HW2 significantly increased. The HFC significantly decreased. The remainder of the waveform descriptors were not consistently changed as the ICP increased.

When the changes in the ICP waveform descriptors during the plateau wave and as refractory intracranial hypertension developed were compared only a few minor differences were found. Both groups had similar increases in PA and the amplitude of the FW and HW2. The amplitude of HW4 and HW5 consistently increased in the plateau wave group, but remained unchanged or decreased in the patients with refractory intracranial hypertension. The k ratio consistently decreased and the slope increased in the plateau wave group, but not in the patients with refractory intracranial hypertension. None of these differences were significant. Only changes in the HFC were significantly different in the 2 groups. The HFC increased in the patients in the plateau group, but decreased in the patients with refractory intracranial hypertension.

At the time that clinical signs of tentorial herniation developed in the patients with refractory intracranial hypertension, the ICP was slightly higher, and BP tended to be lower, resulting in a CPP of approximately 41 mmHg. The remainder of the physiological parameters, including the $SjvO_2$ were unchanged.

Table 1. Summary of ICP waveform descriptors during plateau waves in 42 patients and in 11 patients as refractory intracranial hypertension developed

Time period	Plateau wave (n = 42 patients)			Refractory intracranial hypertension (n = 11 patients)					
	Pre-plateau wave	Peak of plateau wave	Post-plateau wave	No clinical changes			Herniation	Decreased SjvO2	CPP <15
				ICP <20	ICP 20–30	ICP >30	ICP >30	ICP >30	ICP >30
Number of observations	42	42	41	8	10	10	11	6	11
	Physiological parameters			Physiological Parameters					
ICP	13.3 ± 0.9	33.1 ± 1.2[a]	13 ± 0.9	16.1 ± 0.7	24.5 ± 0.6[b]	35.6 ± 0.9[b]	41.6 ± 4.0[b]	52.0 ± 6.5[b]	49.2 ± 7.0[b]
HR	92.3 ± 3.1	105.7 ± 3.5[a]	94.9 ± 2.9	99.5 ± 6.5	93.7 ± 6.6	87.7 ± 7.2	102.3 ± 8.7	97.6 ± 7.8	94.1 ± 3.8
MAP	92.1 ± 2.1	110.0 ± 3.8[a]	93.9 ± 2.3	101.1 ± 4.8	87.5 ± 6.4	91.3 ± 9.2	82.5 ± 5.0[b]	76.8 ± 5.7[b]	62.6 ± 3.7[b]
SjvO2	68.2 ± 1.8	72.8 ± 1.8[a]	69.9 ± 1.7	75.2 ± 4.0	70.4 ± 3.6	72.3 ± 5.2	69.8 ± 4.6	42.3 ± 3.9[b]	75.6 ± 6.5
SaO2	98.1 ± 0.3	97.1 ± 0.9	98.5 ± 0.1	98.4 ± 0.4	98.1 ± 0.3	98.3 ± 0.5	98.6 ± 0.3	97.3 ± 1.0	94.6 ± 2.1
ETCO2	28.8 ± 1.6	36.5 ± 1.9[a]	31.5 ± 2.0	29.2 ± 2.4	23.1 ± 1.6	26.8 ± 2.0	24.8 ± 1.7	28.1 ± 4.8	29.6 ± 5.1
	ICP parameters derived from the pulse amplitude			ICP parameters derived from the pulse amplitude					
PA	5.0 ± 0.4	10.4 ± 0.8[a]	5.1 ± 0.4	6.0 ± 1.0	7.7 ± 1.0	10.4 ± 1.1[b]	10.5 ± 1.5[b]	10.9 ± 3.6	3.9 ± 1.9
PAICP	0.52 ± 0.09	0.34 ± 0.03	0.50 ± 0.05	0.39 ± 0.08	0.32 ± 0.04	0.29 ± 0.03	0.26 ± 0.04	0.22 ± 0.06	0.24 ± 0.11
PR ratio	1.64 ± 0.13	1.89 ± 0.24	1.76 ± 0.15	1.42 ± 0.23	1.73 ± 0.24	3.13 ± 0.89	2.16 ± 0.26	2.97 ± 0.70	1.91 ± 0.36
slope	0.47 ± 0.04	0.86 ± 0.08[a]	0.49 ± 0.05	0.50 ± 0.12	0.65 ± 0.12	0.63 ± 0.11	0.68 ± 0.11	0.65 ± 0.27	0.31 ± 0.10

	ICP parameters derived from the Fourier transform			ICP parameters derived from the Fourier transform					
FW	1.06 ± 0.01	2.51 ± 0.33[a]	1.11 ± 0.11	1.47 ± 0.32	2.00 ± 0.28	3.07 ± 0.43[b]	2.94 ± 0.53	2.94 ± 0.95	1.11 ± 0.38
HW2	0.47 ± 0.04	0.93 ± 0.16[a]	0.50 ± 0.04	0.52 ± 0.11	0.68 ± 0.10	0.99 ± 0.10[b]	0.91 ± 0.15	1.26 ± 0.54	0.50 ± 0.21
HW3	0.32 ± 0.03	0.44 ± 0.06[a]	0.33 ± 0.03	0.31 ± 0.07	0.37 ± 0.07	0.54 ± 0.13	0.49 ± 0.10	0.37 ± 0.13	0.28 ± 0.09
HW4	0.23 ± 0.03	0.39 ± 0.05[a]	0.23 ± 0.03	0.21 ± 0.06	0.18 ± 0.02	0.26 ± 0.06	0.27 ± 0.06	0.23 ± 0.11	0.32 ± 0.17
HW5	0.20 ± 0.02	0.33 ± 0.04[a]	0.18 ± 0.02	0.21 ± 0.07	0.19 ± 0.04	0.19 ± 0.03	0.16 ± 0.03	0.23 ± 0.10	0.09 ± 0.03
%FW	46.4 ± 1.5	53.8 ± 1.8[a]	46.6 ± 1.6	53.6 ± 4.9	58.3 ± 2.5	60.3 ± 4.0	61.5 ± 2.8	59.5 ± 3.3	46.3 ± 4.5
%HW2	21.0 ± 1.0	19.9 ± 0.9	22.2 ± 1.0	19.6 ± 1.5	19.5 ± 1.5	19.9 ± 1.3	19.1 ± 1.4	24.8 ± 2.7	22.0 ± 2.4
%HW3	14.5 ± 0.8	9.8 ± 0.5[a]	14.2 ± 0.6	12.5 ± 2.6	11.3 ± 1.4	10.7 ± 2.2	10.2 ± 1.8	7.9 ± 0.8	13.5 ± 1.6
%HW4	9.5 ± 0.6	8.3 ± 0.7	9.2 ± 0.6	7.3 ± 1.5	5.6 ± 0.6	5.2 ± 1.0	5.8 ± 1.0	3.9 ± 0.7	13.9 ± 6.8
%HW5	8.6 ± 0.7	8.1 ± 1.1	7.9 ± 0.7	7.0 ± 1.7	5.3 ± 0.5	3.8 ± 0.5	3.4 ± 0.3	4.0 ± 0.4	4.3 ± 0.6
HFC	7.71 ± 0.12	7.95 ± 0.13[a]	7.70 ± 0.10	8.28 ± 0.19	7.74 ± 0.21	7.39 ± 0.18[b]	7.38 ± 0.19[b]	7.69 ± 0.29	7.38 ± 0.14[b]
k ratio	0.72 ± 0.04	0.55 ± 0.04[a]	0.73 ± 0.06	0.59 ± 0.11	0.46 ± 0.05	0.48 ± 0.07	0.51 ± 0.12	0.54 ± 0.08	0.68 ± 0.05

[a] different from pre-plateau wave
[b] different from ICP <20
different from ICP >30, no clinical changes

At the time that CBF began to drop, the ICP was even higher and blood pressure was lower, resulting in a CPP of approximately 25 mmHg. The $SjvO_2$ decreased to 42 ± 4%, reflecting the CBF decrease in response to the low CPP.

As neurological deficits due to the refractory intracranial hypertension developed and as the $SjvO_2$ indicated a drop in CBF, there were no significant changes in the ICP waveform compared to the previous time period. When cerebral perfusion dropped to very low values, there were significant changes in the ICP waveform descriptors. The PA decreased, the amplitude of FW and the percent of the total power contained in the FW decreased, and the slope markedly decreased.

Discussion

The differences in the physiological parameters (especially the $SjvO_2$ response) between the 2 types of ICP increases support the hypothesis that the increase in intracranial pressure has different underlying pathophysiologies. During a plateau wave the increase in ICP is caused by primary vasodilation of cerebral vessels, while as refractory intracranial pressure develops due to worsening cerebral edema or to a mass lesion, the vasodilation of cerebral vessels is a compensatory mechanism attempting to maintain cerebral blood flow in the face of a decreasing CPP.

The lack of more clear-cut differences in the ICP waveform descriptors as the ICP increases illustrates the lack of specificity in the present generation of indices. The changes are relatively similar regardless of the cause of the ICP increase, perhaps indicating that vasodilation has occurred, but not suggesting the cause.

References

1. Avezaat CJJ, Van Eijndhoven JHM, Wyper DJ (1979) Cerebrospinal fluid pressure and intracranial volume-pressure relationships. J Neurol Neurosurg Psych 42:687–700
2. Bray RS, Sherwood AM, Halter JA, et al. (1986) Development of a clinical monitoring system by means of ICP waveform analysis. In: Miller JD, Teasdale GM, Rowan JO, Galbraith SL, Mendelow AP (eds) Intracranial Pressure VI, Springer, Berlin Heidelberg New York Tokyo, pp 260–264
3. Chopp M, Portnoy HD (1980) Systems analysis of intracranial pressure. Comparison with volume-pressure test and CSF-pulse amplitude analysis. J Neurosurg 53:516–527
4. Dearden NM, Miller JD (1989) Paired comparison of hypnotic and osmotic therapy in the reduction of intracranial hypertension after severe head injury. In: Hoff JT, Betz AL (eds) Intracranial Pressure VII. Springer, Berlin Heidelberg New York Tokyo, pp 474–481
5. Hirai O, Handa H, Ishikawa M, et al. (1984) Epidural pulse waveform as an indicator of intracranial pressure dynamics. Surg Neurol 21:67–74
6. Robertson CS, Narayan RK, Contant CF, et al. (1989) Clinical experience with a monitor of intracranial compliance. J Neurosurg 71:673–680
7. Szewczykowski J, Sliwka S, Kunicki A, et al. (1977) A fast method of estimating the elastance of the intracranial system. A practical application in neurosurgery. J Neurosurg 47:19–26

8. Takizawa H, Gabra-Sanders T, Miller JD (1987) Changes in the cerebrospinal fluid pulse wave spectrum associated with raised intracranial pressure. Neurosurgery 20:355–361
9. Wilkinson HA, Schuman N, Rugiero J (1979) Nonvolumetric methods of detecting impaired intracranial compliance or reactivity. J Neurosurg 50:758–767

Effects of Heart Rate on the Shape of the Intracranial Pressure Wave and Related Parameters

C.F. Contant, Jr., C.S. Robertson, R.K. Narayan, C. Hayes, and R.G. Grossman

Department of Neurosurgery, Baylor College of Medicine, Houston, TX, USA

Introduction

Changes in the shape of the intracranial pulse wave have been used to estimate cerebral compliance [2] and have been related to outcome after head injury [6]. The changes in the complex shape of the intracranial pulse wave that occur with changes in ICP have been analyzed by decomposing the pulse wave into its component frequencies using the Fast Fourier Transform (FFT) [3, 6], as well as by using simpler measures such as pulse amplitude and slope [1]. We have observed that changes in heart rate have a powerful effect on the shape of the intracranial pulse wave, and have studied these changes using an on-line computerized monitoring system which is described elsewhere in this volume [4].

Methods

Recording of ICP and Variables Examined

A ventriculostomy and pressure transducer or a fibre-optic catheter within a ventriculostomy was used to record the ICP and intracranial pulse wave. The amplitude spectrum and periodogram were obtained using the FFT. The High Frequency Centroid (HFC), which has been shown to be related to outcome [6], was defined as the amplitude weighted-average frequency between the frequencies 4 and 15 Hertz (Hz), and is written as:

$$\mathrm{HFC} = \frac{\sum\limits_{\mathrm{freq}=4}^{\mathrm{freq}=15} \mathrm{frequency} \times \mathrm{amplitude}}{\sum\limits_{\mathrm{freq}=4}^{\mathrm{freq}=15} \mathrm{amplitude}}.$$

The HFC was used to examine the response of the brain to the higher frequencies in the ICP wave. Two types of changes in HFC can be caused by changes in the heart rate. As the heart rate increases, its fundamental frequency and the frequencies of the harmonics increase. These are transmitted to the ICP wave. The position of the harmonics in the 4–15 Hz window increases, and the HFC increases. With increasing heart rate some of the higher harmonics exit the upper portion of the window, and some of the lower harmonics enter the lower portion. Therefore, the relationship of heart rate to the HFC becomes non-linear. A major change occurs as the second harmonic enters the window at 120 beats per minute. This type of change is a mathematical artifact induced by the form of the HFC, and other indices using fixed frequency windows are subject to the same artifact. A second type of change, however, reflects actual changes in the shape of the wave. As the heart rate changes, the amplitudes of the fundamental and harmonic waves may not remain constant. Changes in the harmonics which occur with changes in heart rate will have an effect on the HFC. Figure 1 displays the behavior of the HFC as the heart rate increases, assuming no change in the amplitudes of the harmonics.

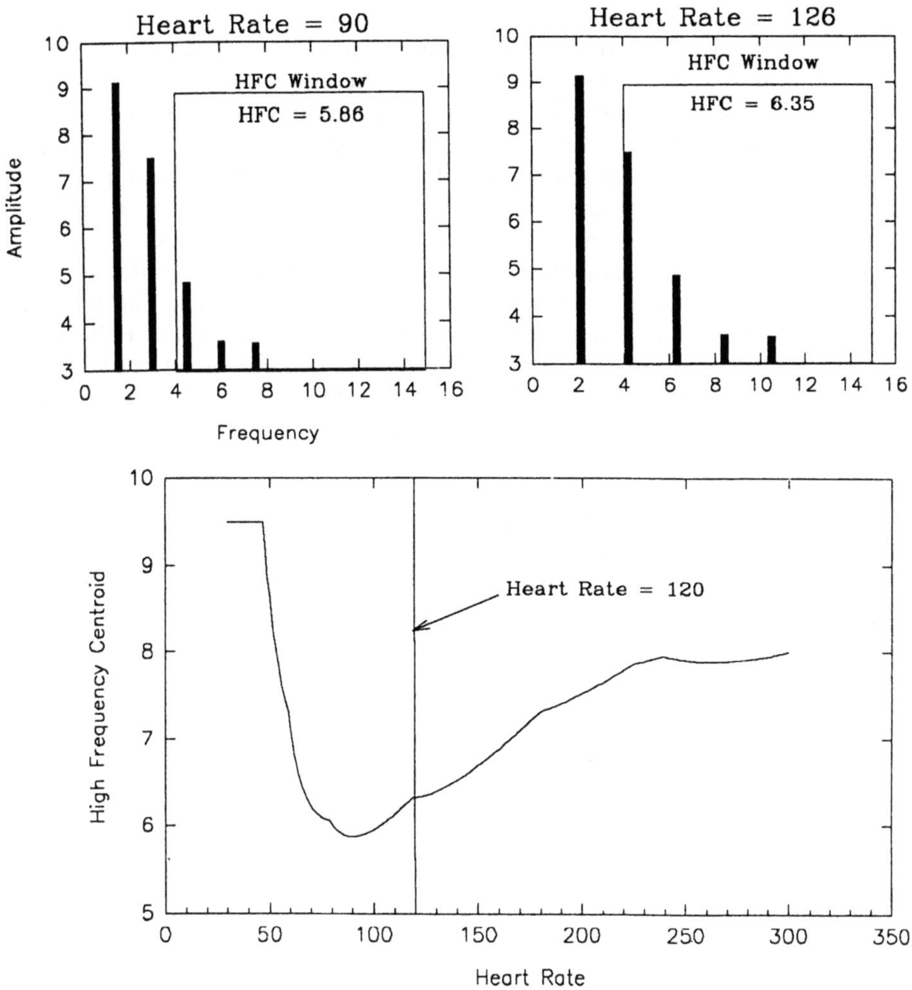

Fig. 1. a Relationship of HFC to heart rate. Position of harmonics as heart rate changes. **b** High frequency centroid as a function of heart rate derived using above harmonics

The amplitudes of the fundamental wave (FW) and the second through fifth harmonics (HW2, HW3, HW4, HW5) were obtained from the FFT. The total variation in the five harmonics, as defined by the sum of the periodogram at each harmonic, was calculated. The percent that each harmonic contributes to this total was calculated by dividing the contribution of each harmonic by the total. The percent of the variation that is found in the 9–16 Hz window is calculated by dividing that portion of the periodogram by the total percent below 20 Hz.

The K-ratio [8] is an index of deviation from a pure sinusodial wave, and is calculated as

$$\text{K Ratio} = \frac{\sqrt{HW2^2 + HW3^2 + HW4^2 + HW5^2}}{FW}$$

This index increases as the amplitudes in the harmonics increase relative to the amplitude of the fundamental wave.

Directly measured indices of the wave shape were obtained as well. The pulse amplitude is the difference of the systolic and diastolic pressures of the ICP wave. The pulse amplitude-respiratory ratio is the pulse amplitude divided by the variation in the diastolic ICP as it changes with respiration. The pulse amplitude/ICP ratio is the pulse amplitude divided by the mean ICP of the wave. Slope is defined as the maximum rate of change of the upgoing part of the ICP wave, and is measured in units of change in pressure per time.

The heart rate was calculated by identifying the number of QRS complexes in the EKG and dividing by the length of time of the sample. The mean ICP was calculated from the same waves that were analyzed for the FFT indices. The mean arterial pressure was obtained from a catheter in the radial artery. Perfusion pressure was calculated by subtracting the ICP from the mean arterial pressure. The end-tidal carbon dioxide concentration ($ETCO_2$) was acquired from a Novametrix capnograph.

Additional physiologic measurements not collected by the computer system were made at the time of cerebral blood flow determinations. The partial pressure of carbon dioxide (PCO_2) was measured with a Corning blood gas analyzer, and the pressure volume index (PVI) was measured by withdrawal of a small amount of CSF and measuring the change in pressure associated with the change in volume, from which the index is calculated [7]. Cerebral blood flow (CBF) was measured using the Kety-Schmidt nitrous oxide method. Cerebral vascular resistance was calculated from the CBF and perfusion pressure. The pulse volume was determined by dividing the CBF by the heart rate, and is an estimate of the average cerebral pulse volume during the course of the measurement of CBF.

Statistical Methods

Relationships between heart rate and the indices of ICP wave shape and other variables on heart rate were examined with the restricted maximum likelihood method [5]. This technique allows for a regression to be performed that fits a separate regression line to each individual, and then forms a weighted average of these regressions. It also adjusts the estimates of the variance to account for multiple observations from the same patient. The model fit for these analyses allowed person-specific differences in the intercept, but forced a common slope. This model is expressed as y = *intercept* + *coefficient* × *heart rate* (*in beats per minute*) + *individual offset*. Significance tests were performed using linear contrasts.

Selection of Patients

Patients were selected for this study on the basis of the availability of data from the thirty minutes preceding or surrounding a cerebral blood flow determination. These data were averaged for each blood flow determination. If the data during that time period were extremely variable or were truncated, the time period following the cerebral blood flow determination was used.

Results

Patient Population

Fifty-six patients were studied. There were 48 men (86%) and 8 (14%) women. The average age was 32.9 years with a range of 16–75 years. The median age was 28, and 24 (44%) of the patients were between 20 and 30. The distribution of injury types was as follows: 22 (39%) subdural hematomas; 10 (18%) epidural hematomas; 8 (14%) contusions; 7 (13%) other injuries, including one subarachnoid hemorrhage; 5 (9%) gun shot wounds; and 4 (7%) intracerebral hematomas. The Glasgow Coma Scale (GCS) score immediately following resuscitation ranged from 3 to 13. Ten (18%) patients scored in the 3–4 range, 8 (14%) scored 5–6, 30 (54%) scored 7–8 category and 8 (14%) scored greater than 8. All patients had a GCS score less than 8 at the initiation of the computer monitoring.

Four hundred and nineteen time periods each approximately 30 minutes long were chosen for analysis. The minimum number of periods was one (4 patients) and the maximum was 31 (1 patient). The majority (57%) of the patients had between 6 and 15 time periods analyzed. The earliest observation was obtained 4 hours after injury, and the latest occurred 302 hours after injury, with the median occurring at 57 hours after injury. The average heart rate was 96 beats per minute.

Regressions

The regression analyses are shown in Table 1. The amplitude of the fundamental frequency decreased significantly with increasing heart rate. The pulse amplitude, pulse amplitude-respiratory ratio and PA/ICP all were negatively related to increased heart rate. The pulse volume demonstrated a strong

Table 1. Results of regressions of indices of ICP wave shape on heart rate using the restricted maximum likelihood method

Variable	Intercept	Coefficient for Heart Rate (beats per minute)	Chi-square
Fundamental Frequency	3.0231	−0.01802	37.84***
Second Harmonic	0.4929	0.00046	0.26
Third Harmonic	0.3762	−0.00075	1.59
Fourth Harmonic	0.2613	−0.00056	1.14
Fifth Harmonic	0.2546	−0.00070	1.71
Percent Fundamental Frequency	68.873	−0.21222	49.31***
Percent Second Harmonic	7.1510	0.15868	79.22***
Percent Third Harmonic	9.8190	0.03631	5.03*
Percent Fourth Harmonic	6.578	0.01658	1.96
Percent Fifth Harmonic	7.6758	−0.00125	0.01
Total Variation	4.4129	−0.01964	24.29***
K-ratio	0.0816	0.00633	45.94***
HFC	8.1649	−0.00272	2.33
Percent of variation in 9–16 Hz	−0.10633	0.01332	25.10***
Pulse Amplitude	7.9446	−0.02602	12.42***
PA/ICP Ratio	0.5619	−0.00203	4.68*
Pulse amplitude-respiratory ratio	3.8025	−0.02200	55.91***
Slope	0.3902	0.00070	0.86
ICP	14.720	0.03390	2.51
Mean Arterial Pressure	97.334	−0.01171	0.06
Cerebral Perfusion Pressure	75.751	−0.02857	0.16
End Tidal CO_2	30.980	−0.02131	0.85
Jugular venous oxygen saturation	68.272	0.02240	0.34
Pulse Volume	1.1680	−0.00696	91.98***
Cerebral blood flow	0.5988	−0.00153	5.26*
Cerebral vascular resistance	1.6502	0.00297	0.79
Pressure Volume Index	23.823	−0.03546	1.00
PCO_2	34.927	−0.04215	7.0**

decrease with increased heart rate. The percent variation of the fundamental frequency and the total variation in the harmonics both decreased significantly with heart rate. The percent of the variation in the second and third harmonics were both significantly higher at higher heart rates. The percent of the variation in the 9–16 Hz window decreased significantly. The K-ratio increased with heart rate. The amplitudes of the remaining harmonics were not significantly related to heart rate, though the third, fourth and fifth harmonics all decreased with increasing heart rate. Of the physiological measurements, the partial pressure of carbon dioxide decreased with increased heart rate, as did the cerebral blood flow. None of the other indices or physiologic measurements were found to be significantly related to heart rate.

To explore the relationship of the HFC to heart rate further, the measurements in which the heart rate averaged between 111 and 130 were selected from the overall data set and divided into two groups, those between 111 and 120, and those between 121 and 130. The mean HFC in the 111–120 group was compared to the mean in the 121–130 group, using the restricted maximum likelihood method. The mean HFC in the 111–120 group was found to be 7.89, and the mean in the 121–130 group was 7.65. This difference was significant at $p < 0.05$, and is consistent with the change in HFC produced by movement of the second harmonic into the HFC window.

Discussion

The relationships detected are consonant with the effects of an increasing heart rate producing a decreasing pulse volume and the expected effect of a decreasing pulse volume on the ICP wave shape. The decreases in pulse amplitude, amplitude of the fundamental frequency, and total variation observed as heart rate increased suggested a reduced pulse volume. However, the analysis of the percent variation in the harmonics indicated that this decrease occurred primarily in the fundamental frequency's contribution, while the percent contribution of the second and third harmonics increased. As a result, the K ratio increased. Because PA/ICP ratio and the pulse amplitude-respiratory ratio are directly proportional to the pulse amplitude, they decrease with increasing heart rate.

The HFC was not found to be significantly related to heart rate, which was a somewhat surprising result. However, the increase in the HFC that is mathematically induced with increased heart rate appears to be offset by the decreases in the amplitudes of the harmonics that are in the 4–15 Hz window. Therefore, the HFC will decrease. The major artifact induced by changing heart rate would then occur at rather specific times, such as when the heart rate crossed the 120 beats-per-minute boundary. The relationship is extremely complex, and use of the HFC should proceed with caution.

These results justify the following conclusions. Heart rate has a significant effect on the indices of the ICP wave shape, and is likely to be operating as a surrogate measure for pulse volume. In those cases where a fixed frequency window is used, as in the HFC, the relationship is complex, as the heart rate has a direct mathematical relationship to the index. Interpretation of changes in all of the indices of ICP wave shape without consideration of pulse volume or heart rate may be misleading. The ability to measure pulse volume or cerebral blood flow continuously would greatly improve our understanding of the mechanisms responsible for the changes observed in ICP wave shape with increasing intracranial pressure.

References

1. Avezaat CJJ, Van Eijndhoven JHM, Wyper DJ (1979) Cerebrospinal fluid pulse pressure and intracranial volume-pressure relationships. J Neurol Neurosurg Psych 42:687–700
2. Bray RS, Sherwood AM, Halter JA, Robertson CS, Grossman RG (1976) Development of a clinical monitoring system by means of ICP waveform analysis. In: Miller JD, Teasdale GM, Rowan JO, Galbraith SL, Mendelow AD (eds) Intracranial Pressure VI. Springer, Berlin Heidelberg New York Tokyo, pp 260–264

3. Chopp M, Portnoy HD (1980) Systems analysis of intracranial pressure. Comparison with volume-pressure test and CSF-pulse amplitude analysis. J Neurosurg 53:516–527
4. Crouch JD, Contant CF, Robertson CS (1993) On-line acquisition and analysis of ICP and physiologic data in the neurosurgical intensive care unit. In: Avezaat CJJ, Van Eijndhoven JHM, Maas AIR, Tans JThJ (eds) Intracranial Pressure VIII. Springer, Berlin Heidelberg New York London Paris Tokyo, Hong Kong Barcelona
5. Laird NM, Ware JH (1982) Random effects models for longitudinal data. Biometrics 38:963–974
6. Robertson CS, Narayan RK, Contant CF, Grossman RG, Gokaslan ZL, Pahwa R, Caram P, Bray RS, Sherwood AS (1989) Clinical experience with a continuous monitor of intracranial compliance. J Neurosurgery 71:673–680
7. Shapiro ER, Marmarou A, Shulman K (1980) Characterization of clinical CSF dynamics and neural axis compliance using the pressure-volume index. Ann Neurol 7:508–514
8. Takizawa H, Gabra-Sanders T, Miller JD (1987) Changes in the cerebrospinal fluid pulse wave spectrum associated with raised intracranial pressure. Neurosurgery 20:355–361

Vascular Mapping of the Intracranial Pulse Wave

E.R. Cardoso, E. Bruni, A.M. Kaufmann, and G.Y. Lohmann, Jr.

Cerebral Hydrodynamics Laboratory and Departments of Surgery and Anatomy, University of Manitoba, Winnipeg, Manitoba, Canada

Introduction

The pulsations originated within the cerebral arteries, microcirculation, and veins influence the configuration of the intracranial pulse wave (ICPW) [2, 3, 5, 6]. Continuous analysis of the ICPW configuration might allow the establishment of correlations are between ICPW components and specific portions of the intracranial vasculature [4].

We investigated the effects of selective cerebral arterial and venous vasodilation on the configuration of the ICPW.

Materials and Methods

Experiments were performed in anesthetized and ventilated cats, maintained under physiological conditions. Anesthesia was induced by intraperitoneal injection of 30 mg/kg body weight of sodium barbital (Nembutal)[1] and maintained by continuous intravenous infusion of approximately 25 mg of sodium barbital per hour. The animals were also paralysed by intravenous injection of 10 mg/kg body weight per hour of gallamine (Flaxedil)[2] and artificially ventilated (Harvard animal respirator). Arterial blood gases were monitored throughout the experiment. Rectal temperature was continuously monitored[3].

Mean pressures and digitized pulse wave measurements of pulse pressure amplitude were obtained from the aorta (SAP), inferior vena cava (CVP), and third cerebral ventricle (ICP). A ratio between the ascending and the total pulse wave duration (ascending time over total time, at/tt) was devised to represent numerically the location of the wave peak on time domain. The at/tt ratios were calculated for the ICPW, SAPW, and CVPW.

Mean and standard errors for all data groups were compared before and after banding by means of two-tailed Student t-test. Regression analysis was used to compare ICPW to SAPW and CVPW changes.

---

[1] Abbott Laboratories LTD, Montreal, Quebec, Canada
[2] Poulene LTD, Montreal, Quebec, Canada
[3] Tec-thermometer, Yellow Springs, OH, USA

Table 1.

	Baseline	Post-banding
	mmHg	mmHg
SAPW	37.48 ± 1.74	35.45 ± 2.5
CVPW	1.4 ± 0.4	4.6 ± 0.75*
ICPW	0.77 ± 0.1	1.6 ± 0.2*
ICPW ratio	0.47 ± 0.03	0.67 ± 0.02*

* $P < 0.001$

First Experiment

In a first experiment 6 animals underwent 25 trials of intermittent pulmonary artery banding, in order to produce cerebral venous hypertension. Values of mean pressure and pulse wave before and during banding were compared.

Second Experiment

In a second experiment 14 cats underwent double-blinded cisternal injections of 1 ml of either placebo or 0.2 mg of Nimodipine[4] under conditions of stable cranioaxial compliance.

Results

First Experiment

Pulmonary banding raised the mean CVP and mean ICP by 3.0 and 1.55 mmHg respectively, and dropped the mean SAP by 27.5 mmHg. These mean pressure changes were accompanied by alterations of amplitude and configuration of the CVPW and ICPW, while the SAPW remained unchanged. Right atrial contractions during pulmonary banding raised the amplitude of the CVPW by 228% and the ICPW amplitude by 117% simultaneously. The SAPW amplitude did not change significantly. There was simultaneous displacement of the wave apex towards the end of wave for the CVPW and ICPW, as the at/tt ratio significantly increased by 0.16 and 0.2 respectively. The configuration of the SAPW remained unchanged, as there was no significant change of the at/tt ratio (Table 1).

[4] BAY E 9736, 10 mg/50 ml, kindly donated by Miles Inc., Pharmaceutical Division, West Haven, CT 06516, USA

Second Experiment

Cisternal Nimodipine produced no changes of mean ICP and CVP, but lowered the mean SAP. Placebo injections did not alter mean pressure values. Nimodipine, but not placebo, produced significant increase of the ICPW amplitude, while CVPW and SAPW remained unchanged. Nimodipine-induced cerebral vasodilatation was responsible for the increases of ICPW amplitude, as they were accompanied by significant increases of cerebral blood volume and cerebral blood flow, of 9.3% and 17.6% respectively ($p < 0.012$ and < 0.025). The ascending ratio of the ICPW decreased significantly from 0.45 ± 0.05 to 0.36 ± 0.04 ($p < 0.0005$) (Table 2).

Discussion

The configuration and amplitude of the ICPW can be altered by the state of craniospinal compliance [1, 7]. Thus, in order to isolate the effects of vascular diameter and eliminate the effects of compliance, measurements of the ICPW should always be taken at the same level of craniospinal compliance [3–5]. Under these conditions, one can search for simultaneous alterations of specific portions of the cerebral vasculature on one hand, and amplitude and configuration of the ICPW on the other.

The findings related to the pulmonary banding experiment indicate that venous pulsations contribute mainly to the late phase of the ICPW, thus suggesting that analysis of the ICPW configuration could be used to monitor cerebral venous hypertension. The findings related to the second experiment showed that cerebral vasodilation raises the amplitude of the ICPW independently of alterations of the venous and arterial pulse waves. Furthermore, cerebral vasodilation produces amplitude increase of the ICPW and shortening of the at/tt ratio, differently from venous hypertension. Our laboratory had previously demonstrated that cerebral vasospasm produces the opposite effect on the ICPW amplitude [2, 3].

Table 2.

	Baseline 1	Placebo	Baseline 2	Nimodipine
	mmHg	mmHg	mmHg	mmHg
SAPW	31.3 ± 3	29.7 ± 3	30.1 ± 3	39.16 ± 3[a]
CVPW	0.32 ± 0.1	0.31 ± 0.1	0.49 ± 0.1	0.54 ± 0.1
ICPW	0.42 ± 0.1	0.5 ± 0.1	0.44 ± 0.1	0.99 ± 0.2[a]
ICPW ratio	0.41	0.35	0.45	0.36[a]
	ml/100 g/min	ml/100 g/m	ml/100 g/min	ml/100 g/min
CBF	35 ± 5.6	32.5 ± 5.3	34.8 ± 6.2	40.7 ± 5.6[a]
	ml/100 g	ml/100 g	ml/100 g	ml/100 g
CBV	0.46	0.44	0.43	0.47[a]

[a] statistical significance

The findings of both experiments indicate that time-domain measurements of the ICPW taken under the same conditions of cerebrospinal compliance can be used to identify changes of specific segments of the cerebral circulation. Our findings also demonstrate that the ICPW configuration on time domain can be mathematically expressed by the at/tt ratio, which describes the position of the wave highest point in relation to its entire duration. Furthermore, the at/tt ratio differentiates numerically amplitude increases of the ICPW caused by cerebral vasodilation from those caused by venous congestion. A ratio greater than 0.5 suggests venous hypertension, while lower ratios associated with cerebral vasodilation. Therefore, our results indicate a somatotopical correspondence between segments of the cerebral vasculature and portions of the ICPW.

Acknowledgements. Project supported by grant from the Canadian Heart and Stroke Foundation. The authors wish to thank Miles Inc. Pharmaceutical for the donation of injectable Nimodipine.

References

1. Avezaat CJJ, Van Eijndhoven JHM (1986) Clinical observations on relationship between cerebrospinal fluid pulse pressure and intracranial pressure. Acta Neurochir 79:13–29
2. Cardoso ER, Reddy K, Bose D (1988) Effect of subarachnoid hemorrhage on intracranial pulse wave. J Neurosurg 69:712–718
3. Cardoso ER, Reddy K, Bose D (1988) Diagnosis of cerebral vasospasm by measurement of the amplitude of the intracranial pulse wave. In Cerebral Vasospasm, RH Wilkins (ed), Raven Press, New York, pp 53–56
4. Cardoso ER, Rowan J, Galbraith S (1983) Analysis of the cerebrospinal fluid pulse wave in intracranial pressure. J Neurosurg 59:817–821
5. Hamer J, Alberti E, Hoyer S, et al. (1977) Influence of systemic and cerebral vascular factors on the cerebrospinal fluid pulse waves. J Neurosurgery 46:36–45
6. Portnoy HD, Chopp M, Branch C, et al. (1982) Cerebrospinal fluid pulse wave form as an indicator of cerebral autoregulation. J Neurosurgery 56:666–678
7. Shigemori M, Tokjutomi T, Kawaba T, Nakashima H, Kuramoto S (1986) Analysis of epidural pressure pulse wave (EDP-PW) and common carotid blood velocity (CBFV) in acute intracranial hypertension. Neurol Res 8:105–109

Changes of Intracranial Pressure and Pulse Wave Form Induced by Various Mechanical Stresses Upon Intracranial Hemodynamics

M. Hashimoto, S. Higashi, K. Tokuda, Y. Yamamoto, and J. Yamashita

Department of Neurosurgery, Kanazawa University, School of Medicine, Kanazawa, Takaramachi 13-1, Kanazawa City 920, Japan

Introduction

The Pulse Wave Form (PWF) of intracranial pressure (ICP) has three fairly consistent components [2, 8, 9]. It has been suggested that its shape depends upon the arterial input, the intracranial contents, and the venous outflow [1, 2, 8]. These intracranial hemodynamics may be modified by vascular reactivity and intracranial compliance [1, 8, 9]. The effect of mechanical stress to intracranial hemodynamics on ICP and PWF was studied to clarify the origin of PWF and its clinical significance.

Materials and Methods

Twenty patients, 14 with subarachnoid hemorrhage, 1 with cerebral infarction, 3 with brain tumor and 2 with aqueductal stenosis underwent ICP monitoring. ICP was recorded with an indwelling ventricular catheter connected to a pressure transducer (P50, Nihon Kohden). Systemic blood pressure (SBP), cerebral perfusion pressure (CPP), and respiration (impedance pneumography) were monitored simultaneously. The patients were subjected to four manoeuvres to change the intracranial hemodynamics:

- bilateral jugular compression for 30 to 60 seconds,
- voluntary hyperventilation for 60 seconds,
- head elevation (30°), and
- Valsalva test (sustained inspiration for 10 seconds).

PWF has three peak components, named P1, P2 and P3 in one cardiac cycle. The change rate of each peak amplitude to mechanical stress was statistically analyzed.

Results

The mean base-line ICP in the 20 patients was 14.2 ± 7.6 mmHg. The mean amplitudes of P1, P2 and P3 were 3.9 ± 1.8 mmHg, 4.53 ± 2.3 mmHg, and

3.3 ± 1.8 mmHg, respectively. The magnitude of the P2 amplitude was significantly higher than that of P1 and P3 amplitude.

Jugular compression (Table 1, Fig. 1A) caused an ICP elevation with a more significant increase of P2 and P3 than P1 amplitude. After release of the manoeuvre, ICP fell rapidly to base-line level and in this phase, P3 amplitude decreased more rapidly than P1 and P2.

Head elevation (Table 1, Fig. 1B) caused a significant decrease of ICP and CPP, and a significant increase of P3 amplitude. Two patients showed a paradoxical rise of ICP similar to plateau waves in head elevation.

Hyperventilation (Table 1, Fig. 2A) caused a significant ICP reduction and a significant reduction of P2 and P3 amplitudes. There were no significant changes of CPP. During the Valsalva test (Table 1, Fig. 2B) sustained inspiration decreased SBP and CPP, and reduced each PWF amplitude progressively from P3 to P1. In the later phase of this manoeuvre, a reactive increase of SBP and CPP were observed with a marked increase of each PWF amplitude. After release of the stress, these phenomena were enhanced with ICP reduction.

Table 1. Changes of intracranial pressure and pulse wave form induced by challenging intracranial hemodynamics. n: sampling number of manoeuvres, d-ICP: the difference of ICP before and after the stress, Px change: the change rate is calculated as (post stress-Px/control-Px; x = 1, 2 and 3). The difference between P1, P2 and P3 was analysed statistically. Statistical significancy is indicated by * at the $p < 0.01$ level and (*) at the $p < 0.05$ level. The given values are means ± standard deviations.

Clinical analysis of ICP pulse wave form changes in intracranial hemodynamic mechanical stress

	Jugular compression	Head elevation	Hyperventilation	Valsalva test
n	29	13	13	13
d-ICP (mmHg) (mean ± SD)	9.086 ± 4.97	-5.038 ± 2.82	-4.770 ± 3.50	2.576 ± 9.32
ICP-amp	P2>P3>P1	P2>P3>P1	P1>>P2>P3	P1>>P2>P3

ICP pulse wave form

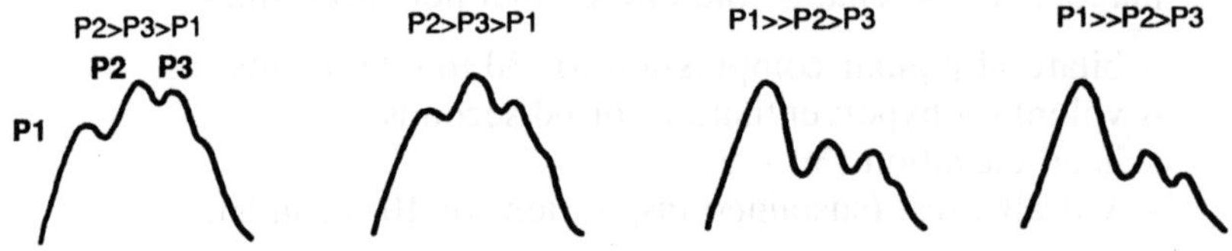

	Jugular compression	Head elevation	Hyperventilation	Valsalva test
Px change (mean ± SD)	P3≥P2 * >P1	P3>P2>P1	P1* > P2=P3	P1* >P2(*) ≥P3
P1/c-P1	1.205 ± 0.24	1.056 ± 0.12	0.842 ± 0.18	1.029 ± 0.17
P2/c-P2	1.521 ± 0.49	1.102 ± 0.19	0.596 ± 0.22	0.526 ± 0.15
P3/c-P3	1.621 ± 0.53	1.323 ± 0.60	0.596 ± 0.15	0.375 ± 0.27
SBP	→	→	→	SAP-amp ↓
CPP	⇓	⇓	→	–
cerebral bulk	⇑	⇑ reactive vasodilatation	⇓ vasoconstriction	⇓ vasoconstriction
Venous out-flow	disturb	~	~	disturb

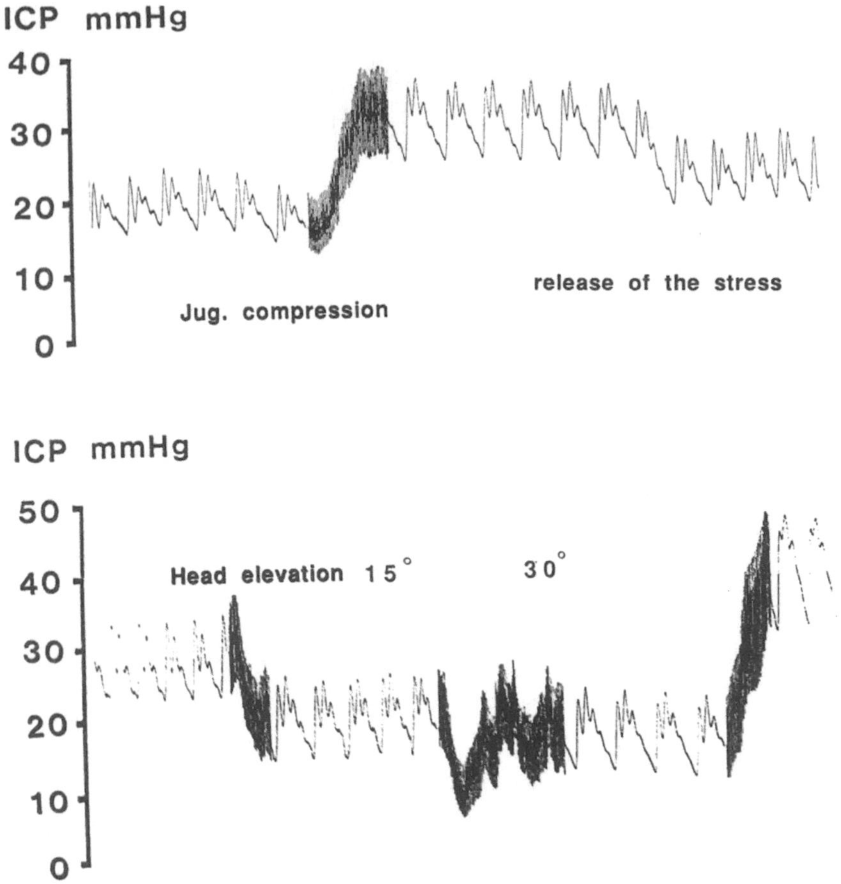

Fig. 1. A The changes of intracranial pulse wave form (PWF) during bilateral jugular compression. Jugular compression causes ICP increase with significant increase of P2 and P3 amplitudes. **B** PWF recordings obtained during head elevation from 0° to 30°. Head elevation causes a mild decrease of ICP, and a significant increase of P3 amplitude. A paradoxical rise of ICP similar to a plateau wave is observed

Discussion

In jugular compression and head elevation, ICP increased significantly as well as the amplitudes of the three PWF peaks. This indicates a decrease of cerebral compliance. In jugular compression it has been shown that venous stasis, and increase of cerebral bulk decreases the compliance [5]. In our study it was observed that the P3 amplitude decreased more rapidly than the other pulse wave amplitudes after release of jugular compression.

In head elevation it has been shown that the decrease of CPP provokes reactive vasodilation and pressure waves [4, 10]. Previous studies by us showed phase differences between P1, P2 and P3 amplitudes during the respiratory cycle [8]. Our data suggest that the generator of the oscillation in P3 amplitude

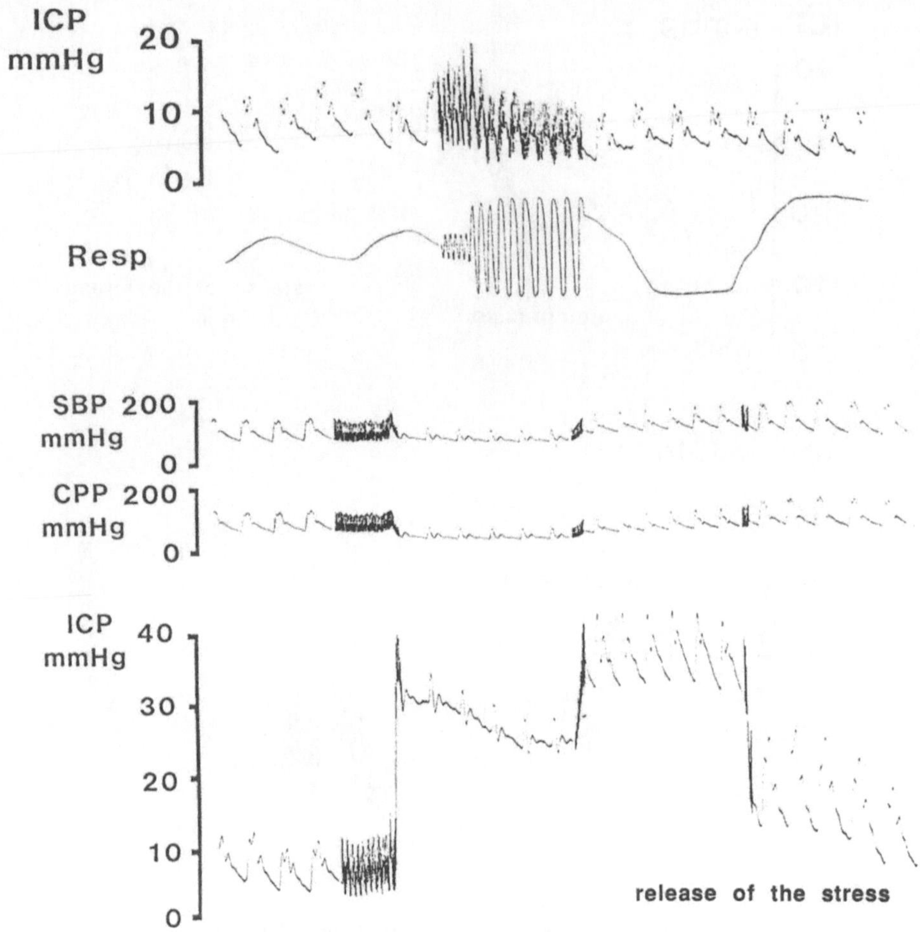

Fig. 2. A The changes of PWF during hyperventilation. Significant reduction of P2 and P3 amplitudes is observed. **B** PWF recording during Valsalva test. Each amplitude is reduced under forced inspiration. The amplitudes increase significantly after release of the stress

is different from that of P1 and P2. It has been suggested that the respiratory cycle of P3 amplitude results from the transmission of venous pressure changes from intrathoracic pressure variations with breathing [3, 7, 8]. From the data of our study it may also be supposed that P2 and P3 components reflect the cerebral blood volume, and P3 is affected directly by the venous system and intrathoracic pressure in these two manoeuvres.

In the hyperventilation study, the change rate of P2 and P3 amplitudes decreased more significantly than that of P1. Since it is known that hyperventilation reduces ICP by vasoconstriction of arterioles, the P2 component may be dependent upon the cerebral compliance [2, 6]. The decrease of P3 amplitude shows that venous circulation may be preserved in this manoeuvre. P1 amplitude may reflect the large intracranial conductive vessels and the vasoconstriction of arterioles.

In the Valsalva manoeuvre, the increased intrathoracic pressure prevented the venous return to the heart and consequently provoked a drop of the cardiac output and arterial hypotension [3]. As a reaction to this arterial hypotension, a tachycardia and a reflex peripheral vasoconstriction occurred. After the release of this stress, reactive vasodilation is initiated by a depressor response due to arterial hypertension [3]. In our study, the amplitude data were sampled in the phase of arterial hypotension, causing peripheral vasoconstriction. Decrease of P2 and P3 amplitude may reflect the relative decrease of cerebral bulk due to decreased cardiac output.

These facts show that the ICP-PWF may be modulated by cerebrovascular reactivity, cerebral compliance and venous circulation in intracranial hemodynamics.

It is concluded that each peak of ICP-PWF has different origins, and that the analysis of PWF provides useful information about intracranial hemodynamics.

References

1. Avezaat CJJ, Van Eijndhoven JH, Wyper DJ (1979) Cerebrospinal fluid pulse pressure and intracranial volume-pressure relationships. J Neurol Neurosurg Psych 42:687–700
2. Cardoso ER, Rowan JO, Galbraith S (1983) Analysis of the cerebrospinal fluid pulse wave in intracranial pressure. J Neurosurg 59:817–821
3. Dardenne G, Dereymaker A, Lacheron JM (1969) Cerebrospinal fluid pressure and pulsatility: An Experimental Study of Circulatory and Respiratory Influences in Normal and Hydrocephalic Dogs. Europ Neurol 2:193–216
4. Durward QJ, Amacher AL, Del Maestro RF, Sibbald WJ (1983) Cerebral and cardiovascular responses to changes in head elevation in patients with intracranial hypertension. J Neurosurg 59:983–944
5. Foltz EL, Aine C (1981) Diagnosis of hydrocephalus by CSF pulse-wave analysis: a clinical study. Surg Neurol 15:283–293
6. Goldensohn ES, Whitehead RW, Parry TM, Spencer TM, Grover RF, Draper WB (1951) Studies on diffusion respiration IX. Effect of diffusion respiration and high concentrations of CO2 on cerebrospinal fluid pressure of anesthetized dogs. Am J Physiol 165:334–340
7. Hamer J, Alberti E, Hoyer S, Wiedemann K (1977) Influence of systemic and cerebral vascular factors on the cerebrospinal fluid pulse waves. J Neurosurg 46:36–45
8. Hashimoto M, Higashi S, Kogure Y, Fujii H, Tokuda K, Ito H, Yamamoto S (1989) Intracranial pressure pulse wave form and its dp/dt analysis of plateau waves. In: Hoff JT, Betz AL (eds) Intracranial Pressure VII. Springer Berlin Heidelberg New York London Paris Tokyo Hong Kong, pp 225–227
9. Hirai O, Handa H, Ishikawa M, Kim S (1984) Epidural pulse waveform as an indicator of intracranial pressure dynamics. Surg Neurol 21:67–74
10. Rosner MJ, Becker DJ (1984) Origin and elevation of plateau waves. J Neurosurg 60:312–324

Analysis of the Intracranial Pressure Waveform by Means of Spectral Methods

J. Berdyga[1], M. Czosnyka[2], Z. Czernicki[1], and M. Williamson[3]

[1] Medical Research Centre, Polish Academy of Science
[2] Warsaw University of Technology, Warsaw, Poland
[3] Pinderfields General Hospital, Wakefield, UK

Introduction

The opinion that the intracranial pressure pulse wave contains information on both cerebrospinal elasticity and autoregulatory reserve seems to be widely accepted [1, 4]. Many authors proposed various methods for the assessment of these phenomena. Calculation of the so-called "high frequency centroid" which contains the concise information on the higher harmonic distortion of the intracranial pressure pulse wave [5], seems to be useful in the intensive care of head injured patients [2].

The aim of this study is to investigate the relationship between the higher spectral components of the ICP pulse wave and the autoregulatory reserve, under various clinical conditions and on the basis of modeling studies.

Material

The material used for the ICP waveform analysis consists of:

- Fifty lumbar infusion tests, in the Children's Health Centre, as a diagnostic procedure in hydrocephalus. The tests were studied in order to investigate the influence of an increase in ICP, caused by the expansion of the CSF volume, on the shape of the pulse wave.
- Five cases with long-term monitoring of ICP (intraventricularly) and cerebral perfusion pressure (CPP), after severe head injury (Pinderfields General Hospital). In this material, the influence of a decrease in CPP on the shape of the pulse wave was studied.

Methods

Two different methods of spectral analysis of the pulse wave were used. The "high frequency centroid" (HFC) method (5) was slightly changed in order to avoid the influence of the heart rate on the value of HFC. This was achieved by an automatic adaptation of the signal sampling rate to the heart rate. In this way, only one pulse wave is included within the time window of the length 128. Then 128 point fast Fourier Transform was used to the power spectrum estimation and further calculations of HFC. Therefore, HFC was expressed, not in frequency units (Hz) but in harmonics of the heart rate, from third to tenth harmonic. The increase in HFC can be interpreted as an increase of the higher harmonic distortion of the pulse wave, irrespective of the heart rate.

The second method was used in the standard software for long-term monitoring in intensive care. The so-called distortion coefficient (DC) was calculated as a power associated with the fundamental component to a power of all higher harmonic components, using standard spectral estimation by means of fast Fourier Transform. DC coefficients were calculated for both ICP waveform (DC1) and arterial blood pressure waveform (DC2).

Finally, some patterns of pulse wave were studied in the computer model of cerebral blood flow and CSF circulation [6].

Results

A specific behavior of HFC was found in the majority of infusion tests. The mean value of HFC on the testing pressure level was 6 ± 0.7. During the gradual increase in ICP, caused by the infusion, a decrease in HFC was observed in 46 cases. The HFC significantly decreased to 3.5 ± 0.4. In 32 cases, an increase in HFC was observed at the end of the infusion when the ICP was considerably elevated. This was obviously correlated with a vasomotor response (Cushing) to the elevated ICP.

In the five head injury cases, characteristic patterns in trends of DC1 and DC2 were observed: DC1 changes proportionally to slow and relatively small changes in ICP after CSF drainage and mannitol administration. This was the case as long as CPP remained above 50 mmHg. When CPP decreased below the lower limit of autoregulation (35–45 mmHg), DC1 started to decrease. DC1 also increased under conditions when DC2 tended to increase: during central vasomotor responses to reduced CPP and during episodes of tachycardia.

Discussion

These results show that the harmonic distortion of the pulse wave is present when slow changes in ICP take place: during infusion tests and in response to mannitol. This phenomenon is caused by the harmonic distortion of the arterial pressure pulse wave, interference of the venous pulse wave and by non-linear effects of the input signals. This means: the arterial and venous pulses are stable but the mechanisms in their transmission influence the shape of the ICP pulse wave. The transmission of the venous pulse wave tends to decrease during intracranial hypertension, whereas the transmission of the arterial pulse increases. This produces a decrease in the harmonic distortion of the ICP pulse

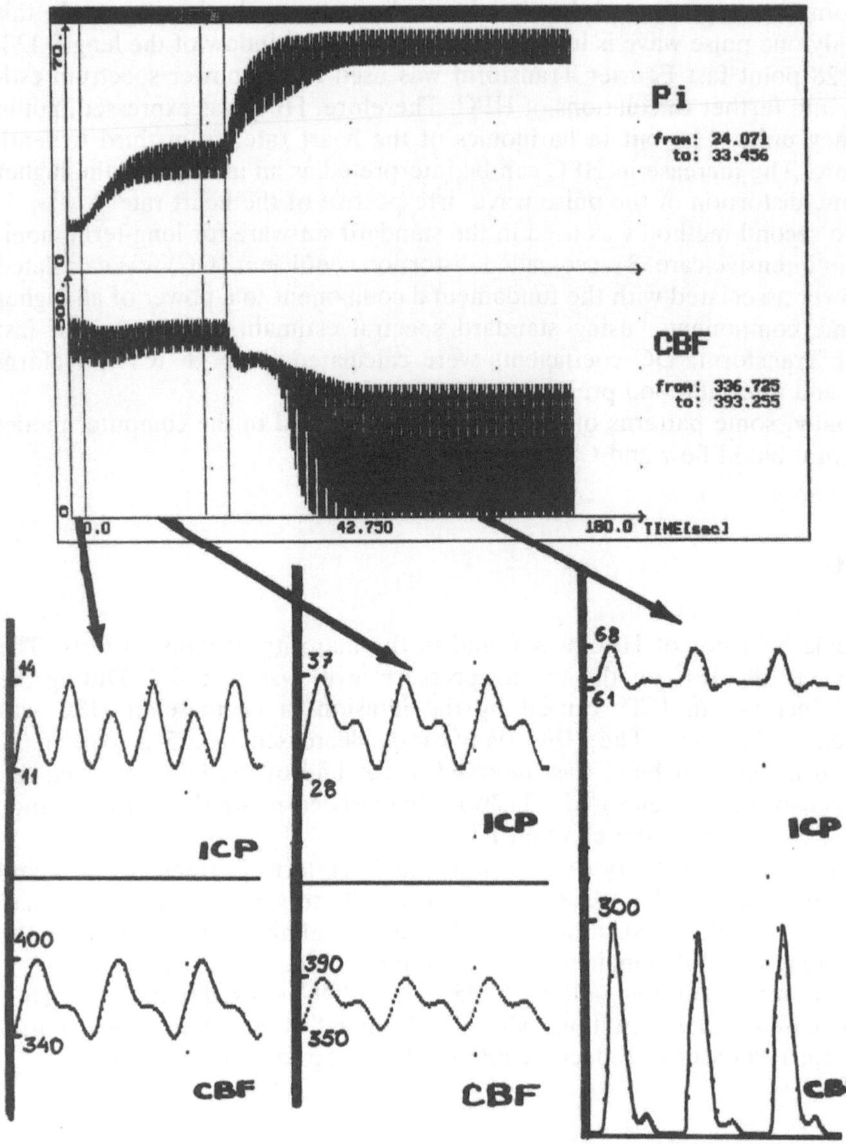

Fig. 1. Simulation of an infusion test by a computer model of cerebral blood flow and CSF circulation

wave. If the harmonic distortion of the arterial pulse wave increases, it is transmitted to the ICP pulse wave. As a result, HFC increases and DC1 decreases during central vasomotor reflexes, during which DC2 tends to increase (Cushing response and tachycardia).

A different situation takes place when the increase in ICP causes a decrease in CPP below the limit of autoregulation. In that case, a strong increase in the harmonic distortion of the ICP pulse wave can be observed. This seems to be caused by non-linear effects of the cerebral blood flow control mechanisms. Such an increase in ICP pulse harmonic distortion is observed in parallel to an increase in the cerebral blood flow pulsatility. The simulation of the phenomena influencing the harmonic distortion of the pulse wave confirms the above observations. They are shown in figure 1. The initial distortion, caused by the interference of the arterial and venous pulses, is high. When the ICP increases, as a result of the simulated CSF infusion, the harmonic distortion significantly decreases. Below the autoregulation limit (CPP $<$ 40 mmHg) the ICP pulse wave distortion decreases. This is evidently correlated with the distorted, pulsatile character of the cerebral blood flow.

Conclusion

The harmonic distortion of the ICP pulse wave contains information on the cerebral autoregulation reserve and on the cause of the elevated ICP. If the autoregulation reserve is sufficient, elevations in ICP caused by changes in brain bulk, produce a decrease in the harmonic distortion. Below the limit of autoregulation, the non-linear effects of cerebral blood flow are responsible for the ICP pulse wave distortion. In many cases this picture can be masked by fluctuations in the shape of the arterial pulse wave, transmitted to the CSF pulse pressure, taking place during central vasomotor reflexes.

References

1. Cardoso ER, Kesava R, Bose D (1988) Effect of subarachnoid hemorrhage on intracranial pulse waves in cats. J Neurosurg 69:712–718
2. Robertson C, Narayan R, Contant C, et al. (1989) Clinical experience with a continuous monitor of intracranial compliance. J Neurosurg 71:673–680
3. Gray J, Rosner M (1987) Pressure-volume index a function of cerebral perfusion pressure. J Neurosurg 67:377–380
4. Takizawa H, et al. (1987) Changes in the cerebrospinal fluid pulse wave spectrum associated with raised intracranial pressure. Neurosurgery 20:355–361
5. Gokaslan Z, Bray RS, Sherwood AM, et al. (1989) Dynamic Pressure Volume Index via ICP Waveform Analysis. In: Hoff JT, Betz AL (eds) Intracranial Pressure VII. Springer, Berlin Heidelberg New York London Paris Tokyo Hong Kong, pp 124–128
6. Czosnyka M, Piechnik S, et al. (1993) The dynamics of Cerebral Blood Flow, Perfusion Pressure and CSF circulation – a modeling study. In: Avezaat CJJ, van Eijndhoven JHM, Maas AIR, Tans JThJ (eds) Intracranial Pressure VIII. Springer, Berlin Heidelberg New York London Paris Tokyo Hong Kong Barcelona

Continuous Analysis of the Intracranial Pressure Waveform as a Method of Autoregulatory Reserve Assessment

P. Laniewski[1], M. Czosnyka[2], W. Maksymowicz[3], and H. Laniewska-Wollk[4]

[1] Department of Anaesthesiology and Intensive Care, Child's Health Centre, [2] Warsaw University of Technology, [3] Department of Neurosurgery, Warsaw Medical Academy, [4] Warsaw Agriculture Academy, Warsaw, Poland

Introduction

During a CSF infusion test a linear relationship can be observed between the amplitude of the ICP pulse wave and the mean ICP. This linear amplitude-pressure characteristic of the intracranial system (ICS) has been documented in many papers and extensively analysed by Avezaat [1]. The origin of this linearity can be explained by the combined effect of the non-linear nature of the capacitance of the ICS and the constant change in cerebral blood volume during each heart beat (ΔCBV). We asked ourselves two questions. The first was, whether this linearity can also be identified during continuous monitoring of ICP. And the second, whether this is another independent parameter describing the nature of the ICS.

Method

To answer these questions, an original algorithm for IBM PC was written [2]. ICP was sampled with a frequency of 18 Hz. The digital power spectrum (128 points) was calculated every 7 seconds. In this way, a fast and accurate method of extraction of the peaks related to pulse wave and respiratory wave, was developed. Furthermore, calculation of the heart rate and the amplitude of the fundamental components of the pulse wave (AMP) and respiratory wave were performed. At the same time, the mean ICP was calculated by digital integration of the signal. A present number of so calculated primary values was stored in the circular buffer to make statistical calculations. The results, such as AMP (mAMP), mean ICP (mICP), mean HR, and the ratio between AMP and ICP (RAP) were stored on floppy-disk. This kind of analysis provides information on the AMP and ICP relationship in two time scales: RAP over a short interval of minutes, and a linear regression model built on the mean values of AMP and ICP (mAMP-mICP) over a period of hours. It should be emphasized that frequency analysis is the best way to avoid the influence of various components of the ICP signal. The loss of higher harmonics during the analysis was not considered a problem, because of the excellent correlation between the fundamental harmonic and the mean ICP, which we had found during infusion tests. The correlation coefficient was 0.965 in a group of 18 consecutive infusions.

Material

The clinical material consists of 70 children, 2–16 years of age, admitted to the Intensive Care Unit after suboccipital craniectomy for posterior fossa tumours (group A) and of 15 comatose (Glasgow Coma Scale score <8) head-injury patients (group B). All patients in group A had a ventricular catheter for external drainage of CSF during the operation and, if necessary, in the post-operative period. The patients were artificially ventilated to maintain an arterial pCO_2 of 30 mmHg. In 18 cases monitoring was continued at the beginning of spontaneous ventilation. In six patients of group B ICP was measured by an epidural sensor. The mean monitoring time was 24 hours.

Results

The mean values and standard deviations of mAMP, mICP, and RAP are presented in Table 1.

The patients in group A and B were in the same range of ICP and the difference in mean ICP was not significant. The amplitude of the pulse wave was significantly higher in group B, as was the slope of the mAMP-mICP relationship (Fig. 1a,b). In group A, the linear mAMP-mICP relationship was only present at mICP below 25 mmHg ($r = 0.996$, $p < 0.001$); the relationship was not linear for the whole range of mICP ($r = 0.25$, $p < 0.365$). In group B, mAMP-mICP was linear for the whole range of mICP ($r = 0.931$, $p < 0.003$). The slope of the relationship was 0.08 in group A and 0.17 in group B. In the control group of 96 infusion tests the slope was 0.37. The RAP value was significantly higher in group B than in group A (Table 1). The dependency of RAP on mICP was different for both groups (Fig. 2a,b). In group B, RAP reached a maximum value at mICP of about 35 mmHg and reached a maximum value at mICP of about 35 mmHg and decreased at a

Table 1.

Group	mAMP		mICP		RAP	
	Mean	SD	Mean	SD	Mean	SD
A	1.3	0.589	25.8	15.182	0.226*	0.089
B	4.82	2.76	32.0	16.583	0.46	0.19

*$p < 0.001$

A

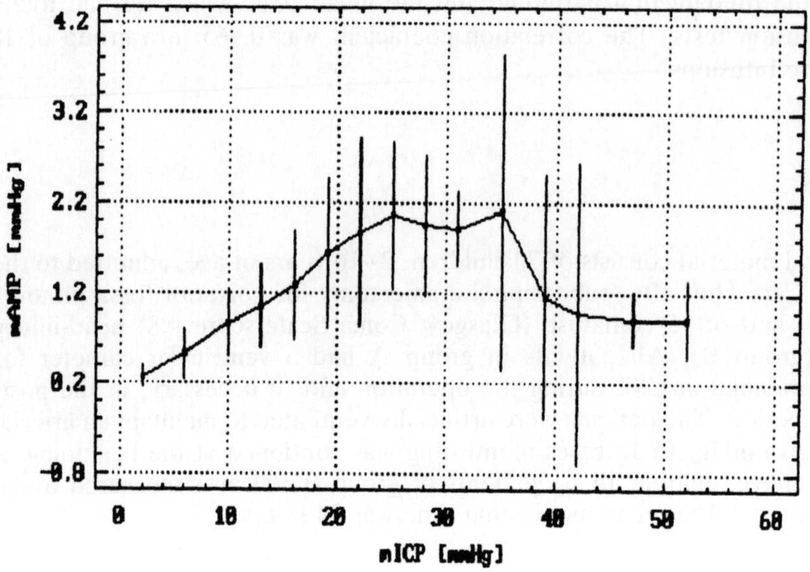

B

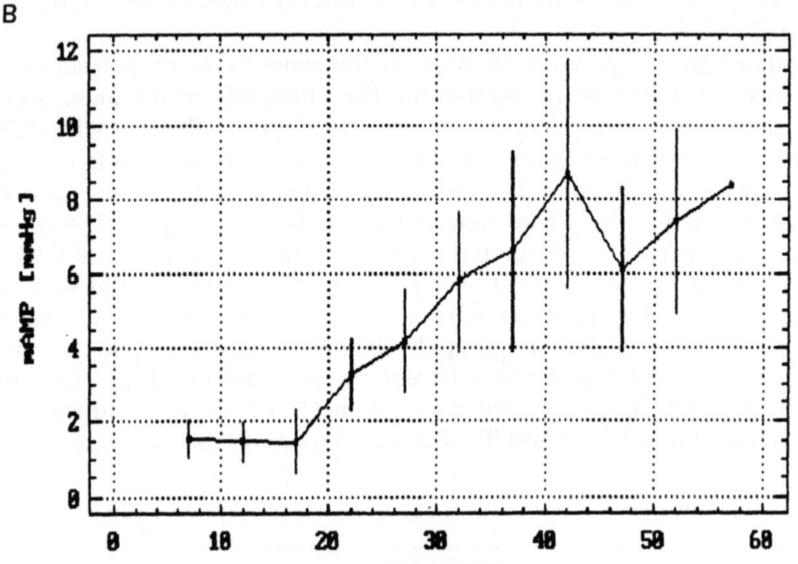

Fig. 1A,B. The relationship between the mean amplitude of ICP pulse wave (mAMP) and the mean intracranial pressure (mICP). The standard deviations are represented by the vertical bars. **A** Group A patients after suboccipital craniectomy. **B** Group B patients: in coma following severe closed head injury

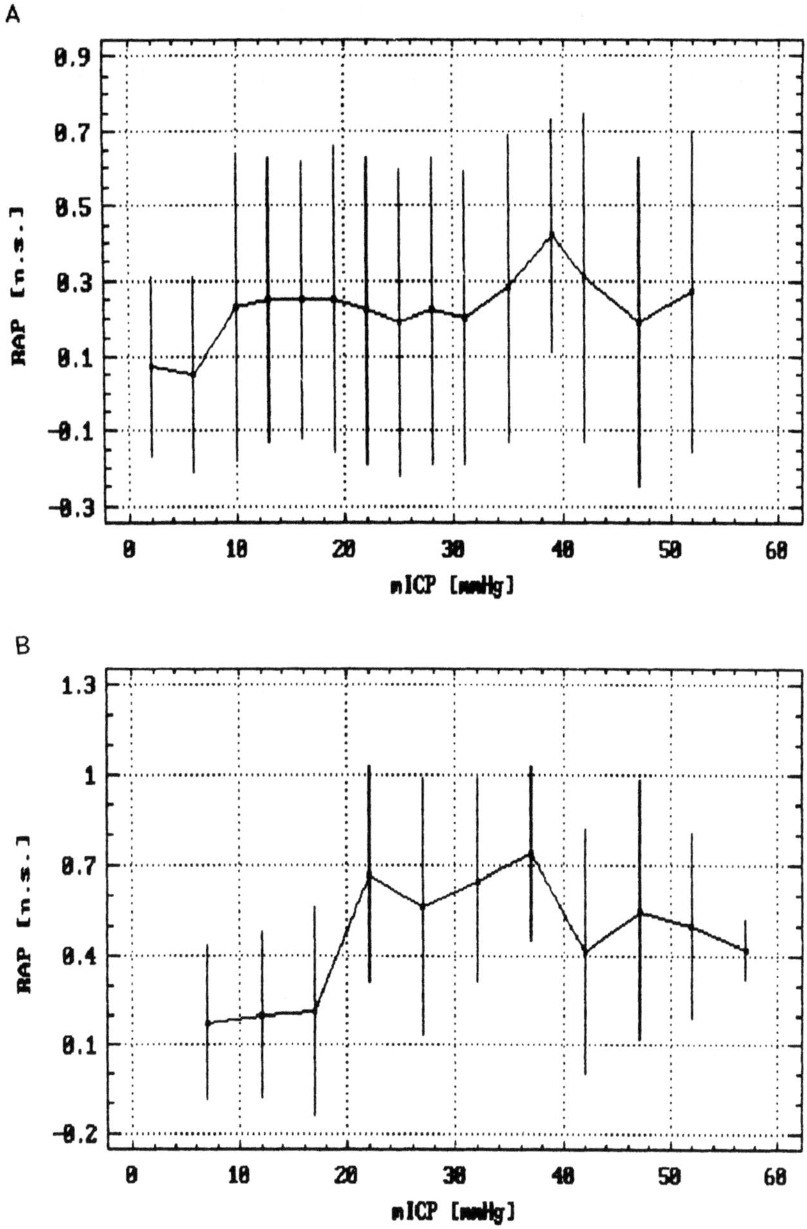

Fig. 2A,B. The relationship of mean AMP/ICP ratio (mRAP) versus mean ICP level calculated for clusters of mAMP and mICP. The vertical bars represent the standard deviations. **A** Group A patients. **B** Group B patients

higher mICP. In group A, RAP was low in the whole range of mICP. It appeared during long term monitoring that RAP can change very fast. When plateau waves were recorded in patients of group B, the tracing of RAP was typical. At the top of a plateau wave an inversion of RAP took place from high

(RAP > 0.8) to low (RAP ≤ 0) (Fig. 3a). The restitution of spontaneous ventilation causing a parallel increase in pCO_2, produced a rise in RAP to a value of about 1 for 1–2 hrs, even when mICP returned to the base-line level (Fig. 3b).

Discussion

The shape of the mAMP-mICP characteristic and the distribution of the RAP values reflect the mechanical properties of ICS and the state of the cerebral

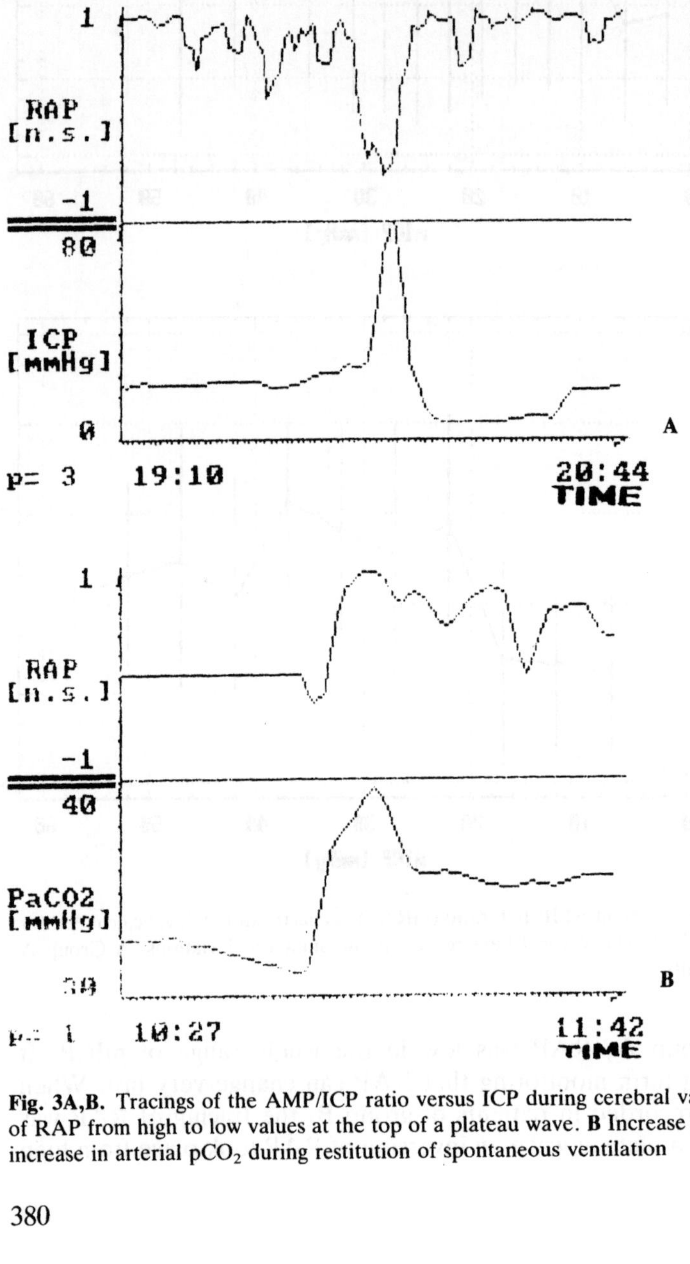

Fig. 3A,B. Tracings of the AMP/ICP ratio versus ICP during cerebral vasodilatation. **A** Inversion of RAP from high to low values at the top of a plateau wave. **B** Increase of RAP concomitant with increase in arterial pCO_2 during restitution of spontaneous ventilation

vascular bed. The slope of this relationship strongly depends on the conditions that affect the mICP level. This thesis is supported by the discrepancy between the slopes found during the infusion tests and continuous monitoring. The dynamic character of mAMP-mICP, the distortion of linearity, especially during plateau waves, and the characteristic response to the increase in pCO_2, support the assumption that the vascular bed plays a dominant role in these phenomena. Certain conditions are necessary to achieve a positive RAP and linear mAMP-mICP characteristics. ΔCBV has to be kept constant by the preserved autoregulation of CBF as well as the balance between inflow and outflow of blood in ICS. The cerebral perfusion pressure must be in the range of autoregulation. Furthermore, ICS elastivity has to be normal or increased in order to guarantee a strong interaction of the various components in the system. This is essential for the filtration of the presumed dependency on "noise". In group A, a low mAMP, flat mAMP-mICP characteristics and a low RAP were observed. This can be interpreted as a consequence of the low elastivity due to the large craniectomy, as well as to vasoconstriction caused by hyperventilation. The increase in RAP due to the increase in pCO_2 supports this assumption. In group B, the elastivity can be assumed to be normal or high. The system was stimulated by a volume process activating vasodilatation, dependent on CBF autoregulation. The decrease in RAP at mICP above 35 mmHg is the average effect of many vasomotor reflexes. A plateau wave is caused by vasodilatation when the ICP is extremely high [4], as a result of which CPP is decreased below the lower limit of autoregulation. At this ICP level the arterial bed is completely dilated and is not able to keep CBF and ΔCBF constant. The observed inversion of RAP can be considered as a consequence of this process. The assumptions presented above, were confirmed in experiments on cats and rabbits. A series of experiments with a digital model of ICS also confirm that these phenomena can be explained on the basis of a physiological interaction of the vascular bed with other components of the intracranial system [3].

References

1. Avezaat CJJ, van Eijndhoven JHM (1984) Cerebrospinal fluid pulse pressure and craniospinal dynamics. Thesis, Erasmus University, Jongbloed en Zoon Publishers, The Hague
2. Czosnyka M, Laniewski P, Batorski L, Zaworski W (1988) A system for ICP processing and interpretation in intensive care. In: Advances in Biomedical Measurement, Plenum Publ Corp, pp 101–109
3. Czosnyka M, Koszewski W, Laniewski P, Maksymowicz W, Paluszek K, Piechnik S, Zabolotny W, Zaworski W (1993) The dynamics of cerebral blood flow, perfusion pressure and CSF circulation – A modelling study. In: Avezaat CJJ, van Eijnhoven JHM, Maas AIR, Tans JTJ (eds) Intracranial Pressure VIII. Springer, Berlin Heidelberg New York London Paris Tokyo Hong Kong Barcelona
4. Rosner MJ (1986) The vasodilatatory cascade and intracranial pressure. In: Miller JD, Teasdale GM, Rowan JO, Galbraith SL, Mendelow AD (eds) Intracranial pressure VI, Springer, Berlin Heidelberg New York Tokyo, pp 137–141

Differential Effect of Hypercarbia and Hypertension on Cerebrovascular Pressure Transmission and Craniospinal Compliance

I.R. PIPER, K.H. CHAN, I.R. WHITTLE, and J.D. MILLER

Department of Clinical Neurosciences, University of Edinburgh, Edinburgh, Scotland

Introduction

Waveform analysis of human cerebrovascular pressure transmission (CVPT) is feasible and certain forms of CVPT are associated with raised ICP [4]. There is experimental and clinical evidence for relationship between CVPT and both cerebrovascular resistance and craniospinal compliance [1, 6]. An increase in arterial PCO2 can cause cerebral vasodilation and thereby alter CVPT. An increase in arterial pressure can produce changes in both craniospinal compliance and cerebrovascular resistance dependent on the state of cerebral autoregulation [2]. The purpose of this experimental study was to observe CVPT under conditions within and beyond the normal limits of cerebrovascular autoregulation, during simultaneous measurement of cerebrovascular resistance and craniospinal compliance. An improved understanding of the relationship between CVPT, craniospinal compliance and cerebrovascular autoregulation may aid the diagnosis and management of raised ICP.

Methods

Twelve cats each weighing between 2.0 and 5.2 kg, were split into a CO2 group ($n = 6$) and a BP group ($n = 6$). Animals were anaesthetised with 1% alpha-chloralose anaesthesia (75 mg/kg IV), given a tracheostomy, intubated and ventilated under positive pressure with oxygen. Muscle paralysis was maintained with pancuronium (0.7 mg IV) given hourly. Ventilator volume was adjusted to maintain the animals normocarbic (PaCO2 35–40 mmHg).

The blood pressure (BP) waveform was recorded using a catheter-tip pressure transducer placed in the descending segment of the thoracic aorta while the ICP waveform was recorded through placement of an optimally damped fluid-filled catheter-transducer system placed in the left lateral ventricle through a 19 gauge 2 inch needle. Cerebrovascular resistance was calculated as the quotient of cerebral perfusion pressure (CPP = BP − ICP) to cerebral blood flow (CBF) where CBF was the average from six cortical sites. CBF was determined through the use of the initial slope index of the hydrogen clearance technique. Craniospinal compliance was calculated from the average intracranial pressure response to four sequential volume injections of 0.05 mls of saline into the cisterna magna using a time averaged short volume pulse response method [5].

Cerebrovascular pressure transmission was determined using Systems Analysis. Systems analysis is a technique whereby an attempt is made to define the physical characteristics of a system using only the system input and output signals (Fig. 1). The assumption is made that the BP waveform is the chief input signal to the cerebrovascular system and the ICP waveform is the output response to that stimulus. The system transfer function is calculated from Fourier analysis of the BP and ICP waveforms and consists of amplitude and phase components. As an example, the first component of the amplitude transfer function was calculated as the ratio of the first cardiac component harmonic in the ICP spectrum to the amplitude of the first cardiac component harmonic in the BP spectrum. This process was repeated for each of the first 6 ICP and BP cardiac component harmonics present in the ICP and BP amplitude spectra. By similar means, the difference between the ICP and BP phase values for each of the measured cardiac component harmonics yielded the phase transfer function. The amplitude transfer function is a measure of how much pressure is transmitted through the cerebrovascular bed at a given frequency. The phase transfer function is a measure of how much a given sinusoidal pressure signal is shifted, with respect to a certain starting phase, as it is transmitted through the cerebrovascular bed (CVB). The amplitude and phase transfer functions allow one to quantify the pressure transmission performance of the CVB, thus providing a basis for comparison between normal and abnormal function. Amplitude harmonics higher than the 6th and phase harmonics higher than the first are not reported as these higher harmonics demonstrate too large a variability between repeated measurements [4].

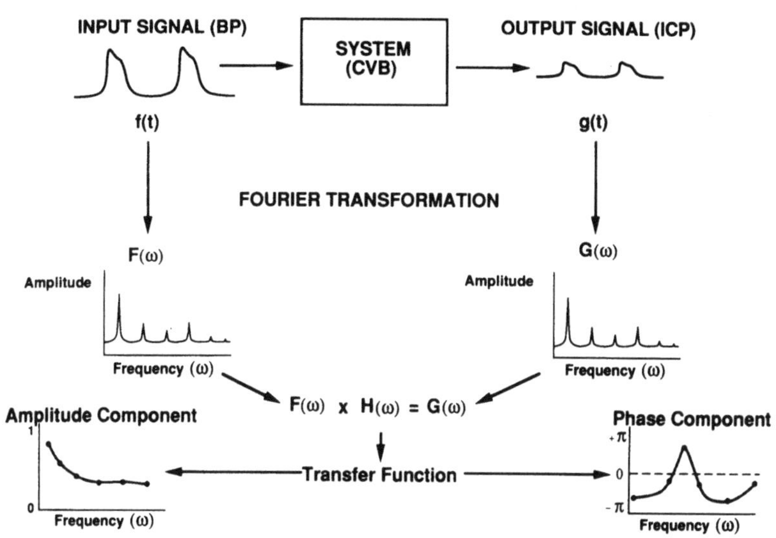

Fig. 1. Systems analysis of cerebrovascular pressure transmission

Protocol

The CVB was challenged by two stimuli in this study, hypercapnia and arterial hypertension. In the CO_2 group of animals the arterial CO_2 tension was raised in two stages with administration of 5% and 10% CO_2 in the inspired gas mixture. In the BP group of animals, arterial hypertension was induced with intravenous infusion (6–40 mls/hour) of Angiotensin II (100 μg/ml) and supplemented as required with Adrenalin (0.2 mg/ml at 10–40 ml/hour). Each level of arterial hypercarbia and hypertension was maintained for 30 minutes. At each stage, four sequential 30 second samples of ICP and BP waveform data were stored to FM magnetic tape for subsequent offline calculation of CVPT, which was immediately followed by four sequential measurements of craniospinal compliance. CBF was then determined through the use of the hydrogen clearance technique, with 10 minutes of hydrogen saturation. Just prior to desaturation, arterial blood gas samples were taken. During the initial slope phase of hydrogen desaturation, BP and ICP were recorded for calculation of the CPP. In one animal, to assess blood brain barrier function post arterial hypertension, 8 ml of a 2% Evans Blue Dye was given intravenously forty minutes before the end of the protocol. The brain was removed and examined for evidence of extravasation of Evans Blue Dye.

Statistical Analysis

Each experiment is a self-paired design. Paired students t-tests were used to test for significant differences.

Results

Induced Arterial Hypercarbia

Figure 2 shows the relationship between CVPT, cerebrovascular resistance and craniospinal compliance before and with two levels of arterial hypercarbia. With 5% CO_2, $PaCO_2$ increased significantly from 35 to 65 mmHg ($p < 0.001$), increasing further still to 99 mmHg with 10% CO_2 ($p < 0.001$). With 5% inspired CO_2, ICP increased significantly from 14 to 24 mmHg ($p < 0.01$). This was associated with a significant decrease in cerebrovascular resistance ($p < 0.001$). With 10% CO_2 cerebrovascular resistance decreased further still ($p < 0.001$) but with no further increase in ICP. Craniospinal compliance decreased significantly with 5% CO_2 ($p < 0.001$) returning towards control levels with 10% CO_2. Compliance with 10% CO_2 was not significantly different from control.

Both low (1st harmonic) and high frequency (4th harmonic) components of the amplitude transfer function increased significantly with 5% CO_2 ($p < 0.001$). Only the first harmonic showed a further increase ($p < 0.05$) with 10% CO_2. The 1st harmonic of the phase transfer function showed a significant

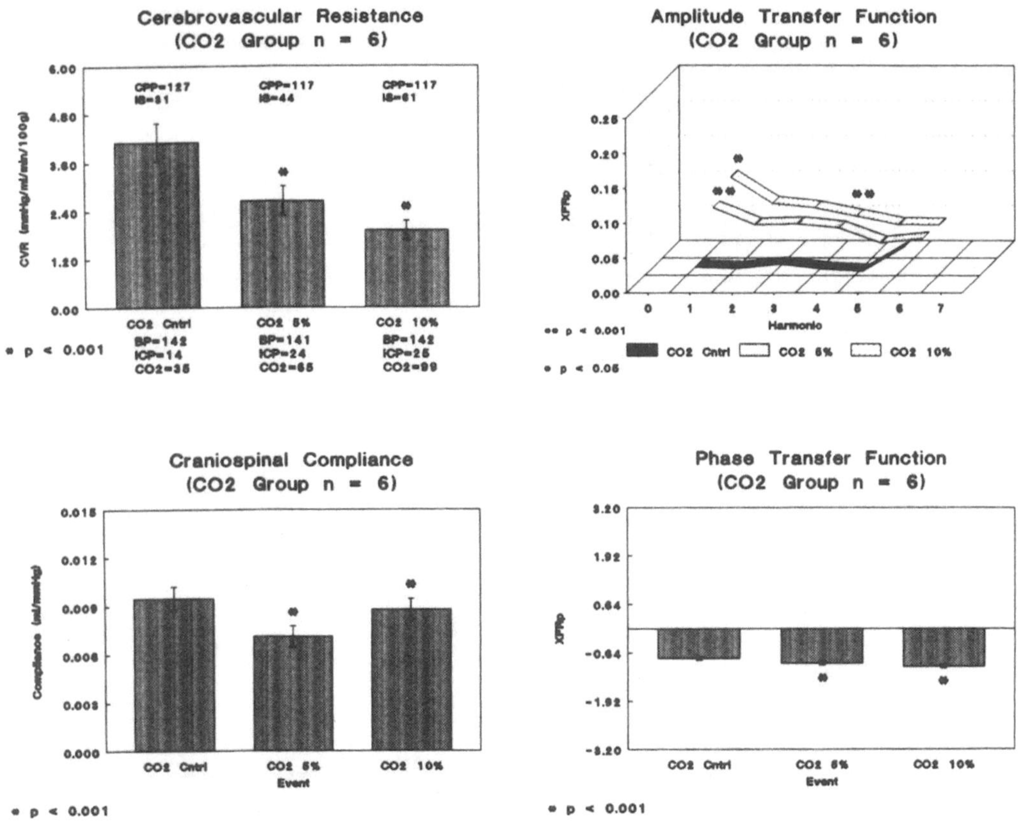

Fig. 2. The relationship between cerebrovascular pressure transmission, cerebrovascular resistance and craniospinal compliance before and with two levels of arterial hypercarbia

increase in phase (more -ve) with 5% CO2, increasing further still with 10% CO2 ($p < 0.001$).

Induced Arterial Hypertension

Figure 3 shows the relationship between CVPT, cerebrovascular resistance and craniospinal compliance before, during and post arterial hypertension. With Angiotension infusion, BP increased significantly from 131 to 195 mmHg ($p < 0.001$). With cessation of Angiotensin infusion BP decreased to 91 mmHg and was significantly different from control levels ($p < 0.001$). During arterial hypertension, ICP increased significantly from 16 to 36 mmHg ($p < 0.001$). This was associated with a significant decrease in cerebrovascular resistance ($p < 0.001$). Post arterial hypertension cerebrovascular resistance increased significantly ($p < 0.01$) but was not significantly different from control. ICP decreased significantly from control levels to 9 mmHg post arterial hypertension ($p < 0.001$). Craniospinal compliance decreased significantly during

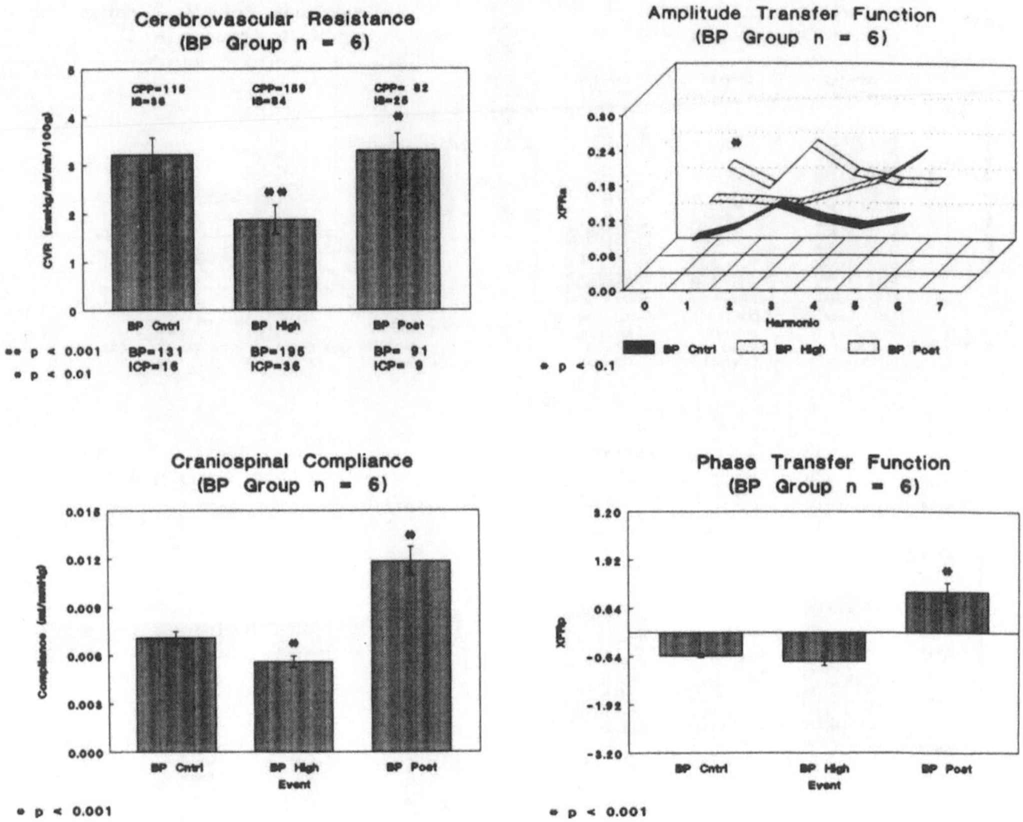

Fig. 3. The relationship between cerebrovascular pressure transmission, cerebrovascular resistance and craniospinal compliance before, during and post arterial hypertension

arterial hypertension ($p < 0.001$). Compliance showed a marked increase above control levels post arterial hypertension ($p < 0.001$).

The 1st harmonic component of the amplitude transfer function increased, but not significantly, during arterial hypertension. The increased first harmonic amplitude post arterial hypertension just failed to reach statistical significance at the 5% level ($p = 0.057$). The 1st harmonic of the phase transfer function during arterial hypertension showed no significant change from control levels and demonstrated a negative phase. Post arterial hypertension there was a marked and significant change towards a positive phase ($p < 0.001$).

Arterial Hypertension and Brain Damage

Coronal slices taken from the brain of the animal injected with Evans Blue Dye show marked extravasation of Evans Blue Dye, both superficially and extending into the full thickness of the cerebral and cerebellar cortex and occasionally spreading to subcortical white matter. In addition to blood-brain barrier breakdown, one animal had blood stained CSF and another had an intraparenchymal haemorrhage located just inferior to the ventricular needle catheter. All animals pupils became fully dilated during severe arterial hypertension and remained fully dilated during the post arterial hypertension stage of the protocol.

Discussion

Arterial hypercarbia causes intracranial vasodilation, predominantly the precapillary arteriolar segment of the cerebrovascular bed [7]. With 5% CO2, the decreased cerebrovascular resistance, increased ICP and decreased craniospinal compliance is consistent with this vasodilation. Interestingly both low and high frequency components of the amplitude transfer function increase under these conditions. The 1st harmonic phase became more negative which in system terms is equivalent to becoming more capacitive or in mechanical terms: less stiff. A decrease in vascular stiffness is consistent with the process of a vasodilatory relaxation in active vascular muscle tone. With 10% CO2 a further decrease in cerebrovascular resistance occurred followed by a further increase in the 1st harmonic of the amplitude transfer function and a more negative 1st harmonic phase. This is consistent with a further vasodilation. Interestingly, with 10% CO2 there was a return towards control levels in craniospinal compliance despite a further vasodilation. The failure of ICP to increase further with 10% CO2 above that of the 5% level supports the data that craniospinal compliance is not decreasing further despite an additional vasodilation. This paradoxical response might be explained by considering that with 10% CO2 there may not be only arteriolar vasodilation but an effect on the intracranial venous system as well. Redistribution of blood to the large and more compliant venous vessels could explain this increase in craniospinal compliance.

The normal upper limit of autoregulation in the cat, under alpha-chloralose anaesthesia and using the H2 clearance technique for measurement of CBF, has been shown to be approximately 160 mmHg [3]. Arterial hypertension induced in the BP group of animals was above this level and is likely to cause a forced vascular distension. During this time the non-autoregulatory decrease in cerebrovascular resistance associated with an increase in ICP and a decrease in craniospinal compliance supports that an arterial vascular distension had occurred. After 30 minutes of severe arterial hypertension, CVPT remained elevated despite a fall in BP below that of control levels. Both CPP and CBF decreased with the latter decreasing proportionally more and consequently cerebrovascular resistance increased and was not significantly different from that of control levels. This latter change suggests that CBF had become pressure passive and that normal autoregulation is either absent or impaired. Mackenzie et al. [3] in a similar study of acutely raised arterial hypertension in cats demonstrated loss of CBF autoregulation, damage to the blood-brain barrier and overdistension of the cerebral resistance vessels. The brain pathology results of the one animal injected with Evans Blue Dye would confirm the breakdown of blood-brain barrier in this preparation.

The two most marked changes at this time are the significant increase in craniospinal compliance above that of control levels and the sudden change in the 1st harmonic phase transfer function from a negative to a positive phase. The changes in craniospinal compliance and system phase seen with the BP group of animals are best understood in electronic terms, where a more negative system phase indicates increased capacitance, and an increase in system phase in a positive direction indicates an increased inductance. In mechanical terms, capacitance is the inverse of elasticity or stiffness i.e. – vascular compliance. Inductance in mechanical terms is equivalent to inertance which is the propensity to resist a movement of mass, the mass in this case being a fluid mass. During the post arterial hypertension stage, the increased phase shift in a positive direction may indicate a greatly increased inertance brought on by the distention of the blood vessels with an increased mass of blood. A possible sequence of events might be that the increased mass of blood, forced in under arterial hypertension, in combination with blood vessels exhibiting reduced tone, results in both greater inertance and increased vascular stiffness, the increased vascular stiffness being the result of increased transmural pressure with raised BP. At this time, the increased vascular stiffness is the dominant factor determining the system phase. When BP is then reduced, the transmural pressure decreases and hence the vascular stiffness decreases. After 30 minutes of severe arterial hypertension, the inertance is now the main determinant of the system phase. The greatly increased craniospinal compliance seen at this time may have resulted from the increased intracranial blood volume in the venous portion of the CVB. An increased blood volume contained within a vasculature that has lost tone will, especially at low transmural pressure, be more readily displaced from the intracranial cavity and therefore result in increased craniospinal compliance. These marked changes in craniospinal compliance and system phase may be interpreted as indicators for a generalized cerebral vasodilation as a consequence of reduced vasomotor tone.

Conclusions

1. Increased cerebrovascular pressure transmission indicates reduced vasomotor tone but does not differentiate between active vasodilation and a non-autoregulatory forced vascular distension.
2. A greatly elevated cerebrovascular pressure transmission in combination with a positive phase shift may indicate a generalized cerebral vasodilation as a consequence of impaired autoregulatory vasomotor tone.

References

1. Bray RS, Sherwood AM, Halter JA, Robertson C, Grossman RG (1986) Development of a clinical monitoring system by means of ICP waveform analysis. In: Miller JD, Teasdale GM, Rowan JO, Galbraith SL, Mendelow AD (eds) Intracranial Pressure VI. Springer, Berlin Heidelberg New York Tokyo, pp 260–264

2. Gray WJ, Rosner MJ (1987) Pressure-volume index as a function of cerebral perfusion pressure. Part 2: The effects of low cerebral pressure and autoregulation. J Neurosurg 67:377–380
3. Mackenzie ET, Strandgaard S, Graham DI, Jones JV, Harper AM, Farrar JK (1976) Effects of acutely induced hypertension in cats on pial arteriolar calibre, local cerebral blood flow, and the blood-brain barrier. Circ Res 39:33–41
4. Piper IR, Miller JD, Dearden NM, Leggate JRS, Robertson I (1990) Systems analysis of cerebrovascular pressure transmission: an observational study in head injured patients. J Neurosurg 73:871–880
5. Piper IR, Miller JD, Whittle IR, Lawson A (1990) Automated time-averaged analysis of craniospinal compliance. Acta Neurochirurgica, [Suppl 51], 387–390
6. Portnoy HD, Chopp M (1981) Cerebrospinal fluid pulse wave form analysis during hypercapnia and hypoxia. Neurosurgery 9:14–27
7. Tuor UI, Farrar JK (1985) Contribution of the inflow arteries to alterations in total cerebrovascular resistance in the rabbit. Pfluegers Arch 403:283–288

A Simulation Study of Wave Transformation Using a Nonlinear Model of Artery and a Physical Model of Intracranial Vascular Bed

H. NISHIMURA and N. YASUI

Department of Surgical Neurology, Research Institute for Brain and Blood Vessels-AKITA, 6-10, Senshu-Kubotamachi, Akita, Japan

Introduction

If hydrodynamic changes in the pressure pulse waveform depend on the condition of the cerebrospinal fluid (CSF) system, we should be able to evaluate that condition by measuring the pattern of the intracranial pressure (ICP) pulse waveform. Although the dependence of the ICP pulse amplitude on the mean ICP can be explained by the nonlinear pressure-volume relationship in the CSF system, changes in the monotonous wave in the ICP pulse waveform, with elevated mean ICP, have not yet been clearly explained. There are some doubts that the deformation of ICP pulse is affected by the pressure-volume relationship. We don't believe that deformation of the ICP pulse (except for pulse amplitude) is related to the CSF pressure-volume relationship. In order to identify the part where the deformation of the ICP pulse waveform occurs, we constructed a cerebrovascular physical model without a venous circulation system. We also designed a nonlinear mathematical model simulating the artery, in order to investigate the genesis and morphology of the ICP pulse waveform.

Method

A physical model of the arterial vascular bed and the cranial closed cavity was constructed using a dializer (Fig. 1). A pulsating flow for input into the dializer was generated from a controlled waterflow using an oscillated magnetic valve. The pressure waveform simulated human arterial blood pressure (Fig. 1a). The fluid pressure outside the hollow-fiber in the dializer was measured as ICP. The mean ICP and the arterial terminal pressure were determined by the height of each siphon. A mathematical model was designed using the nonlinear elastance element of the vessel wall and the inertia element of the blood fluid (Fig. 2a). The model equations were numerically integrated on a Macintosh II computer (Apple Computer Inc.), using the 4th order Runge-Kutta-Gill method.

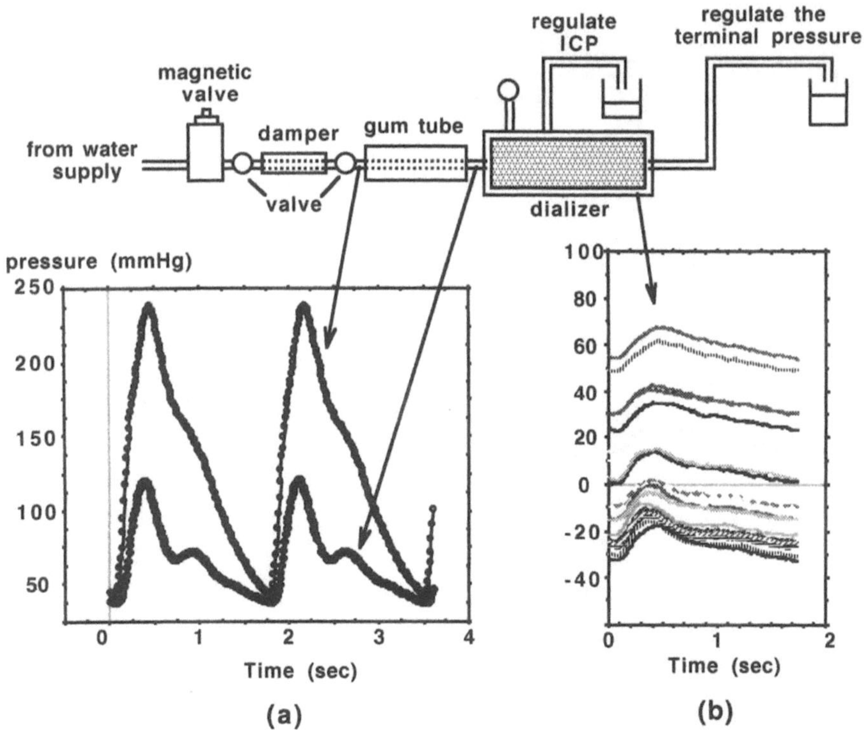

Fig. 1a,b. A physical model of the cerebrospinal fluid system without the venous circulation system. **a** Input pressure waveform into the dializer. **b** The fluid pressure waveform inside the dializer

Results

In the physical model simulation, the fluid pressure waveform inside the dializer was analogous to the human ICP, and the changes in the monotonous pressure pulse were observed with the elevation of ICP (Fig. 1b). But the increase of pressure pulse amplitude was not observed in the human CSF system. The pressure waveform-input into the dializer did not change during the experiment. The same changes in the monotonous pressure pulse wave were computed in the simulation of the mathematical model when the elasticity coefficient of the artery was decreased. Moreover, in the mathematical simulation at the increase of the elasticity coefficient, the artery generated a multi-peak wave when the pressure waves were transmitted through the artery (Fig. 2b).

Conclusion

A wave similar to the human ICP was observed in the physical model. We believe that the model can simulate the cerebrovascular system. The change in

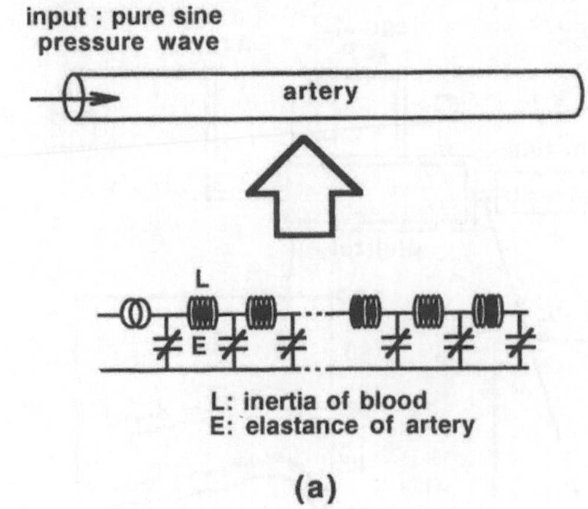

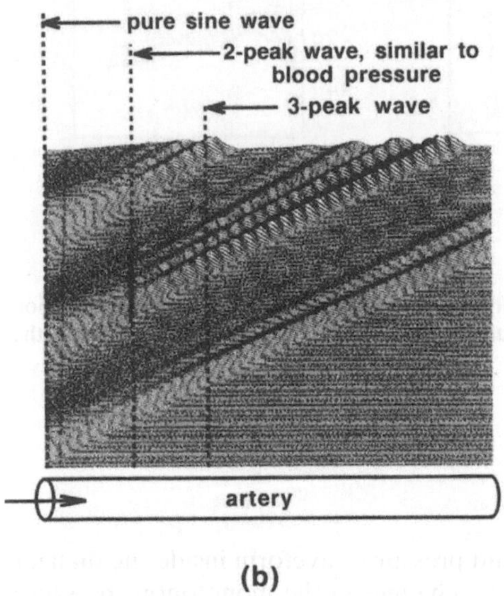

Fig. 2a,b. A mathematical model of the artery and the simulation of the pressure wave. **a** Electrical circuit, analogous to the mathematical model. **b** Simulation of the pressure wave being transmitted in the artery

the monotonous wave, with the elevation of the mean ICP, was observed in the physical model. It is important that the physical model does not include the venous circulation system and does not try to simulate the increase of pressure pulse amplitude. This means that the human arterial circulation system has the ability to change complex waveforms into monotonous waveforms. In the mathematical simulation, it is interesting that the multi-peak waves are generated in the artery when the elasticity coefficient of the artery is increased. This pressure phenomenon is not caused by a resonance of the pressure wave in the vessel but is caused by a dispersion of the wave, in order for large amplitude waves to be transmitted faster than small amplitude waves. We conclude that the change in the ICP pulse waveform, except for the pulse amplitude, occurs within the artery when pressure waves are transmitted in the artery.

References

1. Czosnyka M, Wollk-Laniewski P, Batorski L, Zaworski W (1988) Analysis of Intracranial Pressure Waveform During Infusion Test. Acta Neurochir (Wien) 93:140–145
2. Cardoso ER, Rowan JO, Galbraith S (1983) Analysis of the cerebrospinal fluid pulse wave in intracranial pressure. J Neurosurg 59:817–821
3. Hirai O, Handa H, Ishikawa M (1982) Intracranial pressure pulse waveform: Consideration about its origin and methods to estimating intracranial pressure dynamics. Brain Nerve (Tokyo) 34:1059–65
4. Marmarou A, Shulman K, Rosende RM (1978) A nonlinear analysis of the cerebrospinal fluid system and intracranial pressure dynamics. J Neurosurg 48:332–344
5. Ursino M (1988) A Mathematical Study of human intracranial hydrodynamics. 1: The cerebrospinal fluid pulse pressure. Ann Biomed Eng 16:379–401
6. Ursino M (1988) Mathematical Study of human intracranial hydrodynamics. 2: Simulation of Clinical Tests. Ann Biomed Eng 16:379–401

Computer Analysis of Intracranial Pressure Pulsatility and Blood Flow Shape During Intracranial Hypertension

M. URSINO[1] and M. GIULIONI[2]

[1] Department of Electronics, Computer Science and Systems, Viale Risorgimento 2, I 40136 Bologna, Italy
[2] Regional Hospital, Neurosurgery Division, Via Abbeveratoia, Parma, Italy

Introduction

The CSF pulse pressure is produced by the pulsating changes in cerebral blood volume which occur within a rigid space, i.e. the craniospinal compartment. Therefore, two main factors affect the transmission of cerebrovascular pulsatility on the intracranial pressure, i.e. the storage capacity of the craniospinal system, usually expressed by the pressure-volume relationship [3], and the compliance of the cerebrovascular bed both of which determine the amplitude of the pulsating changes in cerebral blood volume. However, both these factors may be deeply altered by the action of regulatory mechanisms working on the cerebrovascular bed [1, 2, 5]. In particular, Eijndhoven and Avezaat [1] demonstrated that vasodilation, induced either by hypercapnia or by arterial hypotension, causes an increase in the slope of the relationship between the CSF pulse pressure and the mean intracranial pressure level. The opposite effect was observed during arterial hypertension or hypercapnia.

In order to clarify the relationships between cerebrovascular pulsatility, CSF pulse pressure, intracranial compliance and the action of cerebral blood flow regulatory mechanisms, we have developed an original mathematical model of cerebrovascular and CSF dynamics [4, 5].

Method

The model takes into account the following intracranial phenomena: elasticity of the craniospinal compartment, characteristics of the CSF production and reabsorption processes, compliance of the large cerebral veins, collapsability of the last portion of the intracranial venous vascular bed at its entrance into the dural sinuses and action of CBF regulatory mechanisms on the wall of both intracranial arteries and arterioles.

The model allows the pattern of the ICP pulse amplitude and blood flow shape at the level of basal intracranial arteries to be evaluated during intracranial hypertension, and also following on several maneuvers which alter the values of cerebral blood flow and cerebral blood volume (arterial hypotension and hypertension; blood CO_2 alterations; injection of mock CSF fluid into the cranial cavity).

Results and Comments

Figure 1 shows the simulated time pattern of ICP and CBF at the level of basal intracranial arteries during normocapnia ($PCO_2 \simeq 36$ mmHg) in response to a stepwise decrease in the arterial pressure mean value from 100 to 80 mmHg, performed at the instant $t = 4$ s. The simulations have been performed starting from three different initial ICP levels.

Figure 2 shows the time pattern of the same quantities simulated with the model during hypercapnia ($PCO_2 \simeq 55$–60 mmHg).

The results of Figs. 1 and 2 demonstrate that the ICP pulse amplitude is affected both by the mean ICP level and by the intravasal pressure, as well as by the action of cerebrovascular regulatory mechanisms on cerebral vessel walls. In particular, during hypercapnia, the alterations in ICP pulsatility are imputable both to the rise in the mean ICP level (consequent on the cerebral blood volume rise) and to alterations in vascular pulsatility at the level of small arteriolar vessels. As a consequence, the changes in the Gosling pulsatility

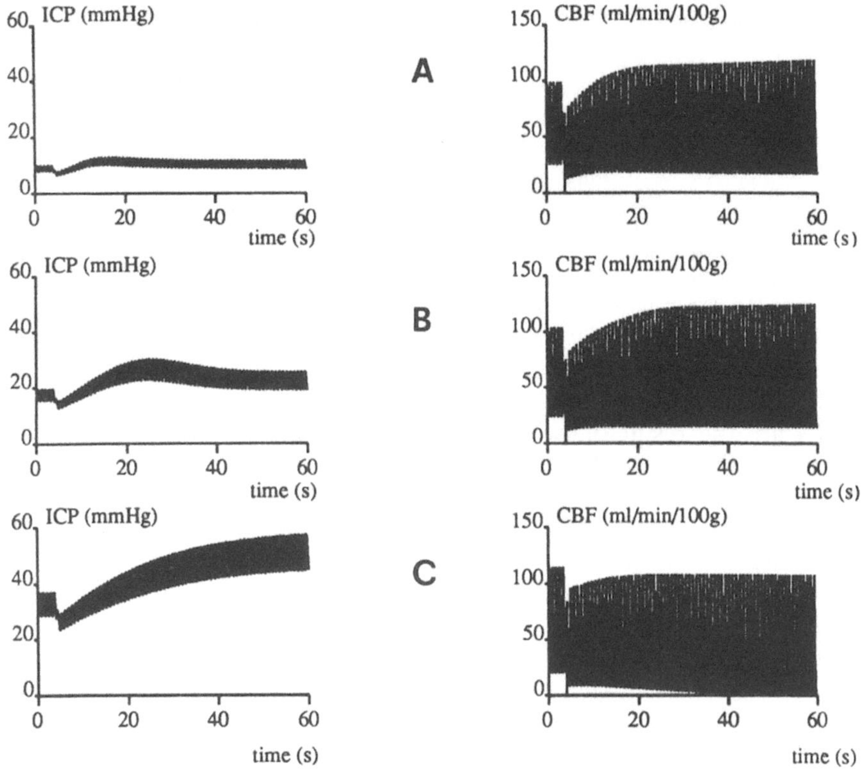

Fig. 1A–C. Time patterns of intracranial pressure and cerebral blood flow per tissue unit weight, simulated with the model in response to a stepwise arterial pressure decrease from 100 to 80 mmHg performed at $t = 4$ s. The simulations have been carried out starting from three different initial ICP levels (cases **A**, **B** and **C**, respectively)

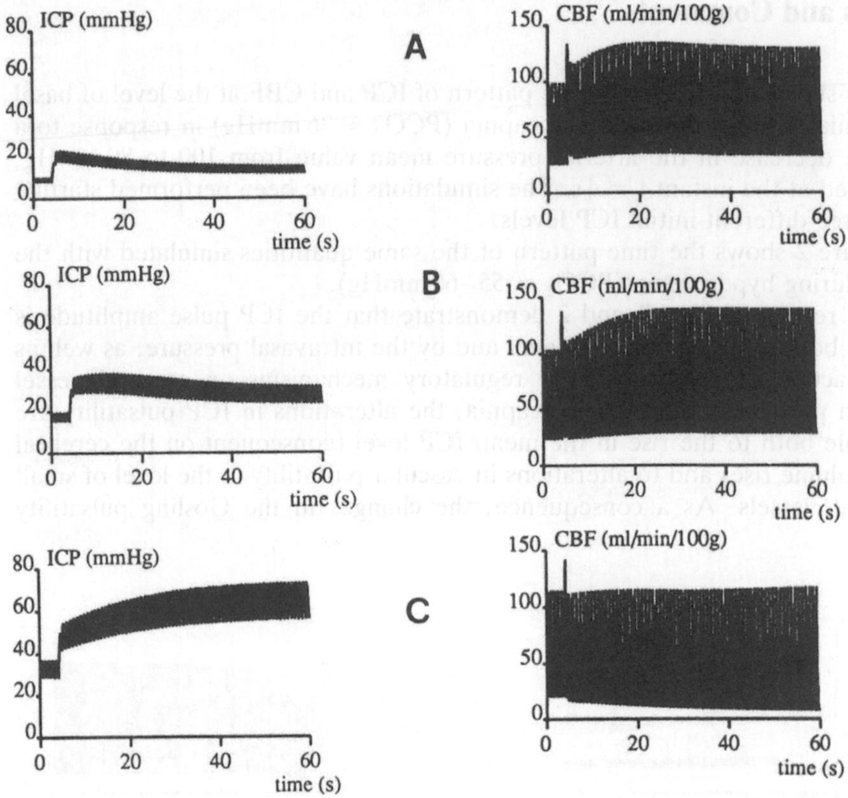

Fig. 2A–C. Time patterns of intracranial pressure and cerebral blood flow per tissue unit weight, simulated with the model in response to an instantaneous arteriolar vasodilation occurring at t = 4 s. This vasodilation is approximately equal to that produced by a change in blood CO_2 from 36 to 55–60 mmHg. The simulations have been carried out starting from three different initial ICP levels (cases **A**, **B** and **C**, respectively)

index are the result of two opposite factors, i.e. the increase in mean CBF level, and the CBF pulse amplitude increase. The latter is especially imputable to a rise in the CBF systolic value. By contrast, during arterial hypotension, also the increase in cerebral basal artery pulsatility becomes relevant, owing to the sharp transmural pressure decrease. In this condition the changes in the CBF mean level are less important (at least within the autoregulatory range) and the Gosling pulsatility index is mainly influenced by changes in CBF pulse amplitude (increase in the systolic value and decrease in the diastolic one).

References

1. Eijndhoven JHM, Avezaat CJJ (1986) Cerebrospinal fluid pulse pressure and the pulsatile variation in cerebral blood volume: an experimental study in dogs. Neurosurgery 19:507–522
2. Giulioni M, Ursino M, Alvisi C (1988) Correlations among intracranial pulsatility, intracranial hemodynamics and transcranial Doppler wave form: literature review and hypothesis for future studies. Neurosurgery 22:807–812

3. Marmarou A, Shulman K, Lamorgese J (1975) Compartmental analysis of compliance and outflow resistance of the cerebrospinal fluid system. J Neurosurg 43:523–534
4. Ursino M (1988) A mathematical study of human intracranial hydrodynamics. Part 1: the cerebrospinal fluid pulse pressure. Ann Biomed Eng 16:379–401
5. Ursino M, Di Giammarco P (1991) A mathematical model of the relationship between cerebral blood volume and intracranial pressure changes: the generation of plateau waves. Ann Biomed Eng 19:15–42

Influence of Intracranial Components on Epidural Pulse Pressure

M. Mase, H. Nagai, Y. Ueda, T. Matsumoto, and K. Kamiya

Department of Neurosurgery, Nagoya City University Medical School, 1-Kawasumi, Mizuho-cho, Mizuho-ku, Nagoya 467, Japan

Introduction

It is well known that the pulse pressure (PP) of the intracranial pressure pulse wave increases with rising intracranial pressure (ICP). However, the PP at the same ICP value is not always identical in various intracranial pathologies. The present study was performed to clarify the changes of PP with alterations in intracranial components (water content of brain tissue, blood and cerebrospinal fluid).

Materials and Methods

Twenty-two adult mongrel dogs of both sexes, weighing from 8 to 12 kg, were included in this study. Anesthesia was induced by intravenous injection of thiopental sodium (10 mg/kg body weight) and maintained with intermittent intramuscular injection of ketamine hydrochloride (10 mg/kg). After endotracheal intubation, the dogs were mechanically ventilated. The right femoral vein was cannulated to paralyze the animals by continuous infusion of alcuronium chloride (0.3 mg/kg/hr) and saline. The right femoral artery was cannulated and connected to a pressure transducer to monitor the arterial blood pressure (ABP). Arterial blood was sampled intermittently; $PaCO_2$ (35 ± 3 mmHg) and PaO_2 (>100 mmHg) were maintained within physiological limits by ventilator adjustment. Body temperature was maintained at approximately 37°C using a heat pad.

The epidural pressure (EDP) pulse wave was measured with a Toyota pressure transducer which was placed epidurally through a burr hole in the right parietal region. EDP and ABP pulse waves were recorded by a data recorder. While recording the data, the endotracheal pressure was equalized with the outside air pressure by removing the respirator for 5 seconds, in order to prevent respiratory effect on EDP. The data from 2 to 4 seconds after the removal were sampled and analyzed with a minicomputer. The interval between each sampling of data was more than 5 minutes to keep arterial blood gases within normal limits. The mean EDP and the mean ABP were calculated by adding one third of the pulse pressure to the diastolic pressure. The pulse pressure (PP) of EDP pulse wave was measured from the bottom to the highest peak of the pulse wave. The mean PP was calculated by averaging 20 PP readings. EDP and PP were evaluated statistically with a two-tailed unpaired t-test in the following groups.

Control Group

ICP was elevated by increasing the volume of cerebrospinal fluid (CSF) ($n = 5$). A 21-gauge needle was introduced percutaneously into the cisterna magna and normal saline was slowly injected.

Edema Group

ICP was elevated by ischemic brain edema ($n = 11$). Ischemia was induced by electro-coagulation of the right anterior cerebral artery and by clipping the right middle cerebral artery and right internal carotid artery transorbitally. The brain was reperfused for 6 hours after 2 hours of ischemia. The orbit was sealed with bone cement to prevent CSF leakage. Water content of the brain was measured by the wet-dry weight method after sacrifice.

Hypercapnia Group

ICP was elevated by increasing the cerebral blood volume (CBV) in the state of hypercapnia ($n = 6$). Hypercapnia was produced by reducing the tidal volume of the respirator.

Results

Water Content

Water content of the ischemic hemisphere (78.31 ± 1.49%) tended to be larger than that of the intact hemisphere (77.30 ± 1.11%, mean ± SD, $p < 0.09$).

$PaCO_2$

$PaCO_2$ of the hypercapnia group (53.6 ± 5.7 mmHg) was higher than that of the other groups ($p < 0.0001$). There was no significant difference in $PaCO_2$ between the edema group (35.2 ± 1.1 mmHg) and the control group (34.7 ± 0.7 mmHg, mean ± SD).

Arterial Blood Pressure (ABP) and Heart Rate (HR)

There was no significant difference in all groups in mean ABP and the ABP pulse amplitude. HR of the hypercapnia group at about 15 to 30 mmHg of mean EDP tended to be smaller than that of the other groups at the same EDP.

EDP and EDP Pulse Pressure (PP)

PP increased linearly with rising EDP in all groups when EDP was from about 10 to 35 mmHg. PP in the edema group was smaller, and PP in the hypercapnia group larger, than PP in the control group at the same EDP value (Fig. 1). The slope of the regression equation of EDP and PP in the edema group (0.061 ± 0.030) was smaller ($p < 0.01$), and that in the hypercapnia group (0.334 ± 0.098) larger ($p < 0.001$), than that in the control group (0.107 ± 0.015, mean ± SD).

Discussion

The relationship between ICP and PP is determined by many factors, such as intracranial elasticity, the compensatory faculty of the craniospinal system, cerebrovascular tonicity, the magnitude of transient increase in CBV, the

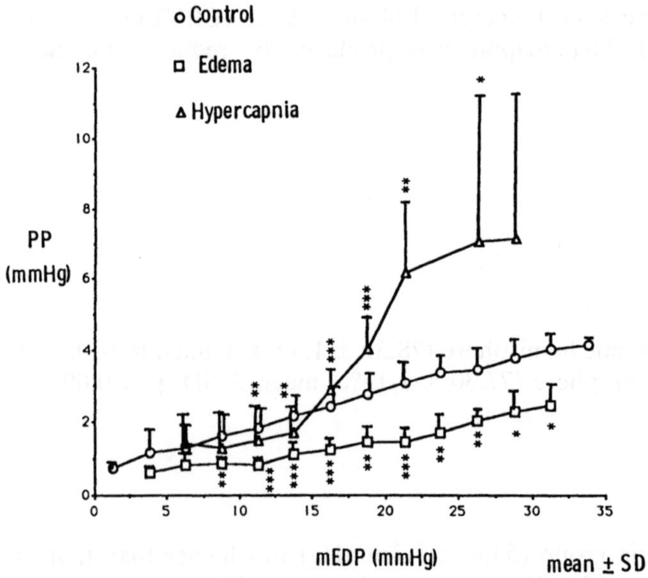

Fig. 1. Pulse pressure (PP) of epidural pressure (EDP) increased with rising mean epidural pressure (mEDP), and PP in the edema group was smaller, and PP in the hypercapnia group larger, than PP in the control group at the same EDP value. *$p < 0.05$, **$p < 0.005$, ***$p < 0.0005$

resistance of venous and CSF outflow from cranium, etc. However, unless there are marked cardiovascular disorders, the ICP pulse wave, especially the PP, closely correlates with the elasticity of the craniospinal system, provided the ICP is under 30 mmHg [5]. Therefore, the increase of PP with rising EDP in the control group correlates with changes of the elastance of the craniospinal cavity by cisternal saline injection.

In the present study, PP in the hypercapnia group was larger than that in the control group at the same EDP, which corresponds to many reports. Cerebral arteriolar vasodilation and increase of the pulsatile change of CBV explain the larger PP in the hypercapnia group [2].

It became apparent that PP in the edema group was smaller than that in the control group at the same EDP value. We previously reported two possibilities to account for the reduced PP in brain edema [4]. The first is decreased volume of the pulsatile vascular bed because of brain edema, which increases tissue pressure, resulting in a mechanical compression of the cerebral vascular bed and reduced cerebral blood flow (CBF) [3].

The second possibility is the damping of ICP pulse transmission by brain edema. In experimental cold injury of the brain, the Young modulus of slightly edematous brain and central necrotic tissue is smaller than that of normal brain tissue [1]. The energy of ICP pulsation may be absorbed by distortion, resulting in smaller PP.

The volume of intracranial components (brain, CSF and CBV) alters in various intracranial conditions. Brain edema indicates an increase in water content of the brain tissue. In summary, PP in the state of increased water content of the brain is smaller, and PP in the state of increased CBV larger, than PP in the state of increased CSF volume, and so are the slopes of the corresponding regression equations. We would like to conclude that PP is easily affected even at the same ICP value with different intracranial components.

It may be impossible to speculate on intracranial pathologies merely by the absolute value of PP, because the ICP pulse wave is affected by many factors. However, by measuring ICP continuously, we may to some extent be able to infer what changes might be taking place intracranially from the changes in PP and the slope of the regression equation.

References

1. Aoyagi N, Masuzawa H, Sano K, et al. (1980) Compliance of the brain. Brain and Nerve 32:47–56
2. Avezaat CJJ, van Eijndhoven JHM, Wyper DJ (1980) Effects of hypercapnia and arterial hypotension and hypertension on cerebrospinal fluid pulse pressure and intracranial volume-pressure relationships. J Neurol Neurosurg Psychiat 42:222–234
3. Iannotti F, Hoff JT, Schielke GP (1985) Brain tissue pressure in focal cerebral ischemia. J Neurosurg 62:83–89
4. Mase M (1990) Changes in epidural pulse pressure in brain oedema following experimental focal ischaemia. Acta Neurochir, Suppl 51:391–393
5. Matsumoto T, Nagai H, Kasuga Y, et al. (1986) Changes in intracranial pressure (ICP) pulse wave following hydrocephalus. Acta Neurochir (Wien) 82:50–56

Systolic Cerebral Blood Inflow (SCBI) as a CBF-Index Estimated with ICP Wave-Change in CBF and SCBI During Mannitol Infusion

A. Wachi, K. Sato, O. Tsuji, K. Bandoh, and M. Ito

Department of Neurosurgery, Juntendo University, Tokyo, Japan

Introduction

The ICP wave is closely related to the pulsatile intracranial blood flow. The objectives of this study are:

1. to estimate the pulsatile inflow by analyzing pulse wave and pressure-volume relationship in an experimental model using a pulsatile pump and to compare the Estimated Inflow Volume with the Actual Inflow Volume in this system,
2. to compare systolic cerebral blood inflow (SCBI) with cortical CBF during mannitol infusion in patients with subarachnoid hemorrhage.

Materials and Methods

Model Experiment

A model system for evaluating pressure-volume relationship, pulse waves and flow volume was established. A rigid container (500 ml) representing the human cranial cavity was connected to another bottle (500 ml) with a buffering capacity which could be changed by increasing or decreasing the air volume. A scaled cylinder accumulates the actual flow volume through the system. A motorized pump generates a pulsatile flow and the pulse pressures are recorded with a transducer (P50, Gould INC.) and a strip-chart recorder (Nihon Koden, INC).

Stepwise bolus injections with 0.1 ml of saline were performed to determine the pressure-volume relationship within this system. If one systolic inflow volume in one cycle is regarded as one bolus volume injection for calculation of the pressure-volume relationship, the inflow volume can be estimated when the pressure-volume relationship is given. Thus, Estimated Inflow Volume can be expressed as follows:

$$EIV = K \times (\text{pulse amplitude}) \times (\text{pulse rate})$$

(EIV: Estimated Inflow Volume, K: coefficient of pressure-volume relationship).

Clinical Study

The CSF pulse wave was monitored through a ventricular catheter with a conventional transducer (P50, Gould INC.) in 5 patients with aneurysmal subarachnoid hemorrhage. Frontal cortical CBF was also continuously recorded by a thermo-gradient CBF meter (Nihon Koden Co). After bolus manipulation test for calculation of the Pressure-Volume Index [1], the ICP, pulse amplitude and pulse rate were recorded. Assuming that the pressure-volume curve is constant during the period of data acquisition, SCBI (ml/min) can be expressed as follows:

$$\text{SCBI (ml/min)} = \text{PVI} * \sum_{n=1}^{HR} [\log(Pn/Pn - 1)]$$

(HR: heart rate, Pn: sequential number of each peak of pulse waves from the first wave peak to the last, Pn − 1: sequential number of each bottom pressure of the pulse waves from the first wave bottom to the last.

Mannitol, 1.5–2.0 g/kg, was administered to the patients when the ICP was above 25 mmHg for at least 3 minutes. Three sequential values of SCBI (pre-administration, 30 and 120 minutes after mannitol infusion) were calculated when mannitol was administered.

Results

Model Experiment

The pressure-volume relationship of this system was not exponential, but linear. The Estimated Inflow Volume (EIV) was significantly ($p < 0.99$), linearly correlated with the Actual Flow Volume (AFV). In high buffering status, the relationship was EIV = 3.67 × AFV − 1.13, and in low buffering status: EIV = 0.91 × AFV − 3.07. Therefore, the Estimated Inflow Volume was greater than the Actual Flow Volume when the buffering capacity was high.

Clinical Studies

The relationship between SCBI and CBF was exponential ($CBF = 28.8 \times 10^{1.06e\text{-}3SCBI}$) and it was statistically significant ($r = 0.69$, $p < 0.02$) in 12 studies (Fig. 1). The average CBF prior to mannitol infusion was 50.1 ± 12.1 ml/min/100 g, it increased to 70.9 ± 13.8 ($p < 0.05$) 30 minutes after mannitol, and decreased to 49.3 ± 7.0 ml/min/100 g (N.S.) after 120 minutes. SCBI was 213 ± 27 ml/min, it increased to 387 ± 56 ($p < 0.001$) 30 minutes after mannitol and returned to 220 ± 21 ml/min (N.S.) after 120 minutes.

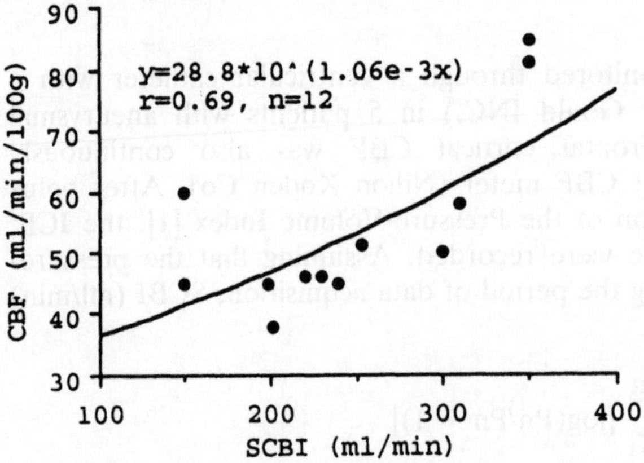

Fig. 1. Correlation between SCBI and CBF was exponential (CBF = $28.8 \times 10^{1.06e\text{-}3SCBI}$) and it was statistically significant ($r = 0.69$, $n = 12$, $p < 0.02$)

Discussion

It has already been described that relative changes of CBF can be estimated by relative changes of ICP pulse wave and pressure-volume relationship during vasospasm in patients with subarachnoid hemorrhage due to ruptured cerebral aneurysm [2]. However, it was found that the percent change of CBF and SCBI were not always equal. It is speculated that two factors are responsible for this dissociation in percent change of CBF and SCBI. First, the results of our physical model indicate that the change in pressure buffering capacity may strongly influence the Estimated Inflow Volume, which is larger than the Actual Flow Volume when the buffering capacity is high. Since mannitol has been reported to increase CBF and the pressure buffering capacity [3, 4], the results of the model experiment may account for the disagreement in the percent change between CBF and SCBI during mannitol infusion.

Secondly, the flow character is another factor which may attribute to this dissociation. It is expected that non-pulsatile flow yields a lower SCBI than pulsatile flow, even if the two flow rates are equal. This can be easily explained by the equation of SCBI which includes a factor of pulse amplitude. We conclude that, clinically, SCBI is not only a valuable index of CBF, but also an index indicating whether the flow is pulsatile or not.

References

1. Marmarou A (1973) A theoretical model and experimental evaluation of the cerebrospinal fluid system (Thesis). Drexel University
2. Wachi A, Ito M, Sato K, Tsuji O, et al. (1990) Change in Systolic Cerebral Blood estimated by the ICP waves in patients with vasospasm. In: Sano K, Takakura K, Kassel NF, Sasaki T (eds) Cerebral Vasospasm, University of Tokyo Press, pp 46–49

3. Johnston IH, Harper AM (1973) The effect of mannitol on CBF. An experimental study. J Neurosurg 38:461–471
4. Miller JD, Leech P (1978) Assessing the effects of mannitol and steroid therapy on intracranial volume pressure relationship. J Neurosurg 43:274–281

Dynamic Response of Subdural Screw Bolt for Intracranial Pressure Measuring

A. BIESTRO[1], C. KADOWAKI[2], T. SHIOGAI[2], M. NUMOTO[2], and K. TAKEUCHI[2]

[1] Center of Intensive Treatment, Hospital de Clínicas of Montevideo, CP 11600 Urugay
[2] Department of Neurosurgery, Kyorin University, Medical School, Mitaka City, Tokyo, Japan

Introduction

The subdural screw bolt, with all its variations [1, 2, 3], remains a common method for ICP monitoring in clinical practice and experimental studies [2, 4, 5, 6]. Since the first report by Vries et al. [1], many authors have tried to improve the static performance of this device. When the lumen is occluded by brain tissue, or a blood clot, the ICP tends to be underestimated when the pressure is high [7]. Regardless of the occlussion and the resulting falsely low pressure reading, the CSF pulsations are preserved. Some workers have produced modified versions of the original screw [2, 3]. Dearden et al. [2] and Shields et al. [9] have designed infusion and flush techniques to solve this problem.

Recently, attention has been paid to the dynamic properties of ICP monitoring devices, because of increasing interest in spectral analysis of the ICP pulse wave [10]. The dynamic response of the subdural screw bolt has not been studied yet. This paper deals with in-vitro frequency analysis of the subdural screw in two different ways.

Materials and Methods

A disposable Philly Bolt (Philadelphia Med. Specialities, Inc., Laurel Spring, NJ. U.S.A., size: 4,5 cm length and 2.9 mm internal diameter) and a disposable transducer, type Gould DT 12 (Viggo-Spectrament Co., Oxnard, Calif., U.S.A.) were used. The device was tested in two different ways: 1. the bolt connected to the transducer by means of a non-compliant tubing (length: 50 cm and internal diameter: 2.5 mm) and a three-way stopcock, as is the daily practice in most centers, and 2. the bolt connected directly to the transducer. Both settings were tested in the frequency range of 1 Hz to 32 Hz. For the purpose of this study a special mechanical pump was used, made at our laboratory, to generate a constant pressure within the range of 1–32 Hz.

Results

Figure 1 shows the results for the system with the tubing interposed between bolt and transducer. The frequency response at 8 Hz is 160% and gradually decreases above 15 Hz until 32 Hz where it is 20%. Figure 2 shows the results of the direct coupling test. The response is flat until 26 Hz and increases up to 160% at 32 Hz.

Discussion

In spite of the problems with regard to the static response, the subdural screw continues to be widely used for ICP monitoring. The reasons are that the device is very easy to introduce and to remove, is durable and economical. ICP pulse wave spectral analysis seems to be a promising method in clinical ICP monitoring. However, this method is meaningless if the ICP data are not correctly acquired. A proper system for ICP waveform analysis should include

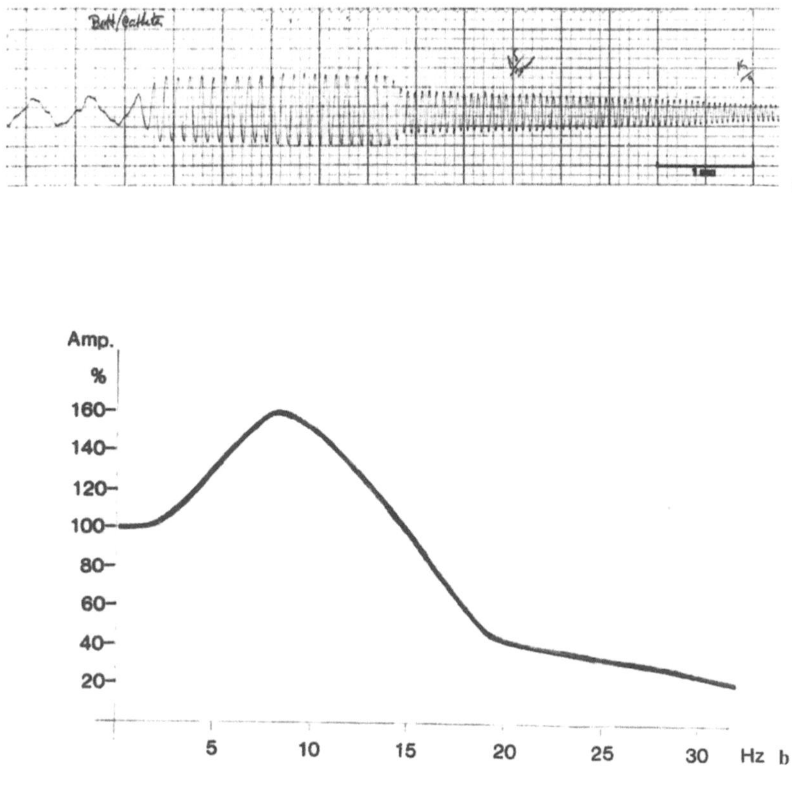

Fig. 1a,b. Screw bolt with tubing (50 cm). **a)** Polygraphic recording. Note variable response. **b)** Plot of amplitude versus frequency. Note considerable distortion below 20 Hz

a

b

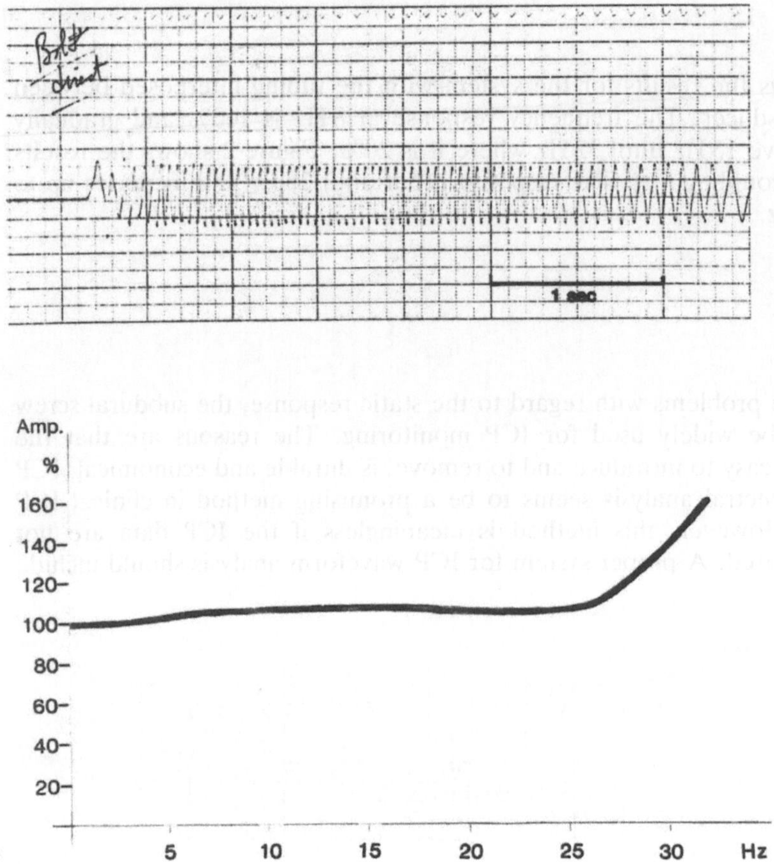

Fig. 2a,b. Screw bolt direct. **a** Polygraphic recording. **b** Plot of amplitude versus frequency. Note uniform response until 26 Hz

accurate frequency responses up to 20 Hz at least, so that the 5th harmonic of the pulse wave is included. It has been pointed out that the fluid filled tubing systems are inadequate for ICP pulse analysis due to the considerable distortion of the waveform in the frequency range of the system [10]. In this study we have shown that a subdural screw bolt directly connected to a disposable transducer displays uniform responses up to 26 Hz. We believe that the rigid structure, the wide diameter and the short length of the connecting channel are the most likely explanations for the good response. Another advantage of this system is that it eliminates the necessity to readjust the zero level when the position of the patient is changed.

References

1. Vries JK, Becker DP, Young HF (1973) A subarachnoid screw for monitoring intracranial pressure. Technical note. J Neurosurg 39:416–419
2. Dearden NM, McDowall DG, Gibson RM (1984) Assessment of Leeds device for monitoring intracranial pressure. J Neurosurg 60:123–129
3. Landy HJ, Villanueva PH (1984) An improved subarachnoid screw for pressure monitoring. Technical note. J Neurosurg 61:606–608
4. Moss E, Gibson JS, McDowall DG, et al. (1983) Intensive management of severe head injuries. A scheme of intensive management of severe head injuries. Anaesthesia 38:214–225
5. Broaddus WC, Pendleton GA, Delashaw JB, et al. (1989) Differential intracranial pressure recordings in patients with dual ipsilateral monitors. In: Hoff JT, Betz AL (eds) Intracranial Pressure VII. Springer, Berlin Heidelberg New York London Paris Tokyo Hong Kong, pp 41–44
6. Miller J, Peeler DF, et al. (1987) Supratentorial pressures. Part I. Differential pressures. Neurol Res 9:193–197
7. Mendelow AD, Rowan JO, Murray et al. (1983) A clinical comparison of subdural pressure measurement with ventricular pressure. J Neurosurg 58:45–50
8. Miller JD (1989) Measuring ICP in patients. Its value now and in the future? In: Hoff JT, Betz AL (eds) Intracranial pressure VII. Springer, Berlin Heidelberg New York London Paris Tokyo Hong Kong, pp 5–15
9. Shields GB, Garretson HD, et al. (1983) Accurate intracranial pressure monitoring. In: Ishii S, Nagai H, Brock M (eds) Intracranial Pressure V. Springer, Berlin Heidelberg New York Tokyo, pp 124–126
10. Gaab MR, Heissler HE, Ehrart K (1989) Physical characteristics of various methods for measuring ICP. In: Hoff JT, Betz AL (eds) Intracranial pressure VII, Springer, Berlin Heidelberg New York London Paris Tokyo Hong Kong, pp 16–21

Analysis of Periodic Waveforms of Brain Element Oscillations

E.A. BUNT[1] and K. LEWER ALLEN[2]

[1] Rand Afrikaans University, Johannesburg, South Africa
[2] Formerly Head of Department of Neurosurgery, University of the Witwatersrand, Johannesburg, South Africa

Introduction

For the complete analysis of the complex waveforms (assumed sinusoidal) apparent from a CAT scan investigation of brain movement and density [1, 2] and in brain pressure and compliance data revealed by the infusion technique [3], where more than one waveform may be present, a straightforward analytical procedure involving the determination of frequencies, amplitudes and phase differences is required. The frequency determination method set forth by Worthing and Geffner [4] is extremely time-consuming and for preference requires an advance estimate of the frequencies present. The method set forth here is direct; it relies on numerical procedures readily available in the STATGRAPHICS computer routine [5], and leads to the determination of frequency, amplitude and phase differences of as many sinusoidal waveforms as may be identified. The procedure facilitates testing the hypothesis of periodicity underlying natural rhythms.

Procedure

Assuming natural brain periodic waveforms for the variation of, for example, compliance, pressure, geometry (size) or parenchymal density, to be sinusoidal, we have equations of the form

$$a_1 \sin(\omega_1 t + \phi_1) + a_2 \sin(\omega_2 t + \phi_2) + a_3 \sin(\omega_3 t + \phi_3) + \ldots = A.$$

This involves unknown amplitudes a, unknown values of ω (where $\omega = 2\pi T$, T being a wave period), and unknown phase angles ϕ. Available data were examined by a STATGRAPHICS program to provide T_1, T_2, $T_3 \ldots$ and the necessary values of A were selected from the data to solve for the remaining unknowns a_1, a_2, $a_3, \ldots$ and ϕ_1, ϕ_2, ϕ_3. The resulting composite equation may then be used to synthesise a waveform for comparison with the original waveform.

A check of this procedure is shown in Fig. 1. The equation (Worthing and Geffner 1959) corresppronding to the original waveform illustrated in Fig. 1a is

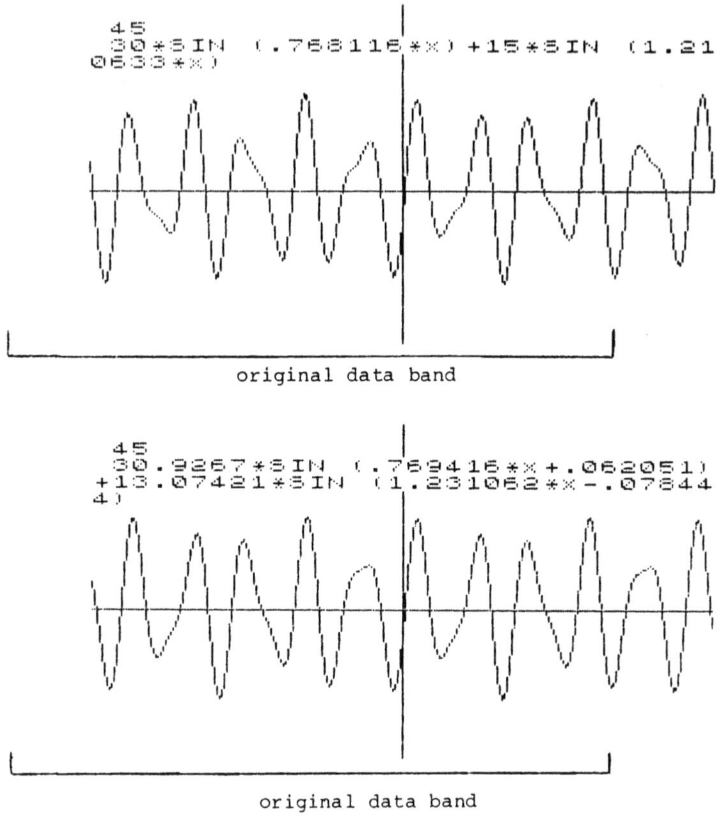

a

b

Fig. 1a,b. Check of method, **a** Original waveform, **b** synthesised waveform

$$f(t) = 100 \sin (2\pi t/8.18 - 2°) + 50 \sin (2\pi t/5.19 - 2°)$$

Here the amplitudes are respectively 100 and 50; the periods are 8.18 and 5.19 s and the phase angles are both −2°. Using the method devised, the deduced equation is

$$f(t) = 103.089 \sin (2\pi t/8.166 = 3.555°) + 43.581 \sin (2\pi t/5.104 - 4.94°)$$

This is considered satisfactory.

Analysis of Brain Parameter Data

Evidence of wave motion in parenchymal density and ventricular distance [1, 2] led to 19 cases of pressure and (derived) compliance data obtained by the infusion method also being examined for periodicity. In contrast to the combination of pure sinusoidal waves illustrated in the check of the method of analysis illustrated above, it was not expected that biologically derived data would yield such regular waveforms in view of the long duration (of the order of 1/2 h) of many of the clinical investigations – during which time rhythms

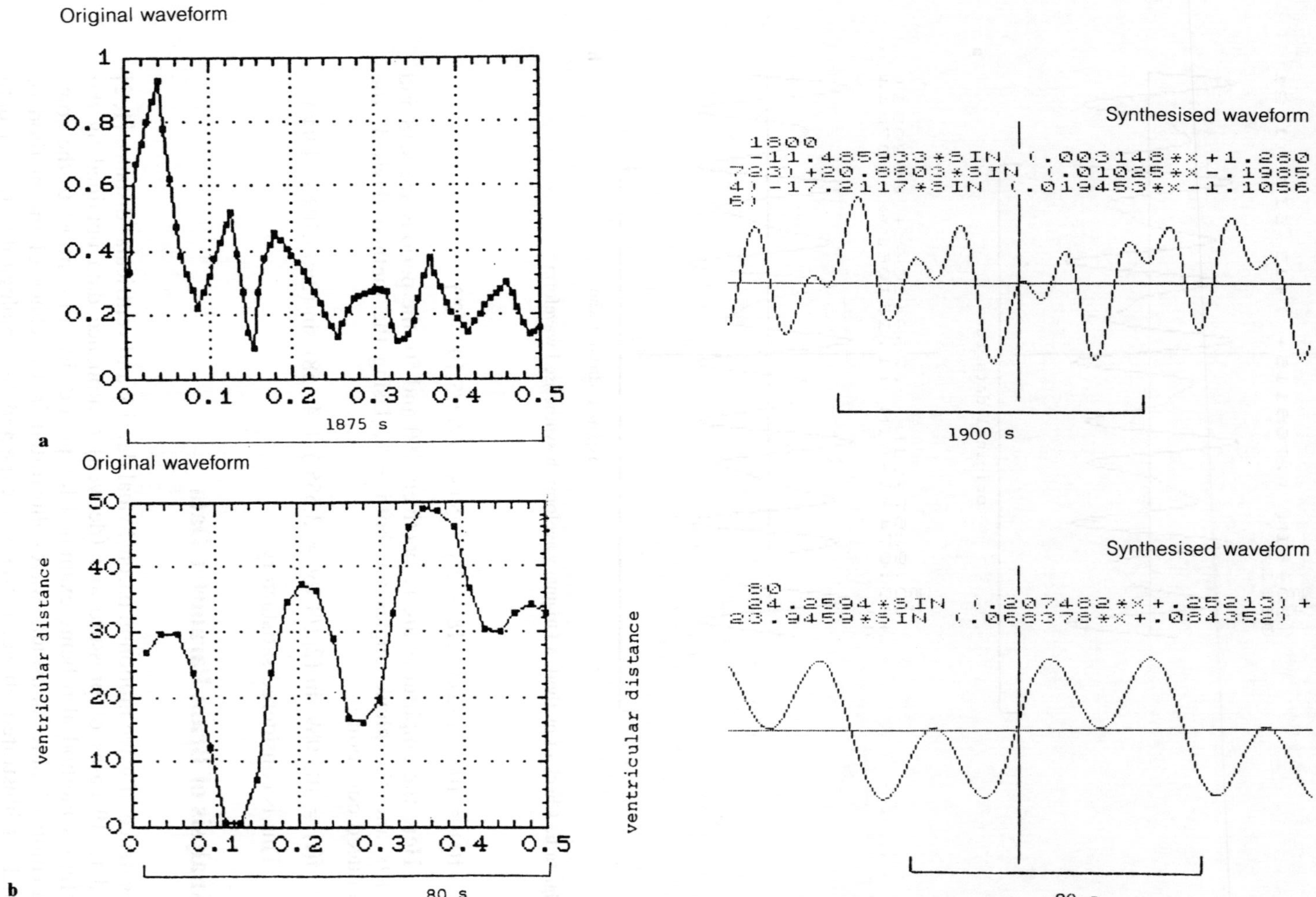

Fig. 2a,b. Applications of method. **a** Waveforms for compliance, **b** waveforms for ventricular distance could change appreciably. (However, short "runs" of up to 2 min in duration typical of the density and ventricular distance data obtained from repeated CAT scans could only be less than satisfactory for purposes of periodographic analysis.)

The compliance wave pattern shown in Fig. 2a is that of a near-normal patient, with wave periods of 1996, 613 and 323 s. The synthesised wave only shows rough agreement in the main repetition rate. The ventricular distance wave motion shown in Fig. 2b was deduced from a series of radiographs of a normal subject aged 22 years.

Conclusion

A mathematical technique devised to analyse data containing non-harmonic periodic functions (supposed sinusoidal) has been employed to analyse experimental brain data involving the parameters of pressure, compliance, ventricular distance and parenchymal density to give frequencies, amplitudes and phase angles.

The results show that the technique is more successful for analysing and subsequently synthesising long "runs" (but these results may be affected by frequency variations within the run). Data from sequential CAT scans – where only a few data points were necessarily available – were least successful from the point of view of agreement between analysis and subsequent reconstruction of waveforms. However, the method is suitable for a wide range of applications.

Summary

A method of analysing periodicity data such as that representing brain pressure, compliance, geometrical variations or parenchymal density to provide equations having amplitude, frequency and phase components is given, together with examples of applications.

References

1. Allen KL, Bunt EA (1979) Computerised tomography study of human brain movement, Paper 82.1, Combined Meeting of XII International Conference on Medical and Biological Engineering and V International Conference of Medical Physics, Jerusalem
2. Allen KL, Bunt EA (1985) Rhythmic brain movement and density variations shown by rapid sequential CT scanning in the human subject. In: Miller JD, Teasdale GM, Rowan JO, Galbraith SL, Mendelow AD (eds) Intracranial Pressure VI. Springer, Berlin Heidelberg New York Tokyo
3. Allen KL, Bunt EA (1988) Slow oscillation of compliance and pressure rate in the naturally closed cranio-spinal system. In: Hoff JT, Betz AL (eds) Intracranial Pressure VII. Springer, Berlin Heidelberg New York London Paris Tokyo Hong Kong
4. Worthing AG, Geffner J (1959) Treatment of Experimental Data, New York, Wiley, p 294
5. STATGRAPHICS, STSC Inc., 2115 E Jefferson St, Rockville, MD 20852, USA

Cyclic CSF Pressure Waves Causally Relate to Systemic Arterial Blood Pressure

M.J. Rosner

University of Alabama at Birmingham, USA

Introduction

We have previously observed CSF pressure waves to be a function of unstable cerebral perfusion pressure (CPP) interacting with intracranial hypertension. This interaction has required intact autoregulation in order to describe the findings which we have reported. In developing the vasodilatory cascade model of ICP pressure wave generation, it became clear that any stimulus capable of decrementing CPP would lead to the generation of a CSF pressure wave and activation of the cascade model. However, when cyclic CSF pressure waves occurred, we suspected that the only etiology was likely to be variations in the systemic arterial blood pressure.

In approaching this problem, we found it necessary to define a model which allowed definition of exactly what was meant by a CSF pressure wave in order to allow quantification. Our observations had also suggested that the so called "A" and "B" waves would be qualitatively similar if not identical.

Hypotheses

A. A model could be defined to describe both "A" and "B" CSF pressure waves.
B. "A" and "B" waves would be qualitatively identical.
C. Cyclic "A" and "B" waves would always relate to SABP change.
D. "A" and "B" waves would differ primarily in the rate at which SABP changes evolved.

Methods

Analysis of 50 ICP recordings primarily representing traces derived from head injury patients but including brain tumor and other diagnoses associated with intracranial hypertension was carried out. These recordings involved the simultaneous recording of systemic arterial blood pressure, intracranial pressure (frontal ventriculostomy in all cases), and the simultaneous calculation and display of cerebral perfusion pressure. Most recordings were carried out in patients pharmacologically paralyzed with stable $PaCO_2$.

The points of analysis were defined as

A: High CPP: Baseline value
B: The next lowest ICP point
C: The next lowest CPP
D: The next highest ICP
E: The next highest SABP
F: The highest CPP

At point A, the time was set arbitrarily to zero. The values of SABP, ICP and CPP were recorded. The time at which point B occurred was then recorded, again with recording of SABP, ICP and CPP. Similarly, all through the next four points through a total of six, we recorded the time at which the defining event occurred. Previous work suggested that lowest SABP and lowest CPP usually occurred together though lowest CPP was the better defining event.

The waves were additionally classified as being either of the "A" or "B" wave type. This information was then entered into a statistical software package (Systat). Multiple statistical analyses were carried out including analysis of variance of differences between the types of waves.

Results

Table 1 lists the pressure values and times at which each event occurred for "B" waves. Table 2 gives similar information for "A" or plateau waves. Both plateau and "B" waves were well described.

The increment from time A to time B was associated with a decrement in systemic arterial blood pressure accompanied by a decrement in intracranial pressure. The latter reduction in ICP was inadequate to neutralize the SABP fall and a net reduction in CPP occurred.

From point B to point C, SABP stabilized with only minimal decrement and, in some cases, a slight increment. However, this was inadequate to reverse the decrement in CPP which continued to fall substantially through this

Table 1. "B" waves

Condition	Point	SABP ± SD (mmHg)		ICP ± SD (mmHg)		CPP ± SD (mmHg)		TIME ± SD (secs)	
High CPP: Baseline	A	116	16	33	10	83	12	000	00
Next ICP Low	B	103	16	28	8	75	12	19	29
Next CPP Low	C	100	14	41	10	59	11	57	47
Next ICP High	D	117	15	49	11	68	11	63	48
Next SABP High	E	122	16	43	12	79	15	73	52
Next CPP High	F	118	16	32	10	86	13	104	85

Table 2. Plateau wave (X ± SD)

Condition	Point	SABP ± SD (mmHg)	ICP ± SD (mmHg)	CPP ± SD (mmHg)	TIME ± SD (secs)
CPP High: Baseline	A	115 ± 11	26 ± 8.5	90 ± 9.8	0 ± 0
Next ICP Low	B	102 ± 14	25 ± 6.2	77 ± 14	160 ± 150
Next CPP Low	C	99 ± 12	37 ± 11	62 ± 15	670 ± 400
Next ICP High	D	108 ± 14	42 ± 15	66 ± 15	700 ± 390
Next SABP High	E	121 ± 10	36 ± 16	85 ± 18	780 ± 460
Next CPP High	F	116 ± 11	25 ± 8.5	91 ± 12	835 ± 450

period of time. ICP rose and accounted for most of the CPP decrement. At point C, a sharp increment in SABP occurred which began to restore CPP. ICP rose instantly (zero latency) but not enough to decrement or hold down the CPP. At point D, the blood pressure rise continued but more slowly. The ICP rise ceased and began to decrement and the combination of both increased CPP further.

At point E, the blood pressure stabilized or began to decrement slightly; primarily because of continued reduction in ICP, and CPP continued to increase slowly toward baseline values.

This same pattern occurred in plateau waves. Analysis of variance suggested the differences between "B" and plateau waves were in the initial ICP. "B" wave initial ICP was 33 vs. 26 mmHg ($p = 0.012$) for the plateau wave. The initial CPP for the "B" wave was 83 mmHg vs. 90 mmHg for the plateau wave ($p = 0.071$). The other pressure difference was the greater increase in the blood pressure/ischemic response for the "B" wave. Both points occurred at about the same SABP/CPP (100 ± 2.4 vs. 99.2 ± 3.0 mmHg SABP; 59 ± 1.9 vs. 62 ± 3.6 mmHg CPP) but then increased to 117 ± 2.5 mmHg for the "B" wave vs. 108 ± 3.3 for the plateau wave ($p = 0.048$).

Most consistently however, were the time course differences between the "B" and "A" wave. These were 3 to 10 times longer between each point for the plateau vs. the "B" wave ($p \ll 0.001$).

Discussion

We feel that this analysis is consistent with the concept that the same qualitative set of points defined in terms of SABP, ICP, or CPP can be used to describe both "A" and "B" waves. The analysis suggests that the waves are qualitatively identical, differing primarily in the rate at which these changes evolved. Plateau wave changes evolve much more slowly than "B" waves.

Further analysis suggests that from point A to B, systemic arterial blood pressure is slowly drifting downward or decrementing. Unpublished results from our laboratory suggest that this is due to gradually decreasing catecholamine levels and decreasing vasoconstrictor tone. As a result, CPP falls to low levels. Because the rate of fall is great in many circumstances, the ICP passively decrements through this phase. Point B to C can be considered a vasodilator cascade phase where the SABP stabilizes, the ICP, however, responds to the low CPP with an active increment in ICP. Sympathetic tone may begin to increase during this phase but more commonly stabilizes.

Point C represents initiation of the ischemic response or a Cushing response characterized by massive sympathetic discharge. The rapidly increasing SABP increases CPP and the ICP passively increases. The latter increase is not sufficient to maintain the low CPP and allows it to increment. At point D, ICP is maximal but SABP continues to rise due to the continued sympathetic activity which is beginning to peak. CPP passes the vasoconstrictor threshold of autoregulation for a period *long enough* to allow vasoconstriction to occur and the ICP begins to decline even though SABP is still rising.

At point E, the SABP has reached its maximum and begins to stabilize toward baseline levels. This can be considered a late vasoconstrictor phase where the ICP continues to decrement even though SABP declines slightly, the net result is an increase in CPP throughout this period. The cycle terminates here, but may begin again if catecholamine metabolism or sympathetic activity once again decay allowing decrements in SABP/CPP to develop.

This system clearly represents a negative feedback loop which appears to function to maintain a relatively narrow range of CPP. This cycle can be aborted by low dose catecholamines which prevent the decrement in SABP or, in fact, essentially any agent or series of treatments which allow CPP to remain stable. This latter situation is not always good since treatments and drugs such as barbituates which allow CPP to remain stable but in a low range may potentiate continued cerebral ischemia.

In conclusion, we find no qualitative difference between "B" waves and plateau waves. The cyclic nature of these waves appears to be due to a negative feedback loop based on mechanisms which function to maintain CPP within a relatively narrow range. We find this model consistent with the previously published model of the vasodilatory cascade supporting the interaction between SABP, ICP, and CPP which when applied to the generation of CSF pressure waves, suggests that autoregulation is present and the latency of the autoregulatory response must be considered to understand each phase of the wave.

Lastly, the therapeutic implications of this analysis are far reaching.

References

1. Rosner MJ (1987) Cerebral Perfusion Pressure: The Link Between Intracranial Pressure and Systemic Circulation. In: Cerebral Blood Flow: Physiologic and Clinical Aspects, James H, Wood MD (ed) pp 425–448
2. Rosner MJ, Becker DP (1984) The origin and evolution of plateau waves: experimental observations and a theoretical model. J Neurosurg 60:312–324
3. Rosner MJ, Daughton S (1990) Cerebral perfusion pressure management in head injury. J Trauma 30:933–941
4. Rosner MJ, Newsome HH, Becker DP (1984) Mechanical brain injury: the sympathoadrenal response. J Neurosurg 61:76–86

Changes in Jugular Bulb Oxygen Saturation and Associated Changes in Intracranial Pressure

C. Rafferty[2,3], G.M. Teasdale[1], R. Bullock[1], W. Fitch[3], and P. Farling[2]

[1] Departments of Neurosurgery and [2] Neuro-anaesthesia, Institute of Neurological Sciences, and [3] University Department of Anaesthesia, Royal Infirmary, Glasgow G31 2ER, Scotland

Introduction

Brain metabolism after human head injury has been studied infrequently. This is because PET scanning methods are difficult to apply to acutely ill patients, and because global techniques have been limited in their validity. Global assessment of brain metabolism requires measurement of cerebral blood flow and cerebral arteriovenous oxygen difference ($AVDO_2$). Until recently, these measurements were possible only on an intermittent basis. However knowledge of continuous cerebral oxygen extraction is increasingly recognised to be an important guide for treatment [3]. Thus, excessive hyperventilation may induce ischaemia due to vasoconstriction, and this can be detected from a widening $AVDO_2$. The diagnosis of "luxury perfusion" or hyperaemia is also made more reliable by the demonstration of a low $AVDO_2$. Recent technical developments have led to methods which can continuously monitor the oxygen saturation of arterial and jugular venous blood. Continuous jugular venous oxygen saturation monitoring is now in use as a monitor of brain function in head injured patients in several neurosurgical centres [1].

The oxygen content of blood, under normal physiological conditions, is dependent upon the haemoglobin concentration and its degree of oxygen saturation (O_2 Content $= Hb \times 1.39 \times SO_2 + [0.003 \times PO_2]$). With a constant haemoglobin and arterial oxygen saturation, continuous in vivo jugular venous oxygen saturation monitoring produces a continuous arteriovenous saturation difference that reflects the arteriovenous oxygen difference ($AVDO_2 = Hb \times 1.39\ [1 - SjO_2]$).

We have assessed the value of jugular bulb oxygen saturation monitoring using the fibre optic Oximetrix SO_2 system, and report our initial findings on 15 patients. In this report we have focused on:

1. Factors affecting the jugular venous O_2 saturation value;
2. Frequency of changes in the jugular venous oxygen saturation and their association with changes in intracranial pressure.

Patients and Methods

Fifteen severely head injured patients, with a median Glasgow Coma Score of 7 (Range 4–10) had ICP and jugular saturation continuously monitored for a total of 1300 hours. In 12 patients, head injury was due to a road traffic accident; 2 were due to falls and 1 to an assault. Four of the patients had a diffuse injury on CT scan with brain swelling and 11 had a focal lesion or haematoma (3 subdural haematomas, 4 extradural haematomas, 2 intracerebral haematomas, 1 intracerebral and extradural haematoma, and 1 patient with all three lesions). The patients were monitored over periods ranging from 24 hours to 7 days with a mean duration of 3.6 days. Ten patients were monitored within 24 hours of their head injury and in the remaining five, monitoring was commenced within hours of deterioration. Their ages ranged from 12 to 66, with a mean of 33 years.

All patients were ventilated with an ICP over 25 mmHg on admission to the ICU. In patients with a coagulopathy or haemodynamic instability, insertion of the jugular bulb catheter was delayed until the patient was stable. The internal jugular vein was cannulated at the level of the cricoid cartilage in a cephalad direction, with a percutaneous introducer sheath. The fibreoptic catheter was advanced through the sheath until the tip was lying in the jugular bulb, or higher and the position was confirmed with a lateral cervical spine X ray. There were no complications from insertion of the catheter.

Jugular venous oxygen saturation was measured using reflectance spectrophotometry, through the disposable fibreoptic catheter, using triple wavelength light. The jugular oxygen saturation value and the light intensity level were displayed on a screen, and trends of both values were printed. All saturation recordings were verified against a printout of the light intensities from the Oximetrix sensor unit.

Intracranial pressure was measured using a Camino 420 ICP monitoring system in nine patients, and a fluid filled ventricular catheter was used in six. The ICP waveform was recorded continuously on time marked paper with a Gould chart recorder, which also recorded jugular venous oxygen saturation, and mean arterial pressure.

Changes in saturation greater than 5% were noted and compared to changes in ICP greater than 10 mmHg.

Results

Extracranial Factors

Fifteen percent of the SJO_2 results were lost as a result of inappropriate light intensities, probably due to impingement of the catheter lumen against the vein wall. This was often a consequence of movement of the patient during nursing manoeuvres, particularly movement of the neck towards the side of the catheter. This could be greatly reduced by using a pneumatic bed.

The SJO_2 increased by up to 12% when a high arterial oxygen tension was induced by preoxygenation prior to physiotherapy (PaO_2 of 500 mmHg).

Saturation Transients

The total number of significant transients (>5% change in SJO_2) was 1195, (mean per patient = 80). The number of transients per patient per day ranged from 6 to 35. There was a difference between patients as well as a difference on different days for the same patient. The most constant accompaniments of SJO_2 transients (Fig. 1) were changes in ICP, and/or MABP. Table 1 relates the increases and decreases in saturation to the pattern of accompanying changes in ICP. The most common event was an increase in SJO_2 with a concurrent increase in ICP.

ICP Changes

Figure 1 shows the relationship between ICP and SJO_2. Table 2 relates increases in ICP to the associated saturation transients. The increases in ICP were accompanied by increases in saturation in 67% of the recordings. Only 11% of the increases in ICP were accompanied by a *decrease* in the SJO_2. The decreases in SJO_2 that occurred with increases in ICP were seen when the baseline ICP was high, and when the jugular saturation was low, implying that O_2 delivery was jeopardised by high ICP.

A value for the change in SJO_2 per mmHg change in ICP was derived by dividing the mean change in saturation by the mean change in ICP. To exclude small transient changes only sustained changes in ICP of more than 5 minutes were included. Changes in saturation values showed a 5 fold range from 0.35 to 1.75%/mmHg change in ICP.

Table 1. Percentage frequency of jugular bulb saturation transients (SJO_2) (>5% change over baseline) in relation to ICP changes (>10 mmHg)

	n	Increase in ICP (%)	No change in ICP (%)	Decrease in ICP (%)
Increased SJO_2	931	69	29	2
Decreased SJO_2	264	40	37	23

Table 2. Increases in ICP and associated saturation changes

	ICP changes	Increase in SJO_2	No change in SJO_2	Decrease in SJO_2
Total	961	642	213	106
Percentage	100	67	22	11

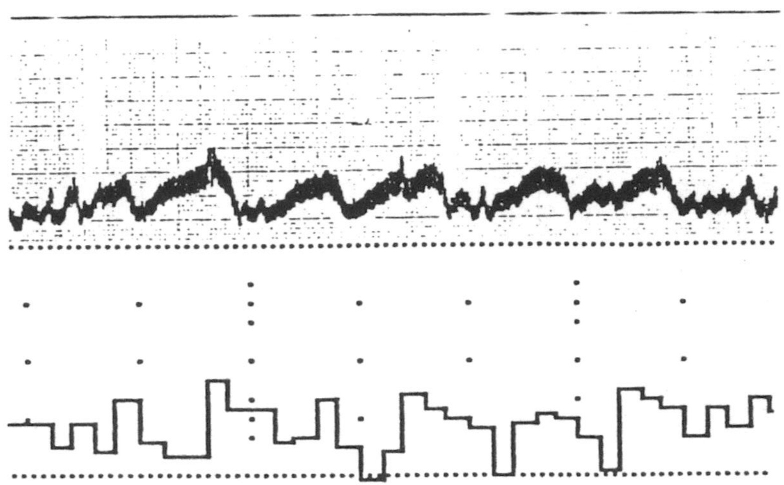

a

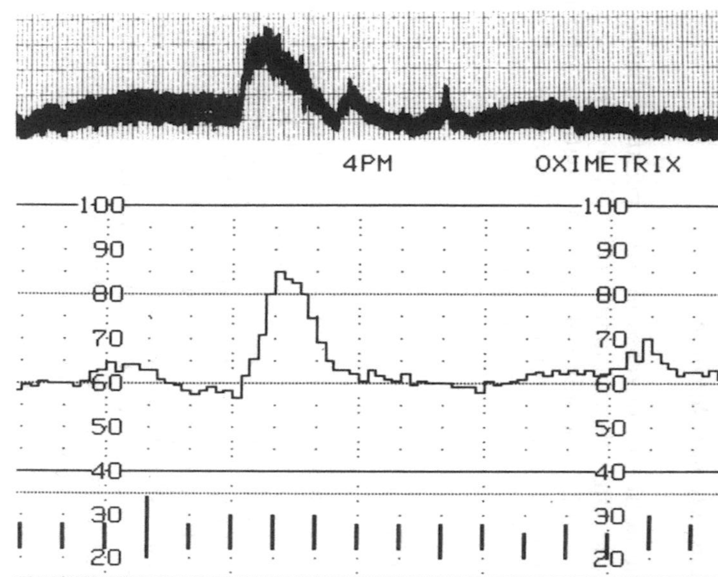

b

Fig. 1. **a**ICP wave ("B-type") top and associated simultaneous jugular venous saturation transients. **b** Spontaneous large ICP increase (*top*) and associated jugular venous oxygen saturation increase

SJO_2 *Transients and Outcome*

When the degree of increase in SJO_2 per unit change in ICP, was compared to outcome after three months (Fig. 2) a large % saturation increase was associated with a poorer outcome. All patients who died had a change in saturation/mmHg ICP greater than 0.5 units while all the patients with a good outcome had a value less than 0.5.

Discussion

Our experience shows the need to exclude technical factors and extracranial factors before assuming that a change in SJO_2 can be attributed to an intracranial event. Technical problems may arise from changes in the light intensity levels caused by movement of the catheter tip, movement of the patient, or damage or kinking of the fibreoptic catheter (Table 3).

The pathophysiological factors which affect the SJO_2 value may arise from intracranial or extracranial events. Extracranial factors may cause a change in the oxygen content, thereby affecting oxygen delivery, to produce changes in the SJO_2. Hypoxia and anaemia reduce the oxygen delivery while preoxygenation can increase it.

Table 3. Factors affecting the observed saturation value

Technical	Light intensity	High
		Low
		Erratic
Pathophysiological	Extracranial	Haemoglobin
		FiO_2
		Hypoxia
		Blood Pressure

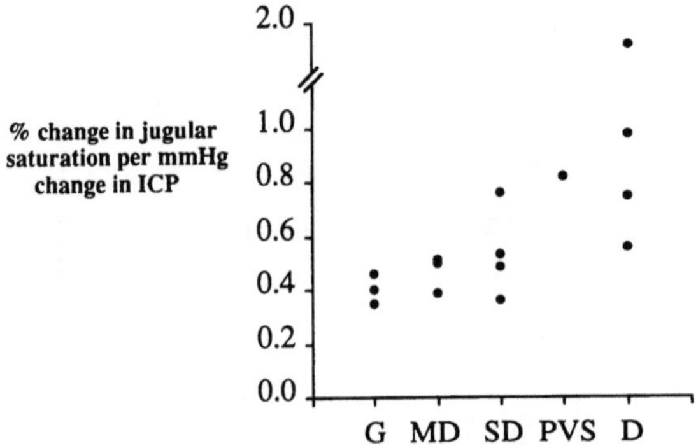

Fig. 2. Relationship between the magnitude of increase in jugular venous oxygen saturation per mmHg ICP rise, and outcome, three months after head injury

ICP increases, in the form of "B-waves", or isolated spontaneous transients (Fig. 1) were the major changes associated with changes in SJO_2 recordings.

The most common event was an increase in SJO_2 with an increase in ICP (Tables 1, 2). This may have been the result of an increase in arterial blood pressure, leading to an ICP rise in patients with reduced autoregulation. These changes tended to occur less often when the patient was sedated under muscle relaxants, and ventilated. Decreases in SJO_2 were rare when CPP was adequate but became more common with the development of high ICP, and a low SJO_2. This pattern was particularly marked in those patients who progressed to brain death. The number of SJO_2 transients and their character depends upon the therapy the patient receives, the severity and nature of injury, and the time after injury.

Engberg et al. [2] have shown changes in $AVDO_2$ occuring with changes in blood pressure in patients likely to have impaired autoregulation. Our simultaneous recordings of blood pressure, ICP and SJO_2, showed concurrent changes in all three parameters occuring at the same time. Autoregulatory control of CBF is disturbed in the majority of severely head injured patients. Increases in blood pressure with diminished autoregulation could thus increase the cerebral perfusion pressure (CPP) and increase cerebral blood flow thereby increasing the oxygen delivery and the SJO_2.

We have shown that continuous SJO_2 monitoring is a practical technique for assessment of global cerebral oxygen delivery. It requires careful interpretation and further development. Transient increases and decreases in the SJO_2 occur simultaneously with increases in ICP, which may be caused by blood pressure changes.

The major implications of this data are that events related to haemodynamic changes and to a lesser extent ICP changes appear to overshadow changes related to cerebral metabolism. In order to derive accurate and representative $AVDO_2$ data, which depict changes in cerebral metabolism, it will therefore be necessary to perform carefully timed and frequent data sampling, at time points when SJO_2 recordings indicate that the "baseline" SJO_2 value is stable.

Previous studies using intermittent sampling must therefore be interpreted with caution.

References

1. Andrews PJD, Piper JR, Dearden NM, Miller JO (1990) Secondary insults during intrahospital transport of head injured patients. The Lancet 335:327–330
2. Engberg M, Melsen NC, Herlevsen P, Haraldsted V, Cold GE (1990) Changes of blood pressure and cerebral arteriovenous oxygen content differences with and without bupivocaine scalp infiltration during craniotomy. Acta Anaesthesiol Scand 34:346–349
3. Robertson CS, Narayan RK, Gokaslan ZL, Pahwa R, Grossman RG, Caram P, Allen E (1989) Cerebral arteriovenous oxygen difference as an estimate of cerebral blood flow in comatose patients. J Neurosurg 70:222–230

Spontaneous Fluctuations in Cerebral Blood Flow as a Cause of B Waves

D.W. Newell[1], R. Aaslid[1], R. Stooss[2], and H.J. Reulen[2]

[1] Department of Neurological Surgery, University of Washington, Seattle, WA, USA
[2] Department of Neurosurgery, University of Bern, Bern, Switzerland

Introduction

The exact mechanism responsible for B waves is unclear, however it has been attributed to cerebral blood flow (CBF) fluctuations, thought to be secondary to respiratory variations during abnormal breathing patterns in neurosurgical patients [6]. Transcranial Doppler (TCD) monitoring of blood flow velocity has demonstrated velocity fluctuations at frequencies similar to those of B waves in head injured patients and also in normal subjects [5, 8, 9]. Recording of TCD and intracranial pressure (ICP) signals simultaneously has demonstrated synchronous variations in both parameters [5].

Utilizing a new method we employed TCD ultrasonography [1] and digital signal processing to allow continous recording of velocity signals from the middle cerebral artery (MCA), simultaneously along with other physiologic parameters. This technique allowed comparison of the MCA velocity and these parameters during B waves of the ICP.

Methods

Simultaneous monitoring of arterial blood pressure (ABP), MCA velocity, ICP, and end tidal CO_2 ($EtCO_2$) was performed on 20 patients with a diagnosis of closed head injury. A total of 150 continuous recordings were obtained, for intervals of between 15 minutes and 2 hours. All patients were intubated, artificially ventilated. Mean age of the patients was 35 years with a range of 17–59 years. There were 17 males and 3 females. Glasgow coma score on admission averaged 6 with a range of 3–10. Continuous $EtCO_2$ signals were obtained using side port sampling with an infrared CO_2 detector. A 2 MHz transcranial Doppler with a transducer fixed by a head band was used to monitor the MCA trunk at a depth between 50–60 mm. The maximum blood flow velocity (V_{max}) spectral outline signal was then taken as an analog signal as described previously [2], and processed with the 3 other analog signals (ABP, ICP, $EtCO_2$) through an analog to digital converter. The extracranial internal carotid artery velocity was recorded simultaneously with ABP, ICP, and $EtCO_2$ during ICP waves in 5 of the head injury patients. This was accomplished using a handheld 2 MHz probe which was set at a depth of 50 mm and aimed from the angle of the mandible toward the foramen lacerum.

Recordings were also taken of MCA velocity and $EtCO_2$ in a group of 10 healthy volunteers. Five male and 5 female subjects were chosen (average age 31 years, range 20–43 years). Continuous recording was performed from the left MCA for 1 hour with the subjects supine.

Results

Continuously monitored tracings, were at least 1 hour in duration in 69 of the 150 recordings. In 38 of the 69 recordings (55%), repeating fluctuations (waves) in the MCA velocity were observed at a frequency of 0.5–2/minute lasting at least 2 minutes. These velocity waves were completely synchronous with waves in the ICP tracing. They sometimes were irregular in their frequency and other times displayed a quite regular frequency. They were always in phase with the ICP waves.

Fourier analysis was performed on all 4 simultaneously recorded parameters (ABP, MCA velocity, ICP, and $ETCO_2$) during selected intervals of waves, to determine their relationship to each other. It was found that during typical waves, the MCA velocity and ICP showed the same frequency amplitude relationship, which was not shared by the ABP and $ETCO_2$. Figure 1a illustrates typical velocity waves and B waves, and Figure 1b illustrates Fourier analysis showing the ventilator frequency which affects all 4 parameters, and the velocity wave frequency at which ICP is affected but no changes in ABP or $ETCO_2$ are seen.

The maximum velocity wave amplitude observed in a head injury patient was 49% of the average mean velocity during the fluctuations. The average velocity wave amplitude for the group analyzed during the maximum wave activity was 23.1% $\pm$ 8.05 (SD) of the average mean velocity.

The amplitude of the ICP fluctuation in response to a given velocity wave amplitude appeared to be dependent on the ICP. A regression analysis was performed between the average ICP and the amplitude of the ICP divided by the percent velocity wave amplitude to correct for the input signal. This revealed a close relationship between the degree of ICP fluctuation for a given relative amplitude in the velocity fluctuation, and the ICP ($r = 0.81$, $p < 0.001$) (Fig. 2).

An additional recording was recently obtained on a head injury patient not included in the original analysis, using a 2 channel TCD. This permits simultaneous velocity recording from both MCA's. Velocity fluctuations in both MCA's were completely synchronous with one another and in phase with the ICP B waves.

Velocity recordings in 5 of the patients from the extracranial internal carotid artery during B waves of the ICP revealed simultaneous fluctuations in the velocity which were synchronous with the ICP fluctuations.

Brief episodes of MCA velocity fluctuations, lasting at least 2 minutes were seen in 7 of 10 (70%) normal volunteers. These waves were similar in

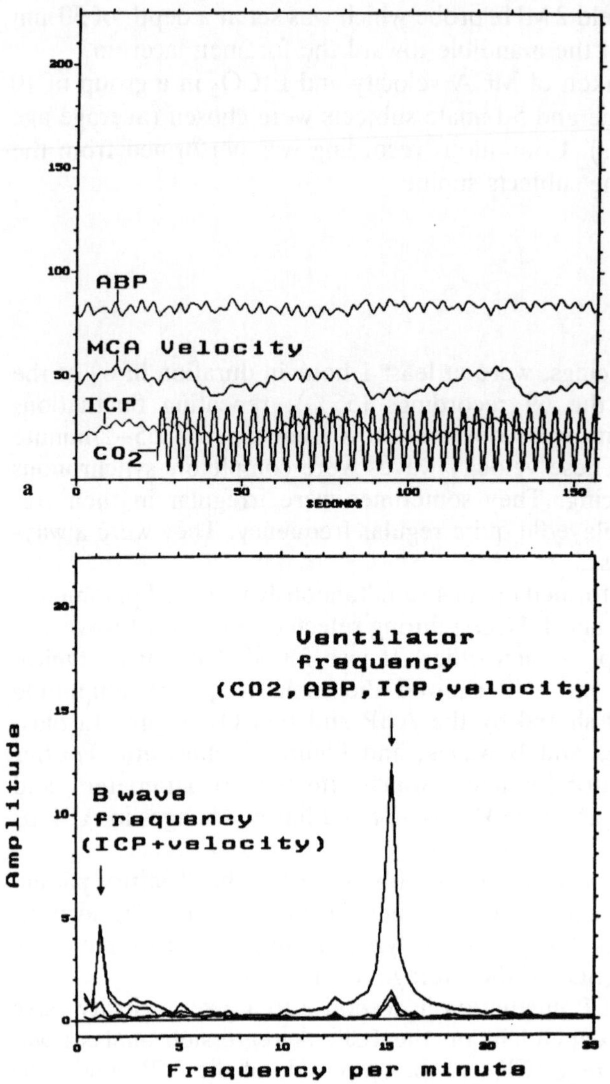

Fig. 1. a Illustration of typical velocity fluctuations which occurred during B waves in the ICP which were independent of changes in ABP or CO_2 concentration. (ABP, ICP, CO_2 in mmHg. MCA velocity in centimeters/second). **b** Fourier analysis of the frequency of repeating waves in the recorded parameters, showing the velocity and ICP waves at a frequency of 1.3 per minute, and no changes at this frequency in the ABP and CO_2. The respirator frequency is seen at between 15 and 16 cycles per minute, and there is an effect on all 4 parameters

character, frequency, and amplitude to those seen in the head injury patients, but tended to occur for shorter durations. The maximum amplitude in this group was 41% of the average mean velocity versus a maximum of 49% in one of the head injury patients. The average velocity wave amplitude for the group during the maximum wave activity was 29.0% ± 7.73 (SD) of the average mean velocity. This value was slightly higher than the head injury group but did not reach statistical significance by the Students t test ($0.05 < p < 0.1$).

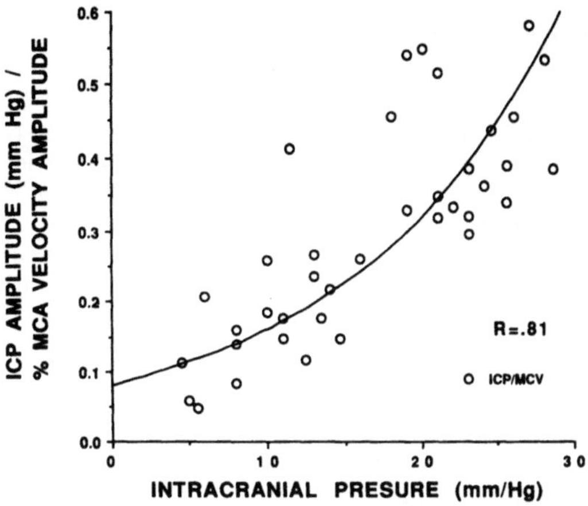

Fig. 2. Regression curve illustrating the relationship between the degree of ICP fluctuation for a certain percentage fluctuation in MCA velocity, and the average ICP ($r = 0.81$, $p < 0.001$)

Discussion

Periodic fluctuations in the MCA velocity can be most easily explained by fluctuations in the CBF. CBF fluctuations are caused by a phasic dilation and contraction of the small regulating arteries (vasomotor waves). Vasomotor waves in turn produce fluctuations in cerebral blood volume, which finally are reflected in the ICP. This interpretation is supported by experiments reported by Auer et al. [3], who observed pial vessels oscillating in synchrony with ICP variations using a pial window preparation in cats. These pial arteries were observed to oscillate at frequencies between 0.5–2 per minute and thus correspond to the present findings and previous descriptions of B waves in the ICP [6].

The exact cause of the fluctations in cerebral blood flow causing B waves is unknown. Some investigators have suggested that a mechanism intrinsic to the arterial smooth muscle cells in the regulating arteries is responsible [3]. Others have postulated that an intrinsic brainstem pacemaker which alters other physiologic parameters as well as cerebral blood flow at a regular frequency, is responsible [4, 7]. The finding of synchronous fluctuations of blood flow in both MCA's suggests a central control mechanism. It was clearly observed that these vasomotor waves can occur despite a constant CO_2 concentration.

The finding of a variable B wave amplitude at different ICP for a given degree of fluctuation in cerebral blood flow velocity can be most easily explained by variations in intracranial compliance at different intracranial pressures.

References

1. Aaslid R, Markwalder TM, Nornes H (1982) Noninvasive transcranial Doppler ultrasound recording of flow velocity in basal cerebral arteries. J Neurosurg 57:769–774
2. Aaslid R, Lindegaard KF, Sorteberg W, et al. (1989) Cerebral autoregulation dynamics in humans. Stroke 20:45–52
3. Auer LM, Sayama I (1983) Intracranial pressure oscillations (B-waves) caused by oscillations in cerebrovascular volume. Acta Neurochir 68:93–100
4. Higashi S, Yamamoto S, Hashimoto M, et al. (1989) The role of vasomotor center and adrenergic pathway in B-waves. In: Hoff JT, Betz AL (eds) Intracranial Pressure VII. Springer, Berlin Heidelberg, New York London Paris Tokyo Hong Kong, pp 220–224
5. Lundar T, Lindegaard KF, Nornes H (1990) Continuous recording of middle cerebral artery blood velocity in clinical neurosurgery. Acta Neurochir 102:85–90
6. Lundberg N (1960) Continuous recording and control of ventricular fluid pressure in neurosurgical practice. Acta Psychiatr Scand, Suppl 149:1–193
7. Maeda M, Takahashi K, Miyazaki et al. (1986) The role of the central monoamine system and the cholinoceptive pontine area on the oscillation of ICP "pressure waves". In: Miller JD, Teasdale GM, Rowan JO, Galbraith SL, Mendelow AD (eds) Intracranial pressure VI. Springer, Berlin Heidelberg New York, Tokyo, pp 151–155
8. Mautner-Huppert D, Haberl RL, Dirnagl U, et al. (1989) B waves in healthy persons. Neurol Res 11:194–196
9. Nakatani S, Ozaki K, Hara K, et al. (1989) Simultaneous monitoring of ICP and Doppler sonogram on the middle cerebral artery. In: Hoff JT, Betz AL (eds) Intracranial Pressure VII. Springer, Berlin Heidelberg, New York London Paris Tokyo Hong Kong, pp 113–115

Postural Changes

Changes in Cerebral Hemodynamics with Head Elevation in Head-Injured Patients

Z. Feldman, M.J. Kanter, C.S. Robertson, C.F. Contant, M.A. Sheinberg, R.K. Narayan, and R.G. Grossman

Department of Neurosurgery, Baylor College of Medicine, Houston, TX, USA

Introduction

Elevated intracranial pressure (ICP) or inadequate cerebral perfusion pressure (CPP) and cerebral blood flow (CBF) are common causes of secondary brain damage in head-injured patients. In patients with elevated ICP it is a common practice to position the patient in bed with the head elevated above the heart. Kenning et al. reported that elevating the head to 45° or 90° significantly reduced ICP [1]. However, some studies suggest that head elevation may also lower the CPP. Rosner et al. have emphasized the importance of adequate CPP and have provided physiological and clinical evidence suggesting that CPP is maximal with patients in the horizontal position, even though ICP is usually higher in this position [6–9]. As the maintenance of adequate CBF is the primary rationale for maintaining adequate CPP in patients with increased ICP, we have studied the changes in CBF, as well as changes in ICP, CPP and other cerebral and systemic physiologic parameters induced by changes in head position in patients with head injury.

Methods

Twenty-two head-injured patients admitted to the Neurosurgical Intensive Care Unit at Ben Taub General Hospital between January 1990 and January 1991 were studied. Patient characteristics are listed in Table 1. Within 72 hours after injury, two consecutive sets of physiological measurements were performed. In the first 13 patients the initial set of measurements was performed at 30° of head elevation; in the subsequent nine patients the initial set was taken at 0°. After the initial set of measurements, the patient's head elevation was changed and, forty-five minutes later, a second set of measurements was done. Measurements were made of CBF, using the Kety-Schmidt N_2O technique (2); ICP; arteriovenous oxygen difference ($AVDO_2$); cerebral metabolic

Table 1. Patient characteristics

Category		Number
1. Sex	Male	19
	Female	3
2. Age	Mean 35 years; range: 18–75	
3. Pathology	Subdural hematoma	8
	Cerebral contusion	5
	Intracerebral hematoma	2
	Epidural hematoma	2
	Diffuse axonal injury	2
	Gunshot to the head	2
	Traumatic subarachnoid hemorrhage	1
4. Initial GCS	3–5	3
	6–8	14
	9–12	5
5. Outcome	Good recovery	6
	Moderately disabled	7
	Severely disabled	5
	Vegetative state	1
	Dead	3

rate of oxygen ($CMRO_2$); oxygen saturation in the jugular bulb ($SjvO_2$); cerebral vascular resistance (CVR); $paCO_2$; paO_2; arteriovenous difference of lactate (AVDL); and mean arterial pressure (MAP). MAP was measured via a radial artery catheter with the transducer zeroed at the level of the foramen of Monro, as an estimate of the mean carotid pressure (MCP) which was then used for calculation of the CPP.

Differences were computed by subtracting the value obtained when the patient was flat from the value obtained when the head of the patient was elevated to 30°. These differences were evaluated using the paired t-test. Comparisons among subgroups of patients were made using analysis of variance of the individual differences.

Results

The mean values for the MCP and ICP were significantly lower at 30° of head elevation than at 0°: 84 ± 15 mmHg vs. 90 ± 15 mmHg for MCP, and 14 ± 7 mmHg vs. 20 ± 8 mmHg for ICP. The mean values for CPP and CBF were unaffected by head elevation: CPP was 70 ± 18 mmHg at 30° and 70 ± 19 mmHg at 0°, and CBF was 47.8 ± 16.9 ml/100 gm/min at 30° and 48.9 ± 20.4 ml/100 gm/min at 0°. None of the other parameters showed a statistically significant change with a change of head elevation. The results were not affected by whether the head was at 30° or 0° for the initial measurements.

Linear regression revealed a significant relationship between the ICP level at 0° and the amount of change in ICP after head elevation ($r = -0.5890$). The higher the ICP was in the horizontal position, the greater the reduction in ICP was at 30° of head elevation. Comparison of the effect of head elevation on ICP in the six patients who had ICP higher than 25 mmHg with the effect observed in the other 16 patients revealed that the greater decrease in ICP observed in the patients with elevated ICP was significant. The reduction in ICP with head elevation was -10 ± 6 mmHg in these six patients, compared with -4 ± 9 mmHg for the remaining 16 patients ($p < 0.05$). In these six patients the ICP fell from a mean of 31 at 0° to 20 at 30°.

Although CBF was unchanged with head elevation when the data for all 22 patients were averaged, there were five patients in whom CBF fell by more than 5 ml/100 gm/min with head elevation. In these five patients, CBF fell from a mean of 67.2 ± 26 ml/100 gm/min at 0° to 50.7 ± 16.5 ml/100 gm/min at 30° ($p < 0.05$). Further analysis of these patients revealed that in four of them the lower CBF at 30° was still within the normal range for CBF (>35 ml/100 gm/min). Only in one of the five patients did the CBF drop below 35 ml/100/min (from 37 to 25 ml/100 gm/min). This patient had a low CPP at both 0° and 30°; 59 and 50 mmHg, respectively. Interestingly, the ICP rose marginally in this patient with head elevation from 12 mmHg at 0° to 14 mmHg at 30°. Other than the suggestion that a low CPP may be associated with a fall in CBF with head elevation, the five patients in whom head elevation produced a decrease in CBF of more than 5 ml/100 gm/min had no distinguishing features.

Discussion

The ideal head position for patients with head injury has been disputed in recent years. Rosner et al. have provided evidence that plateau waves are triggered by a fall in CPP [7], and that maintaining CPP above 70–80 mmHg prevented plateau waves. In patients with intracranial hypertension, they advocated keeping the patient's head at 0° of elevation and using fluid expansion or pharmacological means to maintain CPP [8, 9]. Our data indicate that even though the MCP is lower at 30° of head elevation than at 0°, CPP and CBF are not significantly altered in most patients by head elevation to 30°.

We have also demonstrated a direct relationship between the ICP level and the change in ICP after head elevation. Our data suggest that in patients with normal ICP head position does not greatly affect ICP and that these patients can be positioned either horizontally or with the head elevated to 30°. However, when the ICP is increased, head elevation is very effective in reducing the ICP. This phenomenon is apparently due to 1) hydrostatic displacement of the cerebrospinal fluid (CSF) from the cranial cavity to the spinal subarachnoid space [1], and 2) facilitated venous outflow from the brain [3, 10]. The contributions of CSF displacement and changes in venous volume to the reduction in ICP in head-injured patients after head elevation may depend upon the relative size of each of the intracranial compartments at the time of head elevation [4, 10]. In patients with elevated ICP, the intracranial compliance decreases [4, 5], and smaller changes in intracranial volume, as those produced by CSF displacement, will produce greater changes in ICP.

Although the overall results of the present study show no effect of head elevation on CBF, one must bear in mind that our measurements are of global CBF and that regional areas of decreased CBF may exist in the presence of normal global blood flow measurements. Only in one patient did the CBF fall to ischemic levels after head elevation, and the vasodilatatory cascade suggested by Rosner et al. seemed to be demonstrable [6, 7]. This patient's low CPP (59 mmHg) emphasizes once more the importance of maintenance of adequate levels of CPP.

The results of the present study suggest that, in general, head-injured patients with elevated ICP should be maintained with the head elevated to 30°, which will produce a fall in ICP without a significant decrease in CBF in the majority of these patients.

References

1. Kenning JA, Toutant SM, Saunders RL (1981) Upright patient positioning in the management of intracranial hypertension. Surg Neurol 15:148–152
2. Kety SS (1951) The theory and application of the exchange of inert gas at the lungs and tissues. Pharmacol Rev 3:1–41
3. Magnaes B (1978) Movement of cerebrospinal fluid within the craniospinal space when sitting up and lying down. Surg Neurol 10:45–49
4. Maset AL, Marmarou A, Ward JD, et al. (1987) Pressure volume index in head injury. J Neurosurg 67:832–840
5. Miller JD (1983) Significance and management of intracranial hypertension in head injury. In: Ishii S, Nagai H, Brock M (eds) Intracranial Pressure V. Springer, Berlin Heidelberg New York Tokyo, pp 44–53
6. Rosner MJ (1985) Vasodilatatory cascade and intracranial pressure. In: Miller JO, Rowan JO, Galbraith SL, Mendelow AO, Teasdale GM (eds) Intracranial Pressure VI. Springer, Berlin Heidelberg New York Tokyo, pp 137–145
7. Rosner MJ (1987) Cerebral perfusion pressure: link between intracranial pressure and systemic circulation. In: Wood JH (ed) Cerebral Blood Flow Physiologic and Clinical Aspects. McGraw-Hill, New York, pp 425–448
8. Rosner MJ, Coley IB (1986) Cerebral perfusion pressure, intracranial pressure, and head elevation. J Neurosurg 65:636–641
9. Rosner MJ, Daughton S (1990) Cerebral perfusion pressure management in head injury. J Trauma 30:933–941
10. Toole JF (1968) Effects of change of head, limb, and body position on cephalic circulation. N Engl J Med 279:307–311

Effects of Postural Changes on Epidural Pressure and Cerebral Perfusion Pressure in Patients with Serious Intracranial Lesions

A. Yoshida, T. Shima, Y. Okada, T. Yamada, and H. Kurino

Departments of Critical Care Medicine and Neurosurgery, Chugoku Rousai Hospital,
1-5-1 Hiro-Tagaya, Kure City, 737-01, Japan

Introduction

Body position is known to be one of the most important factors affecting intracranial pressure (ICP). Patients with raised ICP have been commonly cared for in a heads-up position to minimize ICP, whereas little attention has been directed toward the postural influence on cerebral perfusion pressure (CPP). In an effort to clarify the optimal posture maximizing CPP, we examined in this study the effect of head elevation and neck flexion and/or extension on ICP and CPP.

Clinical Material and Methods

The study was performed on 19 consecutive patients with serious intracranial lesions, aged 16 to 73 years. They comprised five patients with closed head injury and 14 with stroke. In all patients, respiration was controlled by volume-cycled ventilator.

ICP was measured by epidural transducer (Ladd/Steritek) and systemic arterial blood pressure (SABP) was simultaneously monitored at the level of the external auditory meatus. CPP was calculated as the difference between SABP and epidural pressure (EDP).

At first, patients were placed horizontally in the supine position without any rotation or flexion of the neck. Then, the upper part of their bodies was elevated from zero to 45 degrees by 15-degree increments. At each increment of elevation the measurements were performed in two positions: the head was tilted at a steep angle from the neutral position (head-tilt position), and the head was elevated about 10 cm from the neutral position with pads under the occiput (sniffing position). In each posture, EDP and SABP were recorded for two minutes after a 5-minute stabilization period.

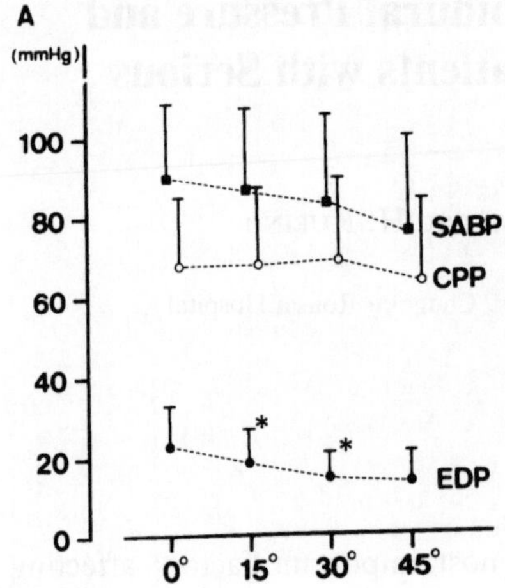

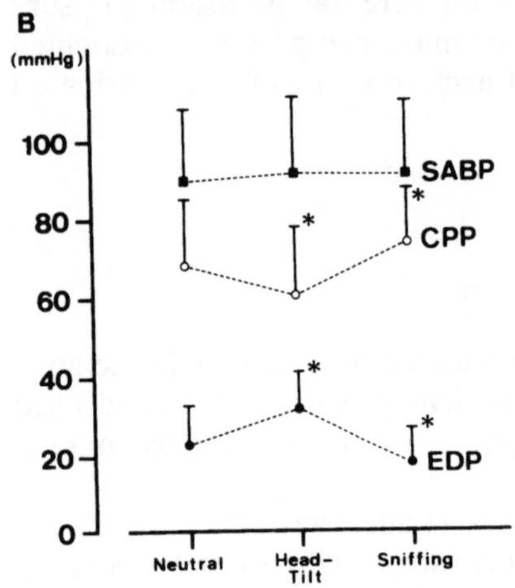

Fig. 1A,B. Postural changes of the mean EDP, mean SABP and mean CPP in 19 patients. **A** Elevation of the upper part of the bodies. Head position was kept in the neutral position. **B** Conversion of head-positions. Elevation of the upper part of the bodies was 0°. (mean ± SD, *$p < 0.01$)

Results

Although the mean EDP and SABP decreased simultaneously with progressive elevation of the upper part of the body (Fig. 1a), the mean CPP changed in each patient (Fig. 2).

The head-tilt position produced a significant elevation in EDP and a decrease in CPP, whereas the sniffing position provided a significant reduction in EDP and an increase in CPP (Fig. 1b). The minimum EDP was obtained at the 30° sniffing position in 12 patients, 15° sniffing in four, and 0° sniffing in the

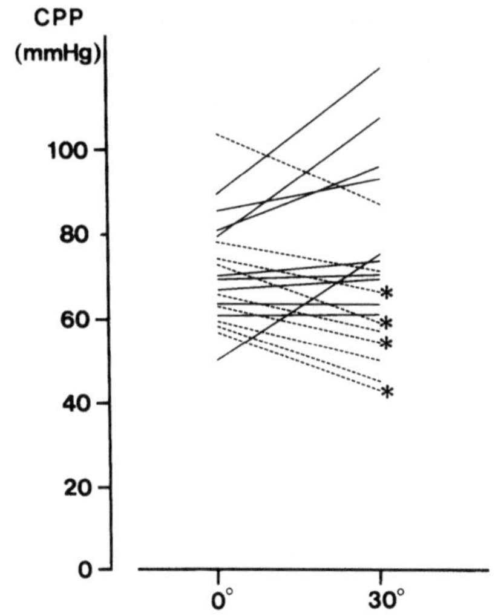

Fig. 2. The individual response of the mean CPP to elevation of the upper part of the bodies from 0° to 30°. Head position was kept in the neutral position. (*patients with the administration of barbiturates)

remainder. The maximum CPP was recorded at the 0° sniffing position in 10 patients, 15° sniffing in six, 30° sniffing in two, and 0° neutral in the other one.

Discussion

Durward et al. reported that elevation of the head to 15° and 30° could minimize ICP without generating a significant reduction in CPP [1]. However, Rosner et al. stressed that any elevation of the head of the bed was associated with a decrease in CPP [2]. Our study demonstrated that the changes in CPP through elevation of the upper part of the body were different in each patient. Namely, CPP reduction was prominent in those patients with low initial CPP, hypovolemia or barbiturate therapy. These results suggest that these patients should not be cared for by elevating their upper bodies.

Considerable attention has been directed toward the effect of neck rotation on ICP [3], but few investigations have been performed concerning the effect of flexion and/or extension of the neck. In our study, a significant elevation in EDP was observed in the head-tilt position, and a consistent reduction in EDP with an increase in CPP was demonstrated in the sniffing position. Although the precise mechanism underlying the EDP reduction in the sniffing position is unclear, hydrostatic displacement of venous blood and cerebrospinal fluid out of the cranial cavity might be facilitated in this posture. Because of its minimal effect on SABP, the sniffing position was considered to be particularly beneficial in the management of intracranial hypertension.

In conclusion, the optimal posture in patients with intracranial hypertension should be individualized by maximizing CPP as obtained from simultaneous monitoring of both ICP and SABP.

References

1. Durward QJ, Amacher AL, Del Maestro RF, et al. (1983) Cerebral and cardiovascular responses to changes in head elevation in patients with intracranial hypertension. J Neurosurg 59:938–944
2. Hulme A, Cooper R (1976) The effects of head position and jugular vein compression (JVC) on intracranial pressure (ICP). A clinical study. In: Becks JWF, Bosch DA, Brock M (eds) Intracranial pressure III. Springer, Berlin Heidelberg New York
3. Rosner MJ, Coley IB (1986) Cerebral perfusion pressure, intracranial pressure and head elevation. J Neurosurg 65:636–641

Positive End-Expiratory Pressure in Supine and Sitting Positions: Its Effects on Intrathoracic and Intracranial Pressures

M. Montolivo[1], S. Lodrini[1], F. Fiacchino[2], and F. Pluchino[2]

[1] Department of Neuroanesthesia and Intensive Care, and [2] Department of Neurosurgery, Neurological Institute, Via Celoria 11, 20133, Milan, Italy

Introduction

PEEP is considered a safe method for prevention of air embolism, the major risk of surgery performed in the sitting position [3, 4, 5]. PEEP-effects are mediated by a reduced venous outflow from the cephalic compartment with a consequent increase in intracranial pressure (ICP) [1, 2].

Methods and Results

In 10 patients with closed sutures, harbouring a posterior fossa tumor with untreated hydrocephalus (Table 1), we studied under general anesthesia and muscle relaxation the effects of a gradual increase of PEEP (from 0 to 15, by steps of 5 mmH_2O) on intrathoracic (central venous catheter) and intracranial (ventricular catheter) pressures, both in supine and sitting positions.

In the supine neutral position there was a gradual and linear increase both in intrathoracic and intracranial pressures (Fig. 1). In the sitting operative position, with the head flexed and/or rotated, the thoracic pressure, without and with PEEP was much lower than in the supine position. ICP, however, varied in 3 different ways (Fig. 2):

1. no changes: 5 patients (marked □)
2. moderate increase: 2 patients (marked ○)
3. rapid and dangerous increase: 3 patients (marked ▲) all with transependymal CSF absorption and 2 with papilloedema (Table 1)

Conclusions

1. Even with PEEP, intrathoracic pressure is very low and is often not transmitted to the cephalic compartment when the patient is in the sitting position. We must carefully check the central venous pressure because in these conditions the risk of air embolism is real.

Table 1. Clinical and radiological characteristics of our 10 patients

No	Response group	Age	Diagnosis	Papilloedema	Hydrocephalus	Transependymal absorption
1	□	24	Astrocytoma	no	yes	no
2	□	60	Hemangioblastoma	no	yes	no
3	□	60	Meningioma	no	yes	no
4	□	38	Hemangioblastoma	no	yes	no
5	□	44	Medulloblastoma	no	yes	no
6	○	14	Chordoma	no	yes	no
7	○	19	Medulloblastoma	no	yes	no
8	▲	7	Astrocytoma	yes	yes	yes
9	▲	60	Neurinoma	yes	yes	yes
10	▲	15	Astrocytoma	no	yes	yes

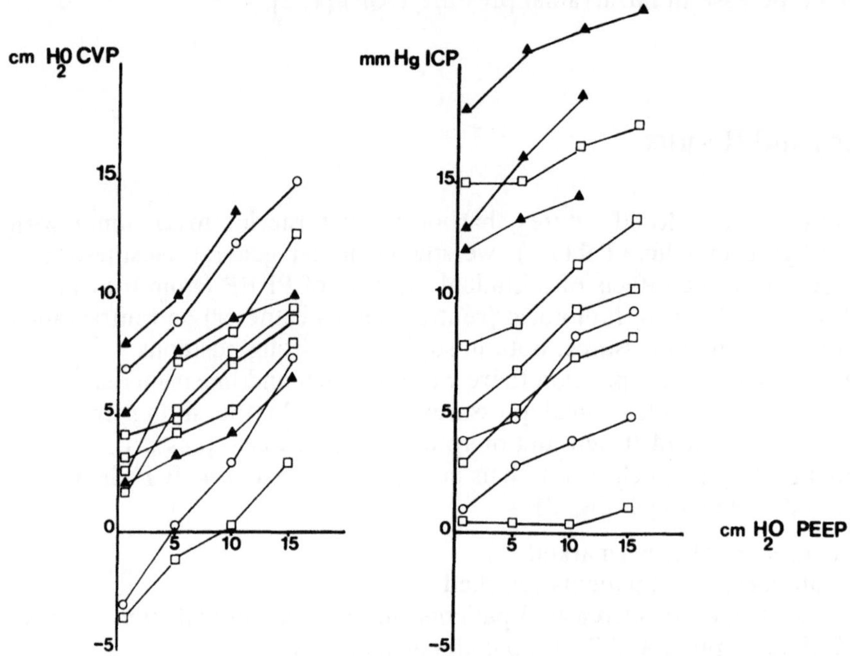

Fig. 1. CVP (*left*) and CIP (*right*) responses to increasing PEEP with patients in supine neutral position. (For explanation of symbols, see text)

2. In patients with papilloedema and radiological signs of increased ICP, the association of flexion-rotation of the head and institution of PEEP can cause a sudden rise in CSF pressure in the sitting position; extreme flexion rotation must be avoided and preoperative withdrawal of CSF is mandatory.

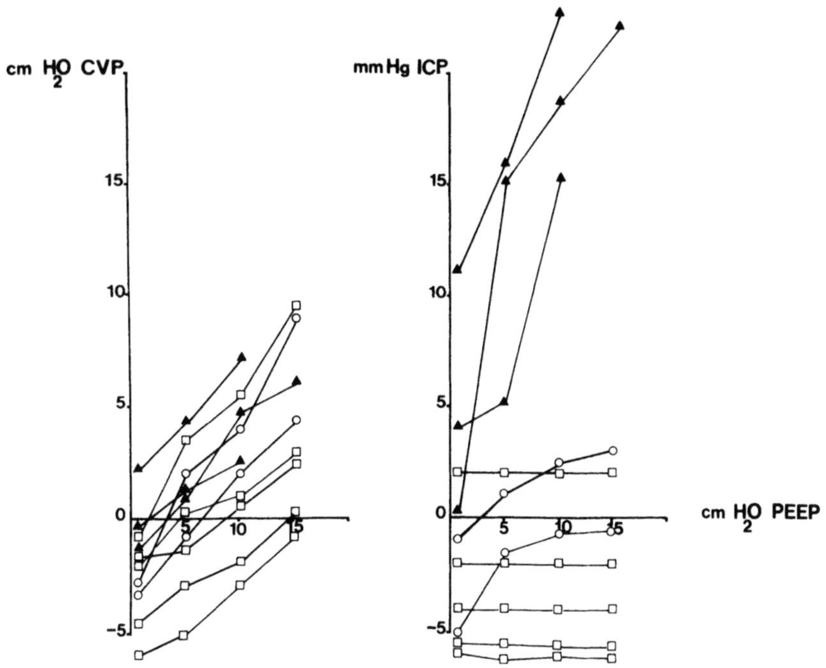

Fig. 2. CVP (*left*) and ICP (*right*) responses to PEEP of patients in the sitting operative position

References

1. Burchiel KJ, Steege TD, Wyler AR (1981) Intracranial pressure changes in brain injured patients requiring PEEP ventilation. Neurosurgery 8:443–449
2. Frost EAM (1977) Effects of PEEP on intracranial pressure and compliance in brain-injured patients. J Neurosurg 47:195–200
3. Matjasko J, Petrozza P, Cohen M, Steinberg P (1985) Anesthesia and surgery in the sitting position. Neurosurgery 17:695–702
4. Standefer M, Bay JV, Trusso R (1984) The sitting position in neurosurgery. Neurosurgery 14:649–658
5. Voorhies RM, Fraser RAR, Van Poznak AV (1983) Prevention of air embolism with PEEP. Neurosurgery 12:503–506

Panel 2
Cerebrovascular Dynamics

Moderator: G. Teasdale

Members: C. Anile, E.R. Cardoso, N.M. Dearden,
C.S. Robertson and M.J. Rosner

TEASDALE, opening the panel discussion, commented that whilst ICP is the theme that binds us together, the interest in ICP really started as a side issue of cerebral blood flow (CBF). Today, many of the posters are looking at new ways of trying to estimate CBF, both experimentally and in patients. By means of various forms of pulse wave analysis we are trying to extract more information for the same price we pay for measuring the pressure. We are perhaps trying to replace ICP by assessing intracranial vascular dynamics. Many papers dealt with measuring flow velocity by transcranial Doppler (TCD) and other papers with methods of measuring tissue flow from laser Doppler. We are trying to get information about the oxygen metabolism of the brain by looking at jugular oxygen content and also at tissue pO_2 or CSF pO_2. Measurements under stable conditions can tell us something, but perhaps not as much as when the system is pertubated. So, many studies involve pertubations of the system by changing blood pressure or blood gases. Some of the studies concern not only the events while an insult is developing, but also after it has been reversed, perhaps a very critical period.

DEARDEN raised some issues about the TCD methodology. The first thing to consider is the fact that TCD is measuring the flow velocity and that may produce its major restrictions as to the interpretation of what it means in terms of CBF. How reliable is this technique, how much practice does someone need in order to get reproducible readings? How reproducible are the data that someone can get within a patient and between patients? Can we do comparisons between patients as well as within patients? Should we monitor TCD continuously or intermittently and which vessels should we insonate and should we insonate more than one vessel at one time? Should we be measuring other things at the same time? And, finally, what do we intend to achieve? Is the aim of the use of this technique to replace perhaps more invasive techniques in an effort to try to extrapolate some information? What level of middle cerebral artery flow velocity, which is what most people seem to have been measuring, is normal? When it is abnormal, what does it mean? An increase in flow velocity can occur as a result of an increase in flow or as a decrease in flow associated with a narrowing of the insonated vessel. How can we tell these two things apart if we are only using TCD or do we need other measurements as well? There seems to be very little cross-validation at the moment and perhaps we can't answer many of these questions until we have that information. And then, finally, what is the effect of ICP on CBF velocity, what is the effect of cerebral perfusion pressure on CBF velocity? Can Doppler give us some information about the adequacy of CBF in relation to cerebral metabolism? These seem to be many of the issues that have been raised by the posters.

McGraw thought that by measuring TCD, it was important to realize that one is measuring vessel flow which is quite different from saturation flow. It had always been his contingent that if you can measure both of them, the difference between them is probably the more valuable parameter.

Marmarou commented that their interest in TCD was really to try to identify some reactivity measurements attempting to correlate transcranial Doppler velocities with CBF. It provides a rapid non-invasive way of testing the reactivity of the vessels after pertubation of the system. The problem is that, in head injury, there is a tendency over time for the velocity to increase, speaking about day three and day four. A poster presented at the recent AANS-conference by the UCLA-group very clearly identified vasospasm as being a characteristic of the head-injured patient and confirmed the vasospasm by angiographic evidence. Since about 50% of head-injured patients have sub-arachnoid haemorrhage, it would not be unexpected not to have some degree of vasospasm. The other issue deals as to whether or not one can or should continuously monitor. Well, then you get into the problem of which side. We have found cases in which, if we induced hypercapnia or hypocapnia and if we were insonating the right middle cerebral artery, we got a reactivity, on the left side not. So, we believe that in terms of TCD, it does have a role in head injury, it does provide a non-invasive method of reactivity, but there are problems when you attempt to relate transcranial flow directly to CBF.

Rosner commented that the Doppler looks at flow in a tube. It is a velocity, but it also represents the integral of everything happening downstream, which may include hyperaemia, high blood flows as well as low blood flows. It is basically the same problem that exists with the Xenon-technique. You may have a completely ischaemic area of one cc surrounded by a much larger volume of hyperaemic tissue and, as a result, you measure an increase in flow. The same problem exists with all of the integrating measurements of jugular bulb oxygen saturation and so forth. Because you integrate the entire hemisphere or the brain and produce a single number, which in fact includes a very pathological tissue as well as tissue which is reacting normally to that pathology, you run a major risk when you lump it all together, and the possibility of making wrong decisions is present.

Traystman compared TCD with CBF measured by microspheres in an animal model. They had been looking at the reactivity of the vessels, the increase of flow with carbondioxyde, hypoxia and reduction in blood pressure. It had been found that the reactivity of the vessels could be told just as easily with the TCD as with the CBF-measurement with microspheres. The delta changes were quite similar whereas it had been difficult to measure absolute blood flows. Trying to measure absolute flows with the TCD, even knowing the vessel diameter and then computing the flow, had not really correlated very well with the absolute flow measurements, particularly at the high and low values of flow. If one is just interested in an absolute flow change, a delta change, under a variety of conditions in the patient or in an animal, probably the TCD is O.K. to do so. If you then take it off the patient and try to come back again, as in the animal models, you will again get differences that are difficult to explain. You've got to be exactly in the same spot, you've got to be in the same geometric form of the insonation of the vessel. He concluded that measuring reactivity changes with TCD works quite well in the laboratory.

MENDELOW stated that he was in agreement with Dearden, Rosner and Marmarou in that TCD really only measures velocity. It doesn't measure blood flow and it doesn't measure diameter. They had embarked on a series of repeated measurements in more than 20 severe head injuries in New Castle very enthusiastically and had found no correlation with anything at all. This was perhaps because their patients were in a stable environment in the intensive care unit. According to his opinion, the interesting thing from the paper from Edinburgh was that the only real dropping of velocity seems to be when perfusion pressure drops below 50 or 60 mmHg. If we use TCD, how can we possibly tell whether it is measuring flow or diameter? The only reliable correlation which has been shown is that it reflects a drop in perfusion pressure.

MEIXENSBERGER gave an additional comment to the methodological problems of TCD blood flow velocity and CBF. They had done a series of examinations in patients with subarachnoid haemorrhage, in whom they had performed a direct correlation between CBF and TCD of the middle cerebral artery and they had found no correlation between global CBF or hemispheric CBF measured by the Xenon-method and the mean velocity of the middle cerebral artery. As far as CO_2 reactivity was concerned, they had found a good correlation. He thought that the CO_2 reactivity in TCD is the better parameter in the diagnostic of the cerebral vascular status of the patient.

DEARDEN agreed with the reservations stated on interpreting TCD. Most of the posters, not all of them, seemed to have found that cerebral perfusion pressure correlated better with flow velocity than anything else. The question of whether the relationship is linear or curvilinear, depends on the people analyzing the data. The big problem is that in a patient with a normal flow velocity at a cerebral perfusion pressure below 50 or 60 mmHg, you cannot detect spasm at least unless you do waveform analysis, which obviously has not yet been validated. This is because you do not record excessively high velocities if your input driving pressure is inadequate to give you a high enough CBF. And clearly, if you have a narrowed vessel, your actual flow may be low, but your flow velocity high. Conversely, you may have a dilated vessel with a relatively high CBF, but a normal or low flow velocity. Unless waveform analysis has a benefit, one has to use TCD with caution and only in the presence of other methods of monitoring, so that one can interpret what a change in flow velocity actually means.

The next issue raised by TEASDALE was waveform analysis, which can be seen as an attempt to get more information than one can get from simply looking at the raw data.

ROBERTSON gave an overview of the posters dealing with this subject. She backgrounded her comments by saying that there are two clinical applications for waveform analysis. The first is to try and estimate the compliance of the brain. There has been a number of parameters that have been thought to indicate the compliance of the brain. The second application is to try to understand the different underlying pathophysiologic mechanisms. The discussion on the different flow velocities with TCD and the contribution of waveform analysis to these problems is illustrative. She mentioned the poster by Piper et al. describing how to measure the amplitude transfer functions in ICP. This group had studied a large number of head-injured patients and looked at the real artery to ICP amplitude transfer function. The patients had been divided into four groups that were thought to correlate with different underlying pathophysiologies. Four patterns of amplitude transfer function could be clearly distinguished: an overall flat frequency response, an elevated low frequency response with a flat high frequency response, an elevated high frequency response and a flat low frequency response and, finally, a fourth group with both high and low frequency responses. The second and the fourth patterns were most often associated with raised ICP. She thought that the methodology should be discussed because the data had been taken from experimental studies where the carotid artery pressures had been used to calculate the amplitude transfer function, whereas in the clinical study the radial artery pressures had been used.

PIPER from Edinburgh answered that this was one of the basic methodology questions which they had not fully answered yet. They had tried to look at the effect of the site of blood pressure measurement on the variation in the amplitude transfer function. Experimentally they had been able to study simultaneous measurements from the radial artery, the abdominal aorta and the carotid artery and they had indeed observed clear differences in the waveform between the different sites. The point they had been trying to make was that, although there are differences between the harmonic components that make up these waveforms at different sites, the variations in the amplitude of these harmonics were still rather small in comparison to the gross changes that had been detected in patients. All they had been trying to do was to see whether this technique could be applied clinically for the detection of some forms of pressure transmission that might have some relevance to therapy for raised ICP.

CARDOSO in relation to the waveform analysis, commented that a word of caution should be made regarding input signals. Obviously, if one is using wave analysis as a reflection of cerebrovascular volume or reactivity, one can not neglect the veins. But even if one is using wave analysis for measurement of compliance, the venous pulse has also to be taken into account. Marmarou had a poster which addressed that very same problem from a completely different perspective, which is the contribution that veins may have to ICP and cerebrovascular pathophysiology in general. Despite whatever the venous pressure is, there is a contribution, an input signal from a retrograde pressure pulse that goes from the vein, enters the head and contributes finally to the configuration of the ICP pulse wave. Unfortunately, in the clinical situation we don't know much at all of what that pulsation might be.

TEASDALE remarked that the computation of transfer functions is technically demanding and drew attention to simple work on the ICP tracing itself and the centroid.

ROBERTSON: this is an interesting question. We have been looking at the centroid. There is a big influence of heart rate on the measurement and there is an artifact caused by the fact that we picked a fixed window to measure the centroid from. I think that this new method for calculating the centroid has basically moved the window based upon the heart rate and this eliminates the at least mathematical artifact of the harmonics moving in and out of the window.

The third issue raised by TEASDALE was the best posture for nursing the patient.

CARDOSO reviewed the posters on posture and thought it fascinating that at this day and age we cannot decide on what position to manage our patients. We have gone to the moon and explored the universe and this seems such a simple question. It might be that it is not that simple. When you are dealing with the position of the head, you should take into account the venous pressure (it seems like I am obsessed with veins today). If you raise the head above 45°, in most people you will get a negative pressure, which is in some way helping blood to pass through the head. The poster by Kanter et al. from Houston reported a study in which, for the first time, CBF measurements using the Kety-Schmidt N_2O-technique were done at 30° and 0° of head elevation. Cerebral perfusion pressure did not increase consistently with the head flat and there was no difference in the CBF of these patients in the elevated or horizontal positions. However, ICP did increase consistently in the flat position and, therefore, it was concluded to be probably safest to continue to nurse head-injured patients at 15–30° of head elevation.

ROSNER commented that in talking about venous pressure, there is a big difference between sagittal sinus pressure and cerebral venous pressure. The sagittal sinus is a semi-rigid structure in which you cannot generate negative pressures. It is not the same pressure as the cerebral venous pressure. In fact, the reason why the giraffe survives so nicely is because he is hypertensive when he raises his head. And if that is not allowed, and Patterson of MCV did a lot of that original work, they die. So, you got to be hypertensive when your head is up. The cerebral venous pressure is very close to the ICP. That is why we can calculate a global perfusion pressure which is not always accurate when it comes to micro-areas of high tissue pressure. The venous blood is probably the first volume to be displaced as CSF gets displaced more slowly. The patients with high ICP are not the ones who are likely to be most helped, in terms of ICP control, by encouraging the venous drainage, as they have already displaced most of their venous blood. So, it is in the people with low ICP in whom you are most likely to see the greatest reduction in ICP by raising the head. The head position does not basically matter in that group. In the ones who have a difficult ICP problem, you get much less of reduction and in fact you may trigger-off a plateau wave.

MARMAROU commented that the poster by Kanter et al. indicates that, at least with the nitrous-oxyde method, there is no change in CBF with the change of head position. However, they did measure a statistically reduced level of ICP and there were ICP's in their patients of up to 35 mmHg. He believed that, on the basis of the results of that poster, in nursing our patients we should keep their heads elevated.

CHOKSEY referring to the comments made by Rosner, said that the question of blood flow through collapsible tubes was already addressed by Hold in 1941. It took about 40 years for this knowledge to permeate itself into neurosurgery. For a system with collapsible tubes in a closed and ridged container, the outflow pressure, that is the pressure inside the sagittal sinus, is completely irrelevant to the amount of flow that you get through the system. The flow is actually determined by the pressure in the last half to one cm of the bridging veins. A reduction of the venous pressure makes no difference at all to the blood flow. Actually, we have the technology for sorting out this very problem, because we have a CBF monitor which will give us the answer as to what the optimum position for each patient is.

Closing the session, TEASDALE went back to what the theme of the first ICP meeting was, at the end of which a series of standards as to the way of talking about ICP, the ways of measuring it and ways of describing it were agreed upon. Presently, we need to do the same thing for a lot of things that are being used alongside ICP.

Bayer Round-Table Discussion on Methodology of Head Injury Trials

Moderator: J.D. Miller

Initial Assessment, Interim Monitoring and Final Outcome in Clinical Studies of Head Injury

G.M. Teasdale

University Department of Neurosurgery, Institute of Neurological Sciences, Southern General Hospital, Glasgow, Scotland

Studies that are well conducted, rigorously analysed and reliably reported are increasingly needed to determine the value of the range of potentially beneficial agents available now and in the forseeable future [14]. Head injuries are very common but there are many different mechanisms of injury and great variations in severity. Therefore, the criteria for entry of patients to the study must be well defined in advance, both to ensure internal consistency and to enable comparison with other reports. Events during the trial need to be monitored, not only in order to determine if an agent has adverse side effects, often the prime concern of the parent company, but to seek also for clues to the mechanisms of injury and how these are affected by the treatment. Assessments of outcome must be made at a time that is appropriate biologically and socially but also convenient for the purposes of acquiring the data in a reasonable time period.

Initial Selection and Characterisation of Head Injuries

One of the first decisions is the age range of patients. Many studies are restricted to adults, yet children make up almost a half of head injuries attending hospital and death from trauma is a leading cause of loss of life in this age group. Different injuries produce different types of damage; an obvious distinction is between gun shot wounds and "closed" injuries, but amongst the latter there are important distinctions between those resulting from high velocity impacts e.g. road traffic accidents and those from a simple assault or fall. The presence of associated multiple injuries is another important factor.

The assessment of severity of brain damage is of over-riding importance in ensuring well characterised and well balanced studies. This depends principally upon clinical assessments of features such as the level of consciousness [11, 12], of brain stem reflexes [3] and of focal neurological deficits. Investigations can provide information both about the type of damage and its severity. CT scanning is particularly valuable because the technique is now widely available and routinely employed in head injuries [13]. Measurement of intracranial pressure, of cerebral blood flow and metabolism, cerebral electrical activity and of biochemical indices of brain damage also characterise the severity of an injury but are less routinely available.

It is increasingly important to decide at what time after injury severity should be assessed. Traditionally this has been at the time of "admission", but this may be on first arrival to a hospital or subsequently, on admission to the Neurosurgical Unit. Systemic factors such as shock, and hypoxia, or the effects of alcohol and other drugs may lead to erroneous over estimates of the severity of damage; some studies therefore base admission on the "post-resuscitation" state but this is clearly liable to vary considerably both within a study and between centres. Assessments that are made too soon may either over estimate the severity of injury or under estimate it in patients who subsequently deteriorate from intracranial complications. In a large international series [7, 8] severity was assessed only after the patient had been in coma for 6 hours but this is now increasingly difficult to determine because of the widespread use of paralysis and ventilation. Indeed, with this treatment now being commenced before admission to hospital it may be that future studies will have to be based upon the patient's last known clinical condition, before the administration of paralysing and relaxing agents and commencement of ventilation.

Most studies focus upon "severe" head injuries but it is important to appreciate that these can be defined in different ways. The simplest definition is a patient that does not obey commands [1, 2]. More rigorous definition of coma requires that the patient also does not open his eyes or produce intelligible words [11]. This approximates to a Glasgow coma score of 8 but it is important to realise that such a score can be made up in a number of different ways; some 15% of patients with a score of <8 are not in coma by the full definition. Persistence of coma for 6 hours implies a severe injury, unresponsive to initial resuscitation and excludes some 15–20% of patients in coma at the time of admission to hospital [8]. These different definitions produce quite different outcomes but very similar outcomes when the same definition is applied in different centres [14].

The problems resulting from the loss of clinical assessment were apparent in the first randomised trial of nimodipine in head injuries [1]; at the time of admission to the Neurosurgical Unit, 49% of the patients were intubated and by the time of admission to the trial 69% of patients were intubated and therefore their verbal performance could not be assessed. Treatment given before arrival at the Neurosurgical Unit can influence the subsequent observations. In a study conducted in different British Neurosurgical Units the proportions of patients in coma who had been intubated and ventilated before arrival at one of three Neurosurgical Units were 38%, 50% and 71%; intriguingly, there was a parallel increase in proportion of patients considered to be in coma for 6 hours after admission to Neurosurgery: 72%, 88%, 94%.

The type of brain damage may be inferred from the mechanisms of injury, from clinical observations, from the findings of CT scanning or operation. The most fundamental distinction lies between focal and diffuse forms of damage [5]. Focal lesions include contusions, haematomas, infarctions and localised brain swelling. Diffuse damage results from diffuse axonal injury due to shearing forces, from diffuse cerebral ischaemia, and diffuse brain swelling. However, with a "diffuse" injury there is important distinction between patients whose CT scan shows signs of raised intracranial pressure (obliteration of the 3rd ventricle and basal cisterns) [13] and those without such features. A simple, relevant division of types of injury therefore is into 3 categories, operated intracranial haematoma (death or vegetative state in approximately 40% of cases) diffuse injury, with raised intracranial pressure (death or vegetative in 50–60% of patients) and diffuse injury without raised pressure (death or vegetative state in 20% of cases).

Monitoring during the course of the study provides information about the pattern and rate of recovery and of pathophysiological changes that may be influenced by treatment. More rapid recovery of responsiveness may anticipate an improved outcome at a later stage but this is yet to be established. In monitoring pathophysiological processes the aim is to identify the target mechanism at which the treatment is aimed and to determine if it is affected in the appropriate way. This may be relatively straightforward in the case of a variable such as intracranial pressure in which the effects of treatment can be observed in a single patient or through comparisons of groups of patients. However, it is important to remember that short-term, immediate effects upon a pathophysiological variable may not necessarily lead to an improvement in ultimate outcome. Thus the Richmond group [9] have shown that patients treated with THAM less often have raised intracranial pressure and, when raised, the pressure is more easily controlled but that this did not correlate with an improvement in outcome. The development of appropriate early indices of the mechanisms and severity of traumatic brain damage and of how their response to treatment relates to outcome is a major target for future research.

In the assessment of outcome a number of questions need to be answered. The first is when should outcome be studied? An early assessment, for example mortality at 7 days, has the advantage of providing a rapid index of the response to treatment. However, an apparent difference at this stage may be nullified by the subsequent death of patients who have survived in a vegetative or severely disabled condition. Late assessments are more relevant to the patient's recovery and reintegration into society but can be influenced by factors other than early treatment, e.g. the extent and efficacy of rehabilitation and social support. It has become customary to assess outcome at 6 months after severe head injury, by which time the great majority of survivors have reached a reasonably stable state.

In the assessment of outcome, the choice lies between simple, overall measures and detailed specific investigations of neurological and neuropsychological function. Disability after head injury is largely mental rather than physical and also results mainly from changes in personality, in affect and other behavioural features that are difficult to quantify. Moreover, assessments of the patient's condition by a member of the family are much more relevant and revealing than the patient's own account. A distinction between 2 outcomes is most efficient for statistical purposes and is usually bassed on the outcome scale devised by Jennett and Bond [6]. A distinction between patients who die or survive is relatively clear, and the incorporation with fatal cases of those small number surviving vegetative state has become accepted as a robust definition of a "bad" outcome. However, survival in a severely disabled state is increasingly viewed as an unsatisfactory result. Thus a distinction between dead, vegetative or severely disabled survivors on one hand and moderate to good recovery on the other is increasingly accepted. Nevertheless it must be borne in mind that in some patients the distinction between severe and moderate disability may be subtle and easily missed in the customary, brief neurosurgical out-patient consultation. Allocation of the patient to a favourable outcome category (moderate or good recovery) must only be made after information has been obtained from a relative or other reliable source.

Recommendations

A severe head injury is defined as a patient known not to be obeying commands before the institution of paralysis and ventilation. (This obviates the need to assess eye opening, which is the most variable aspect of response and also the verbal response which may be affected by intubation.) The population thus defined has a statistically convenient distribution of the 2 main divisions of outcome; almost half the patients have an unfavourable outcome, (dead or vegetative state, or severely disabled survival) and half make a moderate or good recovery. Three main subtypes of injury should be described; operated intracranial haematoma, and diffuse injuries with and without CT signs of raised ICP.

References

1. Bailey I, Bell A, Gray J, et al. (1991) A trial of the effect of nimodipine on outcome after head injury. Acta Neurochirurgica 110:97–105
2. Becker DP, Miller JD, Ward JD, et al. (1977) The outcome from severe head injury with early diagnosis and intensive management. J Neurosurg 47:491–502
3. Born JD (1988) Prognostic value and evolution of motor response and brain stem reflexes after severe head injury. Acta Neurochirurgica 91:1–11
4. Eisenberg H, Gary HE, Turner B. CT scan findings in 683 patients with severe head injury. A report from the NIH Traumatic Coma Data Bank. In: ICP VII Eds Hoff & Betz etc, pp 557–559
5. Gennarelli TA, Spielman GM, Langfelt TW, et al. (1982) Influence of the type of intracranial lesion on outcome from severe head injury. J Neurosurg 56:26–32
6. Jennett B, Bond M (1975) Assessment of outcome after severe brain damage (GOS). Lancet i:480
7. Jennett B, Teasdale G, Galbraith S, et al. (1977) Severe head injuries in 3 countries. JNNP 40:291–298
8. Jennett B, Teasdale G, Braakman R, et al. (1979) Prognosis of patients with severe head injury. Neurosurgery 4:283–289
9. Levi L, Wolf AL, Ward JD, et al. (1991) Failure of THAM to improve outcome in patients with severe head injury. A 2 center randomised study. Paper 834 AANS
10. Teasdale E, Cardoso E, Galbraith S, Teasdale G (1984) CT scan in severe diffuse head injury: physiological and clinical correlation. JNNP 47:600–603
11. Teasdale G, Jennett B (1976) Assessment and prognosis of coma after severe head injury. Acta Neurochir 34:45–55
12. Teasdale G, Jennett B (1979) Assessment of impaired coma and consciousness. Lancet ii: 81–84
13. Teasdale G, Teasdale E, Hadley D. CT/MRI Classification of head injury. (in press)
14. Teasdale G, Bullock R, McCulloch J. Pharmacological therapy of head injury. J Neurotrauma (in press)

Lessons in Clinical Trial Design From the Traumatic Coma Data Bank

L.F. MARSHALL and S. BOWERS MARSHALL

Division of Neurological Surgery, University of California Medical Centre, San Diego, CA, USA

In 1979, the San Diego experience with hypnotics was presented for the first time at a meeting in Charlottesville, Virginia. At that time, Professor Bryan Jennett presented a slide which made the following suggestions for the comparisons of new treatments with present methods of care. Suggestions and questions were:

1. Are the patients well matched?
2. Are the treatments well controlled?
3. Had the outcome measures been selected in advance, and are they clear?

These criteria were, and are, the guiding principles of clinical trials. In the few minutes available today, I will attempt to share with you what we have learned in the Traumatic Coma Data Bank, an almost 10 year experience in the United States. Professor Teasdale has already emphasized the importance of traditional factors, including age, severity of injury as measured by the clinical examination, and the time from injury to both pre-hospital and definitive neurosurgical treatment. The importance of these factors has also been clearly demonstrated within the Data Bank, and perhaps, one of the Data Bank's more important contributions is its emphasis on a new classification of brain injury utilizing CT scanning. This classification, is shown in Table 1. There is a progressive increase in mortality as evidence of mass or volume effect increases on the CT scan (Table 2). This confirms in a large series of patients and further amplifies the observations of Teasdale, et al. [6]; van Dongen, et al. [8]; and Toutant, et al. [7], that compression or absence of the mesencephalic cisterns is an ominous prognostic finding, even in patients who appear relatively well clinically. It already has had a direct influence on patient management in the Data Bank centers. Thus, Luerssen, et al., were able to show that a substantial reduction in mortality occurred from the pilot phase to the full-phase Data Bank in these patients and that treatment had begun earlier and was more intense, suggesting that these head injury centers were placing more emphasis on the CT scan than they had previously in deciding when and with what vigor to treat [4]. This policy appears logical as in this group of patients, as shown in Table 3, it is the volume status of the brain, as linked with the highest ICP, that is the most important determinant of outcome as compared to all other CT patterns of brain injury where age and motor score are dominant predictive factors. The rather similar mortalities and outcomes which are seen in Diffuse Injury III and IV when compared with patients with evacuated mass lesions, suggests that these two categories of Diffuse Injury are the non-surgical coun-

Table 1. Diagnostic categories of types of abnormalities visualized on CT scanning

Diffuse Injury I: (No visible pathology)	No visible intracranial pathology seen on CT
Diffuse Injury II:	Cisterns are present with shift 0–5 mm and/or Lesion densities present No high or mixed density lesion >25 cc May include bone fragments and foreign bodies
Diffuse Injury III: (Swelling)	Cisterns compressed or absent with shift 0–5 mm No high or mixed density lesion >25 cc
Diffuse Injury IV: (Shift)	Shift >5 mm No high or mixed density lesion >25 cc
Evacuated Mass Lesion:	Any lesion surgically evacuated
Non-evacuated Mass Lesion:	High or mixed density lesion >25 cc, not surgically evacuated

terpart of the mass lesion group and that treatments which influence intracranial volume in a positive manner might have beneficial effects in these two populations.

The need for a classification of head injury, based on CT scanning, is emphasized by the fact that there were major differences in outcome between the four centers within the Data Bank which were primarily explained by differing populations of these types of injuries. When these variations in CT injury severity were taken into account, the inter-center differences largely disappeared given the fact that post-resuscitation GCS scores in the four centers were very closely matched, indicating that matching on GCS and age alone will be inadequate to be certain that populations are similar. The reliability of the CT scan reading is a critical factor when making such comparisons. The Data Bank utilized one reader in each center and common test CT scans, which were read and used to judge each center's reliability. Issues of difference were discussed and uniform definitions were agreed upon. This led to a high degree of inter-center reliability and is essential in clinical trials of head injury.

In addition to the CT pattern of injury, another critical factor appears to have emerged from the Data Bank experience. In 1988, Chesnut and Marmarou both presented work from the Data Bank demonstrating the critical importance of hypotension on brain injury outcome [1, 5]. This work followed up on previous efforts of Eisenberg, et al. [2], from the pilot Data Bank, where the adverse consequences of shock and hypoxia on severe head injury had been clearly demonstrated. What was unique about these new studies was the dramatic influence of shock occurring both in the pre-hospital as well as in the in-hospital phase and the fact that relatively brief periods of moderate hypotension with systolic blood pressures in the 80's appeared to have such a dramatic and adverse influence on outcome. As this area has been explored in more detail by Blunt, S.B. Marshall, and the other members of the San Diego group, it has become apparent that the influence of shock or perhaps, more appropriately, the reduction of cerebral perfusion pressures to unsatisfactory levels, has a profound influence on head injury outcome. The frequency of late shock (defined as the period more than 9 hours following Data Bank hospital admission) is astoundingly high and in over 80% of the patients is not an

Table 2. Number of patients (percent) by discharge Glasgow Outcome Scale (GOS) and intracranial diagnosis

	Intracranial diagnosis								
GOS (Discharge)	Diffuse injury I No visible pathology	Diffuse injury II	Diffuse injury III (Swelling)	Diffuse injury IV (Shift)	Evacuated mass	Non-evacuated mass	Brain stem injury	Unknown	Total
Good	14	15	5	1	14	1	0	0	50
	(27.0)	(8.5)	(3.3)	(3.1)	(5.1)	(2.8)	(0)	(0)	(7.0)
Moderate	18	46	20	1	49	3	0	1	138
	(34.6)	(26.0)	(13.1)	(3.1)	(17.7)	(8.3)	(0)	(5.9)	(18.5)
Severe	10	72	41	6	72	7	1	0	209
	(19.2)	(40.7)	(26.8)	(18.8)	(26.1)	(19.4)	(33.3)	(0)	(28.0)
Vegetative	5	20	35	6	34	6	0	0	106
	(9.6)	(11.3)	(22.9)	(18.8)	(12.3)	(16.7)	(0)	(0)	(14.0)
Dead	5	24	52	18	107	19	2	16	243
	(9.6)	(13.5)	(34.0)	(56.2)	(38.8)	(52.8)	(66.7)	(94.1)	(32.5)
Total	52	177	153	32	276	36	3	17	746
	(100)	(100)	(100)	(100)	(100)	(100)	(100)	(100)	(100)

Table 3. Potential predictors of mortality for intracranial diagnosis of diffuse injury III (swelling) by predictor P-value and goodness-of-fit P-value

Predictor	Prediction P-value	P-value Goodness-of-fit[a]
Highest ICP (first 72 hours)	<0.001	0.038
Pupil reactivity (post-resuscitation)	<0.001	0.610
Lowest ICP (first 72 hours)	0.023	0.930
Best Motor (post-resuscitation)	0.510	0.970
Age	0.680	0.970

[a] By the Hosmer-Lemeshow test, P-value for each row for model fit including predictors in its row and above (the higher the P-value, the better the fit)

agonal terminal event. Rather, it is occurring at a time of active intervention. While the frequency of intracranial mass lesions is higher in the late shock group when compared to the no-no-no group, this is not the only variable operating here. What is of particular interest is the fact that in the patients with Diffuse Injury, the frequency of the different CT classifications is rather similar, but that one episode of shock in this population appearing to have similar severities of injury, based both on CT and on initial GCS, has a profound influence on outcome. Thus, it would appear to be appropriate in future clinical trials to record the frequency time course and severity of shock or reductions in cerebral perfusion pressure when outcomes are analyzed. Studies do not need to be stratified, according to the presence or absence of shock because this event is often late and patients must be randomized before. However, failure to recognize the heterogenous nature of head injury and new factors which influence this heterogeneity may well yield false conclusions regarding the efficacy or lack thereof of certain pharmacological and other treatments. Given the fact that many of the agents that are now being tried for the treatment of severe head injury such as Nimodipine and the aminosteroids appear to have an effect by protecting neurons from ischemia, it is logical to conclude that such a stratified analysis will be essential. Our demonstration that patients with Diffuse Injury and no evidence of shock throughout their entire course have a mortality of less than 10% indicates that it is most unlikely that a pharmacologic treatment can or will be shown to be effective in this population where the outcome is so good already. Thus, a particular emphasis on identifying specific groups at high risk of an adverse outcome should be a feature of all future clinical trials. Other factors which have an adverse outcome and which are frequent in head injury should also not be forgotten. Subarachnoid hemorrhage, which occurs in almost one-half of all severe head injuries, is a significant independent predictor of adverse outcome, as demonstrated by Eisenberg, et al. [3]. Thus, the likelihood that both focal and global ischemia occur in head injury appears to be extremely high, and this is yet another factor which may well need to be taken into account.

Clearly, there is a danger in developing more and more small cells within large clinical trials. One can wind up with studies in which the number of patients to test the basic hypothesis is far too small, and nothing will come out of a major clinical effort. Nevertheless, some attention to major risk factors and important variables prior to study initiation are more likely to yield appropriately targeted trials, and the possibility of detecting a successful effective treatment will be improved. Just as it is inappropriate to overstate the efficacy of an agent when a very small effect is noted, it is inappropriate to understate the importance of an agent's efficacy in a sub-population of patients, particularly those at high risk. As the overall poor outcome from severe head injury in most major advanced societies has been reduced to approximately 35% and has not changed materially over the last decade in experienced institutions, more strategic targeting of therapy and of clinical trials is imperative.

References

1. Chesnut RM, Marshall LF, Klauber MR, Blunt BA, Baldwin N, Eisenberg HM, Jane JA, Marmarou A, Foulkes MA. The role of secondary brain injury in determining outcome from severe head injury: Analysis of the frequency of occurrence and impact on outcome of hypotension and hypoxia and their interactions with severe multiple trauma in severely brain injured patients. Submitted to JAMA
2. Eisenberg HM, Cayard C, Papanicolaou A, Weiner R, Franklin D, Jane J, Grossman R, Tabaddor K, Becker DP, Marshall LF, Kunitz S (1983) The effects of three potentially preventable complications on outcome after severe closed head injury. In: Ishii S, Nagai H, Brock M (eds) Intracranial pressure V. Springer, Berlin Heidelberg New York Tokyo, pp 549–553
3. Eisenberg HM, Gary HE Jr, Turner B, Jane JA, Marmarou A, Marshall LF, Young HF, and the NIH TCDB Writing Group (1989) CT scan finding in 683 patients with severe (GCS $\leqslant$ 8) closed head injury: A report from the NIH Traumatic Coma Data Bank. In: Hoff JT, Betz AL (eds) Intracranial pressure VII. Springer, Berlin Heidelberg New York London Paris Tokyo Hong Kong, pp 557–559
4. Luerssen TG, Hults KR, Klauber Mr, et al. (1989) Improved outcome as a result of recognition of absent or compressed cisterns on admitting CT scan. In: Hoff JT, Betz AL (eds) Intracranial pressure VII. Springer, Berlin Heidelberg New York London Paris Tokyo Hong Kong, pp 598–602
5. Marmarou A, Anderson RL, Ward JD, Choi SC, Young HF, Eisenberg HM, Foulkes MA, Marshall LF, Jane JA: Impact of ICP instability and hypotension on outcome in patients with severe head trauma. J Neurosurg (submitted)
6. Teasdale E, Cardoso E, Galbraith S, et al. (1984) CT scan in severe diffuse head injury: physiological and clinical correlations. J Neurol, Neurosurg and Psychiatry 47:600–603
7. Toutant SM, Klauber MR, Marshall LF, et al. (1984) Absent or compressed basal cisterns on first CT scan: Ominous predictors of outcome in severe head injury. Neurosurg 61:691–694
8. van Dongen KJ, Braakman R, Gelpke GJ (1983) The prognostic value of computerized tomography in comatose head-injured patients. J Neurosurg 59:951–957

Consequences for Trials of Variations in the Management of Severe Head Injuries

B. JENNETT

Professor of Neurosurgery, Institute of Neurological Sciences, University of Glasgow, Glasgow, Scotland

In most surgical specialties there are wide variations in what surgeons do for the same kinds of patient. Reporting studies of surgical variations between adjacent counties of New England, and between New England and old England and other European countries, Wennberg concluded that these differences reflected the practice styles or surgical signatures of different surgeons [6]. In his view wide variations in practice indicate professional uncertainty about the effectiveness of, or necessity for, those interventions that are used at very different rates.

Variations may occur between different places, or in one place between different time periods; and sometimes between different professionals in the same place and at the same time. Variations in the early care of head injuries may also reflect the influence of different disciplines (e.g. trauma surgeons, anaesthetists and neurosurgeons), because one or other of these may be the dominant decision-maker in different places, or at different stages in management. Several factors influence the balance of activity between those who see the head injured patient first and the regional neurosurgeons who see him later. These include geographical distance, the availability of neuro-imaging facilities in other hospitals and the willingness of other surgeons to operate on the head. There are still some countries where local surgeons are encouraged to make burr holes and then to arrange rapid transfer to the neurosurgeon.

Variations therefore apply not only to what is done in neurosurgical units but also to what occurs before that – both what is done, and the interval between injury and arrival at a neurosurgical unit. When the transfer policy for the Glasgow neurosurgical unit was changed not only did the number of head injuries admitted each year double, but the proportion that came within six hours of injury also doubled. Even within the same country, however, this interval can vary considerably between places.

A striking change in recent years in many places is the proportion of patients who are already intubated by the time they reach a neurosurgical unit, some of whom are also paralysed, sedated and ventilated. This can make it difficult to identify which patients are severely injured, and to grade their severity. To assume that all patients who arrive on a ventilator at the neurosurgical unit are severely injured will almost certainly result in including some patients who would not have been so categorised by the criterion of being GCS <8 after initial resuscitation. This is because some aggressive anaesthetists or paramedics at the roadside or at the first hospital insist on the need for such interventions for some less severely injured patients. Professor Braakman tells me that the European Nimodipine study confirms that this occurs in several places. Compared with series based on stricter entry criteria, the inclusion of such less severely injured patients will lead to better outcomes for the series as a whole.

It might be expected that once in the NSU treatment would be more consistent – after so many years of systematic studies of head injury management. However, we have reported wide variations in the management of severe head injuries between Glasgow, the Netherlands and two centres in California [3]. No one country was consistently more active or aggressive than another; indeed the greatest single difference was between the tracheostomy rates in Los Angeles and San Francisco. In spite of these variations the mortality rate for injuries who were well-matched for age and severity was similar in all four places, as was the distribution of outcomes in survivors.

A recent study of four UK neurosurgical units between 1986 and 1989 showed somewhat less variation than in the three countries study, but the use of intracranial pressure monitoring varied from 0 to almost 70% [5]. In the multicentre Nimodipine trial only 6 of 21 European centres were found to be using intracranial pressure monitoring, according to Professor Braakman. Although not a therapeutic modality, those who often use such monitoring presumably consider that it makes management more effective, while those who seldom do presumably consider that the advantages are often outweighed by the risk of complications. There was no striking difference in the mortality rates in the four UK centres, in spite of the variations in management.

Doctors looking after critically ill patients tend to have strong views about what should be done, even if these opinions are not based on good evidence that these interventions are definitively beneficial. The more a trial protocol constrains the choices of clinicians, the more likely is it that cases will either be excluded from the trial, or will be included with protocol violations, which may not always be declared. A compromise has to be struck between too tight and too close a protocol.

An advantage of minimal constraints is that it provides an opportunity to discover what management variations occur in practice. It may also make it possible to assess the influence on outcome of certain interventions, or of therapeutic packages, by comparing the outcomes in groups of similar patients who were treated differently. Because the basis of demonstrating efficacy is to show an outcome better than predicted without the therapy under test, similarity between patients should mean that they were predicted to have similar outcomes. Analysing the consequences of the chance variations in the use of therapies is a legitimate first stage in assessing the value of modalities that are already in common use, but are not always employed [1].

False claims for benefit from certain interventions or therapeutic packages arise from one or more of three methodological errors. The probability of a poor outcome without the specified intervention may be over-estimated, particularly if the case mix is biased towards less severe injuries. Or the hazards of the intervention may be under-estimated, or even unacknowledged. Or the assessment of efficacy may be based on small numbers, on inadequately matched cases, or on unsatisfactory statistical methods. It is also necessary to show that any improved outcome observed is significant in degree. Also that it is not confined to laboratory parameters but is of definite benefit to patients. And that a significant percentage of patients do so benefit.

In 1980 we reported that steroids had been of no benefit in the international study of some 1200 cases, about half of whom had received these drugs by the free choice of their doctors [3]; this has subsequently been confirmed by several randomised trials. Another example of this application was the study of 8000 head injuries in 41 US hospitals, between which management and mortality varied widely – from many times more and many times less than predicted [4]. However, this difference in mortality applied only to the low risk cases (<10% predicted mortality). The mortality for severely injured patients was little better in the best than in the worst hospitals. This indicates the importance of ensuring that severity of injury is similar in groups of patients used to test efficacy.

Such studies of outcome in patients treated differently by chance may indicate which interventions ought to be the focus of formal clinical trials, and which patients should be chosen. They make preliminary stratification of patients possible, so that planned trials need much smaller numbers of cases than if all patients were included. Without such choice of patients any benefit to one group might be obscured by the large number who are so severely or so mildly injured that treatment would not be expected to influence their outcome. That could be very valuable as more drugs are developed that need to be evaluated, at the same time as the incidence of severe head injury in many developed countries is slowly falling as preventive measures take effect.

When variations are wide it is almost certain that the use of some treatment modalities are often inappropriate. This is not only because they do not improve outcome, but because they also add unjustifiable hazard and/or expense. We should therefore hesitate to regard these variations as a welcome sign of the diversity of opinion and practice among neurosurgeons, and between them and their colleagues in other disciplines [2]. Instead we should ask whether they are not disturbing differences, and seek to devise protocols that minimise inappropriate interventions and thus reduce variations that cannot be justified.

References

1. Jennett B (1987) Assessment of a technological package using a predictive tool. Int J Tech Assess in Health Care 3:335–38
2. Jennett B (1988) Variations in surgical practice: welcome diversity or disturbing differences. Br J Surg 75:630–31
3. Jennett B, Teasdale G, Fry J, et al. (1980) Treatment for severe head injury. J Neurol Neurosurg Psychiat 43(4):289–95
4. Klauber RM, Marshall LF, Leurssen TG, et al. (1989) Determinants of head injury mortality: importance of the low risk patient. Neurosurgery 24:31–36
5. Teasdale G, Murray L, Jennett B (1991) Unpublished report to the MRC on a study of severe head injuries: 4 UK neurosurgical units
6. Wennberg JE (1984) Dealing with medical practice variations; a proposal for action. Health Affairs 3:6–32

Practical Problems During the Nimodipine Head Injury Trial II

R. Braakman

Department of Neurosurgery, Erasmus University Rotterdam, NL-3015 GD Rotterdam, The Netherlands

The aim of both randomized, prospective and double blind Bayer Nimodipine Head Injury studies is to establish whether the intravenous administration of Nimodipine reduces the occurrence of an unfavourable outcome after severe head injury and increases the rate of independent survival. Six centres participated in HIT I, the British-Finnish cooperative study, the number of patients enrolled totalling 351. On entry into the trial within 24 hours of injury the patients were not obeying commands. Nimodipine was administered intravenously at a rate of 2 mg per hour, for 7 days.

The hypothesis to be tested was that Nimodipine administration might reduce the unfavourable outcome after 6 months (death, vegetative state or severe disability) from 50% to 35% and increase the rate of independent survival (moderate disability and good recovery) from 50% to 65%. The results of this study show that the increase in favourable outcome was in fact far less, only 4% (effectively 8% if considered in relation to the 50%), and not statistically significant. The study did not exclude a modest, but clinically useful, advantage of treatment [2].

The Nimodipine Head Injury study II enjoys participation from 21 centres distributed over 13 European countries. Eligible for entry are patients not obeying commands. It is also a 7-days parallel, double-blind, multicentre study of Nimodipine versus placebo with a follow-up of 6 months.

The intravenous infusion of the test drug should be initiated as soon as possible and not later than 12 hours after the patient fails to obey commands (Table 1).

In such a controlled study we have to find an equilibrium between a feasible hypothesis, the number of cases required, and the optimal period that the study can last (2–3 years). HIT I demonstrated that it was very unlikely that a 15% increase in independent survival would be achieved. Proof of a 5% increase in favourable outcome would hardly be interesting for clinicians. Moreover, to prove such a 5% increase would require the participation of thousands of patients. This is not feasible, because such a study would take too long to complete.

In HIT II, the hypothesis is that the unfavourable outcome might be reduced from 50% to 40% and hence the independent survival rate increased from 50% to 60%.

The enrolment of patients ceased on the first of July 1991 and the results of this study will be available in the first half of 1992.

Table 1. The design of the Nimodipine HIT II study

– 13 countries
– 21 centres – 800 patients
– not obeying commands (n.o.c.)
– Nimodipine 2 mg/hr iv for 7 days initiated less than 12 hrs after n.o.c.
– 6 months outcome

Table 2. The reasons why patients were eligible but not enrolled

– investigator not informed
– investigator not available
– cardiovascular instability
– under influence of drugs
– no informed consent
– time of injury uncertain
– "too many patients in I.C."
– no particular reason

Assuming a 50% rate of severe outcome in the control group, a reduction to 40% of severe outcome with a 5% level of statistical significance and a power of 80%, the study would require about 400 patients per group; this is an acceptable number.

Prior to embarking on the study, the representatives of the centres estimated the number of patients they expected to include within a 2-year period. Half of them greatly overestimated – by more than 100% – the number they actually enrolled. Of the number conservatively expected to be enrolled, about 30% will actually enter the study.

Not all patients eligible for the study are necessarily enrolled. The reasons are mentioned in Table 2, in a declining frequency. At the present stage, with over 800 patients enrolled, 160 (20%) were eligible but not included.

Although the enrolment criterion of not obeying commands was required in all centres, mortality and morbidity differed greatly between the various centres. This confirmed our expectation that a lack of homogeneity exists in such large multicentre designs. This is due to differences in geography and referral policy. Such designs can, therefore, only be employed when the nature of the trial is pragmatic and not explanatory.

Despite personal visits to most centres on more than one occasion by the two principal investigators, and although a full-time datamanger and at least one physician was employed in every country as local trial monitor, we came across a relatively large number of *protocol violations*; these are mentioned in Table 3.

The most common violations were

– an intensive care doctor prescribed a calcium antagonist for reasons which were not obvious.

Table 3. Distribution of protocol violations

>12 hrs not obeying commands	15
Calcium antagonists given	23
Follow-up too late or not at all	10
Obeying commands	6
<80% test drug	7
barbiturate coma	5
miscellaneous	12
	85

– enrolment took place although more than 12 hours had passed since the onset of the state of not obeying commands.
– follow-up was performed too late or not at all.

In our protocol the principles of *informed consent* in the current revision of the Helsinki declaration were implemented. Informed consent in unconscious patients is an example of emergency consent, where the initial consent has to be given by the relatives. The relatives, or necessary legal representatives, were given ample opportunity to inquire about details of the trial, etc.

Different European countries hold quite varying views concerning informed consent. In some countries even obtaining informed consent is considered to be an avoidable nuisance. Most European doctors and patients, however, agree that obtaining informed consent is problematic because patients or relatives do not fully understand the implications of a formal clinical trial [3].

The real motivation for the patient or his family to give consent lies in fear and a willingness to do anything that has even the slightest appearance of contributing to the recovery. It is clear that very different and sometimes perhaps even abusive procedures have been used in our and in other trials to obtain what is called "informed consent" [1].

Obtaining informed consent is part of *good clinical practice* (GCP). GCP and its criteria are far more common and developed in the United States than in Europe. This term means: a standard by which clinical trials are designed, implemented and reported so that there is public assurance that the data are credible, and that the rights, integrity and confidentiality of subjects are protected.

On the first of July, 1991, such GCP rules for trials and medicinal projects became mandatory in the European community [4]. These detailed requirements have been published in an extensive document. They concern the protection of trial subjects and consultation of Ethics Committees, the responsibilities of the sponsor, the monitor and the investigator, the data handling by the investigator and monitor, the filing of data, the language used, the statistical approach and guarantee of quality. This recent document was not available 2 years ago when we embarked on HIT II.

Nevertheless, our study, approved by the FDA, meets these requirements [5]. Future clinical trials will have to meet all the requirements mentioned in this document and, consequently, good clinical practice will become more important than many of us realize today [6].

In *assessing outcome*, the distinction between patients who are dependent and classified as severely disabled, and those patients with a marked degree of moderate disability, is not easy. In quite a number of cases the review committee, who checked all outcome forms, wondered whether the patient was classified in the correct category. Sometimes the investigator changed the categorization after our comment. This means that a patient may be transferred from the unfavourable to the favourable category or vice versa and that this may completely change the outcome of the study. A consistent, well described distinction is essential for a study like this one. I wonder whether the distinction in HIT I and in HIT II, between SD (unfavourable) and MD (favourable), is the best distinction available to study drug-efficacy.

It has been shown – yet again – after the enrolment of 800 patients, that the very critical and conscientious *review committee*, consisting of at least three neurosurgeons who do not only review all case report forms, but also all inital CT's and outcome forms, is indispensable for such a multicentre trial.

Despite all our efforts, it was impossible to omit all protocol violations and other shortcomings of our study and this will remain a challenge. But we do believe that on the whole the study is well designed and well performed and fulfills a pivotal role.

References

1. Abramson NS, Meisel A, Safar P (1986) Deferred consent. JAMA 255:426–471
2. Bailey I, Bell A, Gray J, et al. (1991) A trial of the effect of Nimodipine on outcome after head injury. Acta Neurochirurgica 110:97–105
3. Brahams D (1989) Incompetent adults and consent to treatment. Lancet 11 Febr
4. Good Clinical Practice: EG Note for Guidance verabschiedet (1990) Pharm Ind 52:1475
5. FDA Guideline for the monitoring of clinical investigations (issued under 21 CFR 10.90) (1988) FDA Maryland
6. Knowles N (1988) Good clinical practice in Europe. PJB Publications Ltd. Richmond

Session V: Head Injury

Chairmen: B. Jennett and D.A. Hovda

Experimental

Concussive Brain Injury Produces a State of Vulnerability for Intracranial Pressure Perturbation in the Absence of Morphological Damage

D.A. Hovda, H. Badie, S. Karimi, S. Thomas, A. Yoshino, T. Kawamata, and D.P. Becker

Division of Neurosurgery, UCLA School of Medicine, Los Angeles, CA 90024-6901, USA

Introduction

Following a fluid percussion (F-P) brain injury the cells in the brain go into a state of vulnerability during which, if they sustain a second, typically nonlethal insult, they die. This has been previously described in the rat [3] where a F-P injury was followed in 1 hour by a 6 min forebrain ischemic insult. Cells within the CA1 region of the hippocampus that normally survive both insults independently, now die when the insults are administered in close temporal proximity.

In a F-P model using the rat we have previously described that although there is no cell death following a diffuse F-P insult, cells are exposed to pronounced ionic shifts of potassium [4] and calcium [1]. This ionic perturbation is responsible for the marked derangement in glucose metabolism typically seen following this injury [5, 8]. We have proposed that this period of post-traumatic metabolic derangement may delineate a period of time during which the brain would be compromised in its ability to respond to a second insult [2].

To examine this question we have begun a series of studies to determine the effect of a second F-P when it is sustained during the first few hours after a concussive brain injury. For the current work both histological and physiological studies were employed.

Methods

Male Sprague Dawley rats (250–300 g) were subjected to either a single or a double lateral F-P (3.5–4.2 atm) using ethrane anesthesia (1.5%). For the double insults a period of 1 or 2 hours separated the two F-Ps. The F-P device used in the current study has been described in detail [3, 6]. However, it should be emphasized that we employ an extension tube of 20 cm interconnecting the injury cap on the animal to the F-P devise to assure a diffuse – concussive type, rather than a localized – contusion type of injury [7].

Two series of animals were used, one to address the changes in intracranial pressure (ICP) using a Camino Catheter and the other for extensive quantitative histology. For the ICP measurements the catheter was inserted into the brain parenchyma and ICP was monitored continuously pre- and post-injury. For quantitative histology animals were sacrificed 10 days following injury and cresyl violet stained coronal (40 um) sections were studied using light microscopy. Cells within the cerebral cortex and hippocampus were counted and drawn with the use of a camera lucida drawing tube. Cross sectional areas for each cell were determined using a computer assisted image analysis system (JAVA, Jandel Scientific).

Results

Following a single insult the animals experienced a period of apnea (mean = 9.7 ± SD 4.2 sec) and unconsciousness (mean = 33.3 ± SD = 16.0 sec) where consciousness was defined as when the animal exhibited a paw pinch reflex. Measurements of ICP indicated an increase from a mean of 6.2–7.2 mmHg prior to injury to a peak level between 43.8–65.8 with the increase in ICP lasting for as long as 10 min (Fig. 1 and 2). Histological analysis indicated that there was no loss of cells or change in cellular cross sectional area within either the cerebral cortex or underlying hippocampus.

In animals who experienced a second insult at 1 or 2 hours, the duration of apnea and unconsciousness was markedly increased (mean apnea time; 1 hour

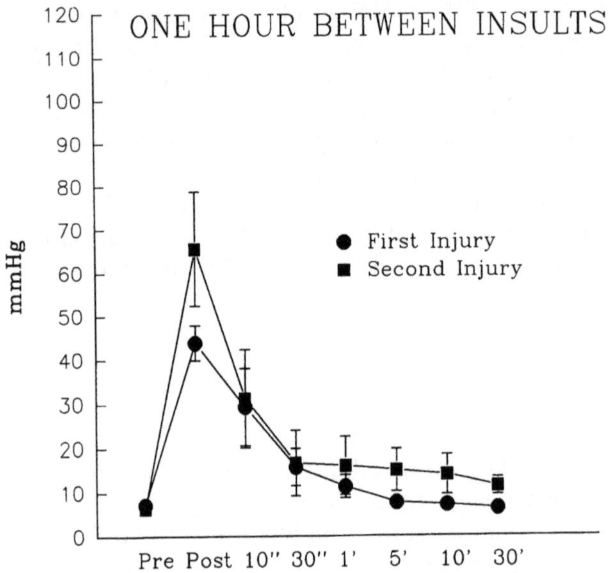

Fig. 1. Mean (± SEM) intracranial pressure (mmHg) for animals pre- and post-injury for both the insults spaced at one hour

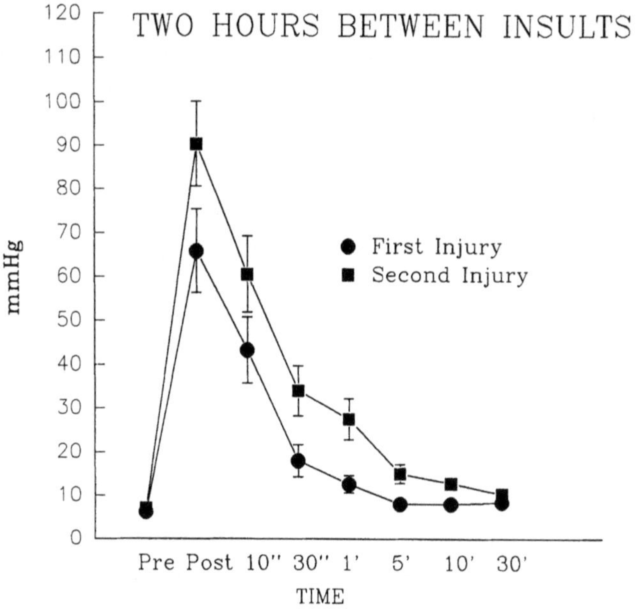

Fig. 2. Mean (± SEM) intracranial pressure (mmHg) for animals pre- and post-injury for both the insults spaced at two hours

= 18.0 ± SD 12.0 sec; 2 hours = 33.3 ± SD = 19.4). Measurements of ICP indicated that it also was markedly increased following the second insult and that this ICP increase was sustained for a much longer period of time. Levels of ICP following a second insult delayed for 1 hour reached a mean peak level of 65.5 mmHg. Levels of ICP following a second insult delayed for 2 hours reached a mean peak level of 90.3 mmHg. Following either the 1 or 2 hour delayed insult ICP remained significantly increased ($p < 0.05$) for as long as 20 min in some animals (Fig. 1 and 2).

Histological analysis in animals who sustained a double insult indicated that the second injury resulted in the development of contusions. These lesions were typically formed at the grey/white boarder, varied in size and demonstrated the extent of cell death typically seen following a second insult.

Discussion

The results from this work indicated that a single F-P injury resulted in a slight increase in ICP without evidence of cell death. Others have repeatedly shown that F-P injury results in the formations of contusions [6]. We attribute this difference to our use of an extension tube which modifies the fluid pulse prior to delivery to the extracellular space [7].

Even though the single insult in the current paper does not result in cell death, the brain appears to be compromised in its ability to respond to a second traumatic insult. This is exemplified in both an increase in the duration of apnea and unconsciousness as well as the pronounced increase in both degree and extent of ICP. Finally, the second insult often results in the formation of contusions and cell death which attests to the vulnerable state of the brain following injury.

We propose that although not morphologically damaged following a single concussive insult, cells are metabolically disrupted during a period of time, during which they are vulnerable to a second insult.

Acknowledgements. We wish to thank Ms. N. Balady and Ms. S. Cristeuscu for their technical assistance. This work was supported by USPHS RO1 NS27544, the Annie Laurie Aitken Charitable Trust, the Lind Lawrence Foundation, and the World Boxing Council.

References

1. Fineman I, Hovda DA, Kawamata T, Yoshino A, Becker DP (1990) Calcium accumulates for at least 48 hours following fluid percussion brain injury in the rat. Soc Neurosci 16:778–778
2. Hovda DA, Becker DP, Katayama Y (1991) Secondary injury and acidosis. J Neurotrauma (In Press)
3. Jenkins LW, Moszynski K, Lyeth BG, Lewelt W, Dewitt DS, Allen A, Dixon CE, Povlishock JT, Majewski TJ, Clifton GL, Young HF, Becker DP, Hayes RL (1989) Increased vulnerability of the mildly traumatized rat brain to cerebral ischemia: the use of controlled secondary ischemia as a research tool to identify common or different mechanisms contributing to mechanical and ischemic brain injury. Brain Res 477:211–224
4. Katayama Y, Becker DP, Tamura T, Hovda DA (1990) Massive increases in extracellular potassium and the indiscriminate release of glutamate following concussive brain injury. J Neurosurg 73:889–900
5. Kawamata T, Katayama Y, Hovda DA, Yoshino A, Becker DP (1992) Administration of excitatory amino acid antagonists via microdialysis attenuates the increase in glucose utilization seen following concussive brain injury. J Cereb Blood Flow Metab 12:12–24
6. Mclntosh TK, Vink R, Noble L, Yamakami I, Fernyak S, Soares H, Faden AI (1989) Traumatic brain injury in the rat: Characterization of a lateral fluid-percussion model. Neuroscience 28:233–244
7. Thomas S, Yoshino A, Hovda DA, Becker DP (1991) Adaptation of the fluid percussion device reduces the formation of contusions in a model of traumatic brain injury. Soc Neurosci 17, 166 (Abstract)
8. Yoshino A, Hovda DA, Kawamata T, Katayama Y, Becker DP (1991) Dynamic changes in local cerebral glucose utilization following cerebral concussion in rats: Evidence of a hyper- and subsequent hypometabolic state. Brain Res 561:106–119

Cerebral Blood Flow and Glucose Metabolism Following Experimental Head Injury

K. SHIMA[1], A. MARMAROU[2], N. ROSHIMAE[1], H. UMEZAWA[1], N. WAKOH[1], and H. CHIGASAKI[1]

[1] Department of Neurosurgery, National Defense Medical College, 3-2 Namiki, Tokorozawa, Saitama 359, Japan. [2] Division of Neurosurgery (Department of Surgery), Medical College of Virginia, Virginia Commonwealth University, Richmond, VA 23298, USA

Introduction

We have as yet very little information on the changes of local cerebral blood flow (lCBF) and glucose metabolism (lCGU) in the early posttraumatic period in closed head injury. Because of the difficulty in measuring CBF soon after head injury, the reported alterations of lCBF after the injury reveal wide variations, ranging from very low to pronounced hyperemia.

The objective of the present study was to detect the changes in lCBF, lCGU and neuronal damage during the acute phase of concussive closed head injury in the rat.

Materials and Methods

Male Sprague-Dawley rats weighing 300–450 g were anesthetized with 1.5–2% halothane in O_2 delivered by a closely fitting face mask. After the reflection of scalp, a stainless steel disc, 10 mm in diameter, was secured on the skull of the midway area between the bregma and lambda. Following catheterization, the animals were immobilized by a loose-fitting plaster cast around the hindquaters to facilitate blood sampling for autoradiographic studies. The physiological condition of each rat was assessed by measurements of rectal temperature, blood pressure, hematocrit and blood gases.

After discontinuing halothane inspiration, the animal was placed on a foam bed. The head injury was delivered by dropping a brass cylinder (450 g) from the plexiglass tubing positioned above the steel disc on the skull. Two levels of the injury were selected by varying the height of the weightdrop; moderate injury from 1 meter and severe injury from 2 meters.

Following head injury, the animal was restrained and the autoradiographic studies were done as follows. Fifteen min and 4 h after the injury, 100 μCi/kg of ^{14}C-iodoantipyrine (^{14}C-IAP) was infused for 30 sec and arterial blood samples were taken every 5 sec to assess ^{14}C activity. At 30 sec the rat was decapitated. The brains were rapidly removed, frozen, cut into 20 μm-thick sections, and subjected to autoradiographs. LCBF was calculated according to Sakurada et al. [4]. LCGU was measured using the technique designed by Sokoloff et al. [5]. Hundred μCi/kg ^{14}C-2-deoxyglucose (^{14}C-DG) was injected intravenously. Timed blood samples were taken for analysis of ^{14}C activity and glucose concentration. The animals were decapitated 40 min or 4 h after trauma, respectively 30 min or 45 min after the injection of ^{14}C-DG. Autoradiographs were prepared in the same manner as for ICBF, and ICGU was calculated using the lumped constant for the normal rat determined by Sokoloff et al. [5]. LCGU was assessed only in the animals subjected to moderate injury.

Posttraumatic neuronal damage was determined by ^{45}Ca autoradiography [1]. Rats subjected to trauma were injected with 100 μCi/100 g ^{45}Ca either 10 min, 1 day, 3 days, 7 days and 10 days after trauma. The ^{45}Ca was allowed to circulate for 4 h, and the brains were removed and autoradiographed in the same manner as for ICBF.

Traumatic changes of blood-brain barrier (BBB) permeability were assessed by intravenous injection of Evans blue (2% in saline) at 5 min pre- or post-injury.

Results

Eleven of 29 (37%) animals injured at the high level deteriorated within a few minutes with apnea and rapidly decreasing blood pressure, and died. All animals at low-injury level survived. Subarachnoid hemorrhage around brain stem was observed in about 40% of moderate injury and in about 80% of severe injury. Macroscopic intraparenchymal hemorrhage was not found in any animals of both injury groups. There was no visible extravasation of Evans blue in the brains of all animals measured at 15 min or 4 h post-injury. The abnormal accumulation of ^{45}Ca was not seen by 72 h after moderate injury and 4 h after severe injury. The mean arterial blood pressure (MABP) rapidly increased by 29% in moderate injury, 60% in survivors of severe injury and 77% in nonsurvivors of severe injury over each baseline value, and returned to baseline values within 30 sec in both levels of injury.

Compared with mean values of sham-operated control rats ($n = 3$), moderate injury resulted in mean ICBF increases of 44% in substantia nigra ($p < 0.05$); and 10–15% in hypothamus, septal nucleus and pontine gray (NS), while there were decreases of ICBF in many others (Fig. 1). In the moderate injury group, there was a tendency for variedly changed ICBF to return to control values by 4 h after the injury.

In severe injury, ICBF was markedly decreased throughout widespread areas, and none of the areas measured showed any increases in LCBF.

At 40 min post-injury, ICGU showed a significant decrease in all structures examined and the percent changes from control values was more than those of ICBF. At 4 h post-injury, there was an insignificant recovery of 5–35% in ICGU in all regions studied excluding hippocampus and mamillary body.

Discussion

Several investigations of cerebral blood flow and metabolism following experimental head injury have been carried out. Nilsson et al. [3], using the impact

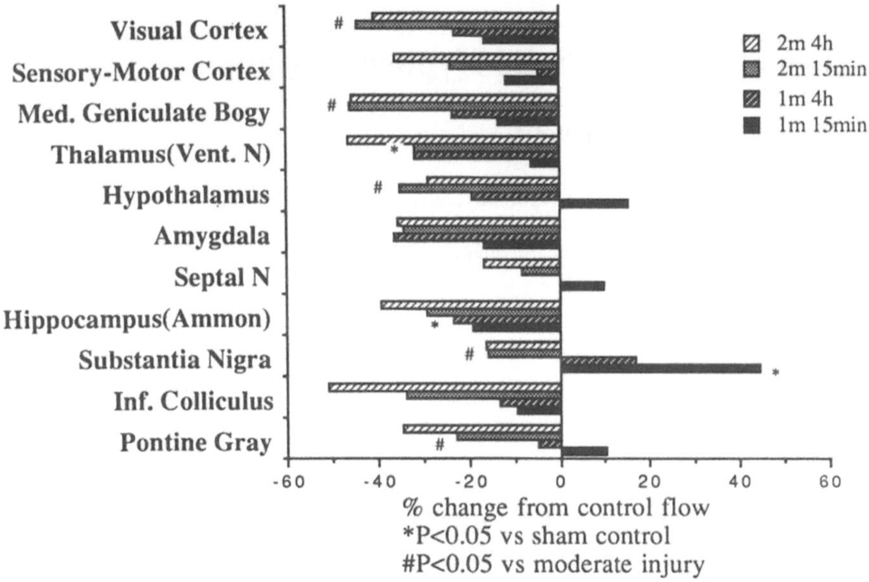

Fig. 1. Percent changes in ICBF following trauma

acceleration model in rats, similar to the present study, found an increase in ICBF in the midbrain and in the central regions of the hemisphere, but not in the superficial gray matter immediate and 30 min after the trauma. Langfitt et al. [2] found the secondary increase in intracranial pressure following an initial transient rise coincident with the impact. They hypothesized that the secondary rise was due to cerebrovascular dilatation and a consequent rise in cerebral blood volume. The structures with an increase in ICBF following concussive brain injury located in the brain stem and diencephalon correspond to the areas to be considered as the neural center of vasomotor activity.

Our results show a marked reduction of CBF and depressive metabolism in severe closed head injury. The result is more consistent with the clinical experience.

References

1. Dienel GA (1984) Regional accumulation of calcium in postischemic rat brain. J Neurochem 43:913–925
2. Langfitt TW, Tannanbaum HM, Kassell NF (1966) The etiology of acute brain swelling following experimental head injury. J Neurosurg 24:47–56
3. Nilsson B, Dick A, Ecklöf B, et al. (1989) Regional blood flow in the brain and in the cervical cord in experimental head trauma. In: Langfitt TW, McHenry Jr LC, Reivich M, Wollman H (eds) Cerebral circulation and metabolism. Springer, Berlin Heidelberg New York, pp 109–112
4. Sakurada O, Kennedy C, Jehle J, et al. (1978) Measurement of local cerebral blood flow with [^{14}C]-iodoantipyrine. Am J Physiol 234:H59–H66
5. Sokolloff L, Reivich M, Kennedy C, et al. (1977) The [^{14}C]deoxyglucose method for the measurement of local cerebral glucose utilization: Theory, procedure, and normal values in the conscious and anesthetized albino rat. J Neurochem 28:897–916

Effect of Posttraumatic Hypoventilation

K. SHIMA[1] and A. MARMAROU[2]

[1] Department of Neurosurgery, National Defense Medical College, Tokorozawa, Saitama 359, Japan
[2] Division of Neurosurgery, Medical College of Virginia, Richmond, VA 23298, USA

Introduction

Respiratory depression and resulting posttraumatic apnea are consistent observations in both clinical and experimental brain injury. Several reports clearly identify the deleterious consequence of hypoxia upon outcome from severe brain injury [3].

A previous report from our laboratory described the metabolic derangement produced by combining experimental trauma and hypoventilation [1]. The objective of this study was to determine the pathophysiology of posttraumatic hypoventilation.

Materials and Methods

Eighteen adult cats (2.5–4 kg) were anesthetized with intravenous chloralose (20 mg/kg), ventilated and maintained normocapnic. Animals were subjected to 3.1 ± 0.1 atm. (mean ± SEM) temporal fluid percussion injury [4]. Immediately following fluid percussion injury, the animals were randomly divided into two groups: Group 1 received trauma alone and Group 2 was subjected to trauma followed immediately by 30 min of controlled hypoventilation. The ventilator was adjusted to maintain pO2 at 32.4 ± 1.2 mmHg for 30 min, then returned to normal. A catheter inserted into the cisterna magna provided continuous monitoring of intracranial pressure (ICP) and bolus injection for pressure-volume index (PVI). Auditory brain-stem responses (ABR) were recorded from electrodes placed at the vertex and earlobe with monoaural click stimulation. Local cerebral blood flow (CBF) was measured with the hydrogen-clearance technique. Thirty minutes before sacrifice, each cat was injected with a 2% Evans blue solution. Eight hours after the brain injury, the animals were sacrificed, and then the brains were removed for measurement of brain water content by gravimetric analysis [2].

Results

Cannulation of cisterna magna was possible at 2 hours post-injury for measurement of ICP and PVI. Time courses of ICP and PVI are shown in Table 1. In

Table 1. Responses of ICP and PVI

	2	3	4	5	6	7	8(h)
Trauma alone							
ICP (mmHg)	13.3	12.8	14.0	14.9	15.1	15.7	18.5
	(0.9)	(1.1)	(0.8)	(1.3)	(1.4)	(2.5)	(4.0)
PVI (ml)	0.83	0.70	0.87	0.78	0.71	0.71	0.62
	(0.1)	(0.1)	(0.1)	(0.2)	(0.1)	(0.1)	(0.1)
Trauma and hypoventilation							
ICP (mmHg)	14.7	15.0	16.7	21.2	25.1	30.5	33.8
	(1.7)	(1.8)	(1.6)	(3.2)	(5.4)	(7.2)	(9.4)
PVI (ml)	0.76	0.65	0.59	0.57***	0.59**	0.54*	0.51
	(0.1)	(0.1)	(0.1)	(0.0)	(0.1)	(0.1)	(0.1)

Mean (SEM); *$p < 0.05$, **$p < 0.01$, ***$p < 0.001$ vs. trauma alone

Group 1 animals, the ICP increased 40% (13.3 to 18.5 mmHg). Group 2 animals showed a pronounced increase in ICP from 4 hours after head injury and the ICP increased 130% (14.7 to 33.8 mmHg) by 8 hours. The PVI in Group 1 averaged 0.83 ml at 2 hours post-injury and 0.62 ml at 8 hours. The PVI in Group 2 decreased from 0.76 ml to 0.51 ml, which was significantly lower than that of Group 1 from 5 hours post-injury ($p < 0.001$).

Immediately following brain injury, peaks II, III, and IV demonstrated a transient and marked suppression. Five of 9 cats in Group 2 showed the disappearance of peak V. The latency of peak IV in Group 2 was significantly longer than that in Group 1 for 2–6 hours post-injury.

Two hours after the injury, the CBF significantly decreased by 60% in Group 1 and 40% in Group 2 of the pre-injury levels. The CBF in Group 1 animals gradually returned to 73% by 8 hours following trauma. However, the low CBF in Group 2 animals persisted in each hemisphere until the end of the experiment.

Group 2 animals developed significantly increased tissue water content throughout the brain, compared with the control values. The water content in Group 2 was the most pronounced in the injured hemisphere, with a water content of 72.8 ± 0.4% by weight in the white matter along the axis of impact, which was significantly higher than that in Group 1. The water content in the brain-stem was also significantly higher bilaterally.

Discussion

The present study shows that posttraumatic hypo-ventilation exacerbates further neuronal damage after trauma and produces more extensive brain edema. The reduction of brain compliance due to the rapid increase in ICP was seen at 5 h after trauma combined with hypoventilation. Andersen et al. [1] used the same trauma plus hypoventilation model as in the present study and found a more pronounced metabolic derangement, compared with the results in animals subjected to fluid-percussion trauma alone [5]. The CBF in trauma combined with hypoventilation remained at critically low levels of 20 ml/100 g/min until the end of the experiment. It is reasonable to presume that posttraumatic hypoventilation produces cerebral ischemia which exacerbates the neuronal damage following trauma. These results suggest that respiratory depression of relatively short duration following traumatic brain injury is a severe secondary insult and contributes to a poor prognosis.

References

1. Andersen BJ, Unterberg AW, Clarke GD, Marmarou A (1988) Effect of posttraumatic hypoventilation on cerebral energy metabolism. J Neurosurg 68:601–607
2. Marmarou A, Tanaka K, Shulman K (1982) An improved gravimetric measure of cerebral edema. J Neurosurg 56:246–253
3. Miller JD, Sweet RC, Narayan R, et al. (1978) Early insults to the injured brain. JAMA 240:439–442
4. Shima K, Marmarou A (1991) Evaluation of brain-stem dysfunction following severe fluid-percussion head injury to the cat. J Neurosurg 74:270–277
5. Unterberg AW, Andersen BJ, Clarke GD, Marmarou A (1988) Cerebral energy metabolism following fluid-percussion brain injury in cats. 68:594–600

The Role of LTC_4 in the Development of Post-Traumatic Intracranial Hypertension

J.B.G. Ghajar, P.S. Barie, P. Peterson, and R.J. Hariri

Cornell University Medical Center, Department of Surgery, Department of Pathology, New York, NY, USA

Introduction

A complex series of pathophysiologic events follow the initial transfer of mechanical energy in traumatic brain injury, and constitute the secondary phenomena which are responsible for the development of intracranial hypertension. Elevation of intracranial pressure is the hallmark of post-traumatic cerebrovascular dysfunction, and reflects some combination of vasomotor dysfunction and vascular permeability abnormalities which result in a net increase in the total intracranial volume. Considerable evidence exists in the literature which demonstrates that following mechanical brain injury, local and regional abnormalities in perfusion occur, characterized by either hyperemia or ischemia [1, 7]. It remains unclear, however, which of these dysfunctional vascular states is responsible for the irreparable tissue damage which occurs in the first 96 hours following injury. Obviously, the goal of therapeutics aimed at preserving potentially viable brain tissue following injury is centered around optimizing oxygen and substrate delivery to the salvagable tissue and interrupting the propagation of pathophysiologic events which subject the brain to secondary ischemic injury.

Recently, we have demonstrated that human glial cells in culture are capable of generating leukotrienes following mechanical injury [4, 6]. These compounds have also been identified in brain in association with other forms of injury [5, 9]. The specific role of these compounds in the pathophysiology of TBI remains, as yet, controversial. Attempts at elucidating the precise stimulus for cerebrovascular dysfunction following TBI has focused attention on the possibility that vasoactive mediators released from injured or dying cells may influence vascular function. This would be strikingly similar, mechanistically, to the series of events which lead to the increase in tissue perfusion and development of tissue edema characteristic of classical inflammation. Based on our recent observations, we propose that mechanical brain injury is followed by an organ-specific inflammatory response, modulated, at least in part, by the glial cell population of the brain. Furthermore, we propose that this inflammatory response is propagated by glial cell elaboration of leukotrienes which cause both vasomotor and permeability changes in the injured brain characterized by the development of intracranial hypertension. To evaluate this hypothesis we compared the effect of exogenously administered leukotriene C4 (LTC4) to an experimental model of TBI on the development of intracranial hypertension in miniature swine. In addition, we examined the appearance of LTC4 in cerebrospinal fluid from animals subjected to mechanical brain injury as well as compared the histologic features of these two forms of experimental brain injury.

Materials and Methods

Sexually mature female Yucatan Miniature Swine (Charles River Laboratories) (n = 16) were employed in these studies. Animals were maintained in accordance with policies of the institutional animal use and care committee.

Animals were premedicated with xylazine and ketamine, intubated and induced with Forane. Animals were then ventilated with a mixture of Forane 2%, Oxygen 23% and Nitrogen 75%, to achieve blood gases in the normal range for this species. Animals were placed supine and left femoral artery and vein were then cannulated with 12 gauge polyethylene catheters for blood pressure monitoring and arterial sampling and venous access, respectively. The right subclavian vein was cannulated as above, for central venous pressure monitoring. A midline cystostomy was performed for urine output monitoring. Animals were then placed in the prone position and heads immobilized in a plexiglass frame. A sagittal incision was then made through the scalp and the margins retracted laterally. A 14 mm burrhole was made in the right frontal bone for placement of a hollow stainless steel coupler to the fluid percussion injury device. Bilateral anterior ventriculostomies were performed for intracranial fiberoptic pressure monitoring (Camino Labs, San Diego, CA.) and ventricular CSF access respectively. A sagittal sinus catheter was placed for sampling of sagittal sinus blood. A rectal temperature probe (Yellow Springs Instruments) was placed and animals core temperature maintained at 37 C by external heating lamps and use of warmed intravenous solutions. Central venous pressure was maintained within baseline levels (3–7 mmHg) and urine output was maintained at 0.5–1 ml/kg/hour by continuous intravenous infusion of lactated ringers solution.

Following surgical preparation, animals were allowed to equilibrate for a 1 hour period. Baseline arterial blood gases were obtained and every 15 minutes thereafter. The following physiologic variables were continuously monitored by an analog to digital conversion computerized data acquisition system: arterial blood pressure (ABP), central venous pressure (CVP), intracranial pressure (ICP), inspired oxygen concentration (FiO2), expired forane concentration (FeForane), end tidal carbon dioxide (ETCO2).

Animals were divided into 3 groups: Group I (n = 6) were subjected to a 7 atmosphere right frontal fluid percussion injury using the method of Sullivan [7], modified for use in our laboratory [3]; Group II (n = 5) were subjected to a single intraventricular bolus administration of 100 nanograms of LTC4 (Sigma Chemicals) in 0.2 ml of phosphate buffered saline (PBS) vehicle administered over 1 minute; Group III (n = 5) were animals which underwent identical surgical preparation and a 0.2 ml intraventricular bolus of PBS alone.

Animals were monitored for a period of six hours. Ventricular CSF was recovered at 3 and 6 hours and assayed for the presence of LTC4 by enzyme-linked immunoassay (Cayman Chemical Corp.) Animals were sacrificed and brains perfusion fixed with neutral buffered formalin and removed for histologic evaluation. Representative sections of right and left frontal lobe were employed in this evaluation. Pathologic examination was done in a blinded fashion. Histopathologic features were graded and scored.

Results

Ventilatory parameters, as well as arterial blood gases, did not significantly vary between the 3 groups of animals. Mean arterial blood pressure was also comparable between groups (Fig. 1). Following experimental mechanical injury (Group I) animals developed significantly increased ICP, compared to pre-injury levels, within 6 hours (9 ± 5 vs. 30 ± 11 mmHg, $p < 0.05$). This intracranial hypertension was also significantly greater than that seen in animals subjected to surgical sham preparation (Group III) (30 ± 11 vs. 10 ± 4, $p < 0.05$). Moreover, animals in Group II showed a similar development of intracranial hypertension over the same time period (6 ± 4 vs. 32 ± 6) when compared to baseline, as well as when compared to sham (32 ± 6 vs. 10 ± 4, $p < 0.05$).

Histologic analysis of frontal lobe sections demonstrated evidence of a meningovasculitis in both groups I and II, characterized by increased microcirculatory inflammatory cells, predominantly polymorphonuclear leukocytes (PMN), with margination, diapedesis and the intraparenchymal presence of

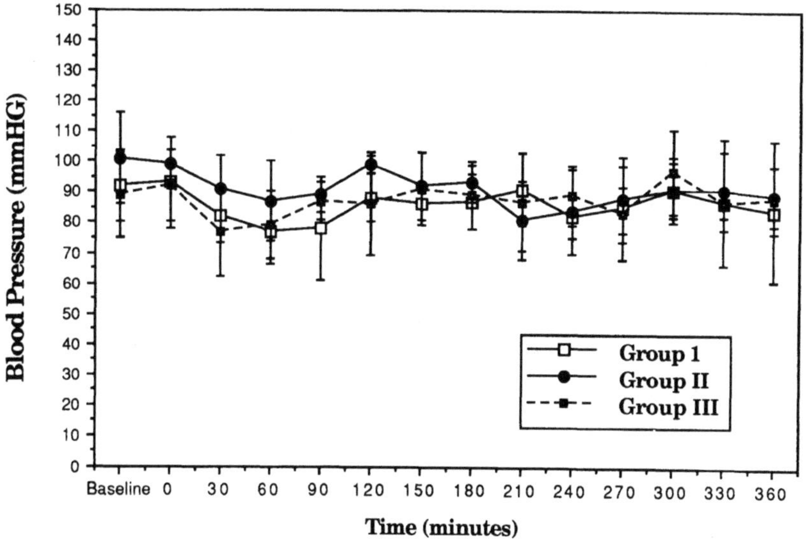

Fig. 1. Mean arterial blood pressure

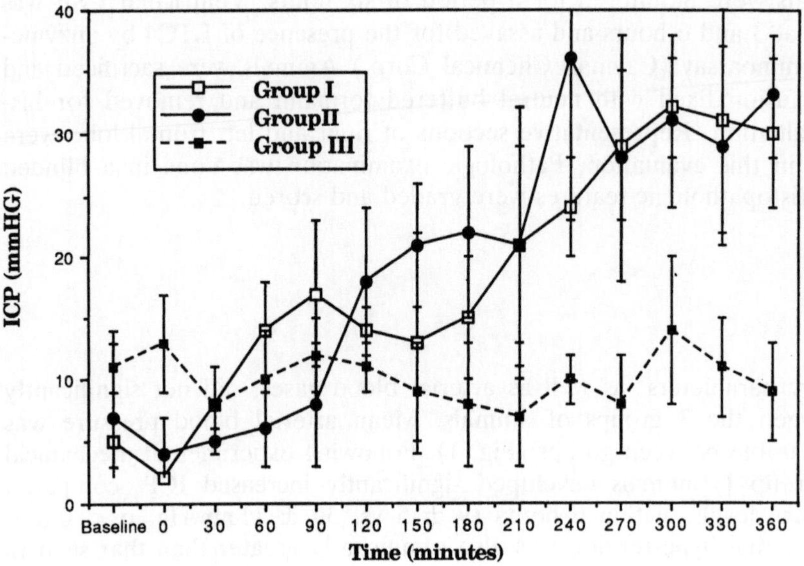

Fig. 2. Intracranial pressure

PMN. Subarachnoid thrombosis was seen in both groups I and II in right frontal lobe sections. No such inflammatory response was seen in group III.

Cerebrospinal fluid levels of LTC4 as measured by enzyme-linked immunoassay demonstrated the presence of this eicosanoid at both 3 and 6 hours following fluid percussion injury. It was not detectable in CSF from group III at any time.

Discussion

The complex pathophysiologic events which are precipitated by mechanical insults to the brain appear to ultimately subject this organ to ischemic injury [2]. Based on previous work which has demonstrated the ability of glial cells to generate inflammatory eicosanoids following injury, we have chosen to view these events as an organ specific inflammatory response. The cerebrovascular dysfunction which accompanies TBI could be accounted for by the elaboration of a mediator or mediators which influence both permeability and vasomotion. To evaluate our hypothesis that LTC4 is responsible for these cerebrovascular changes we examined the effect of exogenously administered compound on intracranial pressure and histopathology and compared it to experimental mechanical injury.

Our findings indicate that intraventricular LTC4 results in the development of intracranial hypertension acutely, which is similar to the time course of changes seen in response to mechanical injury. Moreover, the histological features of mechanical brain injury in our model show evidence of the development of an intense inflammatory cell recruitment and subsequent intraparenchymal migration of blood borne PMN. This is virtually indistinguishable from that response seen after the administration of exogenous LTC4. In addition, LTC4 is detectable in CSF after experimental mechanical injury.

These findings support our hypothesis that mechanical brain injury initiates an organ specific inflammatory response which is characterized by both the development of a meningovasculitis and intracranial hypertension, and is mediated, at least in part, by LTC4. This warrants further examination of this phenomenon as an inflammatory disorder, with specific attention to the role of glial cell elaboration of classical vasoactive mediators.

References

1. Enevoldsen EM (1976) Dynamic changes in regional CBF, intraventricular pressure, CSF pH and lactate levels during the acute phase of head injury. J Neurosurg 44:191–214
2. Graham DI, Adams JH (1978) Ischemic brain injury in fatal head injuries, J Neurol Sci 39:266–269
3. Hariri RJ, Ghajar JBG, Cohen DS, Fiamengo SA, Emery JM, Jones WG, Minei JP (1989) Intracranial hypertension following traumatic brain injury associated with shock and resuscitation, Surg Forum 40:483–485
4. Hariri RJ, Ghajar JBG, Patterson RH (1989) Human glial cell production of lipoxygenase-generated eicosanoids: A potential role in the pathophysiology of vascular changes following traumatic brain injury. The Journal of Trauma 29.9:1203–1210
5. Kiwak KJ, Moskowitz MA, Levine L (1985) Leukotriene production in gerbil brain after ischemic insult, subarachnoid hemorrhage, and concussive injury. J Neurosurg 62:865–869
6. Shepard SR, et al. (1990) Leukotriene production by human glia. Acta Neurochirurgica 51: 58–60
7. Sullivan HG (1976) Fluid percussion model of mechanical brain injury in the cat. J Neurosurg 45:520–534
8. Tornheim PA, McLaurin RL (1981) Acute changes in regional brain water content following experimental closed head injury. J Neurosurg 55:407–413
9. Wolfe I (1985) Involvement of arachidonic acid metabolites in experimental brain injury. Identification of lipoxygenase products in brain. Clinical studies on prostacyclin infusion in acute cerebral ischemia. Adv Prosta, Thrombox, Leuko Res 15:585–588

Changes in Cerebrovascular Permeability and Excitatory Amino Acid-Mediated Cellular Swelling Following Experimental Concussive Brain Injury

Y. KATAYAMA[1,2], D.P. BECKER[1], and T. TAMURA[1]

[1] Division of Neurosurgery, UCLA School of Medicine, UCLA, Los Angeles, CA 90024, USA
[2] Department of Neurological Surgery, Nihon University School of Medicine, Tokyo 173, Japan

Introduction

Changes in cerebrovascular permeability following experimental traumatic brain injury have been described previously employing various intravascular tracers [4]. However, the time courses and actual significance of such changes have not yet been determined. We monitored the changes in concentration of intravascularly administered ^{14}C-sucrose in the extracellular space (ECS), using microdialysis [1–3], as a measure of the cerebrovascular permeability.

Materials and Methods

Since the sucrose in the ECS is not taken up by the brain cells or capillaries for the most part, the blood-to-ECS transfer constant (K_1) of intravascularly administered ^{14}C-sucrose is given by the equation:

$$K_1 = Ce \cdot Ve/Cpdt$$

where Ce, Ve and Cp represent the concentration in the ECS, the ECS volume and the arterial plasma concentration, respectively. In order to detect changes in K_1, both Ce and Ve, in addition to Cp, have to be determined.

Determination of the ECS Volume

Dialysis probes were placed in the rat hippocampus [1]. The probes were perfused for 20 min with ^{14}C-sucrose (10 mM). Since the sucrose in the ECS is not taken up by either cells or capillaries, ^{14}C-sucrose can be regarded as an ECS marker. The probes were subsequently perfused (5 μl) with Ringer solution without ^{14}C-sucrose, and the dialysate concentrations of ^{14}C-sucrose ([^{14}C-sucrose]$_d$) were determined with a scintillation counter (Experiment 1). When water moves from the ECS to the cells (cellular swelling and shrinkage of the ECS volume), the marker concentration within the ECS increases because the ECS marker does not move into the cells but is left behind. Thus, a decrease in Ve can be demonstrated as an increase in [^{14}C-sucrose]$_d$ pre-perfused into the ECS.

Determination of the Cerebrovascular Permeability

In a separate group of animals, ^{14}C-sucrose was administered systemically. Probes were perfused with Ringer solution without ^{14}C-sucrose, and [^{14}C-sucrose]$_d$ and arterial plasma concentration of ^{14}C-sucrose were determined with a scintillation counter (Experiment 2). An increase in [^{14}C-sucrose]$_d$ in this experiment would indicate either an increase in K_1 or a decrease in Ve. If the increase in [^{14}C-sucrose]$_d$ was caused by a decrease in Ve, the magnitude and time course of the increase should be the same as those for the increase observed in Experiment 1. Thus, changes in K_1 can be evaluated by comparing the increases in [^{14}C-sucrose]$_d$ in Experiments 1 and 2.

Injury Induction and Pharmacological Modification

Traumatic brain injury was induced by fluid-percussion (2–4 atm) [1–5]. The dialysis probe was temporarily withdrawn at the moment of injury and repositioned in the same place immediately after the injury. The effects of kynurenic acid (KYN), a broad spectrum antagonist of excitatory amino acids, were tested by administering KYN in situ through the dialysis probe.

Results

Immediately after injury induction, an increase in [^{14}C-sucrose]$_d$ was observed in Experiment 1 (Fig. 1A). This indicated that cellular swelling and a decrease in Ve during the initial several min had occurred. Such changes were not induced by repositioning of the probe alone in the case of sham-injury (Fig. 1A). At 3–5 min after injury induction, [^{14}C-sucrose]$_d$ returned to a level which did not differ from the [^{14}C-sucrose]$_d$ following sham-injury. The increases in [^{14}C-sucrose]$_d$ were inhibited by KYN (10 mM) (Fig. 1A).

Only a very low radioactivity was detected from dialysate before injury in Experiment 2. Immediately after injury induction, an increase in [^{14}C-sucrose]$_d$ was also observed in Experiment 2 (Fig. 1B). Such an increase was not observed in the case of sham-injury which involved only repositioning of the probe (Fig. 1B). [^{14}C-sucrose]$_d$ remained elevated in Experiment 2 ($p < 0.02$) even after the increase in [^{14}C-sucrose]$_d$ in Experiment 1 had subsided. The increase in [^{14}C-sucrose]$_d$ in Experiment 2 was not significantly inhibited by KYN (Fig. 1B).

Discussion

The increase in [^{14}C-sucrose]$_d$ was not remarkably different between the Experiments 1 and 2, indicating that the major component of the increase in [^{14}C-sucrose]$_d$ in Experiment 2 (Ce) was due to a decrease in ECS volume

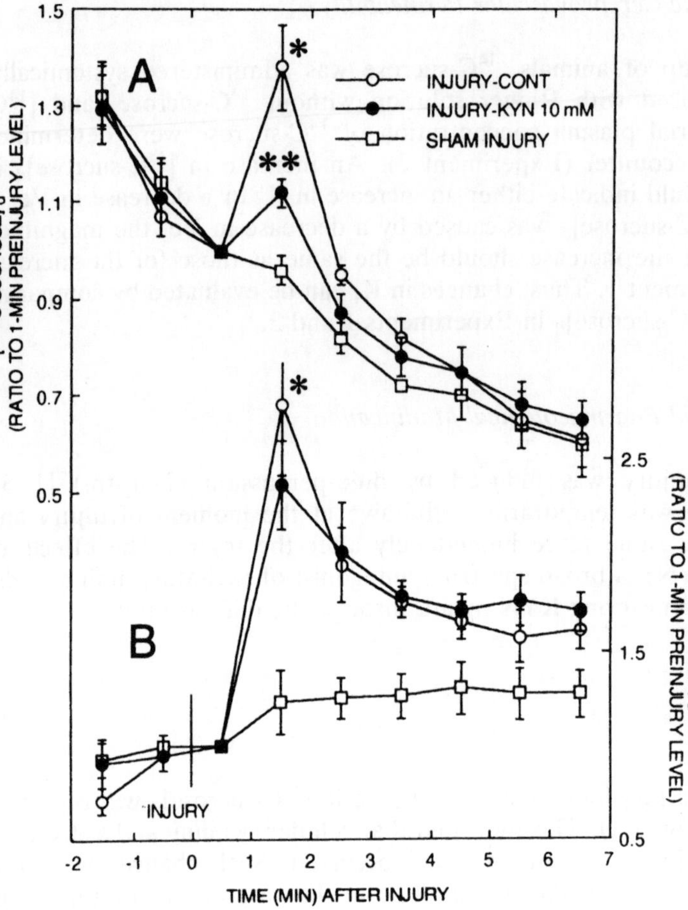

Fig. 1. Changes in [^{14}C-sucrose]$_d$ (ratio to 1-min preinjury level) after injury. **A** Experiment 1, in which ^{14}C-sucrose was preperfused into the ECS through the dialysis probe. **B** Experiment 2, in which ^{14}C-sucrose was administered systemically. The responses were delayed for 1 min corresponding to the dead space (5 μl) of the dialysis system. *$p < 0.02$ as compared to sham injury. **$p < 0.02$ as compared to control injury

(Ve) [1]. It appears, however, that a certain amount of sucrose had entered into the ECS from the blood immediately after injury, since [^{14}C-sucrose]$_d$ remained elevated in Experiment 2 even after the increase in [^{14}C-sucrose]$_d$ in Experiment 1 had subsided. This inference is consistent with the previous observations employing various intravascular tracers [4].

Excitatory amino acid antagonist inhibited both the cellular swelling and massive ionic fluxes occurring simultaneously [2]. This indicates that cellular swelling is caused by water movement along with excitatory amino acid-mediated ionic fluxes [3]. The present data suggest that the increase in cerebrovascular permeability occurs at approximately the same time. Since excitatory amino acids do not appear to be involved in the increase in cerebrovascular permeability, these two phenomena are thought to be induced by independent mechanisms. The simultaneous occurrence of water movement from the ECS into the cells and an increase in cerebrovascular permeability, however, may contribute to the elevated intracranial and interstitial pressure observed during this same period [5].

Acknowledgment. This work was supported by NIH Grant NS27544 (USA).

References

1. Katayama Y, Becker DP, Tamura T, Ikezaki K (1990a) Early cellular swelling in experimental traumatic brain injury: A phenomenon mediated by excitatory amino acids. Acta Neurochir, Suppl 51:271–273
2. Katayama Y, Becker DP, Tamura T, Hovda D (1990b) Massive increase in extracellular potassium and indiscriminative glutamate release after concussive brain injury. J Neurosurg 73:889–900
3. Katayama Y, Cheung MK, Alves A, Becker DP (1989) Ion fluxes and cell swelling after experimental traumatic brain injury: The role of excitatory amino acids. In: Hoff JT, Betz AL (eds) Intracranial pressure VII. Springer, Berlin Heidelberg New York London Paris Tokyo Hong Kong pp 584–588
4. Povlishock JT, Becker DP, Sullivan HG, Miller JD (1978) Vascular permeability alterations to horseradish peroxidase in experimental brain injury. Brain Res 153:223–239
5. Wako N, Shima K, Marmarou A (1989) Time course of brain tissue pressure in temporal fluid percussion injury. In: Hoff JT, Betz AL (eds) Intracranial pressure VII. Springer, Berlin Heidelberg New York London Paris Tokyo Hong Kong pp 593–597

Lack of Relationship Between Hippocampal Cell Loss and ICP After Experimental Head Injury

M.J. KOTAPKA[1], T.A. GENNARELLI[1], D.I. GRAHAM[2], and J.H. ADAMS[2]

[1] Division of Neurosurgery, University of Pennsylvania, Philadelphia, PA, USA
[2] Department of Neuropathology, University of Glasgow, Glasgow, Scotland

Introduction

Hippocampal damage in non-missile head injury has traditionally been considered a manifestation of hypoxic brain damage associated with decreased cerebral perfusion pressure (CPP) secondary to raised intracranial pressure (ICP) [6]. This report examines hippocampal damage in experimental acceleration head injury in which ICP and CPP were monitored.

Methods

Details of this method of injury have previously been reported [4, 5]. 54 anaesthetized non-human primates were monitored for ICP and arterial blood pressure prior to injury. Animals were subjected to a single controlled non-impact acceleration injury. Animals were reanaesthetized at varying times (2 hours to 8 weeks) after injury and were perfusion fixed with FAM. Comprehensive neuropathologic examination was performed on 6 mm thick coronal brain slices. Representative histologic sections of the hippocampus at the level of the lateral geniculate body were assessed for overt neuronal loss and irreversible ischemic damage. This experiment was approved by the University of Pennsylvania Institutional Animal Care and Use Committee and conforms to all relevant guidelines.

Results

Histologic examination of the 54 animals subjected to acceleration injury revealed hippocampal damage in 32 animals (59%). Lesions always involved the CA-1 subfield of the hippocampus and were bilateral in 24 animals.

The number of animals with major pathologic findings were as follows: subdural hematoma = 23 (43%); intracerebral hematoma = 8 (15%); contusions = 34 (63%); diffuse axonal injury = 16 (30%). Hypoxic brain damage in sites other than the hippocampus was present in 7 animals. Only 5 animals (9%), had evidence of pressure necrosis of the parahippocampal gyrus (PHG),

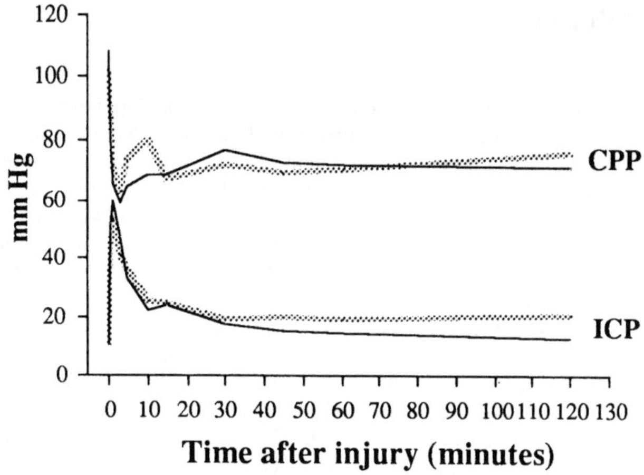

Fig. 1. Relationship of ICP and CPP to hippocampal damage in 49 primates subjected to acceleration injury. Damage was noted in 30 subjects (·.·.·.·) and absent in 19 (——). See text for details

a finding known to correlate with high ICP during life [1]. Pathologically, these animals had large subdural hematomas associated with marked mass effect.

The mean maximal ICP for the 5 animals with PHG necrosis was 133 mmHg. The mean minimal CPP for these animals was 15 mmHg. The 49 animals without PHG necrosis had a mean maximal ICP of 62 mmHg and a mean minimal CPP of 54 mmHg. 30 of the 49 animals without PHG necrosis had hippocampal damage. The temporal relationships of ICP and CPP in the 49 animals without pathologic evidence of high ICP is presented in figure 1.

Discussion

The hippocampus is known to be selectively vulnerable to a wide variety of hypoxic insults [3]. The traditional explanation for traumatically induced hippocampal damage has involved increased ICP leading to reduction in CPP which in turn results in hypoxic brain damage [6]. In the present study, maximal elevations of ICP were modest in the 49 animals without pathologic evidence of high ICP, 30 of whom sustained hippocampal damage. The ICP profiles of these 49 animals are similar to those noted in animals subjected to acceleration injury without resulting brain damage [2, 4].

The results of this study indicate that hippocampal damage in acceleration brain injury is not related to markedly abnormal ICP or globally reduced CPP. Possible mechanisms include local microcirculatory disturbances, inherent properties of affected neurons that lead to selective vulnerability, or pathologic excitation involving amino acid neurotransmitters.

References

1. Adams JH, Graham DI (1976) The relationship between ventricular fluid pressure and the neuropathology of raised intracranial pressure. Neuropath Appl Neurobiol 2:323–332
2. Adams JH, Graham DI, Gennarelli TA (1982) Neuropathology of acceleration induced head injury in the subhuman primate, in: Head Injury: Basic and Clinical Aspects RG, Grossman PL, Gildenberg (eds) Raven Press New York, pp 141–150
3. Brierley JB, Graham DI (1984) Hypoxia and vascular disorders of the central nervous system, in: Greenfiels's Neuropathology, 4th ed. Adams JH, Corsellis JAN, Duchen LW (eds) Edward Arnold: London, pp 125–207
4. Gennarelli TA, Segawa H, Wald U, Czernicki Z, Marsh K, Thompson C (1982) Physiologic response to angular acceleration of the head, in : Head Injury: Basic and Clinical Aspects, Grossman RG, Gildenberg PL (eds). Raven Press New York, pp 129–140
5. Gennarelli TA, Thibault LE, Adams JH, Graham DI, Thompson CJ, Marcincin RP (1982) Diffuse axonal injury and traumatic coma in the primate. Ann Neurol 12:564–574
6. Graham DI, Adams JH, Doyle D (1978) Ischemic brain damage in fatal non-missile brain injuries. J Neurol Sci 39:213–234

Computerized Tomography and Magnetic Resonance Imaging

CT Scan Predictors of Intracranial Hypertension After Head Injury

Z. Feldman, C.S. Robertson, Ch.F. Contant, R.K. Narayan, and R.G. Grossman

Department of Neurosurgery, Baylor College of Medicine, One Baylor Plaza, Houston, TX 77030, USA

Introduction

The need exists for objective criteria for the use of intracranial pressure (ICP) monitoring in head injured patients [2]. The initial CT scan taken soon after the arrival of the head injured patient to the hospital can provide important information as to whether ICP monitoring is needed. A normal CT scan has been associated with low incidence of intracranial hypertension in head injured patients [1, 3, 4, 5]. An abnormal admission CT scan was found by Narayan et al. to be correlated with an increased incidence of intracranial hypertension in head-injured patients: 53% of patients with hypodense lesions and 63% of patients with hyperdense lesions had elevated ICP [4]. Other CT scan features as midline shift and perimesencephalic cistern compression, have also been found to be associated with elevated ICP [6, 7]. Our goal in this study was to identify within the group of head-injured patients with abnormal admission CT scans subgroups of patients with elevated ICP.

Methods

One hundred fifty four patients who were admitted to the neurosurgical intensive care unit at Ben Taub General Hospital, after severe head injury between July 1, 1989 and January 1, 1991, had an abnormal admission CT scan and underwent ICP monitoring. The admission CT scans of these patients, obtained with a G.E.9800 scanner, were categorized according to the presence of the following pathological conditions:

1. Intracerebral hematomas (ICH)
2. Extra-axial hematomas
3. Cerebral contusions
4. Subarachnoid hemorrhage (SAH)
5. Midline shift
6. Basal cistern (BC) compression.

Intracranial hypertension was defined as an ICP value of 21–30 mmHg for 2 consecutive hours or more, 31–40 mmHg for 30 minutes or more or, > 40 mmHg for 10 minutes or more. The pathological findings on the initial CT scan were correlated with the highest ICP values obtained on days 1 to 3 after admission.

Results

Patient characteristics are listed in Table 1. Hypodense lesions (focal edema and diffuse swelling) were associated with elevated ICP in 46% of patients. Hyperdense lesions taken as a group (cerebral contusion, ICH, epidural hematoma (EDH), subdural hematoma (SDH), and SAH were associated with intracranial hypertension in 71% of the patients. The presence of midline shift was associated with elevated ICP in 79% of patients, and perimesencephalic cistern compression in 77% of patients. The association between the risk of intracranial hypertension and specific pathological findings on CT scan are shown in Fig. 1.

Significant differences were found within the different pathologies when factors as cisternal compression and additional pathologies were considered. Patients with cerebral contusion without basal cistern compression had a risk of 58% for an elevated ICP, while when basal cistern compression was present, the risk rose to 82%. Intracerebral hematoma was associated with intracranial hypertension in 55% of the patients when the basal cisterns were not compressed. Once the basal cisterns were compressed, the incidence of elevated ICP rose to 100% in these patients ($p < 0.05$ Chi square = 5.646). EDH, when present as a single pathology was associated with elevated ICP in 53% of the patients. But when either SDH, ICH, cerebral contusion or SAH was also present the incidence of intracranial hypertension rose to 88% ($p < 0.05$ Chi square = 4.069). The incidence of elevated ICP in patients with SDH and SAH

Table 1. Patient characteristics

Category		Number	Percent
1. Age	Mean 31; range 14–91		
2. Sex	Male	133	86.4
	Female	21	14.6
3. Primary Pathology	Hypodense lesions	13	8.5
	Cerebral contusions	33	21.4
	Intracerebral hematoma	19	12.3
	Epidural hematoma	29	18.8
	Subdural hematoma	49	31.8
	Traumatic SAH	11	7.2
4. Initial GCS	3–5:	43	27.9
	6–8	68	44.2
	9–13	34	22.1
	14–15	9	5.8

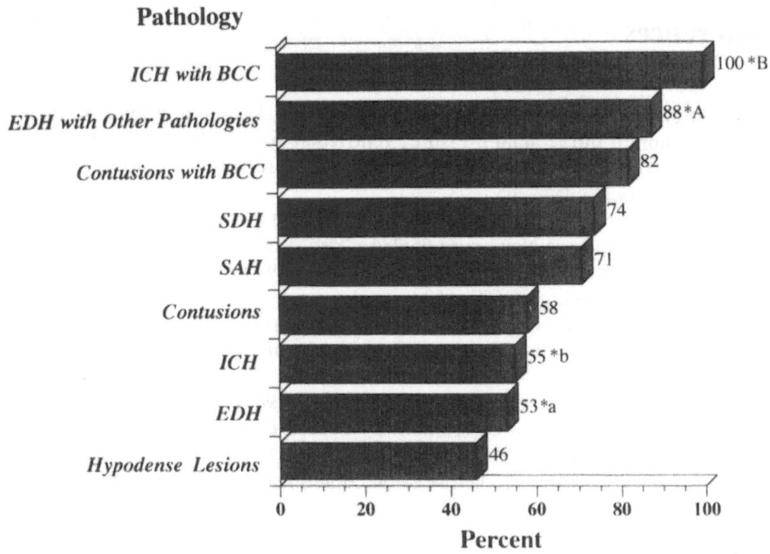

Fig. 1. The association between the risk of intracranial hypertension and specific pathological findings on CT scan. Only the differences between isolated epidural hematoma and epidural hematoma combined with other lesions, and between intracerebral hematoma and intracerebral hematoma with basal cistern compression reached statistical significance (*). *EDH*, epidural hematoma; *ICH*, intracerebral hematoma; *SAH*, subarachnoid hemorrhage; *SDH*, subdural hematoma; *BCC*, basal cistern compression

was not different with or without basal cistern compression and the overall incidence of intracranial hypertension in these groups was 74% and 71% respectively. The presence of midline shift did not significantly change the incidence of intracranial hypertension within the different categories.

Discussion

In the present series, we found a high incidence of abnormal CT scans after head injury as compared to the incidence reported in the literature (1, 3, 4). We found a significant difference between the occurrence of intracranial hypertension in patients with EDH with additional pathologies when compared to EDH alone, and between patients with ICH and basal cistern compression compared to ICH alone. The incidence of elevated ICP in cases of ICH and EDH associated with BCC and other pathologies is so high as to warrant ICP monitoring when these conditions are detected on the admission CT scan.

References

1. Holliday PO III, Kelly DL, Ball M (1982) Normal computed tomograms in acute head injury: Correlation of intracranial pressure, ventricular size, and outcome. Neurosurgery 10:25–28
2. Kanter MJ, Narayan RK (1991) Intracranial pressure monitoring. Neurosurgery Clinics of North America 2:257–265
3. Lobato RD, Sarabia R, Rivas JJ, et al. (1986) Normal computerized tomography scans in severe head injury. J Neurosurg 65:784–789
4. Narayan RK, Kishore PRS, Becker DP, et al. (1982) Intracranial pressure: to monitor or not to monitor. J Neurosurg 56:650–659
5. Snoek J, Jennett B, Adams H, et al. (1979) Computerised tomography after recent severe head injury in patients without acute intracranial hematoma. J Neurol Neurosurg Psychiat 42:215–225
6. Teasdale E, Cardoso E, Galbraith S, et al. (1984) CT scan in severe diffuse head injury: physiological and clinical correlation. J Neurol Neurosurg Psych 47: 600–603
7. Toutant SM, Klauber MR, Marshall LF, et al. (1984) Absent or compressed basal cisterns on first CT scan: ominous predictors of outcome in severe head injury. J Neurosurg 61:691–694

Revaluation of Closed Head Injury: Comparative Study of MR and CT

N. Kojima[1], N. Tamaki[2], T. Kondoh[2], S. Hisahiko[2], A. Ishikawa[2], T. Nagashima[2], M. Fujiwara[1], and S. Matsumoto[2]

[1] Department of Neurosurgery, Fujiwara Hospital, Fukuchiyama, Japan
[2] Department of Neurosurgery, Kobe University, School of Medicine, Kobe, Japan

Introduction

The purpose of this study is to define the respective roles of MR and CT in detecting acute and chronic head injury and to revaluate the radiopathological features of closed head trauma. CT has contributed to the management of patients with head trauma, but has not been able to provide adequate information about some types of head injury. This is particulary the case in patients with parenchymal cerebral contusions or extraparenchymal intracranial abnormalities. In this report, we systematically evaluated and compared the CT and MR findings of acute and chronic head trauma to determine the relative sensitivities of both methods for detecting a more complete spectrum of traumatic lesions.

Materials and Methods

During a period of 36 months, 116 patients with closed head trauma underwent both CT and MR examinations in our hospital. All had CT scanning as their initial investigation. MR was performed on a 0.35 T superconducting magnet. T1- and T2-weighted images were obtained with spin-echo (SE) pulse sequences. Axial scans were taken in all patients, supplemented with sagittal or coronal views in selected cases. Patients were divided into the following three groups: 1) Fresh head trauma (70 cases). MR scans were obtained within 10 days after trauma in 60 patients. Ten patients were examined subacutely (11 to 30 days after injury). 2) Chronic subdural hematoma (27 cases). All patients underwent CT and MR before operation. 3) Chronic head trauma (19 cases). The interval from injury to MR evaluation was 1 month to 15 years. Contrast-enhanced MR images were taken in 25 patients of fresh head trauma and 1 patient of chronic head trauma after the administration of gadopentate dimeglumine.

Results

Fresh Head Trauma

The most common type of traumatic lesion was brain contusion. Sixty out of 70 patients had brain contusions. Seventy-two contusions were identified in the

Table 1. MR findings of accompanied lesions of corpus callosal injury and Glasgow outcome scale

Type of injury	No. of patients					
	Total	GR	MD	SD	VS	D:GOS
Cortical/subcortical hematoma	16	4	3	3	2	4
Cortical contusion	10	3	2	3	1	1
Brain stem injury	8	1	2	2	1	2
White matter injury	7	2	3	1	1	0
Basal ganglia injury	6	1	2	1	1	1
Intraventricular hemorrhage	11	3	2	1	2	3
Subarachnoid hemorrhage	9	4	0	1	2	2
Subdural hematoma	9	4	0	1	2	2
Epidural hematoma	3	0	0	1	1	1

GR, good recovery; MD, moderate disability; SD, severe disability; VS, vegetative state; D, dead

frontal lobe in 35 patients on MR, while CT demonstrated 57% of these lesions. MR revealed 53 temporal (CT, 43%), 21 parietal (CT, 67%), 19 occipital (CT, 53%), and 6 cerebellar contusions (CT, 17%). The incidence of hemorrhagic lesions and bilateral involvement was 80% and 46% in the frontal lobe, 71% and 2% in the temporal lobe, 71% and 13% in the parietal lobe, 53% and 13% in the occipital lobe, respectively. Brain contusions were present in multiple lobes in 40 out of 60 patients. Due to its high sensitivity and multiplanar imaging capability, MR identified more clearly the location and extension of contusion and edema than CT, because cerebral contusions tended to occur at the undersurface or lateral aspect of frontal and temporal lobes. Generally speaking, CT provided more superior delineation of hemorrhagic components during the acute phase of trauma ($<$ 3 days). In evaluating subacute contusions MR was more informative than CT. On MR, injury to the corpus callosum was detected in 18 patients with fresh head trauma and in 3 patients with chronic trauma. CT showed callosal lesions in only 6 cases. The splenium or body was the most common area of involvement. In the majority of cases MR was superior to CT in identifying the associated lesions, suggesting that callosal injury occurred not only as diffuse axonal injury but also as focal injury. (Table 1). Brain stem injuries were located in the midbrain of 8 patients on MR, which were never seen on CT. Such brain contusions, including those in the corpus callosum, basal ganglia, hemispheric white matter, and brainstem may be categorized as of white matter shear injuries [5]. MR was the most sensitive for assessing this pathology. Acute subdural hematomas were identified in 28 patients. MR was superior to CT in demonstrating thin subdural hematomas in 20 patients. There were 12 cases of extradural hematomas, which were visible on MR and CT. MR was more useful when the hematomas were located at the vertex or in the posterior fossa. CT had a significant advantage over MR in the detection of subarachnoid hemorrhage in 22 patients.

Chronic Subdural Hematoma

In 8 cases, MR taken just before the operation showed hypo- or isodense on T1-weighted images and hyperdense on T2-weighted images. Their CT's exhibited high density areas mixed with isodensity areas. In the remaining 19 cases clots appeared hyperdense on both T1- and T2-weighted images, showing iso- or slightly hypodense on CT. The variety of signal intensities on MR may reflect the stage of hematoma. MR was more sensitive than CT in identifying chronic subdural hematoma.

Chronic Head Trauma

Nineteen chronic cases had sequelae of brain contusions, which were appreciated as porencephaly or encephalomalacia with focal atrophy and ventricular dilatation. MR was found to be equal or superior to CT in demonstrating these chronic changes.

Enhancement in the area of brain contusion was noted in 17 of 25 patients with fresh head trauma on contrast-enhanced MR. These patients tended to have more severe injuries. Chronic cases did not show enhancement.

Discussion

MR has significant advantages over CT in evaluating patients with closed head trauma. However, CT is still superior for showing hemorrhagic components during the acute phase of trauma [2, 3, 4] when decisions regarding surgery should be made. MR is particularly superior to CT in detecting the much more prevalent nonhemorrhagic consequences of trauma. MR showed that brain contusions were often multiple and sometimes bilateral. As brain contusions were likely to occur at the undersurface or lateral aspect of the frontal and temporal lobes, CT often failed to visualize these lesions because of streching artifacts from bone at the base of the skull. Traumatic lesions in the corpus callosum, deep white matter and brain stem are the specific features of diffuse axonal injury [1]. The radiopathological characteristics of this entity were well assessed by MR. It is suggested that these lesions could occur not only as diffuse axonal injury but also as combined injuries with focal lesions. MR detected a more complete spectrum of closed head trauma than did CT. These advantages of MR may be the key to more accurate prediction of the prognosis of closed head trauma.

References

1. Adams JH, Graham DI, Murray LS, Scott G (1982) Diffuse axonal injury due to non-missile head injury in humans: an analysis of 45 cases. Ann Neurol 12:557–563
2. Gentry LR, Godersky JC, Thompson B, Dunn VD (1988) Prospective comparative study of intermediate-field MR and CT in the evaluation of closed head trauma. AJNR 9:91–100
3. Hesselink JR, Dowd CF, Healy ME, Baker LL, Luerssen TG (1988) MR imaging of brain contusions: a comparative study with CT. AJNR 9:269–278
4. Snow RB, Zimmerman RD, Gandy SE, Deck MDF (1986) Comparison of magnetic resonance imaging and computed tomography in the evaluation of head injury. Neurosurgery 18:45–52
5. Zimmerman RA, Bilaniuk LT, Gennarelli T (1978) Computed tomography of shearing injuries of the cerebral white matter. Radiology 127:393–396

CT and MRI Evaluation of Traumatic Brain Edema and its Biochemical and Hystological Correlates

A.I. Svadovsky, A.A. Potapov, L.B. Likhterman, M.L. Demchuk, A.V. Moshkin, and G.F. Dobrovolsky

Burdenko Neurosurgical Institute, Fadeev-Str. 5, Moscow 125047, Russian Federation

Introduction

CT and MRI data allow the visualization of post-traumatic brain edema in patients. Investigations conducted over the past 10–15 years were largely experimental, some dealing with the clinical aspects of this problem including vasogenic edema (VE). It is known that CT shows VE as a perifocal zone of low density, but it is not clear whether CT and MRI can show the clearance of edematous fluid (EF) of vasogenic edema into the ventricular system (VS). Biochemical markers indicating the degree of brain parenchyma damage still remain to be identified. Blood brain barrier (BBB) permeability in severe head injury requires further study as well as the controversial role of pathogenic lipid peroxydation (LP).

Material and Methods

Thirty-nine patients with severe head injury (GCS 6–10, mean 8) were examined. The patients were divided into two groups. Group A consisted of 23 patients with cerebral contusions and/or intracerebral hematomas of considerable size. Group B consisted of 16 patients with small cortical/subcortical lesions or shearing injury, in some cases accompanied by extracerebral hematomas. MRI was performed with a strength of 0.02 T in T-2 mode (SE – 1500/150 msec). The dynamics of perifocal vasogenic edema (PVE) were investigated using both CT and MRI. The level of the stable end product of LP-malone dialdehyde (MDA) in CSF and the BBB permeability, applying the $\frac{\text{Albumin CSF mg/l}}{\text{Albumin plasma g/l}}$ ratio (Ka) introduced by K. Felgenhauer, were also studied. With regard to the level of MDA, the patients were divided into comatose (GCS $\leqslant$ 7) and non-comatose (GCS $\geqslant$ 8) patients.

Results

Analysis of the CT data showed in eight cases of group A PVE formation in the first 24 hours after injury. From the second day after trauma CT showed the hypodense route leading from the PVE to the adjacent parts of VS. MRI performed on 16 patients of both groups showed a high intensity signal (HIS) corresponding with the PVE and the hypodense route on CT. The phenomenon of "break-off" and disappearance of the route was observed both on CT and MRI a few weeks later (Fig. 1). Group B patients did not show any signs of communication between PVE and VS. Post mortem examination in two cases of group A demonstrated VE in the white matter and disruption of the ependyma where the hypodense zone surrounding the contusions was in contact with the ventricular wall (Fig. 2).

Tables 1 and 2 present the results of the MDA examinations. The data show that during the first days after injury the MDA content in CSF in group A was significantly higher ($p < 0.001$) than in group B. At the same time,

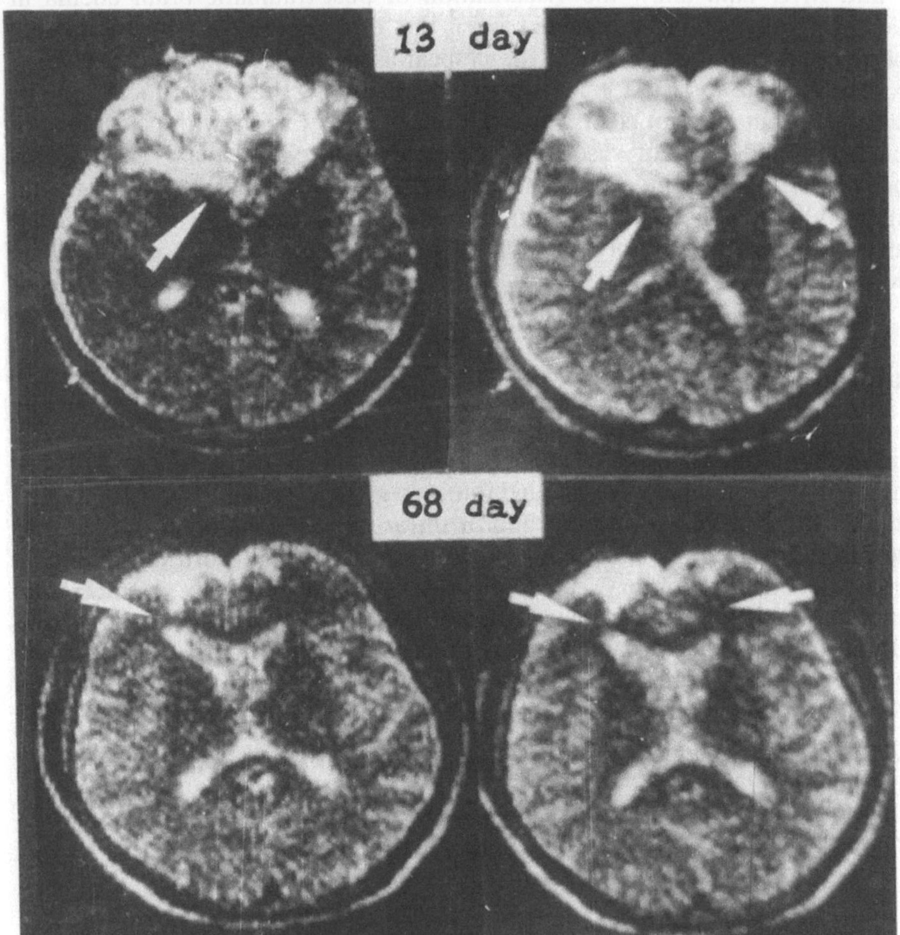

Fig. 1. MRI of patient with marked cerebral contusions in frontal lobes. Upper: arrows show communication of HIS with the apex of the anterior horn. Lower: arrows show the "break-off" phenomenon

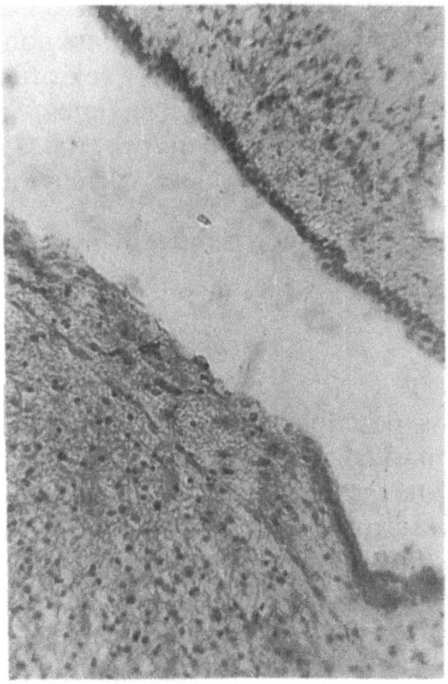

Fig. 2. Destruction of ependyma at the place of contact between the hypodensity zone surrounding V-contusion and ventricular wall (magnification 250x)

Table 1. Mean MDA values in CSF obtained during the first 10 days after injury in patients of group A and B

	MDA value in nM/ml (mean ± SD)
Normal values	0.09 ± 0.03 $n = 3$
Group A	0.76 ± 0.09 $p < 0.001$ $n = 11$
Group B	0.27 ± 0.04 $p < 0.01$ $n = 15$

Table 2. Mean MDA values in CSF of comatose and non-comatose patients

	MDA value in nM/ml (mean ± SD)
GCS ≤ 7	0.56 ± 0.11 $p_1 < 0.01$ $n = 8$
GCS ≥ 8	0.44 ± 0.08 $p_1 < 0.01$ $p_2 > 0.05$ $n = 18$

p_1, deviation from the normal value; p_2, difference between the two groups

MDA levels in CSF were not significantly different between comatose and non-comatose patients. The BBB permeability for albumin in the first week after trauma was considerably higher (mean Ka values more than five times) in group A patients compaired to group B patients (more than two times). Analysis of Ka and MDA relationships in CSF showed a close correlation between the parameters ($R = 0.68$; $p < 0.01$).

Discussion

The perifocal zone of low density on CT is described in the literature as perifocal or lobe edema. The V-form of marked cerebral contusions and hematomas on CT and at autopsy are well known. Reulen [1, 2] assumed a clearance of vasogenic edema into VS. This was explained by the existence of a tissue pressure gradient permitting EF spread through the white matter into the ventricular system. In our view, the connection of PVE with adjacent parts of VS on CT and MRI proves the clearance of EF into VS. The "break-off" and disappearance phenomena mean the "turn in" of the second phase of reabsorption of EF and products of brain tissue destruction. High MDA levels in CSF in focal injury can explain its elimination with EF into VS. Such one-way transport can exist only in the presence of pressure gradients from the vascular compartment to the tissue and then to VS. This is confirmed by the close correlation between Ka and MDA. In small cortical/subcortical lesions the pressure gradient is insufficient to force edematous fluid to the ventricular system. The difference in BBB permeability between group A and group B patients implies a different degree of VE involvement in diffuse and focal brain injury.

According to these results, MDA as a marker of severe brain damage may also have a secondary effect on brain tissue in the area of EF circulation. This is supported by the histological picture of VE and the destruction of ependyma where the ventricular wall is in contact with the edematous route.

References

1. Reulen H-J, Graham R, Spatz M, et al. (1977) Role of pressure gradients and bulk flow in dynamics of vasogenic brain edema. J Neurosurg 46:24–37
2. Reulen H-J, Tsuyumu M, Tack A, et al. (1978) Clearance of edema fluid in cerebrospinal fluid. J Neurosurg 48:754–764

Post-Traumatic Ventricular Enlargement in the Traumatic Coma Data Bank: Incidence, Risk Factors, and Influence on Outcome

R.M. Chesnut[1], T.G. Luerssen[3], M. van Berkum-Clark[1], L.F. Marshall[1], M.R. Klauber[2], B.A. Blunt[2], and the Traumatic Coma Data Bank Investigators*

[1] Division of Neurological Surgery and [2] Department of Community and Family Medicine, 225 Dickinson Street, University of California, San Diego Medical Center, San Diego, CA 92103-1990, USA
[3] Division of Neurosurgery, 702 Barnhill Drive, Indiana University Medical Center, Indianapolis, IN 46202-5200, USA

Introduction

Post-traumatic ventricular enlargement (PTVE) is a known consequence of head injury. However, its incidence and factors associated with its occurrence have not been well delineated in the severely head injured patient. We have investigated PTVE int the Traumatic Coma Data Bank (TCDB) to define its incidence, risk factors, and impact on outcome in severely head injured patients.

Materials and Methods

The Traumatic Coma Data Bank was a four center North American study of severe head injury from 1984–1987. Epidemiologic, clinical, radiographic, and outcome information was prospectively acquired on 1039 severely head injured patients. Severe head injury was operationally defined as a Glasgow Coma Scale (GCS) score of eight or less occurring on admission (post-resuscitation) or during the ensuing 48 hours. Patient outcome was determined by the last recorded Glasgow Outcome Scale (GOS) score.

There were 1030 patients entered into the TCDB. Of these, 284 did not survive resuscitation or suffered a gunshot wound to the brain. In an additional 248 patients, data necessary for our analysis was incomplete, leaving 498 patients suitable for inclusion in this study. For this group, the median time from injury to last recorded GOS for survivors was 456 days.

* This work was supported by the Traumatic Coma Data Bank (TCDB) under Contracts NO1-NS-3-2339, NO1-NS-3-2340, NO1-NS-3-2341, NO1-NS-3-2342, NO1-NS-6-2305 from the National Institute of Neurological Disorders and Stroke (NINDS). The TCDB Manual of Operations, which includes the TCDB data forms, is available from the National Technical Information Service (NTIS), U.S. Department of Commerce, 5285 Port Royal Road, Springfield, VA 22161 (NTIS Accession No. PB87 228060/AS).

Protocol CT scans were obtained upon admission and on post-injury days 3, 7–10, 90 (3 months), and 180 (6 months). PTVE was defined as bilateral ventriculomegaly in a patient whose initial CT scan(s) evidenced no ventricular enlargement. CSF infection was defined as CSF pleiocytosis and positive bacterial cultures. For analysis as a risk factor, subarachnoid hemorrhage (SAH), intraventricular hemorrhage (IVH), or CSF infection must have been diagnosed prior to PTVE.

The decision to shunt a patient with PTVE was made on an individual basis and left to the discretion of the physician. Shunting was performed when the clinical and radiographic picture appeared to indicate obstructive hydrocephalus (HCP). Factors favoring shunting were progressive PTVE, periventricular lucency as evidence of trans-ependymal fluid migration, compression of cortical sulci, or arrest or reversal of a patient's post-injury recovery.

Homogeneity of a relationship between categories of patients was tested using interaction terms in polychotomous logistic regression models [4]. Chi-square analysis with Yates' Correction was used for comparison of outcomes between patients with or without PTVE. The 1% level was used for statistical significance.

Results

Of the 498 patients without admission ventriculomegally, 27 (5.4%) developed PTVE. CT scanning performed prior to the study revealing PTVE had shown SAH in 12 patients (44%) and IVH in 16 patients (59%). Four patients (15%) had CSF infection prior to developing PTVE. Three patients developed CSF infection subsequent to PTVE.

The post-injury interval preceding appearance of PTVE is illustrated in Figure 1. The exact time of diagnosis of PTVE was missing in one patient,

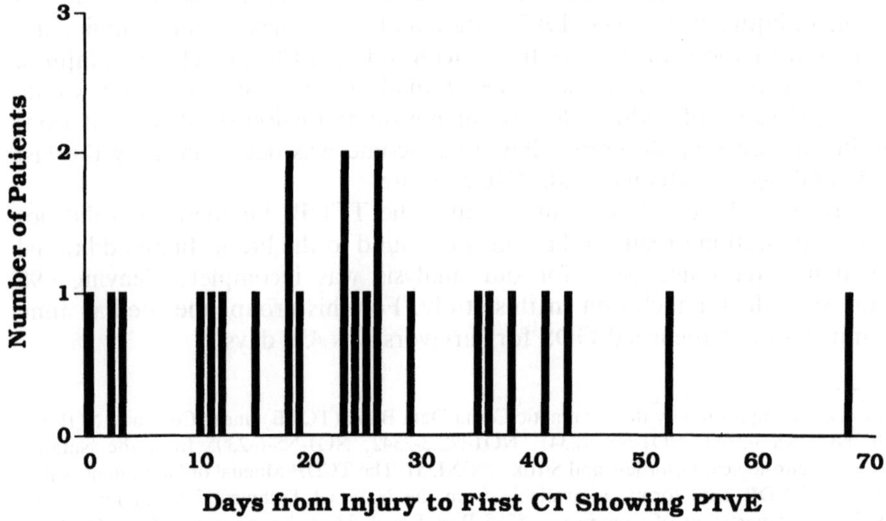

Fig. 1. Time course of appearance of post traumatic ventricular enlargement (PTVE)

leaving 26 for time analysis. Six of 26 cases (23%) appeared within 2 weeks; 23 of 26 cases (88%) appeared within 6 weeks.

Logistic regression analysis of risk factors, including age, admitting CT scan diagnosis, SAH, IVH, and CSF infection, showed that IVH ($p = 0.0028$) was a significant predictor of PTVE while SAH ($p = 0.36$) and CSF infection ($p = 0.42$) were not.

For all patients with IVH, 18 (9.7%) developed PTVE. For all patients with CSF infection, 7 (15.2%) developed PTVE. SAH was seen on 232 CT scans (47.3%) but only 12 (5.2%) of these patients developed PTVE. All of the patients in the PTVE group that had CSF infections also had IVH and 9 of the 12 patients with SAH (75%) also had IVH.

Patients with PTVE fared significantly worse on the Glasgow Outcome Scale than those without PTVE (Table 1a [$\chi^2 = 13.04$; $p = 0.0015$]). The relative risk of death or vegetative outcome was about the same for the two groups; among non-vegetative survivors, however, those without PTVE had an estimated 8.7-fold better chance of a good outcome than those with PTVE.

In all, 17 of 27 patients (63%) underwent CSF shunting procedures. The presence of IVH was associated with shunting in 12 of 17 patients (71%); one third (6/18) patients with IVH, however, did not require shunting. Notably, there was no significant difference in outcome between patients with or without shunts (Table 1b [$\chi^2 = 0.338$; $p = 0.561$]) despite several individual patients showing notable post-shunting improvement. Analyzing the effect of shunting on patients with IVH or SAH only also revealed no significant differences in outcome between shunted and non-shunted patients ($\chi^2 = 0.500$; $p = 0.48$ for both analyses) although the N values were very small in both instances.

Table 1a. TCDB data: Glasgow outcome score by presence or absence of post-traumatic ventricular enlargement (PTVE)

Status of ventricles	Number of patients	% Total patients	Outcome percent		
			Good	Moderate or severe	Vegetative or dead
Total Cases	498	100.0	28	40	32
PTVE	27	5	4	70	26
No PTVE	471	95	29	38	33

Table 1b. TCDB data: Glasgow outcome score in shunted vs non-shunted patients with post-traumatic ventricular enlargement (PTVE)

Presence of shunt	Number of patients	% Total patients	Outcome percent		
			Good	Moderate or severe	Vegetative or dead
Total Cases	498	100.0	4	70	26
Shunted	17	63	6	65	29
Not Shunted	10	37	0	80	20

Discussion

Literature estimates of PTVE range from 2.8–64% [1–3, 5, 6]. Unfortunately, most estimates are confounded by being retrospective analyses of patients with varying definitions of head injury lacking repeated CT imaging data. This study is a first attempt to study PTVE in prospectively and serially collected patients with strictly defined severe head injury. These TCDB data suggest the following conclusions:

1. PTVE occurs in approximately 5.4% of severely head injured patients. These patients have significantly poorer outcome than comparable patients without PTVE.
2. PTVE may appear at significantly delayed post-injury intervals. Although 88% appeared by 6 weeks, less than 25% was apparent within 2 weeks. We suggest that PTVE should be suspected for at least up to 3 months in patients who remain in coma, arrest their post-injury recovery, or do not meet expected rehabilitation goals.
3. There is a significant correlation between IVH and the development of PTVE. SAH and CSF infection were not found to be statistically correlated but the patient groups in these risk categories were small. Certainly the finding that 15.2% of patients with CSF infection developed PTVE suggests that infected patients should be considered at significant risk, particularly if they also evidence IVH.
4. Shunting patients with PTVE due to HCP did not improve their overall course as compared to non-shunted patients (although resulting in notable improvement in some individuals). Shunting was performed based on combined clinical and CT data per routine post-injury care at each institution. The implication is not that the PTVE patients should not be shunted; rather, our diagnostic acumen at determining which patients may benefit from shunting is wanted. Part of the difficulty certainly lies in our inability to accurately gauge the relative roles of HCP and atrophy in producing PTVE in individual patients [1, 5]. MRI imaging, radionuclide cisternography, ICP monitoring, or clinical response to trial drainage of CSF by lumbar puncture may be useful adjunct studies.

References

1. Gudeman SK, Kishore PR, Becker DP, et al. (1981) Computed tomography in the evaluation of incidence and significance of post-traumatic hydrocephalus. Radiology 141:397–402
2. Hawkins TD, Lloyd AD, Fletcher GI, Hanka R (1976) Ventricular size following head injury: a clinico-radiological study. Clin Radiol 27:279–89
3. Kishore PR, Lipper MH, Miller JD, Girevendulis AK, Becker DP, Vines FS (1978) Post-traumatic hydrocephalus in patients with severe head injury. Neuroradiology 16:261–5
4. Hosmer DW, Lameshow S (1989) Applied Logistic Regression. John Wiley and Sons, New York
5. Pedersen KK, Haase J (1973) Isotope liquorgraphy in the demonstration of communicating obstructive hydrocephalus after severe cranial trauma. Acta Neurol Scand 49:10–30
6. Roberson FC, Kishore PR, Miller JD, Lipper MH, Becker DP (1979) The value of serial computerized tomography in the management of severe head injury. Surg Neurol 12:161–7

Secondary Rise of Intracranial Pressure Following Severe Head Injury

A. Unterberg[1], K. Kiening[1], P. Schmiedek[2], and W. Lanksch[1]

[1] Department of Neurosurgery, Universitätsklinikum Rudolf Virchow, Free University of Berlin, 1000 Berlin 65, Germany
[2] Department of Neurosurgery, Klinikum Großhadern, Ludwig-Maximilians-University, 8000 München 70, Germany

Introduction

Intracranial pressure is frequently increased, following severe head injury. Usually intracranial hypertension is maximal one to three days following trauma [5]. Sometimes, however, severely injured patients develop a later, second rise of intracranial pressure following the initial peak. There are only few reports about long term observations of ICP following trauma [3, 5]. Thus, the purpose of this study was (a) to analyze different types of ICP courses following trauma, (b) to characterize the secondary rise of intracranial pressure and (c) to search for possible causes.

Clinical Material and Methods

In this study those patients were closely analyzed who were admitted to the Neurosurgical Intensive Care Unit of the Klinikum Großhadern in Munich during a three-year period. These were 90 patients whose Glasgow Coma Score (GCS) on admission was seven or less for at least 24 hours. Intracranial pressure was monitored in 53 patients. Except for four cases, intracranial pressure was increased, i.e. higher than 20 mmHg, during the following observation period (n = 49). Treatment of intracranial hypertension included head elevation, external CSF drainage, mild hyperventilation, diuretics (mannitol and furosemide) and a barbiturate coma in selected cases.

Results

Posttraumatic Courses of ICP

The courses of intracranial pressure of the 49 patients with a significant posttraumatic intracranial hypertension were characterized as follows:

1. In 15 patients (15/49) we observed a transient ICP increase with a maximum of intracranial hypertension on day one to day three following trauma.
2. In six patients (6/49) there was a longlasting increase of intracranial pressure, i.e. ICP was increased for more than four days following trauma.
3. A steadily increasing ICP indicating massive posttraumatic brain swelling was documented in 13 patients (13/49).
   These three categories were regarded as "typical" patterns of ICP following trauma which are wellknown for some time.
4. In a fourth category, 15 patients (15/49) are summarized revealing a "secondary" rise of intracranial pressure. Yet, these 15 patients are 28% of all monitored patients, or about 17% of the whole group.

Secondary Rise of ICP

The secondary rise of ICP following trauma is defined as follows:
At first, ICP is increased in these patients following trauma, but can be controlled by treatment. A first peak of intracranial hypertension is observed during the first to third postraumatic day. Subsequently, ICP decreases for at least 12 hours. Later, ICP increases again, in spite of aggressive pharmacological treatment, including barbiturate coma, i.e. ICP becomes uncontrollable (see also Fig. 1).

The 15 patients with a "secondary" rise of ICP following severe head injury were 3 to 67 years old. Most of them were younger patients between 16 and 25 years of age. Predominant neuropathological lesions were multiple contusions in seven cases and an acute subdural hematoma in five cases. The clinical outcome of this group of patients is extremely bad. Six months after trauma, seven patients were dead, one patient is in a vegetative state, four had survived severely disabled, one moderately disabled and only two had a good recovery, according to the Glasgow Outcome Score (GOS). Thus, the outcome of patients with a secondary rise of intracranial pressure is significantly worse compared to the outcome of patients without such a complication.

The secondary rise of intracranial pressure starts between day three and day 10 post trauma. During this episode the ICP increased to 30 up to 90 mmHg. Always, a clinical deterioration coincided with the secondary rise.

Possible Causes

By looking for possible causes of this phenomenon, posttraumatic hypoxia was suspected to play a major role [2, 6]. This severe complication was found in 60% of respective patients, only.

Nevertheless, the thorough analysis of all patients revealed some other possible causes. A delayed traumatic intracerebral hemorrhage (DTICH) with perifocal edema was observed in three patients [3]. In two patients a cerebral vasospasm was documented as evidenced by cerebral angiography and transcranial Doppler sonography (TCD), in one patient a severe adult respiratory distress syndrome (ARDS) with significant hypoxia and in another patient a pronounced hyponatremia [1, 3, 7]. In seven patients the secondary ICP rise coincided with a pronounced leukocytosis, which was not associated with apparent infections or sepsis. A typical example of such an ICP pattern is given in Fig. 1. Sometimes leukocytosis is a prominent finding after severe head injury [8]. It is most pronounced, however, 10 to 12 days post trauma. Interestingly, leukocytosis associated with a secondary rise of ICP appeared earlier, usually on day four to six post trauma and was not related to episodes of infections or sepsis [4]. Up to this point it is not clear whether the leukocytosis observed preceded the secondary rise of ICP, or whether it followed shortly after.

Only in three patients there was no correlation of the secondary ICP peak and any other pathological finding. Whereas vasospasm, hyponatremia and ARDS-related hypoxia can easily explain secondary intracranial hypertension, the correlation between leukocytosis and intracranial hypertension remains to be clarified.

Summary and Conclusions

The secondary rise of intracranial pressure following severe head injury is of great importance for the clinical outcome. There are some possible causes for

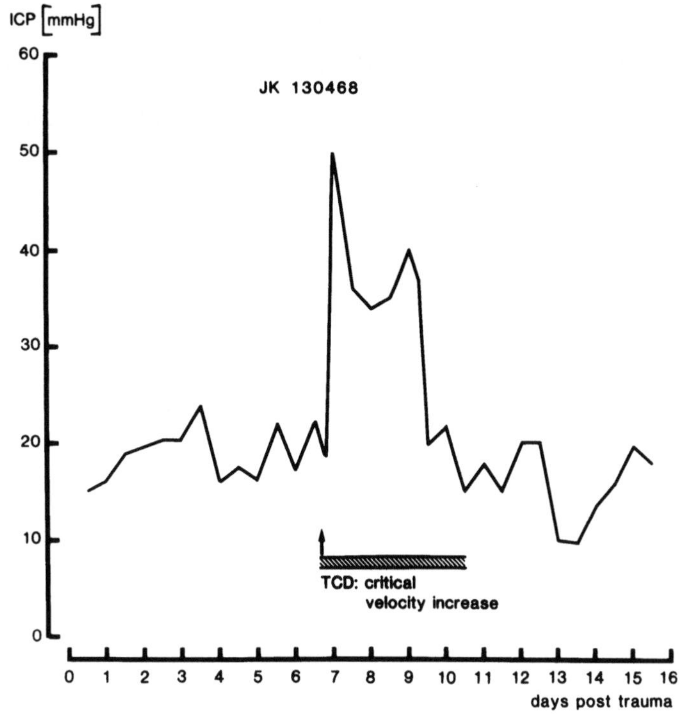

Fig. 1. Typical course of a secondary rise of intracranial pressure accompanied with a significantly elevated white blood cell count in a 12-year old girl with multiple contusions

this phenomenon: The secondary rise of intracranial pressure may be caused by delayed hemorrhage, vasospasm, hyponatremia, hypoxia, or may correlate with leukocytosis. There are only a few cases in which the secondary ICP peak can be prevented. Nevertheless a prominent leukocytosis in the early post-traumatic period appears to be a warning signal for a secondary rise of ICP. Consequently, monitoring of intracranial pressure following severe head injury should be prolonged.

Acknowledgements. The assistance of J. Kopetzki and G.-H. Schneider is gratefully acknowledgded.

References

1. Arieff AI, LLach F, Massry SG (1976) Neurological manifestations and morbidity of hyponatremia: correlation with brain water and electrolytes. Medicine 55:121–129
2. Baethmann A, Go KG, Unterberg A (1987) Mechanism of secondary brain damage. Plenum, New York
3. Cooper PR (1982) Head injury. Williams & Wilkins, Baltimore/London, pp 212, 221–223, 335–336
4. Gamache FW, Ducker TB (1982) Alterations in neurological function in head-injured patients experiencing major episodes of sepsis. Neurosurgery 10:468–472
5. Johnston IH, Johnston JA, Jennett B (1970) Intracranial-pressure changes following head injury. Lancet 1:433–436
6. Miller JD (1987) Relevance of primary and secondary brain damage for outcome of head injury. In: Baethmann A, Go KG, Unterberg A (eds) Mechanism of secondary brain damage. Plenum, New York, pp 323–328
7. Wilkins RH, Odom GL (1970) Intracranial arterial spasm associated with craniocerebral trauma. J Neurosurg 32:626–633
8. Young AB, Ott LG, Beard D, Dempsey RJ, Tibbs PA, McClain CJ (1988) The acute-phase response of the brain-injured patient. J Neurosurg 69:375–380

Characteristics of ICP of Head Injury in the Elderly

S. Kobayashi, H. Yokota, and S. Nakazawa

Department of Neurosurgery, Nippon Medical School, Tokyo 113, Japan

Introduction

It is well known that the outcome after head injury is related to the patient's age and score on the Glasgow Coma Scale (GCS) [1, 3]. On the other hand, the value of monitoring of the intracranial pressure (ICP) in patients with severe head injury has been well documented [2, 5, 6, 8, 9, 10]. Teasdale et al. [10] suggest that ICP measurement is useful in all head injury patients with mass lesions, occult hematoma, postoperative swelling and in patients with a normal CT scan and any of the following risk factors: abnormal motor responses, hypotension, or over 40 years old. Little specific information is available concerning ICP monitoring of head injury in the elderly. This study presents the clinical aspects and characteristics of ICP in the elderly, head injured population.

Patients and Method

Observations of clinical signs, computerized tomography (CT), serial CT scanning (SCT), and continuous monitoring of ICP were undertaken in 112 cases of head trauma in the elderly (over 60 years old) out of 876 cases of acute head injury during an 8-year period. ICP was measured by a subarachnoid catheter [2]. Among the 112 cases there were five patients who "talked and died" [4, 7]. Consciousness state on admission was defined according to the Glasgow Coma Scale and clinical outcome was scored using the Glasgow Outcome Scale (GOS): good recovery (GR), moderate disability (MD), severe disability (SD), persistent vegetative state (PVS) and dead.

Results

There were 84 men and 28 women, ranging from 60 to 83 years in age (mean: 68.0 years). GCS on admission was 3 in 15 cases, 4 in 11 cases, 5 in 7 cases, 6 in 13 cases, 8 in 4 cases and 9–15 in 56 cases. Fifty percent of our patients had severe head injury, which means a GCS on admission less than 8. Initial CT findings in these 112 patients were placed in one of the following categories: epidural hematoma (8%), subdural hematoma (38%), cerebral contusion (26%), intracerebral hematoma (15%), diffuse cerebral swelling (2%), intraventricular hemorrhage (4%), subarachnoid hemorrhage (27%), pneumocephalus (5%) and no abnormal findings (29%). Subdural hematoma, cerebral contusion and subarachnoid hemorrhage were the most common findings. Diffuse cerebral swelling, a very common finding in the younger age group, was uncommon. During SCT, there were new findings in 36 of 53 cases. These new findings were classified into seven types: decreased density collection in the subdural space (34%), ventricular dilatation (6%), intracerebral hematoma (33%), intraventricular hemorrhage (6%), extracerebral hematoma (4%), edema (8%) and infarction (2%). Common findings on SCT in our series were decreased density collection in the subdural space and intracerebral hematoma (so called "delayed traumatic intracerebral hematoma").

The ICP was monitored in 28 cases. Initial ICP (Table 1) was divided into 4 groups: ICP 0–10 mmHg in 7 cases, ICP 11–20 mmHg in 9 cases, ICP 21–40 mmHg in 8 cases and ICP over 41 mmHg in 4 cases. The initial ICP was below 20 mmHg in 16 cases (57%). The course of the ICP was divided into three groups: ICP remained below 20 mmHg (Group I), ICP rose above 20 mmHg but was controlled by therapy (Group II) and ICP rose above 20 mmHg but could not be controlled by therapy (Group III). The outcome

Table 1. Initial ICP and outcome

ICP (mmHg)	Glasgow outcome scale			Total
	GR/MD	SD/PVS	Dead	
0–10	1	5	1	7
11–20	2	2	5	9
21–40	1	2	5	8
41–	0	0	4	4
Total	4	9	15	28

Table 2. Course of ICP and outcome

ICP Course	Glasgow outcome scale			Total
	GR/MD	SD/PVS	Dead	
I	2	0	0	2
II	2	9	0	11
III	0	0	15	15
Total	4	9	15	28

ICP, intracranial pressure
I, ICP remained below 20 mmHg; II, ICP rose above 20 mmHg but was controlled by therapy; III, ICP rose above 20 mmHg but could not be controlled by therapy

was GR and MD in Group I (2 cases), GR/MD (2 cases) and SD/PVS (9 cases) in Group II (11 cases); all 15 patients in Group III died.

Even if the ICP was controlled by treatment, the outcome of the patients whose ICP was over 20 mmHg was poor. Our criteria for severe head injury patients who "talk and die" are: a verbal score greater than 3 and a total GCS score greater than 9, excluding patients with a lucid interval due to epidural hematoma. The ages of these 3 male and 2 female patients ranged from 63 to 75 years. They had the following GCS scores: 10 in 1 case, 11 in 2 cases, 13 in 1 case and 14 in 1 case. Skull fractures were observed in 4 of these patients. The initial CT scan showed cerebral contusion in all cases, traumatic subarachnoid hemorrhage in 4 cases and subdural hematoma in 3 cases. SCT could be obtained in all cases: delayed traumatic intracerebral hematoma was found in 4 patients and subdural hematoma in one patient. As far as the outcome of these patients at three months after injury is concerned, 4 had died and one was severely disabled. The outcome of the whole group of elderly head injury patients at three months after trauma was: GR/MD in 66 cases (59%), SD/PVS in 17 cases (15%) and dead in 29 cases (26%).

Discussion

It has been emphasized that intensive care is necessary in the management of severe head trauma. Monitoring of ICP is an useful practice commonly performed in head injury patients whose CT scans show mass lesions, occult hematoma or postoperative swelling [10]. ICP monitoring of patients with head injury has been extensively studied and elevated ICP within 72 hours of injury appears to be a predictor of poor outcome [6, 9]. It is well known that the prognosis is worse when ICP exceeds 40 mmHg [5]. In this case, the capillary blood flow, and venous flow in particular, are disturbed, possibly resulting in venous engorgement followed by brain swelling. Recently, Ross et al. [8] measured ICP in 114 cases with head injury (over 65 years old). They confirmed that an ICP greater than 20 mmHg predicts a poor outcome in elderly patients. In this series, the ICP was monitored in 28 cases. Even when the ICP is controlled by treatment, the outcome of the aged patients whose ICP is over 20 mmHg is poor. ICP monitoring is thus helpful in determining the likely outcome of patients with head injury, particularly when they are over 60 years old.

References

1. Jennett B, Teasdale GM, Braakman R, et al. (1979) Prognosis of patients with severe head injury. Neurosurgery 4:283–289
2. Kobayashi S, Nakazawa S, Yano M, et al. (1983) The value of intracranial pressure (ICP) measurement in acute severe head injury showing diffuse cerebral swelling. In: Ishii S, Nagai H, Brock M (eds): Intracranial Pressure V. Springer, Berlin Heidelberg New York Tokyo, pp 527–531

3. Luerssen TG, Klauber MR, Marshall LF (1988) Outcome from head injury related to patient's age – A longitudinal prospective study of adult and pediatric head injury. J Neurosurg 68:409–416
4. Marshall LF, Toole BM, Bowers SA (1983) The National Traumatic Coma Data Bank. Part 2: Patient who talk and deteriorate. Implications for treatment. J Neurosurg 59:285–288
5. Miller JD, Butterworth JF, Gudeman SK, et al. (1981) Further experience in the management of severe head injury. J Neurosurg 54:289–299
6. Pitts LH, Kaktis JV, Juster R, et al. (1980) ICP and outcome in patients with severe head injury. In: Shulman K, Marmarou A, Miller JD, et al. (eds) Intracranial pressure IV. Springer, Berlin Heidelberg New York, pp 5–8
7. Reilly PJ, Adams JH, Graham DI, et al. (1975) Patients with head injury who talk and die. Lancet 2:375–377
8. Ross AM, Kobayashi S, Pitts LH (1989) ICP in the elderly head injury population. In: Hoff JT, Betz AL (eds) Intracranial Pressure VII. Springer, Berlin Heidelberg New York London Paris Tokyo Hong Kong, pp 570–674
9. Seelig JM, Klauber MR, Toole BM, et al. (1986) Increased ICP and systemic hypotension during the first 72 hours following severe head injury. In: Miller JD, Teasdale GM, Rowan JO, et al. (eds) Intracranial pressure VI. Springer, Berlin Heidelberg New York Tokyo, pp 675–679
10. Teasdale GM, Mendelow AD, Galbraith S (1986) Causes and consequences of raised intracranial pressure in head injuries. In: Miller JD, Teasdale GM, Rowan JO, et al. (eds) Intracranial pressure VI. Springer, Berlin Heidelberg New York Tokyo, pp 3–8

Transporting and Monitoring the Head-Injured Patient*

D. Deyo[1], P. Brockenbrough[2], R. Briggs[2], P. Fatouros[3], Neuroscience I.C.U. Staff[1], and A. Marmarou[1]

[1] Division of Neurosurgery, and [2] Department of Respiratory Care, [3] Department of Radiology, Medical College of Virginia, Richmond, VA, USA

Introduction

Patients with severe brain injury may be at risk during intrahospital transport to imaging facilities [1]. Specialized studies such as stable xenon measurements of cerebral blood flow by computerized tomography (CTCBF) and brain water mapping by magnetic resonance (MRI) imaging require even longer durations in excess of 2 hours away from the intensive care setting. Knowledge of ICP and systemic parameters is critical to reducing risks of complication. Equally important, the maintenance of blood gases at normal levels is essential to preventing either brain ischemia induced by over aggressive manual ventilation or excessive rise in ICP caused by hypoventilation.

The objective of this research was to develop a mobile transport cart with suitable monitoring equipment [2] and ventilatory support [3] to maintain patient stability during prolonged absence from the intensive care setting.

Methods

Study Population

Severely injured patients scheduled for CTCBF or MRI investigations were included in the study (Table 1). A transport team consisting of a physician, ICU nurse, respiratory therapist and research fellows transferred the patient to the cart and performed the appropriate equipment calibrations prior to transport. This included calibration of ICP and BP transducers which were switched from the bedside monitor to the transport monitors.

Mobile Transport Cart

The nonmagnetic stretcher[a] was equipped with a rechargeable battery pack[b] capable of providing continuous power to monitoring equipment during actual

* This research supported in part by NIH grant 5RO1NS19235, the Richard Roland Reynolds Research Laboratories, and NIDRR grant H133B88029.

Table 1.

Study Population	
Sex (M:F)	16:3
Age (yrs.)	
mean (±SD)	28.8 ± 14.8
median	24
range	15–73
Glasgow Coma Score	6.11 ± 2.12
Primary Diagnosis:	
Closed Head Injury	17
Subdural Hematoma	6
Epidural Hematoma	3
Intracerebral Hematoma	2

transport. The monitoring equipment consisted of modules for measurement of systolic, diastolic and average blood pressure, intracranial pressure (VFP) from a ventricular catheter, heart rate, respiratory rate[c], end tidal pCO_2, and oxygen saturation[d]. A gas driven, MRI compatible ventilator[e] accompanied the stretcher.

Data Collection

The systemic parameters and ICP were collected at hourly intervals 4 hours prior to transport and 4 hours following return to the intensive care unit. These values were monitored from the bedside monitor by a VAX computer located in the Neuroscience ICU. Hourly values for each parameter were averaged to determine the degree of instability resulting from transport using the cart.

Results

Patient transport proceeded smoothly and without complication. In one patient, tubing from the ventilator was inadvertently pinched while mounting the MRI head coil. This was detected by the oxygen sensing alarm and the tube readjusted within 30 seconds by the technician. In several patients, it was necessary to treat elevated ICP by either drainage or mannitol during the course of the 2 hour absence from the intensive care unit. Recognition was easily accomplished by the neuroscience nurse observing the monitors while in the MRI or CT suite. The ICP and systemic parameters remained stable after transport as shown in Figs. 1, 2 and 3. The cart remains free of any required maintenance and the battery pack and monitors have performed without incident.

[a] Atomic Products MRI Stretcher, [b] TrippLite Battery Backup System, [c] Hewlett-Packard 4-Channel Patient Monitor, [d] Criticare Pulse Oximeter-End Tidal CO_2, [e] Monaghan Ventimeter

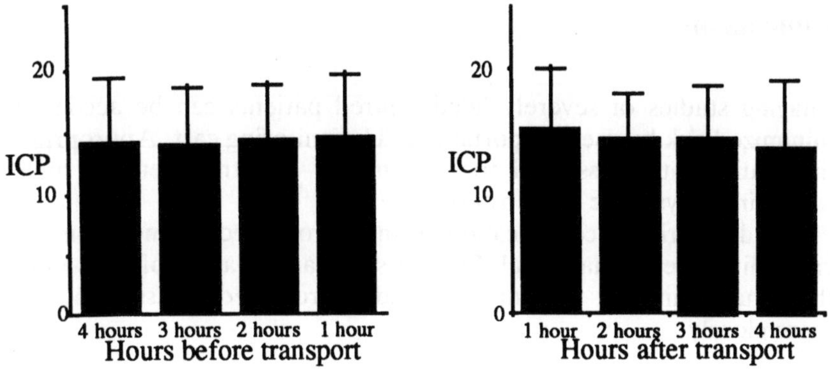

Fig. 1. Intracranial pressure: before and after transport

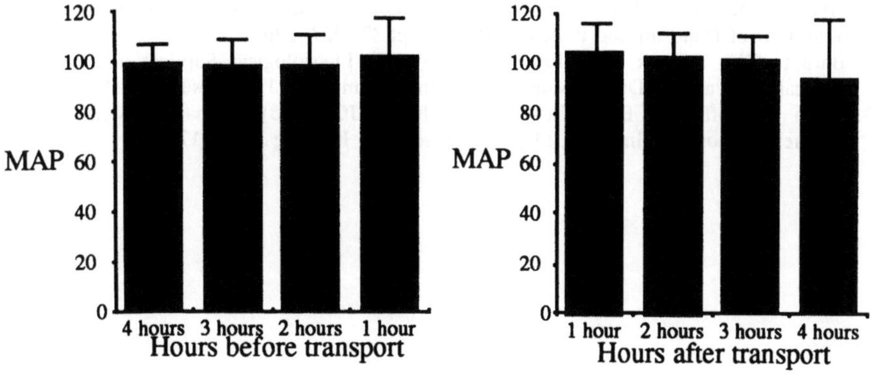

Fig. 2. Mean arterial pressure: before and after transport

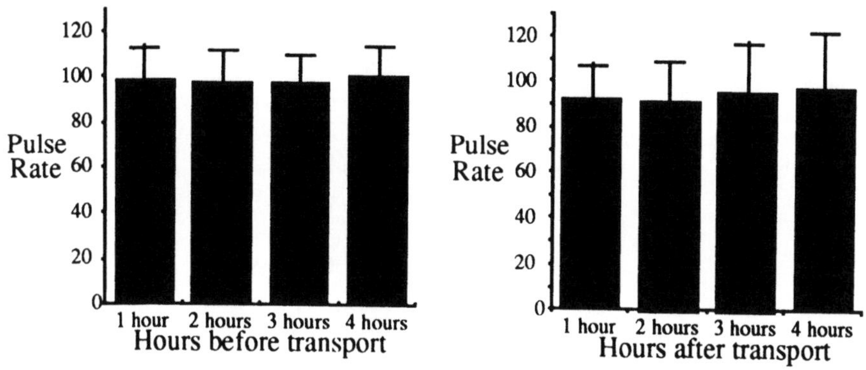

Fig. 3. Pulse rate: before and after transport

Conclusion

Imaging studies of severely head injured patients can be accomplished with minimized risk by use of a portable ICU monitoring cart. Appropriate monitoring equipment is essential for recognition and treatment of high ICP and maintaining systemic homeostasis.

Reduced risk of complication during a prolonged absence from the intensive care unit is the ultimate goal. Further study and analysis of data aquired during the actual transport and imaging study is required to assess patient stability more closely.

References

1. Andrews JD, Piper IR, Dearden NM, Miller JD (1990) Secondary Insults During Intrahospital Transport of Head-injured Patients, The Lancet 335:327–330
2. Barnett GH, Ropper AH, Johnson KA (1988) Physiological Support and Monitoring of Critically Ill Patients During Magnetic Resonance Imaging, J Neurosurg 68:246–250
3. Dunn V, Coffman CE, McGowan JE, Ehrhart JC (1985) Mechanical Ventilation During Magnetic Resonance Imaging, Magnetic Resonance Imaging 3:169–172

Intracranial Pressure Monitoring in Multidisciplinary Care Unit

R. Alberti, A. Biestro, M. Cancela, and B. Borovich

Department of Intensive Care Medicine and Department of Neurosurgery, Hospital de Clínicas of Montevideo, Av. Italia s/n., Montevideo, Uruguay

Introduction

Brain injury is an *alteration of anatomic structures and functions* [3]. As a whole, it can compromise the one more than the other, but its clinical expression is an *interaction of lesions*. One of the more important characteristics of these lesions is that they present dynamic processes. Beside this damage, there are other factors like age, clinical status on admission and "vacuum" therapeutics which establish the prognosis.

In this study we want to verify the following hypotheses: 1) the lesional patterns are the result of multiple pathologies, and 2) the lesional patterns and their dynamic changes are very important in the prognosis of these patients.

Materials and Methods

Between 1989 and 1991 we studied 47 patients in a polivalent intensive care unit. The criterion for entry into the study was: Glasgow coma scale (GCS) 8 points or less.

We classified these patients by their pathology in 2 groups: A) included 35 patients: thirty with closed injuries and five with gunshot wounds. B) included 12 patients: three intra-cranial infections, three subarachnoid hemorrhage, two strokes post cardiac surgery, two eclampsias, one brain tumor and one dural arteriovenous malformation.

Thirty patients with closed injuries were studied by CT scan. They showed the following lesions: 1) diffuse axonal injury (DAI); 2) brain swelling (BS); 3) single or multiple hemorrhagic contusion; 4) intraventricular hemorrhage and 5) epidural hematoma. They were classified in: a) *pure patterns*: only one type of lesions; b) *combined patterns*: two or more types of lesions. The changes of these lesions were: enlargement, appearance of new lesions (brain edema, cerebral infarction, ventricular enlargement, delayed hematomas) and their combinations. Intracranial pressure (ICP) was measured by means of subdural Richmond screw (39 cases), subdural catheter (6 cases) and intraventricular catheter (3 cases). The ICP was considered normal when 15 mmHg or less; high controllable (HC) between 15–40 mmHg; and high uncontrollable (HU) when it was 40 mmHg or more.

Results

Group A

1. Head Injuries

DAI. Three patients between eighteen and thirty-four years. GCS was 4,5 and 7. All of them had normal ICP. Two patients showed moderate disability (MD) in the follow-up and the third showed persistent vegetative status (PVS). The CT study did not show changes in the lesional patterns.

BS. Three patients; one patient had bihemispheric swelling, the other two presented subdural lamina and unilateral swelling underneath. Their age was between twenty and fifty-one. GCS was 4,6 and 6. ICP was HU in two patients and HC in the other one. All died. We established lesional enlargement in the serial CT controls.

Hemorrhagic Contusion. Five cases, all of them unilateral lesions. Their age was between nineteen and fifty-five. GCS was 6,6,6,7 and 7. ICP was HC in three cases and HU in two of them. The last two patients died; two of the remaining three patients recovered with MD, the other one with SD. The lesional patterns of all the patients showed enlargement of brain contusion and appearance of hypodensity around them.

Combined Patterns

DAI and BS. Included three patients between fourteen and twenty years of age. GCS was 4,7 and 7. ICP was normal in one of them and HC in the other two. GOS was MD in two and PVS in another. On follow-up, CT scan showed enlargement in the BS and appearance of an hypodense brain area.

DAI, BS and Intraventricular Hemorrhage. Two cases, twenty-seven and fifty-six years of age. GCS was 4 and 6. ICP was normal in one of them and HC in the other one. Both of them died. Again, the follow-up showed enlargement in the BS and appearance of an hypodense brain area.

DAI, BS and Hemorrhagic Contusion. Eleven cases; ten showed bilateral injury; their ages were between nineteen and fifty-one. GCS was 3,4,4,4,5,6,7, 7,7 and 8. ICP was HC in ten cases and HU in one. Six of them died and the remaining five recovered with MD. The lesional patterns showed enlargement of the hemorrhagic contusion and BS. Hypodense brain area appeared around these lesions.

BS, Hemorrhagic Contusion and Epidural Hematoma. Three cases between twenty and thirty-five years. GCS was 4,5 and 6. ICP was HC in two cases and HU in one. Two of them died and the other one recovered with SD. All of them underwent surgical evacuation. The lesional patterns of all these patients showed hemorrhagic brain contusion enlargement and appearance of hypodense brain lesions underneath the epidural hematoma.

Group B

2. Gunshot Wounds

Five cases between twenty-one and forty-seven years of age; all of them with bihemispheric traject. CT patterns were hemorrhagic lesions.

Among eleven patients we found: two strokes with the same CT patterns. Normal ICP was seen in one case and HU in the other one. Two cases with eclampsia had CT scan compatible with BS; one of them showed normal ICP and the other one HC.

Discussion

Brain injury is a multifactorial process of primary and secondary lesions [1, 4]. In our series, the multiple patterns accounted for 63% of the cases. Pure patterns were seen in 36%. CT scan patterns showed dynamic changes in 90%. We have found that it is difficult to classify these patients because in most cases they show combined patterns. It is often difficult to know which is the main lesion in the prognosis of these patients. These morphological modifications change the physiopathological behavior of the patients, for example increasing ICP. We have found a close correlation between the clinical deterioration and the CT scan patterns. We think that the management and the prognosis of these patients will be improved if we follow lesional patterns and their changes [2]. We also compared GOS, age, GCS and ICP and we did not find any difference with other studies [5]. The rate of mortality was 53%.

References

1. Becker DP (1989) Common themes in head injury. In: Becker DP, Gudeman SK. Textbook of head injury. Saunders, Philadelphia, pp 1–22
2. Gennarelli TA, Spielman GM, Langfitt TW, et al. (1982) Influence of the types of intracranial lesion on outcome from severe head injury. A multicenter study using a new classification system. J Neurosurg 56:26–32
3. Miller JD, Becker DP (1982) General principles and pathophysiology of head injury. In: Youmans J (ed) "Neurological surgery" vol 4, Saunders, Philadelphia
4. Miller JD (1986) Relevance of primary and secondary brain damage for outcome of head injury. In "Mechanisms of secondary brain damage". Plenum, New York
5. Saul TC, Ducker TB (1982) Effects of intracranial pressure monitoring and agressive treatment of mortality in severe head injury. J Neurosurg 56:498–503

Intracranial Pressure Related to Sleep

A. Yokota, K. Kohshi, and H. Kajiwara

Department of Neurosurgery, University of Occupational and Environmental Health, Kitakyushu 807, Japan

Introduction

To clarify the characteristics of changes in intracranial pressure (ICP) relating to sleep phenomena, the correlation between the pressure waves, sleep cycles and clinical conditions of patients was investigated by analysis of simultaneous overnight recordings of ICP and electroencephalography (EEG).

Clinical Materials and Methods

Overnight recordings of both ICP and EEG were conducted on 85 neurosurgical patients with intracranial hypertension and/or ventriculomegaly. ICP was measured by ventricular or spinal fluid pressure in all but 3 cases, with the patient in the supine position using calibrated straingauge transducers referenced to the external auditory meatus. ICP was recorded polygraphically with impedance pneumography and heart rate in all patients and with systemic arterial pressure and end-tidal CO_2 in some. EEG was recorded together with electro-oculogram (EOG) and electromyogram in all patients. All the data obtained simultaneously from ICP and EEG recording systems were stored on magnetic tape for further analysis.

Overnight profiles of ICP and sleep stages were diagrammed for each patient. Pressure waves were classified into 5 types according to the level of resting pressure and pattern of appearance [1, 2], and their correlation with sleep cycles and clinical conditions of the patients were investigated. Changes in ICP during sleep were studied in patients whose sleep stages were clearly scored.

Results

Pressure Waves and their Clinical Correlations

A-(plateau) waves (type 1) appeared in 15 patients with long-standing intracranial hypertension and episodic B-waves (type 2) appeared in 22 patients with chronic hydrocephalus. When these episodic pressure waves appeared, the patients were conscious and sleep cycles including stage REM were observed. Persistent, high pressure B-waves (type 3) were seen in 15 stuporous patients with acute and subacute phases of intracranial hemorrhage. The EEG of these patients showed alternate appearances of light sleep and waking rhythms in accordance with cyclic oscillations of B-waves which coincided with a periodic, apneic respiratory rhythm. Markedly regular B-waves of moderately high pressure (type 4) appeared continuously in 12 patients who were severely impaired in consciousness and were in acute and subacute phases of intracranial hemorrhage. B-waves of this type were also highly correlated with apneic respiratory rhythms. EEG showed continuous slow activities and sleep stages were not scored in these patients. No characteristic clinical features were found in 21 patients whose ICP remained within normal range without pressure waves throughout the recording (type 5).

ICP Changes During Sleep

ICP changes in accordance with sleep stages were clearly observed in patients with A-waves (type 1) and with episodic B-waves (type 2). On many occasions ICP in the light sleep stages (Stage I, II) was higher than that in the deep sleep stages (Stage III, IV), but ICP in Stage III remained as high as that in Stages I and II in some cases. However, ICP in stage IV was always lower than that in the other sleep stages. In REM sleep, ICP rose abruptly, forming A-waves and episodic B-waves in the majority of cases.

Correlation Between Pressure Waves and REM Sleep

In patients with A-waves, 88.9% of the total number of A-waves appeared in accordance with REM sleep, and the rest occurred during waking or in Stage II. On the other hand, REM was associated with A-waves at a rate of 91.8%, or with B-waves in this group. In patients with episodic B-waves, 95.1% of episodic B-waves occurred during REM sleep, and only 4.9% appeared in Stage II and during waking. REM accompanied episodic B-waves at a rate of 75.0%, while other REM occurred without any pressure changes. The initiation of a REM stage on EEG, which proceeded the EOG discharges characteristic of REM by 1 to 2 minutes, usually occurred 1 to 2 minutes prior to the initiation of A-waves or just at the ascending phase of the plateau (Fig. 1). Episodic B-waves also occurred 1 to 2 minutes after the initiation of REM.

Discussion

The clinical significance of pressure waves is related to whether pressure waves appear episodically or continuously. Episodic pressure waves are seen in patients with long-standing intracranial hypertension who are conscious and have

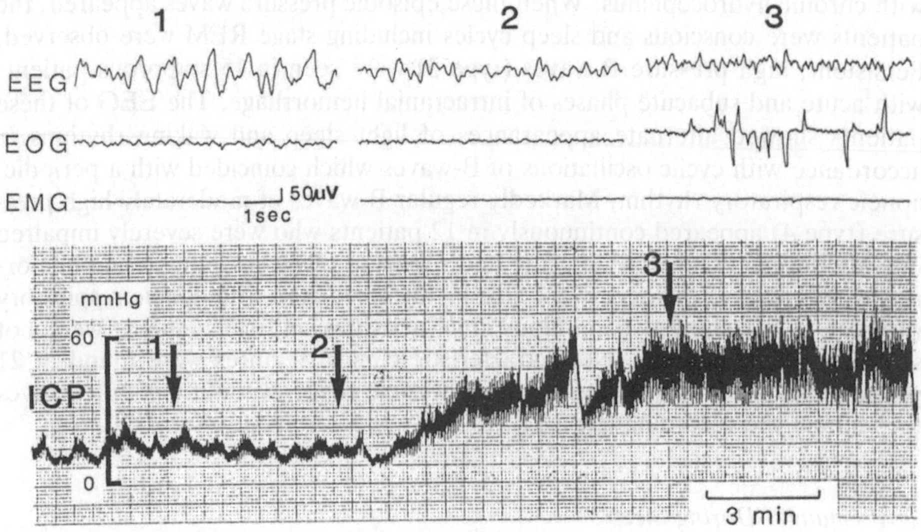

Fig. 1. Time relation between the initiation of REM and pressure wave in a patient with A-wave. REM stage characterized by EOG discharge (*3*) appears markedly at the plateau of A-wave, however, REM stage scored on EEG (*2*) begins about 2 minutes prior to the ascending slope of A-wave

sleep cycles. In these patients, ICP changes during REM sleep are characterized by the frequent appearance of episodic pressure waves, rather than by gradual elevation of the resting pressure. A high correlation between REM sleep and episodic pressure waves occurred quantitatively as well as temporally in this study, suggesting a causal relationship between them. The episodic pressure waves are assumed to be induced by intracranial conditions in REM sleep, when increased brain activity and reduced sympathetic tone occur simultaneously. On the other hand, the continuous pressure waves appearing in high coincidence with periodic, apneic respiratory rhythm are seen in patients with acute and subacute intracranial hypertension whose consciousness is disturbed. These continuous pressure waves appearing in conditions which interfere with normal sleep cycles are thought to be regulated by the same mechanism causing the periodic respiratory rhythm.

References

1. Yokota A, Matsuoka S, Ishikawa T, Kohshi K, Kajiwara H (1989) Overnight recordings of intracranial pressure and electroencephalography in neurosurgical patients. Part I: Intracranial pressure waves and their clinical correlations. J UOEH 11:371–381
2. Yokota A, Matsuoka S, Ishikawa T, Kohshi K, Kajiwara H (1989) Overnight recordings of intracranial pressure and electroencephalography in neurosurgical patients. Part II: Changes in intracranial pressure during sleep. J UOEH 11:383–391

Edema, Hemodynamics and Oxygenation

The Contribution of Brain Edema to Brain Swelling*

A. Marmarou, P. Fatouros, M. Yoshihara, K. Bandoh, C.B. Zerate, D. Deyo, P. Brockenbrough, Neuroscience ICU Nursing Staff, and H.F. Young

Richard Roland Reynolds Neurosurgical Research Laboratories, Division of Neurosurgery, Medical College of Virginia, Richmond, VA, USA

Introduction

The deleterious effect of raised ICP following traumatic brain injury has been well recognized. However, it remains unclear whether the primary disruption of volume homeostasis and subsequent development of pressure is caused by brain edema or vascular engorgement. Primary traumatic swelling usually involves both hemispheres and in the more recent data obtained from the traumatic coma data bank (TCDB), of 595 patients studied, 31% of patients showed evidence of brain swelling [1]. Heretofore, it has not been possible to assess the contribution of increased water because of methodological problems in volume assessment. However, the recent introduction of magnetic resonance (MR) methods and the inherent sensitivity of changes in relaxation time to brain water has led to the development of quantitative methods capable of determining spatial distribution of edema non-invasively [2, 3].

The objective of this study was to determine the contribution of brain edema to the swelling process in severely head injured patients using the magnetic resonance imaging methods.

Methods

Study Population

Severely brain injured patients (GCS 8 or less), were transported to the MRI suite utilizing a special cart (see elsewhere in this volume) equipped for monitoring ICP, Blood Pressure (BP), Heart Rate (HR) and oxygen saturation and an MR compatible gas driven ventilator for maintaining patients normocapnic. A total of 19 patients were studied, with gender, age and primary diagnosis

* This work was supported by a NIDRR Grant No. H133B80029

Table 1. Study population (n = 19)

Gender	M:F	15:4
Age (yrs)		
	Mean	25.1
	SD	17.6
	Range	15–50
Primary Diagnosis		
Closed head injury		9
Subdural H.		5
Contusion		2
Epidural		3

described in Table 1. Studies were performed within the first 5 days post injury and targeted ideally for 72 hours post injury as MRI scheduling permitted.

MRI Methodology

Following stabilization of patients in the magnet, a rapid T1 scan was accomplished for purposes of selecting the brain slice for study. After slice selection, four inversion recovery scans were obtained at a repetition time (TR) of 4.0 seconds, echo time of 28 msec and inversion times (T1) of 250, 600, 1000 and 1700 msec respectively. Following these scans a multi-echo spin sequence was performed with TR = 4.0 seconds. The selection of the inversion recovery pulse sequence were arrived at after extensive studies of calibration standards of known relaxation rates, and results of previous animal studies. The result of this effort produced water maps in which the enhancement was directly proportional to tissue water content expressed in gmH_2O/gm tissue. From these water maps, total brain water was measured in each patient and the percentage edema and volume computed.

Results

All studies were conducted with no complication. Average study time was approximately 1.5 hours. Patients were returned to the ICU and stability of ICP and BP remained stable throughout the transfer period. Water maps were analyzed by obtaining a global tissue measure of brain edema with careful attention to excluding CSF spaces. The increase in brain water content of head injured patients averaged 1.74% gmH_2O/gm tissue ±0.86 S.D measured within 5 days post injury. The average time post injury equaled * days. The increase in edema water ranged from 0.10 to 3.41% for the study group. Volume change (cc) attributed to the increased water was calculated based on a an estimated average brain weight of 1400 gm and is summarized in Table 2.

Although the measurement time was targeted for 72 hours, the actual time of study varied and allowed us to plot the distribution of percent volume

Table 2. Contribution of edema to brain swelling volume in severe injured patients

	Swelling %	Volume
Patients	19	1400 gm (Est.)
Range	0.13–4.4%	18.2–62.0 cc
Average	2.22%	31.1 cc
SD	1.11%	15.5 cc

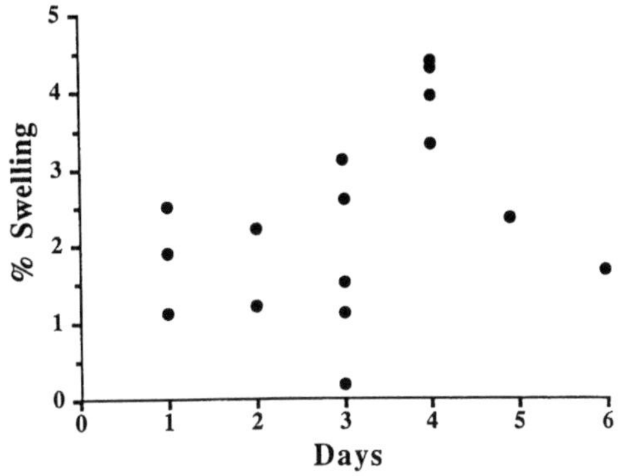

Fig. 1. Percent swelling due to edema in head injured patients

swelling vs. time post injury for this cohort. (Fig. 1). The maximal edema volumes were found at 4 days post injury. Interestingly, there was no direct correlation of ICP or PVI at time of study with the edema volumes measured in this study group.

Discussion

These studies show that edema develops and contributes significantly to the brain swelling following traumatic injury. The maximal increase in edema water measured in this study equaled 3.41% representing an estimated increase in volume of 4.4% or 62 cc. Heretofore, it has not been possible to quantify the amount of brain water increase in severely injured patients. Now, with the development of these MR methods, we remain optimistic that the dynamics of the swelling process can be ascertained with reasonable accuracy.

We anticipated a correlation between swelling volume and ICP. This was not the case as the degree of swelling in this patient group was within the pressure/volume reserve of each patient. This became more clear as we examined the average ICP for these patients and we found that ICP was only moderately increased for the first 72 hours post injury.

Table 3. Average daily ICP – MRI cohort

	Day 1	Day 2	Day 3
ICP mmHg	13.8	15.4	15.1
SD	5.4	3.9	3.8

The bias of patient selection in this preliminary study was due in part to our reluctance to transfer the more severely injured patient from the ICU for a period of 2.0 hours or more, particularly those patients in whom ICP management was difficult. This problem has now been solved with our development of the ICU transport cart where ventilatory parameters can be adjusted and elevated ICP treated appropriately.

In conclusion, brain edema contributes up to 4.4% total swelling volume in head injured patients. This volume can be accommodated with moderate increase in ICP and highest edema values were measured 3 to 4 days post injury.

References

1. Eisenberg H, Gary H, Jane J, et al. (1988) CT scan findings in a series of 595 patients with severe closed head injury: A report from the NIH traumatic coma data bank. Annual Meeting of the American Association of Neurological Surgeons Toronto, Ontario April 24–28
2. Fatouros P, Marmarou A, Kraft K, et al. (1991) In vivo brain water determination of T1 measurements: Effect of total water content hydration fraction and field strength. Magn Reson Med 17:402–413
3. Marmarou A, Fatouros P, Ward, et al. (1990) In Vivo measurement of brain water by MRI. Brain Edema VIII. JH Reulen, A Baethmann, J Fenstermacher, A Marmarou, M Spatz (eds) Acta Neurochirurgica supplementum 51:261–262, by Springer-Verlag

Cerebral Blood Volume in Acute Head Injury: Relationship to CBF and ICP

G.J. Bouma[1,3], J.P. Muizelaar[1], R. Schuurman[3], P. Fatouros[2], and A. Marmarou[1]

[1] Division of Neurosurgery and [2] Department of Radiology, Medical College of Virginia, Virginia Commonwealth University, Richmond, VA, USA
[3] Department of Neurosurgery, Academic Medical Center, University of Amsterdam, Amsterdam, The Netherlands

Introduction

Uncontrollable high ICP due to brain swelling is the single most important factor determining mortality from severe head injury [6, 7]. Yet, it is uncertain what the exact cause of posttraumatic brain swelling is, and no satisfying treatment for this problem exists. Theoretically, brain swelling may be caused by increased brain water content (edema), or by cerebrovascular engorgement with increased cerebral blood volume (CBV). While brain edema has been extensively studied both experimentally and clinically, relationships between cerebrovascular status and ICP have so far mostly been studied by cerebral blood flow (CBF) measurements [8]. However, it has become clear that CBF and CBV are not linearly related [3, 9], especially under pathologic conditions, and thus, CBF measurements alone may not be sufficient to fully comprehend the vascular contribution to raised ICP. To date, only scant data on post-traumatic CBV have been reported [4]. This may at least in part be due to the fact that thus far, no practical method for measuring CBV in humans has been available. Although measures of CBV can be reliably obtained by PET or SPECT, these techniques are difficult to implement in critically ill and unstable patients, additional equipment is required, and necessary transportation of the patients may interfere with acute treatment. Nonetheless, as appropriate therapeutic management depends on precise identification of the cause of increased ICP, determination of CBV in the acute stage of severe head injury may be an important adjunct to the clinician.

In the present study, we have evaluated the role of CBV in acute head injury, using a recently developed method which allows rapid determination of CBV during any regularly obtained CT scan. Specifically, we have examined the relationships between CBV and CBF on one hand, and between CBV and ICP dynamics on the other. We were also interested in the temporal course pattern of these parameters.

Clinical Materials and Methods

Simultaneous determinations of CBF and CBV were made in comatose head-injured patients who underwent CT scanning for diagnostic purposes during the first week after injury. All patients were intubated, artificially ventilated and well oxygenated (pO_2 > 80 mm Hg), and were hemodynamically stable (systolic blood pressure >100 mm Hg) during the studies. Vital signs, oxygen saturation, and expiratory CO_2 were continuously monitored. An intraventricular catheter was inserted for determination of ICP and pressure-volume index (PVI).

All studies were performed on a General Electric 9800 CT scanner. CBF was measured by the stable xenon-enhanced CT technique (Xe-CT) as described in detail elsewhere [10]. A gasmixture containing 32% stable xenon was administered through a volume-cycled respirator for 4.5 minutes. No significant rise in ICP was observed during xenon-inhalation.

Determination of CBV was performed by independent measurement of cerebrovascular mean transit time (MTT) immediately following the Xe-CT CBF study, using rapid sequential ("dynamic") CT scanning [1]. Synchronous with an i.v. bolus-injection of 50 cc iodine contrast (Omnipaque 300) through a large-bore catheter, ten CT scans with a scan time of 2.0 sec and minimum interscan delay of 2.3 sec were performed at the same level for which CBF was previously determined. The raw data were segmented into three images per scan, and a time vs. density curve was obtained for each hemisphere. The curve was fitted to a gamma-variate function using a minimum chi-square procedure in a repetitive approach. Details of the procedure have been described previously [2].

Results

A total of 45 determinations of CBF and CBV were performed in 35 patients. In 15 of these patients, CBV was measured during the first CT scan obtained on admission to the hospital, on average 3.6 hours after injury. The average CBV value in these 15 cases was 4.8 ± 1.2 ml/100 g (range: 2.8 to 7.1 ml/100 g), which did not differ significantly from the mean CBV value obtained at later intervals after injury (Table 1). Mean CBF, however, was significantly lower early after injury (Table 1). These effects could not be attributed to differences in pCO_2. In general, CBV and CBF correlated poorly (Fig. 1). Three patients died within 24 hours after admission. On admission, all three had very low

Table 1. Cerebral blood flow (CBF), cerebral blood volume (CBV), and arterial pCO_2 in relation to the time after injury at which measurements were obtained. Values are mean ± SD

hours post injury	no. of studies	CBF (ml/100 g.min^{-1})	CBV (ml/100 g)	pCO_2 (mm Hg)
<12	15	34.5 ± 12.4*	4.8 ± 1.2	34.1 ± 7.4
12–24	4	48.6 ± 10.2	5.4 ± 1.2	34.8 ± 3.4
>24	26	44.7 ± 11.8	5.1 ± 1.5	37.7 ± 7.2

* $p < 0.05$, Student-Newman-Keuls test

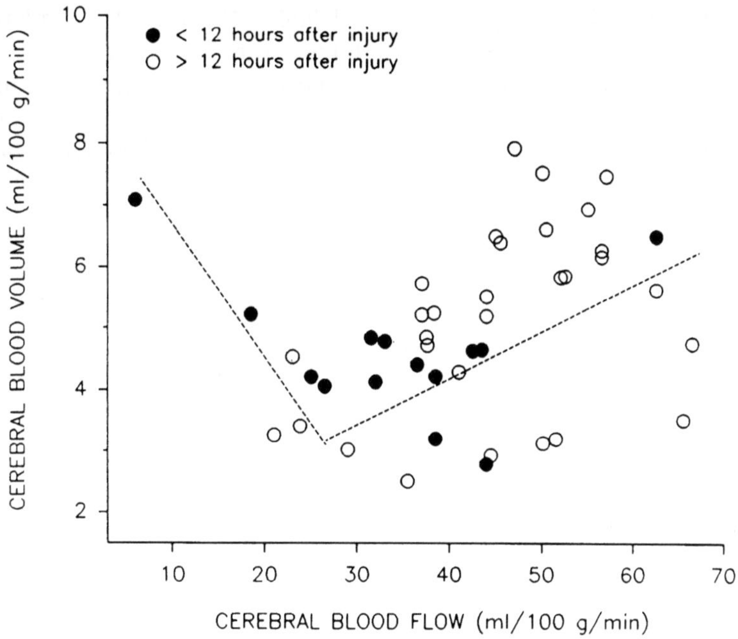

Fig. 1. Plot of cerebral blood volume (CBV) vs. cerebral blood flow (CBF). Fifteen measurements were performed within 12 hours after injury (filled circles). Below CBF of 30 ml/100 g . min^{-1}, an inverse trend between CBV and CBF was found (dashed line)

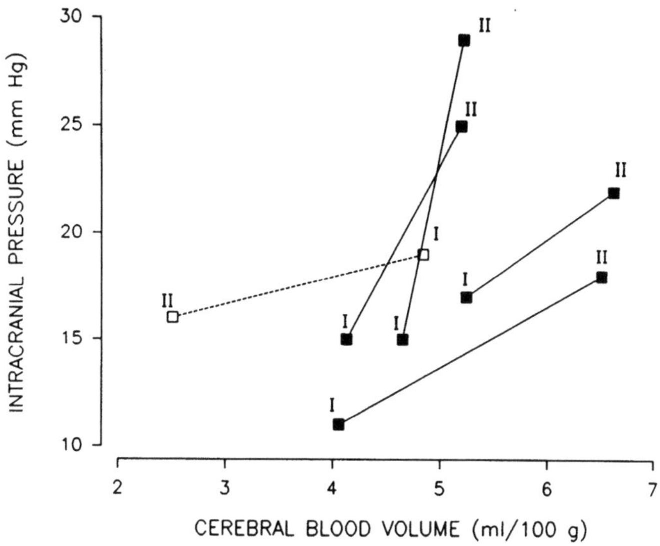

Fig. 2. Temporal course of CBV and relationship with ICP in five patients in whom CBV was measured both on admission (I), and at approximately day 3 after injury (II). In 4 of 5 patients both CBV and ICP had increased (filled squares), while in the fifth patient both parameters had decreased (open squares)

CBF (17 ± 8 ml/100 g . min^{-1}) and high CBV (5.7 ± 1.2 ml/100 g), with high opening ICP (>40 mm Hg). When these three patients are omitted, there was a general trend for CBV to increase during the first three days after injury. This is illustrated by 5 patients in whom CBV was measured both on admission and at follow-up at approximately 3 days after injury (Fig. 2). In all but one, CBV had increased concomitant with a rise in ICP. In the fifth patient, both CBV and ICP were slightly lower. Overall, the correlation between CBV and ICP was weak. Although patients with the lowest CBV values consistently also had low ICP (Table 2), CBV values were not predictive of ICP in individual cases (Fig. 3A). However, the volume buffering capacity of the intracranial space, as indicated by the pressure-volume index (PVI) was markedly reduced in patients with higher CBV. The inverse correlation between CBV and PVI was more consistent (Fig. 3B) and statistically significant ($r = 0.69$, $p < 0.001$).

Table 2. Mean ± SD of cerebral blood flow (CBF), intracranial pressure (ICP), and pressure-volume index (PVI) at various levels of CBV

CBV	no. of studies	CBF (ml/100 g.min^{-1})	ICP (mm Hg)	PVI (ml)
<4.0	10	40.3 ± 13.0	14.3 ± 3.2	24.4 ± 3.1
4.0–5.2	15	37.2 ± 10.1	25.6 ± 10.6	21.0 ± 4.9
>5.2	20	45.6 ± 13.6	21.4 ± 8.9	17.1 ± 5.4

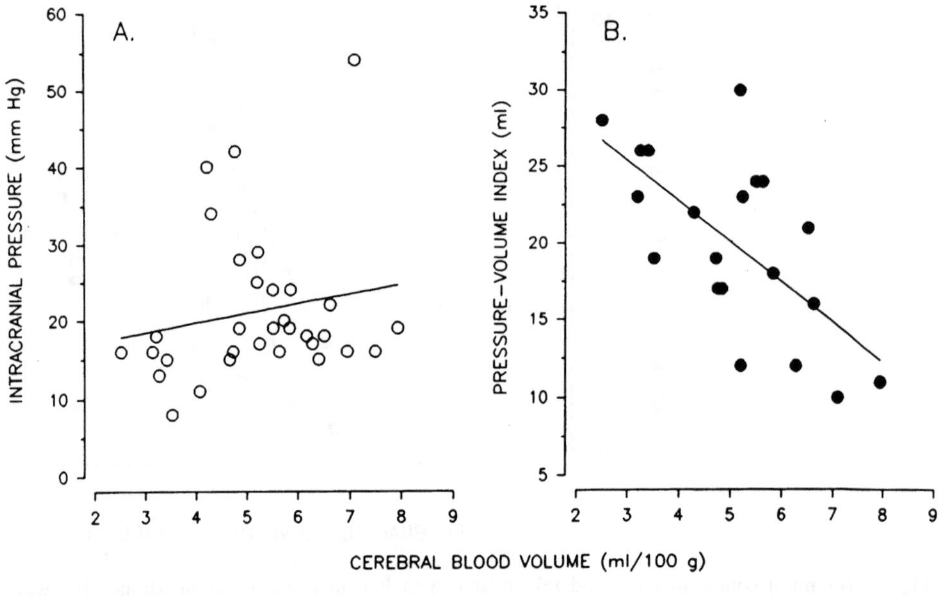

Fig. 3. Plot of ICP vs. CBV in 32 patients (**A**) and CBV vs. PVI in 21 patients (**B**). Only a weak (non-significant) positive correlation between CBV and ICP was found. The correlation between PVI and CBV was statistically significant ($r = 0.69$, $p < 0.001$)

Discussion

This study demonstrates that CBV measurements in severely head-injured patients are feasible, even in the very acute stage, and that these data may provide some important insight into the pathophysiology of raised ICP. The lack of correlation between CBF and CBV underscores the importance of measuring CBV apart from CBF. The inverse correlation between CBF and CBV at lower levels of CBF appears to be consistent with autoregulatory vasodilation of the microcirculation, and concurs with previous findings [3, 9]. Although the average CBV in this series of head-injured patients did not differ from reported normal values [5], the wide variety that was found points to the many different and uncontrolled mechanisms (ischemia, swelling, loss of autoregulation), that may occur and affect cerebrovascular status. The scatter seen on the CBV vs. ICP plot (Fig. 3A) may be explained by two mechanisms. First, many other factors aside from CBV (e.g. edema, hemorrhage) influence ICP, the extent of which was not analyzed in this study. Second, ICP is never allowed to run its course in head-injured patients, but is instead vigorously treated when it rises above certain levels (usually 20 mm Hg). Nonetheless, the marked inverse correlation between CBV and PVI suggests that increased CBV contributes to increased brain stiffness and may lead to more difficult ICP control.

References

1. Axel L (1980) Cerebral blood flow determination by rapid sequence CT, a theoretical analysis. Radiology 137:679–686
2. Bouma GJ, Fatouros PP, Muizelaar JP, Stringer WA, Marion DW, Marmarou A (1991) Determination of cerebral blood volume by simultaneous Xenon-CT CBF measurement and intravenously enhanced dynamic CT. In: Yonas H (ed) Proceedings of the International Congress on Stable Xenon/CT CBF. Raven Press, New York, in press
3. Grubb RL, Raichle ME, Eichling JO, Gado MH (1977) Effects of SAH on cerebral blood volume, blood flow, and oxygen utilization in humans. J Neurosurg 46:446–453
4. Kuhl D, Alavi A, Hoffman EJ, Phelps ME, Zimmerman RA, Obrist WD, Bruce DA, Greenberg JH, Uzzell BP (1980) Local cerebral blood volume in head injured patients. Determination by emission computed tomography of 99mTc-labeled red cells. J Neurosurg 52:309–320
5. Leenders KL, Perani D, Heather JD, Buckingham P, Healy MJR, Gibbs JM, Wise RJS, Hatazawa J, Herold S, Beaney RP, Brooks DJ, Spinks T, Rhodes C, Frackowiak RSJ, Jones T (1990) Cerebral blood flow, blood volume and oxygen utilization. Normal values and effect of age. Brain 113:27–47
6. Marmarou A, Anderson R, Ward JD, Eisenberg HM, Jane JA, Marshall LF, Young HF (1989) The Traumatic Coma Data Bank: Monitoring of ICP. In: Hoff JT, Betz AL (eds) Intracranial Pressure VII. Springer, Berlin Heidelberg, New York London Paris Tokyo Hong Kong, pp 549–551
7. Miller JD, Butterworth JF, Gudeman SK, Faulkner JE, Choi SC, Selhorst JB, Harbison JW, Lutz HA, Young HF, Becker DP (1981) Further experience in the management of severe head injury. J Neurosurg 54:289–299
8. Obrist WD, Langfitt TW, Jaggi JL, Cruz J, Gennarelli TA (1984) Cerebral blood flow and metabolism in comatose patients with acute head injury. J Neurosurg 61:241–253

9. Sabatini U, Celsis P, Viallard G, Rascol A, Marc-Vergnes JP (1991) Quantitative assessment of cerebral blood volume by single-photon emission computed tomography. Stroke 22:324–330
10. Yonas H, Wolfson SK, Gur D, Latchaw RE, Good WF, Leanza R, Jackson DL, Jannetta PJ, Reinmuth OM (1984) Clinical experience with the use of xenon-enhanced CT blood flow mapping in cerebral vascular disease. Stroke 15:443–450

Intracranial Compliance and Cerebral Hemodynamics in Head-Injured Patients

C.S. Robertson, Z. Feldman, C.F. Contant, R.K. Narayan, and R.G. Grossman

Baylor College of Medicine, One Baylor Plaza, Houston, TX 77030, USA

Introduction

Pressure Volume Index (PVI) and Volume Pressure Response (VPR) have been used as a measure of intracranial compliance. PVI is defined as the volume of CSF that would have to be infused to raise the ICP ten-fold. Normal PVI is 26 ml [6]. Less than 13 ml is considered to indicate reduced volume buffering capacity. VPR is defined as the change in ICP with the infusion of 1 ml of CSF. Normal VPR is <2 mmHg [5]. Greater than 5 mmHg is considered to indicate reduced volume buffering capacity. Some experimental studies have suggested that PVI is altered by hemodynamic factors, such as cerebral perfusion pressure (CPP) [3, 5]. We have investigated the relationship of PVI to cerebral hemodynamics and to the severity of intracranial hypertension in head-injured patients.

Methods

Patient Characteristics and Management

Forty-four patients admitted to the Neurosurgical Intensive Care Unit at Ben Taub General Hospital between July 1, 1989 and April 30, 1991 had serial measurements of cerebral blood flow (CBF) and metabolism and of cerebral pressure-volume relationship during the acute phase of injury (1–10 days postinjury). Mean ICP and mean blood pressure (MAP) were collected continuously by a bedside computer. Measurements of cerebral perfusion pressure (CPP), PVI, VPR, CBF, and cerebral vascular resistance (CVR) were obtained every 8 hours during the period that the ICP was monitored. Initial measurements were obtained within the first 24 hours of injury when possible. A total of 375 measurements of CBF, or an average of 8.5 per patient (range 1–22 per patient) were obtained. The majority of the measurements were made in the first 5 days after injury. On 269 of these occasions a measurement of PVI was obtained. The volume of CSF injection or withdrawal was 1.0 ml on 245 occasions such that a VPR could be calculated.

CBF was measured by the nitrous oxide saturation method. CVR was calculated by the equation:

$$CVR = \frac{MAP - ICP}{CBF}$$

The mean value for CBF in normal adults with this method is 0.5 ml/gm/min. CVR is normally 0.016 mmHg/ml/gm/min.

PVI was calculated from the ICP change to a bolus injection or withdrawal of a known volume of CSF from the lateral ventricle, by the equation:

$$PVI = \frac{V}{\log P_p/P_0}$$

where V = volume injected or withdrawn (ml), P_p = peak ICP after injection (mmHg), and P_0 = baseline ICP before injection (mmHg). A series of 3 PVI estimations were made and averaged for each value. When the volume of CSF injected or withdrawn was 1.0 ml, VPR was also calculated.

The severity of intracranial hypertension was quantitated by using the values of the mean ICP, averaged over the preceeding 30 minute period, and the ICP treatment score for that 8 hour period. The ICP treatment score is a measure of the intensity of treatment required to control the ICP. The ICP treatment score ranges from 0 to 17. In general, an ICP treatment score ≥6 indicated the requirement of mannitol for increased ICP, while an ICP treatment score of >10 indicated the administration of barbiturates.

Statistical Analysis

The individual measurements were analyzed and, in addition, because there were varying number of observations per patient, the average values of the individuals measurements for each patient were analyzed. The physiological parameters (CBF, CVR, CPP, ICP, MAP) were related to PVI and to VPR by regression analysis. Differences in the physiological parameters by the severity of intracranial hypertension and by the level of CBF were sought by analysis of variance followed by a t-test.

Results

Relationship of ICP and PVI, VPR

Nineteen patients had a normal ICP or mild intracranial hypertension (ICP < 20 mmHg and ICP treatment score <8). Fifteen had increased ICP that required treatment with sedation, paralysis, hyperventilation, mannitol, and CSF drainage (ICP treatment score ≥8). Ten had fatal intracranial hypertension. The average values for the other measured physiological variables are summarized in Table 1.

PVI was highest in patients with fatal intracranial hypertension, averaging 18.6 ± 1.5 ml. The typical pattern of PVI in the patients with fatal intracranial

Table 1. Relationship of severity of intracranial hypertension to PVI and VPR

Parameter	Severity of intracranial hypertension			ANOVA
	None/Mild	Moderate/Severe	Fatal	p Value
Number of Patients	19	15	10	
CBF (ml/100g/min)	49.8 ± 2.9	48.6 ± 2.8	38.6 ± 3.8	0.055
CVR (mmHg/ml/100 gm/min)	1.9 ± 0.1	1.7 ± 0.1	1.5 ± 0.1	0.17
ICP (mmHg)	12 ± 1	19 ± 1	30 ± 3	<0.001
ICP Treatment Score	2.2 ± 0.3	7.3 ± 0.5	9.9 ± 1.0	<0.001
CPP (mmHg)	78 ± 2	71 ± 3	54 ± 7	<0.001
MAP (mmHg)	91 ± 2	90 ± 2	82 ± 5	0.12
PVI (ml)	12.7 ± 1.2	14.1 ± 0.7	18.6 ± 1.5	0.005
VPR (mmHg)	1.7 ± 0.2	2.5 ± 0.2	3.8 ± 0.4	<0.001

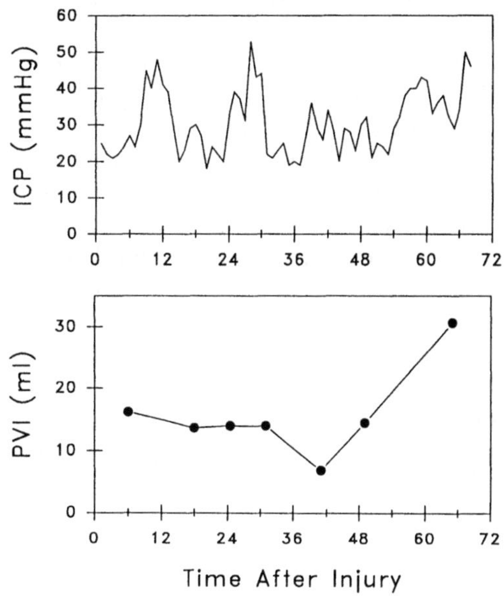

Fig. 1. Tracing of ICP and PVI in a patient who developed refractory intracranial hypertension after evacuation of a subdural hematoma. The PVI gradually decreased to a low of 7 just before the patient clinically deteriorated. Later, after the ICP became refractory to treatment, the PVI increased to more normal values

hypertension is shown in Fig. 1. PVI was only slightly decreased in the first 12 hours postinjury, but decreased to very low levels during hours 12–48, and then increased back to near normal levels as the ICP became refractory to treatment. VPR, in contrast, was directly related to ICP ($n = 44$, $r = 0.73$, $p < 0.001$), and was significantly higher in patients with fatal intracranial hypertension, averaging 3.8 ± 0.4 mmHg compared to 2.5 ± 0.2 mmHg and 1.7 ± 0.2 mmHg in patients with moderately elevated and normal ICP, respectively.

Table 2. Relationship of PVI and VPR to CBF group

Parameter	CBF group			ANOVA
	Reduced	Normal	Elevated	p Value
Number of Patients	9	13	22	
CBF (ml/100g/min)	33.3 ± 2.6	40.6 ± 2.4	56.1 ± 1.7	<0.001
CVR (mmHg/ml/100 gm/min)	2.1 ± 0.2	1.9 ± 0.2	1.5 ± 0.1	0.013
ICP (mmHg)	22 ± 4	17 ± 2	18 ± 2	0.42
ICP Treatment Score	7.2 ± 1.9	5.5 ± 1.1	5.1 ± 0.6	0.37
CPP (mmHg)	64 ± 8	67 ± 5	74 ± 2	0.21
MAP (mmHg)	84 ± 5	86 ± 3	92 ± 2	0.12
PVI (ml)	13.3 ± 1.8	14.8 ± 1.5	14.8 ± 1.9	0.71
VPR (mmHg)	3.4 ± 0.5	2.2 ± 0.3	2.2 ± 0.2	0.045

Relationship of CBF and PVI, VPR

Twenty-two patients had an elevated CBF, averaging 56.1 ± 1.7 ml/100 gm/min, 13 had a normal CBF, averaging 40.6 ± 2.4 ml/100 gm/min, and 9 had a reduced CBF, averaging 33.3 ± 2.6 ml/100 gm/min. The average values for the other measured physiological variables are summarized in Table 2. CVR was inversely related to the CBF, averaging 1.5 ± 0.1 ml/100 gm/min/mmHg in the patients with an elevated CBF, compared to 1.9 ± 0.2 ml/100 gm/min/mmHg and 2.1 ± 0.2 ml/100 gm/min/mmHg in the patient with a normal and reduced CBF, respectively. ICP, ICP treatment score, MAP, CPP were not different among the 3 groups.

While PVI was not significantly different among the 3 CBF groups, VPR was inversely related to CBF ($n = 44$, $r = -0.40$, $p < 0.01$) and was significantly higher in the patients with a reduced CBF, 3.4 ± 0.5 mmHg, compared to 2.2 ± 0.3 mmHg in the patients with a normal CBF and 2.2 ± 0.2 mmHg in the patients with an elevated CBF.

Discussion

Intracranial compliance, as measured by a bolus injection or withdrawal of CSF from the ventricles, is a complex physiological parameter. Several practical difficulties limit the clinical usefulness of the parameter.

First, PVI or VPR measurements can only be obtained when a ventriculostomy catheter can be placed. Patients with markedly compressed ventricles had ICP monitoring by methods other then a ventriculostomy and were not included in this study.

Secondly, PVI was not linear with ICP throughout the ranges of ICP seen in the patients studied, and was actually highest in the patients with fatal intracranial hypertension. This is similar to observations in experimental studies in which PVI or VPR plateaued or returned toward more normal values as ICP exceeded 30–60 mmHg [1, 2].

Finally, PVI and VPR are associated with changes in CBF and CVR. The lowest PVI values and the highest VPR values, indicating reduced intracranial compliance, were found in patients with low CBF and high CVR.

References

1. Avezaat CJJ, van Eijndhoven JHM, Wyper DJ (1979) Cerebrospinal fluid pulse pressure and intracranial volume-pressure relationships. J Neurol Neurosurg Psych 42:687–700
2. Chopp M, Portnoy HD (1980) Systems analysis of intracranial pressure: comparison with volume-pressure test and CSF-pulse amplitude analysis. J Neurosurg 53:516–527
3. Gray J, Rosner JM (1987) Pressure volume index: Part II. The effects of low cerebral perfusion pressure and autoregulation. J Neurosurg 67:377–380
4. Miller JD, Pickard JD (1974) Intracranial volume-pressure studies in patients with head injury. Injury 5:265–260
5. Rosner MJ (1987) Cerebral perfusion pressure: The link between intracranial pressure and systemic circulation. In: Wood JH (ed) Cerebral Blood Flow: Physiologic and Clinical Aspects, McGraw-Hill, New York, pp 425–448
6. Shapiro K, Marmarou A, Shulman K (1980) Characterization of clinical CSF dynamics and neural axis compliance using the pressure-volume index. I. The normal pressure-volume index. Ann Neurol 7:508–514

Cerebral Perfusion Pressure Management of Head Injury

M.J. Rosner and S.D. Rosner

University of Alabama at Birmingham, USA

Introduction

Previous work has demonstrated a causal relationship between unstable cerebral perfusion pressure (CPP) and the development of intracranial pressure (ICP) waves [3]. The genesis of this CPP instability has usually (though not exclusively) been decrements in systemic arterial blood pressure (SABP). A simple model termed the "Vasodilatory Cascade" has been developed which demonstrates the interrelationships which lead to the complex interaction of SABP, ICP, and CPP [5]. More importantly, the "Cascade" model in a more complex form leads directly to a model which helps interrelate both positive and negative aspects of many therapeutic modalities and their effect upon the whole system. From this understanding, a model upon which therapy [6] can be based has been developed and serves as the basis for the current report.

Hypotheses

CPP management will be associated with

1. Prevention of "Malignant Intracranial Hypertension"
2. Improved survival

Methods

I. Frontal Ventriculostomy
   ICP Monitoring
   Therapeutic CSF drainage-drained prn to maintain CPP $\geq$ 70 torr.

II. Ventilation
   Muscle paralysis
   $PaO_2 \geq 70$ ($SaO_2 \geq 90\%$)
   $PaCO_2$ 35–40 torr
   Reserve "hyperventilation" for acute situations

III. Phenylephrine used to Maintain CPP $\geq$ 70 Tor
   – try to limit <4 μg/kg/min
   – Dopamine 2 μg/kg/min to protect renal function.

IV. Mannitol
   0.5–1.0 gm/kg/prn CPP < 70 torr
   – try to limit to q4h
   – replace diuresis cc/cc if patient euvolemic
V. Hydration
   – Euvolemia
   – Maintain CVP 8–10 torr, PCWP 12–15 torr
   – Avoid
     Overhydration
     Positive Na^+ balance
   – Pack red cells, concentrated (25%) albumin used frequently
   – Many IV orders: I = O + losses to avoid wide swings in hydration
   – Daily weights
VI. Patients nursed flat
VII. CCP level:
   Start ≥ 70 torr
   Increase as needed to eliminate pressure waves and minimize ICP
   May require CPP 90–100 torr in acute situation.
VIII. Nutritional support withheld until ICP controlled by CSF drainage alone.

Results

Overall mortality in this series of 98 patients with severe head injury was 29% (Table 2) and average GCS was 5 (Table 1). Equally important was the very low rate of persistent vegetative state (3%) accompanied by a 55% rate of favorable outcome.

Approximately 20% of the deaths represent deaths due to progressive intracranial hypertension; many of these included management errors. Another 20% represented gross management error. Forty percent were "non-cerebral" deaths and the remainder were due to elective withdrawal of support.

Discussion

CPP management has shown itself to improve mortality and probably morbidity [6]. ICP deaths have typically accounted for ≥50% deaths after head injury in

Table 1. Patients with traumatic brain injury of GCS ≤ 7

n =	98
Age	27.4 ± 12.0 years
GCS	5.00 ± 1.35
CSF lactate	4.35 ± 3.15 mmol/L
Multiple injury	50%
Operative mass lesion	24%

No patient entered if GCS > 7 by 24 hours post-injury

Table 2. Outcome

GCS (entry)	n	Died (%)	Morbidity (GOS)[a] 2	3	4	5	Total (%)
3	18	10–56	1	3	2	2	8–44
4	20	7–35	1	3	6	3	13–65
5	18	7–39	0	2	4	5	11–61
6	28	4–14	1	0	3	20	24–86
7	14	1–7	0	3	2	8	13–93
Total	98	29–29	3	11	17	38	69–71

[a] GOS 2 = Persistent vegetative state
GOS 3 = Severe impairment
GOS 4 = Moderate impairment
GOS 5 = Essentially normal activity and work

Table 3. Comparison of "traditional" vs. "CPP management"

Modality	Traditional ICP therapy	CPP Management
Position flat [4]	Elevate HOB ≥30°	HOB = 0°: Patient
Fluids	2/3 Maintenance BUN 35 mg%	Hydrate normally I = O + losses
Hypertension	Prevent – use sedatives – use antihypertensives – use blockers – avoid stimulation	Facilitate – vascular expansion – vasopressors – active stimulation
Mannitol [5] patient	Osmolality 310–320 Replace 2/3 diuresis	Normal osmolality Replace cc/cc if euvolemic I = O + losses
Barbiturates depressants	Burst suppression	Avoid-cardiac
Hyperventilation	pCO_2 25–28 torr	pCO_2 35–40 torr – "Bag" acutely only

previous series and this "malignant intracranial hypertension" has yielded very slowly if at all to traditional ICP management. The regimen presented here deviates significantly from the "traditional" management schemes and is, in fact, incompatible with most components (Table 3) of "standard" ICP management. However, our results have been consistently better than most prior reports [1, 2] and the techniques are now used throughout our intensive care unit for all ICP "problems" [4, 5]. We feel that nearly 50% of the deaths are potentially avoidable and mortality can be reduced further. More importantly, morbidity is at least as good and probably better than that of previous reports and again, can probably be further reduced.

Conclusion

1. CPP management has resulted in greatly improved control and markedly reduces the occurrence of "malignant" intracranial hypertension.

2. Mortality has been reduced to <50% compared to "traditional" treatment regimes used for management of traumatic brain injury.
3. At a minimum, these results bring into question the tenets of "traditional" ICP management techniques.

References

1. Colohan WMA., Gross CR, Torner JC, et al. (1989) Head injury mortality in two centers with different emergency medical services and intensive care. J Neurosurg 71:202–207
2. Gennarelli TA, Spielman GM, Langfitt TW, et al. (1982) Influence of the type of intracranial lesion on outcome from severe head injury. J Neurosurg 56:26–31
3. Rosner MJ, Becker DP (1984) The origin and evolution of plateau waves: experimental observations and a theoretical model. J Neurosurg 60:312–324
4. Rosner MJ, Coley I (1986) Cerebral perfusion pressure, intracranial pressure, and head elevation. J Neurosurg 65:636–641
5. Rosner MJ, Coley I (1987) Cerebral perfusion pressure: A hemodynamic mechanism of mannitol and the post mannitol hemogram. Neurosurgery, 21:147–156
6. Rosner MJ, Daughton S (1990) Cerebral perfusion pressure management in head injury. J Trauma 30:933–941

Intracranial and Cerebral Perfusion Pressure Monitoring in the Head Injured Patient: Which Index?

A.D. Mendelow[1], D.A. Allcutt[2], I.R. Chambers[3], A. Jenkins[1], P.J. Crawford[2], and H. Sultan[2]

[1] Department of Surgery (Neurosurgery), University of Newcastle Upon Tyne, [2] Regional Neurosciences Centre, and [3] Regional Medical Physics Department, Newcastle General Hospital, Westgate Road, Newcastle upon Tyne NE4 6BE, England

Introduction

For patients with severe head injury it is well known that intracranial pressure (ICP) and cerebral perfusion pressure (CPP) correlate with outcome. McGraw et al. [5] have shown that the length of time at a prevailing level of CPP correlates with outcome and that a CPP of 80 mmHg and above is also associated with a better outcome. Although it is accepted that the lower limit of autoregulation for cerebral blood flow (CBF) is 50 mmHg in normal animals [3], this level may be insufficient to maintain an adequate CBF in patients with severe head injury who have disturbed autoregulation.

With automated recording of ICP and CPP it becomes possible to analyse the average length of time at any particular level of ICP and CPP. The problem is knowing the time duration over which a particular level is important. There are different ways of analysing pressures in relation to time: it is important to avoid including artefactual changes as occur during suction (with regard to ICP) and during blood gas sampling (from arterial pressure lines). We have developed software which avoids including such artefacts [1] and the pressures so obtained need to be evaluated in relation to outcome.

The aim of the present study therefore was to determine which was the most valuable index of ICP and CPP for patient management in those in whom the outcome was known six months after the head injury.

Patients and Methods

Outcome was determined at six months using the Glasgow Outcome Scale [4] in seventy-nine patients with severe head injury. The range over which such outcomes could be accurately determined was from twelve to thirty-two weeks. Intracranial pressure and mean arterial blood pressure were measured in all these patients over periods ranging from three to one hundred and sixty-eight hours. Intracranial pressure was measured with the Camino subdural screw in forty-one patients and with a ventricular catheter in the thirty-six patients. Arterial pressure was measured via an arterial line. Cerebral perfusion pressure was calculated electronically and displayed continuously [1], as was ICP and mean arterial blood pressure (MABP). The CPP was derived from the difference between ICP and MABP and stored on a Psion Organiser as described elsewhere [1]. The data so derived was down loaded for subsequent analysis which allows an algorithm built into the software to exclude artefacts produced by coughing and suction (for ICP) and disconnection of the arterial line (for MABP). This analysis has been evolved over the last few years and the data presented here were derived from the most recent analysis of the raw data.

In this analysis we have defined "minimum ICP" or "maximum ICP" as the average minimum or maximum value over a two minute period. "Average minimum CPP" or "average maximum ICP" were the lowest or highest values respectively over a sixty minute period. "Independent" outcome was used to describe those patients who made a good recovery or who were moderately disabled; "poor" outcome included those patients who were severely disabled, vegetative or dead [4].

Levels of ICP were divided into those of less than 30 mmHg and 30 mmHg and above, these being clearly defined limits that are well accepted indications for clinical intervention [2]. Similarly, CPP levels were divided into those below 50 mmHg and those of 50 mmHg and above, these limits being the commonly regarded lower limit for autoregulation of cerebral blood flow.

Results

Of the seventy-nine patients, thirty-six became independent and forty-three had a poor outcome. Maximum (two minutes) ICP was below 30 mmHg in seventeen patients and thirteen of them became independent. By contrast, average maximum ICP was below 30 mmHg in forty-six patients and twenty-four of them became independent. Modal ICP was below 30 mmHg in sixty-nine patients and thirty-four of them became independent (Table 1). Chi squared analysis of this table showed that only maximum (two minutes) ICP was significant (Chi squared = 8.34, $P < 0.01$), the two other parameters not reaching significance.

Average minimum CPP (sixty minutes) was below 50 mmHg in twenty patients and only three of them became independent. Minimum CPP (two minutes) was below 50 mmHg in fifty-one patients and nineteen of them became independent. Modal CPP was below 50 mmHg in seven patients and only one of them had an independent outcome (Table 2). In this one patient it

Table 1. ICP and outcome

Outcome	Maximum (2 mins)		Average max (60 mins)		Modal	
	<30	≥30	<30	≥30	<30	≥30
Independent	13	23	24	12	34	2
Poor	4	39	22	21	35	8
X^2	8.34		1.94		3.02	
P <	0.01		NS		NS	

Table 2. CPP and outcome

Outcome	Minimum (2 mins) <50	≥50	Average min (60 mins) <50	≥50	Modal <50	≥50
Independent	19	17	3	33	1	35
Poor	32	11	17	26	6	37
X^2	4.01		10.09		3.03	
P <	0.05		0.01		NS	

Table 3. Rank order of significance

		X^2	P <
Average Minimum	CPP	10.09	0.01
Maximum	ICP	8.34	0.01
Minimum	CPP	4.01	0.05
Modal	CPP	3.03	NS
Modal	ICP	3.02	NS
Average Maximum	ICP	1.94	NS

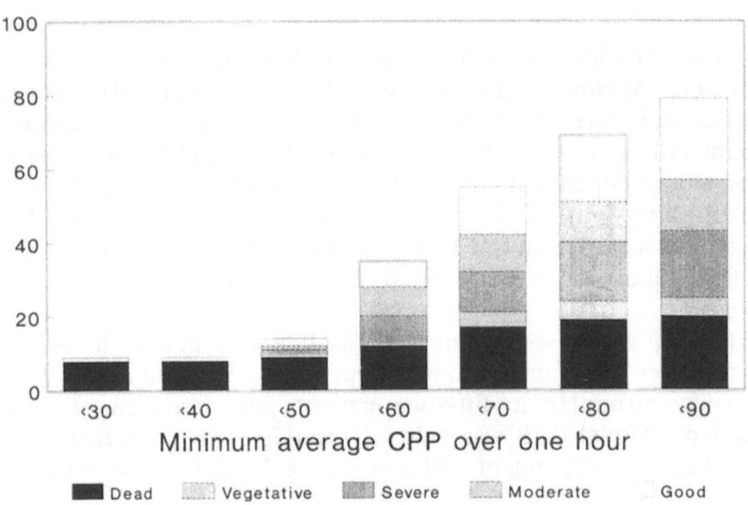

Fig. 1. Cummulative frequency of the number of patients (Y Axis) with minimum average CPP over 1 hour below each 10 mmHg Cohort

was thought that the ICP was reading artificially high, but because the Camino cannot be recalibrated in situ, this could not be confirmed. It was therefore felt that this patient should still be included in the analysis as having a low CPP.

The best Chi squared value was for average minimum (sixty minutes) CPP (Chi squared = 10.09, P < 0.01) and this represents the most significant variable of the six analysed in this study. The rank order of the Chi squared

Table 4. Change of management from 1987–1991. Average minimum CPP (60 min) and outcome

	Early period (1987, 1988, 1989)		Later period (1990, 1991)	
Outcome	<50	≥50	<50	≥50
Independent	3	17	1	15
Poor	12	14	6	11
	Low CPP = 33%		21%	
	Independent = 44%		49%	

values is given in Table 3, where it can be seen that the average minimum (sixty minutes) CPP correlated best with outcome. Maximum ICP (two minutes) was next best. Average maximum (sixty minutes) ICP was the least useful index.

Analysis of the individual (10 mmHg intervals) levels of average minimum CPP (over sixty minutes) suggests that the higher pressures were associated with a better outcome (Fig. 1). Routine display of CPP in all intensive care and high dependency beds became available in January 1990. There were 33% of patients with a low CPP before then compared with only 21% since then (Table 4). Similarly, independent outcomes increased from 44% to 49%. The numbers are too small to permit statistical analysis.

Discussion

Our data suggests that CPP averaged over an hour is the best predictor of outcome from head injury of the six parameters defined in the present study. When this parameter was analysed at each 10 mmHg interval of CPP, it appeared that levels of average minimum CPP of 80 mmHg or higher were associated with an independent outcome. This observation is in agreement with that of McGraw et al. [5]. The difficulty is to determine whether the higher levels of CPP were the reason for improved outcome or whether they simply reflect patients that were more stable haemodynamically and that had lower levels of ICP.

Because a policy of maintaining CPP in excess of 50 mmHg became progressively more accepted over the years that the study was conducted, it is more likely that maintenance of higher CPP would have contributed to better outcome more frequently in the later period. Since routine display of CPP on the monitoring apparatus became available in January 1990, the frequency of low CPP has dropped and the proportion of independent outcomes has increased although the numbers are probably too small to draw firm conclusions at this stage. This observation suggests that greater awareness of CPP in head injured patients does result in higher average values, and that this is associated with improved outcome. Larger numbers of patients would be required to confirm this observation but it would be difficult to go back to earlier forms of management. The suggestion therefore is that higher CPP is causally related to outcome rather than a simple association.

The data could also be criticised because we have selected only two time periods: two minutes and sixty minutes. However, shorter periods are more likely to be marred by artefact. Longer periods can be evaluated from the modal value, but, in general, this was less useful for both CPP and ICP. There seems therefore to be little justification for taking periods of greater than one hour into consideration.

Despite these reservations, average minimum CPP over sixty minutes gave the best predictor of outcome.

There is no perfect way to analyse ICP and CPP data that has yet been agreed, but we suggest that minimum average CPP over a sixty minute period is a clinically useful measurement that correlates with outcome and may lead to improved care of the severe head injured patient.

Acknowledgements. Our thanks go to Miss A Robinson for her preparation of the manuscript.

References

1. Chambers IR, Clark A, Kane PJ, Mendelow AD (1993) Continuous Monitoring and Recording of Cerebral Perfusion Pressure. In: Avezaat CJJ, van Eyndhoven JHM, Maas AIR, Tans JThJ (eds) Intracranial pressure VIII. Springer, Berlin Heidelberg New York London Paris Tokyo Hong Kong Barcelana
2. Galbraith S, Teasdale GM (1982) Head Injuries. In: RCG Russell (ed) Recent Advances in Surgery, Churchill Livingstone, Edinburgh, 71–84
3. Harper AM (1966) Autoregulation of Cerebral Blood Flow: Influence of the Arterial Blood Pressure on the Blood Flow Through the Cerebral Cortex. J Neurol, Neurosurg, Psychiat, 29:398–403
4. Jennett B, Bond M (1975) Assessment of Outcome After Severe Brain Damage. Lancet 1, 480
5. McGraw CP (1989) A Cerebral Perfusion Pressure Greater Than 80 mmHg is More Beneficial. In: Hoff JT, Betz AL (eds) Intracranial Pressure VII. Springer, Berlin Heidelberg New York London Paris Tokyo Hong Kong, pp 839–841

Relationship Between Cerebral Oxygenation and Perfusion Pressure in Acute Brain Injury

J. Cruz[1], M.E. Miner[2], S.J. Allen[3], W.M. Alves[1], and T.A. Gennarelli[1]

[1] Division of Neurosurgery and Head Injury Center, University of Pennsylvania, 3400 Spruce St., Philadelphia, PA 19104, USA,
[2] Division of Neurologic Surgery, Ohio State University, Columbus, OH 43210, USA,
[3] Department of Anesthesiology, University of Texas, Houston, TX 77030, USA

Introduction

When we proposed clinical monitoring and management of the arteriojugular oxygen difference [1–4], we coined the term "oligemic cerebral hypoxia" to define hypoxia in the presence of normal arterial oxygenation, but excessively reduced cerebral blood flow (CBF) in relation to cerebral oxygen consumption ($CMRO_2$). We have extensively monitored the arterio-jugular bulb difference in oxygen content ($AJDO_2$) in acute severe brain trauma, and managed the $AJDO_2$ in conjunction with intracranial pressure (ICP), as a means of optimizing global CBF in relation to $CMRO_2$ and ICP [2]. We had previously found an excellent inverse relationship between mean regional CBF values and the $AJDO_2$ in acute severe brain trauma [6], and confirmed the interrelationships among CBF, $CMRO_2$, and $AJDO_2$, which can be expressed by the equation: $AJDO_2 = CMRO_2/CBF$. It then became clear to us that the $AJDO_2$ represented the proportionality variable which could be monitored and managed, in order to optimize the global $CMRO_2$/CBF ratio. Such optimization could not be accomplished by CBF measurements alone.

Over the years, we have simplified $AJDO_2$ monitoring and management by assessing the arterio-jugular bulb difference in oxyhemoglobin saturation, which we termed cerebral extraction of oxygen (CEO_2). The CEO_2 is a more practical calculation than the $AJDO_2$, and also reliably measures the global $CMRO_2$/CBF ratio. The present work is an outgrowth of our previous experience, in which we devised a mathematical means of directly assessing the relationship between global cerebral oxygen extraction (CEO_2) and perfusion pressure (CPP). A new concept of cerebral hemodynamic and metabolic physiology, cerebral hemodynamic reserve (CHR), was born from this experience.

Clinical Material and Methods

Twelve adults with acute severe closed brain trauma were prospectively evaluated. The Glasgow Coma Scale [7] scores were in the range of 4 to 6, and the admission computerized tomography (CT) scans of the head disclosed predominantly severe diffuse brain swelling, with markedly reduced cerebrospinal fluid spaces. All patients underwent continuous monitoring of the systemic arterial pressure (SAP), ICP, expired PCO_2 (P_ECO_2), arterial and jugular bulb oxyhemoglobin saturation (SaO_2, SjO_2). The CPP was monitored as the difference between mean SAP and ICP, and the CEO_2 as the difference between SaO_2 and SjO_2. The SaO_2 and SjO_2 were recorded from No. 4 French fiberoptic oximetry catheters placed, respectively, into a femoral artery and the right jugular bulb. The SAP was recorded from the femoral arterial catheter. P_ECO_2 was recorded from an infrared monitor. The multivariate monitoring system has been previously described [3, 4].

The normal ranges for SaO_2 and SjO_2 are, respectively, 93.9% ± 2% and 61.8% ± 7.4% [5]. From these norms we calculated the CEO_2 values and estimated a normal range of 31.6% ± 7.8%. The above values are means ± 2 SD, and relate to a normocapnic arterial PCO_2 in the range of 40 mmHg. A CEO_2 < 24% is consistent with global cerebral hyperperfusion relative to $CMRO_2$ (luxury perfusion); a CEO_2 in the range of 24% to 40% is consistent with adequate $CMRO_2$-CBF coupling; and a CEO_2 > 40% is consistent with global cerebral hypoperfusion relative to $CMRO_2$ (oligemic cerebral hypoxia) [1, 2, 4]. The CHR was assessed during periods of spontaneous ICP elevations in the presence of constant P_ECO_2 and SaO_2, and virtually constant SAP, with normal SAP and SaO_2 values. The CHR was calculated as the relative change in CEO_2 over the relative change in CPP, from two time points: baseline (initial), and the point of maximum ICP recording (final) just prior to ICP treatment (at 20 mmHg or higher). The following equation was used to calculate the CHR:

$$CHR = [(CEO_{2(F)} - CEO_{2(I)})/CEO_{2(I)}]/[(CPP_{(F)} - CPP_{(I)})/CPP_{(I)}]$$

where (I) and (F) stand, respectively, for initial and final values. The CHR was considered preserved if ⩾ zero, and compromised if < zero. A total of 34 observations were carried out in the 12 patients, over the initial 48 hours posttrauma. The CHR was assessed 16 times during the initial 24 hours (day 1), and 18 times over the following 24 hours (day 2). Each patient underwent at least one assessment of the CHR on each day. Two-tailed t-test and the paired Chi-square (McNemar's test) were used for statistical analysis. A p value of ≤ 0.05 was considered significant. Data are presented as means ± SD. Since all observations were carried out during the course of profound hyperventilation for ICP control below 20 mmHg, the recorded (actual) CEO_2 values were subsequently corrected for normocapnia (PCO_2 of 40 mmHg), in order to estimate the natural occurrence of cerebral luxury perfusion or otherwise. We adopted a CEO_2 correction of 3% per unit change in PCO_2 [6].

During the study period, ICP management for control below 20 mmHg involved a cumulative treatment protocol, which has been previously described [4]. Therapeutic hyperventilation was adjusted (optimized) according to the recorded CEO_2 values; that is, in the presence of normal SaO_2, abnormally low SjO_2 values (⩽54%) were to be avoided whenever possible. This was usually accomplished by increasing the PCO_2 and administering intravenous mannitol boluses. Under these circumstances, mannitol not only decreased the ICP but also further increased the SjO_2 towards the normal range [4]. After the study period, follow-up head CT scans showed no evidence of cerebral infarction.

Results

In the 34 observations, the P_ECO_2 was in the range of 20 ± 1.4 mmHg. The CHR was in the range of -3.1 to 1.75, being preserved 9 times (26.5%) in 6 of the patients, and compromised 25 times (73.5%) in 10 of the patients. The average ICP increase was 5.8 ± 1.5 mmHg, from 14.2 ± 2.7 to 20 ± 2.6 mmHg ($p < 0.0001$). The corresponding CPP decrease was -6.3 ± 2.2 mmHg, from 79.5 ± 7.6 to 73.2 ± 8 mmHg ($p < 0.0001$). The CEO_2 decreased or remained unchanged (preserved CHR) 9 times in 6 of the patients, in the range of 30% to 39%, and it increased (compromised CHR) 25 times in 10 of the patients, in the range of 37.2% ± 4.5% to 41.5% ± 5.2%. On day 1, the CHR was compromised 12 times in 10 of the patients. In these 10 patients, a significant CHR improvement was found on day 2, the respective mean CHR values on days 1 and 2 being -1.73 and -0.46 ($p < 0.002$). However, no significant differences between the two days were found for the P_ECO_2, for the initial and final CPP, and for the initial and final CEO_2 (Table 1). Although not statistically significant, there was a mean decrease of 11.6% in the final CEO_2 on day 2, compared with day 1.

The initial CEO_2 was above 40% in only 3 of the 34 observations, and from 24% to 40% in the remaining 31. None of the monitored CEO_2 values was below 24%. These findings indicated that the therapeutic hypocapnia was optimized in the vast majority of the observations, accounting for adequate $CMRO_2$-CBF coupling. However, the final CEO_2 values (at maximum ICP) were above 40% in 17 of the 34 observations, indicating that although the ICP increases were relatively small, they induced cerebral oligemic hypoxic changes. These were usually very brief (a few minutes), because mannitol was promptly administered to lower the ICP, and it simultaneously increased the SjO_2 towards normal (normalizing the CEO_2). When the above described CEO_2 values were corrected for normocapnia, the initial CEO_2 was below 24% in all 34 observations, consistent with cerebral luxury perfusion. The corrected final CEO_2 was also below 24% in 33 of the 34 observations, and within the normal range in one occasion. None of the corrected CEO_2 values was above 40%. These large differences in the distribution of uncorrected and corrected CEO_2 values were highly statistically significant ($p < 0.00001$).

Discussion

CHR assessment represents a novel methodology and technique for evaluating the relationship between global cerebral oxygenation and perfusion pressure. It allows dynamic quantification of the effects of ICP increases upon the cerebral oxygenation, due to impairments of net tissue perfusion. Such an information cannot be obtained from CBF measurements, which do not disclose the metabolic status or consequences of cerebral hypoperfusion, insofar as cerebral oxygenation is concerned. Our findings demonstrated that cerebral oxygenation may be compromised due to decreases in CPP occurring well within its normal range. This finding appears to be of paramount importance, as it demonstrates that the CPP alone may not be a reliable indicator of adequate tissue perfusion and oxygenation, at least during profound hyperventilation.

The vast majority of patients presented with compromised CHR on day 1. However, the CHR significantly improved on day 2, suggesting an improved tolerance of the cerebral hemodynamics to ICP increases after 24 hours post-trauma. Such an improvement was most likely due to a decrease in the final CEO_2 on day 2, which, although not statistically significant, could physiologically explain the CHR improvement. Indeed, the final CEO_2 was the variable in which the largest change (a decrease of nearly 12%) was found between days 1 and 2. Such a change could have been due to a decrease in the $CMRO_2$ or an increase in CBF, in response to the ICP increases. Since $CMRO_2$ decreases in the presence of normal CPP are highly unlikely, the most likely explanation for the CEO_2 decrease on the second day would have been an increase in CBF. The latter, occurring in response to an ICP increase (CPP decrease), would strongly suggest an improved autoregulatory response to ICP changes, occurring on day 2, and representing an apparently spontaneous change. However, a beneficial effect on the CHR due to the cumulative use of mannitol over time could not be definitely ruled out.

The decreases in global cerebral oxygenation (SjO_2) directly attributed to relatively small ICP increases were somewhat unexpected. In fact, the CPP changes were well within its normal range, so that a better autoregulatory response to the ICP increases could be expected on day 1. However, this was observed only on day 2 (to our knowledge, a finding not previously reported). We believe the above described findings were due to the fact that CBF was invariably decreased (by optimized hypocapnia), therapeutically matched with the expected decrease in $CMRO_2$ in the presence of coma [6]. In addition, such CBF reduction was found in patients whose admission head CT findings strongly suggested increased intracranial "tightness". Thus, the relatively subtle ICP changes associated with small SjO_2 (and CEO_2) variations were, nevertheless, sufficient to result in mild to moderate (although brief) cerebral oligemic hypoxic changes. Thus, the CHR allowed estimation of the effects of increased intracranial "tightness" upon the cerebral hemodynamics and oxygenation. To our knowledge, such information cannot be obtained from any other currently available methodology or technique.

Table 1. Physiological variables in 10 patients

Variable	Day 1	Day 2	p Value
CHR	-1.73 ± 0.6	-0.46 ± 1	<0.002
P_ECO_2 (mmHg)	20 ± 1.9	20 ± 1.2	1 (NS)
$CPP_{(I)}$ (mmHg)	82 ± 7	79 ± 9	0.33 (NS)
$CPP_{(F)}$ (mmHg)	75 ± 7	72 ± 11	0.51 (NS)
$CEO_{2(I)}$ (%)	37 ± 5.5	36 ± 4.8	0.58 (NS)
$CEO_{2(F)}$ (%)	43 ± 6	38 ± 6.3	0.08 (NS)

Values are means ± standard deviation. NS = not statistically significant.

Since the CHR represents a new concept in neurophysiology, potential applications of the present work may be expected, possibly involving a broad spectrum of areas of clinical and basic research, in a variety of acute, predominantly diffuse brain insults. Initially aimed at studies of physiology and pathophysiology, CHR may also prove useful in assessing new therapeutic modalities.

Acknowledgements. This work was supported in part by Grants R49/CCR303687-02 from the Center for Environmental Health and Injury Control of the Centers for Disease Control, and NS-08803-19 from the National Institute of Neurological Disorders and Stroke.

The authors thank Randall F. Wiser, M.S.E., for help in statistical analysis.

References

1. Cruz J, Allen SJ, Miner ME (1985) Hypoxic insults in acute brain injury. Crit Care Med 13:284
2. Cruz J, Miner ME (1986) Modulating cerebral oxygen delivery and extraction in acute traumatic coma. In: Miner ME, Wagner KA (eds) Neurotrauma. Treatment, Rehabilitation, and Related Issues, ed. 1. Butterworths, Boston, pp 55–72
3. Cruz J (1988) Continuous versus serial global cerebral hemometabolic monitoring: applications in acute brain trauma. Acta Neurochir 42 (Suppl):35–39
4. Cruz J, Miner ME, Allen SJ, Alves WM, Gennarelli TA (1990) Continuous monitoring of cerebral oxygenation in acute brain injury: injection of mannitol during hyperventilation. J Neurosurg 73:725–730
5. Gibbs EL, Lennox WG, Nims LF, Gibbs FA (1942) Arterial and cerebral venous blood. Arterial-venous differences in man. J Biol Chem 144:325–332
6. Obrist WD, Langfitt TW, Jaggi JL, Cruz J, Gennarelli TA (1984) Cerebral blood flow and metabolism in comatose patients with acute head injury. Relationship to intracranial hypertension. J Neurosurg 61:241–253
7. Teasdale G, Jennett B (1974) Assessment of coma and impaired consciousness. A practical scale. Lancet 2:81–84

Multimodality Monitoring of Intracranial Pressure Therapy After Severe Brain Injury

K.H. Chan, N.M. Dearden, and J.D. Miller

Department of Clinical Neurosciences, University of Edinburgh, Scotland, EH4 2XU

Introduction

Uncontrolled intracranial hypertension remains an important cause of mortality and morbidity after severe brain injury. Controversies surrounding ICP treatment include the relative importance of lowering ICP or preserving CPP although the optimal level of CPP in severely brain injured patients is not known.

Transcranial doppler (TCD) allows noninvasive continuous monitoring or changes in intracranial blood flow velocity [1]. Continuous recording of jugular bulb venous oxygen saturation (SJO2) reflects the global ratio of cerebral oxygen supply to consumption, allowing detection of states of hypoperfusion [2]. The present study aims to define the roles of TCD and SJO2 as monitors of the effects of ICP reduction therapy following severe brain injury.

Methods

Twenty-two patients with severe brain injury who received therapy for raised ICP and/or reduced CPP were studied. Patients were managed according to a standard protocol that included artificial ventilation, muscle paralysis and sedation with continuous infusions of pancuronium and phenoperidine respectively. Arterial pressure, ICP, arterial oxygen saturation (SaO2) by pulse oximetry and end-tidal carbon dioxide concentration were recorded continuously. In 17 patients, SJO2 was measured continuously by the Oximetrics 3 system (Abbott Laboratories, Chicago, USA) following percutaneous retrograde insertion of a Shaw 40 cm catheter into the jugular venous bulb on the side of the predominant venous drainage [2].

Patients were ventilated to an end-tidal carbon dioxide level of 3.5–4.5 kpa and PaO2 $>$ 13 kpa (SaO2 $>$ 95%). After remediable causes for intracranial hypertension had been excluded, therapy was provided if ICP rose above 25 mmHg, or when CPP fell below 60 mmHg. Treatment modalities employed included intravenous mannitol ($n = 23$), thiopentone ($n = 19$), CSF drainage ($n = 4$) and raising the blood pressure with inotropic agents when CPP was compromised by systemic hypotension ($n = 3$). Therapy for raised ICP was considered to be successful when ICP fell below 20 mmHg, accompanied either by an increase or preservation of CPP above 60 mmHg.

Transcranial Doppler (Medasonics, California, USA) sonography was first performed within 24 hours of admission according to the method described by Aaslid [1]. Continuous monitoring of MCA velocity was accomplished by mounting the ultrasound probe in a head band during ICP treatment. The temporal window was used and the MCA insonated at the depth which gave the highest velocity. Measurements of TCD timed-mean velocity and pulsatility index (PI) (defined as peak-systolic minus end-diastolic divided by timed-mean velocities) and SJO2 were taken at the points of maximum decrease of CPP before treatment and maximum increase of CPP after therapy had been initiated. A change in any monitoring parameter was defined as the post-treatment minus the pretreatment values. Statistical analysis was performed by linear correlation regression.

Results

Forty-nine treatment responses were recorded. SJO2 was monitored during 39 of these treatments. There was significant correlation between CPP and PI ($r = -0.846$, $p < 0.001$) and SJO2 ($r = 0.651$, $p < 0.001$) before and after therapy. Sequential linear regression analysis of CPP versus PI and SJO2 yielded breakpoint values at CPP of 70(PI) and 68(SJO2) mmHg. Below these CPP breakpoints, PI progressively increased ($r = -0.941$, $p < 0.0001$) and SJO2 decreased ($r = 0.837$, $p < 0.0001$) with falling CPP. Above the breakpoints, CPP did not correlate with either PI or SJO2. There was no relationship between ICP and PI or SJO2. Correlations between changes in CPP and alterations in mean velocity, PI and SJO2 were always better than with changes in ICP (Table 1).

Of the 49 treatment responses recorded, 39 were considered successful and 10 failure. Therapy always reduced ICP, but the response to therapy depended upon the pretreatment level of CPP. When pretreatment CPP levels were below 60 mmHg, CPP alteration showed linear correlation with changes in PI ($r = -0.767$, $p < 0.001$) and SJO2 ($r = 0.677$, $p < 0.001$) but not with mean flow velocity ($r = 0.062$, $p = NS$), although mean velocity always rose to some extent with increasing CPP. If pretreatment CPP exceeded 60 mmHg, a rise in CPP correlated only with an increase in mean velocity ($r = 0.501$, $p < 0.05$) during successful treatment.

Table 1. Relationships between changes in CPP/ICP and alterations in monitored parameters during therapy for raised ICP

Alterations in	CPP change	ICP change
MCA velocity	$r = 0.605$, $p < 0.001$	$r = -0.25$, $p = NS$
SJ02	$r = 0.873$, $p < 0.001$	$r = -0.679$, $p < 0.001$
PI	$r = -0.85$, $p < 0.001$	$r = -0.637$, $p < 0.001$

Seven of the 10 unsuccessful responses were associated with hypnotic therapy; CPP decreased due to a fall in MAP despite some improvement in ICP. This was accompanied by decreases of mean flow velocity and SJO2, and an increase in PI. The remaining three failed responses followed mannitol therapy, although CPP, SJO2 and mean velocity increased, and ICP and PI decreased to a minor extent.

Summary of Results

1. Treatment always reduced ICP to some extent in this series. If CPP increased, PI fell and SJO2 rose, up to CPP breakpoints of 70(PI) and 68(SJO2) mmHg. Above these CPP breakpoints such changes did not continue.
2. Changes in CPP correlated better than alterations in ICP with changes in PI, mean velocity and SJO2.
3. Successful treatment resulted in rises of velocity and SJO2 and fall of PI when pretreatment CPP was below 60 mmHg.
4. Successful treatment was not associated with changes in PI and SJO2 when pretreatment CPP exceeded 60 mmHg.
5. Failed treatment was usually with hypnotics. MAP was reduced in association with decreases in CPP, ICP, SJO2, flow velocity and increases in PI.

Discussion

Since the introduction of ICP monitoring into the management of head injury, attention has focused largely on therapeutic reduction of ICP, irrespective of the level of CPP. Cerebral blood flow (CBF) and oxygen supply are critically related to CPP after severe head injury [5]. Therapeutic elevation of compromised CPP should improve CBF and cerebral oxygen supply. Since change in MCA velocity is proportional to alteration in CBF, during TCD recording, an increase in CBF will be associated with a rise in mean flow velocity and a reduction in PI [3]. However, measurement of CBF does not define the relationship between cerebral oxygen supply and consumption. If SaO2, haemoglobin concentration and the position of the oxygen dissociation curve remain unaltered, the SJO2 may be used to monitor the ratio of global cerebral oxygen supply to oxygen consumption [4]. Relative hypoperfusion occurs when SJO2 falls below 54%, while elevation above 75% signifies global hyperaemia [6, 8]. During successful ICP therapy, elevation of CPP should improve cerebral oxygen supply over consumption leading to a rise in SJO2. Whether ICP reduction therapy influences primarily CBF (mannitol), CPP (CSF drainage) or CBF and cerebral metabolism (CMRO2) (thiopentone), the overall effect on CBF to CMRO2 ratio may be ascertained from SJO2. Recording of MCA velocity during ICP therapy should help interpretation of SJO2 findings when therapeutic agents which affect both CBF and CMRO2 are used.

The physiological goal of autoregulation is to maintain an adequate CBF to meet tissue metabolic demands [7]. Cerebral resistance vessels are sensitive to both metabolic stimuli and changes in CPP [7]. If autoregulation is preserved, the effects on CPP manipulation will depend on the threshold level below which cerebral oxygen supply becomes compromised. At CPP levels below this threshold, elevation of CPP should improve cerebral oxygen delivery associated with increases in SJO2 and mean velocity and reduction in PI. Once the lower autoregulatory CPP threshold is surpassed, however, elevation of CPP would not further improve cerebral oxygen supply.

Failed therapy associated with falls in CPP occurred only after hypnotic administration; mean flow velocity reduced, PI increased and SJO2 decreased to levels of relative hypoperfusion.

Analysis of the overall relationship between CPP and either PI or SJO2 during ICP treatment demonstrated linear correlation when pretreatment CPP was below 70 mmHg. Above this value, PI and SJO2 were unaltered when CPP rose. This may indicate preservation of autoregulation and suggests ICP therapy after severe head injury should raise and keep CPP above 70 mmHg to ensure adequate cerebral oxygen supply. Our observations raise the question as to whether ICP therapy is appropriate when CPP exceeds 70 mmHg if PI is low and SJO2 normal.

CPP response correlated better than ICP change with alterations in mean velocity, PI and SJO2 during ICP treatment. This suggests that CPP is the crucial parameter to monitor. Continuous recording of CPP, PI and SJO2 during ICP therapy may permit identification of patients with preserved autoregulation and indicate the critical threshold above which CPP should be maintained. On average, this is 70 mmHg for severely head injured patients, higher than has been previously thought.

References

1. Aaslid R, Markwalder TM, Nornes H (1982) Noninvasive transcranial doppler ultrasound recording of flow velocity in basal cerebral arteries. J Neurosurg 57:769–774
2. Andrews PJD, Dearden NM, Miller JD (1991) Jugular bulb cannulation; description of a technique and validation of a new continuous monitor. Br J Anesth (In press)
3. Bishop CCR, Powell S, Rutt D, Browse NL (1986) Transcranial doppler measurements of middle cerebral artery blood flow velocity: A validation study. Stroke 17:913–915
4. Gilbert J (1989) Estimation of cerebral blood flow by cerebral venous oxygen difference. J Neurosurg (letter) 71:790–791
5. Miller JD (1985) Head injury and brain ischemia. Implications for therapy. Br J Anaesth 57:120–129
6. Obrist WD, Langfitt TW, Jaggi JL, Cruz J, Gennarelli T (1984) Cerebral blood flow and metabolism in comatose patients with acute head injury. Relationship to intracranial hypertension. J Neurosurg 61:241–253
7. Paulson OB, Strandgaard S, Edvinsson L (1990) Cerebral autoregulation. Cerebrovascular and Brain Metabolism Reviews 2:161–192
8. Robertson CS, Narayan RK, Gokaslan ZL, Pahwa R, Grossman RG, Caram P, Allen E (1989) Cerebral arteriovenous oxygen difference as an estimate of cerebral blood flow in comatose patients. J Neurosurg 70:222–230

CPP and SJO_2 with ICP Reduction Therapy After Severe Head Injury

S. Midgley, N.M. Dearden, and J.D. Miller

Department of Clinical Neurosciences, University of Edinburgh, Western General Hospital, Crewe Road, Edinburgh, Scotland

Introduction

After head-injury cerebral metabolic rate ($CMRO_2$) is reduced [2]. Cerebral blood flow (CBF) may be increased, normal or decreased. According to the Fick Principle, the relationship between global $CMRO_2$ and CBF can be described by measurements of the arterio-jugular venous oxygen content difference ($AJDO_2$). Thus, $AJDO_2 = CMRO_2/CBF$. The $AJDO_2$ = Haemoglobin × 1.39 × (Arterial oxygen saturation – Jugular bulb venous oxygen saturation)/100. It is now possible to monitor the Jugular bulb venous oxygen saturation (SjO_2) continuously using the "Oximetrix 3" system with a fibre-optic catheter placed high in the jugular bulb [1, 3]. If arterial oxygen saturation (SaO_2), haemoglobin concentration and the position of the haemoglobin dissociation curve remain constant, SjO_2 is proportional to $CBF/CMRO_2$ · SjO_2 above 75% represents luxury perfusion, while below 54% increased oxygen extraction signifies hypoperfusion [4]. This study examines the effects of both hypnotic and osmotic treatments of raised intracranial pressure (ICP) on cerebral perfusion pressure (CPP) and SJO_2 after severe head injury.

Methods

Nine patients who had suffered severe head injury (post resuscitation Glasgow Coma Score below 9 without eye opening) were managed according to a standard regime including artificial ventilation under sedation (phenoperidine) and paralysis (pancuronium). PaO_2 was maintained above 15 kPa and $paCO_2$ between 3.0–4.0 kPa. All patients had continuous monitoring of ICP (subdural "Cordis" catheter or "Camino" tissue pressure), blood pressure (radial or femoral artery), biparietal brain electrical activity ("Cerebral Function Monitor"), SjO_2 ("Oximetrix 3" system with a 40 cm Shaw opticath), SaO_2 and end tidal CO_2. Intracranial pathology was classified as focal (unilateral swelling or mass lesion) or diffuse from the admission CT. If ICP rose above 25 mmHg during the first 48 hours post injury or 30 mmHg thereafter, once remediable causes were excluded, patients were given either thiopentone 4 mg/kg over 5 minutes through a central venous catheter or mannitol 0.5 g/kg iv over 15 minutes. A subsequent increase in ICP was treated with the other agent.

The blood pressure (BP), ICP, CPP (mean BP-mean ICP) and SjO_2 were automatically recorded at 1 minute intervals by microcomputer. Treatment was considered successful if CPP was increased or maintained at or above 60 mmHg and ICP was reduced to 20 mmHg or less. Data was analysed from the start of drug administration to the time of minimum ICP using correlation regression analysis and Fisher's exact probability test (2 tail) with $p < 0.05$ considered significant. A change in a parameter is defined as the value at the epoch studied minus the value at the start of treatment.

Results

Nine patients (8 male 1 female) age range 17–58 years received treatment with both agents within 72 hours of admission. Thiopentone was given first in 6 patients. Five patients suffered focal and four diffuse brain injury. Mannitol was successful in 7 patients (4 focal 3 diffuse) and thiopentone was successful in four patients (1 focal 3 diffuse) ($p = 0.50$). CPP was below 60 mmHg at the start of 6 mannitol and 3 thiopentone treatments. SJO_2 never exceeded 75% at the start of therapy and was less than 54% before 3 mannitol and 4 thiopentone administrations. CPP rose during all 9 mannitol and 6 thiopentone treatments while SJO_2 was increased after all mannitol administrations but fell during 3 of the thiopentone treatments in which CPP rose. SJO_2 fell in 2 of the 3 thiopentone treatments in which CPP also fell.

Mannitol Treatment

There was statistical significance but clinical poor correlation between SJO_2 and CPP ($r = -0.298$ $p < 0.001$). There was good correlation between SJO_2 and ICP ($r = -0.572$ $p < 0.001$). Change in SJO_2 correlated with change in CPP ($r = 0.335$ $p < 0.001$) and alteration in ICP ($r = -0.162$ $p < 0.001$) (Fig. 1).

When only successful reponses to mannitol were analysed there was a significant relationship between SJO_2 and CPP ($r = 0.181$ $p = 0.001$) and ICP ($r = -0.580$ $P < 0.001$). Change in SJO_2 correlated with both change in CPP ($r = 0.658$ $p < 0.001$) and alteration in ICP ($r = -0.520$ $p < 0.001$) (Fig. 2).

Thiopentone Treatment

There was no relationship between SJO_2 and either CPP or ICP. Change in SJO_2 correlated with change in CPP ($r = 0.442$ $p < 0.001$) and alteration in ICP ($r = 0.344$ $p < 0.001$) (Fig. 1).

When data from only successful treatment was analysed there was a significant relationship between SJO_2 and both CPP ($r = 0.507$ $p < 0.001$) and ICP ($r = 0.244$ $p = 0.027$). Change in SJO_2 correlated with change in CPP ($r = 0.421$ $p < 0.001$) and alteration in ICP ($r = 0.331$ $p = 0.002$) (Fig. 2).

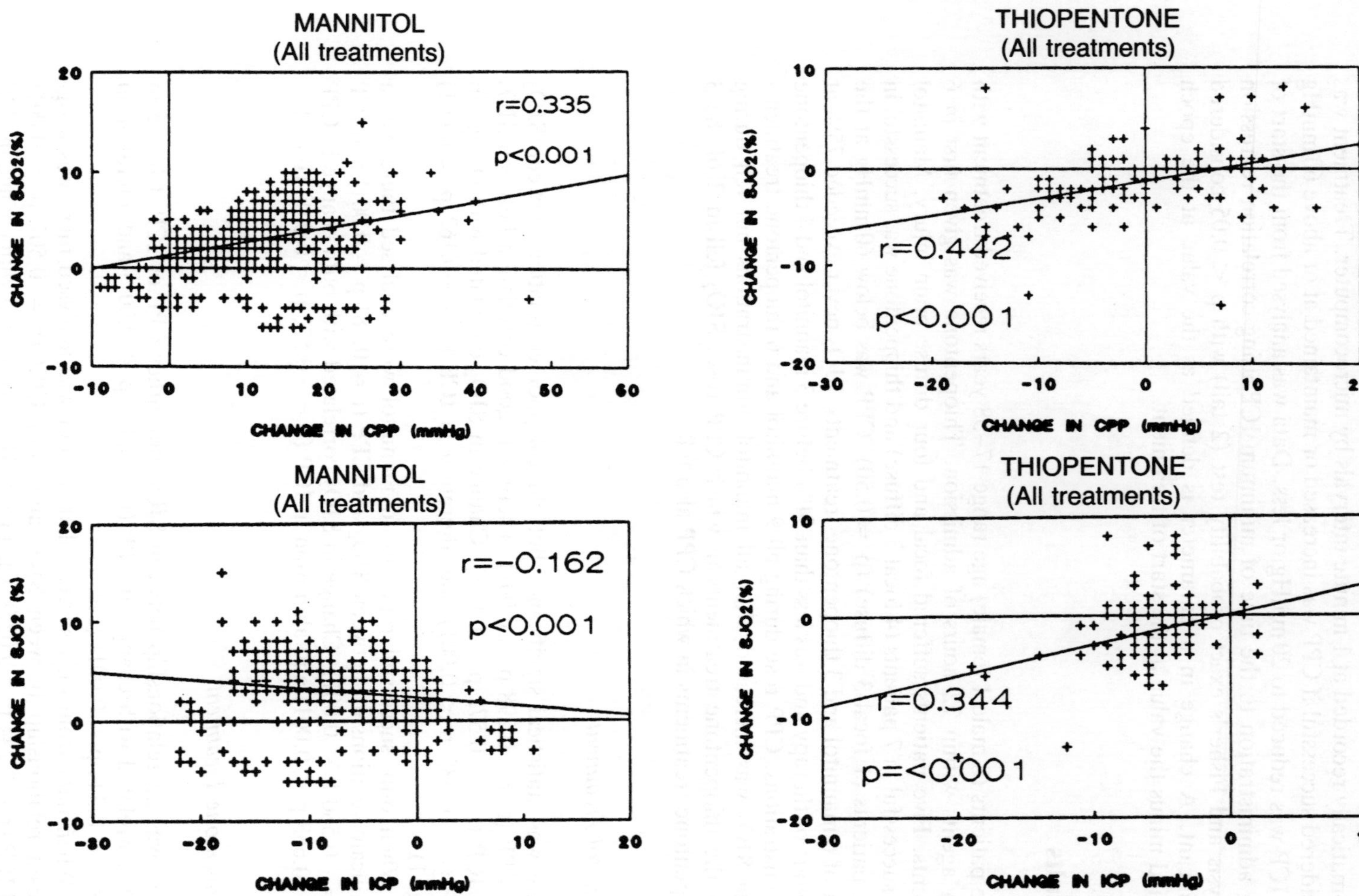

Fig. 1. Plot of change in SJO2 v's change in CPP and change in ICP for all treatments

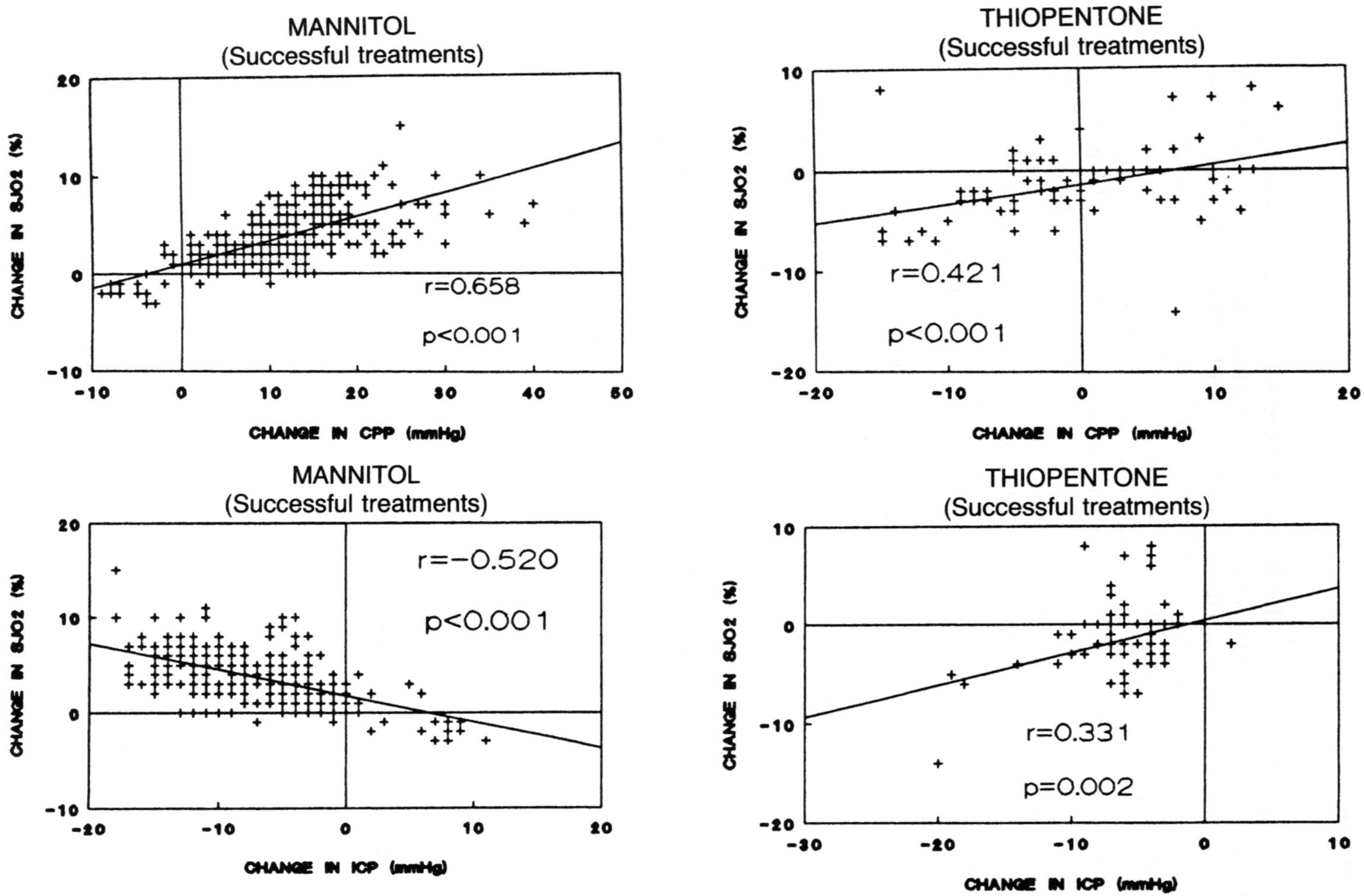

Fig. 2. Plot of change in SJO2 v's change in CPP and change in ICP for successful treatments only

Discussion

Intracranial hypertension following severe head injury leads to compromised CPP, reduced cerebral oxygen delivery and ischaemia which is associated with increased mortality and morbidity [4]. Reduction of ICP has not however, been shown to improve outcome. If ICP reduction therapy is to be beneficial it should be used selectively and only continued if CPP is preserved or raised until cerebral oxygen delivery is adequate. Specific ICP reducing treatment should only be given after avoidable causes have been corrected. Mannitol is reported to be of greatest efficacy after focal head injury, in patients with CPP below 70 mmHg and with preserved pressure autoregulation associated with normal cerebral arterio-venous oxygen content difference [7]. Hypnotic therapy appears most effective following diffuse head injury especially in association with cerebral hyperaemia (SJO_2 > 75%) [5]. Our observations concur with these reports.

Mannitol has effects on cerebral blood flow and brain water content while thiopentone reduces cerebral metabolism and often systemic blood pressure thereby lowering cerebral blood flow. Continuous measurement of SJO_2 allows the effects of different methods of ICP reduction on the ratio of global cerebral oxygen delivery to consumption to be ascertained throughout treatment. This enables rapid detection of cerebral hypoperfusion. The level of CPP below which this exists may also be determined.

We found a poor relationship between CPP and SJO_2 before commencing treatment. Hypoperfusion (SJO_2 < 54%) was met at both extremes of CPP (<50 and >90 mmHg). Although hyperventilation may have explained hypoperfusion in some patients a CPP above 60 mmHg may still be inadequate. With mannitol an increase in CPP was associated with an increase in SJO_2.

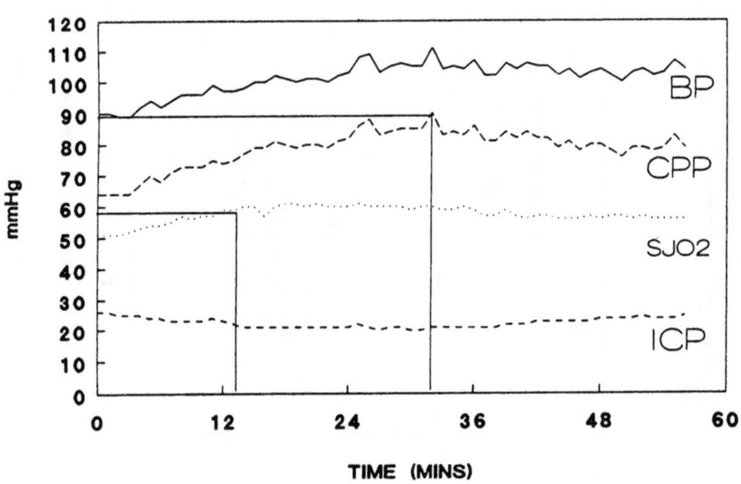

Fig. 3. Plot of BP, CPP, SJO2 and ICP during mannitol treatment. SJO2 rises to a plateau at 14 minutes, CPP continues to rise until 30 minutes post treatment

However, increasing CPP during thiopentone administration was associated with both increases and decreases in SJO_2. CPP occasionally fell during ICP reduction after thiopentone in conjunction with no change or a fall in SJO_2, even if, at the time of maximum reduction in ICP, therapy was considered successful. For both treatments, whether successful or not the change in CPP correlated better with change in SJO_2 than change in ICP. The CPP response is therefore the more important parameter to monitor.

During successful treatment with mannitol, SJO_2 initially increased and then remained unchanged while CPP continued to rise in some patients, suggesting autoregulation was intact and that above this threshold level further increase in CPP did not improve cerebral oxygen delivery (Fig. 3).

In conclusion, increasing CPP was always associated with rising SJO_2 during mannitol therapy. During thiopentone therapy increasing CPP was associated with falls in SJO_2 making CPP an unreliable guide to the success of therapy. If CPP falls during thiopentone therapy, SJO_2 may or may not decline. Continuous monitoring of SJO_2 allows modification to the administration of ICP reduction treatments, both to avoid hypoperfusion and to ascertain the CPP above which cerebral oxygen delivery is not further improved.

References

1. Andrews PJD, Dearden NM (1990) Validation of the Oximetrix 3 for continuous monitoring of jugular bulb oxygen saturation after severe head injury. Comparison with IL 282 in vitro cooximeter. Br J Anaesthesia 64:393–394
2. Cold GE (1978) Cerebral metabolic rate of oxygen ($CMRO_2$) in acute phase brain injury. Acta Anaesth Scand 22:249–256
3. Dearden NM (1991) Jugular bulb venous oxygen saturation monitoring in the management of severe head injury. Current Opinion in Anaesthesiology 4:279–286
4. Miller JD (1985) Head injury and brain ischaemia-implications for therapy. Br J Anaesthesia 57:120–129
5. Obrist WD, Langfitt TW, Jaggi JL, Cruz J, Gennarelli TA (1984) Cerebral blood flow and metabolism in comatose patients with acute head injury. J Neurosurg 61:241–253
6. Robertson CS, Narayan RK, Gokaslan ZL, Pahwa R, Grossman RG, Caram P, Allen E (1989) Cerebral arteriovenous oxygen difference as an estimate of cerebral blood flow in comatose patients. J Neurosurg 70:222–230
7. Rosner MJ, Coley I (1987) Cerebral perfusion pressure. A haemodynamic mechanism of mannitol and the post mannitol haemogram. Neurosurgery 21:147–156

Diffuse Axonal Injury

ICP Monitoring of Severe Diffuse Axonal Injury

S. KOBAYASHI, H. YOKOTA, and S. NAKAZAWA

Department of Neurosurgery, Nippon Medical School, Tokyo 113, Japan

Introduction

In acceleration/deceleration injuries of the head, large forces produce widespread destruction of axons in the white matter of the cerebral hemispheres and brain stem.

Recently, this kind of injury has been described as so-called "diffuse axonal injury (DAI)" [2, 3, 5]. There is increasing evidence from human and experimental studies that the most important factor governing the outcome in head injury is severity of DAI. This report presents the clinical aspects and ICP monitoring of DAI in severe head injury.

Patients and Method

We have experienced 18 cases of severe DAI which showed post-traumatic coma for more than 24 hours with brainstem dysfunction and CT findings resembling those of "shearing injuries of the cerebral white matter" [10], which are bilateral cerebral swelling with ventricular and cisternal compression, eccentric hemorrhage in the corpus callosum, subarachnoid hemorrhage, and the absence of a specific focal mass lesion, as well as small focal hemorrhage in the brain stem and in the white matter of the cerebral hemisphere. ICP was monitored by the subarachnoid catheter method [4]. Consciousness state on admission was defined according to the Glasgow Coma Scale (GCS) and clinical outcome was scored using the Glasgow Outcome Scale (GOS): good recovery (GR), moderate disability (MD), severe disability (SD), persistent vegetative state (PVS) and dead.

Results

The consciousness levels on admission were 6 or less on GCS and all cases showed clinically primary brain stem injury. The main type of head trauma

Table 1. Intracranial pressure on admission

ICP on Admission (mmHg)	No. of Patients
0–10	4
11–20	7
21<	2
Total	13

Table 2. Course of intracranial pressure and outcome

ICP Group	Glasgow Outcome Scale			Total
	GR/MD	SD/PVS	Dead	
I	0	4	0	4
II	0	6	0	6
III	0	0	3	3
Total	0	10	3	13

ICP, Intracranial pressure
I, ICP remained below 20 mmHg; II, ICP rose above 20 mmHg but was controlled by therapy; III, ICP rose above 20 mmHg but could not be controlled by therapy

resulted from road traffic accidents (83%). Skull fractures were found in only 5 cases (28%). These findings suggest that acceleration/deceleration injury produced severe DAI in these patients. Small parenchymal hemorrhagic lesions on initial CT were in the basal ganglia (7 cases), corpus callosum (4 cases), pons (4 cases), midbrain (3 cases) and thalamus (2 cases). Extraparenchymal hemorrhagic lesions included intraventricular hemorrhage (6 cases) and subarachnoid hemorrhage (6 cases). ICP was monitored in 13 cases. Table 1 presents the ICP on admission. Initial ICP was below 20 mmHg in 11 cases (85%). The course of ICP was divided into three groups (Table 2): ICP remained below 20 mmHg (Group I); ICP rose above 20 mmHg but was controlled by therapy (Group II); ICP rose above 20 mmHg and could not be controlled by therapy (Group III). The outcome in (Group) Group I (4 cases) and Group II (6 cases) was SD and/or PVS; all 3 patients in Group III died. Two autopsied cases of severe DAI (acute case and chronic case) showed remarkable congestion and edema in the deep part of the frontal white matter.

Microscopic examination revealed marked axonal degeneration including axonal retraction balls in the corpus callosum, in the internal capsule and in the white matter of the brain stem. GOS of the 18 patients at 3 months after the trauma was SD in 5 cases (28%), PVS in 6 cases (33%) and dead in 7 cases (39%).

Discussion

In acceleration/deceleration injuries of the head, widespread damage to axons in the white matter has been a well recognized pathological process for a long time [1, 2, 7, 8, 9]. These pathological alterations of the white matter were first described in detail by Strich [8]. Subsequently, many neuropathologists reported these pathological changes using different names: "shearing injury" [7, 9], "diffuse damage of immediate impact type" [1], and "diffuse white matter shearing injury" [10]. Recently, Adams et al. reported 45 cases with DAI [2]. They described the "triad" associated with DAI, such as focal lesions in the corpus callosum and in the dorsolateral quadrant (or quadrants) of rostal brain stem, and microscopic evidence of diffuse damage to axons. The CT findings of DAI were first demonstrated by Zimmerman et al. [10]. They reported 8 cases in which there appeared to be a marked discrepancy between the CT appearance and the clinical state. These patients showed deep coma and special CT findings like bilateral cerebral swelling with ventricular and cisternal compression, eccentric hemorrhage in the corpus callosum, subarachnoid hemorrhage, and the absence of a specific focal mass lesion, as well as small focal hemorrhage in the brain stem and in the white matter of the cerebral hemisphere. In our series, parenchymal hemorrhagic lesions were seen in the basal ganglia (39%), midbrain (17%) and corpus callosum (24%). The incidence of the small focal hemorrhage in the corpus callosum is less than that reported by others [6, 10]. Recently, Lobato et al. [6] emphasized the importance of the CT findings of DAI in their new CT classification of severe head injury. There are not many reports dealing with ICP in patients with DAI. Only one out or 8 patients (13%) reported by Zimmerman et al. developed delayed increased intracranial pressure.

In our series, 11 cases out of 13 (85%) had an ICP of below 20 mmHg, and 9 cases (70%) developed raised ICP for some period. These results of ICP measurement indicate that pathological changes in the cerebral hemispheres and brain stem of DAI were primarily caused by the initial impact, and not secondarily by the increased intracranial pressure. Diffuse axonal injury remains a great problem, and makes a major contribution to long-term disability after head injury.

References

1. Adams JH, Mitchell DE, Graham DI, et al. (1977) Diffuse brain damage of immediate impact type. Its relationship to primary brain stem damage in head injury. Brain 100:489–502
2. Adams JH, Graham DI, Murray LS, et al. (1982) Diffuse axonal injury due to non-missile head injury in humans: An analysis of 45 cases. Ann Neurol 12:557–563
3. Gennarelli TA, Thibault LE, Adams JH, et al. (1982) Diffuse axonal injury and traumatic coma in the primate. Ann Neurol 12:564–574
4. Kobayashi S, Nakazawa S, Yano M, et al. (1983) The value of intracranial pressure (ICP) measurement in acute severe head injury showing diffuse cerebral swelling. In: Ishii S, Nagai H, Brock M (eds) Intracranial Pressure V. Springer, Berlin Heidelberg New York Tokyo, pp 527–531

5. Langfitt TW, Gennarelli TA, Orbist WD, et al. (1982) Prospects for future in the diagnosis and management of head injury: pathophysiology, brain imaging, and population-based studies. Clin Neurosurg 29:353–376
6. Lobato RD, Cordobes F, Rivas JJ, et al. (1983) Outcome from severe head injury related to the type of intracranial lesion. A computerized tomography study. J Neurosurg 59:762–774
7. Peerless SJ, Rewcastle NB (1967) Shear injuries of the brain. Can Med Assoc J 96:577–582
8. Strich SJ (1956) Diffuse degeneration of the cerebral white matter in severe dementia following head injury. J Neurol Neurosurg Psychiatry 19:163–185
9. Strich SJ (1961) Shearing of nerve fibres as a cause of brain damage due to head injury. Lancet 2:443–448
10. Zimmerman RA, Bilaniuk LT, Gennarelli TA (1978) Computed tomography of shearing injuries of the cerebral white matter. Radiology 127:393–396

Diffuse Traumatic Axonal Injury: a Longitudinal Study

E.P. Sganzerla[1], G. Tomei[1], F. Servadei[2], P.M. Rampini[1], P. Guerra[1], and F. Tiberio[1]

[1] Institute of Neurosurgery, University of Milano, Milano, Italy
[2] Department of Neurosurgery, O. Bufalini, Cesena, Italy

Introduction

Patients who immediately lose consciousness after acceleration-deceleration injuries of the head and whose CTs are characterized by the presence of small hyperdense lesions in the corpus callosum and/or paramedian white matter and/or upper brainstem are generally considered as affected by diffuse axonal injury (DAI). The presence of scattered haemorrhages in the white matter of cerebral hemispheres and posterolateral mesencephalon (tissue tear haemorrhages) would be considered by many authors as a hallmark of severe axonal damage, predictive of less than optimal outcomes.

To define clinical and physiopathological characteristics of these patients, we longitudinally studied all patients admitted to our intensive care during the period January 1980–December 1990 whose clinicoradiological aspects fitted the diagnosis of severe DAI.

Patients and Methods

Among all severe head-injured patients (GCS <8, >24 hrs) admitted to the Intensive Care Unit (ICU) of the Institute of Neurosurgery of the University of Milano in the period January 1980–December 1990, we selected for this study only patients with immediate and prolonged loss of consciousness after trauma whose CTs clearly showed shearing injuries considered typical of DAI. Patients with CT signs of diffuse brain swelling (i.e. obliterated basal cisterns and third ventricle and generalized reduction of subarachnoid spaces) or with associated focal intracranial mass lesions other than deep white matter haemorrhages were excluded from this study.

Injury severity was defined summing up the score of single categories considered by the Glasgow Coma Scale, while outcome was categorized by the Glasgow Outcome Scale (GOS). Daily neurological assessments were made during the acute stage of trauma. Particular attention was given to the presence of clinical signs of brainstem lesion (eye signs, reflex oculomotor activity).

All patients had been treated with a standard regimen: mechanical ventilation with tidal volumes, respiratory frequencies and Fio2s adjusted to obtain mild hypocapnia and normoxia (Paco2 30–32 Torr, Pao2 > 90 Torr). Weaning procedures (spontaneous breath + CPAP), preceding definitive removal of the endotracheal tube, were started as soon as possible, in order to minimize pulmonary complications (usually when patients regained vigilance, i.e. eye opening, spontaneous and/or after painful stimuli).

EEG was recorded bedside with an 8 channel pen recorder using standard references (4 traces per hemisphere).

Multimodality evoked potentials (SEPs, VEPs and BAEPs) were obtained with an Amplaid MK3 apparatus.

ICP monitoring was done by means of a ventricular catheter inserted in the right frontal horn of a lateral ventricle, connected to a Statham P23 pressure transducer and a pen recorder. Measures to reduce ICP were started only when stable trends of increasing ICP (>20 Torr) were observed. Further hyperventilation, CSF drainage, diuretics, osmotics were then introduced stepwise, according to the ICP.

Results

Fifty-two patients satisfying our strict selection criteria ("pure" DAIs) have been observed during the period under consideration. Most patients were severely injured with GCS admission scores of 4 in 29%; 5 in 48%; 6 in 5.8% and 7 in 17%. Decerebrate and/or decorticate postures were thus present at admission in 77% of the patients.

Eye Signs

Only 2 patients (3.8%) presented with clearcut clinical signs of brainstem damage with internuclear ophthalmoplegia evidenced by the otovestibular caloric reflex (disconjugate tonic eye deviation). Slight anisocoria was present in 38.5% of the patients, never associated with CT or ICP monitoring signs of secondary brainstem lesion. In a recent case, acute MRI evidence of a pathological magnetic signal intensity in the posterolateral region of the upper brainstem (brainstem contusion) might explain the frequent observation of this pupillary abnormality in patients with traumatic DAI. Bilateral miosis, nevertheless, was the most frequent pupillary abnormality, observed in 61.5% of our patients.

EEG, recorded in 25 patients of this series, would indicate that the most characteristic tracing of DAI is a biphasic, reactive tracing, recorded in 56% of the patients.

Multimodality Evoked Potentials

Multimodality evoked potentials confirmed the clinical observation of the rarity of significant brainstem damage. BAEPs indeed never evidenced severe brainstem damage. Unilateral reduction of the amplitude of wave V and prolonged wave I–V interpeak latency were the only abnormality observed in individual patients.

Prolongation of CCTs (SEPs and VEPs) observed in most patients seems to relate to the predominant white matter damage known to affect these patients, whereas the absence of cortical responses correlated with poor functional outcomes in 2 patients (PVS).

Intracranial Pressure

Intracranial pressure was recorded in 18 patients. Increases of ICP towards intracranial hypertension were recorded in only one patient. Intracranial hypertension was associated with ventricular dilatation and CSF hypertension complicating intraventricular bleeding. Control of CSF hypertension and reduction of ventricular size were immediately obtained with continuous CSF withdrawal through the indwelling ventricular catheter, against opening pressures of 10 mmHg to avoid ventricular collapse and too rapid ICP variations. In all other patients in whom ICP was continuously recorded, it remained within normal ranges (<20 mmHg in 66% and <10 mmHg in 28%). ICP increases, thus, do not characterize these patients and ICP was not a predictor of outcome. Therefore, subsequent patients were not submitted to routine ICP monitoring.

Outcome

6 patients of this series died (mortality = 11.5%). In 4, death was secondary to septic complications and in 2 to massive pulmonary embolism, notwithstanding DVT prophylaxis with subcutaneous calciheparin. No death was due to intracranial traumatic complications. Clinical evolution was characterized in the majority of patients of this series by the slow recovery of consciousness, usually after a transient period of vegetative state. Vigilance reappeared in all patients after a mean time of 10 days (median 7.5 days). Only two patients (3.8%) of this series remained in a permanent and irreversible vegetative state, having resumed crude vigilance after prolonged coma (>3 weeks). One of them died after 5 years of PVS. In analyzing the clinical characteristics of the acute posttraumatic stage of these two patients, it appears that from the very beginning they showed peculiarities if compared to the other patients of the series, i.e.: pathological otovestibular reflexes (internuclear ophthalmoplegia), bilateral extensor reactions to pain persisting for >72 hrs (at variance with the usual improvement of motor reactions in patients with GCS 4 on admission within 48–72 hrs) and eventually resulting in tetraplegia; vigilance was resumed >3 weeks after injury and absent or severely demodulated cortical responses were obtained by SEPs. More caudal deterioration with clinical signs of brainstem damage seems to be associated with an extensive damage of supratentorial white matter, not compatible with the resumption of useful consciousness. Outcome was fair in the remaining patients with Good Recovery in 10 (19.2%), Moderate Disability in 29 (59.6%), Severe Disability in 3 (5.8%).

No correlation was found between number and location of tissue tear haemorrhages and outcome.

MRI Examinations

MRI examinations were available at follow-up controls in 20 pts. Increases of ventricular dimension due to reduction of brain bulk and thinning of corpus callosum were the most characteristic signs of previous traumatic DAI. In individual patients, focal signal intensity alterations of the white matter, almost identical with those described for patients with multiple sclerosis, were seen.

Conclusions

In patients with "pure" DAI mortality should be very low as the main causes of death are extracranial, potentially avoidable, complications. The hazard of hospital acquired infections should be particularly considered if aggressive management protocols are used.

Increases of intracranial pressure are seldom observed in DAI patients when no signs of brain swelling are present on CT. The two categories of trauma patients should therefore always be strictly distinguished when comparing series of patients with "diffuse brain damage" in order to avoid misunderstandings in the interpretation of contrasting results. The only possible cause of intracranial hypertension in DAI seems to be CSF hypertension due to progressive posthaemorrhagic hydrocephalus. ICP monitoring should not be routinely considered for these patients. Notwithstanding initial injury severity (GCS 4 or 5) and an usually slow recuperation stage, with more or less prolonged periods of PVS, a fair outcome can be predicted for the majority of these patients. Although most will present with neuropsychological and/or neurological deficits at follow up controls, the majority will be able to reach a state of moderate disability according to GOS within 1 year after trauma.

Clinical evidence of brainstem damage in the acute stage of trauma (Internuclear ophthalmoplegia, prolonged decerebration eventually followed by tetraplegia, prolongation of coma >3 weeks) is predictive of a permanent vegetative state.

Reduction of brain bulk and focal signal intensity alterations, similar to those observed in other leukoencephalopaties, are characteristic late MRI aspects in DAI patients.

References

1. Adams JH, et al. (1982) Diffuse axonal injury due to nonmissile head injury in humans: an analysis of 45 cases. Ann Neurol 12:557
2. Sganzerla EP, et al. (1989) Clinicoradiological and therapeutic considerations in severe diffuse traumatic brain injury in children. Child's Nerv Syst 5:168

3. Tomei G, et al. (1988) Etude clinicoradiologique de la lésion cérébrale diffuse post-traumatique. Agressologie 29:267
4. Wilberger JE, et al. (1990) Acute tissue tear haemorrhages of the brain: computed tomography and clinicopathological correlations. Neurosurgery 27:208

"Pure" Diffuse Axonal Injuries with Multiple Lesions on CT-Scan: Analysis of 20 Consecutive Patients

F. SERVADEI[1], A. PASINI[2], G. VERGONI[2], S. MALTONI[3], and D. ZAPPI[3]

[1] Division of Neurosurgery, [2] Department of Neuroradiology, and [3] Intensive Care Unit, Ospedale M. Bufalini, Cesena, Italy

Introduction

Diffuse axonal injury (DAI), widespread damage to the axons of the white matter, was first observed by Strich [8] in a group of patients affected by post-traumatic dementia. Other observations followed defining the macroscopic and microscopic [2] pathology of DAI. Until recently, the diagnosis of DAI has been confined to neuropathological investigations. Adams et al. [1], in 1982, reported a typical clinical course (coma of immediate onset, slow recovery rate and, at that time, poor prognosis). In 1978, Zimmerman [10] demonstrated with a first generation CT the macroscopic pathological hallmarks of DAI (small hemorrhagic lesions without mass effect in the corpus callosum, upper brainstem, cortico/nuclear medullary junction, parasagittal areas) in 8 patients. More accurate investigations with high resolution CT [6] and with MRI allow a radiological diagnosis of DAI in an increasing number of patients.

Methods and Results

From May 1989 to February 1990, 100 consecutive cases of severe head injury (GCS $\leqslant$ 8) were admitted to our intensive care unit. Twenty-five patients presented radiological (CT scanner Somatom DRH2, Siemens Manufact, slices at 4 mm) signs of DAI in "typical" areas. Five patients were exluded from the study ("pure" DAI) because of the presence of associated brain swelling (compression of the third ventricle and/or the basal cisterns) at some stage on CT. Our material, therefore, consists of 20 patients. Each patient harboured at least 2 small hemorrhagic lesions: there were 2 lesions in the brainstem, 10 lesions in the corpus callosum, 3 lesions in the periventricular area, 8 lesions in the basal ganglia, 22 lesions at the cortico-medullary junction and 7 gliding contusions. In 2 cases (both with a lesion in the corpus callosum and in the cortico-medullary junction), the first CT examination was normal and only a control examination (24 hours later) showed a hemorrage. We observed an associated subarachnoidal hemorrage in 6 cases and an intraventricular bleeding in 2 cases.

In 2 more patients, both lesions were present. A skull fracture was detected in 7 patients. There were 16 males and the mean age was 27.8 years (from 6 to

47 years). All patients were victims of road traffic accidents, mainly related to motor-car crash (15 out of 20). The onset of coma was immediate in all of our patients and on admission the mean GCS was 6.1 (from 4 to 8 without eyes opening). Only 2 of our patients had pupillary abnormality (one dilatated pupil). In no case herniation was the cause of this abnormality. During their stay in the intensive care unit, 6 patients showed motor patterns of decerebrate rigidity or combined decerebrate rigidity. In 8 cases an increased sympathetic activity was observed. The patients opened their eyes from day 8 to day 21 after injury and started to speak from day 23 to day 72. Intracranial pressure was monitored in 17 patients and never exceeded 25 mmHg. At the follow-up (at least 6 months after trauma) there were 3 deaths (2 related to respiratory failures and 1 sudden death on day 7), 3 cases of severe disability, 4 cases of moderate disability and 10 cases of good recovery.

Discussion

DAI is due to a rotational acceleration mechanism [5] usually related to high speed road accidents. The radiological diagnosis of DAI was first reported by Zimmerman in 1978 [10]. He observed 8 cases (out of 286 head injuried patients) with "shearing injuries of the cerebral white matter". DAI patients with CT signs were seen in 20% of all severe head injuries by Cordobes [3] and in 28, 2% by Uzzell [9]. In our material, if we add to the 25 cases 3 cases with associated extracerebral collections and 8 cases with single lesions on CT scan, (excluded, since the diagnosis of DAI is doubtful in the presence of a single lesion) [2], we reach 34% of all severe head injuries. In 1982, Gennarelli [4] found that 37% of patients in a group of 1107 severe head injuries were affected by diffuse brain lesion as defined only by the absence of mass lesion. In the period of observation (May 1989 to February 1990), we admitted only 4 cases of immediate comatose patients after head injury with a normal CT. One of these, in spite of persistent normal examinations, showed on NMR a contusion of the corpus callosum. NMR can, therefore, be useful in DAI but only in a minority of patients. In the vast majority of cases (34 out of 38 in our experience) the hallmarks of DAI are identified by high resolution CT. No correlation could be found in our material between outcome and a) location of the lesion b) presence of associated intraventricular and subarachnoidal blood. However, all the three severely disabled cases presented at least one lesion in the basal ganglia producing a severe degree of paresis. Studies based on clinical material of DAI showed poor outcome (death and persistent vegetative state) in 64% [3], in 52% [9], and from 29% to 63% [5] of the patients. Diffuse injury with coma lasting more than 24 hours was identified as the most severe type of lesion in trauma patients, together with subdural hematoma [4]. In contrast, severe head-injury patients with a normal CT had a very good outcome (only 10.8% poor outcome) [7]. We believe that the "bad reputation" concerning outcome of DAI patients is due to the radiological identification of only a small minority of cases, the most severe ones. Meanwhile, the inclusion of cases with associated intracranial lesion and/or brain swelling worsened the prognosis as shown by Levi [6]; 85% of DAI who died had an associated intracranial lesion. If we consider only "pure" DAI with a clear radiological diagnosis the outcome is good (14 out of 20 patients) in spite of a very slow recovery (18 cases were still in "prolonged coma" 3 weeks after trauma). In Adams' report [2], most DAI can be identified only with a post-mortem microscopic examination. We believe that patients with DAI have homogeneous clinico-radiological features. If the diagnosis is made with high resolution CT with thin slices and if we exclude cases with associated intracerebral lesions and brain swelling, the outcome is moderately good in spite of a slow recovery.

References

1. Adams JH, Graham DI, Murray LS, Scott G (1982) Diffuse axonal injury due to non missile head injury in humans: an analysis of 45 cases. Ann Neurol 12:557–563
2. Adams JH, Doyle D, Ford I, et al. (1989) Diffuse axonal injury in head injury: definition, diagnosis and grading. Histopathology 15:49–59
3. Cordobes F, Lobato RD, Rivas JJ, et al. (1986) Post-traumatic diffuse axonal brain injury. Analysis of 78 patients studied with computed tomography. Acta Neurochirurgica 81:27–35
4. Gennarelli TA, Spielman GM, Langfitt TW, et al. (1982) Influence of type of intracranial lesion on outcome from severe head injury. J Neurosurg 56:26–32
5. Gennarelli TA (1987) Cerebral concussion and diffuse brain injuries. In: Cooper PR (ed) Head Injury, Williams and Wilkins, Baltimore, pp 108–124
6. Levi L, Guildburd JN, Lemberger A, et al. (1990) Diffuse axonal injury: analysis of 100 patients with radiological signs. Neurosurgery 27:429–432
7. Lobato RD, Sonabia R, Rivas JJ, et al. (1986) Normal computerized tomography scans in severe head injury. J Neurosurg 65:784–789
8. Strich SJ (1956) Diffuse degeneration of the cerebral white matter in severe dementia following head injury. J Neurol Neurosurg Psychiatry 19:163–185
9. Uzzel BP, Dolniskas CA, Wiser RF, Langfitt TW (1987) Influence of lesions detected by CT on outcome and neuropsychological recovery after severe head injury. Neurosurgery 20: 396–402
10. Zimmerman RA, Bilaniuk LT, Gennarelli T (1978) Computed tomography of shearing injuries of the cerebral white matter. Radiology 127:393–396

Diffuse Axonal Injury: Changes of Cerebral Blood Flow, Intracranial Pressure and Evoked Potentials

C.K. PARK, Y.K. HONG, K.S. CHO, M.W. BAIK, J.K. KANG, and C.R. CHOI

Department of Neurosurgery, Catholic University Medical College, Seoul, 137-040, Korea

Introduction

There are various types of diffuse brain damage as a consequence of nonmissile head injury, but it is likely that widespread tearing of nerve fibers occurs at the moment of injury in most of these patients. A number of synonyms have been proposed to denote this type of brain damage. Recently, "diffuse axonal injury (DAI)" was preferably used and the concept of DAI has been well recognized not only pathologically [1] but also clinically [2]. However, the details of its clinical features and its influence on prognosis remain to be elucidated. This prospective study was done to investigate the relationship of ICP, cerebral blood flow (CBF) and changes of multimodality evoked potentials (MEPs) with outcome in patients with DAI.

Method

A total number of 25 consecutively hospitalized head injured patients with DAI CT lesions [3] were included in this study. Subdivision of the patients into three grades was made, based on clinical features [2]: mild (n = 5), moderate (n = 12) and severe DAI (n = 8). Fifteen of these patients underwent continuous ICP monitoring, and all patients were subjected to MEPs examinations and CBF measurements with single-photon emission computerized tomography (SPECT). ICP was monitored during the first 7 days, CBF was measured two times: one examination within three days after the accident and the other one 3 to 4 weeks later; MEPs were examined on the first day of admission and then once or twice a week for 4 weeks. The outcome was evaluated with the Glasgow Outcome Scale (GOS) at 3 months postinjury.

Results

A significant difference ($X^2 = 16.4$, $P < 0.05$) between the grades of DAI and GOS was observed (Table 2). Poorer outcomes occurred in the patients with severe DAI, but there was no death in any grade of the patients.

Table 1. Clinical features

	DAI grades		
	Mild (n = 5)	Moderate (n = 12)	Severe (n = 8)
Time course of ICP			
Continuous normal		4/8	6/7
IICP, therapy needed		2/8	1/7
IICP, therapy not needed		2/8	
CBF by SPECT at admission			
Normal	3		
Focal hypoperfusion	2	6	4
Diffuse hypoperfusion		7	5
MEPs at admission			
Normal	4	3	
Abnormal SEP	1	6	8
Abnormal VEP		7	8
Abnormal AEP		2	8

Table 2. 3 month outcome: results from DAI grades and changes of CBF and MEPs

	Glasgow outcome scale			
	Good recovery	Moderate disability	Severe disability	Vegitatitive state
DAI grades*				
Mild (n = 5)	4	1		
Moderate (n = 12)	5	6	1	
Severe (n = 8)		2	5	1
CBF, 3 months postinjury (n = 16)**				
Diminished previous hypoperfusion area (n = 8)	5	3		
Enlarged previous hypoperfusion area (n = 7)		3	3	1
Hypoperfusion in the periventricular white matter (n = 6)		1	4	1
MEPs, follow-up for 3 weeks**				
Normal (n = 7)	6	1		
Completely recovered (n = 5)	2	2	1	
Partially recovered (n = 10)	1	7	2	
Not recovered (n = 3)			2	1

* $p < 0.05$; ** $p < 0.01$ (Chi-Square test)

Continuous monitoring of ICP was carried out in eight of the patients with moderate DAI and in seven of the patients with severe DAI (Table 1). 67% of the patients monitored were in the normal range of ICP throughout the period of monitoring. 20% of them showed increases of ICP from 3 to 5 days following the injury and required aggressive therapy. The remaining 13% showed intermittent increases of ICP, which recovered spontaneously to the normal range without any specific management. Time course of ICP had no relationship with the severity of DAI ($X^2 = 2.68$, $P = 0.613$).

On the initial CBF measurement by SPECT (Table 1), all patients but three with mild DAI showed focal and/or diffuse hypoperfusion, which was poorly correlated with the findings of CT scan. In sixteen patients, follow-up SPECT was carried out a month later (Table 2). In 50% of these patients, the hypoperfusion areas observed at the initial SPECT were diminished and good outcomes occurred. In contrast, the other 50% had the findings of an enlarged hypoperfusion area and/or of newly developed hypoperfusion area in the white matter around the lateral ventricles, even though there was no corresponding ventriculomegaly on CT and their outcomes were poorer ($X^2 = 24.2$; $P < 0.001$).

On the initial MEPs (Table 1), all patients but four with mild DAI and three patients with moderate DAI, showed abnormal findings. In moderate DAI, major changes were noted in somatosensory evoked potentials (SEP) and/or visual evoked potentials (VEP), but in severe DAI all modalities of evoked potentials including brainstem auditory evoked potentials (AEP) were seriously changed. On serial examinations of MEPs (Table 2), the degree of recovery in MEPs was highly related to the outcome at 3 months postinjury ($X^2 = 24.4$; $P < 0.001$).

Discussion

Analysis of the outcome of the patients reveals that patients with severe DAI have the poorest outcome. Severe DAI is prolonged coma of more than 24 hours with brain stem signs. Brain stem signs are the most ominous findings predicting a poor outcome in head injured patients. However, it appears that the degree of injury in the white matter is also an important contributing factor. This is supported by our observations that the patients with hypoperfusion in the white matter areas and/or without recovered MEPs had poorer outcome. Good recoveries obtained in 42% of moderate DAI patients in spite of prolonged coma of more than 24 hours are due to the fact that widespread injury of the white matter occurred to a less severe degree. In conclusion, the present study suggests that the severity of DAI is decided at the moment of trauma and depends upon the degree of injury in the brain stem and the white matter of the cerebral hemisphere. On the other hand, intracranial hypertension is less responsible for its severity. Serial examinations of MEPs and SPECT could be a useful tool to monitor the clinical course and to predict outcome of the patients with DAI.

Acknowledgement. This work was supported by Catholic Medical Center, Seoul.

References

1. Adams JH, Graham DI, Murray LS, Scott G (1982) Diffuse axonal injury due to nonmissile head injury in humans: an analysis of 45 cases. Ann Neurol 12:557–563
2. Gennarelli TA (1987) Cerebral concussion and diffuse brain injuries. In: Cooper PR (ed) Head injury, 3rd edn. Williams & Wilkins, Baltimore London Los Angeles Sydney, pp 108–124
3. Zimmerman RA, Bilaniuk LT, Gennarelli TA (1978) Computed tomography of shearing injuries of the cerebral white matter. Radiology 127:393–396

Session VI: Control of ICP

Chairmen: J.D. Miller and J.B. North

Hyperventilation

Ischemic Insult Due to Manual Ventilation in Head Injured Patients with Intracranial Hypertension

F. Procaccio, G. Menasce, L. Sacchi, F. Conci, C. Betto, R. Fontana, and L. Boselli

Reparto di Neurorianimazione, Ospedale Niguarda-Ca'Granda, Milano, Italy

Introduction

Manual Hyperventilation (MHV)

Manual hyperventilation by Ambu bag is usually and frequently performed during nursing procedures, chest physiotherapy and interhospital transport of severely head injured patients.

As a fall in ICP is easily obtained, bagging has been widely used in ICUs as a first-line intervention to control intracranial hypertension. Unfortunately, a fall in mean arterial pressure (MAP), due to impaired venous return and reduced cardiac output, is often present during MHV. In a previous retrospective study undesirable reductions in cerebral perfusion pressure (CPP) were observed in 40% of baggings [7].

Acute hypocapnia causes cerebral vasoconstriction, a decrease in cerebral blood flow (CBF), blood volume (CBV) and ICP, but also respiratory alkalosis with a leftward shift of the hemoglobin dissociation curve.

In comatose brain injured patients with reduced CBF, mechanical hyperventilation may provoke cerebral oligemia [2, 5].

Although CBF and cerebral oxygen metabolism (CMRO2) monitoring are not clinically available, indirect but relevant information may be obtained from continuous recordings of the EEG, using a *Cerebral Function Monitor* (CFM), and *jugular bulb oxygen saturation* (SjO2). Arteriojugular difference in oxygen content provides a good measure of the global CBF/CMRO2 relationship [3, 8, 9]; its continuous monitoring through SjO2 permits to detect short periods of CBF inadequacy.

The lower border voltage of the CFM trace correlates with the minimum level of cortical electrical activity and mirrors different degrees of cortical metabolic depression [6].

In comatose head injured patients CMRO2 is usually reduced; in contrast, CBF may be increased, excessively decreased or adequate to the metabolic demand [5]. When CBF is low, the oxygen uptake by the brain is maintained at its normal level by an increase in the oxygen extraction from the blood in proportion to the fall in CBF, as shown by a fall in SjO2. If the increase in oxygen extraction can no longer counterbalance the fall in CBF, a decrease in the cerebral uptake and metabolic rate of oxygen occurs. Cerebral oligemia is reflected consistently in a decrease in cortical electrical voltage and an increase in periods of EEG suppression, particularly in the arterial boundary zones, where the CFM electrodes are located [1].

The *aim of this study* was to examine the effect of manual hyperventilation on CPP, SjO2 and cortical electrical activity in comatose head injured patients with intracranial hypertension.

Patients and Methods

Ten comatose patients with severe head injury were studied (Table 1). The median age was 22. All the patients were mechanically ventilated to achieve a PaCO2 between 3.3 and 4.5 KPa and a SaO2 > 95%. EtCO2 (infrared capnometer) and SaO2 (pulse oximeter) were continuously monitored. Patients were sedated by continuous infusion of diazepam (0.05–0.1 mg/kg/h) and intermittent i.m. opiates. Normovolemia was preserved on the basis of continuous monitoring of central venous pressure and fluid balance. Blood was given to maintain hematocrit higher than 30%.

A chart recorder run at 18 cm/h provided a continuous recording of arterial blood pressure (ABP) (arterial catheter), ICP (intraventricular or subdural catheter), CFM output (standard biparietal electrodes with reference at Cz), SjO2 (right jugular Opticath fiberoptic catheter, Oximetrics 3 oximeter).

Protocol

When the ICP increased to more than 20 mmHg, manual hyperventilation (Ambu bag; FiO2 = 0.4–0.5) was performed for 1 minute by nurses of the

Table 1. Details of patients

Pt	Sex	Age	Type of lesion	Admission GCS	Outcome 3 months	Day of study	Bagging n = 51
1	F	20	DAI	5	SD	2–4	5
2	M	22	DAI	6	MD	2–5	7
3	M	12	DAI	4	SD	4	3
4	F	17	Laceration	5	D	5	2
5	M	16	Swelling	4	D	2	4
6	M	41	Subdural	6	SD	2–6	12
7	M	59	Subdural	4	D	2–5	7
8	F	31	Laceration	4	MD	4–6	5
9	M	25	Laceration	7	GR	2–4	4
10	M	22	Laceration	7	GR	3–4	2

DAI, diffuse axonal injury

Neuro ICU to obtain a decrease in ICP. SaO2 (95–100%) remained unchanged during bagging in all the cases.

Mean ICP, MAP, CPP, SjO2, ETCO2 and minimum voltage of the CFM trace (in millimetres above the $0\,\mu V$ baseline for statistical processing) were measured 2 minutes before MHV, at the point of maximum change in ICP during MHV and within 3 minutes after.

Paired arterial, mixed venous and jugular bulb SO2 PO2, PCO2 and pH were measured at the same points on 10 occasions.

In this prospective study 51 baggings by 5 different nurses were considered; occasions accompanied by the administration of any drug and during which any stimulating procedure had occurred, were excluded. Mean values ± SEM are reported. Wilcoxon's signed-rank test, Fisher's exact test and Pearson's correlation coefficient were used.

Results

Mean basal values and changes during and after MHV are shown in Table 2. ICP decreased in 90% (Percentage change in ICP = −27.5 ± 3.2%) but MAP fell in 53% of the occasions. Consequently, CPP decreased in 35%. ETCO2 fell in 86% and SjO2 in 90%. There was a correlation between the change in ETCO2 and the change in SjO2 ($r = 0.57$, $p < 0.0001$).

Prior to bagging, CPP was lower than 60 mmHg in 1/3 of the occasions; SjO2 was never below 55% and in the range 55–60% in 1/4. SjO2 fell below 55% during bagging in 1/3 of the occasions.

There was a significant correlation between the absolute change in ICP and basal ICP ($r = -0.56$, $p < 0.0001$) but no correlation was demonstrated between the percentage change in ICP and basal CPP, ETCO2 and SjO2. Only a weak correlation was present between the change in SjO2 and pre-MHV ICP ($r = -0.42$, $0.001 < p < 0.005$).

At the end of bagging, ICP showed a rebound in 37% and CPP was lower than pre-MHV in 41%. The lower voltage of the CFM trace decreased in 18%. This ischemic effect occurred more frequently (32% against 3%, $p < 0.01$) in the group ($n = 22$) in which pre-MHV CPP was lower than 60 mmHg or SjO2 lower than 60%.

Table 2. Effects of manual hyperventilation (MHV)

		Pre-MHV		Max change	within 3 min
ICP	(mmHg)	22.7 ± 1.8	*	−6.6 ± 1.0	22.9 ± 2.1
MAP	(mmHg)	95.7 ± 2.9	*	−6.0 ± 2.0	95.2 ± 2.8
CPP	(mmHg)	72.9 ± 3.4		0.6 ± 1.9	72.3 ± 3.5
ETCO2	(mmHg)	27.8 ± 0.4	*	−7.0 ± 0.6	27.7 ± 0.4
SjO2	(%)	70.2 ± 1.2	*	−7.0 ± 0.8	69.1 ± 1.6

mean value ± SEM * = $p < 0.005$ Wilcoxon's Test

When pre-MHV CFM minimum voltage was not severely depressed (higher than 4 μV), a decrease in voltage never occurred in the pre-MHV CPP > 60 mmHg & SjO2 > 60% group (n = 17).

A decrease in CFM voltage occurred in 40% when pre-MHV CPP was higher than 60 mmHg and CFM higher than 4 μV but SjO2 was lower than 60% (compensated hypoperfusion).

Discussion

Manual hyperventilation is a simple model to evaluate the relationship between treatment and pathological dynamics of acute cerebral lesion. To obtain control of ICP by reducing CBF without decreasing metabolic demand may aggravate pending ischemic damage.

The results of this study suggest that bagging may induce repeated and unnoticed cerebral oligemic insults. For this reason the Ambu bag should be used very carefully and probably avoided in the intensive care of severe brain injuries.

The method of bagging was often inadequate. With critically low CPP the risk of an ischemic insult became much higher when unpredictable reductions in arterial pressure occurred, probably due to excessive rate of ventilation, increased intrathoracic pressure and reduced venous return.

Independent from basal PaCO2, an abrupt fall in PaCO2 and SjO2 occurred during bagging, both confirmed by arterial and jugular gas analyses. In 18% a decrease in CFM lower border voltage suggested that the reduction in CBF had caused a secondary oligemic reduction in cortical metabolism. This effect frequently occurred when a low SjO2 and a preserved electrical cortical activity indicated a state of global *compensated hypoperfusion* [8].

A severely depressed EEG with increasing periods of suppression, as indicated by a CFM minimum voltage lower than 4–5 μV, may have masked more frequent oligemic insults. This was suspected when a low SjO2 and a severely depressed CFM indicated a state of *non compensated hypoperfusion*. On those occasions SjO2 had very low values during bagging (Fig. 1). On the contrary, no changes in SjO2 were seen when a high basal SjO2 and an extremely depressed CFM indicated a cerebral infarct with a global impairment of CO2 reactivity.

The ICP rebound observed in 37% of cases after the end of bagging might have been caused by the autoregulatory dilatation in response to decreased MAP or by both the hyperemic rebound, due to the oligemic insult with impairment of autoregulation, and the venous engorgement with increased CBV, due to hampered venous return.

Different states of CO2 reactivity and autoregulation might have influenced the results of the study. A positive correlation between CO2 reactivity, the effect of barbiturate treatment and clinical outcome has been demonstrated [4]; thus the observation of the effect of acute hyperventilation on jugular bulb oxygen saturation could offer simple but relevant clinical information.

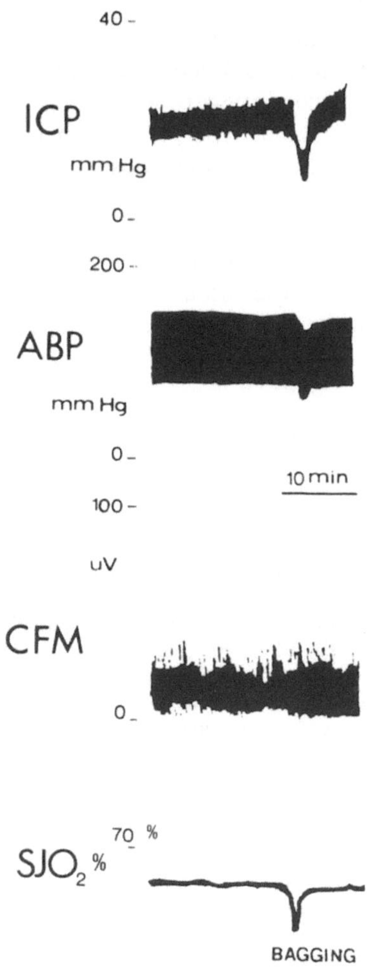

Fig. 1. Polygraphic recording of intracranial pressure (ICP), arterial blood pressure (ABP), Cerebral Function Monitor (CFM) and jugular bulb oxygen saturation (SjO2) in a mechanically ventilated brain injured patient (female, 20 yrs; GCS = 5, diffuse cerebral lesion).

Basal CPP was higher than 60 mmHg but CFM was severely depressed (<4 μV) and SjO2 was lower than 60%.

Bagging caused a transient decrease in ICP and ABP and an abrupt fall in SjO2 below 45%. ETCO2 fell from 3.7 to 2.3 KPa.

After bagging, a rebound in ICP occurred and SjO2 remained lower than basal value. No changes in the lower border voltage of the CFM were evident

Conclusions from this study cannot be extended to mechanical ventilation, in which timing and magnitude of induced physiological changes are different. Nevertheless, SjO2 [3, 9] and CFM continuous monitoring could be useful to indicate and modulate hyperventilation therapy in clinical brain injury.

Conclusions

Accurate treatment of avoidable factors, preservation of an adequate CPP and CBF and qualified intensive nursing could prevent intracranial hypertension and secondary cerebral ischemic damage in most patients.

Manual hyperventilation is not an adequate treatment for raised ICP. In this study bagging caused repeated cerebral oligemic insults and frequently precipitated a compensated hypoperfusion (SjO2 $< 60\%$ & CFM $> 4\,\mu V$) into ischemia.

Continuous monitoring of CPP, SjO2 and CFM may improve the knowledge on the effects of treatment and offer a reliable guide for nursing procedures and therapy to avoid iatrogenic ischemic insults.

References

1. Brierley JB, Prior PF, Calverley J, Jackson SJ, Brown AW (1980) The pathogenesis of ischaemic neuronal damage along the cerebral arterial boundary zones in papio anubis. Brain 103:929–965
2. Cold GE (1989) Does acute hyperventilation provoke cerebral oligaemia in comatose patients after acute head injury? Acta Neurochir 96:100–106
3. Cruz J, Miner ME, Allen SJ, et al. (1990) Continuous monitoring of cerebral oxygenation in acute brain injury: injection of mannitol during hyperventilation. J Neurosurg 73:725–730
4. Nordstrom CH, Messeter K, Sundbarg G, et al. (1988) Cerebral blood flow, vasoreactivity and oxygen consumption during barbiturate therapy in severe traumatic brain lesions. J Neurosurg 68:424–431
5. Obrist WD, Langfitt TW, Jaggi JL, Cruz J, Gennarelli TA (1984) Cerebral blood flow and metabolism in comatose patients with acute head injury. J Neurosurg 61:241–253
6. Prior PF (1985) EEG monitoring and evoked potentials in brain ischaemia. Br J Anaesth 57:63–81
7. Procaccio F, Martani L, Friolo R (1990) Effect of manual ventilation on ICP, CPP and EEG in severely head injured patients. Intensive Care Med 16:S77
8. Robertson CS, Narayan RK, Gokaslan ZL, et al. (1989) Cerebral arteriovenous oxygen difference as an estimate of CBF in comatose patients. J Neurosurg 70:222–230
9. Sutton LN, McLaughlin AC, Dante S, et al. (1990) Cerebral venous oxygen content as a measure of brain energy metabolism with increased intracranial pressure and hyperventilation. J Neurosurg 73:927–932

Is There a Risk to Induce Ischemia by Hyperventilation Therapy?

J. MEIXENSBERGER[1], A. BRAWANSKI[1], I. DANHAUSER-LEISTNER[2], M. HOLZSCHUH[1], and W. ULLRICH[1]

[1] Department of Neurosurgery and [2] Anaesthesiology, University of Würzburg, 8700 Würzburg, Germany

Introduction

Therapeutic hyperventilation is a tool in the treatment of raised intracranial pressure. Thereby, the decrease of intracranial pressure is produced by a decrease of the cerebral blood volume following vasoconstriction of the pial vessels and arterioles. On the other hand, secondary ischemic brain damage influences outcome of head injured patients. Therefore, we were interested in the following issues:

1. Is there a risk of inducing a drop in CBF, causing ischemic brain damage, by hyperventilation therapy?
2. Can this risk vary in the time course after head injury?

Patients and Methods

Twenty-eight head injured patients (20 male, 8 female, mean age 32.6 ± 20.4 years) were studied during day 1–14 after brain injury in the Neurointensive Care Unit. All patients were conservatively treated by sedation and automatic ventilation. Besides continous epidural and arterial pressure monitoring, serial CT scans were performed to evaluate form and extent of the brain lesion over time.

A mobile unit for bedside measurements (Novo Cerebrograph 10a) with ten detectors, five placed over each hemisphere, was utilized for CBF measurements using the intravenous ^{133}Xenon method. As a measure of CBF we used the Initial Slope Index (ISI) [5] calculated by a bicompartimental model [3].

We performed fifty-eight rest CBF studies (mean $PaCO_2$: 30.4 ± 2 mmHg) and fifty activation studies after $PaCO_2$ changes (mean change 6.5 mmHg). We calculated mean global resting CBF and determined global CO_2-reactivity as change in CBF per 1 mmHg change in $PaCO_2$. We assumed an upper normal limit for global CBF of 35 ml/100 g min (ISI) [2, 4] and a normal limit for CO_2 reactivity of 0.75 ml/100 g min per 1 mmHg change in $PaCO_2$ [1].

Results

Under therapeutic resting conditions ($PaCO_2$: 30.4 ± 2 mmHg (mean ± SD) we distinguished a group with reduced CBF (54% of our cases) and a group with hyperemia (46% of our cases) according to the Obrist classification [4]. The global CBF was calculated as 42.4 ± 4.4 ml/100 g/min (ISI) in the hyperemia group; the group with reduced CBF had a mean CBF of 28.9 ± 4.1 ml/100 g/min (ISI). The global CBF CO_2 reactivity varied in the course of time after the brain injury. A reduced or inverse CBF CO_2 reactivity could mostly be detected in the first eight days after trauma. Totally 56% of our cases showed an intact global CBF CO_2 reactivity. However, we found in 44% of cases a disturbance of CBF CO_2 reactivity. A correlation between absolute global resting CBF values and CBF CO_2 reactivity did not reach statistical significance (r = 0.27). Finally, we selected a risk group (cases with reduced CBF and intact CBF CO_2 reactivity), where increased hyperventilation (25 mmHg ± 1.6 SD) led to low CBF values on the borderline of ischemia (21.9 ± 4.1 ml/100 g/min (ISI)). In 24% of our cases we found such a risk of induced ischemia. Figure 1 summarizes the effects of increased hyperventilation in the hyperemia group and in the group with reduced CBF.

A

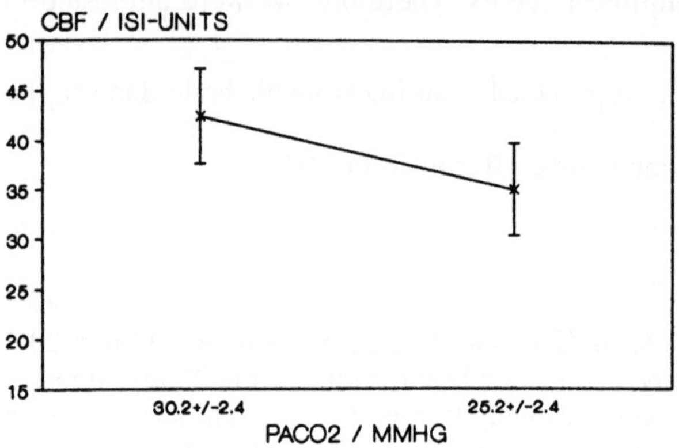

B

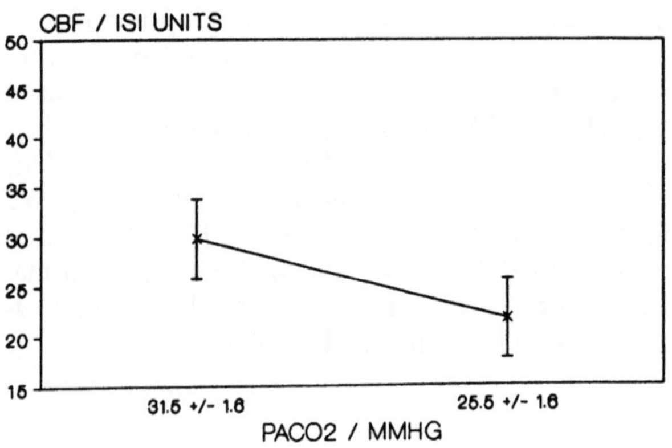

Fig. 1A,B. Effect of increased hyperventilation on global CBF in the hyperemia group **A** and the group with reduced CBF **B** with normal CBF-CO2-reactivity. Values are given as mean ± SD. Number of cases hyperemia group n = 16, group with reduced CBF n = 12

Conclusion

Analyzing our data regarding global CBF under induced hypocapnia to about 30 mmHg $PaCO_2$, we rarely found reduced absolute flow values close to the borderline of ischemia. However, we could exclude a group of patients who will be at risk of ischemia under such treatment: hyperventilation of patients with reduced CBF and intact CBF CO_2 – reactivity can reduce CBF to ischemic levels. This risk varies and increases if CO2 reactivity is normal during the time after injury. Therefore, we should reflect critically upon the duration and extent of hyperventilation therapy.

References

1. Maximilian VA, Prohovnik I, Risberg J (1980) The cerebral hemodynamic response to mental activation in normo- and hypercapnia. Sroke 11:342–347
2. Messeter K, Nordström CH, Sundberg G, et al. (1986) Cerebral hemodynamics in patients with acute severe head trauma. J Neurosurg 64:231–237
3. Obrist WD, Thomson HK Jr, Wang HS, et al. (1975) Regional cerebral blood flow estimated by ^{133}Xenon inhalation. Stroke 6:245–256
4. Obrist WD, Langfitt TW, Jaggi JL, et al. (1984) Cerebral blood flow and metabolism in comatose patients with acute head injury. J Neurosurg 61:241–253
5. Risberg J, Ali Z, Wilson EM, et al. (1975) Regional cerebral blood flow by ^{133}Xenon inhalation. Preliminary evaluation of an initial slope index in patients with unstable flow compartments. Stroke 6:142–148

Effects of Mannitol Treatment on Cerebral Water Content

A.M. KAUFMANN and E.R. CARDOSO

Cerebral Hydrodynamics Laboratory, Health Sciences Clinical Research Centre, Winnipeg, Manitoba, Canada

Introduction

Mannitol treatment is useful in the acute management of intracranial hypertension. However, the pharmacokinetics of mannitol administration and associated longterm effects on cerebral water content have not previously been established. In this study, we investigated single- and multiple-dose mannitol treatment in a feline vasogenic edema model. The alterations of water content in normal and edematous white matter regions were determined.

Methods

Cold-injury cerebral edema was produced in 23 anesthetized cats, and was traced by intravenously administered Evan's blue dye. One hour later, treatment group animals received either a single dose or five four-hourly doses of 0.33 g/kg intravenous mannitol, infused over 15 minutes each. Four hours following the last dose, cerebral water contents were determined by the gravimetric technique [2, 3, 4]. Control group animals were similarly assessed, also five or twenty-one hours post-injury. An independent Student's t-test was used to compare results in mannitol treatment groups and their respective time-matched control groups, as well as to assess physiological variables. Differences were considered significant for p smaller than 0.05, and variations from the mean are given as standard errors.

Results

The overall mean arterial blood pressure was unaffected by single or multiple injections of mannitol. Oxygenation, carbon dioxide tension, and body temperature were also maintained within normal physiological ranges throughout the experiment. Furthermore, there was no difference in serum sodium, osmolality, and fluid balance between treatment and control groups.

The average water content of non-edematous white matter was 68.9 ± 0.2% and 69.6 ± 0.2% at 5 and 21 hours following the cold-injury. Neither single or multiple doses of mannitol produced any significant alteration of these values, as measured four hours after the last dose (Fig. 1). The water content of edematous white matter was significantly greater than in non-edematous regions, and was 84.2 ± 1.0 and 83.3 ± 0.2 in the 5 and 21 hour control groups (Table 1). Single-dose mannitol treatment produced no significant change of water content (Fig. 2). However, multiple-dose mannitol treatment was associated with a further 3% increase in edematous water content ($p = 0.0034$).

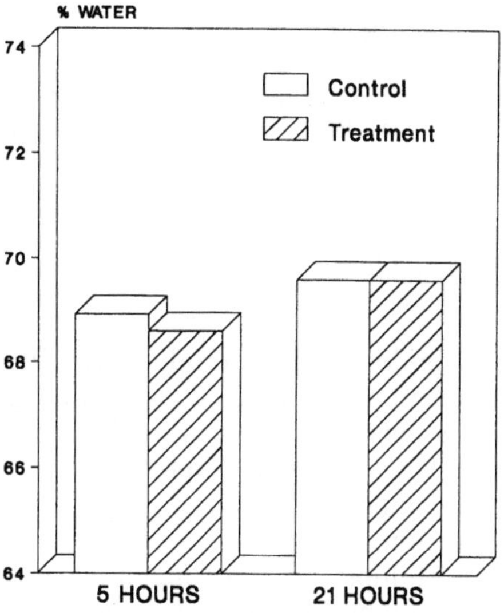

Fig. 1. Water content of non-edematous white matter: no significant change at 5 and 21 hours following the cold-injury, and no significant change produced by single or multiple mannitol doses

Table 1. Cerebral water content (white matter)

Water Content (%)	Non-Edematous	Edematous
5 Hours:		
Control	68.9 ± 0.2	84.2 ± 1.0
Single dose	68.6 ± 0.2	83.3 ± 0.8
21 Hours:		
Control	69.6 ± 0.2	83.3 ± 0.2
Multiple-doses	69.6 ± 0.4	86.2 ± 0.5*

* $p < 0.005$

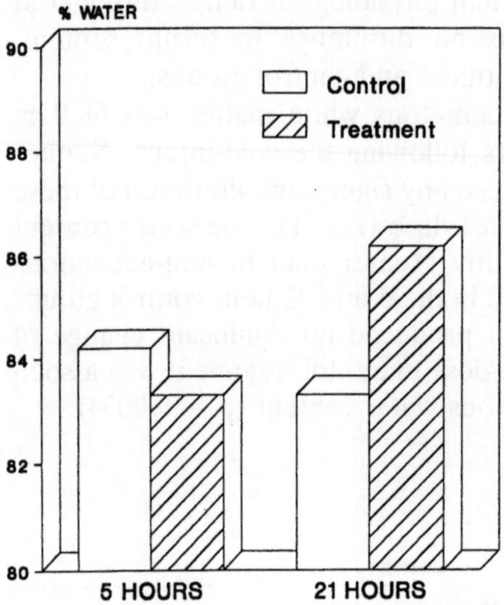

Fig. 2. Water content of edematous white matter: no significant change produced by single-dose mannitol at 5 hours following the cold-injury, while multiple mannitol doses significantly raised the water content by an additional 3% ($p = 0.0034$)

Discussion

Single-dose mannitol reduces cerebral bulk by osmotic dehydration. An osmotic gradient is established between high plasmatic and low cerebral concentrations, which promotes the efflux of water across the intact blood-brain barrier [5]. However, the cerebral dehydration is a transient effect, and we found no significant reduction of cerebral water content four hours post-mannitol injection.

Multiple doses of mannitol are often employed for treatment of patients with cerebral edema. However, there exist concerns that mannitol may extravasate through damaged blood-brain barrier, and accumulate in edematous regions. It has been speculated that the osmotic gradient between plasma and brain may thus become reversed, and thereby promote the influx of water and increase cerebral edema [1]. Although this "rebound" effect of mannitol treatment has not been shown to occur following a single dose, we have demonstrated such an exacerbation of cerebral edema following five 0.33 g/kg doses of mannitol. Further investigations are required to determine whether the regional increase of water content related to multiple-dose mannitol has adverse effects upon local tissue pressure, perfusion and function.

In summary, our results are in agreement with previous observations that single-dose mannitol does not increase vasogenic edema. There is no doubt that its clinical use for transient reduction of the cerebral bulk is justified. However, we also observed that repeated mannitol injections lead to an increased cerebral water content in edematous regions. These results suggest that use of multiple-dose mannitol in clinical practice should be reconsidered. The beneficial effects must be weighed against the potentially adverse effects of the exacerbated cerebral edema.

Acknowledgements. Project funded by grant from the Department of Surgery, University of Manitoba. We wish to thank Mrs. Monica Dajic for technical assistance, Mr. Tony Gauthier for technical advice, and Mrs. Karla Patterson for typing of the manuscript.

References

1. Klatzo I (1967) Neuropathological aspects of brain edema. J Neuropath Exp Neurol 26:1–14
2. Marmarou A, Poll W, Shulman K, Bhagavan H (1978) A simple gravimetric technique for measurement of cerebral edema. J Neurosurgery 49:530–537
3. Marmarou A, Tanaka K, Shulman K (1982) An improved gravimetric measurement of cerebral edema. J Neurosurg 56:246–253
4. Nelson SR, Mantz M-L, Maxwell JA (1971) Use of specific gravity in the measurement of cerebral edema. J Appl Physiol 30:268–271
5. Pappius HM, Dayes LA (1965) Hypertonic urea: Its effect on the distribution of water and electrolytes in normal and edematous brain tissues. Arch Neurol 13:395–402

Pharmacokinetic Analysis of Mannitol in Relation to the Decrease of ICP

H. TAKAGI, M. TANAKA, T. OHWADA, and F. TOMONAGA

Department of Neurosurgery, Yamato City Hospital, Yamato, Kanagawa, Japan, School of Pharmaceutical Science, Kitasato University, Sagamihara, Kanagawa, Japan

Introduction

Mannitol has been used for the reduction of raised intracranial pressure (ICP) for years, however, the most effective dose and the method of administration have remained controversial [2, 3]. One of the reasons is that the pharmacokinetics of mannitol has not been clearly understood in relation to the changes of mannitol concentration and serum osmolality and the decrease of ICP after the mannitol administration [1].

In this paper, we shall report the pharmacokinetics of mannitol analyzed by 2-compartment method assisted by computer, and discuss the correlations of these parameters with the changes of ICP.

Materials and Methods

Fifteen adult cats, average weight 3.7 kg, were anesthetized with intraperitoneal administration of pentobarbital (30 mg/kg), intubated and mechanically ventilatated with room air using a Harvard respirator. Mean arterial blood pressure and central venous pressure were monitored continuously. Arterial blood gases were examined and $PaCO_2$ was maintained at 30 torr.

The cats were placed in a stereotaxic head holder and bilateral frontal burr holes were made. Small rubber balloons filled with sterile water were inserted epidurally, one of which was used to raise the ICP and the other to monitor the ICP. The cisterna magna was cannulated to measure the cisterna magna pressure for a reference of epidural pressure. The cats were divided into 3 groups (5 cats in each group). 10%, 20% and 30% concentrations of mannitol were made and administrated intravenously at a rate of 0.667/kg/min within 15 minutes in each group of cats. The 10%, 20% and 30% mannitol administrations are equal to 1g/kg, 2g/kg and 3g/kg mannitol within 15 minutes infusion, respectively. In each group, mannitol concentration (mg/dl), serum osmolality (mOsm/kg), Glucose (mg/dl), BUN (mg/dl), Creatinine (mg/dl), Na (mEq/L), K (mEq/L), Cl (mEq/L) were sequentially examined for 120 minutes.

Pharmacokinetics of mannitol is known to fit best to the 2-compartment model analysis, so that parameters were analyzed according to the description of Yamaoka [4] assisted by personal computer, PC-9801Vm (NEC). Integral values of mannitol concentration difference, subtracted from the Central compartment (Cc) to the Peripheral Compartment (Pc), were calculated and the correlation with the changes of ICP was examined.

Results

After the intravenous administration of mannitol at a rate of 0.667 ml/Kg/min, mannitol concentration and extrinsic serum osmolality took the same time course showing the bi-exponential curve with distribution and elimination phases in each mannitol group (Fig. 1).

Mannitol pharmacokinetic parameters are shown in Table 1. $t_{1/2}\ \alpha$ (distribution half-time) of 30% mannitol group was smaller than that of other groups, but $t_{1/2}\ \beta$ (elimination half-time) was similar in each mannitol group. Vd (distribution volume) was highest in 10% mannitol group. AUC (Area Under the blood Concentration time) was significantly different for each group. The correlation coefficients of the integral values of mannitol concentration difference between the Cc and the Cp and the ICP levels for 120 minute were r = 0.2210 (10%), r = 0.6012 (20%) and r = 0.8421 (30%). Although, there was a tendency of the correlation coefficient to increase with increasing mannitol concentration, there was no strong correlation between them. On the other hand, during mannitol administration (15 min), there was a strong positive correlation between them (10% r = 0.9030, 20% r = 0.8469, 30% r = 8621). A stronger correlation was noticed when the ICP reached the lowest

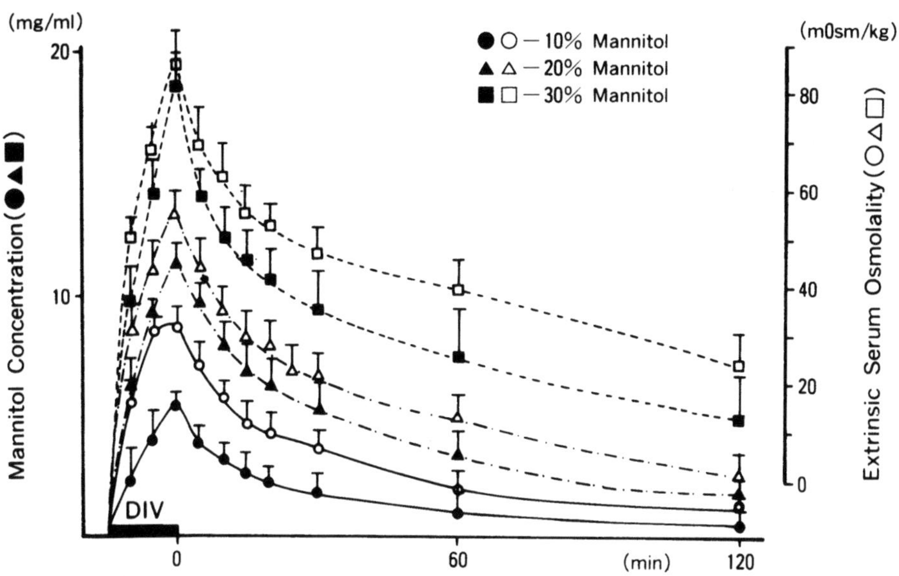

Fig. 1. Time course of mannitol concentration and extrinsic serum osmolality. Extrinsic serum osmolality = Actual serum osmolality − {18.6Na (mEq/l) + Glucose (mg/dl)/18 + BUN (mg/dl)/2.8} DIV: duration of mannitol administration

Table 1. Mannitol pharmacokinetic parameters in cats

	10% Mannitol	20% Mannitol	30% Mannitol
P(1) (g/l,min)	0.4685 ± 0.101*	0.6409 ± 0.307*	1.6629 ± 0.590
$t_{1/2}\ \alpha$ (min)	7.96 ± 4.25	7.75 ± 4.65	3.70 ± 2.79
$t_{1/2}\ \beta$ (min)	103.33 ± 40.24	60.23 ± 13.18	87.09 ± 19.07
Vc (l/kg)	0.1189 ± 0.0350	0.1221 ± 0.0237	0.0847 ± 0.0234
Vp (l/kg)	0.2357 ± 0.1059	0.0863 ± 0.0332	0.1206 ± 0.0166
Vd (l/kg)	0.3546 ± 0.1331**	0.2084 ± 0.0237**	0.2053 ± 0.0287**
K_{21} (min^{-1})	0.0357 ± 0.0330**	0.0560 ± 0.0240**	0.0942 ± 0.0410**
K_{12} (min^{-1})	0.0598 ± 0.0482**	0.0416 ± 0.0250**	0.1535 ± 0.0978**
Ke (min^{-1})	0.0332 ± 0.0162	0.0252 ± 0.0109	0.0231 ± 0.0082
AUC (min, mg/ml)	221.07 ± 85.47*	594.07 ± 98.97*	1146.79 ± 264.24*

* significant difference form each other, $p < 0.05$, (each group, n = 5 ± SD)
** significant difference between 10% and 30%, 20% and 30%, $p < 0.05$
$P(1) = Ko(\alpha - K_{21})/Vc(\alpha - \beta)$, Ko: infusion rate constant, $t_{1/2}\ \alpha$: distribution half-time, $t_{1/2}\ \beta$: elimination half-time, Vc: central compartment volume, Vp: peripheral compartment volume, Vd: steady-state distribution volume, K_{21}: first order rate constant form peripheral compartment to central compartment, K_{12}: first order rate constant from central compartment to peripheral compartment, Ke:elimination rate constant, AUC: area under the mannitol concentration time

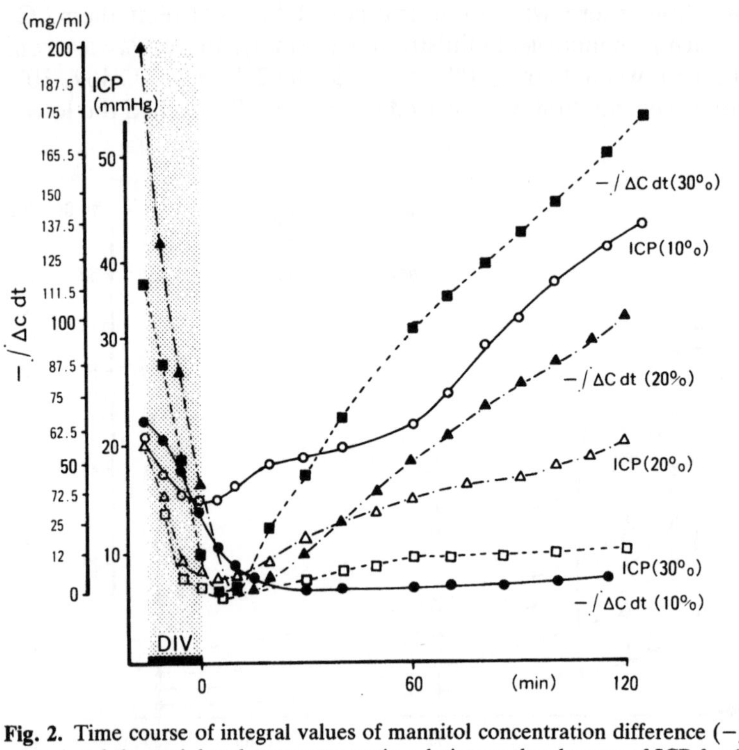

Fig. 2. Time course of integral values of mannitol concentration difference ($-\int \Delta cdt$) between the central and the peripheral compartment in relation to the changes of ICP for 120 minutes. Shaded area indicates the duration of the strong positive correlation between them. DIV: duration of mannitol administration

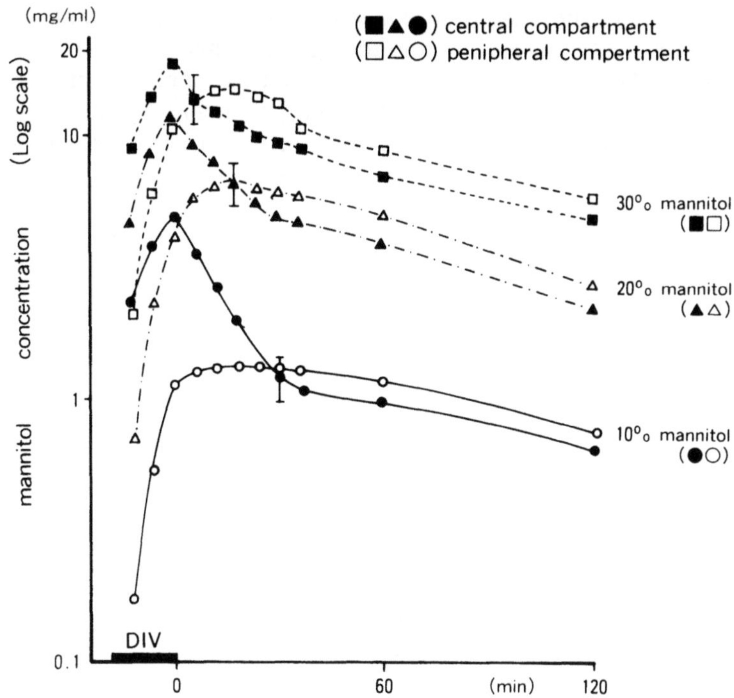

Fig. 3. Time course of mannitol concentration of the central and the peripheral compartment. Short vertical line indicates the time when the mannitol concentration difference between the two compartments equals zero. DIV: duration of mannitol administration

level (10% r = 0.9286, 20% r = 0.9038, 30% r = 0.9061). The results are shown in figure 2 as shaded area. The time for the mannitol concentration difference between the Cc and the Cp to disappear, became shorter as the administrated mannitol concentration increased (Fig. 3). It showed a strong reversed correlation (r = 0.9943) to the time when the ICP reached the lowest level.

Discussion

The disposition of pharmacokinetic parameters in cats was similar to that reported in dogs and humans [1]. Elimination half-time of mannitol was almost the same in each mannitol group indicating that the elimination of mannitol is independent of the administrated mannitol concentration. On the other hand, distribution half-time was faster in 30% mannitol group, indicating that the equilibrium of mannitol concentration between plasma and extracellular fluid is reached faster in high concentration of mannitol administration. This is also supported by the finding that the time for the disappearance of the integral values of mannitol concentration difference between the Cc and the Pc became shorter as the administrated mannitol concentration increased. In our experiment, the mannitol concentration and the serum osmolality changed proportionally in each mannitol group. This result contrasts with previous reports [1]. It has been emphasized that the speed of mannitol administration is playing an important role [2, 3], in producing the uncoupling of the time to reach the highest mannitol concentration and the time to reach the highest serum osmolality [1]. In our experiment, volume and infusion time of each mannitol group were the same, and only the concentration was different. This may be the reason why our data showed synchronous changes of mannitol concentration and serum osmolality. It was an unexpected result that there was no strong correlation between the integral values of mannitol concentration difference between the Cc and the Pc, and the changes of ICP, if they were matched during 120 minutes. However, there was a strong positive correlation between them, if they were matched during the time the mannitol was infused, and even more strongly, if they were matched during the time that the ICP reached the lowest level. The time for the mannitol concentration difference between the Cc and the Pc to disappear showed a strong reversed correlation with the time to reach the lowest ICP level. These results suggest that the driving force to decrease the raised ICP by mannitol administration is produced by the mannitol concentration difference between plasma and extracellular fluid, that is the difference of serum osmolality, during the mannitol infusion. The faster the mannitol concentration difference between plasma and extracellular fluid equilibrates, the stronger and the longer the reduction of ICP. Thus, not only the dose (g/kg) of mannitol, but also the speed (g/kg/min) of administration is the determining factor to decrease the raised ICP.

References

1. Cloyd JC, Synder BD, Cleeremans B, Bundie SR (1986) Mannitol pharmacokinetics and serum osmolality in dogs and humans. J Pharmacol Exp Ther 23:301–306
2. Marshall LF, Smith RW, Rausher LA, Shapiro HM (1978) Mannitol dose requirements in brain injured patients. J Neurosurg 48:169–172
3. Roberts PA, Pollay M, Engles C, Pendleton B, Reynolds E, Stevens FL (1987) Effect on intercranial pressure of furosemide combined with various dose and administration rates of mannitol. J Neurosurg 66:440–446
4. Yamaoka K (1984) Method of pharmacokinetic analysis by personal computer. Nanzando, Tokyo

The Early Role of Mannitol-Induced Hemodynamic Changes in the Control of Intracranial Hypertension

M. Abou-Madi[1], D. Trop[1], and P. Ravussin[2]

[1] Department of Neuro-Anesthesia, Montreal Neurological Institute and Hospital, McGill University, Montreal, Quebec, Canada
[2] Centre Hospitalier Universitaire Vaudois, University of Lausanne, Lausanne, Switzerland

Introduction

Mannitol is frequently given to patients with critically raised intracranial pressure (ICP). Transient rises in ICP occur after mannitol infusion in patients with brain tumours and normal ICP [3]. In contrast, it has recently been demonstrated, in experimental animals [1] and in humans [6], that a bolus of mannitol rapidly reduces ICP in subjects with intracranial hypertension. It has also been suggested that the initial effects of mannitol on ICP derive from vascular rather than osmotic properties of the drug [2]. The present study was conducted to elucidate the relationship between ICP and the hemodynamic changes, following the rapid infusion of mannitol in two groups of patients: those with a normal ICP and those with an elevated ICP.

Material and Methods

Study Group

With institutional approval, five comatose patients (2 males and 3 females), aged 24–68 years (mean 48 ± 18.6 SD) who were given mannitol boluses for the control of intracranial hypertension, were studied. Two of these patients had sustained a major head injury and three had suffered a massive subarachnoid hemorrhage. In all five cases, 0.5–1.0 g/kg dose of a solution of 20% mannitol was rapidly infused over a period of 5 minutes. ICP was continuously transduced (Ladd M1000 pressure monitor) and recorded (Ladd Medilogic recorder) using the external auditory meatus as the zero reference point. Baseline circulatory data included heart rate (HR), mean arterial pressure (MAP), central venous pressure (CVP), mean pulmonary artery pressure ($\underline{PAP}$), pulmonary capillary wedge pressure (PCWP) and cardiac output (CO). Total peripheral resistance (TPR) and pulmonary vascular resistance (PVR) were calculated in dynes/sec/cm5. ICP and hemodynamic measurements were recorded 2, 5 and 15 minutes after the beginning of the 5-minutes infusion.

Control Group

Six patients (3 male and 3 female), aged 22–68 years, (mean 40.8 ± 18.8 SD), scheduled for intracranial tumour surgery and presenting with normal ICP served as controls.

Following the induction of general anesthesia, CSF pressure was continuously measured from an 18-gauge spinal malleable needle introduced between the third and fourth lumbar intervertebral space, mannitol 1 g/kg was infused and ICP and hemodynamic measurements were recorded as in the study group. Data were analysed using analysis of variance and Dunnett's modified t-test for multiple comparisons. P values <0.05 were considered to be significant.

Results

The results are presented in Table 1.

Study Group (n = 5)

15 mannitol infusions (2–5 per patient) given during the first 48 hours, were analysed. Means from each patient were determined; the data represent mean values of the means. In all patients, ICP significantly decreased without any initial increase ($p < 0.05$). The systemic hemodynamic response to mannitol

Table 1. Mean changes in ICP (mmHg), MAP (mmHg), HR (beats/min), CVP (mmHg), PAP (mmHg), PCWP (mmHg), CO (L/min), TPR (dynes.sec.cm^{-5}), PVR (dynes.sec.cm^{-5}) ± SEM, in group I (control group) and group II (study group) following a rapid infusion of manitol 0.5–1 g.kg^{-1} over 5 minutes

Parameters	Groups	Baseline	2 min of infusion	End of infusion	15 min
ICP	I	8.7 ± 0.8	9.8 ± 0.7	11.7 ± 0.8*	6.7 ± 0.3
	II	31.6 ± 1.5	26.5 ± 1.3*	18.9 ± 0.6*	13.0 ± 1.0*
MAP	I	82.7 ± 1.9	80.8 ± 2.0	79.7 ± 2.0	86.7 ± 2.7
	II	104 ± 2.8	98.2 ± 3.3	97.2 ± 3.4	95.2 ± 2.1
HR	I	75.1 ± 2.2	76.3 ± 2.2	78.4 ± 2.3	78.2 ± 2.1
	II	70.2 ± 3.9	69.5 ± 3.6	72.3 ± 3.9	72.7 ± 3.7
CVP	I	5.0 ± 0.3	7.6 ± 0.7*	9.3 ± 0.7*	6.8 ± 0.3
	II	7.9 ± 0.7	10.2 ± 0.8*	11.6 ± 0.6*	9.8 ± 0.8
$\overline{\text{PAP}}$	I	15.7 ± 1.0	19.0 ± 1.4*	21.5 ± 1.4*	19.2 ± 1.4
	II	17.1 ± 1.1	19.8 ± 1.2	22.2 ± 1.3*	20.1 ± 1.3
PCWP	I	5.8 ± 1.5	10.0 ± 1.7*	12.0 ± 1.5*	9.2 ± 1.2
	II	10.6 ± 1.0	13.9 ± 1.2	14.8 ± 1.1*	12.8 ± 1.0
CO	I	5.1 ± 0.2	5.8 ± 0.3	6.4 ± 0.3*	6.1 ± 0.1
	II	5.2 ± 0.6	7.6 ± 0.9*	8.7 ± 0.8*	6.7 ± 0.8
TPR	I	1225 ± 54	1028 ± 72	890 ± 57*	1059 ± 45
	II	1606 ± 177	1006 ± 111*	822 ± 75*	1118 ± 118
PVR	I	152 ± 17	122 ± 17	118 ± 16	132 ± 12
	II	103 ± 13	69 ± 10	73 ± 9	96 ± 12

* $p < 0.05$ within group

consisted of an early, statistically significant decrease in TPR which closely correlated with the early decrease in ICP ($p < 0.05$). Immediate decrease in MAP was also observed. ($p < 0.1$). HR remained unchanged. A significant increase in CVP, PAP PCWP and CO ($p < 0.05$) accompanied the drop in ICP, MAP and TPR.

Control Group (n = 6)

ICP increased during the infusion of mannitol, reached a peak at 5 minutes, and then gradually decreased ($p < 0.05$). The systemic hemodynamic response to mannitol consisted of a less significant and more gradual decrease in MAP and TPR. HR, CVP, PAP PCWP, and CO changes paralleled those of the study group.

Discussion

This study confirms in humans what has lately been demonstrated in a canine model of intracranial hypertension [2]. Mannitol given rapidly has several direct effects on the blood and the vasculature which may affect the ICP. Mannitol decreases peripheral vascular resistance by both direct and histamine-related vasodilatation [4]. The sum of these effects is a dose-related decrease in MAP with a concomittent increase in CO, CVP, cerebral blood flow (CBF) and volume (CBV). The effects on TPR and MAP, however, significantly differed between the 2 groups. In patients with normal ICP a modest fall of TPR and MAP was observed after mannitol; as for the initial rise in ICP, it could have resulted from the transient increase in CVP, CBF and CBV.

In contradistinction, the study group demonstrated a precipitous drop in ICP, TPR and MAP after mannitol, which vasodilatatory action and effect on resistance was very pronounced in the thightly constructed vessels of patients presenting with an increased ICP. As intracranial hypertension cancels out the capacity of the cerebral vasculature to autoregulate, any change in MAP is transmitted to ICP, with MAP itself being regulated by changes in CO and TPR. Similar rises in CO and CVP were noticed in both groups, although patients with increased ICP demonstrated a greater fall in TPR. This caused the MAP to decrease significantly more than in the control group and the ICP to drop without an initial increase. An alternative explanation for the early opposing effects of mannitol on ICP, observed in the 2 groups of subjects, may be sought in the analysis of the effect of arterial and venous pressure transmission on ICP. Under normal conditions, as the rate of pressure transmission is small, it can be neglected and ICP is considered to be mainly determined by venous pressure. However, in the presence of high ICP values, the ICP is essentially determined by the transmitted arterial blood pressure to the CSF, i.e. by the systemic blood pressure [5].

Conclusion

Our data indicate that rapid administration of relatively large doses of mannitol is safe in the presence of intracranial hypertension and suggest that the initial effect of the drug is reflecting for a large part hemodynamic changes.

References

1. Abou-Madi M, Trop D, Abou-Madi N, Ravussin P (1987) Does a bolus of mannitol initially aggravate intracranial hypertension? A study at various $PaCO_2$ tensions in dogs. Br J Anesth 59:630–639
2. Abou-Madi N, Katz J, Abou-Madi M, Trop D (1989) Effects of mannitol-induced hemodynamic changes on intracranial pressure responses in dogs. In: Hoff JT, Betz AL (eds) Intracranial pressure VII. Springer, Berlin Heidelberg New York, London Paris Tokyo Hong Kong, pp 463–465
3. Cottrell JE, Robustelli A, Post K, Turndorf H (1977) Furosemide and mannitol-induced changes in intracranial pressure and serum osmolality and electrolytes Anesthesiology 47:28–30
4. Findlay SR, Dvorak AM, Kagey-Sobotka A, Lichtenstein LM (1981) Hyperosmolar triggering of histamine release from human basophils. J Clin Invest 67:1604–1613
5. Ikeyama A, Maeda S, Ito A, Banno K, Nagai H, Foruse M (1978) The analysis of the intracranial pressure by the concept of the driving pressure from the vascular system. Neurochirurgia 21:43–53
6. Ravussin P, Abou-Madi M, Archer D, Chiolero R, Freeman J, Trop D, DeTribolet N (1988) Changes in CSP pressure after mannitol in patients with and without elevated CSF pressure. J Neurosurg 69:869–876

A Comparison Study Between Mannitol and Glycerol Therapy in Reducing Intracranial Pressure

R.J. Smedema, M.R. Gaab, and H.E. Heissler

Neurochirurgische Klinik, Medizinische Hochschule, Konstanty-Gutschow-Straße 8, D-3000 Hannover 61, Germany

Introduction

Intracranial hypertension is pharmacologically usually treated with osmotic diuretics [3]. Intravenous (iv) mannitol is most used [5]. Glycerol is an alternative osmodiuretic, which is effective both by the oral and iv route and gives nutritional support. Its main problem, hemolysis, can be avoided by reducing concentration and infusion rate [5]. The aim of this study was to compare the effectiveness of mannitol iv with oral and intravenous glycerol.

Clinical Material and Methods

We studied 14 patients (9 males, 5 females; ages: 21 to 55 years), who were all sedated and slightly hyperventilated (pCO_2 of 30–35). Diagnoses: severe head injury: 7, supratentorial tumor extirpation: 7. Intracranial pressure monitoring: miniaturized epidural pressure transducer (12 patients), ventricular catheter (2 patients). Systemic blood pressure, fluid balance, serum electrolytes and glucose were monitored. The following *regimens* were applied at random when ICP exceeded 25 mmHg: 1) mannitol 20% 0.5 g/kg iv in 30 min; 2) glycerol 10% 0.5 g/kg iv in 60 min; 3) glycerol 85% 0.7–0.75 g/kg oral (with equal volume of 0.9% saline). Analyzed trials: 102. Results were considered significant at $p < 0.05$ level. Additionally we determined changes in serum osmolality and drug concentration at short intervals in a separate group of 5 neurosurgical patients.

Results

Figure 1 shows the results for the following time-lags: 1) from starting treatment to the first visible ICP reduction, 2) from starting treatment to the lowest recorded pressure, 3) from starting treatment to the point, where ICP had returned to the initial level. Only in case of the third time-lag one of the therapy groups had a significant better result: with oral glycerol the duration of action was longer.

Figure 2 depicts the maximal reduction in ICP. The mean values for all 3 therapy groups differed statistically significant.

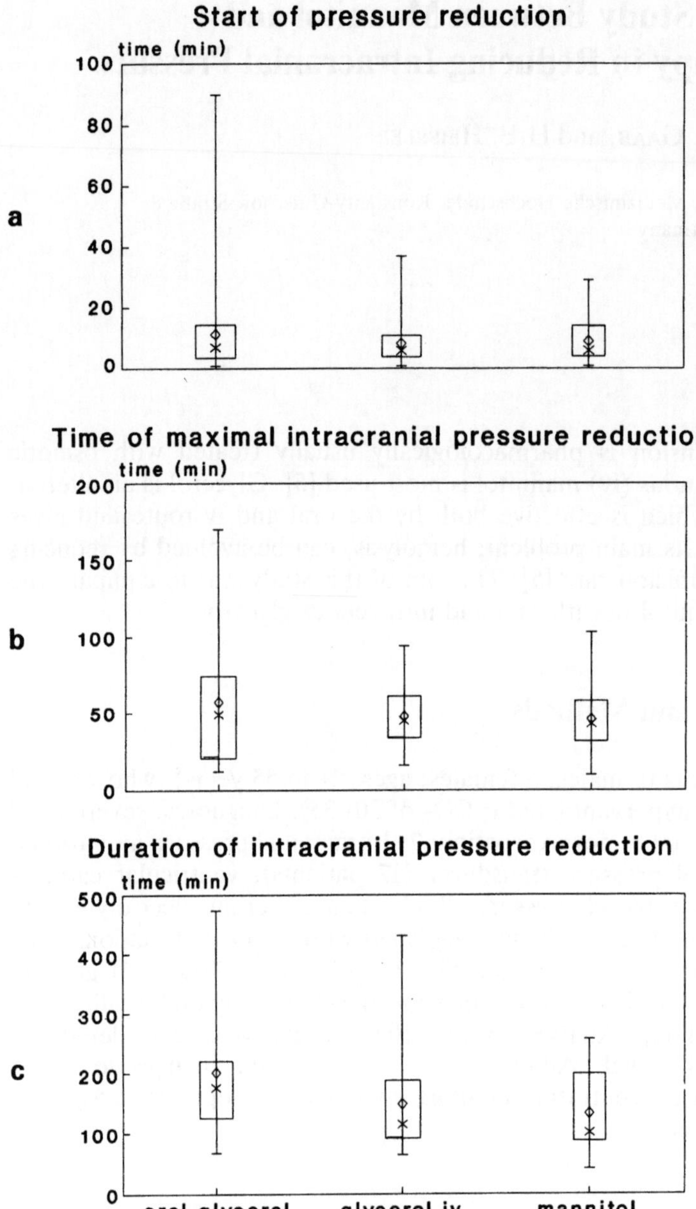

Fig. 1a–c. For data representation a boxes and whiskers graph is used, in which the mean is represented by a diamond and the median by an x. The box depicts the range from the first to the third quartile. The whiskers cover the range from the minimum to the maximum value. Start of ICP reduction, **a**: no significant difference. Time from starting treatment to the lowest recorded pressure, **b**: no significant difference. Duration of ICP reduction, **c**: significant results for oral glycerol only

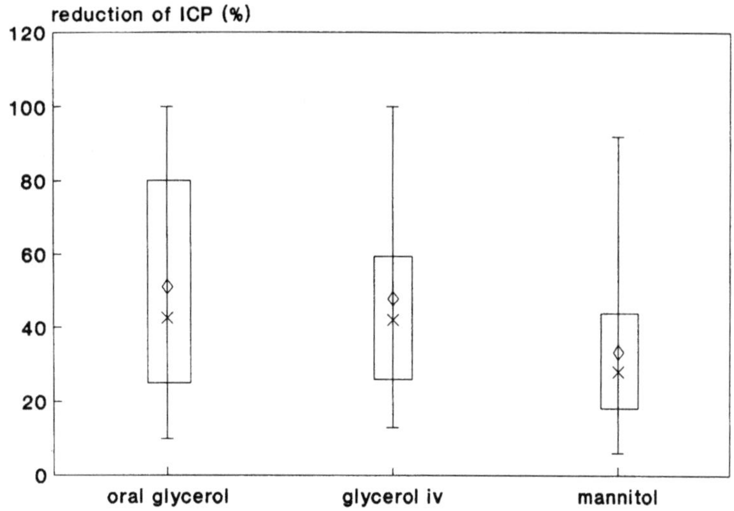

Fig. 2. Maximal ICP reduction: significant better results for oral and intravenous glycerol

The use of glycerol during the trials was not complicated by hemolysis. The *measurement* of *serum osmolality* and *drug concentration* during therapy showed a maximal rise in osmolality of 8 to 15 mosm/l (mannitol iv), 6 to 12 mosm/l (glycerol iv) and 14 to 25 mosm/l (oral glycerol). Maximal achieved serum drug concentrations were: 198 mg/dl mannitol, 70 mg/dl glycerol (iv group) and 160 mg/dl (oral group).

Discussion

When using osmotherapy we give small dosages, e.g. 0.5 g/kg mannitol in 30 minutes [1]. The changes in serum drug concentration and osmolality in this study support the idea that a rise in serum osmolality of about 10 mosm/l is sufficient to reduce ICP [4]. We compared the effects of an equivalent dose of mannitol and glycerol iv and found better pressure reduction for glycerol iv, in contrast to MacDonald and Uden [3]. The duration of ICP reduction was equally long in accordance with these authors. Oral glycerol caused with the same slope of pressure decrease a significantly larger pressure reduction and a longer duration of action. These results may be explained by the amount of osmoles given in each therapy regimen [2].

Conclusions

Comparing the effects of 10% glycerol iv, with 85% oral glycerol and 20% mannitol iv, we observed a greater and/or longer lasting pressure reduction when using the glycerol solutions.

References

1. Gaab MR, Bushe KA (1981) Die Behandlung der intrakraniellen Drucksteigerung. Intensivbehandlung 1981, 1:34–52
2. Hase U, Reulen HJ (1980) Wirkung von Sorbit und Mannit auf den intrakraniellen Druck. Neurochirurgia 23:205–211
3. MacDonald JT, Uden DL (1982) Intravenous glycerol and mannitol therapy in children with intracranial hypertension. Neurology 32:437–440
4. Marshall LF, Smith RW, Rauscher LA, Shapiro HM (1978) Mannitol dose requirements in brain-injured patients. J Neurosurg 48:169–172
5. Quandt CM, Reyes RA de los (1984) Pharmacologic management of acute intracranial hypertension. Drug Intelligence and Clinical Pharmacy 18:105–112

A Pilot Study on Postoperative ICP Control by Glycerin Combined with Lidocaine or Nitroglycerin

A. HIRAYAMA, S. YAMASAKI, and K. MIYATA

Division of Surgical Neurology Chifune Hospital, Tsukuda 2, Nishiyodogawa Osaka 555, Japan, and Department of Neurosurgery Takatsuki Hospital, 1-3-13, Kosobe, Takatsuki 569, Japan

Introduction

During our neurosurgical postoperative management, which inevitably enabled us to take closer observation on each patient, we had noticed that lidocaine and nitroglycerin, originally used to control cardiovascular problems, decreased ICP significantly, although this is reported by a few authors only [1, 4, 5]. This prospective study was carried out to evaluate the benefit from lidocaine and nitroglycerin combined with conventional dosages of glycerin in postoperative ICP control.

Patient Population and Methods

While in group A of 7 patients, steroids (Dexamethasone 5–10 mg intravenous injection, 3 times a day) were used together with glycerin (glycerin and fructose solution, maximum glycerin 200 g/day), in group B and C of 14 patients, lidocaine was administered to 7 patients and nitroglycerin to the remaining 7 during 2 weeks postoperatively. Lidocaine (10% solution) was intravenously administered by a continuous infusion pump at the rate of 1.5–3 mg/min but less than 300 mg/hr. Nitroglycerin (500 μg/ml solution) was also intravenously administered at the rate of 3–7 μg/kg/min but less than 25 mg/hr.

Although the protocol of the study was approved by a committee of our hospital administration board, the indication and dosage of the lidocaine and nitroglycerin was within precise and meticulous cost guidelines set by the Japanese National Health Insurance system.

Results

Group A (glycerin plus steroid): ICP decreased gradually in all cases in comparison with preoperative ICP, although statistically nonsignificant in 2 cases with higher ICP. The ICP in this group of patients was 38.6 ± 1.4 mmHg before the procedure, 2 hours after surgery. The decrease of the ICP, after 24 hours of the 5 cases, was 30.3 ± 4.8 mmHg.

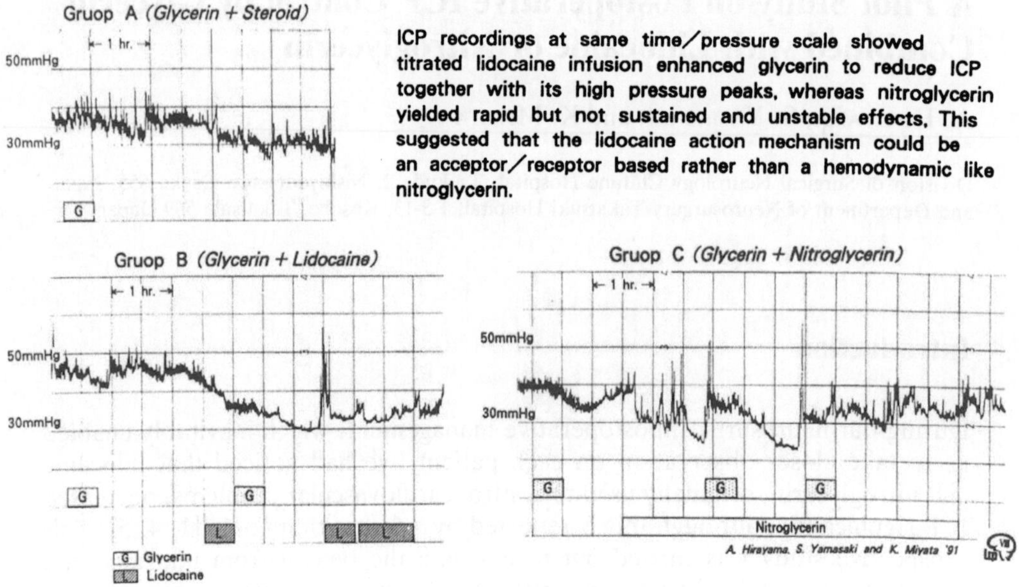

Fig. 1. Pressure recording with Lidocaine and Nitroglycerin accompanied by Glycerin

Group B (glycerin plus lidocaine): ICP decreased in association with a reduction of high ICP spike episodes. There was an increase in the dose required at later stages. The ICP in this group of patients was 37.8 ± 4.4 mmHg and the change in 24 hours was down to 28.9 ± 6.8 mmHg.

Group C (glycerin plus nitroglycerin): ICP decreased rapidly in 5 cases from 38.1 ± 2.8 mmHg to 30.7 ± 2.9 mmHg after 24 hours.

Discussion

Lidocaine has a depressant effect on the central nervous system [1]. A tolerance was developed in group B as shown by the figures. This suggests that its mechanism of action can be the same acceptor and receptor binding as with benzodiazepins. A similar delayed effect of lidocaine was already experienced by the authors in the case of continuous intraventricular administration in their "Therapeutic Hydrocephalus" treatment as previously reported [3].

Nitroglycerin relaxes vascular smooth muscle. Its hemodynamic picture is dominated by action on small postcapillary vessels because of its effects on cadiac output. In group C patients, the mean systemic arterial pressure was usually decreased, irrespective of the presence or absence of acquired tolerance. The mechanism of nitroglycerin action was hemodynamic as far as the ICP is concerned.

Summary

This pilot study showed that, in selected cases, nitroglycerin in continuous use with glycerin solution can be a potent tool in postoperative ICP control, whereas lidocaine in properly titrated dosage is better than the conventional use of glycerin alone particularly in topical use.

References

1. Bedford RF, Persing JA, Poberskin L, et al. (1980) Lidocaine or thiopental for rapid control of intracranial hypertension. Anesth Analg 59:435–437
2. Bradley PB (1989) Introduction to neuropharmacology, 1st edn. Butterworth, London, pp 119–120
3. Hirayama A, Yamasaki S (1989) Therapeutic hydrocephalus for postoperative delayed coma patients. In: Bhatia R, Bhatia S (eds) Book of Abstract 9th International Congress of Neurological Surgery. New Delhi, pp 370
4. Khayata M, Arbit E, DiResta GR, Lau N, Galicich JH (1989) ICP Reduction by Lidocaine: Dose response curve and effect on CBF and EEG. In: Hoff JT, Betz AL (eds) Intracranial Pressure VII. Springer, Berlin Heidelberg New York London Paris Tokyo, Hong Kong, pp 490–496
5. Rout A, Padmanabhan V, Rout D (1987) Role of lignocaine anesthesia in neurosurgery. In: Merry G (ed) Proceedings of the seventh asian australian congress of neurological surgery Brisbane, pp 184

Effect of Hypertonic-Hyperoncotic Solutions (HHS) on Increased Intracranial Pressure after a Focal Brain Lesion and Inflation of an Epidural Balloon

R. HÄRTL[1], L. SCHÜRER[1], C. DAUTERMANN[2], F. RÖHRICH[1], S. BERGER[1], R. MURR[3], K. MESSMER[1], and A. BAETHMANN[1]

[1] Institute for Surgical Research Departments of [2] Neurosurgery and [3] Anaesthesiology, Ludwig-Maximilians-University, Klinikum Großhadern, 8000 München 70, Germany

Introduction

Many trauma victims with hemorrhagic shock sustain head injury in addition to their peripheral injuries. As in other patients with shock, rapid resuscitation is lifesaving under these conditions. Small volumes of hypertonic-hyperoncotic solutions have been successfully used in severe hemorrhage for prompt restoration of the cardio-vascular function [3, 4]. The effects of this method, of small volume resuscitation, on the general circulation, are well understood, while little is known about its effects in the central nervous system. Among others, it is very important to obtain information on the effects or side effects, respectively, of treatment with the hypertonic-hyperoncotic solution on the intracranial pressure in the presence of a damaged blood-brain barrier and intracranial mass.

In the present investigation we have studied the effects of a small bolus of intravenous 7.2% saline/10% Dextran 60 on the intracranial pressure after traumatic brain injury and inflation of an epidural balloon as an intracranial mass.

Methods

New Zealand rabbits were anaesthetized with a-chloralose, tracheotomized and mechanically ventilated. Catheters were then introduced into the abdominal aorta and vena cava inferior for monitoring of arterial and venous pressure, for sampling of blood and infusion of fluids and drugs. The head was positioned in a stereotactic frame. An epidural screw was inserted through a 2 mm burr hole in the right hemicranium for continuous measurement of ICP. A cranial window was prepared over the left cerebral hemisphere and the epidural balloon was introduced.

After a control phase of 60 min., the focal lesion was made in the occipital cortex by freezing the tissue with a liquid N2-cooled steel rod (1 cm) for 2 min. The bone was reimplanted and fixed with dental cement. Sixty min later the balloon was inflated. Balloon volume was increased slowly over a period of 30 min until an ICP value of 15 mmHg was obtained. Balloon expansion was then maintained for the duration of the experiment. The first bolus of the small volume resuscitation was given through an ear vein 90 min after induction of the cold lesion, a second bolus was administred about 90 min later.

Results

Intracranial pressure was 3 ± 1 mmHg at baseline and rose radually to 8 ± 1 mmHg 60 min after induction of the cold lesion. The volume of the epidural balloon needed to maintain an ICP of 15 mmHg was approximately 0.27 ml. The infusion of the first bolus of HHS produced a marked reduction of ICP to baseline values. The ICP reached 15 mmHg (pretreatment value) again 88 ± 17 min after start of the infusion. The second bolus of HHS resulted in a less impressive decrease of ICP to 9 ± 1 mmHg. 74 ± 17 min after the start of the second infusion the ICP had again reached 15 mmHg.

Mean Arterial Blood Pressure was 88 ± 3 mmHg at baseline and averaged 83 ± 2 mmHg after infusion of the second HHS-bolus. It was not altered by inflation of the balloon.

As a limitation of the treatment with HHS the high concentration of sodium might be considered, although a small volume is given only. Measurements of the sodium concentration in plasma revealed an increase after infusion by 20 mM/l which, however, was normalized within 30 min. The second bolus of HHS led again to an increase in sodium by 25 mM/l, which was followed by recovery within 60 min thereafter.

The colloid osmotic pressure remained largely unchanged during the whole course of the experiment.

Carbon dioxide remained stable during all experimental phases.

The hematocrit decreased from an average of 40% to values of about 30 ± 1% after the first and 26 ± 1% after the second HHS bolus. This indicates an amount of fluid osmotically mobilized of approximately 27 and 25 ml, respectively, per 100 ml of blood volume.

Discussion

The current study demonstrates the effect of a small volume of resuscitation fluid containing hypertonic sodium, chloride and hyperoncotic dextran on the potential to decrease the intracranial pressure caused by an epidural mass and traumatic injury of the brain. Maintenance of an intact blood-brain barrier is paramount for the effectivity of hypertonic solutions to extract water from the brain [5]. On the other hand, it has to be considered that volume expansion by this form of fluid treatment with a hypertonic-hyperoncotic fluid might enhance formation of brain edema in the presence of blood-brain barrier damage [1, 2].

The results of the present study do not provide any evidence to support such a conclusion, however. On the contrary, the intracranial pressure could effectively be lowered for a limited period of time to the baseline value. Then, however, in relationship with the normalization of the osmotic equilibrium, as shown by the normalization of the plasma sodium, ICP was increasing again reaching its maximum at 80 or 90 min after treatment.

It is concluded that small volume resuscitation by hypertonic-hyperoncotic solutions which are highly effective to normalize cardiac output in hemorrhagic shock does not pose any risk in the presence of an open blood-brain barrier and intracranial mass. On the contrary, the current findings demonstrate that the intracranial pressure is acutely lowered, although the treatment cannot prevent the secondary increase caused by the persistence of the intracranial mass. Since patients with head injury are liable to develop ischemic lesions in the brain from a general circulatory failure, the method of shock treatment by the current resuscitation fluid might be adventagous to inhibit this important manifestation of secondary brain damage.

References

1. Gunnar WP, Jonassen O, Merlotti G (1988) Head Injury and Hemorrhagic Shock: Studies of the Blood Brain Barrier and Intracranial Pressure after Resuscitation with Normal Saline Solution, 3% Saline Solution, and Dextran-40. Surgery, No 103:398–407
2. Gunnar WP, Merlotti GJ, Jonasson O, Barrett J (1986) Resuscitation from Hemorrhagic Shock. Ann Surg Vol 204, No 6:686–692
3. Kramer GC, Perron PR, Lindsey DC, Ho HS, Gunther RA Boyle WA, Holcroft JW (1986) Small Volume Resuscitation with Hypertonic Saline Dextran Solution. Surgery Vol 100, No 2:240–247
4. Kreimeier U, Messmer K (1987) New Perspectives in Resuscitation and Prevention of Multiple Organ System Failure. In: Baethmann A, Messmer K (eds): Surgical Research: Recent Concepts and Results. Springer, Berlin-Heidelberg
5. Shackford SR (1990) Fluid Resuscitation in Head Injury. J Intensive Care Med 5:59–68

A Prospective Randomized Clinical Trial of Tromethamine (THAM) and its Effect Upon Outcome in Severe Head Injury

A.L. Wolf[1], L. Levi[1], A. Marmarou[2], J.D. Ward[2], D. Rigamonti[1], J.P. Muizellar[1], S. Choi[2], H.F. Young[2], and W. Robinson[1]

[1] Division of Neurological Surgery, Shock Trauma Center, University of Maryland, Baltimore, MD, USA
[2] Division of Neurosurgery, Medical College of Virginia, Richmond, VA, USA

Introduction

Tromethamine (THAM) has experimentally proved more effective than bicarbonate in resolving cerebral and cerebral spinal fluid (CSF) acidosis [5], which can irreversibly damage otherwise potentially viable brain cells, especially after head trauma [1, 2, 5, 6]. Clinically, THAM has been safely used in a wide variety of applications including head injury studies because it is not metabolized to any extent and is mainly excreted by the kidney. In the current trial, sustained hyperventilation was excluded and a prospective randomized study of THAM vs conventional treatment was implemented to evaluate the effect of THAM in the management of head injured patients using GOS as a primary endpoint. A second objective was to determine the effect of THAM in control of ICP.

Materials and Methods

During a period of 18 months each patient who had acute head injury (GCS $\leq$ 8 after resuscitation), aged 16–75 years, and was admitted to either MCV or the Shock Trauma Center (STC) of Maryland, was potentially enrolled into the study. Exclusions included pregnancy, chronic renal failure, admission creatinine clearance of 30 or less, requirement for massive blood transfusions, major visceral injury, or gunshot wound. In addition, any patient with a GCS score of 3 for whom only supportive measures were to be undertaken or failure to obtain consent was also excluded. Each patient was assigned for each treatment group by the opening of an envelope from two sets of envelopes each according to the motor score of the patient. The clinical parameters of these groups were matched in terms of age, sex, number with surgical mass lesions, number in each GCS stratum, mean GCS, and first ICP measurement.

All patients were intubated and artificially ventilated over the first few days. The pCO_2 level in all patients was maintained in the 33 ($\pm$ 2) mmHg range. ICP was monitored by ventricular catheter or Camino fiberoptic bolt; attempts were made to keep ICP below 20 mmHg by the following intervention sequence: skeletal muscle paralysis with Pavulon and sedation with morphine, intravenous mannitol, hyperventilation to levels of $PaCO_2$ of 28–30 mmHg, CSF drainage, and when these measures failed to control ICP elevation above 20 mmHg lasting longer than 30 minutes, barbiturate coma was instituted.

THAM was administered intravenously as a 0.3 M solution. Dosage was calculated by taking the baseline arterial blood gas sample and calculating the amount of base required to raise the Ph to 7.6 by multiplying the body weight by the base deficit. This was given over 2 hours and was followed by a constant infusion of 1 ml/kg/hr for 5 days.

Outcome was analyzed via the Glasgow Outcome Scale in which good outcome was taken as good recovery and moderate disabvility.

Differences between the two groups were analyzed by chi^2 tests, and the variance of the protocol's effect was calculated for covariates, using logistic regression analysis. The high resolution ICP data from MCV included hourly proportions of ICP measurements above 20 mmHg was transformed to arcsin square root for the analysis of covariance.

Results

The first bolus dosage averaged 4.27 cc/kg/hour (range, 1 to 11 cc/kg/hour) and was given at a median time of 354 min postinjury (range, 83 to 720 min). Rate of complications was similar in both groups.

Forty-five (25 in the control group – 32.9%, 20 in the THAM group – 27.4%) died in the initial hospitalization period (median, 3 days postinjury; range, 1 to 91 days postinjury). Overall, there was no difference in any time in the outcome between patients in the control and THAM groups.

ICP data showed that patients in the THAM group had fewer episodes of ICP elevation than those in the control group; in fact only 18.2% of the first 48 hourly measurements were above 20 mmHg in the MCV THAM patients compared to 34.2% of the measurements of the control group ($p < 0.05$). The rate of patients needing hyperventilation was significantly higher among the control group and the mean pCO_2 beginning on day 4 was significantly lower compared to all the patients in the THAM group ($p < 0.05$). Further, formal barbiturate coma was required for control of ICP in 18.42% of the patients in the control group versus 5.48% of those in the THAM group ($X^2 = 4.71$, $p < 0.05$). Uncontrollable elevated ICP was the main cause of death in 73.7% and 36.4%, respectively ($p < 0.05$).

Discussion

The control and THAM groups in this study, consisting of 79 and 76 randomly and prospectively assigned patients, respectively, were matched in terms of most of the clinical variables known to affect outcome, including age, GCS score, signs of brainstem dysfunction, presence of surgical mass lesions, and occurrence of prehospital insults (such as hypoxia and hypotension). Our analysis showed no overall difference in GOS between control and THAM

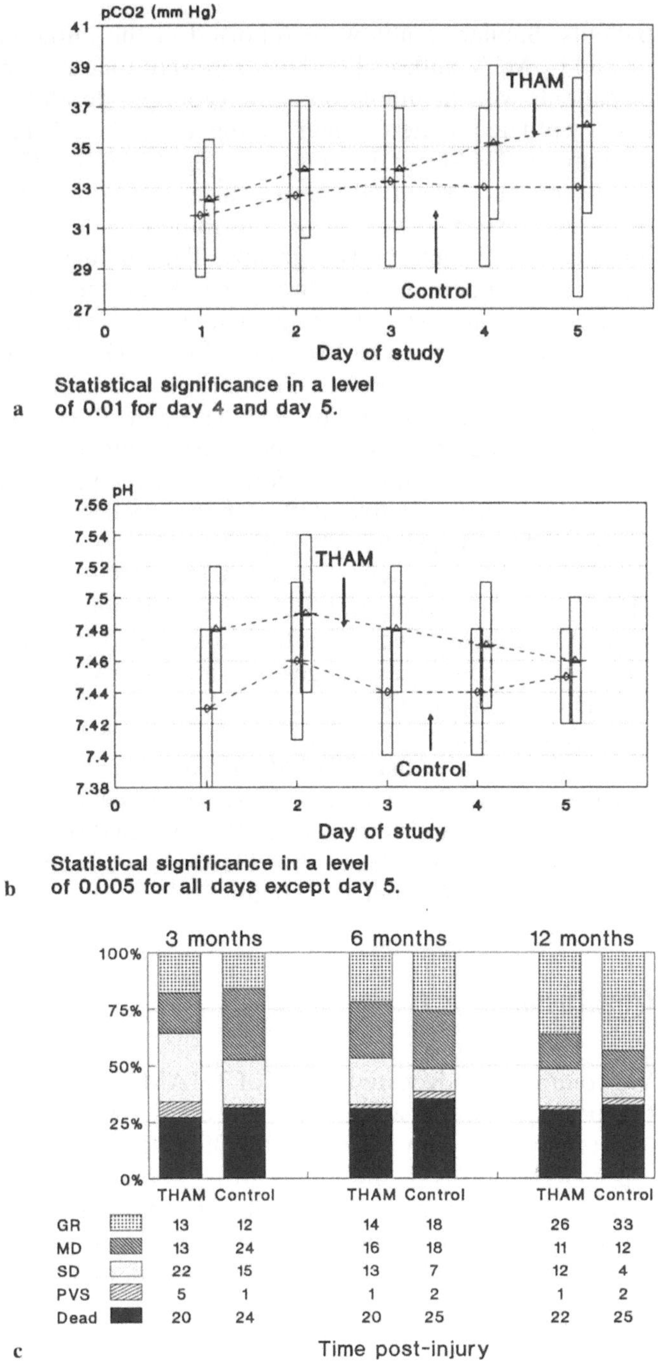

Fig. 1. **a** pCO_2 levels during the study days in both control and THAM groups. Patients in the THAM group exhibited less effect from hyperventilation after day 3 when the difference was statistically significant. **b** The pattern of blood pH values also demonstrated THAM's alkalotic effect and the difference between the two groups was significant through day 4 of drug administration. **c** Outcome after 3, 6, and 12 months for both control and THAM groups

patients. Similar results were reported in the initial clinical THAM trial conducted by MCV authors [7]. They reported that at 3 and 6 months, the number of patients with favorable outcome (good/moderate) was significantly lower in hyperventilated patients than in the control and THAM groups. However, outcome of THAM patients was not significantly different from control.

In the study reported herein, variations in the drug dosage and the timing of its administration may have contributed to the lack of significant difference in outcome between the two groups. The loading dose varied greatly between patients, although it was always less than the total recommended loading dosage [4]. The mean loading dose in this study was 4.27 cc/kg/hr versus reported dosages of up to 16 cc/kg/hr [3, 4]. The protocol expectation of pH up to 7.6 was not accomplished in either the control or the THAM group. The timing of drug administration was also crucial as long-standing elevated ICP and brain tissue acidosis were shown to adversely affect the outcome.

A statistically significant difference between the two groups in the measures to manage uncontrollable ICP and the need for barbiturate coma (18.42% versus 5.48%, respectively) was observed ($p < 0.05$). This observation is consistent with improved management of ICP reported by others [4]. The MCV analysis of temporal ICP data collected continuously revealed a significant treatment effect upon the transformed ICP response ($p < 0.018$) after adjusting for covariates, suggesting that THAM may be beneficial in preventing the elevation of ICP.

The mechanism by which THAM reduces ICP is not clearly understood. One explanation is that THAM increases the CSF capacity of buffering pH changes with $PaCO_2$ changes. This would be reflected in improved volume pressure status and attenuated ICP fluctuation. Experimental studies of traumatic injury have shown that THAM was effective in reducing brain edema as measured by gravimetric technique [8].

Conclusions

We continue to advocate the use of THAM as an adjunct to other measures in the presence of persistent ICP elevation, especially if the patient requires hyperventilation with P_aCO_2 below 30 mmHg. Additional studies are needed, especially in terms of the timing of its application (earlier), the dosage to be used (higher), its use as a possible prophylactic measure for patients with severe head injuries, and its potential use for patients with less severe head injuries (GCS scores of 8 to 10). Careful monitoring of renal function is advocated.

References

1. Akioka T, Ota K, Matsumoto A, Iwatsuki K, Doi A, Okao S, Ninomiya K, Nishimoto A (1976) The effect of THAM on acute intracranial hypertension. An experimental and clinical study. In: Beks JWF, Bosch DA, Brook M (eds): Intracranial Pressure III. Springer, Berlin Heidelberg New York Tokyo, pp 219–223
2. Gaab M, Knoblich OE, Sphor Al(1980) Effects of THAM on ICP, EEG and tissue edema parameters in experimental and clinical brain edema. In: Shulman K, Marmarou A, Miller JD, Becker DP, Hochwald GM, Brock M (eds) Intracranial Pressure IV. Springer, Berlin Heidelberg New York Tokyo, pp 664–668
3. Gaab MR, Seegers K, Goetz C (1989) THAM (Tromethamine, "Tris-Buffer"): effective therapy of traumatic brain swelling? In: Hoff JT, Betz AL (eds) Intracranial Pressure VII. Springer, Berlin Heidelberg New York London Paris Tokyo Hong Kong, pp 616–619
4. Nahas GG (1963) The clinical pharmacology of THAM [tris(hydroxymethyl) aminomethane]. Clin Pharmacol Ther 4:784–803
5. Rosner MJ, Becker DP (1984) Experimental brain injury: successful therapy with the weak base, tromethamine. J Neurosurg 60:961–971
6. Rosner MJ, Elias KG, Coley I (1989) Prospective randomized trial of THAM therapy in severe brain injury: preliminary results. In: Hoff JT, Betz AL (eds) Intracranial Pressure VII. Springer, Berlin Heidelberg New York London Paris Tokyo Hong Kong, pp 611–615
7. Ward JD, Choi S, Marmarou A, Muizelaar JP, DeSalles A, Becker DP, Kontos HA, Young HF (1989) Effect of prophylactic hyperventilation on outcome in patients with severe head injury. In: Hoff JT, Betz AL (eds) Intracranial Pressure VII. Springer, Berlin Heidelberg New York London Paris Tokyo Hong Kong, pp 630–633
8. Yoshida K, Marmarou A (1991) Effects of thromethamine and hyperventilation on brain injury in the cat. J Neurosurg 74:87–96

Correction of CSF Acidosis and Craniospinal System Viscoelastic Parameters with Intrathecal THAM

M. KUKLANE, J. EELMÄE, M. ROOSE, and A.E. KAASIK

Department of Neurology and Neurosurgery, 2 L. Puusepp Street, 202400 Tartu, Estonia

Introduction

Cerebral injury and hypoxia produce extracellular lactic acidosis which can have severe secondary effects on the brain and hinder its recovery. Amelioration of brain acidosis and increased ICP by systemic buffering agents has been proposed as a method of treatment [1, 2, 5, 7]. As presumed by B.K. Siesjö [6], administration of base via the CSF route may also ameliorate CSF and cellular acidosis and so improve the conditions for survival or revival of cell function and structure.

The aim of this study was to investigate the possibility of the correction of CSF acidosis and craniospinal system viscoelastic parameters with intrathecal administration of trishydroxyaminomethane (THAM).

Materials and Methods

The study was carried out on 26 patients after severe head injury and brain infarction (Reaction Level Scale – RLS85 – greater than 3) during the first 36 hours after admission to the intensive care unit of Tartu University Hospital. Mean age of patients was 49.2 ± 18.7 and score of RLS85 6.0 ± 1.3. All patients were managed by a standard protocol that emphasized early surgical evacuation of intracerebral hematomas, controlled ventilation and monitoring of CSF pressure. Routine medications, except for barbiturates, were used to control CSF pressure. Computerized tomography (CT) scans were performed as soon as possible after stabilization. In lumbar CSF, internal jugular venous and arterial blood samples pH, pCO_2, pO_2, BE, lactate, pyruvate, lactic dehydrogenase (LDH), gammaglutamyltranspeptidase (GGT) were analyzed before, one and 24 hours after intrathecal administration of 5 ml 0.3 M THAM. Enzymatic activity was recorded using photocolorimeter Spekol and suitable kits from Boehringer. Acid-base parameters were determined with a Radiometer.

CSF pressure was measured through a lumbar catheter by the registration system (Transducer MP-4, Amplifier RP-3, both of them Nihon-Kohden and chartwriter PS-1-02). Using the repeated bolus infusion test method the craniospinal system (CSS) viscoelastic parameters were calculated; elastance (E), pressure-volume index (PVI) and resistance to CSF absorption (R).

Table 1. Changes in CSF, internal jugular venous and arterial blood pH, pCO_2 (mmHg), BE, lactate (mmol/l), CSF pyruvate (mmol/l), LDH and GGT activity (I.U.), CSF pressure (mmHg), craniospinal system (CSS) E (mmHg/ml), PVI (ml), R (mmHG/ml/min) after THAM administration (Mean ± SD)

		Before THAM	Time (hours) after THAM 1	24
CSF	pH	7.224 ± 0.089	7.636 ± 0.022*	7.351 ± 0.017*
	pCO_2	36.2 ± 3.1	16.0 ± 4.8*	35.3 ± 4.0
	BE	−12.3 ± 3.9	0.06 ± 4.9*	−6.8 ± 4.0*
	Lactate	3.8 ± 1.5	4.0 ± 1.5	4.9 ± 1.8**
	Pyruvate	227 ± 79	339 ± 76	249 ± 80
	LDH	140 ± 119	136 ± 117	159 ± 129
	GGT	3.3 ± 1.9	3.5 ± 1.9	3.4 ± 1.8
Arterial blood	pH	7.401 ± 0.086	7.422 ± 0.069	7.421 ± 0.068
	pCO_2	28.5 ± 2.8	28.7 ± 2.6	29.4 ± 2.7
	BE	−5.7 ± 4.4	−4.9 ± 4.6	−4.8 ± 3.7
	Lactate	1.7 ± 0.5	1.8 ± 0.4	1.6 ± 0.6
Internal jugular venous	pH	7.348 ± 0.061	7.371 ± 0.048	7.366 ± 0.052
	pCO_2	35.1 ± 3.0	34.4 ± 3.1	35.5 ± 2.7
	BE	−7.0 ± 4.6	−5.3 ± 4.3	−5.0 ± 4.5
	Lactate	1.8 ± 0.5	2.0 ± 0.4	1.8 ± 0.7
CSF	pressure	15.5 ± 6.1		13.5 ± 7.4
CSS	E	2.7 ± 1.3		2.1 ± 1.3
	PVI	11.4 ± 4.3		12.6 ± 5.4
	R	2.8 ± 1.9		2.5 ± 1.6

$^*p < 0.01$; $^{**}p < 0.05$

Results

The data of this study are presented in Table 1. One hour after the intrathecal administration of THAM, CSF pH increased, pCO_2 decreased. BE in CSF normalized or was alkaline. Twenty-four hours after THAM administration, higher CSF pH and lactate values were detected. No statistically significant changes were observed in arterial and internal jugular venous blood acid-bace, metabolites values and enzymes activity. However, higher pH values in internal jugular venous blood and CSF LDH activity were detected after THAM administration.

The effect of THAM on viscoelastic parameters of CSF was a normalization of elastance, but rapid decrease of CSF pressure and increase of PVI were not observed.

Discussion

The study showed that intrathecal administration of THAM causes pH alkaline shift and normalization of BE in the CSF. As THAM accepts hydrogen, it shifts the $CO_2-HCO_3^-$ equilibrium towards bicarbonate and lowers pCO_2. In addition, we found the CSF pH to be higher even 24 hours after THAM administration. In the same time, a remarkable decrease in CSS elastance, together with increased lactate, LDH and pyruvate values were detected. As previously shown [3, 6], evidence exists that raising extracellular pH may enhance lactic acid efflux from cells. From this point of view we can speculate that elevated lactate in CSF after THAM administration appears to be due to the lactate efflux from cells to the extracellular space. Since 30% of THAM is in the non-ionized form, it can cross the membranes and directly affect also intracellular acidosis [4]. Concerning this, it seems highly probable, that such therapy could be beneficial in cases of persisting ischemia due to stroke or trauma with cellular edema.

Summary

The effect of THAM after intrathecal administration was studied in 26 patients with severe CSF acidosis. It was concluded that THAM causes CSF pH alkaline shift and secondary efflux of lactate and increase of LDH activity, resulting in a decrease of CSS elastance and a reduction of the risk of ICP elevation.

References

1. Akioka T, Ota K, Matsumoto A, Iwatsuki K, Doi A, Okao S, Nimomiya K, Nishimoto A (1976) The effect of THAM on acute intracranial hypertension. An experimental and clinical study. In: Beks JWF, Bosch DA, Brock M (eds) Intracranial pressure III. Springer, Berlin Heidelberg New York, pp 219–223
2. Gaab MR, Knoblich OE, Spohr A, Bonecke H, Fuhrmeister U (1980) Effect of THAM on ICP, EEG and tissue edema parameters in experimental and clinical brain edema. In: Shulman K, Marmarou A, Miller JD, Becker DP, Hochwald GM, Brock M (eds) Intracranial pressure IV. Springer, Berlin Heidelberg New York Tokyo, pp 664–668
3. Mainwood GW, Worsley-Brown P (1975) The effects of extracellular pH and buffer concentration on the efflux of lactate from frog sartorius muscle. J Physiol London 250:1–22
4. Nahas GG (1963) The clinical pharmacology of THAM [tris(hydromethyl)aminomethane]. Clin Pharmacol Ther 4:784–802
5. Rosner MJ, Becker DP (1984) Experimental brain injury: successful therapy with the weak base, tromethamine. With an overview of CNS acidosis. J Neurosurg 60:961–971
6. Siesjö BK (1984) Administration of base via the CSF route: a clinically useful treatment of cerebral acidosis? Intens Crit Care Digest 3:5–9
7. Yoshida K, Marmarou A (1991) Effect of tromethamine and hyperventilation on brain injury in cat. J Neurosurg 74:87–96

Comparison of Thiopentone and Propofol at Two Rates of Intravenous Administration in Severely Head Injured Patients

P.J.D. Andrews[1], N.M. Dearden[2], and J.D. Miller[1]

[1] University Departments of Clinical Neurosciences and [2] Anaesthesia, University of Edinburgh, Western General Hospital, Crewe Road, Edinburgh, EH4 2UX Scotland

Introduction

During intensive care management of severely head injured patients undergoing IPPV sedation may be administered, to obtund paroxysmal ICP rises during therapeutic manoeuvres, and to treat persistently elevated ICP. The recently reintroduced intravenous anaesthetic, 2, 6 di-isopropyl phenol (Propofol), has attracted attention as a sedative in ICU both for general critical care patients and head injured patients [1, 3]. Propofol causes a decrease in CBF and CBV and is therefore of potential value in treatment of intracranial hypertension after severe head injury [6, 8]. However, there is concern that CBF is reduced more than CMR resulting in desaturation of cerebral venous blood [7, 8].

The aim of this study was to compare the effect of rapid versus slow infusion of Propofol and Thiopentone, administered over 20 seconds and 120 seconds on BP, ICP, CPP and jugular venous saturation ($SjvO_2$) as a measure of the ratio between $CMRO_2$ and CBF. Propofol 1.5 mg/kg was compared with Thiopentone 4 mg/kg.

Patients and Methods

This study was approved by the Lothian Health Board ethics of medical research committee. After informed consent had been obtained, ten severely head injured patients (GCS < 9) with untreated ICP less than 20 mmHg were studied. The mean age was 26 (17–41 years) and the average weight 62.1 kg (49–76 kg). Patients were ventilated to $PaCO_2$ 3.5–4.0 kpa and managed according to a standard regime. Continuous recordings of radial arterial pressure (BP), ICP (subdural Camino pressure monitor), arterial oxygen saturation (pulse oximetry), $SjvO_2$ (Oximetrix 3) [7], end tidal CO_2 (Datex capnograph) and biparietal cerebral electrical activity (cerebral function monitor; CFM) were made (only those patients with CFM lower edge voltage >5 uV were included in the study).

Vasoreactivity to CO_2 was determined by adding and removing one standard length of dead space ventilator tubing, $PaCO_2$ changing by 0.5 Kpa. Only those patients with preserved vasoreactivity were studied.

An aqueous 2.5% solution of Thiopentone or 1% Propofol emulsion was used and the effect of the hypnotic administration observed thereafter for 30 minutes or until return to pre-treatment values (whichever was greater).

The study had a structured randomised crossover design and treatments included. 1) A rapid infusion of hypnotic drug injected manually over 20 seconds, via the CVP line and flushed in with normal saline. 2) Slow infusion over 120 seconds administered by a Harvard double syringe driver. Start of hypnotic infusion was the moment when the CVP lumen dead space was calculated to have been flushed with hypnotic and the end was two minutes later.

Statistics

Data were analysed by paired Wilcoxon's rank sum test (W Test), Kolmogorov-Smirnov two sample test (KS) and two way analysis of variance (ANOVA) as appropriate.

1. Paired comparisons were made of the maximum changes in BP, ICP, CPP and $SjvO_2$ following hypnotic drug administration (paired W-test).
2. Throughout the 30 minute study period recordings were made every 30 seconds of physiological variables and subsequently the change from baseline of these variables calculated. In the case of CPP, change was assessed against a baseline of 60 mmHg. Differences were analysed using paired W test.
3. Kolmogorov-Smirnov two sample test was employed to assess the difference in distribution of the change in variables over 30 minutes between the infusion groups.
4. Integrated reductions in the physiological parameters were calculated for the 30 minute period of study and compared using W test.

* $P < 0.001$; ** $P < 0.05$; NS, not significant at 5% level; SD, Standard Deviation.

Results

Assessment was made of possible differences in the starting values of the physiological variables and CFM lower border voltage by ANOVA. There was no significant difference in the starting values of any of the variables in the four study groups. Routine transcranial doppler ultrasound showed cerebral vasospasm to be absent in these study cases.

There was some reduction in arterial pressure, ICP, CPP and $SjvO_2$ in all four treatment groups. When comparing *rapid infusion of Propofol*, *Pr*, and *Thiopentone*, *Tr*, Pr caused a significantly greater maximum decrease in mean arterial pressure (W test*). Over the 30 minutes of administration the total reduction in mean blood pressure was also greater in Pr group, but did not reach sigificance at 5% level (W test, KS test). The integrated reductions were similar (Fig. 1). Duration of effect was similar.

Significantly greater maximum reduction in mean ICP occurred with Tr (W test*), however, ICP reduction was similar when assessed over the entire period of study (W test, KS test) (Fig. 1). Integrated reductions of ICP and duration of effect were similar.

Maximum reduction in CPP was significantly greater in the Pr group (W test**) (Fig. 2). Evaluation over 30 minutes showed a greater decrease in CPP in Pr group but was not significant at 5% level (W test, KS test). Integrated reductions and duration of effect were similar.

Maximum decreases in $SjvO_2$ were similar. $SjvO_2$ fell in both groups and was sustained in Pr group for the period of study being significantly greater than Tr (W test*, KS test*). The integrated reduction was greater in Pr group (W test*) (Fig. 2). Duration of $SjvO_2$ reduction was longer in Pr group.

When given by slow infusion (Propofol slow infusion, Ps, and Thiopentone slow infusion, Ts) Ps caused a significantly greater maximum decrease in mean arterial pressure (W test*); mean BP change over 30 minutes, integrated reduction and duration of effect were similar (Fig. 1).

Maximum reduction in mean ICP was similar, however, analysis over the entire period of study established that the decrease in ICP was significantly greater in Ps group (W test**, KS test**). Analysis of the integrated reduction confirmed this finding. The duration of effect on ICP was similar (Fig. 1).

Greatest reduction in CPP was in Ps group (W test*). Average CPP over 30 minutes did not decrease below 60 mmHg in Ts group and integrated reduction (Fig. 2) was significantly greater in Ps group. Duration of effect was greater in Ps group (W test, NS).

Maximum $SjvO_2$ reduction was similar in both groups. $SjvO_2$ reduction assessed over the entire period of study was significantly less in Ps group (W test**, KS test*). The integrated reduction was significantly smaller in Ps group (W test*, Fig. 2). Duration of effect was similar in both groups.

Discussion

Propofol caused a greater decrease in blood pressure than Thiopentone. The rate of administration of both agents affected the magnitude of the decrease in blood pressure. This BP effect was reflected by the change in cerebral perfusion pressure. Although all four treatments resulted in a decrease in CPP, Thiopentone by slow infusion caused the smallest reduction in CPP, the average CPP for this group did not fall below 60 mmHg.

The patients in this study had intact vasoreactivity to $PaCO_2$ and maintained brain electrical activity and, therefore, were in the sub-group most likely to respond favourably to hypnotic drug therapy. Pinaud and others found Propofol to cause a small decrease in ICP in their group of 10 severely head injured patients with starting ICP less that 15 mmHg and postulated ICP reduction with this agent was mainly BP dependent [4, 5]. These results may be related to poor brain electrical activity as all had low Glasgow Coma Scores

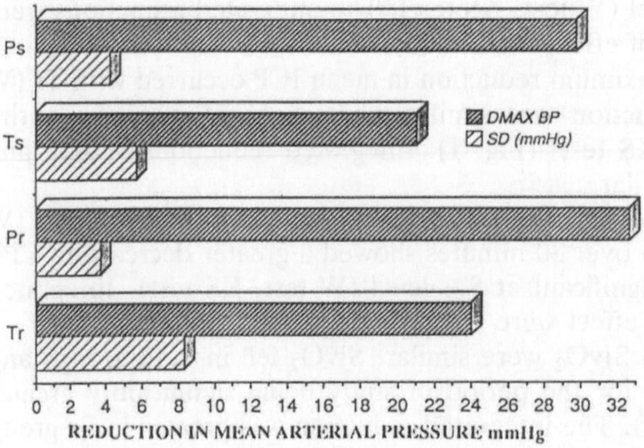

	Tr	Pr	Ts	Ps
AUC median	-557	-765	-533	-772
IQR (25-75%)	-205 -659	-657 -865	-262 -616	-557 -805

AUC = mmHg secs x 10^3

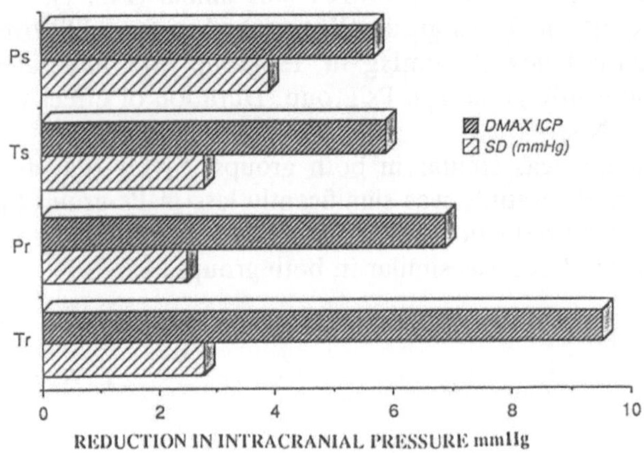

	Tr	Pr	Ts	Ps
AUC median	-49	-97	-53	-151
IQR (25-75%)	-18.9 -105	-8.7 -165	-27.9 -99	-18.9 -207

AUC = mmHg secs x 10^3

Fig. 1. Effect of Propofol and Thiopentone on blood pressure and intracranial pressure by the two rates of infusion. The effect on BP was greater with Propofol when compared within rate, BP effect was similar within drugs. The effect on ICP is superior with slow infusion of Propofol. (), standard deviation, [], interquartile range, IQR. Dmax, maximum pressure change from pre-treatment values = mmHg, $SjvO_2$ = % saturation. AUC, integrated reduction = area under the curve, mmHgsecs * 10^3 or $\%SO_2$ * 10^3, AUC, median value for the integrated reduction

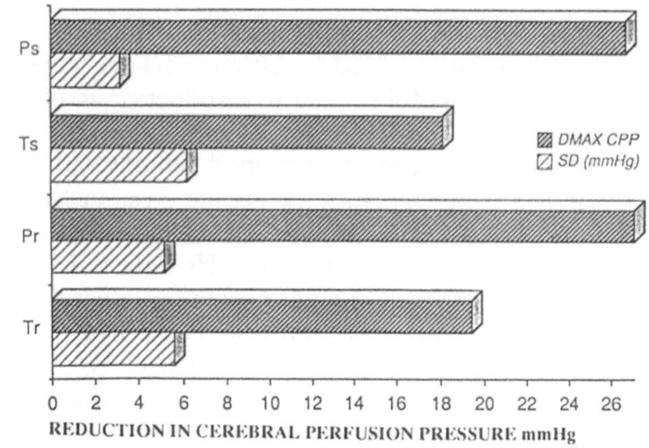

	Tr	Pr	Ts	Ps
AUC median	-191	-437	-39	-316
IQR (25-75%)	-4.5 -527	-0.3 -630	0 -58	-108 -443

AUC = mmHg secs x 10^3

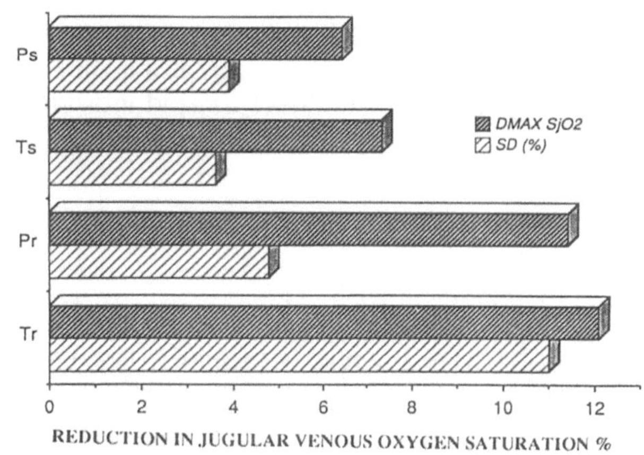

	Tr	Pr	Ts	Ps
AUC median	-29	-139	-50	-6.7
IQR (25-75%)	-10 -162	-22.1 -199	-21 -155	-3.6 -33

AUC = $\%SO_2$ secs x 10^3

Fig. 2. Effect of Propofol and Thiopentone on cerebral perfusion pressure and jugular venous saturation. Pr and Ps caused significantly greater decreases in CPP when compared within rate. The integrated reduction in CPP was less in Ts when compared within rate and within drug. $SjvO_2$ reduction was similar when compared within rate. The greatest reduction in $SjvO_2$ was in Pr. (), standard deviation, [], interquartile range, IQR. Dmax, maximum pressure change from pretreatment values = mmHg, $SjvO_2$ = % saturation. AUC, integrated reduction = area under the curve, mmHgsecs * 10^3 or $\%SO_2$ * 10^3, AUC, median value for the integrated reduction and had, until 12 hours before the study, received Thiopental by infusion further decreasing $CMRO_2$. Other workers have found a significant reduction in ICP with Propofol related to a reduction in $CMRO_2$, an increase in CVR [2, 6] and reduction in EEG [8].

In our experience a sustained increase in CPP in severely head injured patients invariably results in an increase in $SjvO_2$ provided $PaCO_2$ remains constant. $SjvO_2$, reflecting the ratio CBF/CMR, was least adversely affected in the Propofol slow infusion group. However, if CPP exceeds 60 mmHg, as in Ts group, $SjvO_2$ may not increase provided pressure autoregulation is intact. With the exception of the results from Pinaud [4, 5] other workers have shown a greater reduction in CBF than $CMRO_2$ [6, 7, 8], the peak effect occurring within 30–120 seconds of starting the Propofol and this is in agreement with our findings.

There is, therefore, a discrepancy between the CPP and $SjvO_2$ data in the two slow infusion groups, the best CPP response being in the Ts group and best ICP and $SjvO_2$ effect in the Ps group. When considering a therapeutic intervention in head injured patients cerebral hypoperfusion (detected by a decrease in $SjvO_2$ below normal) must be avoided. Of the treatments compared in this study, Propofol by slow infusion was most likely to avert increased cerebral oxygen extraction and compensated hypoperfusion despite causing decreases in BP and CPP.

Administration of hypnotic drugs for sedation or ICP reduction therapy should be by slow infusion possibly using zero order kinetics preferably while monitoring both CPP and $SjvO_2$. Rapid infusion is to be avoided.

References

1. Grounds RM, Lalor JM, Lumley J, Royston D, Morgan M (1987) Propofol infusion for sedation in intensive care: preliminary report. British Medical Journal 294:397–400
2. Herregods L, Verbeke J, Rolly G, Colardyn F (1988) Effect of propofol on elevated intracranial pressure, preliminary results. Anaesthesia 43:107–109
3. Newman LH, McDonald JC, Wallace PGM, Ledingham IMcA (1987) Propofol infusion for sedation in intensive care. Anaesthesia 42:929–937
4. Pinaud M, Lelausque JN, Fauchoux N, Chattanneau A, Chomarat P (1989) Effects of Propofol on cerebral haemodynamics and metabolism in patients with head trauma. Anaesthesiology 69, no 3A, (A 569)
5. Pinaud M, Lelausque JN, Chattanneau A, Fauchoux N, Menegalli D, Souron R (1990) Effects of Propofol on cerebral haemodynamics and metabolism in patients with brain trauma. Anaesthesiology 73:404–409
6. Ravussin P, Guinard JP, Ralley F, Thorin D (1988) Effect of propofol on cerebral spinal fluid pressure and cerebral perfusion pressure in patients undergoing craniotomy. Anaesthesia 43: 37–42
7. Stephan H, Sonntag H, Schenk HG, Koholhausen S (1987) Effects of propofol on cerebral blood flow, cerebral metabolic rate, and cerebral vascular reactivity. Anaesthetist 36:60–65
8. Vandesteene A, Trempont V, Engelman E, Deloof T, Focroul M, Schoutens A, de Rood M (1988) Effect of propofol on cerebral blood flow and metabolism in man. Anaesthesia 43: 42–43, suppl.

Propofol vs. Thiopental for the Control of Elevated ICP in Head Injured Patients

F. Merlo[1], P. Demo[1], T. Moretti[1], A. Digito[1], S. Barbacini[1], M. Visentin[1], and A. Landi[3]

[1] Department of Anaesthesia and Intensive Care Unit, and [2] Department of Neurosurgery, General Hospital, 36100 Vicenza, Italy

Introduction

In patients with severe brain injury the control of intracranial pressure (ICP) has considerable importance for survival and outcome. The first treatments usually include head elevation, hyperventilation, sedation and the use of steroids and hyperosmolar solutions. In cases where such treatment is not sufficient to control the rise of ICP, drugs such as barbiturates, etomidate, althesin and midazolam have been used, given their ability to decrease ICP by reducing the volume of cerebral blood. Recently, propofol, a new anaesthetic intravenous agent, the cerebrovascular effects of which seem to be similar to those of barbiturates, has also been used [4]. The aim of the present study is to evaluate the results of the administration of a single bolus of propofol compared to thiopental to control ICP in patients with severe head injury.

Patients and Methods

Ten patients, six men and four women aged between 18 and 64 years (average age 39) admitted to I.C.U. with brain injury and in coma ranging from 4 to 6 on the Glasgow Coma Scale, had their ICP monitored epidurally using a fiberoptic probe. All patients were on controlled ventilation in order to keep $PaCO_2$ at 30 mmHg and all were sedated with flunitrazepam (1 mg.i.v. every 4–6 hrs) and fentanyl (0.05–0.10 mg/h). In addition three patients were treated with a rapid infusion of 20% mannitol (0.2–0.3 gr/kg 4–6 times a day). When ICP remained constantly above 20 mmHg despite the above treatments, we injected a bolus of propofol (1.5 mg/kg. i.v.) over 30 seconds avoiding the simultaneous use of drugs that could influence the results. One hour later and at similar ICP levels, we administered a bolus of thiopental of 3 mg/kg. Before the administration of the drugs (baseline) and after 1-2-5-10-15 and 30 minutes, we measured the Systolic Arterial Pressure (SAP), Mean Arterial Pressure (MAP), Heart Rate (HR) and ICP; then we calculated the Cerebral Perfusion Pressure (CPP) according to the equation CPP = MAP − ICP. Statistical analysis was done using Student-T test (Paired) and multiple analysis of variance. $P < 0.05$ was considered statistically significant. All values were expressed as mean ± S.D.

Results

Before the administration of propofol the average values of the parameters examined were: SAP 147 ± 21 mmHg, MAP 87 ± 9, HR 81 ± 15, ICP 28 ± 6 and CPP 59 ± 9 mmHg. Almost identical values were found just before the infusion of thiopental, in particular ICP was 29 ± 6 and CPP 59 ± 10 mmHg. After the injection of propofol SAP and MAP decreased significantly ($p < 0.05$) within the first 10 minutes while, after the bolus of thiopental, MAP decreased only at the first minute. Over the same period HR increased more markedly after propofol than after thiopental. Both drugs were effective in lowering ICP significantly ($p < 0.05$) in the first five minutes after administration: there was no difference between the effect of propofol and thiopental. CPP was unchanged after the bolus of thiopental, whereas it decreased in the first minutes after propofol but this was not statistically significant (Fig. 1). It should be pointed out, however, that in four patients, during the first five minutes, CPP decreased to approximately 45 mmHg after propofol, rising to initial levels at the following measurements.

Discussion

After the first positive experiences in patients undergoing craniotomy, different dosages of propofol have been used in the treatment of patients with isolated cerebral lesions [1] and with severe head injury [3]. Some authors observed a significant change of the level of MAP, ICP and CPP after propofol, depending on the dosage of the drug and the basal level of ICP. They emphasized that in

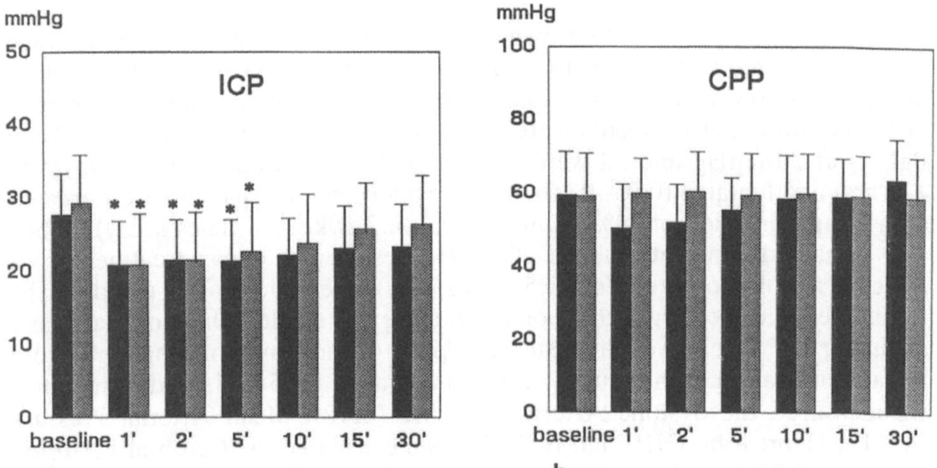

Fig. 1a,b. Effects of propofol (filled bars) and thiopental (hatched bars) administration on ICP (**a**) and CPP (**b**) in ten brain injured patients. Values are expressed as mean ± S.D. $^*p < 0.05$.

head injured patients with ICP > 20 mmHg, propofol (2 mg/kg) reduced MAP and ICP, without influencing CPP [5], in contrast with a previous report by Herregods et al. [3]. Very few studies investigated the effects of propofol on ICP in comparison with thiopental, especially in cases with preexisting increased ICP. Hartung noted after 1 mg/kg propofol and subsequently 2 mg/kg thiopental comparable effects of the two drugs on ICP and CPP, but blood pressure was markedly reduced by propofol and slightly by thiopental [2]. Our data confirm that propofol has an efficacy similar to thiopental in lowering ICP in patients with head injury and that it significantly decreases blood pressure in the first minutes after administration. CPP does not undergo statistically significant changes. We can conclude that both propofol and thiopental can be used in head injured patients with elevated ICP, but the marked cardiovascular side effects of propofol must be taken into consideration.

References

1. Hartung HJ (1987) Beeinflussung des intrakraniellen Druckes durch Propofol (Disoprivan). Erste Ergbnisse. Anaesthesist 36:66–68
2. Hartung HJ (1987) Intracranial pressure in patients with craniocerebral trauma after administration of propofol and thiopental. Anaesthesist 36:285–287
3. Herregods L, Verbeke J, Rolly G, Colardyn F (1988) Effects of propofol on elevated intracranial pressure. Anaesthesia 43S:107–109
4. Stephen H, Sonntag H, Schenk HD, Kohlhausen S (1987) Einfluss von Disoprivan (Propofol) auf die Durchblutung und den Sauerstoffverbrauch des Gehirms and die Co2-Reaktivitat der Hirngefasse beim Menschem. Anaesthesist 36:60–65
5. Weinstabl C, Mayer N, Hammerle AF, Spiss CK (1990) Effekte von Propofolbolusgaben auf das intrakranielle Druckerhalten beim Schaedel-Hirn-Trauma. Anaesthesist 39:521–524

Comparison of Sodium Nitroprusside and Labetalol on the Intracranial Pressure of Cats

S. Thiagarajah, E. Lear, and I. Azar

Beth Israel Medical Center, 16 Street @ First Avenue, New York, NY 10003, USA

Introduction

The commonly used antihypertensive agent sodium nitroprusside (SNP) increases intracranial pressure and causes tachycardia [1]. Labetalol (La) is also an antihypertensive agent with α and β advenergic blocking activity [2], but how it affects intracranial pressure in comparison to SNP has yet to be determined. We, therefore, compared the effect of La and SNP on the intracranial pressure and heart rate of cats.

Materials and Methods

Twenty cats (2.5–3.5 kg) were anaesthetized with isoflurane, the trachea was intubated and the lungs ventilated with a Harvard animal respirator. Femoral vessels were cannulated. The cats were placed in the sphinx position using a stereotactic frame with the interaural plane 127 mm above the level of the chest. The scalp and the underlying muscles were dissected and a 5 mm hole trephined in the left parietal area. A 7-French gauge catheter was inserted to the subarachnoid space and connected to a pressure transducer to allow the continuous monitoring of ICP. Ten cats were allocated to each of two groups. In one group, normal ICP (N-ICP) was maintained. In the other group, a 5-mm hole was trephined in the right parietal area and a 10-French gauge Foley catheter was placed in the extradural space. The balloon of Foley catheter was inflated slowly with incremental volumes (0.1–0.2 ml) of water at 5-min intervals until the ICP reached 27 + 2 mmHg and remained constant (AI-ICP). All trephined holes were made airtight with bone wax.

Anaesthesia was maintained with nitrous oxide in 30% oxygen and 0.5% isoflurane. Mean arterial pressure, heart rate (HR), ICP, ECG and endtidal carbon dioxide concentration were monitored continuously. $PaCO_2$ was maintained at 30 $\pm$ 2 mmHg (normocarbia for cats 28–32 mmHg); $PaCO_2$ was maintained slightly greater than 100 mmHg, pH at 7.35 ± 0.5. Rectal and brain temperatures were maintained at 37 ± 0.5 C.

After one hour of stabilization, the dose of La or SNP that decreased the blood pressure of each cat by approximately 30% was first determined, and this predetermined dose was infused for 5 minutes. La was administered to five of the normal intracranial pressure cats and to five with artificially increased intracranial pressure. An equal number of cats with normal intracranial pressure and artificially increased intracranial pressure were infused with SNP. Before and during infusion of the vasodilators, blood pressure, electrocardiogram and highest intracranial pressure were recorded. Measurements were taken at end expiration, and the zero-level for ICP measurements was referenced at external auditory meatus. Intragroup differences were analyzed by the student's paired t-test and intergroup difference by analysis of variance. P values less than 0.05 were considered significant.

Results

All experimental procedures strictly adhered to American Association for Accreditation Laboratory Animal Standards, and the protocol was approved by the Animal Use Committee of the hospital.

The results are summarized in Table 1. Labetalol did not affect the ICP of cats with normal ICP or of those with increased ICP. SNP increased the ICP of cats with normal ICP from 6 mHg to 7 mHg which was statistically significant but was within normal ICP range. In the group with increased ICP, SNP increased the ICP from 28 mHg to 40 mgHg, a significant increase. The blood pressure in all groups decreased by about 30%. The base line ICP and the BP were satistically not different in the two groups. Labetalol decreased the heart rate in all animals significantly, where as SNP increased the heart rate significantly.

Table 1. Blood pressure (BP) and intracranial pressure (ICP) in mmHg and heart rate HR in beats per minute

Normal ICP (n = 10)				
	Before –	Labetalol	Before –	SNP
BP	105 ± 7	*70 ± 8	110 ± 5	*75 ± 5
ICP	6 ± 0.3	6.2 ± 0.6	6 ± 0.2	7 ± 0.2
HR	162 ± 18	*147 ± 20	159 ± 20	*178 ± 12
Increased ICP (n = 10)				
	Before –	Labetalol	Before –	SNP
BP	112 ± 6	*77 ± 8	108 ± 5	*74 ± 8
ICP	29 ± 0.5	29.5 ± 0.6	28 ± 0.6	*40 ± 0.8
HR	165 ± 16	*146 ± 18	150 ± 12	*170 ± 20

* ($p < 0.05$) significant.

Discussion

Our study indicates that Labetalol does not cause tachycardia or rebound hypertension, nor is it associated with tachyphylaxis. In our experiment, there was no significant increase in intracranial pressure during La infusion for cats with normal or increased intracranial pressure, whereas, sodium nitroprusside increased the ICP of cats with artificially increased ICP. Labetalol has both α and β adrenergic blocking activity, but since the brain's vessels are deficient in α receptors, the blood vessels in the brain do not dilate when labetalol is administered, thus, the minimal effect of labetalol on intracranial pressure. We therefore conclude that if an antihypertensive agent is required in patients with intracranial hypertension, La may be an appropriate drug to select.

References

1. Tinker JH, Michenfelder JD (1976) Sodium nitroprusside: Pharmacology, toxicology and therapeutics. Anesthesiology 45:340–54
2. Weiner N (1975) Drugs that inhibit advenergic nerves and block advenergic receptors. The Pharmacological Basis of Therapeutics. In: Gilman AG, Goodman LS, Gilman A (eds) MacMillan Publishing, p. 197
3. Ganong WF (1987) Circulation through special regions. In: Ganong WF (eds) Review of medical physiology, Lange, California

Cerebral Hemodynamic Response of Sodium Nitroprusside and Esmolol

G.P. Lu, M. Peck, J.A. Gibson, Jr., E.A.M. Frost, and P.L. Goldiner

Department of Anesthesiology, Albert Einstein College of Medicine, 1300 Morris Park Avenue, Bronx, NY 10461, USA

Introduction

Sodium nitroprusside (SNP), an induced hypotensive agent has been shown to be a cerebral vasodilator and increase intracranial presure (ICP) [5, 7]. SNP hypotension has become a frequently used technique for various surgical procedures and during clinical treatment of hypertensive crisis [6].

Esmolol (ES), an ultra short-acting cardioselective beta-adrenergic receptor blocking agent, either alone or in combination with other agents has been used for both treatment of hypertension and to induce hypotension [1, 2]. However, there is little information concerning the effect of ES on brain microcirculation.

The present study was designed to determine the effect of SNP and ES intravenously or topically by simultaneously monitoring internal diameter (ID), and red cell velocity (Vrbc) changes in single pial microvessels and changes in calculated volumetric flow (Q) and ICP.

Materials and Methods

Rats, 200–250 g ($n = 48$) were anesthetized with pentobarbital (30 mg/kg). Femoral arterial blood pressure (BP) was recorded and blood gases and pH were maintained by controlled ventilation via a tracheostomy. Femoral vein was cannulated for infusion of drugs. A left parietal craniotomy with an encapsulated cranial window was prepared for biomicroscopy [4]. Changes in ID of three orders of arterioles (15–50 μm) were measured by image-shearing. In selected arterioles, Vrbc (mm/sec) was measured by dual-slit photodiodes and cross-correlator and Q ($\times 10^{-3}$ mm^3/sec) calculated [3]. ICP was measured through an outlet port of the cranial window.

Result

The infusion of SNP (35 μg/kg/min, 0.02% sol, $n = 20$) resulted in significant fall in BP (53.9%, $p < 0.01$), increases in ICP (22%, $p < 0.05$), arteriolar ID (33%, $p < 0.01$), and Q (48%, $p < 0.01$). Topical application of 0.2 ml of

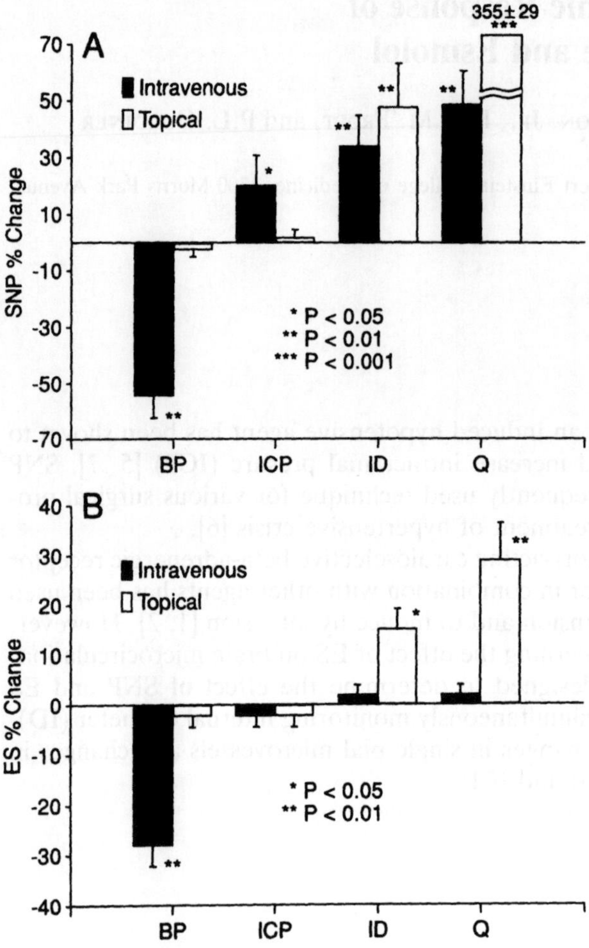

Fig. 1A,B. Bar graph represents blood pressure (*BP*), intracranial pressure (*ICP*), diameter (*ID*) and volumetric flow (*Q*) changes with intravenous and topical *SNP* **A** or *ES* **B**

0.01% solution of SNP (n = 8) resulted in arteriolar dilation (48%, $p < 0.01$) and increase of Q (355 ± 29%, $p < 0.001$) without change in BP (Fig. 1A). The infusion of ES (500 μg/kg, n = 12) bolus resulted in 28% decrease in BP ($p < 0.01$) with 2.5% isoflurane anesthesia. There were no additional changes in either ICP, ID or Q. Topical application of ES (0.01% in 0.2 ml, n = 8) showed increase in ID (15%, $p < 0.05$) and Q (28%, $p < 0.01$) without changes in other parameters (Fig. 1B).

Conclusion

The results show that SNP is a potent vasodilator (intravenously or topically) which also causes intracranial hypertension during infusion. ES alone is not a potent hypotensive agent. The desirable hypotension can be achieved by increasing the isoflurane concentration. However, despite topical vasodilating effect, ES may be a better intravenous agent to choose for patients with critical blood brain perfusion.

References

1. Edmondson R, Del Valle O, Shah N, Wong G, Dwyer D, Matarazzo D, Thorne A, Coffey C, Bedford R (1989) Esmolol for potentiation of nitroprusside-induced hypotension: Impact on the cardiovascular, adrenergic, and renin-angiotensin systems in man. Anesth Analg 69:202–206
2. Gold MI, Sacks DJ, Grosnoff DB, Herrington C, Skillman C (1989) Use of esmolol during anesthesia to great tachycardia and hypertension. Anesth Anal 68:101–104
3. Lipowsky HH, Zweifach BW (1978) Application of the "two-slit" photometric technique to the measurement of microvascular volumetric flow rate. Microvas Res 15:93–101
4. Lu GP, Kaul DK, Feldman SM, Orkin LR, Baez S (1990) Sodium nitroprusside (SNP) hypotension: Intracranial pressure (ICP) and hemodynamics in pial arteriole in the rat. Microcirc Endoth Lymphatics 6:315–341
5. Marsh ML, Aidinis SJ, Naughton KVH, Marshall LF, Shapiro H (1979) The technique of nitroprusside administration modifies the intracranial pressure. Anesthesiology 51:538–541
6. Michenfelder JD, Milde JA The interaction of sodium nitroprusside, hypotension and isoflurane in determining cerebral vascular effects. Anesthesiology 69:870–875
7. Stange K, Lagerkranser M, Solelvi AS (1989) Effect of sodium nitroprusside-induced hypotension on cerebral autoregulation in the anesthetized pig. In: Cerebrovascular Effects of Controlled Hypotension Induced by Adenosine, Isoflurane, and Sodium Nitroprusside. Kongl Carolinski Medico Chirurgiska Institut, Stockholm. V:1

ICP and Systemic Blood Pressure Changes After Administration of Prostaglandin E1 in Acute Stage of SAH

K. KAMIYA, N. YAMASHITA, N. SUGIYAMA, M. OHNO, and H. NAGAI

Department of Neurosurgery, Nagoya City University, Nagoya, Japan

Introduction

We have already experimentally clarified impaired autoregulation and CO_2 reactivity in the acute stage of subarachnoid hemorrhage (SAH). At the 7th ICP meeting, we presented the potential of Nitroglycerin (TNG) infusion to maintain systemic blood pressure (SBP) and its intracranial pressure (ICP). This time, we aimed to clarify the effects of prostaglandin E1 (PGE1) infusion on ICP in the acute stage of SAH, both experimentally and clinically.

Materials and Methods

Animal Experiment

Five Japanese monkeys (Macaca Fuscata) were used. SAH was induced by tearing the anterior cerebral artery (ACA) transorbitally. The detailed procedure was described elsewhere [1]. ICP was measured in the bilateral temporal region extradurally. SBP, Central venous pressure (CVP) and end-tidal CO_2 were measured. PGE1 was injected intravenously (0.5 microg/kg and 1 microg/kg).

Clinical Analysis

Five cases of SAH due to aneurysmal rupture, who were operated within 72 hours after SAH, had their ICP (EDP) monitored after operation. PGE1 (Prostandin 500) was infused continuously to maintain SBP (0.1–0.2 microg/kg/m).

Results

Figure 1 shows original traces of two animals. SBP fell from 100 mmHg to 80 mmHg (Mean SBP) immediately after injection (1 microgram/kg). ICP also decreased to 20 mmHg in accordance with SBP changes.

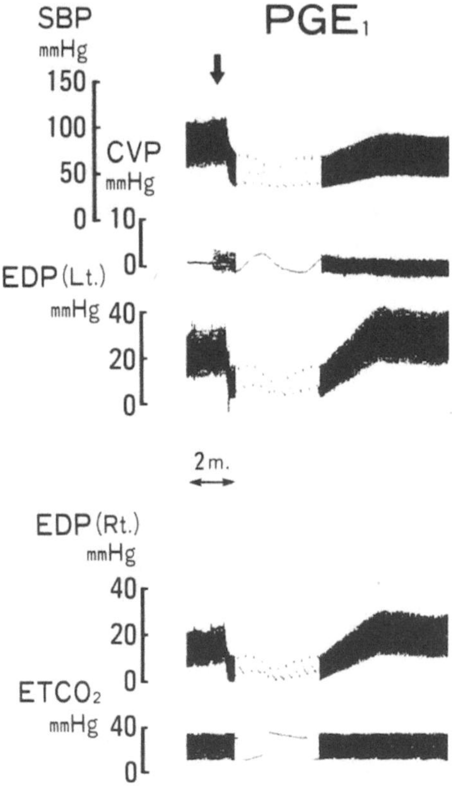

Fig. 1. Original trace of SBP and ICP changes after injection of PGE1 (animal experiment). (1 micro-gram/kg)

Figure 2 shows a typical case of SAH due to MCA aneurysm rupture. SBP was reduced to 120 mmHg mean after continuous infusion of PGE1. ICP values revealed the same pattern as in the experimental work. ICP and SBP rose gradually to pre-infusion levels after PGE1 infusion was stopped.

Discussion

At the previous ICP meeting, ICP VII, we reported that TNG reduced ICP when ICP had been blood pressure dependent, as after SAH. TNG increased ICP under normal conditions. PGE1 is a vasodilating agent acting on peripheral arteries mainly and reduces SBP dose-dependently. This drug does not dilate the cerebral vascular bed with resulting ICP elevation. Olesen reported that r-CBF increased when PGE1 was administered via the carotid artery [2]. It is still uncertain why ICP reduction took place; however, as far as SAH is concerned, reduction of SBP contributed to ICP reduction as did TNG

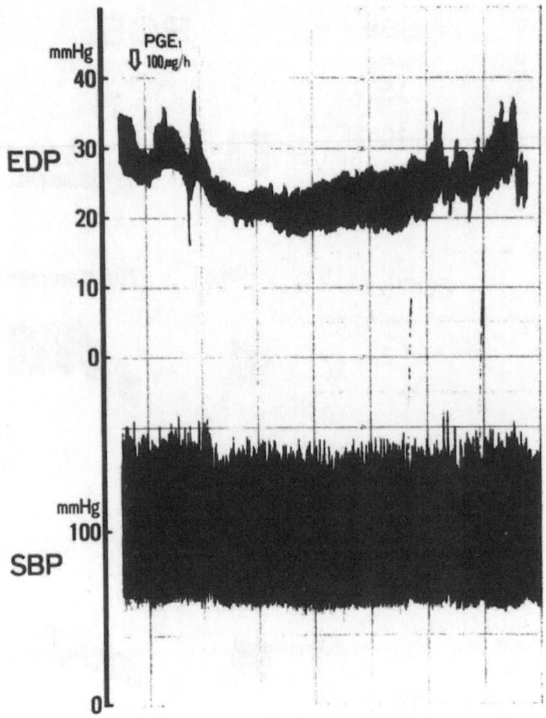

Fig. 2. Original trace of SBP and ICP changes after infusion of PGE1 (clinical case). (0.1 microgram/kg/m)

in the high ICP state. TNG increased ICP when the ICP was normal or slightly elevated. We examined this drug also in the high ICP state (more than 40 mmHg) and moderately high ICP state (around 20 mmHg) experimentally. In both states ICP was reduced corresponding to SBP reduction. We should like to perform further studies on cerebral hemodynamics after intravenous injection of PGE1. This drug might have features which are ideal for application in neurosurgical practice.

References

1. Kamiya K, Kuyama H, Symon L (1983) An experimental study of the acute stage of subarachnoid hemorrhage. J Neurosurg 59:917–924
2. Olesen J (1976) Effect of intracarotid prostaglandin E1 on regional cerebral blood flow in man. Stroke 7:566–569

Influence of Isoflurane on Cerebrospinal Fluid Pressure and Cerebral Blood Flow Velocity

A. Parma[3], E. Calappi[3], R. Massei[1,2], M. Caroli[4], M. Egidi[4], S. Balbi[4], C. Arienta[4], and G. Granata[4]

[1] Department of Anesthesia and Intensive Care, Civic Hospital Lecco (Co), [2] University of Milan, [3] Department of Anesthesia and Intensive Care, [4] Institute of Neurosurgery, University of Milan, Italy

Introduction

Inhalational anesthetic agents cause a reduction in cerebrovascular resistance and, at the same time, an increase in cerebral blood flow (CBF) resulting in a rise of the cerebral blood volume (CBV). Therefore, they induce an increase in intracranial pressure (ICP) that may be hazardous in patients with reduced cerebral compliance.

Since the increase in CBV has been experimentally demonstrated to be smaller with isoflurane compared with halothane and enflurane with 1 MAC at normocapnia [6], we can hypothesize that less changes in CBF occur during anesthesia with isoflurane.

The increase in ICP induced by isoflurane at normocapnia, mainly in patients with high baseline values, can be minimized or abolished by establishing hypocapnia. Conversely, hypocapnia should be established prior to introducing enflurane and halothane in order to avoid ICP increases [4].

Transcranial Doppler (TCD) sonography is a recently introduced non invasive technique to assess blood velocity in the cerebral vessels: cerebral blood flow velocity (CBFV) measurements have been shown to parallel changes in CBF [3].

The aim of the present study is to evaluate the effect of isoflurane on ICP and cerebrovascular reactivity to CO_2 using TCD.

Materials and Methods

Ten patients, ASA class 1 or 2, with supratentorial intracranial tumours, scheduled for neurosurgery, were recruited. The study was approved by the Hospital Ethical Committee and all the patients were informed and consented. Atropine sulphate, 0.007 mg/kg (im), was administered 45 min before induction of anesthesia. Cerebrospinal fluid pressure (CSFP) was evaluated using a lumbar needle. A 20 gauge catheter was inserted into the radial artery, before the Allen test, to measure arterial blood pressure (MABP) and blood gases. Cerebral perfusion pressure (CPP) was calculated as MABP-CSFP. Pressures were recorded in the supine position using a calibrated Statham strain-gauge transducer positioned at the lateral, middle thoracic level (MABP) and external auditory meatus (CSFP). Transducers were connected to a two-channel monitor (Sirecust 404-1, Siemens) and a strip chart recorder. Cerebral blood flow velocity (CBFV) was measured using a TC2-64 transcranial Doppler (EME with a spectrum analyser 64 Fast Fourier Transformation-FFT). Ultrasound signals were of low frequency (2 MHZ), the depth of signal varying between 25 and 135 mm. The probe was positioned on the temporal area between the zygomatic process and the ear. Following induction with Propofol 2 mg/kg and endotracheal intubation with Pancuronium bromide, 0.008 mg/kg, we initiated mechanical ventilation with an inspired gas mixture of 1.28% (= 1 MAC) Isoflurane, 70% air and 30% oxygen. Minute ventilation was set to produce hypocapnia ($PaCO_2$ = 25–30 mmHg) for ten minutes. Afterwards, normocapnia was maintained by adding CO_2 to the inspired gases and monitoring end-tidal CO_2 during the period of recording.

Statistical analysis was performed by SPSS/PC+ (Statistical Package for Social Sciences SPSS Inc). Differences between the means of the continuous variables analyzed were tested by Wilcoxon Matched-pairs Signed-ranks non-parametric test.

Results

The mean values of MABP, CSFP, CBFV, CPP, $PaCO_2$ and Pulsatility Index (PI) [(Systolic-diastolic velocity)/mean velocity] recorded during different time intervals of the study, are summarized in Table 1. In the hypocapnic

Table 1. CSFP, CBFV, MAPB, PaCO2, CPP, PI before (T1), and after Isoflurane 1 MAC administration during hypocapnia (T2) and normocapnia (T3)

	Basal (T1) mean ± SD (median)	sign.*	Hypocapnia (T2) mean ± SD (median)	sign.*	Normocapnia (T3) mean ± SD (median)
CSFP (mmHg)	13.7 ± 5.1 (14.0)	p = 0.012	10.4 ± 4.8 (10.5)	p = 0.005	21.4 ± 9.1 (20.0)
CBFV cm/sec	50.2 ± 11.8 (51.5)	p = 0.005	35.7 ± 9.2 (33.0)	p = 0.005	60.2 ± 18.1 (61.0)
MABP (mmHg)	98.7 ± 6.0 (100.0)	p = 0.005	78.4 ± 7.0 (78.0)	p = 0.313	80.1 ± 7.6 (79.0)
CPP (mmHg)	85.0 ± 7.5 (87.0)	p = 0.007	63.7 ± 16.5 (67.0)	p = 0.073	58.5 ± 5.6 (59.0)
PaCO2 (mmHg)	38.6 ± 1.3 (38.5)	p = 0.005	31.5 ± 2.3 (31.0)	p = 0.005	39.9 ± 2.0 (39.5)
PI	0.80 ± 0.20 (0.90)	p = 0.005	0.92 ± 0.22 (1.01)	p = 0.005	0.56 ± 0.11 (0.53)

* = Wilcoxon pairs

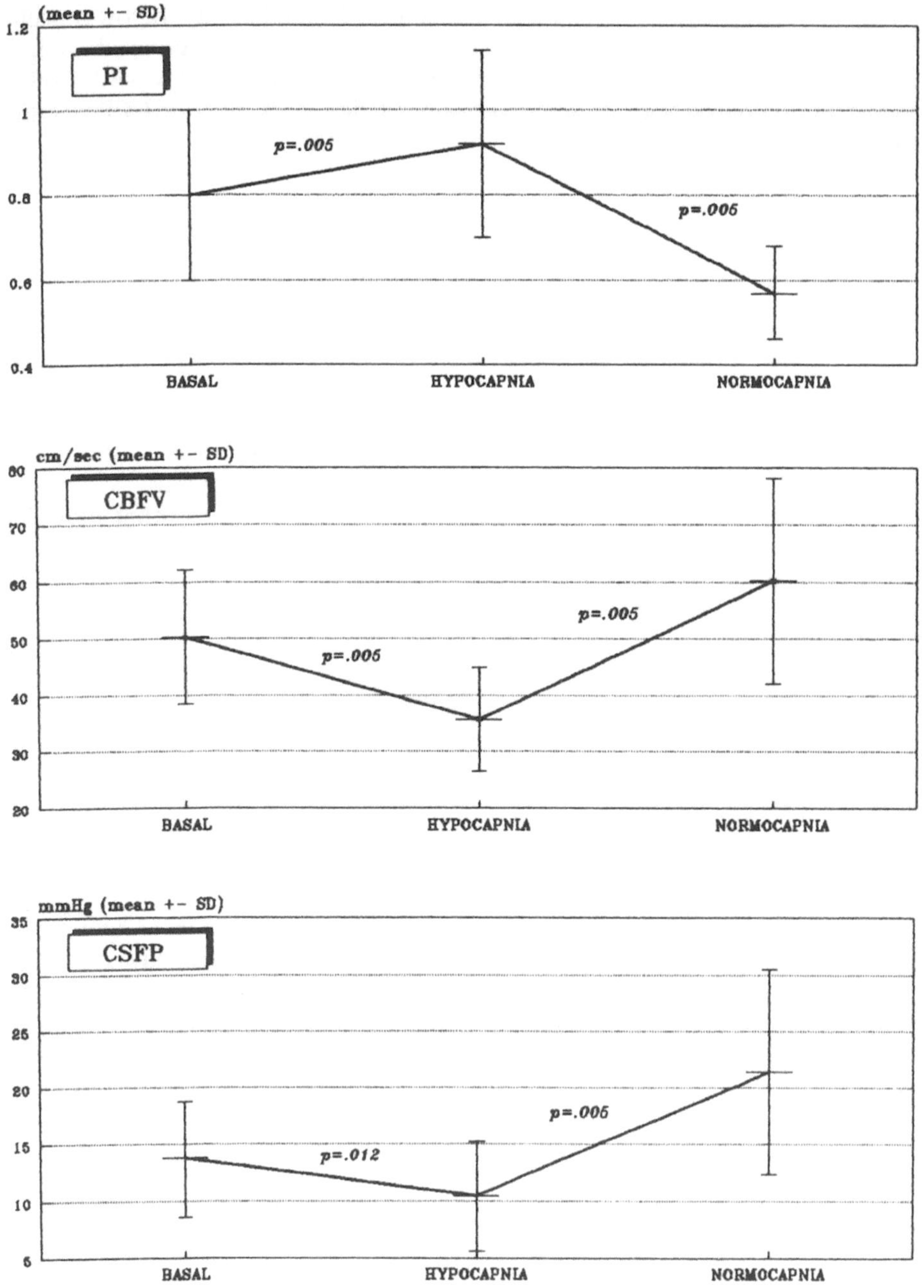

Fig. 1. CSFP and CBFV decrease during hypocapnia with Isoflurane 1 MAC versus PI increase. Reversed changes during normocapnia. Significance was calculated by Wilcoxon Matched-pairs Signed-Ranks nonparametric test

patients MABP, CSFP, CBFV, CPP decreased significantly below baseline values following Isoflurane administration, whereas PI increased. During normocapnia we observed a significant increase of CSFP, CBFV and a reduction of PI compared with hypocapnic values (Fig. 1). A further CPP decrease was also demonstrated.

Discussion

Isoflurane, like other volatile anesthetics, causes a reduction in cerebrovascular resistance and a concomitant increase in CBF, both dose-dependent effects. Cucchiara and Michenfelder (1974) reported not significant changes in CBF at Isoflurane 1 MAC and, conversely, a 60% increase at 1.7 MAC [5].

Our study demonstrates that CSFP is influenced by the use of isoflurane 1 MAC at hypocapnia and that it tends to increase at normocapnia.

These data confirm previous results of Campkin indicating that induction of hypocapnia should prevent the increase in ICP [4].

Studies from Artru et al. (1984) [2] showed that, with normal MABP values, hypocapnia increases cerebrovascular resistances by 82% and reduces CBF by 43%.

The significant increase in CSFP at normocapnia associated with a reduction in MABP induces a decrease in CPP with in our patients (with baseline CSFP elevated values) may reach the critical value of 50 mmHg. Therefore, both the increase in CSFP and the reduction in MABP may limit the use of alogenates as Isoflurane.

TCD data (as an index of CBF) demonstrates that CBFV changes parallel the CSFP changes, suggesting the significant influence of Isoflurane upon cerebrovascular resistance.

According to Giller, TCD can be an effective monitoring technique during neurosurgical operations providing a rapid and noninvasive assessment of autoregulatory capacity and vasodilatory reserve evaluated as response to changes in $PaCO_2$ [7].

Our results underline some fundamental points: 1) rise of CBFV after increase in $PaCO_2$ should prove that cerebrovascular reactivity to CO_2 is maintained during anesthesia with Isoflurane 1 MAC; 2) Isoflurane at this concentration and at normocapnia induces an increase in CSFP; 3) this increase is probably due to diminished cerebrovascular resistance, indirectly demonstrated by PI decline during normocapnia; 4) increase in CSFP and reduction in MABP require a close monitoring of the CPP threshold values.

References

1. Adams RW, et al. (1981) Isoflurane and cerebrospinal fluid pressure in neurosurgical patients. Anesthesiology 54(2):97–99
2. Artru AA, Colley PC (1984) Cerebral blood flow responses to hypocapnia during hypotension. Stroke 15:878–883

3. Bishop CCR, et al. (1986) Transcranial Doppler measurement of middle cerebral artery blood flow velocity. Stroke 17(5):913–915
4. Campkin TV (1984) Isoflurane and cranial extradural pressure. Br J Anaesth 56:1083–1087
5. Cucchiara RF, et al. (1974) The effects of Isoflurane on canine cerebral metabolism and blood flow. Anesthesiology 40:571
6. Eintrei C, et al. (1985) Local Application of Xenon for measurement of regional blood flow (rCBF) during halothane, enflurane and isoflurane anesthesia in man. Anesthesiology 63: 391–394
7. Giller CA (1989) Transcranial Doppler monitoring of cerebral blood velocity during craniotomy. Neurosurgery 25(5):769–776

Isoflurane vs. Nitrous Oxide: Impact on Cerebrospinal Fluid Pressure in Anesthetized Patients with Brain Tumors

R.S. JUNG, R. REINSEL, J.H. GALICICH, and R.F. BEDFORD

Department of Anesthesiology, University of California, Irvine Medical Center, Orange, California; Department of Anesthesiology and Critical Care Medicine and the Neurological Service, Memorial Sloan-Kettering Cancer Center, and Cornell University Medical College, New York, New York; and the Department of Anesthesiology, University of Virginia, Charlottesville, VA, USA

Introduction

Concern has been expressed regarding the use of both N_2O and isoflurane for neurosurgical anesthesia, since these agents cause increases in cerebral blood flow (CBF) [1, 2] that may produce undesirable increases in cerebrospinal fluid pressure (CSFP) [3, 4]. The present study utilizes a randomized, cross-over protocol to identify which of these agents, in equipotent doses, has the least effect on CSFP in brain tumor patients.

Methods

Twenty patients undergoing excision of supratentorial tumors were studied. The protocol was approved by our IRB and informed consent was obtained. Anesthesia was induced with thiopental, 5 mg/kg, in divided doses; vecuronium, 0.1 mg/kg, was used to facilitate endotracheal intubation; ventilation was controlled to maintain end-tidal CO_2 tension ($PetCO_2$) between 30–35 mmHg (Perkin Elmer Mass Spec). Patients were randomized to one of 2 anesthetics: Group 1 = 0.7% end-tidal isoflurane in oxygen, and Group 2 = 70% nitrous oxide in oxygen. Radial arterial and lumbar subarachnoid catheters were placed to continuously monitor blood pressure (BP) and CSFP, respectively; heart rate (HR) was recorded from EKG lead II. Pressure transducers were referenced to the level of the mid-cranium. Prior to surgical incision and during a period of stable BP and CSFP, the initial anesthetic agent was abruptly changed; Group 1 then received 70% nitrous oxide; Group 2 received isoflurane, 1–2% inspired, adjusted to 0.7% end-tidal isoflurane. Fresh gas flow rate was 10 l/min. CSFP, HR and BP were recorded for 20-min. End-tidal N_2O and isoflurane concentrations were tabulated and arterial blood gas tensions were determined just prior to changing anesthetics (T = 0 min) and at the end of the 20 min observation period (T = 20 min). Data were analyzed in two ways: a) changes between T = 0 and T = 20 min were compared within groups using Student's t-test for paired data, and b) repeated measures analysis of variance with orthogonal contrasts was used to compare mean values for CSFP during

Table 1. Measurements at beginning and end of 20 min observation period

	Group 1 (Isoflurane to N_2O)		Group 2 (N_2O to Isoflurane)	
	0 min	20 min	0 min	20 min
CSFP (mmHg)	9.1 ± 1.2	12.3 ± 2.2*	9.5 ± 1.1	9.1 ± 1.4
MAP (mmHg)	87.6 ± 4.9	89.9 ± 3.9	94.2 ± 5.7	87.2 ± 4.0
HR (bpm)	74.7 ± 5.0	70.4 ± 4.6	75.6 ± 3.3	71.8 ± 3.3
$PaCO_2$ (mmHg)	37.0 ± 1.4	34.2 ± 0.9*	35.1 ± 0.9	36.3 ± 1.3
%ET isoflurane	0.68 ± 0.01	0	0	0.71 ± 0.01
%ET N_2O	0	65.6 ± 1.1	67.8 ± 0.5	0

All values = Mean ± S.E. * $p < 0.05$ vs value at T = 0

successive five-minute intervals throughout the observation period. $P < 0.05$ was regarded as significant.

Results

Table 1 summarizes the baseline and final values for measured variables during the 20-min observation period. CSFP increased 33% in group 1, despite a slight decrease in $PaCO_2$. In contrast, there was no changes in CSFP in group 2. ANOVA showed that the changes in CSFP over time varied significantly between the two anesthetic regimens starting with the second 5 min interval after T = 0. Group*Time: $F_{(4,72)} = 4.33$, $p < 0.004$.

Discussion and Conclusions

These data suggest that, at equipotent concentrations, N_2O is more likely than isoflurane to cause increases in CSFP in patients with brain tumors. We conclude that isoflurane is the preferable to N_2O as an inhalational anesthetic for neurosurgical patients with brain tumors.

References

1. Hansen TD, Warner DS, Todd MM, Vust LJ (1989) Effects of nitrous oxide and volatile anesthetics on cerebral blood flow. Br J Anesth 63:290–295
2. Archer DP, Labrecque P, Tyler JL, Meyer E, Trop D (1987) Cerebral Blood Volume is Increased in Dogs during Administration of Nitrous Oxide or Isoflurane. Anesthesiology 67:642–648
3. Henriksen HT, Balslev Jörgensen P (1973) The Effect of Nitrous Oxide on Intracranial Pressure in Patients with Intracranial Disorders. Brit J Anesth 45:486–496
4. Grosslight K, Foster R, Colohan AR, Bedford RF (1985) Isoflurane for Neuroanesthesia: Risk Factors for Increases in Intracranial Pressure. Anesthesiology 63:533–536

Influence of Anesthetic Agents on the Regional Cerebral Blood Flow in Rabbits with a Focal Cerebral Lesion and General Hypoxia*

R. MURR[1], L. SCHÜRER[2], S. BERGER[2], R. ENZENBACH[1], K. PETER[1], and A. BAETHMANN[2]

[1] Institute for Anesthesiology and [2] Institute for Surgical Research, Klinikum Großhadern, Ludwig-Maximilians-Universitaire, 8000 München 70, Germany

Introduction

Secondary brain damage is a major determinant of morbidity and mortality in patients with severe head injury. Shock or hypoxia after trauma are the most important extracerebral factors, which affect outcome [4]. Patients with severe head injury often require anesthesia for diagnostic or surgical procedures. Anesthetic agents may either exert cerebroprotective effects by a decrease of brain metabolism or elevate the intracranial pressure by an increase of cerebral blood flow. We have analyzed the effect of various anesthetic agents on rCBF after a focal cerebral lesion combined with systemic hypoxia.

Methods

New Zealand white rabbits (n = 6 per group) were anesthetized after induction by thiopental either with isoflurane (I) (1 MAC, 2.1 Vol%), fentanyl (F) (1.0 μg/kg b.w. × min for 90 min, thereafter 0.5 μg/kg b.w. × min), thiopental (T) (28.8 mg/kg b.w. × h), or α-chloralose (C) (50 mg/kg b.w.). Mean arterial pressure (MAP), central venous pressure, hematocrit (Hct), and arterial blood gases were monitored by arterial and venous femoral catheters. Animals with isoflurane required infusion of angiotensin II (0.13 μg/kg b.w. × min) to maintain MAP. Four Pt-needle electrodes (75 μm ∅, 1.2 mm length) were impaled into the exposed left cerebral cortex at intervals of 5 mm or 17 mm from the lesion for assessment of rCBF by H_2-clearance. An additional electrode was placed through a burr hole into the contralateral cortex. After control measurements a cold lesion according to KLATZO [3] was induced in the occipital part of the cortex. This was followed 7 min later by arterial hypoxia at an pO_2 of 35 mmHg by apnoe and subsequent hypoventilation. After a hypoxic period of 20 minutes, the animals were transiently hyperventilated at a FiO_2 of 0.7 and infused with bicarbonate to correct the metabolic acidosis. rCBF was assessed at intervals of 15 minutes during the first hour, then every 20 minutes until termination of the experiment 6 hrs after lesion.

* Supported by Deutsche Forschungsgemeinschaft Ba 452/6-7

Results

The MAPs in the posttraumatic period were 70 (I), 77 (F), 78 (T), or 71 (C) mmHg, respectively. Arterial pCO_2 was not different between the groups. Control values and time course of rCBF in the posttraumatic period are shown in Table 1. During hypoxia assessment of rCBF in the lesioned hemisphere was not possible due to distortion of the H_2-curves by spreading depression. rCBF in the contralateral hemisphere increased in this period by 41–115%. After reoxygenation, rCBF decreased by approximately 10 to 20% for 20 to 40 minutes in the hemisphere with trauma in animals with thiopental ($p < 0.01$) or α-chloralose (n.s.). These changes were particularly pronounced in the vicinity of the lesion. In animals with isoflurane, cerebral blood flow after trauma and hypoxia increased by 5–15% in all regions (n.s.), while it remained fairly unchanged with fentanyl anesthesia.

Discussion

During hypoxic episodes, the cerebral perfusion increases to maintain oxygen supply of the brain [1]. In the contralateral hemisphere (without trauma), we found an adequate increase of rCBF during hypoxia. The flow response of the hemisphere with trauma under the hypoxic challenge, however, could not be assessed due to interference of the hydrogen washout curves with spreading depression. Inhalation anesthetic agents such as isoflurane may increase the cerebral blood flow by vasodilation of brain vessels, although cerebral metabolism is reduced [2]. Compared to halothane or enflurane, there is a smaller or no increase of rCBF with isoflurane [8]. Fentanyl in most studies led to a decrease in CBF and cerebral metabolism by 10 to 30% [5]; barbiturates as thiopental are potent cerebral metabolic depressants and reduce CBF and metabolic rate by 20 to 50% [7]. Former experiments with these anesthetic agents have shown an initial, shortlasting hyperemia after a focal lesion with isoflurane and fentanyl in the traumatized hemisphere [6]. Additionally, a persistent increase of flow distant to the lesion was observed in isoflurane anesthesia. rCBF in the vicinity of the lesion was depressed by about 15–35% with I, F, or T, or remained unchanged with C [6]. Currently, no initial hyperemia was found in any of the groups. Furthermore, in isoflurane animals only a small increase of flow was observed within the entire posttraumatic period, which however was not statistically significant. rCBF was moderately, but significantly depressed close to and distant from the lesion. Since with all anesthetic agents the response of rCBF to the trauma combined with hypoxia was markedly different from that in groups with trauma, but without hypoxia, it is concluded, that general hypoxia abolished the specific flow response elicited by any of the anesthetic agents studied. Although the blood pressure was somewhat different between the groups and rCBF in thiopental animals was lower than with isoflurane, the results do not indicate significant protective or adverse effects of the anesthetic agents tested in the presence of a cerebral lesion and general hypoxia.

Table 1. rCBF in rabbits with a focal cerebral lesion and a hypoxic episode of 20 minutes. rCBF was studied for 6 hrs after lesion. Close: 5 mm apart from the lesion; distant; 17 mm apart from the lesion; opposite = contralateral hemisphere. p.L.: post Lesion. rCBF is given in ml/100g × min or percent of control. 6 animals per group were studied

Anesthesia	Measuring site	Control mean ± SEM	Hypoxia % of cont	2 hours p.L. % of control	3 hours p.L. % of control	4 hours p.L. % of control	5 hours p.L. % of control	6 hours p.L. % of control
Isoflurane	Close	54.4 ± 4.6		109.2	97.4	112.9	94.2	110.2
	Distant	60. 1 ± 4.6		110.4	113.4	115.4	108.5	125.2
	Opposite	52.6 ± 1.7	188.1	103.1	91.3	99.2	110.4	117.6
Fentanyl	Close	46.4 ± 2.7		106.8	99.8	96.5	96.0	108.8
	Distant	48.9 ± 2.1		93.6	92.7	96.8	99.4	104.2
	Opposite	43.7 ± 2.5	141.4	112.4	105.8	106.9	109.3	106.8
Thiopental	Close	58.4 ± 2.5		81.9	83.9	75.8	73.8	75.6
	Distant	65.5 ± 3.8		96.4	96.5	92.2	90.5	88.1
	Opposite	39.3 ± 1.5	183.0	110.3	107.0	105.9	104.7	104.4
α-Chloralose	Close	46.7 ± 2.4		86.7	84.4	96.3	88.0	80.5
	Distant	49.8 ± 2.3		85.5	81.0	84.5	89.5	93.1
	Opposite	36.0 ± 2.3	215.9	107.9	112.2	114.8	122.6	123.7

References

1. Cohen PJ, Alexander SC, Smith ThC, Reivich M, Wollman H (1967) Effects of hypoxia and normocapnia on cerebral blood flow and metabolism in conscious man. J Appl Physiol 23:183–189
2. Cucchiara RF, Theye RA, Michenfelder JD (1974) The effects of isoflurane on canine cerebral metabolism and blood flow. Anesthesiology 40:571–574
3. Klatzo I, Piraux A, Laskowski EJ (1958) The relationship between edema, blood-brain-barrier and tissue elements in a local brain injury. J Neuropathol Exp Neurol 17:548–564
4. Levati A, Farina ML, Vecchi G, Rossanda M, Marrubini MB (1982) Prognosis of severe head injuries. J Neurosurg 57:779–783
5. Michenfelder JD, Theye RA (1971) Effects of fentanyl, droperidol, and innovar on canine cerebral metabolism and blood flow. Brit J Anaesth 43:630
6. Murr R, Berger S, Schürer L, Baethmann A (1989) Regional cerebral blood flow and tissue pO_2 after focal trauma: Effects of isoflurane and fentanyl. In: Hammersen F, Messmer K (eds) Cerebral microcirculation. Progr Appl Microcirc, vol 16. Karger, Basel, pp 61–70
7. Nilsson L, Siesjö BK (1975) The effect of phenobarbitone anaesthesia on blood flow and oxygen consumption in the rat brain. Acta Anaesth Scand, Suppl 57:18–24
8. Todd MM, Drummond JC (1984) A comparison of the cerebrovascular and metabolic effects of halothane and isoflurane in the cat. Anesthesiology 60:276–282

Brain Blood Volume and Cerebral Hemodynamics in the Anesthetized Rat

P.A. Roberts, S.C. Kim, P. Tompkins, and M. Pollay

Division of Neurosurgery, University of Oklahoma, HSC, P.O. Box 26307, and V.A. Medical Center, Oklahoma City, OK 73190, USA

Materials and Methods

Adult male rats (400+ grams) were used for all studies. Nembutal anesthesia was induced via intraperitoneal injection at 40 mg/kg and maintained by IV infusion at 8 mg/kg/hr. Induction for Halothane was via inhalation in a bell jar at 2.5% in an 80/20 mixture of breathing air/100% O2. Induction with Forane was likewise in a bell jar at 4% Forane in 100% O2. Maintenance for Halothane and Forane was at 1.5–2% in an 80/20 mix of breathing air/O2. All animals were mechanically ventilated via tracheostomy. Following placement of femoral arterial and venous catheters, animals were placed in a head frame in the sphinx position. For measurement of ICP and determination of PVI's, a 26 gauge needle was inserted into the cisternal space and connected to a Camino fiber optic pressure measuring system. Normocarbic conditions (pCO_2 30–40 mmHg) were obtained using a respirator volume of 2.5 cc and a rate of 60/min. Hypercarbia ($pCO_2 > 40$ mmHg) was achieved by lowering the respirator rate. After stabilization of blood gases and ICP, 10 μl of liquid was injected through a side port via a Hamilton syringe for the PVI measurement.

For the extradural mass experiments small craniectomies were made after placement in the head frame and a blunt, angled 26 gauge needle inserted extradurally and fixed to the skull with super glue. The cannula was connected to a 1 cc syringe filled with the gel. After insertion of the cisternal needle and measurement of control PVI's, gel was slowly infused in 50 μl increments to attain the desired final ICP (15 to 20 mmHg). After stabilization at the higher ICP, experimental PVI's were determined and the animal was loaded with ^{99m}Tc-HSA for blood volume measurement. After equilibration of the HSA with systemic circulation, a reference blood sample was drawn and the animals were killed with a KCl bolus into the venous line. Blood volumes were determined by comparison of radioactivity in weighed brain samples to radio-activity in the reference blood sample.

Results

Group I

For both Nembutal and Halothane, hypercarbia resulted in a significantly increased BBV compared to normocarbic control animals. This increase in

BBV for these agents is reflected in significantly lower PVI and compliance measurements. Hypercarbia with Forane anesthesia caused no measurable increase in BBV and resulted in no change in either PVI or compliance. These results are shown in Fig. 1 (A, B).

Group II

Elevating ICP by extradural mass (ICP 15–20 mmHg) resulted in no measurable effect on BBV. Following elevation of ICP, PVI and compliance were reduced (compared to normal pressure) for all three anesthetics, however, the decrease in brain compliance is attenuated with Forane anesthesia. These results are shown in Fig. 2 (C, D).

Discussion

There are many uncertainties associated with the effect of most commonly used anesthetics on brain blood volume and ICP. This is due in part to a lack of information concerning steady-state BBV, ICP, and compliance [1]. Using thiopental sodium anesthesia in a dog model, we have previously reported an increase in BBV and decrease in PVI and brain compliance with hypercarbia [2]. By documenting the effects of other anesthetics on BBV, PVI and C, the present study adds to our understanding of this dynamic system.

Using a dog model Roberts et al. [3] and Pollay et al. [4] have reported the use of an extradural mass (balloon tip catheter) for the controlled stable elevation of ICP. However, BBV and PVI were not measured in these studies. The present study evaluates the effect of increased ICP through the measurement of BBV, PVI and brain compliance.

Using Nembutal or Halothane anesthesia, either hypercarbia or elevation of ICP by extradural mass has a deleterious effect on cerebral hemodynamics as reflected in brain compliance. Forane anesthesia appears to better maintain cerebral compliance hence offers advantages over either Nembutal or Halothane.

Summary

As part of a larger study involving cerebral hemodynamics and vascular reactivity, brain blood volumes (BBV) were measured in rats anesthetized with either Nembutal, Halothane, or Forane. Pressure volume indices (PVI) were measured through a cisternal needle and compliances (C) calculated. For each anesthetic BBV, PVI, and C were determined under conditions of normo- and hypercarbia (Group I). For both Nembutal ($p < 0.002$) and Halothane ($p < 0.005$), hypercarbia significantly increased BBV. Hypercarbia with Forane anesthesia caused no measurable increase in BBV ($p > 0.4$). Using

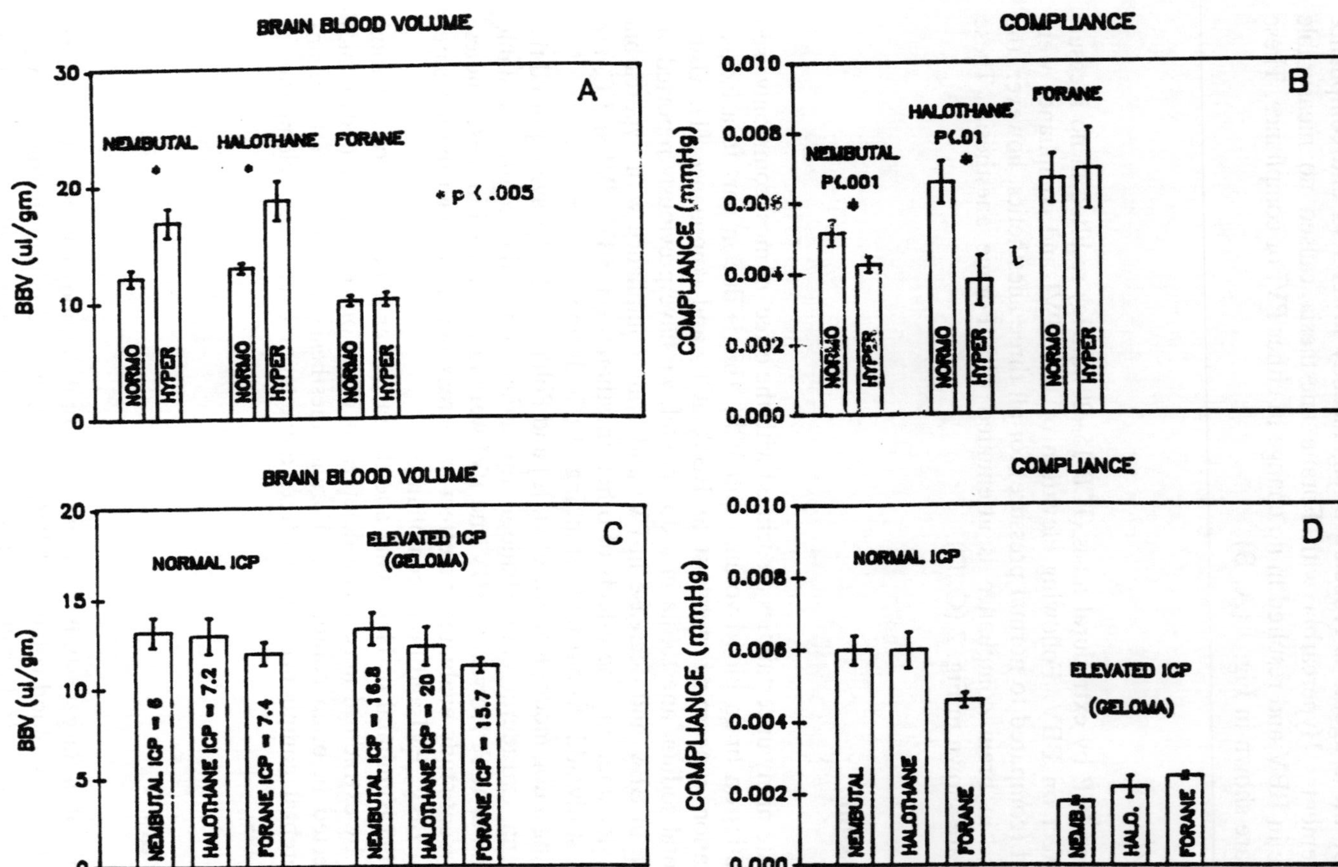

Fig. 1. A,B Brain blood volume and compliance for all three anesthetics, normo- and hypercarbia. **C,D** Brain blood volume and compliance for all three anesthetics, normal and elevated ICP

Nembutal or Halothane, PVI and C were significantly lower with hypercarbia compared to normocarbia. Forane anesthesia resulted in no change in PVI or C during hypercarbia. In another set of experiments these same parameters were evaluated with and without an extradural mass (for the purpose of acutely elevating ICP) (Group II). ICP in the control animals was about 7 mmHg and this was increased to 15–20 mmHg by extradural infusion of a semisolid gel. Under both normal and elevated ICP Forane had the lowest BBV. C was also better for the Forane anesthetized group, although still reduced compared to normal ICP animals. With regard to cerebral hemodynamics (BBV, PVI, C) under conditions of hypercarbia or elevated ICP caused by extradural mass, Forane anesthesia appears to offer advantages over either Nembutal or Halothane.

References

1. Messick JM, Newberg LA, Nugent M, Faust RJ (1985) Principles of neuroanesthesia for the non-neurosurgical patient with CNS pathophysiology. Anesth Analg 64:143–174
2. Pollay M, Roberts PA, Fullenwider C, Stevens FA (1983) The effect of mannitol and furosemide on the blood brain osmotic gradient and intracranial pressure. J Neurosurg 59:945–950
3. Roberts PA, Williams G, Smith S, Stevens FA, Arancibia C, Pollay M (1987) The effect of apnea on brain compliance and intracranial pressure. 8th European Congress of Neurosurgery, Barcelona, Spain, Sept.
4. Roberts PA, Pollay M, Engles C, Pendleton B, Reynolds E, Stevens FA (1987) Effect on intracranial pressure of furosemide combined with varying doses and administration rates of mannitol. J Neurosurg 66:440–446

Flumazenil and ICP Changes During Reversal of Benzodiazepine Sedation

T. CAFIERO[1], P. MASTRONARDI[1], G. GARGIULO[1], B. MAZZARELLA[1], L. STELLA[2], and B. GALLICCHIO[2]

[1]I. Cattedra di Anestesiologia e Rianimazione and [2]Istituto di Neurochirurgia, II. Facoltà di Medicina e Chirurgia di Napoli, Napoli, Italy

Introduction

Benzodiazepines (BDZ) are widely used in premedication, in inducing anesthesia and in ICU as sedative and anticonvulsant agents [2, 3]. BDZ are frequently used in ICU for sedation in patients during CT examination, arterial or venous cannulation and suctioning of secretions. At first diazepam was used and then chlordemethildiazepam, flunitrazepam and recently midazolam which, besides exerting minimal effects on circulation and respiration, also possess more favourable pharmacokinetic characteristics [4]. Since midazolam and flumazenil, a new antagonist of BDZ, have been introduced in clinical practice the therapy of BDZ acute intoxication and the reversal of BDZ-induced sedation are greatly improved. In patients with intracranial pathology it is indispensable to avoid any increase in ICP. In this study we evaluated the influence of flumazenil on ICP either as sole drug administered or as antagonist of BDZ sedation.

Methods

Thirty-five patients, 25 males and 10 females, with a mean age of 46.3 (± 3.7) years and a mean weight of (68.3 ± 5.6) kg, ASA class II, were studied. No patient with hepatic, renal or cardiocirculatory disease or with compromised level of consciousness was included in the study. Patients gave their informed consent to participation in the study. ICP was monitored and continuously recorded for diagnostic or therapeutic purposes. The patients were studied in the supine position with ICP zero reference at the midcranial level. ICP monitoring was carried out via a ventricular catheter connected to a poly graph (Honeywell). The following parameters were monitored throughout the procedure: MAP by Dinamap, heart rate, ECG (lead II) and ETCO2 by Normocap. CPP was calculated as the difference between MAP and ICP. Ventilation was spontaneous or assisted in order to hold normocapnia. Ten patients received flumazenil alone (1.0 mg in 30 sec.) and the remainder received BDZ (midazolam = 15 cases, flunitrazepam = 7 cases, chlordemethildiazepam = 3 cases) and flumazenil as antagonist. The dosages of the BDZ used were: midazolam = 0.2 mg kg-1, flunitrazepam = 0.03 mg kg-1, chlordemethildiazepam = 0.1 mg kg-1. Flumazenil as antagonist was injected in this sequence: 0.3 mg i.v. and then 0.1 mg bolus doses each minute until recovery from sedation was achieved. Finally, patients who received BDZ and flumazenil were divided into two groups as regards the ICP baseline value: below 15 mmHg (15 cases) and above 15 mmHg (10 cases). Statistical comparisons were performed by analysis of Student's test. P = 0.05 was considered to be significant.

Results

As regards the results in patients who received flumazenil as sole drug, all parameters studied were absolutely stable and no significant changes during the study were recorded. In patients with ICP baseline value below 15 mmHg (15 cases) who received BDZ and flumazenil as antagonist no significant changes in ICP and MAP were noted (Fig. 1). In patients with ICP baseline value above 15 mmHg BDZ administration induced a significant decrease in ICP at times T1, T2, T3 and T4 and flumazenil antagonism caused a gradual restoration of the pre-existing awake control value. No significant changes in MAP and CPP were recorded (Fig. 2).

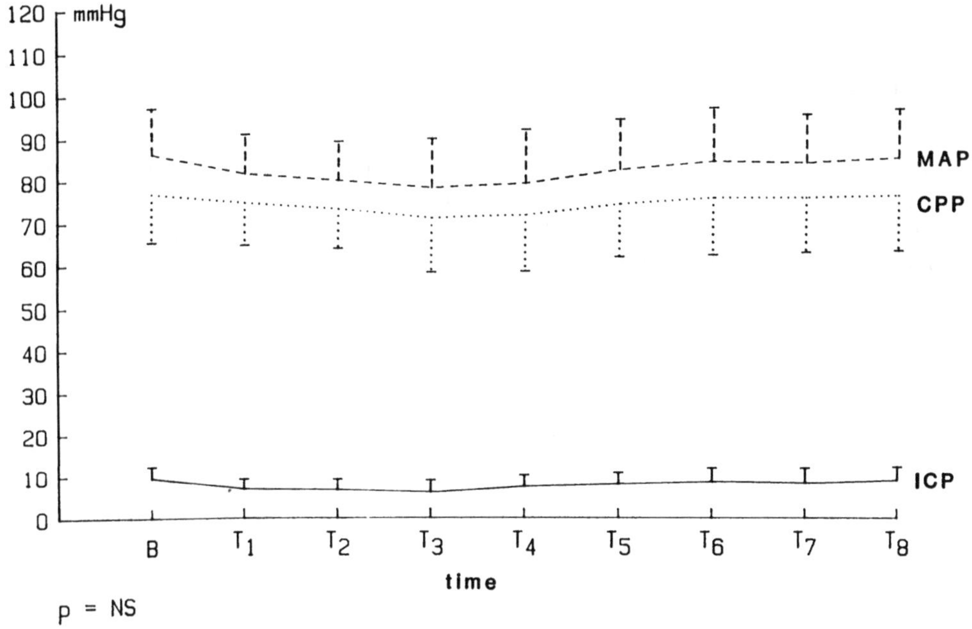

Fig. 1. MAP, ICP and CPP changes after BDZ sedation and flumazenil administration as antagonist in patients with ICP baseline value below 15 mmHg (15 cases). Times B = baseline value; T1, T2, T3 and T4 respectively at 1, 2, 3 and 5 min after BDZ; T5 1 min after flumazenil; T6 at awakening; T7 and T8 respectively 10 and 40 min after T6

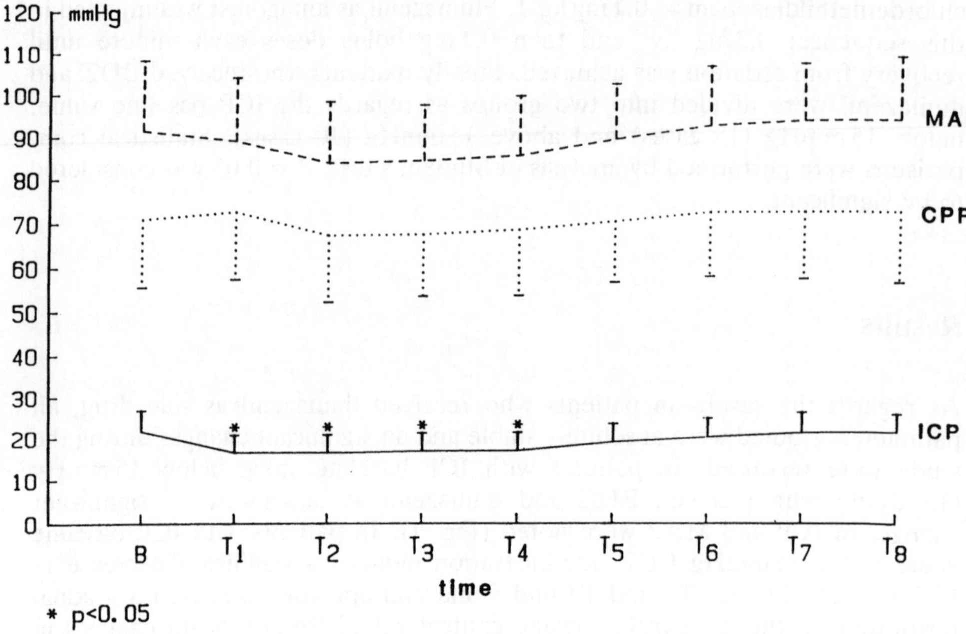

Fig. 2. MAP, ICP and CPP changes after BDZ sedation and flumazenil administration as antagonist in patients with ICP baseline value above 15 mmHg (10 cases). Times B = baseline value; T1, T2, T3 and T4 respectively at 1, 2, 3 and 5 min after BDZ; T5 1 min after flumazenil; T6 at awakening; T7 and T8 respectively 10 and 40 min after T6

Discussion

Concerning the effects of BDZ on ICP, the results confirm the positive action in reducing ICP in patients with intracranial hypertension [6, 7]. Furthermore, BDZ do not alter the cardiocirculatory parameters. Flumazenil possesses no effects on ICP and MAP and can be safely administered in patients, even when there are no BDZ to be antagonized. In agreement with other authors [1], the decrease in ICP was completely antagonized by flumazenil in patients with intracranial hypertension who received BDZ. Reversal of BDZ-induced sedation by flumazenil is not associated with significant haemodynamic responses as demonstrated in previous investigations [5]. Flumazenil effectively antagonized the central effects of the BDZ used and there was no sign of resedation during the observation period of 3 hours after either midazolam or the other BDZ administration. We can conclude that this antagonist is suitable also in patients with decreased intracranial compliance.

References

1. Chiolero RL, Ravussin P, et al. (1988) The effects of midazolam reversal by RO 15-1788 on cerebral perfusion pressure in patients with severe head injury. Inten Care Med 14(3):196–200
2. Kanto J, Klotz U (1982) Intravenous benzodiazepines as anaesthetic agents: pharmacokinetics and clinical consequences. Acta Anaesth Scand 26:554
3. Kapp W (1986) Pharmacology and toxicology of the benzodiazepines. In: Gotz E, Steffens J (eds): Midazolam in Anesthesiology. Editiones ROCHE, Basle, Switzerland, pp 11–22
4. Lauven PM, Stoeckel H (1986) Clinical pharmacokinetics of midazolam. In: Gotz E, Steffens J (eds): Midazolam in Anesthesiology. Editiones ROCHE, Basle, Switzerland, pp 31–40
5. Marty J, Joyon D (1988) Haemodynamic responses following reversal of benzodiazepines-induced anaesthesia or sedation with flumazenil. Europ J Anaesthesia, Suppl 2:167–171
6. Mazzarella B, Mastronardi P, Cafiero T, et al. (1985) Studio randomizzato comparativo tra midazolam e tiopentone per il controllo della PIC. Minerva Anestesiologica 51(7–8):393–396
7. Nugent M, Artru AA, Michenfelder JD (1982) Cerebral, metabolic, vascular and protective effects of midazolam maleate: comparisons to diazepam. Anesthesiology 56:172

Effect of Propofol on Cerebro-Spinal Fluid Pressure in Patients with and without Intracranial Hypertension

P. RAVUSSIN[1], R. TEMPELHOFF[2], P.A. MODICA[2], J.P. GUINARD[1], D. THORIN[1], and J. FREEMAN[1]

[1] Department of Anesthesiology, Centre Hospitalier Universitaire Vaudois, CH-1011 Lausanne, Switzerland
[2] Department of Anesthesiology, Division of Neuroanesthesia, Washington School of Medicine, St. Louis, MO, USA

Introduction

Propofol has been shown to be a suitable agent for neuroanesthesia [2]. It decreases cerebral oxygen consumption ($CMRO_2$) and cerebral blood flow (CBF), and increases cerebral vascular resistance [4]. Intracranial pressure (ICP) decreases as a result of the effects of propofol on cerebral hemodynamics [2]. In this study [2], baseline ICP of the 23 patients before propofol ranged from 6 to 32 mmHg. Accordingly, the present study was designed to evaluate and to quantify prospectively the cerebrospinal fluid pressure (CSFP) decreasing effect of propofol in patients with and without intracranial hypertension (ICH) to determine whether their ICP reacts in the same way to propofol and to the same degree in both groups.

Methods

After institutional ethical approval and informed consent, 21 consecutive adult patients (age 18–71 years, weight 45–79 kg, Glasgow coma score 15) scheduled for elective intracranial surgery, were assigned to 2 groups prior to induction according to their baseline CSFP value: Group I – CSFP $\leq$ 15 mmHg, n = 13; Group II – CSFP > 15 mmHg, n = 8. Patients with cardiac, renal or hepatic disease, or in whom a lumbar drain was not essential, were not studied. Arterial and CSF pressures were measured in the supine position using previously calibrated transducers (Hewlett-Packard Quartz, MK4-04QNWF), referred to the lateral midthoracic line and the external auditory meatus respectively. Mean direct arterial pressure (MAP), CSFP via a 20 G malleable lumbar needle, and cerebral perfusion pressure (CPP = MAP − CSFP) were recorded on an HP 78342A System (Hewlett-Packard Inc., Palo Alto, Los Angeles, USA) just before (baseline) and after a bolus induction dose of propofol $1.6 \pm 0.1\,mg\,kg^{-1}$ (mean ± SEM) followed by a continuous infusion of propofol $97.3 \pm 6.2\,\mu g\,kg^{-1}\,min^{-1}$; since no patient had an intracranial lesion which might have been an obstacle to CSF flow, CSFP changes were taken to indicate ICP changes [5]. Fentanyl $4\,\mu g\,kg^{-1}$, pancuronium $0.1\,mg\,kg^{-1}$ and lidocaine 1.5 mg kg^{-1} were added 2 min after induction (3 min before intubation). FiO_2 was 1 and $P_{ET}CO_2$ was maintained constant during the study. The patients were kept normothermic using a thermal blanket and unstimulated during the first 5 min before intubation. For statistical analysis, analysis of variance (ANOVA) within groups with Scheffe's range test for multiple comparisons was used to compare the baseline findings for CSFP, MAP and CPP with their corresponding values recorded 0.5, 1, 1.5, 2, 3, 4, 5, 6 and 10 min after induction. Unpaired t-tests were applied to compare demographic data, doses of propofol and fentanyl, and cerebral hemodynamics between groups.

Results

Age (54.9 ± 5.2 yrs in Group I vs. 52.6 ± 5.5 yrs in Group II), weight (63.9 ± 3.1 kg vs. 71.2 ± 4.2 kg), type of surgery, induction and maintenance doses of propofol and fentanyl were similar in both groups. Baseline CSFP (18.4 ± 2.0 mmHg vs. 8.1 ± 0.9 mmHg) and MAP (101.0 ± 3.9 mmHg vs. 93.8 ± 3.1 mmHg) were significantly higher in Group II than in Group I and remained significantly higher up to 5 min after intubation (T) ($p < 0.05$, Figs. 1 and 2). After propofol alone, CSFP decreased significantly more in Group II than in Group I by 46 ± 4% vs. 22 ± 2% ($p < 0.01$), with the lowest value at 1 min

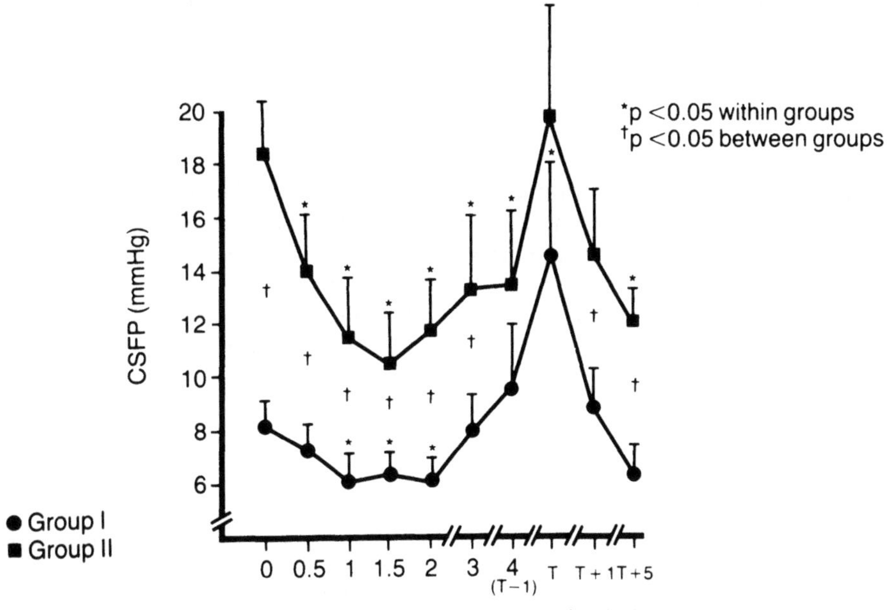

Fig. 1. Effect of propofol on CSFP in Groups I and II; 0 is baseline just before induction and T is orotracheal intubation (mean ± SEM)

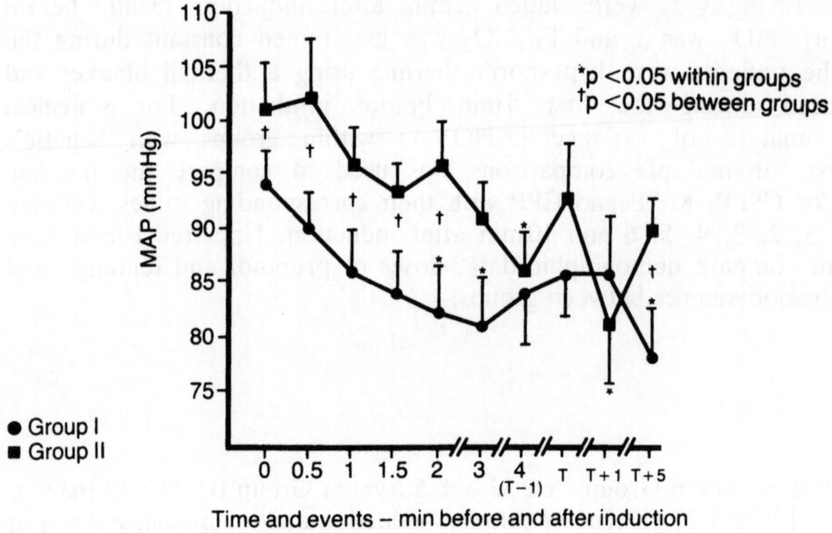

Fig. 2. Effect of propofol on MAP in Groups I and II; 0 is baseline just before induction and T is orotracheal intubation (mean ± SEM)

after induction in Group I and at 1.5 min in Group II ($p < 0.05$, Fig. 1). MAP decreased similarly in Groups I and II, by 13 ± 1% vs. 10 ± 1% with the lowest value at 3 min in Group I and at 4 min in Group II ($p < 0.05$, Fig. 2). CPP in both groups remained above 70 mmHg, even during intubation, when CSFP but not MAP increased significantly above baseline in Group I.

Conclusion

This study demonstrates that the higher the CSFP, the greater the decrease in CSFP after an induction does of a cerebro-vasoconstrictor agent such as propofol, as suggested by the shape of Langfitt's pressure/volume curve and as shown previously for barbiturates [3] and etomidate [1]. In other respects, during induction and after tracheal intubation, CSFP and MAP remain significantly higher in patients with preoperative ICH than in those without.

References

1. Prior JGL, Hinds CJ, Williams J, Prior P (1983) The use of etomidate in the management of severe head injury. Int Care Med 9:313–320
2. Ravussin P, Guinard JP, Ralley F, Thorin D (1988) Effect of propofol on cerebrospinal fluid pressure and cerebral perfusion pressure in patients undergoing craniotomy. Anaesthesia 43 (Suppl):37–41
3. Shapiro HM, Galindo A, Wyte SR, Harris AB (1973) Rapid intraoperative reduction of intracranial pressure with thiopentone. Brit J Anaesth 45:1057–1062

4. Stephan H, Sonntag H, Schenk HD, Kohlhausen S (1987) Einfluss von Diprivan (Propofol) auf die Durchblutung und den Sauerstoffverbrauch des Gehirns und die CO_2-Reaktivität der Hirngefässe beim Menschen. Anaesthesist 36:60–65
5. Takizawa H, Gabra-Sanders T, Miller JD (1986) Analysis of changes in intracranial pressure and pressure volume index at different locations in the craniospinal axis during supratentorial epidural balloon inflation. Neurosurgery 19:1–8

Intracranial Pressure, Pressure-Volume Index and Cerebral Perfusion Pressure During Anaesthesia with Propofol in Neurosurgery

PH. BENDRISS[1], H. LOISEAU[2], H.P. STOÏBER[1], PH. DABADIE[1], and J.P. CASTEL[2]

[1] Départment d'Anesthésie Réanimation IV and [2] Clinique Universitaire de Neurochirurgie, Hopital Pellegrin-Tripode, 33076 Bordeaux Cedex, France

Introduction

Effects of anesthetics on intracranial pressure (ICP) and pressure-volume index (PVI) remain an important matter in neuroanaesthesia. Only few studies dealing with the effects of anesthetics on ICP and PVI in humans are available.

The goal of this prospective study was to evaluate the effects of a Propofol induced anesthesia on ICP and on the PVI in patients suffering from active hydrocephalus.

Clinical Material and Methods

The procedure was performed before ventriculo-peritoneal implantation in 18 patients suffering from chronic (n = 11) or acute hydrocephalus (n = 7).

All parameters were calculated or recorded before and during Propofol anaesthesia.

ICP was recorded through a frontal intraventricular catheter placed under local anesthesia. Duration of ICP recording was about 20 minutes before and during anaesthesia. PVI calculations were carried out 10 minutes after intubation and at the time of a stable period of MAP. PVI was obtained by the bolus injection technique (1 to 5 ml saline isotonic) or by withdrawal bolus technique (1 to 3 ml of CSF) and calculated from formulas proposed by Marmarou [2]. As normal values were considered: <15 mmHg for ICP and $\geqslant 20$ ml for PVI [5]. Cerebral perfusion pressure (CPP) was calculated from Monroe-Kellie's hypothesis. Mean arterial pressure (MAP), heart rate and $ETCO_2$ were continuously monitored. $PaCO_2$ was measured by blood gas analysis and expressed in kilo-pascal (Kpa).

Induction anaesthesia was performed with: 2.4 ± 0.5 mg/kg of Propofol, 0.1 mg/kg of Vecuronium and 2 μg/kg of Fentanyl, then intubation was performed. The lung ventilation was performed with 50% oxygen and nitrogen. The anaesthesia values of $ETCO_2$ and $PaCO_2$ were maintained at preanaesthesia level. Fluid gelatins (500 ml in 15 minutes) were systematically administrated before anaesthesia induction. The maintenance of anaesthesia was obtained by administration of Propofol alone (46 mg/kg/h) immediately after anaesthesia induction.

Statistical analysis used paired Student's test, significant difference threshold was $p \leqslant 0.05$ and values are presented as Mean ± SD.

Results

$PaCO_2$ was considered to have a major influence on PVI through its effect on the cerebro-vascular bed and for this reason 4 patients were excluded because of too large differences between $PaCO_2$ before and during anaesthesia.

Before anaesthesia 8 patients exibited an ICP less than 15 mmHg and 6 patients an ICP over or equal to 15 mmHg. No plateau waves were observed. No stastistically significant differences in ICP were observed between measurements before anaesthesia and during Propofol anaesthesia (14.5 ± 7.7 vs. 15.9 ± 8.8). There was a no statistically significant increase of PVI ($p < 0.06$) (18 ± 6.4 vs. 22.7 ± 8.8) (Fig. 1). There were no statistically significant differences when comparing normal ICP group versus high ICP group for ICP or PVI. However, a significant difference was observed between values recorded before anaesthesia and during Propofol anaesthesia for MAP and for CPP. Results are summarized in Table 1.

Discussion

To our knowledge, this is the first report on the effects of Propofol on intraventricular ICP and PVI in humans. PVI was chosen because it was considered as the most reliable variable to quantify the stiffness of the neuraxis [1]. PVI was considered to be relatively costant and independent of ICP level unlike compliance which is correlated to ICP [1, 3, 5]. The lack of effect of Propofol

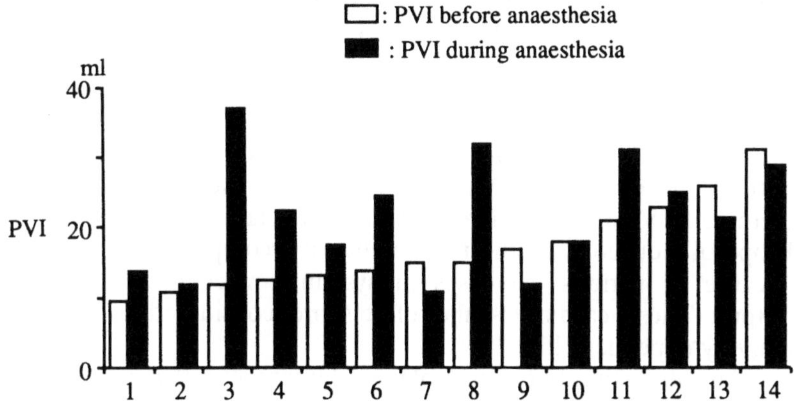

Fig. 1. Evolution of PVI before and during Propofol anaesthesia

Table 1. Analytical results

		Before Anesthesia	During Anesthesia	
Total n = 14		14.5 ± 7.7	15.9 ± 8.8	NS
N ICP n = 18	ICP	9.5 ± 4.3	10.8 ± 4	NS
H ICP n = 6		21.2 ± 5.6	22.8 ± 8	NS
Total n = 14		18 ± 6.4	22.7 ± 8.8	●●●
N ICP n = 8	PVI	15.5 ± 5.8	21.8 ± 9.8	NS
H ICP n = 6		21.5 ± 6	23.9 ± 8	NS
Total n = 14		4.7 ± 0.8	4.5 ± 0.9	NS
N ICP n = 8	PaCO2	4.9 ± 0.7	4.7 ± 0.7	NS
H ICP n = 6		4.3 ± 0.9	4.3 ± 1	NS
Total n = 14		102 ± 18	83 ± 12	***
N ICP n = 8	MAP	104 ± 20	83 ± 8	**
H ICP n = 6		99 ± 16	83 ± 16	*
Total n = 14		88 ± 20	67 ± 14	***
N ICP n = 8	CPP	95 ± 21	72 ± 11	***
H ICP n = 6		78 ± 13	60 ± 16	***

N ICP : normal intracranial pressure; H ICP: high intracranial pressure
Values expressed as in Material & Methods section
*** $p \leq 0.0001$; ** $p \leq 0.001$; * $p \leq 0.01$; ●●●: $p > 0.06$

on the level of ICP found in our study does not confirm previous data in the literature. [3, 4]. The differences in the ICP recording procedures (i.e. lumbar versus frontal catheter) could be the explanation.

An increase in PVI after anaesthesia (but not statistically significant, $p < 0.06$) was observed (Fig. 1). This increase was observed even in the cases of abnormal ICP. At least two explanations can be proposed: the decrease of MAP and a direct effect of Propofol on cerebral vessels leading to a lowering of cerebral blood volume.

Previous studies [1] have reported that PVI is a function of CPP and that an increase in CPP leads to an increase in PVI in normal conditions of autoregulation. Vasoconstriction of cerebro-vascular bed constitute a theoretical explanation for the increased PVI. In conditions of a normal autoregulation a decrease in MAP should cause a vasodilatation of the cerebro-vascular bed leading to a decrease of PVI [1]. Our study shows an increase of PVI even with a significant decrease of CPP due to a decrease of MAP. Our patients never showed MAP values under the autoregulation limits. The increased PVI of our patients cannot be explained by a decreased MAP only. Propofol induced anaesthesias are always accompanied by a decrease in MAP because of various decreases in systemic vascular resistances and cardiac output. These cardio-vascular effects are considered to be dose and rate-delivery dependent [6].

An interesting but non explained feature was that instead of a decreased CPP, PVI remained stable during Propofol anaesthesia even in patients with high levels of ICP. These facts were possibly due to the direct effect of Propofol on the cerebro-vascular bed even if the exact mechanism is still unclear. Propofol is considered to have vasoconstrictive effects of short duration on the cerebro-vascular bed and to have a dose dependent effect on cerebral blood flow [6]. Our methodology of ICP recording could explain these results on PVI, even if we have systematically waited for stable hemodynamic parameters before performing the measurements. At last, increasing PVI could not be explained by changes in $PaCO_2$ in our patients.

These results confirm the safe use of Propofol in the field of neuro-anesthesiology, because even in conditions of profound anaesthesia, this anaesthetic produced neither a increase in ICP, nor a decrease in PVI. Further studies are needed to confirm the favourable effect of this product on PVI and to compare this effect with other anaesthetic drugs.

References

1. Gray WJ, Rosner MJ (1987) Pressure-volume index as a function of cerebral perfusion pressure. Part 1: The effects of cerebral perfusion pressure changes and anesthesia. J Neurosurg 67:369–376
2. Marmarou A, Shulman K, Rosende RM (1978) A nonlinear analysis of the cerebrospinal fluid system and intracranial pressure dynamics. J Neurosurg 48:332–344
3. Ravussin P, Guinard JP, Ralley F, Thorin D (1988) Effect of propofol on cerebrospinal fluid pressure and cerebral perfusion pressure in patients undergoing craniotomy. Anaesthesia 43, suppl: 37–41
4. Ravussin P, Tempelhoff R, Modica PA, Bayer-Berger MM (1991) Propofol vs. Thiopental-Isoflurane for Neurosurgical Anesthesia: Comparison of Hemodynamics, CSF Pressure, and Recovery. J of Neurosurgical Anesthesiology 3, 2:85–95
5. Shapiro K, Marmarou A, Shulman K (1980) Characterization of Clinical CSF Dynamics and Neural Axis Compliance Using the Pressure-Volume Index: 1 The Normal Pressure-Volume Index. Ann Neurol 7:508–514
6. Stephan H, Sonntag H, Schenk HD, Kohlhausen S (1987) Einfluss von Disoprivan (Propofol) auf die Durchblutung und den Sauerstoffverbrauch des Gehirns und die CO_2-Reaktivität der Hirngefässe beim Menschen. Anaesthesist 36:60–65

Succinylcholine, Motor Deficits, Intracranial Hypertension and Potassium Levels in Brain Tumor Patients

M. ABOU-MADI, D. TROP, and K. KARDASH

Department of Neuro-Anesthesia, Montreal, Neurological Institute and Hospital, McGill University, Montreal, Quebec, Canada

Introduction

The use of succinylcholine (Sch) has been eschewed in the setting of upper motor neuron (UMN) weakness of varying etiology, for fear of inducing hyperkalemia and subsequent malignant cardiac arrhythmias. In contrast, it has recently been demonstrated that hyperkalemia following Sch appeared unlikely in patients with brain tumors with or without accompanying motor nerve deficits [3, 4]. These results, however, applied to a patient population free of intracranial hypertension. This study examined whether such a risk exists in the particular setting of brain tumor patients with evidence of UMN lesions and elevation of the intracranial pressure (ICP).

Material and Methods

With institutional approval and informed consent, 20 patients scheduled for elective craniotomy for tumor resection were studied. Ten patients had weakness from UMN lesions and clinical and CT Scan evidence of elevated ICP. The other 10 patients had UMN lesions and no evidence of increased ICP. All patients received dexamethasone and phenytoin preoperatively. The patients' demographic characteristics and preoperative neurological status are detailed in Table 1. On arrival in the operating suite, a peripheral venous cannula and a 20-gauge radial arterial cathether were inserted. A standard lead II ECG was monitored. General anesthesia was induced with a precurarizing dose of d-tubocurarine 0.05 mg/kg, fentanyl 2 mcg/kg, droperidol 0.15 mg/kg, and lidocaine 1.5 mg/kg, followed 3 minutes later with thiopental 5 mg/kg and Sch 1.5 mg/kg. Ventilation was carefully controlled throughout the study period to maintain a constant end-tidal PCO2 around 35 mmHg. Anesthesia was maintained with 50% N20-O2, pancuronium 0.1 mg/kg, and fentanyl increments 2 mcg/kg as required. Arterial blood samples for serum potassium (K+) levels were obtained before induction (baseline) one minute before Sch was administered, and 1, 3, 5 and 10 minutes post-Sch administration. Arterial blood samples for blood gas analysis were obtained at baseline and at 10 minutes post-Sch administration. Changes in serum K+, arterial PCO2 and pH were compared using Bonferroni modified Student's t-test. $P < 0.05$ was regarded as significant.

Table 1. Preoperative demographic characteristics and neurological status of the two groups of patients: Study group (n = 10) with motor deficit and raised ICP. Control group (n = 10) with motor deficit and normal ICP

Study group (motor deficit + raised ICP)					Control group (motor deficit + normal ICP)				
Age	Sex	Wt	Pathology	Deficit	Age	Sex	Wt	Pathology	Deficit
42	M	75	Rt glioma	Lt hemiplegia × 2 wks	66	M	70	Rt glioma	Lt hemiplegia × 2 wks
53	F	50	Lt glioma	Rt hemiplegia × 3 wks	60	M	72	Rt glioma	Lt hemiplegia × 2 wks
62	F	64	Rt glioma	Lt hemiplegia × 2 wks	62	F	64	Rt glioma	Lt hemiplegia × 2 wks
60	M	52	Lt metastatic	Rt hemiparesis × 1 wk	60	M	52	Lt metastatic	Rt hemiplegia × 1 wk
69	M	85	Rt meningioma	Lt hemiparesis × 8 wks	69	M	85	Rt meningioma	Lt hemiparasis × 8 wks
77	M	81	Lt glioma	Rt hemiparesis × 3 wks	40	F	61	Lt meningioma	Rt hemiparesis × 8 wks
60	M	110	Rt glioma	Lt hemiparesis × 3 wks	59	F	70	Rt glioma	Lt hemiparesis × 12 wks
68	M	73	Rt glioma	Lt hemipleglia × 4 wks	77	M	81	Lt glioma	Rt hemiparesis × 3 wks
47	F	67	Lt meningioma	Rt hemiparesis × 2 wks	60	M	104	Rt meningioma	Lt hemiparesis × 2 wks
51	F	58	Lt glioma	Rt hemiplegia × 2 wks	68	M	73	Rt glioma	Lt hemiplegia × 4 wks

Table 2. Serum potassium, arterial pH and PCO_2 before and after succinylcholine (Sch) 1.5 mg/kg in patients with brain tumor, motor deficit and elevated ICP (Study group n = 10) and in patients with brain tumor, motor deficit and normal ICP (control group n = 10) Mean ± SD. No significant ($P < 0.05$) difference in any of the values

		Baseline	1 min before Sch	1 min after Sch	3 min after Sch	5 min after Sch	10 min after Sch
Serum potassium (mEq/L)	Study group	3.74 ± 0.26	3.70 ± 0.33	3.70 ± 0.31	3.80 ± 0.26	3.77 ± 0.29	3.83 ± 0.25
	Control group	3.83 ± 0.25	3,80 ± 0.37	3.78 ± 0.34	3.81 ± 0.29	3.81 ± 0.27	3.86 ± 0.28
Arterial pH	Study group	7.43 ± 0.01					7.44 ± 0.04
	Control group	7.44 ± 0.02					7.42 ± 0.02
Arterial PCO_2 (mmHg)	Study group	38.2 ± 2.51					38.9 ± 2.87
	Control group	37.4 ± 2.42					38.9 ± 2.87

Results

There were no statistically significant differences between the study groups with respect to age, sex or weight. Types of pathology and duration and extent of motor deficit were also comparable. Changes in serum K+, arterial PCO2 and arterial pH are shown in Table 2.

Serum K+ levels never varied significantly from baseline in either groups. The maximum serum K+ increase in any individual patient was 0.3 mEq/L. No significant difference between groups was observed at any time. There was no significant change in arterial pH and PCO2 during the study period within or between the two groups. The ECG complex, monitored during the study period, remained unchanged in all patients.

Discussion

Our findings suggest that intracranial tumors per se, UMN lesions and elevated ICP secondary to them, do not pose a risk for Sch-induced hyperkalemia. In certain disorders, however, such as spinal cord injuries resulting in paraplegia or cerebrovascular accidents accompagnied by hemiplegia, the cause of Sch-induced hyperkalemia appears to be increased chemosensitivity of the muscle membrane following functional denervation due to the development of new receptor sites in extra junctional areas [1]. Prolonged immobility resulting in disuse atrophy with subsequent increased chemosensitivity to Sch has also been suggested as a possible cause of Sch-induced hyperkalemia [2]. All our patients received d-tubocurarine, lidocaine, and phenytoin prior to Sch administration.

Previous reports have shown that d-tubocurarine does not block the hyperkalemia response of Sch in susceptible patients. On the other hand lidocaine and phenytoin both are known to affect cellular membrane ionic stability. However, until the mechanism of this possible protective effect is established, it is impossible to predict its clinical usefulness.

In summary, we have demonstrated that in the setting of planned neuroanesthetic techniques for patients with brain tumors, UMN lesions and intracranial hypertension, the use of Sch does not appear to elevate serum K+ levels.

References

1. Gronert GA, Theye RA (1975) Pathophysiology of hyperkalemia induced by succinylcholine. Anesthesiology 43:89–99
2. Gronert GA, Theye RA (1974) Effect of succinylcholine on skeletal muscle with immobilization atrophy. Anesthesiology 40:268–271
3. Kardash K, Abou-Madi M, Trop D, Delorme M (1989) Succinylcholine, motor deficits and potassium levels in brain tumor patients. Anesthesiology 71:A1139
4. Minton MD, Stirt JA, Bedford RF (1986) Serum potassium following succinylcholine in patients with brain tumours. Can Anesth Soc J 33:328–331

Surgical Decision-Making in Patients with Traumatic Contusion and Intracerebral Haematoma – ICP Monitoring or CT Scanning?

R. BULLOCK and G.T. BLAKE, M.D.

Department of Neurosurgery, Institute of Neurological Sciences, Southern General Hospital, Glasgow G51 4TF, Scotland

Introduction

With the increasing use of CT scanning after head injury, many patients who have intrinsic cerebral mass lesions such as contusion and intracerebral haematoma will present to the neurosurgeon conscious, without prior neurological deterioration [4]. Experience has shown that most of these patients will tolerate their haematomas and recover within the limitations of the extent of the focal damage sustained [5]. However, a minority may deteriorate or die due to raised intracranial pressure because of delayed swelling of the mass lesion or the surrounding brain. Patient selection for prophylactic surgery is, therefore, crucial in this group of patients. We have reviewed the results of ICP monitoring as a means to assist surgical decision-making in a group of 85 patients with traumatic intracerebral haematomas in whom doubt existed about the need for surgical evacuation. We have also retrospectively reviewed the CT scan findings in the same patients in order to formulate guidelines for optimal management of this difficult group of patients.

Patients and Methods

Because of the difficulty in making comparisons between different groups of patients with these heterogeneous lesions, we have confined our analysis to patients with post traumatic intracerebral haematomas which could be measured on the CT scan. From a total of 1079 head injured patients referred to the neurosurgical service of the University of Natal in Durban, South Africa, over three years, (1985–1987) 183 patients (10.1%) were found to have solitary intracerebral haematomas. (Defined on CT as a mass lesion of predominantly high density.) In a further 61 patients, multiple intracerebral haematomas were present. One hundred and fifty nine patients from this group of 244 were treated by immediate craniotomy to evacuate their mass lesion. In the remaining 85, there was no history of deterioration in conscious level or development of new neurological deficit since injury. The need for immediate surgical evacuation of the lesion was in doubt and the patients were therefore selected for prospective ICP monitoring after CT scan.

Four main clinical features were recorded for analysis: conscious level after injury; initial neurological findings; age; delay between injury and ICP monitoring. Outcome was graded according to the Glasgow Outcome Scale based on an outpatient assessment at three months or later. Post mortem examination was performed in all patients who died, and the features of raised ICP were particularly evaluated on the fixed brains.

ICP Monitoring

A subdural cordis cup catheter or a ventricular catheter, and chart recording system were used. The highest mean ICP sustained during any one hour period of monitoring was correlated with other parameters.

CT Scan Analysis

The site (frontal, parietal, temporal or multiple), and the size of the haematoma (the largest measurable diameter) and shift of the midline in millimetres at the level of the third ventricle were all noted from the admission CT scan. Basal cistern status was assessed by grading the pre-mesencephalic cistern as obliterated or not obliterated. In some patients, cistern status could not be assessed and these were deleted from further studies. The extent of cerebral oedema – the low density area surrounding the haematoma was graded on a three point scale of severity (mild = 1; moderate = 2; severe = 3).

Fisher's exact test was used to assess the relationship between basal cistern status and ICP, and multiple linear regression analyses were used to assess inter-relationships between the other parameters.

Both clinical and CT parameters were correlated with outcome using multiple linear regression analysis. The strength of association was taken as proportional to the statistical significance of the correlation co-efficient (r). Students' t values for the correlations between outcome and the variables were calculated (Tables 3 and 4).

Results

The clinical and CT scan features in the 85 patients who underwent ICP monitoring are shown in Table 1.

In 55 patients, ICP was above 30 mmHg and all of these underwent surgical evacuation of intracerebral haematoma. In the remaining 30 patients, ICP remained under 30 mmHg and for this group, the mean ICP was 20 ± 12 mmHg. This group was monitored for 52 ± 39 hours. After ICP monitoring had been discontinued, two patients suddenly deteriorated in conscious level

Table 1. Clinical and CT scan features in 85 patients with traumatic ICH (mean ± SD)

Age (yrs)	29 ± 12
Interval from injury to ICP monitoring (hrs)	26 ± 16
Hemiparesis since injury	49 (58%)
ICP (mmHg) – Haematomas evacuated	42 ± 16
– No initial surgery	20 ± 12
CT Features:	
Maximum Haematoma Diameter	3.8 ± 2 cm
Midline shift (at third ventricle)	2.1 ± 1.7 cm
Basal Cisterns – Effaced	73 (85%)
Not effaced	12 (15%)
Haematoma site – Frontal	42 (49%)
Parieto-temporal	30 (36%)
Multiple	13 (15%)
Surrounding Oedema – Mild	23
Moderate	32
Severe	30

Table 2. Outcome and management in 85 patients with intracerebral haematoma

Outcome	Surgical evacuation	No initial surgery (delayed surgery later needed in 2 patients)
Good result/minimally isabled	26 (47%)	14 (47%)
Moderate disability	11 (20%)	7 (23%)
Dead/Vegetative	18 (33%)	9 (30%)

and CT scans revealed progression of their haematomas. Urgent surgical evacuation was then performed. Eight of the remaining 28 patients died and in three of these, signs of raised ICP such as uncal herniation were found. ICP monitoring thus failed to predict late deterioration or death due to a mass related rise in ICP in five of the 30 patients with an initially low intracranial pressure.

Outcome did not differ significantly between those patients managed by initial surgery and those who underwent ICP monitoring (Table 2).

CT Scan Features

The mean haematoma diameter in the 85 patients was 3.8 ± 2.1 cm, seen on three CT cuts, on average. Haematoma volume was thus about 29 ml. In spite of the moderately large mean size of the lesions, the midline shift was slight −2.1 ± 1.7 mm. This was partially because the majority of haematomas were frontal in situation and therefore unassociated with much midline shift. To assess the relationship between size of haematoma and midline shift, frontal haematomas were therefore separated from those in the parietal and temporal region. For the latter, a significant relationship was found between the haema-

Table 3. Student's t values of correlation coefficients between outcome and CT scan findings

Variable	Site of haematoma		
	All regions (n = 85)	Frontal (n = 42)	Parietal and temporal (n = 30)
Peak ICP	5.37**	4.33**	4.02**
Premesencephalic cistern status	2.94*	1.78	2.98*
Surrounding oedema	2.30*	0.54	2.91*
Haematoma diameter	1.32	0.05	2.92*
Age	1.75	1.60	0.12
Midline shift	1.33	1.01	0.80

*p < 0.01; **p < 0.001

Table 4. Student's t values of correlation coefficient (r) between peak ICP and CT findings

Variable	All regions (n = 85)	Frontal (n = 42)	Parietal and temporal (n = 30)
Premesencephalic cistern status	4.72**	2.60*	2.55*
Surrounding oedema	4.18**	1.58	2.72*
Midline shift	2.20*	1.07	1.95
Haematoma diameter	1.19	0.21	1.88

*p < 0.05; **p < 0.001

toma diameter and midline shift ($r = 0.56$ $p < 0.001$). No such relationship was found for the frontal lesions ($r = 0.162$).

In spite of the failure of ICP monitoring to predict delayed deterioration due to high ICP in 16% of the patients in whom monitoring initially showed low intracranial pressure, ICP was the variable most strongly associated with *outcome* regardless of the haematoma site (Table 3). Effacement of the basal cisterns was significantly associated with bad outcome for lesions in the temporal and parietal regions, but not for frontal lesions, so this sign may be of less value for frontal haematomas. Extensive oedema surrounding an intracerebral haematoma is an indicator of poor outcome, and was the CT abnormality most frequently seen in the five low ICP patients who developed delayed deterioration due to a mass related increase in ICP up to 11 days after injury. Haematoma diameter was associated with outcome for parietal and temporal lesions, but not for frontal ones.

The association between *intracranial pressure* and basal cistern status, midline shift, haematoma diameter and extent of perifocal oedema was tested using multiple linear regression analysis (Table 4). Basal cistern status was the most reliable indicator of raised ICP. Midline shift and haematoma diameter were surprisingly poor indicators of high intracranial pressure. The extent of surrounding oedema was the second most reliable indicator of high ICP. Coma was also significantly associated with the development of high ICP. Table 5 shows the relationship between ICP and basal cistern status. Effacement of the

Table 5. Basal cistern status and ICP (%)

	ICP		
Cistern status	>30 mmHg	<30 mmHg	Total
Effaced	53 (96%)	20 (66.6%)	73
Open	2 (4%)	10 (33.3%)	12
Total	55 (100)	30 (100%)	85

$p < 0.001$ (Fisher's Exact Test)

basal cisterns on the first CT scan correctly predicted raised ICP in 96% of patients, but failed to indicate high ICP in 4%. However, cisterns were also effaced in two thirds of the patients in whom ICP did not exceed 30 mmHg. In three of the five patients who deteriorated or died due to delayed mass related high ICP after an initial period of low ICP on monitoring, basal cisterns were effaced. Effacement of the basal cisterns is thus, a reliable "screening test" for high ICP but with a false positive rate which may be as high as 30–40%. It is however, unlikely that patients with truly raised ICP will *not* have an effaced pre-mesencephalic cistern.

Discussion

In this study we have compared the clinical usefulness of two methods of assessment of ICP in the management of one of the more difficult groups of head injured patients. Our data show that neither a period of ICP monitoring (mean 52 hours) nor information from the CT scan are absolutely reliable in their own right as a basis for clinical decision-making. This may be because raised ICP is a dynamic process which may develop progressively over time. There is evidence that delayed blood brain barrier breakdown develops after focal contusion and intracerebral haematoma to cause brain oedema to be at its maximum after the fifth to seventh day after injury [2]. Early ICP monitoring may therefore, be unlikely to predict this delayed rise with great accuracy. Likewise, the CT scan can only depict intracranial events at one point in time. Our data nevertheless emphasise the value of basal cisterns status as a *predictor* of high ICP in common with other authors [5].

Our data also suggests that severe cerebral oedema surrounding a focal lesion when present on an early CT study is an indicator that raised ICP is likely to occur. When the basal cisterns are uneffaced on an initial CT scan the likelihood of developing delayed ICP rises is low −4% in this study. However, when cisterns are effaced not all patients will have an ICP over 30 mmHg. This may indicate that brain swelling has occurred but that the compensatory processes involving extrusion of CSF from the basal cisterns are sufficient to prevent high ICP from developing. Thus, effacement of basal cisterns on an early CT should be regarded as a "screening test" for high ICP. In a conscious patient with a focal mass lesion open basal cisterns suggest that surgical evacuation and ICP monitoring are not necessary and that careful neurological observation is appropriate management. When the cisterns are effaced, however, management should be more active – when the haematoma is large, surgical evacuation is usually needed. If surgical evacuation is not carried out under these circumstances then ICP monitoring should certainly be used.

The outcome in this group of patients was very favourable in comparison with previous series [1, 4, 5]. We feel that outcome can be further improved by basing the surgical management decisions in this difficult group of patients upon a spectrum of findings from the CT scan and ICP monitoring.

References

1. Becker DP, Miller JD, Ward JD, Choi SC, Lutz HA (1977) The outcome from severe head injury with early diagnosis and intensive management. J Neurosurg 47:491–502
2. Bullock R, Statham P, Patterson J, Wyper D, Hadley D, Teasdale E (1990) The time course of vasogenic oedema after focal human head injury. Evidence from SPECT mapping of blood brain barrier defects. Acta Neurochir, Suppl 51:286–288
3. Galbraith SL, Teasdale GM (1981) Predicting the need for operation in a patient with an occult traumatic intracranial haematoma. J Neurosurg 55:75–81
4. Jamieson KG, Yelland JDW (1972) Traumatic intracerebral haematoma. Report of 63 surgically treated cases. J Neurosurg 37:528–531
5. Toutant SM, Klauber MR, Marshall LF, Toole BM, Bowers SA, Seelig JM, Varnell JB (1984) Absent or compressed basal cisterns on first CT scan: ominous predictors of outcome in severe head injury. J Neurosurg 61:691–694

Spontaneously Disappearing Acute Subdural Hematomas: Conservative Treatment with Intracranial Pressure Monitoring

Y. Katayama, M. Fujii, T. Tsubokawa, S. Miyazaki, T. Yamamoto, and K. Kinoshita

Department of Neurological Surgery, Nihon University School of Medicine, Tokyo 173, Japan

Introduction

It has become increasingly clear that the acute thin subdural hematomas detected in the very early period following trauma can disappear spontaneously within a day [1–6]. We have experienced 10 cases of such hematomas since our initial reports [3]. It seems that the earlier the initial CT scan is taken, the more frequently such hematomas are encountered.

Recognition of this entity has raised a dilemma in the clinical setting as to whether the given hematoma should be operated on or not [1, 2], since some acute thin subdural hematomas do, on the other hand, increase in size rapidly and could therefore lead to disastrous neurological deterioration [7]. We successfully treated a consecutive series of 5 cases of acute thin subdural hematoma detected within 60 min following trauma employing an ICP monitoring and conservative treatment protocol designed prospectively.

Materials and Methods

In order to establish criteria for entry to a conservative therapy, we reviewed 16 cases including those reported in the literature and our own cases. Based on the criteria so obtained, a consecutive series of 5 cases of acute thin subdural hematomas was treated conservatively with ICP monitoring. The purpose of the ICP monitoring was to detect a disastrous enlargement of the hematoma as early as possible if such an increase in size occurred and to control the ICP effectively if an increase in ICP unrelated to hematomas occurred.

Results

Characteristics of Spontaneously Disappearing Acute Subdural Hematomas

The clinical characteristics of a total of 21 cases, including the 5 cases considered below, were analyzed. Although their ages ranged from 3 to 84 years, most cases were between 15 and 30 (12 cases). Injury had often been induced by traffic accidents (11 cases), suggesting high velocity injury. The Glasgow coma scale (GCS) on admission ranged from 3 to 15. Acute thin subdural hematomas were detected mostly within 60 min (13 cases) after injury. A significant decrease in hematoma size was demonstrated at as early as 6 hours after injury (4 cases). It seems, therefore, that the earlier the initial CT scan was taken, the more frequently acute thin subdural hematomas which rapidly disappeared could be detected.

Although hemiparesis and pupillary abnormality were sometimes observed (5 and 4 cases, respectively), these abnormalities were not related to a bad outcome. In contrast, the presence of respiratory disturbance (4 cases) or hypotension (2 cases) was always associated with subsequent death. Cases with GCS values of 8 or less frequently demonstrated early development of unilateral hemispheric swelling (9 cases) or diffuse brain swelling (4 cases) on their CT scans, although only diffuse brain swelling was associated with a high mortality rate. Since hematomas did not explain the low GCS values on admission as well as poor outcome, brain swelling and cardiovascular failure appeared to be responsible for these clinical conditions.

Conservative Treatment of Acute Thin Subdural Hematomas

Based on the above characteristics of spontaneously disappearing acute thin subdural hematomas, 5 cases of such hematomas with the following criteria were treated conservatively: (1) the hematomas were detected within 60 min after injury; (2) the GCS value on admission was 8 or less; and (3) the hematoma did not explain the clinical conditions (Table 1).

The initial CT scans typically revealed an acute thin subdural hematoma and, in most cases, unilateral hemispheric swelling (Fig. 1). The ICP initially

Table 1. Summary of cases of spontaneously disappearing acute thin subdural hematomas with GCS values of 8 or less

Case No.[a]	Age/Sex	Cause of trauma	GCS	Time of initial CT scan	CT findings	Neurological findings	Time of follow-up CT scan[b]	Outcome
2.	20/M	football	8	30 min	unilateral swelling	hemiparesis	8 hours	GR
3.	20/M	traffic accident	5	60 min	unilateral swelling	anisocoria hemiparesis	24 hours	GR
5.	25/F	traffic accident	7	60 min	unilateral swelling	slight hemiparesis	24 hours	GR
6.	37/F	traffic accident	8	60 min	unilateral sweling		18 hours	GR
7.	19/M	traffic accident	8	60 min	frontal contusion		12 hours	GR

[a] Case numbers among 10 cases experienced in our service
[b] Follow-up CT scans always revealed that the hematoma had decreased remarkably in size. GR, good recovery

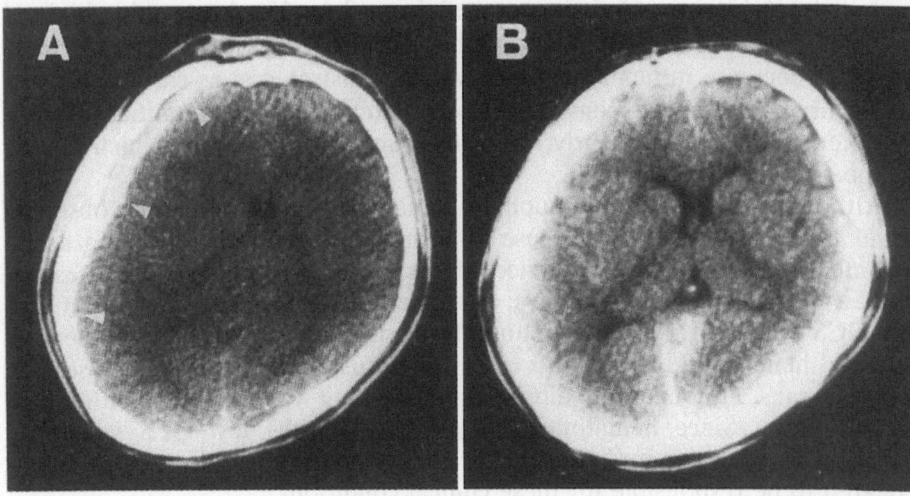

Fig. 1. A representative example of acute thin subdural hematoma (*arrow heads*) detected in the very early period (**A**, 60 min) after trauma, which rapidly disappeared spontaneously (**B**, 18 hrs)

ranged from 15 to 30 mmHg. It remained below 20 mmHg in 3 cases with moderate hyperventilation ($PCO_2 > 23$ mmHg). In 2 cases, the ICP was controlled at below 30 mmHg with intense hyperventilation ($PCO_2 < 23$ mmHg) and barbiturate administration. Even with intense hyperventilation, the oxygen saturation of the jugular vein was maintained at above 65%. hematomas disappeared within 36 hours and good recovery was achieved in all of the 5 cases.

Discussion

It does not seem uncommon for acute thin subdural hematomas detected in the very early period following injury to disappear spontaneously [1–6]. Repeated CT scans and careful observation of the neurological changes have therefore been recommended before undertaking surgical intervention in such cases [1, 2]. ICP monitoring provides an alternative means in cases with a low GCS for deciding whether or not surgical removal of the hematomas is required.

This group of hematomas may constitute part of the so-called "benign" acute subdural hematomas [8]. Their clinical course, however, is not always benign, which suggests that co-existent intraparenchymal lesions may play a significant role in deciding the clinical condition and outcome. A review of 21 cases of spontaneously disappearing acute thin subdural hematomas indicated that low GCS values are often associated with early development of unilateral hemispheric or diffuse brain swelling [3]. The present study revealed that such hemispheric swelling is associated with an elevated ICP. Intensive medical control of the ICP is apparently more important than surgical removal of the hematomas in such patients.

In the cases examined in the present study, an elevated ICP was well managed by hyperventilation. This suggests that the elevation of the ICP is mainly caused by hyperemia. ICP monitoring appears to be a useful guide not only for detecting enlargement of the hematoma but also for controlling ICP medically.

References

1. Aoki N (1990) Acute subdural haematoma with rapid resolution. Acta Neurochir (Wien) 103:76–78
2. Fujioka S, Hamada J, Kaku M, et al. (1990) Rapid resolution of acute subdural hematoma. Report of two cases. Neurol Med Chir (Tokyo) 30:827–831 (in Japanese)
3. Makiyama Y, Katayama Y, Tsubokawa, T (1987) Rapid, spontaneous disappearance of acute suvdural hematoma. Neurosurgery 21:429
4. Nagao T, Aoki N, Mizutani H, et al. (1986) Acute subdural hematoma with rapid resolution in infancy. Case report. Neurosurgery 19:465–469
5. Niikawa S, Sugimoto S, Hattori T, et al. (1989) Rapid resolution of acute subdural hematoma. Report of four cases. Neurol Med Chir (Tokyo) 29:820–824
6. Polman CH, Gijsbers CJ, Heimans JJ, et al. (1986) Rapid spontaneous resolution of an acute subdural hematoma. Neurosurgery 19:446–448
7. Seelig JM, Becker DP, Miller JD, et al. (1981) Traumatic acute subdural hematoma. N Engl J Med 304:1511–1518
8. Singounas EG, Sfakianos G, Sourtzis I, et al. (1990) "Benign" acute subdural hematomas. Acta Neurochir (Wien) 106:140–144

How to Reduce the Ischemic Brain Damage Secondary to Severe Head Injury?

C. ANILE[1], G. MAIRA[1], A. MANGIOLA[1], A. RINALDI[1], P. AMANTE[1], P. PALMA[1], A. DAL LAGO[2], P. POLA[2], and F. DELLA CORTE[3]

[1] Institutes of Neurosurgery, [2] Anaesthesiology and [3] Angiology, Catholic University, Rome, Italy

Introduction

Head injury represents the cause of injury deaths in 50–70% of cases and is the main cause of death in the group under 20 years of age. Brain sequelae are often so severe as to hinder a satisfactory social reintegration. Prevention and control of the extension of the secondary cerebral lesions are important. Ischaemia has been recognized as the common final pathway in post-traumatic brain damage and seems to be mainly due to acute intracranial hypertension and decreased cerebral perfusion pressure (CPP) [3].

The main problem of the so-called intracranial system (ICS), i.e. an incompressible organ contained within a stiff envelope, is represented by the necessity to keep the internal volume absolutely constant in order to maintain an adequate perfusion. In such a system, any change in volume, however small, if not immediately and totally compensated will cause an increase in the outflow resistance. This is mediated by a functional cuff compression mechanism at the distal low pressure segment of the vascular tree, at the level of the so-called Starling resistor [1]. This increase in the outflow resistance will produce a further increase in ICP and, consequently, in cerebral blood volume (CBV), thereby generating and maintaining a vicious circle [2] leading to the disastrous condition of cerebral circulatory arrest. This pathophysiological picture becomes more serious if we consider that the ICS is continuously influenced by a periodic perturbation of its volume due to the rhythmic action of the cardiac pump. It follows that the physiological pulsatile cerebral blood flow is maintained by an exact balance between the inflow (arterial) and outflow (venous) blood volume. In pathological conditions, as after severe brain injury, this mechanism, purely hydraulic in our opinion, can fail and become in itself a pathogenetic factor worsening the effects of the primary cerebral lesion by decreasing CBF.

Material and Methods

To investigate the relevance of this mechanical factor in the prognosis of severe brain injury, a retrospective analysis was made in a series of 26 out of 105 patients in post-traumatic coma (GCS $\leq$ 8) in whom decompressive craniectomy with dural graft was performed because of uncontrollable ICP increase (>40 mmHg).

Of the 26 craniectomized patients, 20 were male and 6 female; the mean age was 31.5 ± 19.6 (range 6 to 85 years). Out of the remaining 79 non-craniectomized patients, 56 were male and 23 female; the mean age was 31.3 ± 22 (range 1 to 82 years). CT examination showed absence of lesions in 13%, diffuse lesions in 35% and focal lesions in 52% of all cases; approximately 50% of this last group were operated on for removal of the lesion. In all patients ICP was monitored by an intraventricular or subdural catheter.

Conservative (or post-surgical) treatment was based on ICP monitoring and consisted of a moderate hyperventilation and osmotherapy when ICP ranged below 20 mmHg; barbiturates were administered when ICP remained constantly above this level. Decompressive craniectomy was performed on one side only: the side was chosen on the basis of clinical signs and/or CT findings. The craniectomy was made as large as possible so as to decompress not only the temporal lobe, as usually stated, but also the brain convexity near to the sagittal sinus in order to eliminate compression over the distal part of the venous vascular bed, the so-called "lacunae laterales", where the hydraulic mechanism of the Starling resistor is to be found. The dura mater underlying the bone flap was totally removed and replaced by a lyophilised dural graft to allow brain displacement without damage.

Together with ICP monitoring, an indirect measurement of the cerebrovascular resistance (CVR) was obtainded by recording the internal carotid artery and middle cerebral artery blood flow velocities, using the Doppler technique.

The outcome was evaluated by the Glasgow Coma Scale, six months after discharge.

Results

In the group of craniectomized patients the mean GCS score on admission was 5.5 and the mean Glasgow Outcome Scale (GOS) was 2; in the non-craniectomized patients the mean GCS score was 5.5 with a mean GOS of 2.8, significantly different ($p < 0.05$) from the former one.

Taking into consideration the mean ICP value recorded during the first 24 hours after admission, it is possible to notice a good correlation with the GCS and GOS score both in the craniectomized (Table 1) and in the non-

Table 1. Mean ICP value recorded in the first 24 hours and GCS-GOS score in the 26 craniectomized patients

No. patients	ICP (mmHg)	GCS	GOS
15	<20	6.214	2.784
9	>20<40	5	1.125
2	>40	4	1

Table 2. Mean ICP value recorded in the first 24 hours and GCS-GOS score in the 79 non craniectomized patients

No. patients	ICP (mmHg)	GCS	GOS
50	<20	5.826	3.478*
22	>20<40	4.9	3*
7	>40	4	1*

* $p < 0.01$

Table 3. Outcome of the 26 craniectomized patients

No. of patients	GOS
4	5
2	4
1	3
2	2
17	1

craniectomized (Table 2) patients. A detail of the GOS for the craniectomized patients is shown in Table 3. Regarding the cerebral hemodynamics study, a constant relationship was observed among changes in the CVR, evaluated by the Doppler technique, the cerebral spinal fluid pulse pressure morphology and the ICP. In particular, brain skull opening induced in all patients an obvious decrease in ICP and CVR, with marked improvement in the CPP and CBF velocity.

Discussion

This study shows that, from the biomechanical point of view, the opening of the skull to the atmosphere in a pathological condition of increasing ICP is able to disrupt the abnormal linkage between the different factors (mainly those due to CVR alterations) which are able to worsen the ischemic brain damage secondary to severe head injury. However, it is very hard to determine from our data indications for performing a decompressive craniectomy in brain injured patients with untreatable intracranial hypertension. The outcome of craniectomized patients does not seem better than that of the non-craniectomized group. However, we must consider that all the patients who showed, during the first 24 hours, a mean ICP value ⩾40 mmHg died, whereas 35% of the craniectomized patients survived and 67% of them were discharged in good condition. This fact could lead to reconsider on the basis of proper ICP monitoring, the therapeutic use of an "obsolete" surgical procedure in order to achieve a sort of "biomechanical brain protection".

References

1. Chopp M, Portnoy HD, Branch C (1983) Hydraulic model of cerebrovascular bed: An aid to understanding of the volume-pressure test. Neurosurgery 13:5–11
2. Rosner MJ (1986) The vasodilatory cascade and intracranial pressure. In: Miller JD, Teasdale GM, Rowan JD, Galbraith SL, Mendelow AD (eds) Intracranial pressure VI, Springer, Berlin Heidelberg New York Tokyo, pp 137–141
3. Takizawa H, Gabra-Saunders T, Miller JD (1987) Changes in the cerebrospinal fluid pulse wave spectrum associated with raised intracranial pressure. Neurosurgery 20:355–361

Toxic Effects of Nutritional Support in the Severely Head Injured Patient

M.J. Rosner and S.D. Rosner

University of Alabama at Birmingham, Birmingham, AL, USA

Introduction

The toxic effects of caloric loading in the face of cerebral ischemia have become well recognized over the last decade as has the association of an ischemic component of the pathological response to severe brain injury. Concurrently, interest in meeting the so called "nutritional needs" of the brain injured has increased. Yet little attention has been paid to the possibility of toxic effects of such nutritional support in traumatically brain injured patients.

We have observed acute elevations in ICP and CSF lactate concentration along with clinical deterioration associated with very early parenteral or enteral nutritional support. Because of these early observations we have pursued a policy of withholding additional nutritional support until intracranial pressure and cerebral perfusion pressure have been controlled by CSF drainage alone. Then alimentation was begun.

With this prospectively established approach we have tested the hypotheses that:

Hypotheses

1. Additional caloric support (nutrition) would be associated with an increase in ICP or effort required (CPP index) for its control.
2. A subset of patients would be identified who, a) Clinically worsened, and/or b) Increased CSF lactate, in association with the institution of alimentation.

Methods

Patients GCS $\leqslant$ 7 on admission. Alimentation begun at 1000 Kcal/day (Dextrose 60%, amino acids 15%, fat 25%; 32 cc/hr or 770 cc/day) when ICP/CPP controlled by CSF drainage). Total intake maintained constant. All patients part of CPP management protocol (CPP $\geqslant$ 70 torr):

Position: Flat, PCO_2 = 35 torr, Pressors used freely, Normovolemia, I = O + insensible.

Daily or qod measures of: CSF Output, CSF Lactate, Mannitol, Phenylephrine, Albumin, Electrolytes, Glucose, Others.

CPP "index" calculated as: index = CSF output (cc) + mannitol (gms) + phenylephrine (mg) + albumin (gm) indexl = CSF output (cc) + mannitol (gm) + phenylephrine (mg).

Results

Table 1 demonstrates representative values for those patients at the outset of alimentation and the four days just prior and following its institution. Note the marked increased in Therapy Indexl by Nday = 4 (168 ± 21 from 127 ± 17). Most of this increase was accounted for by CSF output. Note the increase in serum glucose over the same period (147 ± 10 vs. 129 ± 7). Other parameters tended to remain constant.

In the group where cessation of alimentation was required (Table 2) similar trends were present but more marked. Glucose increased to 148 ± 18 on Nday 1, ICP Therapy Indexl increased to 199 ± 109 from 115 ± 56 with most of the difference contributed by increased mannitol and pressor requirement since the smaller ventricles "clamped down" and allowed less CSF drainage for ICP/CPP control. These changes reverted as alimentation was quickly withdrawn on Nday = 3 and 4.

Overall mortality in the GCS $\geq$ 7 groups was 29% with 3% persistent vegetative state. The outcome in those patients with surgical mass lesions was identical to the "non-operated" medically managed group.

Discussion

Alimentation leads to an increase in the effort necessary to maintain ICP/CPP constant. This increase is frequent in the head injured population though variable; it is severe enough to warrant withholding of nutritional support in the majority of patients until ICP is controlled by CSF drainage. Even then, the response to alimentation may be significant enough to require discontinuation of feeding in 15–20% of patients.

The putative mechanism is caloric loading. While increasing caloric intake may lead to hyperglycemia, the use of insulin or a natural tolerance to increased calories may limit the level of hyperglycemia yet not the adverse response.

In the subset of patients deteriorating to the point we felt it necessary to hold further nutritional support once started, the increase in CSF lactate was 50%. Highly variable, but significant considering the generally decrementing CSF lactate level which accompanied clinical improvement. This trend reversed when alimentation was discontinued.

In addition, these data suggest that alimentation per se, beyond the 1000–1500 Kcal/day delivered via fluids and colloid, is not necessary to achieve good clinical results and may hamper recovery in some.

Table 1. Response to nutritional support. (Overall group)

(Nday[a]) Nutrition day	−4	−3	−2	−1	0	0	2	3	4
GCS	8 ± 0.4	9 ± 0.4	9 ± 0.4	9 ± 0.4	10 ± 0.4	10 ± 0.4	10 ± 0.4	10 ± 0.4	10 ± 0.5
Highest ICP	30 ± 1	28 ± 0.9	28 ± 1	28 ± 0.9	28 ± 1	29 ± 2	29 ± 2	27 ± 2	30 ± 3
SABP[b]	103 ± 2	105 ± 2	104 ± 2	103 ± 1	104 ± 1	105 ± 2	106 ± 2	105 ± 2	106 ± 2
ICP[b]	21 ± 0.6	21 ± 0.6	21 ± 0.6	20 ± 0.6	20 ± 0.7	21 ± 0.8	21 ± 0.9	19 ± 1.1	20 ± 1
CPP[b]	83 ± 2	84 ± 2	84 ± 2	83 ± 1	83 ± 2	85 ± 2	87 ± 2	86 ± 2	87 ± 4
Glucose	135 ± 6	132 ± 6	127 ± 7	119 ± 4	129 ± 7	140 ± 6	149 ± 8	150 ± 9	147 ± 10
Art. Lactate	1 ± 0.1	1 ± 0.2	1 ± 0.1	0.8 ± 0.1	0.8 ± 0.1	0.9 ± 0.1	1 ± 0.1	1 ± 0.1	0.8 ± 0.1
CSF Lactate	2 ± 0.2	2 ± 0.2	2 ± 0.2	2 ± 0.1	2 ± 0.1	2 ± 0.2	2 ± 0.2	2 ± 0.2	2 ± 0.2
NET I&O	267 ± 222	314 ± 145	447 ± 683	643 ± 397	308 ± 134	137 ± 235	310 ± 236	545 ± 107	765 ± 130
CSF Out	108 ± 13	113 ± 12	112 ± 14	119 ± 15	110 ± 16	90 ± 15	101 ± 18	161 ± 24	162 ± 22
CPP Therapy Index I	162 ± 19	160 ± 19	138 ± 18	142 ± 18	127 ± 17	102 ± 16	117 ± 19	165 ± 25	168 ± 21
CPP Therapy Index	205 ± 22	201 ± 22	180 ± 20	183 ± 19	170 ± 19	147 ± 18	151 ± 20	201 ± 26	208 ± 22
Alimentation (KCal)	0	0	0	0	360 ± 40	815 ± 51	1047 ± 65	1285 ± 89	1417 ± 113

[a] Nday 0 = day alimentation was begun – negative "Nday" are days prior to and positive "Nday" values are after alimentation begun
[b] All numbers are mean

Table 2. Response to nutritional support. (Deteriorating group) (n = 6)

Nutrition day	−4	−3	−2	−1	0	1	2	3	4
GCS	8 ± 2	9 ± 2	9 ± 1	8 ± 1	8 ± 1	9 ± 2	9 ± 2	8 ± 1	9 ± 2
Highest ICP	31 ± 2	29 ± 2	28 ± 1	31 ± 2	34 ± 4	46 ± 8	40 ± 5	34 ± 4	304 ± 2
SABP[a]	100 ± 3	101 ± 5	95 ± 3	98 ± 4	102 ± 4	108 ± 6	106 ± 7	102 ± 5	106 ± 7
ICP[a]	21 ± 2	20 ± 2	22 ± 2	21 ± 2	23 ± 2	24 ± 4	25 ± 2	23 ± 2	22 ± 2
CPP[a]	80 ± 5	79 ± 5	77 ± 4	78 ± 3	77 ± 5	82 ± 6	82 ± 6	81 ± 6	84 ± 6
Glucose	150 ± 37	112 ± 4	108 ± 7	100 ± 3	106 ± 9	148 ± 18	134 ± 24	142 ± 17	122 ± 8
Art. Lactate	1 ± 0.2	0.7 ± 0.1	0.8 ± 0.2	0.6 ± 0.1	0.5 ± 0.1	0.6 ± 0.1	0.9 ± 0.1	0.6 ± 0.1	0.8 ± 0.1
CSF Lactate	3 ± 1	3 ± 0.8	3 ± 0.8	2 ± 0.4	2 ± 0.3	2 ± 0.5	3 ± 1	3 ± 1	4 ± 1
NET I&O	362 ± 306	428 ± 407	574 ± 329	−402 ± 347	143 ± 642	−291 ± 334	−402 ± 828	670 ± 405	760 ± 561
CSF Out	112 ± 48	137 ± 43	138 ± 39	128 ± 39	93 ± 38	98 ± 51	62 ± 39	65 ± 30	104 ± 39
ICP Therapy Index I	177 ± 89	226 ± 70	170 ± 52	140 ± 43	115 ± 56	134 ± 72	199 ± 109	130 ± 72	183 ± 95
ICP Therapy Index	232 ± 105	271 ± 72	242 ± 59	203 ± 50	178 ± 45	194 ± 64	274 ± 113	198 ± 69	243 ± 82
Alimentation	0	0	0	0	364 ± 84	907 ± 188	441 ± 278	384 ± 275	126 ± 126

[a] All numbers are mean

Conclusions

1. ICP/CPP "index" increases 50% or more after instituting an additional 1000 Kcal/day as parenteral nutrition. The putative mechanism is caloric loading via glucose.
2. There is a subset of patients more susceptible to these effects which may relate to their "glucose tolerance".
3. Delaying alimentation until CSF drainage alone controls ICP does not deleteriously affect outcome, and brings into question the "dogma" or bias that early alimentation is necessary for a "good" outcome.

References

1. Clifton GL, Robertson CS, Choi SC (1986) Assessment of nutritional requirements of head-injured patients. J Neurosurgery 64:895–901
2. Clifton GL, Robertson CS, Contant CF (1985) Enteral hyperalimentation in head injury. J Neurosurgery 62:186–193
3. Deutschman CS, Konstantinides BS, Ramp S et al. (1986) Physiological and metabolic response to isolated closed head injury: Part I: Basal metabolic state: correlations of metabolic and physiological parameters with fasting and stressed controls. J Neurosurgery 64:89–98
4. Grahm TW, Fadrozm DB, Harrington T (1989) The benefits of early jejunal hyperalimentation in head-injured patients. Neurosurgery 25:729–735
5. Hadley MN, Grahm TW, Harrington T, et al. (1986) Nutritional support and neurotrauma: A critical review of early nutrition in forty-five acute head injury patients. Neurosurgery 19:367–373
6. Rosner MJ, Becker DP (1984) Experimental brain injury successful therapy with the weak base, tromethamine with an overview of CNS acidosis. J Neurosurgery 60:961–971
7. Rosner MJ, Newsome HH, Becker DP (1984) Mechanical brain injury: the sympatho-adrenal response. J Neurosurgery 61:76–85

Panel 3
Head Injury and Control of ICP

Moderator: J.D. Miller

Members: R. Bullock, A.I.R. Maas, L.F. Marshall, A.D. Mendelow, N. Stocchetti

MILLER opened the panel discussion stating that the main topics to be addressed were head injury and therapy for control of raised intracranial pressure. One of the issues that came up, both during the oral and poster sessions, was the concept of secondary insults in magnifying or worsening brain damage. A poster from the Richmond group related to problems occurring during transport of patients, potentially enhancing the possibility of secondary insults. When people are taken to the CT-scan, it must be realized that this is not an entirely safe procedure and the real need for a second CT-scan should be considered, because we may be exposing patients to a risk of problems happening along the way. In fact, during our studies we confirmed that 50% of the patients had one or more insults during transport affecting arterial blood pressure and ICP. Another point of considerable interest is the role of mediators causing secondary insults amplifying brain damage. A large number of posters refer to diffuse axonal injury (DAI). It appears that there is some confusion on the definition of DAI. Are we to use a pathological definition, which is obviously only of value after the patient has died, or should we use the increasingly common CT-based definition. I would like to ask Dr. Marshall to say a few words on this aspect and also Dr. Mendelow.

MARSHALL: the original description of DAI was in a number of patients who were immediately unconscious and, if I could read it quickly from one of these abstracts, patients having DAI have immediate loss of consciousness, prolonged coma and flexion or extension reactions to pain. In pathological studies, median and paramedian shearing injuries are noted. Based on the work of Gennarelli and the Glasgow group, a more broad definition came into being, trying to describe the spectrum of head injury. Two important points should be made: one is the distinction between patients with DAI who have no swelling of the brain and others where there is swelling of the brain and raised ICP. A second important point is the description of whether or not there are hemorrhages in the deep structures of the brain, such as basal ganglia, thalamus and brain stem. Relating to this aspect, we have problems in visualization of the lesions. Of course, the CT-scan is not very suitable for identification of these lesions and you really need to use the MRI, which, however, is cumbersome and relates to the issues of transport already alluded to by Miller. In my opinion, the distinction between swelling and open cisterns and normal brain spaces is clinically quite relevant and can be determined by CT-scan; a more accurate classification, however, does not necessarily require the brain in the bucket, but magnetic imaging. The stated problems in definition explain the great disparity in outcome of patients with DAI: one paper showing no deaths and another showing 60 to 80% mortality.

MENDELOW: one of the problems in definition is caused by the fact that clinicians like to differentiate between focal and non-focal injuries. In practice, all non-focal injuries are often lumped together in the category of diffuse injury. The pathological definition of DAI as already stated is, however, very different with specific CT and MRI criteria. I do think we have a big problem with defining DAI on the basis of neuro-imaging techniques. The MRI is a long way from becoming a routine in head injury, certainly in the United Kingdom. Are we going to call non-focal injury without diffuse axonal characteristics one thing or are we going to call that brain swelling and separate it from the real DAI?

BROCK: if you have no colour t.v. set, you will not be able to watch t.v. in colours. My conclusion is that if you do not have the possibility to detect DAI, you should not talk about it.

PARK: I don't agree that MRI is always necessary. In the cases described in my poster as well as in those described by others, the diagnosis of DAI could be made on basis of the CT-scan showing spotted hemorrhages in the brain stem and basal ganglia. Only when there is a normal CT-scan and the patient remains in a deep comatose state is MRI necessary.

SERVADEI: I think for the diagnosis DAI on CT-scan we should have at least two small scattered hemorrhages, not only one.

NORTH: I would like to support the definition of DAI on a purely pathological basis. We have been comparing magnetic resonance imaging with subsequent neuropathological examinations and also have studies with post-mortem MRI examinations. The MRI imaging modality in our experience comes very close to whole brain slices done by the pathologists.

MILLER: I would like to move on now to the experimental studies on head injury and maybe we could ask Dr. Bullock to say a word or two about that.

BULLOCK: I found the poster on lack of relationship between hippocampal cell loss and ICP after experimental brain injury very interesting. The background is that in patients who died of severe head injury, the neuropathologist finds hippocampal damage even in patients who had low intracranial pressures. In this experimental study, which is a relatively pure model without secondary ischemic insults, there was also evidence of ischemic damage in the hippocampal region. It seems evidence is accrueing that the hippocampus is vulnerable to ischemic insults both by shearing injuries from impact of fluid percusion type in experimental models and by mass lesions such as subdural hematoma.

The exact mechanisms underlying this damage are not clear at this moment, but these aspects seem extremely important for clinicians because of the resulting disturbances of high mental function and neuropsychological abnormalities.

MARSHALL: Dr. Bullock, the poster you commented on used the term hippocampal cell loss. You use the term ischemia. Do you really mean hippocampal cell loss because it is conceivable to have hippocampal damage and cell loss front mechanisms that have nothing to do with ischemic change?

BULLOCK: my view would be that if you can exclude raised ICP as a mechanical cause for deformation and compressive damage, then what else could it be if it is not ischemia.

KOTAPKA: there are a whole series of methods of getting hippocampal damage that have nothing to do with cerebral blood flow in that area. The poster that we presented showed a blood brain barrier defect selectively in the hippocampal area that was gone by an hour. Hippocampal cell loss may occur with no ischemia whatsoever.

BULLOCK: the central hypothesis would be that if the cause is not ischemia, it is probably neurotransmitter driven, the process being initiated by the release of large amounts of neurotransmitters.

MILLER: I think the biggest section of posters relates to issues concerning the control of raised ICP after head injury. There are so many treatments mentioned in the various posters and presentations, that the cynic or sceptic might draw his own conclusions without even reading the titles of the abstracts or even looking at the posters. Perhaps Dr. Maas would like to make some comments about this therapy section.

MAAS: it is really amazing looking at all the posters and hearing the papers to see people doing all different types of modalities of treatment in the severe head injury just lumping them all together. We should not forget that in head injury we have many different pathophysiological entities. There are different causes of raised ICP and I think it is an illusion to think that just one method of treatment or one single drug will work over the entire spectrum of head injury. What I think we should really try to do is to differentiate between the various mechanisms and causes of secondary injury. Is it edema or is it vasodilation that causes raised ICP? Dr. Miller, what are your views on possibilities to differentiate between vasodilation and edema and do you think we could then apply appropriate treatment protocols?

MILLER: the question really is whether to adopt a staircase approach in treatment of raised ICP or to target therapy. In the staircase approach, you start with the simplest treatment first, which is least likely to harm the patient and then as you run out of options you begin to consider treatments that are perhaps more intensive and maybe carry a hazard for the patient. In the targeted approach, you attempt to classify the patients using the monitoring modalities we have, but at this stage I have to say that our possibilities for differentiation are imperfect and we don't yet perfectly understand the significance of things like the pulsatility index on the Doppler. Is a falling jugular venous saturation always bad or may it sometimes be good? Nevertheless, I do think that on the basis of monitoring we should be able to differentiate on mechanisms of raised ICP and target our therapy. Before discussing the particular classes of agents reported on I would like to open up the discussion to the audience.

McGraw: if we are not maintaining an adequate cerebral perfusion pressure above at least 70 mmHg, we probably may need to rethink all those treatments, and the cerebral perfusion pressure really seems to be critical. I think there has been a lot of support for this perhaps during the whole conference. The best perfusion pressure is probably 80, not 70. 70 I consider a minimum and if the perfusion pressure is below this, we are really doing badly.

Miller: to achieve a perfusion pressure of 80, you will in most cases need to push up the blood pressure and in doing this you may be introducing things that are actually difficult to administer and taking us to the upper runs of the staircase.

Nn: does the panel have any views on the choice of medication that should be used to raise blood pressure in an attempt to increase cerebral perfusion pressure? Is there any agreement which pressure agents should be used and whether you should use hypervolemia?

Mendelow: maybe we should approach this from a slightly different point of view; one of the problems has been us concentrating on the ICP and its control at the expense of the blood pressure and cerebral perfusion pressure. Any agent that lowers the blood pressure, will also reduce the ICP. I think we should look very carefully at all the agents used for reducing ICP in terms of perfusion pressure.

Miller: okay, but could you answer the specific question now?

Mendelow: in Newcastle we start with volume loading and if that does not work we will go on to Dopamine, mainly because that is the agent we are familiar with.

Stocchetti: we are following exactly the same policy. The first reason why a patient can be hypotensive is that he is hypovolemic. More than 50% of our patients have extracranial lesions. So first of all, we correct hypovolemia and after that we prefer to use phenylephrine and dobutamine, just like Rosner pointed out this morning. We prefer dobutamine, because we are worried of course about the kidneys.

Baethmann: may I come back to the subject of target oriented versus staircase approach. I think this is a very good distinction and in general one should prefer the target oriented treatment because this means saving neurons and inhibiting secondary loss of neurons. The target might include treatment of DAI. What we are teaching our students currently is symptomatic treatment, inhibiting the rise of ICP and trying to preserve cerebral perfusion. But this is not a specific treatment, this is a symptomatic staircase approach.

NN: I completely disagree. Most of the people sitting here do not do the work in the ICU; the real work is done by people not as highly trained as we are and I think the stepwise approach is the safest one and certainly more easy to train and teach people in. Otherwise, the risk of targeted approach is that people start thinking but do nothing.

MARMAROU: my concern is, as we begin to evaluate the different approaches, we pay little attention to the severity and classification of the injuries. I think we should consider classification in severity and then see how successful we are in managing patients at the 4th, 5th and 6th staircase level.

BROCK: I would like to speak in the same direction Dr. Marmarou just spoke in and make a consensus proposal. One of the prerequisites to perform targeted therapy is that you are able to recognize the target and this meeting has shown what great difficulties there are in some cases to recognize the target. If you consider yourself able to recognize the target in a given case, then certainly you should act targeted, but if you are uncertain the staircase therapy is safer.

MILLER: we have had the pragmatics, we have had the academics and now we have the politician. Right.

NN: I think even now, in 1991, we can adopt a simple targeted approach. We should distinguish between patients who are primarily hyperaemic and those who have primarily brain edema. If you look at the group of patients that have low blood flows, these patients are the ones that are least likely to respond to hyperventilation and most likely to be hurt by it. In fact, the studies which show bad effect of hyperventilation probably concern the patients with low blood flows. So in terms of targeted therapy, I think one fairly simple first step is to try and find out whether globally the patients belong to the low blood flow group in which cases hyperventilation should not be performed and patients with a high blood flow. Obviously, of course we are looking for better guns or better weapons, but right now our options are limited.

MILLER: I'm afraid we have really run out of time now but there is one last message on the therapy side I would like to leave you with and that is: if raised ICP is bad for you, a low arterial blood pressure is even worse. So whatever else we do with our treatments, we should not be jeopardizing the arterial blood pressure.

Session VII: CSF Dynamics

Chairmen: A. Marmarou and P. Janny

The Dynamics of Cerebral Blood Flow, Perfusion Pressure and CSF Circulation – A Modelling Study

M. Czosnyka[1], S. Piechnik[1], W. Koszewski[3], P. Laniewski[2], W. Maksymowicz[3], K. Paluszek[1], P. Smielewski[1], W. Zabolotny[1], and W. Zaworski[1]

[1] Warsaw University of Technology, Institute of Electronics Fundamentals, [2] Children's Health Centre, Intensive Care Unit, [3] Warsaw Medical Academy, Department of Neurosurgery, Warsaw, Poland

Introduction

The first modelling studies on the craniospinal volume compensation were focused on finding the best approximation of the cerebrospinal pressure-volume relationship. An expanded model, explaining the process of the formation, storage and outflow of cerebrospinal fluid [1, 4] was accepted by clinicians as a powerful tool in the examination of hydrocephalic patients.

However, this model cannot be applied directly to the interpretation of the phenomena associated with the changes in the cerebral blood volume. Attempts to integrate CBF and CSF circulation were made in the past [3]. The resulting models proved to be helpful in the understanding of many events involving the compensatory and autoregulatory mechanisms. The objective of this study was the interpretation of the phenomena which couldn't be explained in the previously published models: the dynamic relationship between the intracranial pressure, its pulse wave, the cerebral perfusion pressure, cerebral blood flow and its pulsatility in different states of autoregulation.

This can be done taking into account the mutual relationships between the autoregulation of CBF, CO_2 reactivity of the cerebrospinal vasculars bed, the pressure-dependent venous blood outflow and the non-linear character of the process of CSF storage within the fluid containers.

Material

The results of mathematical simulation were compared with the clinical and experimental results which were carried out in many centers worldwide.

The material includes:

- ICP recordings in children after operations of posterior fossa tumors (53 cases) and in children with head injuries (15 cases) from the Children's Health Centre, Poland.

- pressure-volume studies in children (117 cases – Children's Health Centre) and in adults (126 cases – Clinic of Neurosurgery, Warsaw Medical Academy).
- ICP and CPP (cerebral perfusion pressure) recordings from 83 head injured patients – (Pinderfields General Hospital, Wakefield, UK).
- ICP, CPP, transcranial doppler flow velocity recordings in experimental intracranial hypertension and systemic hypotension in rabbits (11 animals, studied in Wessex Neurological Centre, Southampton, UK).

Method

The model has two input signals: the arterial (P_a) and venous sinuses blood (P_v) pressure. The pressure was chosen as an input drive in order to model the factors influencing CBF.

Three major compartments, able to store an extra cerebrospinal volume, were considered: arterial bed (represented by its compliance C_a), venous bed (compliance C_v) and cerebrospinal fluid volume buffering container, anatomically associated with the reserve of the distensible dural sac (C_i).

The model contains two flow pathways.

The CSF circulatory pathway includes the source of CSF formation, storage, and the resorption mechanisms. The CBF pathway consists of the non-linear cerebral vascular resistance (R_a), including the autoregulatory mechanism, and the resistance to cerebral blood outflow (anatomically represented by the bridging veins).

These two routes of the blood and CSF circulation are coupled to each other by the compliances C_a and C_v.

Assuming that in the electrical equivalence the flow can be expressed by the electrical current and the pressure by the voltage, the hydrodynamic compliances can be modelled by electrical capacitors and the resistances to flow by resistors. The equivalent electrical model is shown in Fig. 1a.

R_a describes the vascular resistance. The autoregulation control is included in the relationship between CPP and R_a (shown in Fig. 1b). The limits for autoregulation indicate the range, where the R_a (CPP) function has a positive slope. Below the lower limit of autoregulation, the closure of cerebral arteries is simulated by the steep increase in R_a.

The resistance to the cerebrospinal venous blood outflow – R_v, depends on the gradient between the cerebral venous blood pressure (P_s) and ICP (P_i). The smaller the gradient is, the greater the resistance. This mechanism represents a collapse of the bridging veins due to the increase in ICP, and presumably plays the decisive role in the development of plateau waves. The capacitance of the arterial bed (C_a) is inversely proportional to its resistance (R_a) – this reflects the rule that the reduction of arterial wall tension, in order to decrease R_a (when autoregulation holds), in parallel increases its compliance.

The cerebral vascular resistance depends additionally on the CO_2 concentration in arterial blood. An increase in $PaCO_2$ produces a decrease in R_a and an increase in C_a.

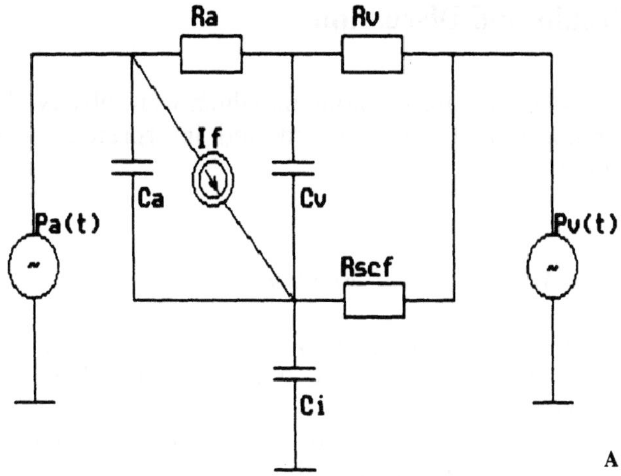

A

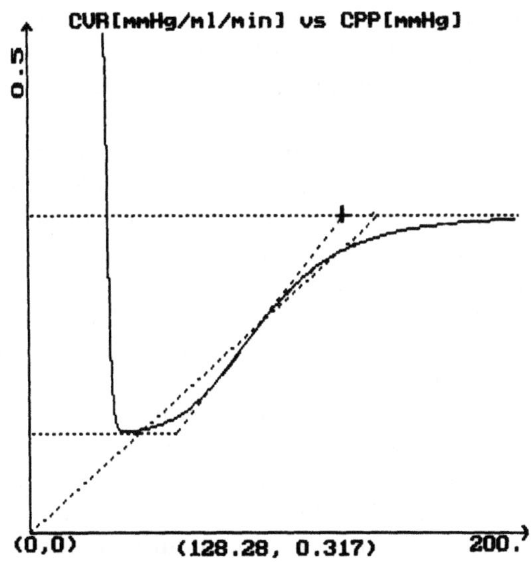

B

Fig. 1. **A** Electrical equivalent circuit of CBF and CSF circulation model. P_a denotes arterial blood pressure, P_v-venous (saggital sinus) pressure. P_i represents ICP and P_s-cerebrospinal venous blood pressure. R_a-cerebral vascular resistance, R_v-resistance of venous outflow, Rcsf-resistance to CSF outflow. C_a, C_v and C_i represent compartmental compliances. **B** Relationship between vascular resistance R_a (y-axis) and CPP (x-axis), representing autoregulation. Limits for autoregulation here are from 40 to 128 mmHg of CPP. Below 40 mmHg R_a increases, as a result of the closure of cerebral arteries

The compliance of the venous bed (C_v) is purely linear, as is the resistance to CSF outflow – RCSF (however the backward flow of CSF is prohibited). The compliance of the CSF fluid containers within the dural sac (C_i), is inversely proportional to ICP above a certain pressure level (named optimal pressure).

The capacitance C_i is the only mechanism which makes the Monroe-Kellie doctrine not valid in the model.

Results and Discussion

The following are phenomena which were observed in clinical or experimental conditions and then studied and interpreted by means of the constructed model.

Pulse Wave-Mean ICP Relationship

The linear relationship between the pulse wave amplitude and the mean ICP is said to be evoked by the non-linear compliance of the cerebrospinal fluid compartment.

The model shows that at least two mechanisms are responsible for this interdependence. Even if the compliance C_i is purely linear, the pulse wave amplitude remains proportional to changes in the ICP level. The explanation for this is that the lowering of CPP increases the transmission of the arterial pressure pulse wave to the cerebrospinal fluid compartment. This is caused by the decrease in R_a and the reciprocal increase in C_a, when the autoregulation holds. This phenomenon can be observed as long as the autoregulatory reserve is sufficient. Therefore, it can be concluded that the positive amplitude-pressure characteristic has its vasomotor origin, apart from the influence of hypothetically monoexponential pressure-volume characteristic of the cerebrospinal fluid space.

The relationship between the intracranial pressure pulse wave amplitude and the mean ICP is distorted in many clinical situations. On the edge, or a little below the CBF autoregulation, the pulse wave amplitude starts to decrease – a phenomenon which can be seen in many clinical cases of severe intracranial hypertension (see Fig. 2a). Until now, this phenomenon has been interpreted as a sign of exhaustion of the autoregulatory reserve. The results of simulation, presented in Fig. 2b, show that in the condition of severe intracranial hypertension (as can be seen during the development of brain oedema – an increase in ICP produces decrease in CPP) the pulse wave amplitude is initially increasing and then starts to decrease – beginning from the mean CPP level of 40 mmHg, which in this case was programmed as the lower limit for the autoregulation. The resulting amplitude-pressure characteristic exhibits the same upper breakpoint as the one observed clinically (compare Fig. 2a and c).

Fig. 2. A Summarized amplitude-pressure characteristic (83 head injured patients) shows the range of proportional amplitude-pressure relationship and the upper breakpoint, interpreted as evidence of loss of autoregulatory reserve. **B** Results of simulation of ICP (Pi-upper trend) and CPP (lower) during modelled increase in brain edema. Pulse wave amplitude increases until CPP systolic reaches a level of 40 mmHg (which was the lower limit of autoregulation in this case). **C** The amplitude (y-axis) versus ICP (x-axis) from the simulation above. The upper breakpoint, above which the amplitude starts to decrease, is at the mean CPP level of 35 mmHg (mean arterial blood pressure was 90 in this case)

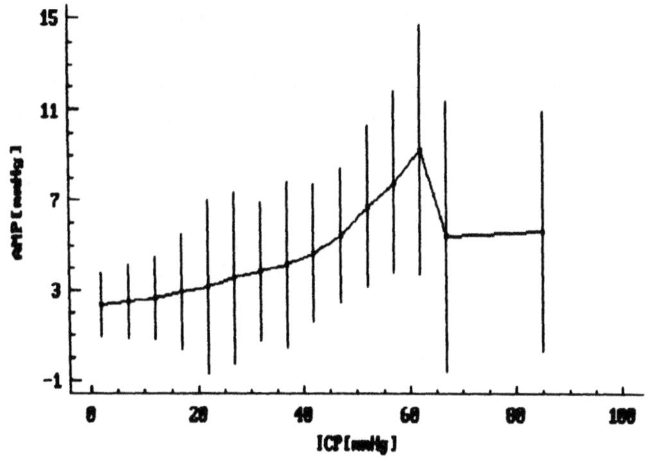

AMP [mmHg]
ICP [mmHg]

A

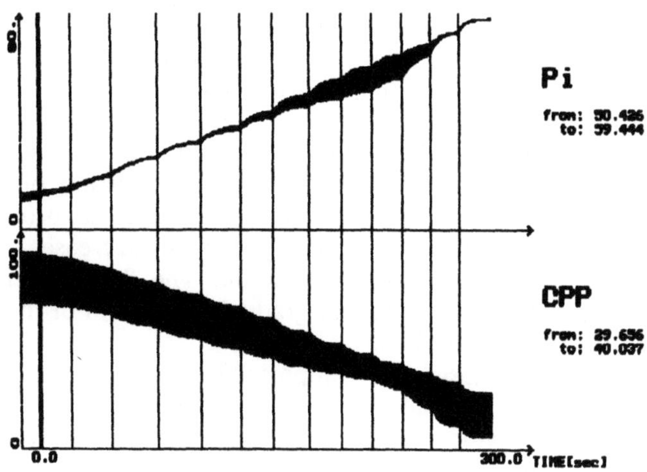

Pi
from: 50.426
to: 59.444
CPP
from: 29.656
to: 40.037
0.0
300.0
TIME[sec]

B

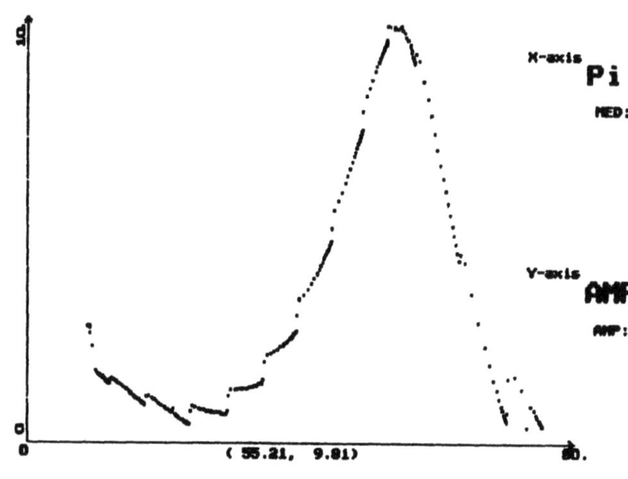

X-axis
Pi
MED:
Y-axis
AMP
AMP:
(55.21, 9.81)

C

Relationship Between CBF, Its Pulsatility and CPP

A comparison of the results of induced intracranial hypertension in rabbits with the results of simulations illustrates the mechanisms involved and explains the gradual increase in CBF pulsatility index, the decrease in blood flow velocity and the increase in the blood flow velocity pulse amplitude.

Experimental recordings are presented in Fig. 3a, as plots of the mean and amplitude of the flow velocity against the decreasing CPP. Mean flow velocity starts to decrease below a CPP of 50 mmHg. At the same level a rapid increase in the amplitude of the flow velocity is observed. The amplitude ceases to increase and reaches the lower breakpoint at a CPP level of about 30 mmHg. The simulation results show a very similar behavior (see Fig. 3b). A decrease in CPP produces first a slight increase in mean CBF and its amplitude and then a decrease in mean CBF – noted when the CPP diastolic reaches a level of 40 mmHg (which was as previously the lower border for the autoregulation). From this point, the rapid increase in CBF pulse wave amplitude is observed. The amplitude starts to decrease when the CPP systolic pressure falls below the autoregulation limit. From this point, the increasing pulsatility index reaches certain saturation and the amplitude of the ICP pulse wave starts to decrease.

The results of the simulation confirm that an increase in the pulsatility index can be considered as a sign of exhaustion of autoregulatory reserve. Moreover, there is a certain "transient zone" as broad as CPP peak-to-peak pressure. The mean flow velocity starts to decrease – pointing out the beginning of the loss of autoregulatation. The flow velocity amplitude ceases to increase when the process of gradual exhaustion of the autoregulatory reserve is already completed.

These conclusions are supported by the results of another simulation, when the CPP was gradually lowered by a decrease of arterial blood pressure. The dynamic behavior of the recorded signals was similar; the mean CBF started to decrease and its pulsatile component started to increase when the CPP diastole reached the lower limit of autoregulation. CBF pulsatile blood flow started to decrease when the systolic CPP exceeded this limit. In these simulations, the specific response of the ICP to the induced variations in arterial blood pressure was recorded. ICP increased in response to the fall in P_a when the autoregulation was intact and decreased when autoregulation was impaired.

Fig. 3. A Plot of mean flow velocity and flow velocity amplitude against cerebral perfusion pressure, recorded in a rabbit, during gradual intracranial hypertension. Flow velocity starts to decrease for CPP below 58 mmHg and the upper breakpoint for the flow velocity amplitude trend is at the level of 38 mmHg. **B** Simulation of gradual intracranial hypertension. Mean CBF (lower trend) starts to decrease when CPP diastole reaches the autoregulation limit (40 mmHg) and the amplitude of the CBF pulsations starts to decrease when the systolic CPP reaches the same level. **C** Simulated relationship of CBF mean and CBF amplitude versus CPP. Lower breakpoint of CBF mean is at CPP = 50 mmHg, and CBFamp at CPP = 30 mmHg. CPP peak to peak was 20 mmHg in this case

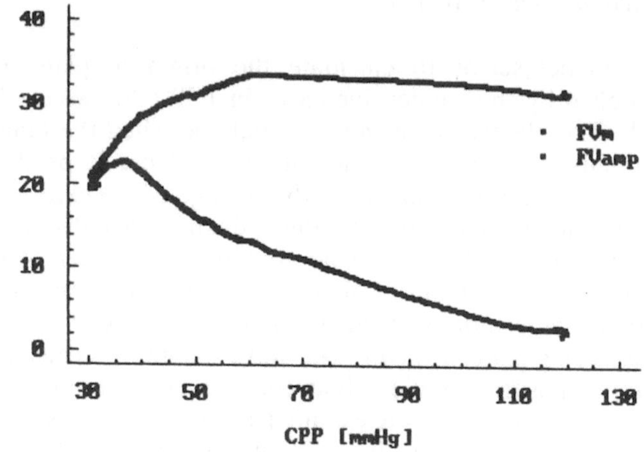
40
30
20
10
0
30
50
70
90
110
130
CPP [mmHg]
FVm
FVamp

A

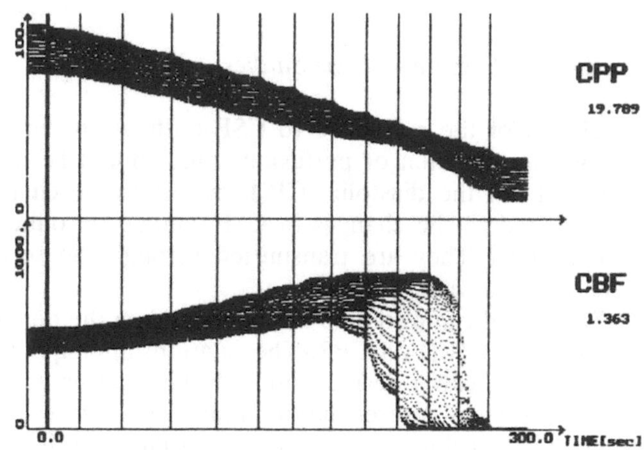
100.
0
1000.
0
CPP
19.789
CBF
1.363
0.0
300.0
TIME[sec]

B

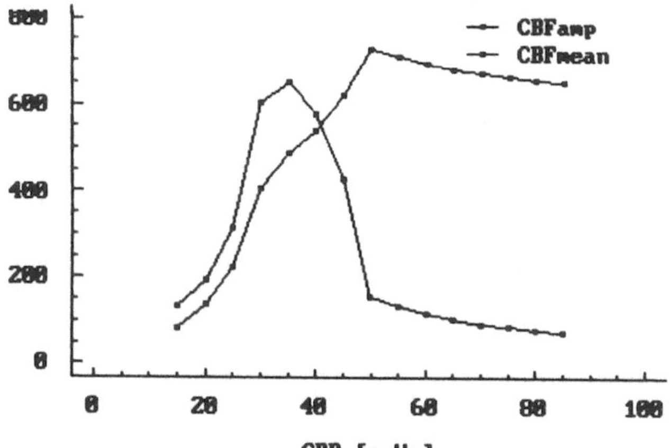
800
600
400
200
0
0
20
40
60
80
100
CPP [mmHg]
CBFamp
CBFmean

C

Origin of Plateau Waves

The model seems to elucidate the origin of plateau waves. They can be modelled by the sudden increases in ICP (Pi), which do not need to be very high. The plateau wave can be simulated when the temporary inversion of the normally positive P_s-P_i gradient takes place. It produces the temporal constriction of the bridging veins, the storage of the extra volume of venous blood, the further increase in ICP, the reduction in CPP, and the arterial vasodilatation. The ICP level must be greater than the cerebrospinal venous pressure P_s during the plateau rise of ICP. This explains why venous (passive) dilatation and not the arterial bed (active) plays the decisive role in the increase in CBV seen during plateau waves. The wave damping is caused by the recovery of the normal, positive gradient between venous bed and CSF pressure. It can be accomplished by an increase in CBF – by central responses (Cushing) or by an autoregulatory reflex (if it is still intact). The formal constraints for the onset of plateau waves are: low cerebrospinal compliance, and weak autoregulation (i.e. the delay in the autoregulatory loop should be long enough).

Remarks on Pressure-Volume Studies

Calculation of the resistance to CSF outflow on the basis of the constant or multiple rate infusion or perfusion study should be made on the basis of the mean and not the diastolic ICP levels. Pulsatile changes of CBV cannot be simply added to the changes in CSF volume introduced during the pressure-volume study. They are transmitted through the serial capacitor C_a, which filters out their mean (dc) level.

The model can also help in understanding the dependence of the pressure-volume index (PVI) on CPP. The relationship is quite complex, but generally PVI increases with a decrease in CPP when autoregulation is intact and starts to decrease when autoregulation is impaired due to a too low CPP. It mainly reflects the contribution of the arterial compliance (C_a) to the total compliance of the cerebrospinal fluid compartment. This disagrees with the studies reported by Gray and Rosner [2].

References

1. Ekstedt J (1978) CSF hydrodynamic studies in man. Journal of Neurol., Neurosurg and Psych 41:345–356
2. Gray J, Rosner M (1987) Pressure-volume index as a function of cerebral perfusion pressure (Part 2). J Neurosurg 67:377–380
3. Hoffmann O (1983) CSF dynamimics: Integration of Pulsatory Components and Autoregulation into Mathematical Model. In: Ishii S, Nagai N, Brock M, Springer, Intracranial pressure Berlin Heidelberg New York Tokyo, pp 169–173
4. Marmarou A (1973) A theoretical and experimental evaluation of the cerebrospinal fluid system. Thesis. Drexel University

Interfering Factors in Cerebrospinal Parameter Estimation

H.E. Heissler, K. Holl, M.R. Gaab, and H. Dietz

Neurochirurgische Klinik, Medizinische Hochschule Hannover, Konstanty-Gutschow-Str. 8, 3000 Hannover 61, Germany

Introduction

Assessment based on the results of volume-pressure tests is often inconsistent with that from clinical and morphological findings. This calls into question the validity of volume-pressure tests as a discriminating examination method. Derived parameters, e.g. PVI, show considerable dispersion and an evident dependence on the injection volume used. With increasing bolus volume craniospinal subsystems, e.g. the cerebrovascular system, are increasingly affected so that autoregulatory mechanisms contribute to unspecific pressure responses. Although there is no alternative to these tests, in our hands these methods bear considerable uncertainties, and lack reproducibility. The object of this project was to investigate the selective properties of the results from an exogenous volume-pressure testing procedure paying particular attention to the effective magnitudes of systematic interfering factors.

Material and Methods

In a retrospective study the results of 88 volume-pressure tests were analysed. These data were rated and data sets were excluded which did not contain pressure measurements at 2, 4 and 8 ml, i.e. within the volume range in which the volume-pressure characteristic was supposed to vary. This reduced the total number of records to 62. All examinations followed the same schedule [3, 4] in patients with CSF circulatory disorders: a series of 1, 2, 4 and 8 ml of saline was rapidly injected into the lumbar CSF space, while the epidural ICP and the lumbar CSF pressure were recorded simultaneously. In some examinations the TCD signal from the MCA was acquired additionally and Diamox administration was used to load the system endogenously. Before the onset of any volume load, the average resting pressure p_0 was determined from the time course and all subsequent pressure changes were related to these values. For each test volume the PVI and the difference Δp between the pressures prior to and immediately after the injection were calculated. To categorize the Δp data records average linkage criterion cluster analysis was carried out on the 62 epidural records previously selected resulting in three clusters (I–III) with distinctive volume-pressure characteristics. All subsequent analyses refer to

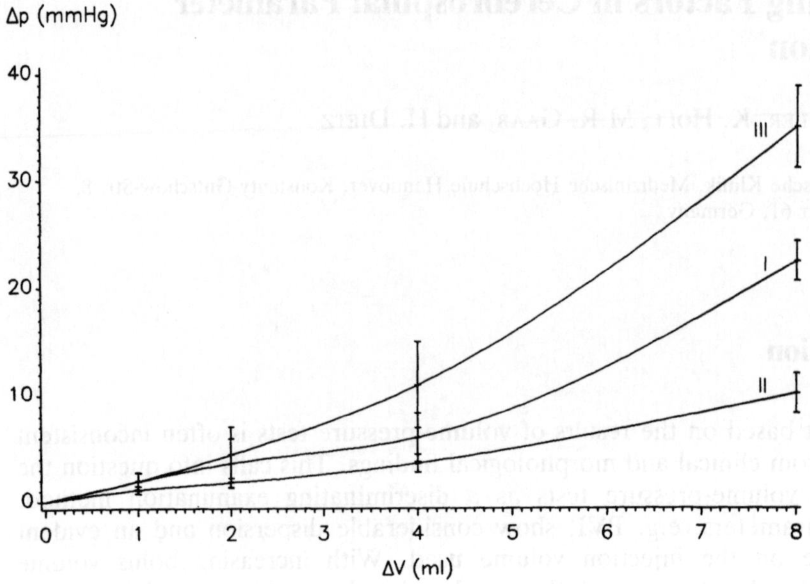

Fig. 1. Volume-pressure diagram and cluster-related spline functions of dynamic elastance. Error bars depict mean Δp and 99% confidence limits

this partition. For each cluster the volume-pressure diagram was constructed, displaying the pressure response (Δp) versus the test volume (ΔV). To estimate the dynamic elastance function exponential LSE regression and cubic spline functions (Fig. 1) were calculated.

Results

A comparison (Wilcoxon test) of the average Δp revealed no statistical differences ($p > 0.01$) for test volumes ranging from 1 to 4 ml for clusters I and III. Otherwise, only significant results were calculated for the pressure responses. Age and resting pressure p_0 as parameters did not reach statistical significance. For 8 ml the pressure responses became strikingly different (Table 1). The regression analyses yielded adequate results in examining the residuals for I and III, confirming the exponential model approach. In II the model fitted poorly, and alternative elastance function approximation seemed to be reasonable. Within the clusters all PVI values varied markedly, and dependence on volume became evident in the range from 1 to 4 ml. Also in this range, the relative coefficient of variation ($CV_r = SEM\sqrt{x}$) took high values always greater than 15%. At 8 ml both all PVI's and CV_r's turned smaller and the averages were similar to those at 1 ml. In III PVI values were least scattered and a consistent estimation of volume reserve was likely. At 8 ml the time course of the epidural pressure transient showed unspecific pressure elevations which reached their maximum amplitude within the range

Table 1. Craniospinal system parameters in hydrocephalus

Cluster	Age	p_o	$\Delta p_{V=1ml}$ PVI	$\Delta p_{V=2ml}$ PVI_2	$\Delta p_{V=4ml}$ PVI_4	$\Delta p_{V=8ml}$ PVI_8	n
I	56[a] 44–73	13.1 ± 1.8[b]	1.9 ± 0.3 21 ± 5[c]	3.6 ± 0.9 33 ± 8	6.0 ± 0.9 41 ± 9	22.5 ± 0.7 23 ± 2	14 [10[d]]
II	50 25–63	15.4 ± 1.4	1.1 ± 0.1 51 ± 9	1.7 ± 0.2 60 ± 9	3.6 ± 0.4 75 ± 14	10.1 ± 0.8 54 ± 7	38 [22]
III	65 51–66	14.0 ± 2.8	1.9 ± 0.3 24 ± 4	4.4 ± 0.9 27 ± 8	10.9 ± 1.4 22 ± 5	35.0 ± 1.4 18 ± 2	10 [8]

Data in bold square represent results from cluster analysis
[a] median age and interquartile limits (years)
[b] mean ± SEM (mmHg)
[c] mean ± SEM (ml)
[d] n $\Delta p_{V=1ml}$

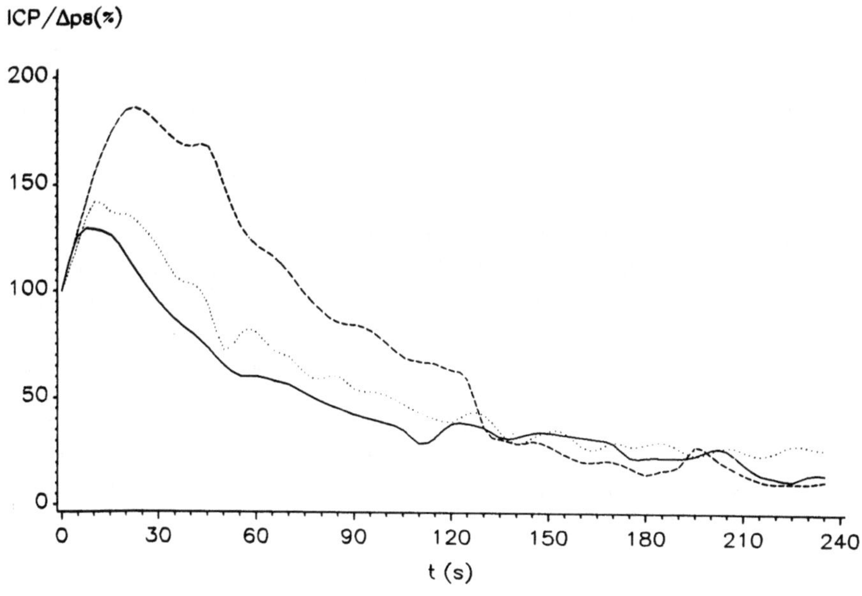

Fig. 2. Average findings of epidural ICP after injection of 8 ml saline. All tracings are shown in normalized percentual units relative to the $\Delta p_{V=8ml}$ for each cluster. (I = dotted, II = solid, III = dashed)

of 10–20 s after the test volume was completely injected (Fig. 2). The average amplitudes of these overshooting pressure were 9 (42%), 3 (29%) and 26 (85%) mmHg for clusters I–III. As an estimate for the pressure decay rate the half life relative to the maximum pressure amplitude was extracted, which proves to be 58 s and 60 s for clusters I and III. In cluster II 43 s was measured.

Conclusions

Based upon the partition into three distinct pressure-volume characteristics, and limited to a volume range from 1 to 8 ml, the data under consideration confirmed the lack of robustness in craniospinal system estimates, e.g. the PVI. This holds true especially for small pressure changes in the low pressure range. Under these circumstances the logarithmic transformation is extremely sensitive to erroneous readings, thus leading to an inconsistent assessment. The more pronounced the amplitude of pressure responses the more reliable the PVI. A reason for this dependence could be found in the system's properties, as the PVI is defined in the framework of closed system theory. Normally, there is a mass transfer through the system and pressure response amplitude is determined by the quality of CSF outflow and compliance. If CSF outflow is reduced then mass transfer is diminished adding to an increased volume storage and the system therefore appears closed. Thus, the effective volume bringing about the pressure response is virtually that being injected. As commonly accepted, unspecific pressure elevations (overshoot) originate from hyperaemia due to autoregulatory responses. Unfortunately, the more selective the pressure response the higher the likelihood and magnitude of such interference. As even for a low pressure response (II) statistically significant pressure overshoots occur, it must be assumed that, in general, unspecific distortion takes place for volume loading per se. Not rarely, the onset of hyperaemia falls concomittantly with the injection phase of a volume load, thence, the pressure response is overestimated and further computations, e.g. the PVI, are affected systematically. To avoid such problems, robust parameters should instead be used. In our hands, the pressure response Δp is a more appropriate parameter because small deviations from a real value are of minor importance for clinical grading. From the data analysed a correlation between the overshoot amplitude and craniospinal volume storage capacity could have been assumed, i.e. any hyperaemic response would increase CSF pressure proportional to the compliant and resistive properties of the craniospinal system [1]. This effect was used intentionally by administering acetazolamide as stimulus for cerebral vasodilation to bring about an endogenous volume load and this resulted in distinct pressure responses in normal and hydrocephalic patients [2].

Acknowledgements. The authors wish to express their gratitude to S. Fischer and S. Noack for technical assistance.

References

1. Benabid AL, De Rougemont J (1984) Non-steady-state analysis of ICP responses to pertubation. In: Shapiro K, Marmarou A, Portnoy H (eds) Hydrocephalus. Raven Press, New York, pp 161–176
2. Holl K, Heissler HE, Nemati N, Gaab MR, Haubitz B, Becker H (1990) Die Wirkung der Acetazolamid-induzierten, endogenen Volumenbelastung des zerebrospinalen Systems auf den intrakraniellen Druck. Neurochirurgia 33:29–36

3. Marmarou A, Shulman K, Rosende RMA (1978) A nonlinear analysis of the cerebrospinal fluid system on intracranial pressure dynamics. J Neurosurg 48:332–344
4. Miller JD, Garibi J, Pickard JD (1973) Induced changes of cerebrospinal fluid volume. Arch Neurol 28:265–269

Elevated Venous Outflow Pressure in Head Injured Patients

A. Marmarou, M.A. Abdelfattah Foda, K. Bandoh, N. Stocchetti, M. Yoshihara, and H.F. Young

Richard Roland Reynolds Neurosurgical Research Laboratories, Division of Neurosurgery, Medical College of Virginia, Richmond, VA, USA

Introduction

The foundation of our understanding of ICP dynamics rests on the assumption that venous outflow pressure, considered the superior saggital sinus, remains constant. As it is further considered that the cortical vein pressure must be slightly higher than ICP to prevent collapse, it follows that a pressure gradient should exist between the cortical veins and saggital sinus [5]. According to this concept, the gradient of pressure is developed along the bridging veins and lateral lacunae.

The objective of this study was to test this theory indirectly by measuring the pressure of the internal jugular bulb (IJ), in patients with raised ICP. If the saggital sinus is at low pressure, in the absence of venous obstruction, the jugular bulb pressure should be a reasonable estimate of the superior saggital sinus pressure.

Methods

Thirty-six patients (25 male and 11 female) with severe head injury [6] (GCS $\leqslant$ 8) were included in this study. Their age ranged between 15 and 81 years with average of 32.3 years. In all patients, catheters were placed in the right jugular bulb and position confirmed with lateral skull films. Front port and side port catheters were used to measure the effect of flow in pressure measurement. Concomitant measures of ventricular fluid pressure (VFP), central venous pressure (CVP) and blood pressure (BP) were also obtained.

Using the bolus injection technique [2, 3], Pressure-Volume Index (PVI) and Resistance for CSF absorption (Ro) were studied once daily for the first five days after injury and average PVI and Ro were then calculated for each patient. In addition, the contributions of CSF (%CSF) and vascular (%VASC.) factors to the elevation of ICP were calculated for each patient according to the following equations [4]:

$$\%CSF = [(Ro \times If - 1.05)/(ICP - 10)] \times 100$$
$$\%Vasc. = [(Pv - 8.5)/(ICP - 10)] \times 100$$

* This work was supported by NIDRR Grant No. H133B80029.

where (ICP) is the measured VFP and (Pv) represents the vascular component of ICP and is equal to VFP during CSF withdrawal at a rate equal to that of CSF formation.

CVP, IJ, VFP, and BP recording over a 24-hour study period was obtained for each patient and two methods of analysis were employed to study these data. In the first, we analyzed the data according to the coefficient of correlation (r) between the IJ and ICP 24-hour temporal course. In the second, the data were studied based upon the degree to which the magnitude of IJ was close to that of VFP. The paired student t-test was used to determine the significance ($p < 0.05$) of ICP-IJ difference in each patient.

Results

The patients were separated into two groups based on the correlation of ICP to IJ; "Good" correlation ($r > 0.5$), and "Poor" correlation ($r < 0.5$) groups. Figures 1A and B are examples of the "Good" and "Poor" groups respectively. We found that the daily average of IJ and ICP was higher in patients where IJ followed the trends of ICP closely. In the "Good" correlation group, however, the difference was not statistically significant. Similarly, P.VI and Ro were not significantly different in these two groups of patients. In contrast, the vascular contribution to ICP elevation was significantly higher ($p = 0.035$) in the "Good" correlation group, while the CSF contribution was higher in the "Poor" correlation group (Fig. 2).

When the data was analyzed according to the ICP-IJ gradient using the paired student t-test, two groups were also identified: those patients in whom IJ was close to ICP ($n = 14$) ($p > 0.05$) and those patients in whom there was a significant ICP-IJ gradient ($n = 22$) ($p < 0.05$). We observed that the PVI was not significantly different between these two groups, however, the Ro was higher in patients with significant "Large" ICP-IJ gradient.

Discussion

Previous studies have shown that the CSF contribution to ICP in severely head-injured patients accounts for approximately 1/3 of ICP rise while the greater component of ICP is attributed to a "vascular" mechanism [4]. These studies were undertaken to further explore the "vascular" component of ICP and to examine the potential contribution of elevatd venous outflow pressure. Our measurements of jugular bulb pressure, although an indirect estimate of sinus pressure, suggest that pressure in the saggital sinus is elevated in approximately 40% of patients. The reasons for sinus elevation are unclear. Under normal condition, venous valves located at the thoracic inlet impede the transmission of intrathoracic pressure to the jugular vein [1]. One possibility is that these valves are not functioning in this group of patients with elevated sinus pressure. Further, increased airway pressure by use of PEEP would contribute to venous

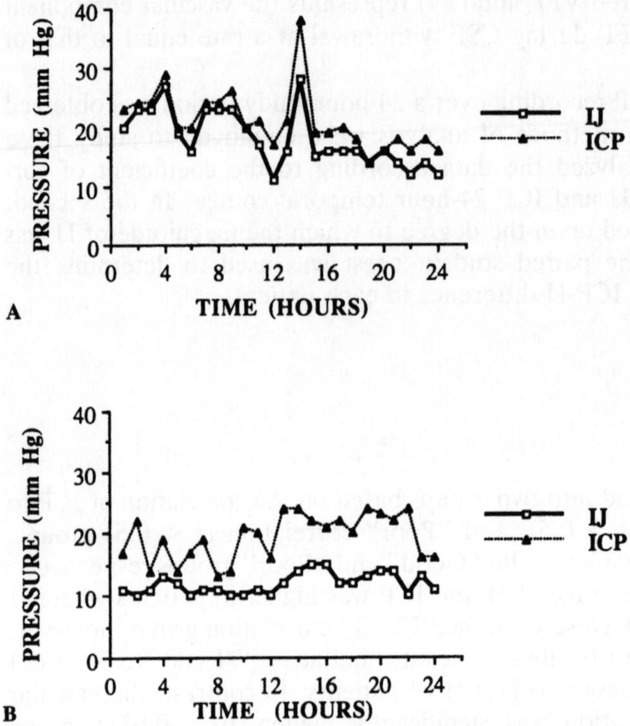

Fig. 1. A Example of ICP and IJ time course in a patient with "Good Correlation" ($r = 0.9$) and "Small" ICP-IJ gradient. We speculate that saggital sinus pressure is elevated in these patients. **B** Example of ICP and IJ time course in a patient with "Poor Correlation" ($r < 0.5$) and "Large" ICP-IJ gradient. We speculate that saggital sinus pressure is near normal and gradient exists along bridging veins and lateral lacunae in these patients

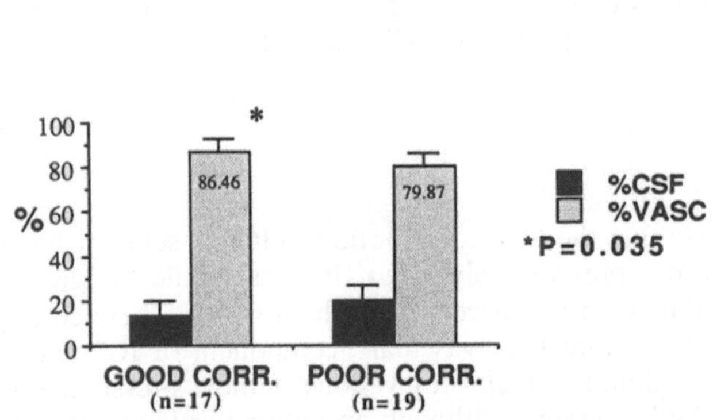

Fig. 2. Percentage vascular contribution to ICP elevation was significantly higher in patients where IJ followed the trends of ICP (Good Correlation Group)

pressure rise in this subset of patients. These studies suggest that venous outflow pressure must be considered when targeting therapy to ICP reduction in severely head-injured patients. Further, that theoretical mathematical models expressing ICP dynamics must now consider the additional complexity of variable dural sinus pressure.

Conclusion

These observations support the notion that saggital sinus pressure is elevated in approximately 40% of severely head-injured patients and that this elevation of venous outflow pressure contributes to raised ICP.

References

1. Fisher J, Vaghaiwalla F, Tsitlik J (1982) Determinants and clinical significance of jugular venous valve competence. Circulation 65:188–192
2. Marmarou A, Shulman K, LaMorgese J (1975) Compartmental analysis of compliance and outflow resistence of the cerebrospinal fluid system. J Neurosurg 43:523–534
3. Marmarou A, Shulman K, Rosende RM (1978) A nonlinear analysis of the cerebrospinal fluid system and intracranial fluid system and intracranial dynamics. J Neurosurg 48:332–344
4. Marmarou A, Maset A, Ward J, et al. (1987) Contribution of CSF and Vascular factors to elevation of ICP in severely head-injured patients. J Neurosurg 66:883–890
5. Rowan J, Johnston I, Harper A, Jennett W (1975) Perfusion pressure in intracranial hypertension. In: Brock M, Dietz H (eds) Intracranial Pressure I. Springer, Berlin Heidelberg New York, pp 165–170
6. Teasdale G, Jennett B (1974) Assessment of coma and impaired consciousness. A practical scale. Lancet 2:81–84

A Finite Element Analysis of Intracerebral Stress Distribution with Viscoelastic Model

S. Hamano[1], T. Nagashima[1], N. Kojima[1], Y. Tada[2], N. Tamaki[1], and S. Matsumoto[1]

[1] Department of Neurosurgery, Kobe University School of Medicine and [2] Department of System Engineering, Faculty of Engineering, Kobe University, Japan

Introduction

The purpose of this study is to characterize the biomechanical property of the brain and to analyze the intracerebral stress distribution by finite element method [3–5] in various pathological conditions.

Materials and Methods

A static Loading Test of Rat Brain and Computer Simulation

Wister rat (250–300 gm) was fixed in a stereotaxic frame and a burr hole was made at the parietal region under anesthesia. Creep curves were obtained by static loadings of 2 gm, 3 gm, and 4 gm at the right parietal region using Biomechanical Spectrometer.

A coronal section of rat brain 1.5 mm anterior to the bregma was used to make a finite element model with 164 triangular elements. Viscoelastic model was applied to the simulation. Time dependent deformation of the brain was simulated under the condition of static loading to the parietal region. Then, the simulated curve was fitted to the curve obtained by the animal experiment so that elastic and viscoelastic modulus of the brain were determined.

Intracerebral Stress Distribution in Various Pathological Conditions

Cases of chronic subdural hematoma and meningioma were selected for the simulation study. Viscoelastic model was applied to the simulation. The elastic and viscous modulus of the brain were those obtained from the animal experiment. Elastic modulus of the falx was tentatively provided 10 times as large as that of the brain.

Chronic Subdural Hematoma. A horizontal (480 elements) and a coronal (206 elements) finite element models were constructed with triangular elements from CT scan and MRI. For the horizontal slice, 10 perpendicular loadings to the brain surface were given to simulate the fronto-parieto-temporal chronic subdural hematoma. Regional cerebral blood flow was measured by SPECT.

Meningioma. A horizontal and a coronal finite element model was constructed from MRI of patients with meningioma. Intracerebral stress distribution was simulated when the perpendicular force was loaded by the tumor. Regional cerebral blood flow was also measured by SPECT.

Results

A Static Loading Test of Rat Brain and Computer Simulation

Elastic and viscous modulus were determined to be 0.418 (kgf/cm^2) and 4.65 ($kgfsec/cm^2$) respectively by fitting the simulated creep curve to the experimental result.

Simulation of Intracerebral Stress Distribution

Chronic Subdural Hematoma. The computer simulation in horizontal slice represented well the displacement of the brain by the chronic subdural hematoma which was observed by CT scan and MRI (Fig. 1, Fig. 2A). The simulated intracerebral stress was mainly distributed in the homolateral hemisphere, and it extended to the central part of the contralateral hemisphere. The stress concentrated just beneath the hematoma and around the falx (Fig. 2C). The area of decreased regional cerebral blood flow coincided with the area of stress concentration in the brain (Fig. 2B,C).

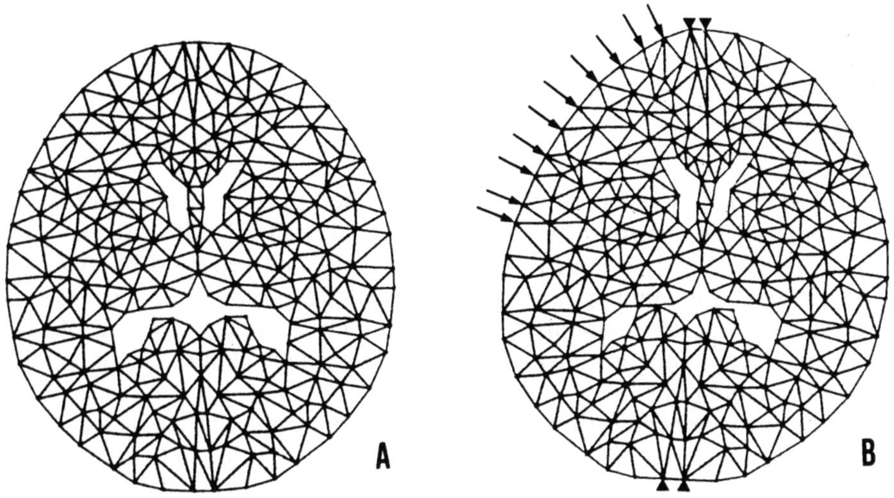

Fig. 1. A The finite element model of the horizontal slice of human brain. **B** The simulated displacement by the chronic subdural hematoma. The arrows represent loading. The arrow heads represent fixed nodes

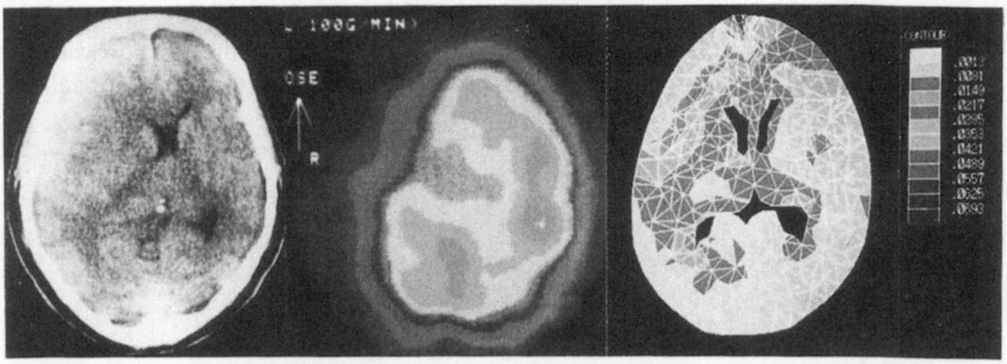

Fig. 2. A CT scan of the case with chronic subdural hematoma. It shows the compressed lateral ventricle with midline shift. **B** Regional cerebral blood flow measured by SPECT. **C** Simulated intracerebral stress distribution. The stress is represented by color grade. Blue means higher stress and yellow means lower stress

The computer simulation in coronal slice also represented the brain displacement by the hematoma. Stress concentration appeared in the brain just beneath the hematoma, around the falx, and in the brain stem. The stress concentration in the brain stem was the remote effect of the hematoma.

Meningioma. The stress concentrated in the brain around the tumor and the ventricle. The regional cerebral blood flow decreased around the tumor and the anterior horn of the lateral ventricle. The area of decreased regional cerebral blood flow coincided with the area of intracerebral stress concentration.

Discussion

The elastic modulus of 0.418 (kgf/cm^2) obtained in the present study approximates the values reported by Galford [2] and Walsh [6]. The viscous modulus of 4.65 ($kgfsec/cm^2$) is much higher than the value reported by Aoyagi [1]. The difference of animal (rat vs. dog) and loading condition (extradural vs. intradural, static vs. dynamic) may cause such a large difference of viscous modulus. Heterogeneous intracerebral stress is generated by brain compression in various conditions.

The stress concentration in the brain parenchyma causes increased interstitial pressure. The simulation by FEM visualized the intracerebral stress distribution and it proved the disturbance of regional cerebral blood flow by intracerebral stress concentration. The remote stress in the brain stem was also revealed in the case of chronic subdural hematoma, which explains brain stem damage by serious brain compression.

References

1. Aoyagi N, Masuzawa H, Sano K, Kihira M, Kobayashi S (1980) Compliance of the brain. Brain Nerve 32:47–56
2. Galford J McElhaney (1970) A visco-elastic property of the brain, J Biomechanics 3:211–221
3. Nagashima T, Tamaki N, Matsumoto S, Seguchi Y, Tamura T (1984) Biomechanics of vasogenic brain edema. Application of Biot's consolidation theory and finite element method. In: Inaba Y, Klazo I, Spatz M (eds) Brain Edema, Springer, Berlin, pp 92–98
4. Nagashima T, Tamaki N, Matsumoto S, Horwitz B, Seguchi Y (1987) Biomechanics of Hydrocephalus: A new theoretical model. Neurosurgery 21:898–904
5. Nagashima T, Shirakuni T, Rapoport SI (1990) A two dimensional finite element analysis of vasogenic brain edema. Neurologia Medico-chirurugica 30:1–9
6. Walsh EK, Alfonso S (1976) Elastic behavior of brain tissue in vivo. Am J Physiol 230:1058–1062

Experimentally Derived Law Governing the Time Relationship of a Pressure-Volume Adjustment in the Human Craniospinal System – a Diagnostic and Management Tool

K. Lewer Allen[1] and E.A. Bunt[2]

[1] Formerly Head of Department of Neurosurgery, University of the Witwatersrand, Johannesburg, South Africa, [2] Rand Afrikaans University, Johannesburg, South Africa

Introduction

In this paper the distinct individuality of pressure-volume behaviour previously shown by Marmarou and Lewer Allen et al. [1, 2] is considered in the extended parameter of time. A series of experiments was launched to study the dynamic response under stress of many specific normal and abnormal individuals – both originally unselected and including cases representative of many clinical problems, including such extremes as chronic low pressure hydrocephalus, Alzheimer's Disease, B.I.H. and N.P.H. This study led to an understanding that the craniospinal system operates to a law PT = C, as defined below and illustrated by a P-T diagram; this was found to apply independently of isolated stress impulses.

Method

The human brain's dynamic response to stress was demonstrated by using a modified infusion technique allowing equilibrium to be found between volume injections in natural time. Experiments were of the order of 2000 s. Telemetric pressure monitoring [3] followed the strain responses with a minimum of opening artifact. Data from 19 patients (24 experiments) were used to plot a parameter $T = t/(V + V_0)\,P$ against a parameter $P = \Sigma \mid \Delta p \mid$. Here t is the total of elapsed times to reach equilibrium pressure after the injection (or withdrawal) of each increment V of fluid. (V_0 is a pseudo-volume having the value of unity to prevent T becoming infinite as $C \rightarrow 0$). P is the summation of magnitudes of pressure changes occurring (whether positive or negative). Thus

$$PT = t/(V + V_0)$$

If PT is a constant C, this equation represents a hyperbola. Experimental data were found to follow such a hyperbola (Fig. 1), the preferred domain of Case 1 (near-normal) being the left (vertical) branch and the knee of the curve; cases operating in "hardness", especially with excess CSF (hydrocephalus) (cf. Case 2) occupy the vertical portion of the curve, and those operating in "softness" (cf. Cases 5, 12, and 18 in the accompanying table) the right (horizontal) portion. The basic curve is also adapted in Fig. 1 to facilitate a quantitative comparison of the operation of the various cases studied. Since C values for the various cases do not differ greatly, the curve for the near-normal Case 1 has been adopted as a "template" and (identical) parallel curves are drawn at suitable arbitrary spacings to plot data representing the other cases studied. From smoothed curves representing rate of pressure change (and noting the existence of a basic wave motion [4]), an indication of the range of slopes of these curves is superimposed on the appropriate hyperbolas.

Findings

1. Pressure-volume-time data for all 19 cases studied, when plotted as P vs. T, closely follow a hyperbolic relationship PT = C (Fig. 1). The excursion on the curve of each case takes place within the range bounded by a mechanism that maintains on demand balanced retention or release of adaptive volumes (CSF or venous blood) – a mechanism that avoids excessive stress build up.
2. The particular location of the range of operation (or the preferred region within it) together with the individuals' excursions about mean positions on the basic hyperbolic curve offers the clinician a comparative guide to pathophysiological behaviour and in turn its classification; these constitute a "tool" which can be used as a guide to clarify "management" of a case.
3. The curve patterns make possible a new dynamic classification of the cases studied (Fig. 2) that extends previous verbal classifications of stress response of cases. All cases represented can be suitably coded (e.g. Normal), Abnormal, Faulty and regions I, II, or III) for more precise description.
4. The graphical representations given are able to reveal the intactness or otherwise of corrective mechanisms and so offer a framework whereby the possibilities of individual case management may be assessed.

Discussion

Normal pulsatile behaviour of the craniospinal system is driven by a vascularly energised wave (VEW) [4, 5]; the VEW would seem to be the main input force (IF) driving the system and maintaining the optimal working property of impedance (Z) for circulatory perfusion. This dynamic balance within the greater law of the curve can also be expressed by Ohm's Law in modification as IF/Z = Flow, thereby giving insight as to the most practical component for modification. The classification shown indicates the presence, absence or latency (or fault) of a corrective mechanism to bring a performance in short or long term into its proper zone on the curve, i.e. $N_{I\,II\,III}$. In A groups the mechanism is effectively lost and must be substituted and monitored for corrective response. When performance is A or F, VEW needs augmenting against a raised inertial Z_{CSF} (NPH) (ventricles enlarged, e.g. Case 5) or raised Z_{venous} (BIH) (ventricles small, e.g. Cases 7 and 12). Correction of the appropriate Z property may augment VEW to assert its lost drive but again if a shunt

Case	Diagnosis		Code
1	Near-normal	N I $II_{i\,ii}$ III	V^n S^n
2	Communicating hydrocephalus – untreated	A III	V> S<
19	Hydrocephalus/N.P.H.	A I III	V> S<
3	Communicating hydrocephalus – closed ventricular catheter	F I II III	V>
11	Post-3rd ventricular tumour		V>
	a. – swinging I.C.P.	F II_{ii} III	V>
	b. – decompressed	F I II_i	V^c
9	Chronic low I.C.P.	N I II III	V^n
8	Post-trauma, paraventricular cysts	A I II III	–
10	Communicating hydrocephalus		
	a. – closed ventricular catheter	N I $II_{i\,ii}$ III	V>
	b. – open ventricular catheter	F I II_i	V^c
16	Communicating hydrocephalus – A/V shunt	F I $II_{i\,ii}$	V>
17	Secondary lymphoma and brain oedema	F II_i	V<
4	Aqueductal stenosis – closed ventricular catheter	F II_i	V>
13	Enlarged ventricles, I.C.P. swinging		
	a. – open catheter	F I II_i	V^c
	b. – closed catheter	F $II_{i\,ii}$	V>
6	Cerebral atrophy – ex vacuo hydrocephalus	F I $II_{i\,ii}$	V> S>
14	Obstructive hydrocephalus – A/V shunt	F I II_i	V>
7	B.I.H. – slit ventricles	F I $II_{i\,ii}$	V< S<
15	Spinal arachnoiditis – headaches	F i II_i	V^n
12	B.I.H. – slit ventricles	AF I II_i	V< S^c
5	N.P.H. – enlarged ventricles	A I II_i	V>
18	Alzheimer degenerative		
	a. – Exp. 1	F I II_i	V> S>
	b. – Exp. 2	A I	V> S>

V, ventricle; S, Sulci; B.I.H., Benign I.C. hypertension; N.P.H., Normal pressure hydrocephalus; <, Attenuated; >, Enlarged; n, Normal; C, Collapsed.

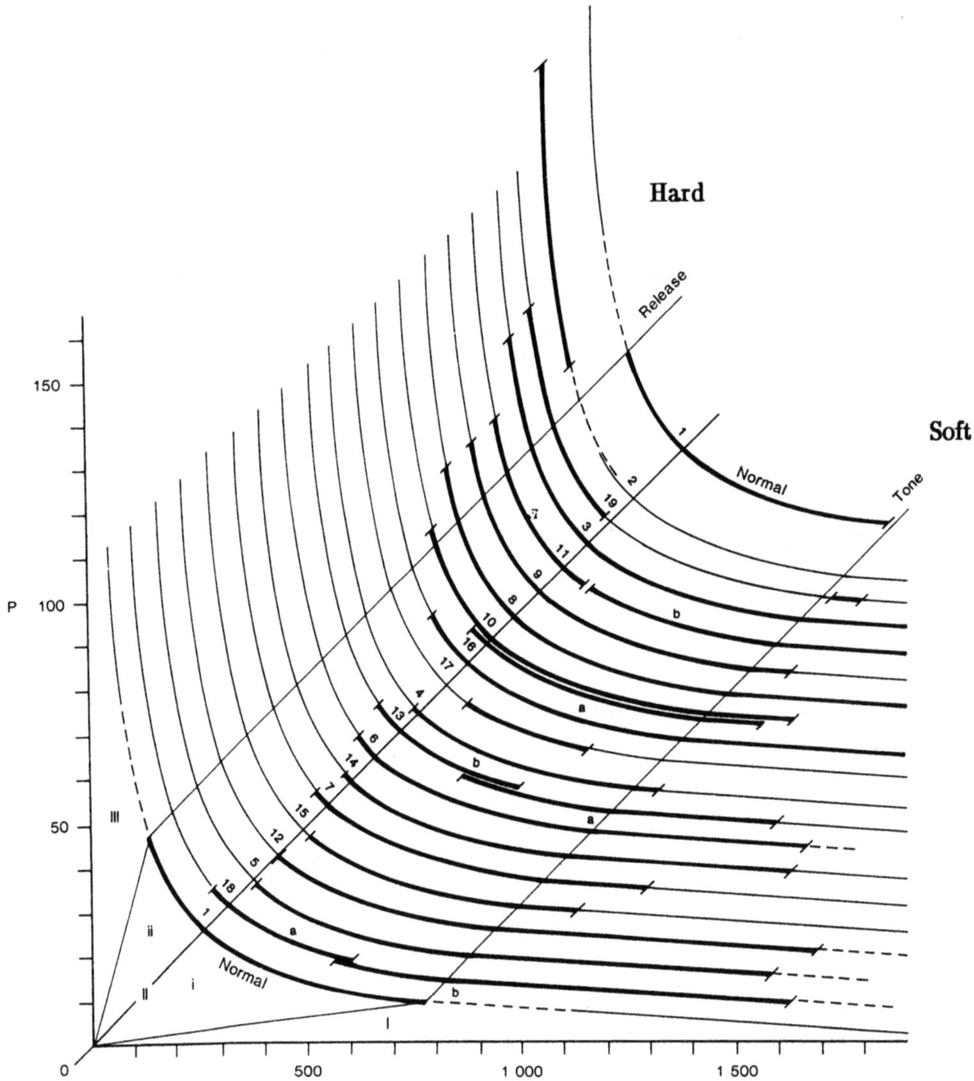

Fig. 1. Hyperbolic relationship

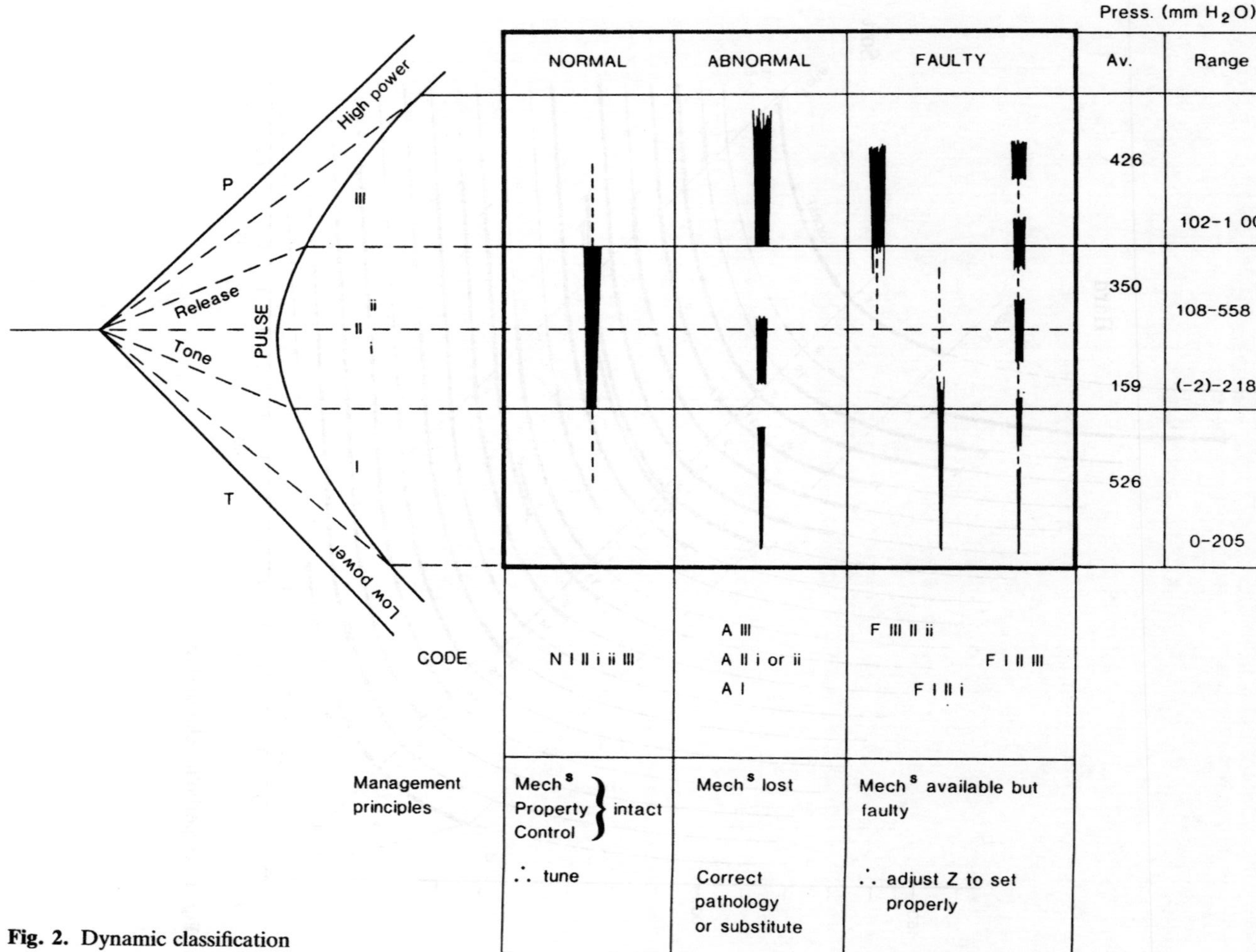

Fig. 2. Dynamic classification

is indiscriminately used in an over-soft situation to reduce Z, VEW cannot be augmented.

Conclusion

The form of representing pressure-volume-time data of the human brain under stress put forward in the form of a hyperbolic graph extends the use of the PVI to characterise individual performance and permits clinical dynamic comparison in actual stress cycles. It is represented as a "tool" for diagnostic classification and management.

References

1. Marmarou A, Shulman K, LaMorgese J (1975) Compartmental analysis of compliance and outflow resistance of the cerebrospinal fluid system. J Neurosurg 43:523
2. Lewer Allen K, Bunt EA (1978) Dysfunctioning of the fluid mechanical craniospinal systems as revealed by stress/strain diagrams. SA Mech Eng 28:159
3. Lewer Allen K (1973) Telemetric monitoring of CSF pressure. J Neurol Neurosurg and Psychiat Dec 922
4. Lewer Allen K, Bunt EA (1986) Rhythmic brain movement and density variations shown by rapid sequential CT scanning in the human subject. In: Miller JD, Teasdale GM, Rowan JO, Galbraith SL, Mendelow AD (eds) Intracranial Pressure VI, Springer, Berlin Heidelberg New York Tokyo, pp 437–440
5. Lewer Allen K, Goldman HI (1967) Phasic pressure characteristics of the cerebrospinal system. SAJ of Surgery, Oct.–Dec. 151

Dynamics and Statics of the Cerebrospinal Fluid: The Classical and a New Hypothesis

M. Bulat

Medical Faculty, University of Zagreb, Zagreb, Croatia

Introduction

According to the classical hypothesis, the cerebrospinal fluid (CSF) is secreted in the cerebral ventricles, it circulates as bulk fluid "downstream" from ventricles along subarachnoid spaces to be absorbed into venous sinuses. Furthermore, increase of intracranial pressure (ICP) and development of hydrocephalus are postulated to be a consequence of obstruction of CSF circulation between these secretory and resorptive sites.

The circulation and absorption of CSF mean by definition the circulation and absorption of the CSF volume (bulk fluid). Since water constitutes 99% of the CSF volume it is apparent that labelled water should be used to demonstrate dynamics of the CSF volume [3]. Any other substance used as marker of CSF dynamics may have half-life and fate in CSF which differs from water and, consequently, it could give a false impression about the behaviour of the CSF volume [3, 4]. In our experiments in cats and dogs we have compared distribution and fate of ^{3}H-water and some other substances both "downstream" and "upstream" in the CSF system.

Fate of ^{3}H-Water in the CSF

After intravenous bolus injection of ^{3}H-water in cats an equilibrium concentration of ^{3}H-water between arterial blood and CSF of cisterna magna is reached in 5 min. On the other hand, half-life of ^{3}H-water in the cisternal CSF is much shorter (5 min) than that of some other substances [6]. Thus, it appears that a rapid free exchange of water between bloodstream and CSF occurs and that any change in concentration of ^{3}H-water in the arterial blood is very soon followed by the same change in the CSF.

During slow infusion of ^{3}H-water in arteficial CSF into the lateral ventricle (1.54 μL/min) of cats, concentrations of ^{3}H-water in the CSF of cisterna magna and arterial plasma very closely follow each other over 4 hours (Fig. 1). ^{3}H-water from the lateral ventricle can reach the arterial bloodstream either by passage into adjacent capillaries or by circulation of CSF via cisterna magna and its entrance into venous sinuses. The fact that the concentration of ^{3}H-water in the cisternal CSF is the same as in arterial plasma speaks against this second possibility, since in such a case, the concentration of ^{3}H-water in

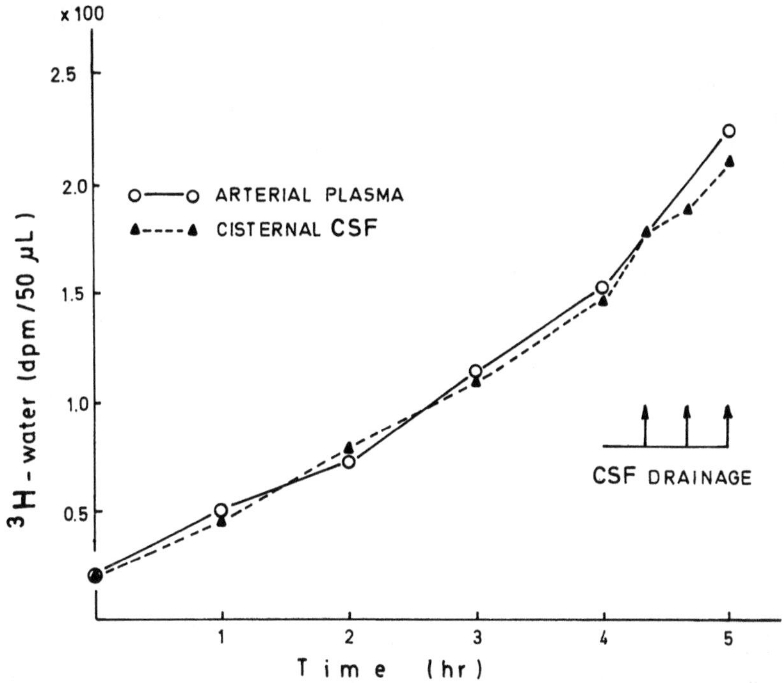

Fig. 1. ^{3}H-water in artificial CSF was continously infused (1.54 µL/min) into lateral ventricle of anesthetized cat (thiopentone sodium, 50 mg/kg i.p.). Samples of cisternal CSF (0.80 µL) were obtained by puncture of cisterna magna at indicated time intervals while during the last hour of experiment CSF was continously drained under negative pressure (−15 cm H_2O below inter-auricular line) and samples collected at 20 min intervals. Samples of arterial blood (0.50 ml) were taken from cannulated femoral artery. ^{3}H-water in 50 µL of cisternal CSF and arterial plasma were measured in Bray's solution

cisternal CSF should be much higher than in arterial blood due to dilution of ^{3}H-water in the large blood compartment. Thus, ^{3}H-water from the lateral ventricle passes into adjacent capillaries and via the vena magna reaches the venous sinuses and the arterial circulation and, thereafter, it enters into all CSF compartments. This interpretation is supported by our additional experiments which showed that the concentration of ^{3}H-water in plasma of venous sinuses was always several times higher than in cisternal CSF and arterial plasma. Furthermore, when CSF was drained from the cisterna magna at a negative pressure for an hour (Fig. 1), the concentration of ^{3}H-water in three sucessive samples of cisternal CSF reflected the concentration of ^{3}H-water in arterial plasma although this drainage should favour a slow flow of the CSF from lateral ventricle to third and fourth ventricles and cisterna magna. Thus, it appears that the exchange of water molecules between ventricular CSF and adjacent capillaries is so rapid that no ^{3}H-water arrives by CSF flow from lateral ventricle to cisterna magna. However, such a flow of ^{3}H-water from lateral ventricle to cisterna magna can be demonstrated when the infusion rate of ^{3}H-water into the lateral ventricle is so high that CSF pressure is increased [5].

After ^{3}H-water was slowly infused for three hours into the cisterna magna of cats, the concentration of ^{3}H-water in the thoracic, lumbar and cortical CSF were the same and equal to that in arterial plasma and much lower than in the cisternal CSF. This speaks against flow of CSF volume (water) from cisterna magna to other CSF compartments, since in such a case the concentration of ^{3}H-water should be higher in these compartments than in arterial plasma (unpublished results).

All data mentioned indicate that there is no flow or circulation of CSF volume (water) between various CSF compartments but that a rapid exchange of water molecules occurs between these compartments and adjacent blood capillaries. Since water constitutes 99% of CSF volume it is obvious that the classical circulation and absorption of CSF volume do not exist. This conclusion, based on experiment with ^{3}H-water, is also supported by experiments with other substances (see below)

Fate of Substances in the CSF

We have observed that ^{3}H-inulin applied into the cisterna magna of dogs is distributed both "upstream" (CSF of lateral ventricle) and "downstream" (lumbar and cortical CSF) [9]. This bidirectional distribution of ^{3}H-inulin along the CSF system can be explained by the CSF pulse waves back and forth and mixing of CSF but not by the classical unidirectional circulation of CSF. Since ^{3}H-inulin is a large molecule which is slowly removed from the CSF (its half-life in CSF is much longer than that of ^{3}H-water [6]), it is not suprising that ^{3}H-inulin reaches all CSF compartments by the CSF pulse waves (Fig. 2).

However, some substances (5-hydroxyindoleacetic acid, iodide) show a limited distribution along the CSF system (Fig. 2) because they are rapidly removed into the bloodstream by active transport so that their half-lives are relatively short in CSF [1, 2]. Thus, it appears that the half-life of a substance in the CSF is an index of its extent of distribution along the CSF system [4]. This idea is supported by our recent observation that ^{3}H-penicillin applied into the cisterna magna of dogs has a short half-life in the cisternal CSF and a limited distribution to remote CSF compartments (cortical, lumbar and ventricular CSF). When active transport of ^{3}H-penicillin out of the CSF was blocked by probenecid, its half-life in the cisternal CSF was doubled and its distribution to remote CSF compartments was much enhanced.

Regulation of the CSF Volume

It is generally assumed that secretion of CSF from the choroid plexuses in the cerebral ventricles and resorption of CSF across the arachnoid villi are the main regulators of CSF volume. Transport of sodium from the choroid plexuses into the CSF followed by osmotically forced water is often mentioned as the main mechanism of CSF secretion. We assume that all ions and sub-

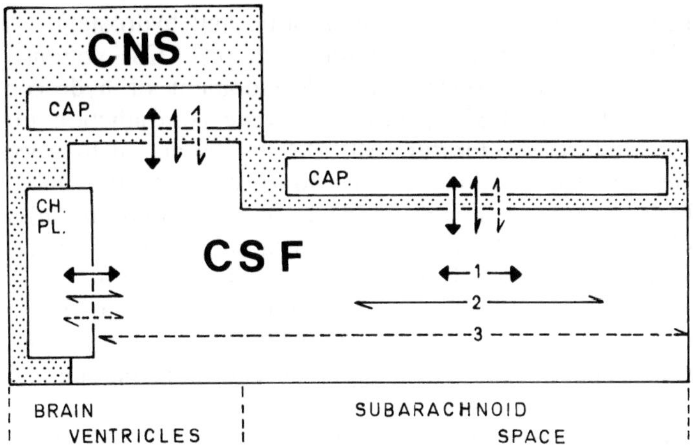

Fig. 2. Scheme of our hypothesis of CSF dynamics. CSF compartments in brain ventricles and subarachnoid space with surrounding CNS parenchyma containing blood capillaries (CAP.) and capillaries of choroid plexuses (CH.PL.) are shown. Water (bidirectional full arrows) exchanges rapidly between CSF and capillaries, has a short half-life in CSF and very limited distribution along CSF spaces (*1*). On the other hand, substances with very restricted passage from CSF to capillaries such as ^{3}H-inulin (bidirectional half-arrows with broken line) have long half-lives in CSF and unlimited bidirectional distribution along CSF spaces (*3*). An intermediate group of substances (bidirectional half-arrows with full line) with relatively limited passage from CSF into capillaries and intermediate half-lives in CSF shows limited distribution along CSF spaces (*2*). Bidirectional distribution of substances along CSF spaces is assumed to be due to bidirectional CSF pulse waves back and forth

stances entering and leaving the CSF are important for the direction of osmotic flow of water between CSF and bloodstream. Since the number of ions and substances entering and leaving the CSF per unit of time is unknown and such a balance sheet is impossible to make at the present time, we are left in the dark concerning the osmotic flow of water across the blood-brain barrier. On the other hand, methods developed to measure "net formation" of CSF volume are not reliable. The most popular ventriculocisternal perfusion method can be criticized on several accounts [7] (Orešković and Bulat, this volume). Since there is no flow of ^{3}H-water from lateral ventricle to cisterna magna (Fig. 1), it is doubtful that "net formation" of CSF exists in the ventricles. After obstruction of the aqueduct of Sylvius in cats, we were not able to record any significant change in the ventricular CSF pressure over several hours which speaks against net formation of CSF in the ventricles.

We presume that hydrostic and osmotic forces are operating between CSF and capillaries located in the choroid plexuses, subependymal and subpial tissues (Fig. 2) and that these forces can regulate the CSF volume and influence ICP in physiological and pathological conditions. Our observation that the concentration of ^{3}H-water is decreased while that of blue dextran is increased in perfusate of the ventricles under enhanced hydrostatic pressure suggests that hydrostatic pressure can regulate the volume of CSF (Orešković and Bulat, this volume). Furthermore, increased osmolality of CSF favours osmotic passage of water into CSF and enhancement of ICP (Klarica et al., this volume). Thus, we believe that an interplay of osmotic and hydrostatic forces operating at the blood-brain barrier is the main regulator of CSF volume.

The classical concept that development of hydrocephalus is due to the obstruction of CSF spaces is in some contradiction to several observations reported in the literature [8]: a) the presence of hydrocephalus of one lateral ventricle with both foramina Monro open, b) the stabilization of obstructive hydrocephalus although the shunt was occluded, and c) secondary obstruction of aqueduct of Sylvius and cortical subarachnoid space during development of hydrocephalus. It is probable that some pathological processes such as meningitis may increase the osmolality of CSF in the ventricles and the ICP (Klarica et al., this volume). It can be speculated that such an osmotic force in ventricular CSF may in some cases lead to development of hydrocehpalus.

Acknowledgements. Supported by U.S.-Yugoslav Joint Board (JFP No. 721) and Ministry of Science and Technology of Republic Croatia.

References

1. Bulat M (1974) Monoamine metabolites in the cerebrospinal fluid: indicators of biochemical status of monoaminergic neurons in the CNS. In: Wolstenholme GE, FitzSimons DW (eds) Aromatic amino acids in the brain, Ciba Foundation Symposium 22, Elsevier, Amsterdam, pp 243–264
2. Bulat M (1977) On the cerebral origin of 5-hydroxyindoleacetic acid in the lumbar cerebrospinal fluid. Brain Res 122:388–391
3. Bulat M (1978) The formation, circulation and absorption of the cerebrospinal fluid. Iugoslav Physiol Pharmacol Acta 14:35–37
4. Bulat M (1980) Biochemical communication of the brain and cerebrospinal fluid. Period Biol 82:257–260
5. Bulat M, Lupret V, Orešković D (1981) Chemistry of the brain and cerebrospinal fluid. Period Biol 83:5–8
6. Lupret V, Orešković D, Klarica M, Bulat M (1985) Half-life and fate of substances in the cerebrospinal fluid. Iugoslav Physiol Pharmacol Acta 21:169–170
7. Orešković D, Bulat M (1988) Critique of perfusion method for calculation of formation and absorption of the cerebrospinal fluid. Iugoslav Physiol Pharmacol Acta 24 [Suppl 6]:309–310
8. Pfeifer T (1987) Hydrocephalus and viral infections. Medicinar 35:87–97
9. Vladić A, Bulat M (1988) Distribution of ^{3}H-inulin by CSF pulsation and body activity into various compartments of the CSF. Iugoslav Physiol Pharmacol Acta 24 [Suppl 6]:489–490

Hydrostatic Force in Regulation of CSF Volume

D. OREŠKOVIĆ[1] and M. BULAT[2]

[1] Department of Experimental Biology and Medicine, "Ruđer Bošković" Institute, Bijenička 54, 41000 Zagreb, Croatia
[2] Department of Pharmacology, Medical Faculty University of Zagreb, Šalata 11, 41000 Zagreb, Croatia

Introduction

The cerebrospinal fluid (CSF) volume is regulated by a balance between CSF formation and absorption. It is generally believed that the increase of hydrostatic pressure enhances absorption of CSF across arachnoid villi into venous blood without affecting CSF formation in brain ventricles. We have recently demonstrated by ventricular perfusion that in isolated brain ventricles augmentation of intracranial pressure (ICP) decreases CSF formation [4]. These data may also suggest that CSF formation and absorption occur in the whole CSF system and that CSF volume is dependent on hydrostatic pressure of CSF. Since only about one fifth of CSF volume is contained inside the brain ventricles, the aim of this study was to investigate by ventriculocisternal perfusion the influence of ICP on the total CSF volume. For calculation of CSF formation (Vf) and absorption (Va) the perfusion of CSF spaces was used as a generally accepted method, with the assumption that the indicator substance in the perfusate does not diffuse into the central nervous system (CNS).

Furthermore, since water represents CSF volume (99% of CSF is water), it can be expected that a change in CSF volume should be reflected by the volume of water. For this reason, perfusion of CSF spaces by radioactive water (^3H_2O) was performed, and the concentration of ^3H_2O in the perfusate at different pressures was monitored. The concentration of ^3H_2O in the perfusate was compared with that of Dextran Blue which is a large molecule (m.w. 2 millions) used as indicator substance for calculation of Vf.

Materials and Method

All experiments were performed with anesthetized (Nesdonal, Specia, Paris; 60 mk/kg i.p.) adult cats of both sexes. The ventriculocisternal perfusion was performed in cats fixed in the stereotaxic instrument [4]. The perfusion solutions with Dextran Blue (Pharmacia, Uppsala) and ^3H_2O (New England Nuclear, Boston, Massachusets; 0.125 mCi/ml) were infused with a perfusion pump (Palmer) at rates of 92.44 or 65.50 μl/min respectively from lateral ventricle to the cisterna magna. ICP was altered by adjusting the outflow tubing above (+10 and +20 cm H_2O) or below (−10 cm H_2O) the auditory meatus which level was taken as zero pressure. After a period of stabilization, 20 minutes samples of perfusate were collected in a glass tube.

The rate of CSF formation (Vf) was calculated according to the equation of Heisey et al. [2] Vf = Vi(Ci − Co)/Co in which Ci and Co are the concentration of Dextran Blue in the inflow and outflow fluid, respectively, and Vi is the perfusion rate. Statistical analysis was performed using Student's t-test.

Results

The results of the outflow concentration of Dextran Blue (Co/Cix100) and Vf during ventriculocisternal perfusion at negative (−10 cm H_2O) and positive (+10 cm H_2O) ICP are shown in Table 1. ICP elevation from −10 to +10 cm H_2O results in a significant increase in outflow concentration of Dextran Blue and substantial decrease in Vf.

A comparison of the behaviour of ^3H_2O and Dextran Blue during ventriculocisternal perfusion at negative (−10 cm H_2O) and positive (+20 cm H_2O) ICP is shown in Fig. 1. The data show that changes in ICP have opposite effects on concentration of ^3H_2O and Dextran Blue; i.e. the elevation of ICP (from −10 to +20 cm H_2O) decreased the concentration of ^3H_2O and increased the concentration of Dextran Blue.

Table 1. Outflow concentration of Dextran Blue (Co/Ci × 100) and the rate of cerebrospinal fluid formation during ventriculocisternal perfusion (rate of perfusion: 65.50 μl/min) at different intracranial pressure (−10 and +10 cm H_2O) in three cats

Pressure	Time (min)	Dextran Blue (Co/Ci × 100)	Vf (μl/min)
−10	80–100	78.97 ± 0.12	18.67 ± 2.66
	100–120	78.57 ± 3.93	22.30 ± 1.93
	120–140	78.60 ± 2.21	21.07 ± 2.61
	140–160	77.37 ± 1.42	22.30 ± 1.93
	160–180	79.13 ± 0.25	19.80 ± 0.69
	180–200	79.90 ± 2.62	19.87 ± 3.01
	(80–200)	78.76 ± 2.02	20.67 ± 2.36
+10	280–300	84.43 ± 3.25	14.20 ± 3.27
	300–320	84.90 ± 2.08	13.47 ± 1.79
	320–340	84.00 ± 3.32	14.57 ± 3.20
	340–360	83.50 ± 1.05	14.87 ± 1.68
	360–380	84.43 ± 2.55	14.87 ± 0.64
	380–400	85.63 ± 3.52	14.20 ± 2.66
	400–420	83.50 ± 0.36	12.70 ± 3.52
	(280–420)	84.33 ± 2.27*	14.12 ± 2.29*

Values are means ± S.D. Differences between outflow concentration of Dextran Blue at −10 and +10 cm H_2O intracranial pressure and between Vf at both pressures under the same conditions are statistically significant (* $p < 0.02$).

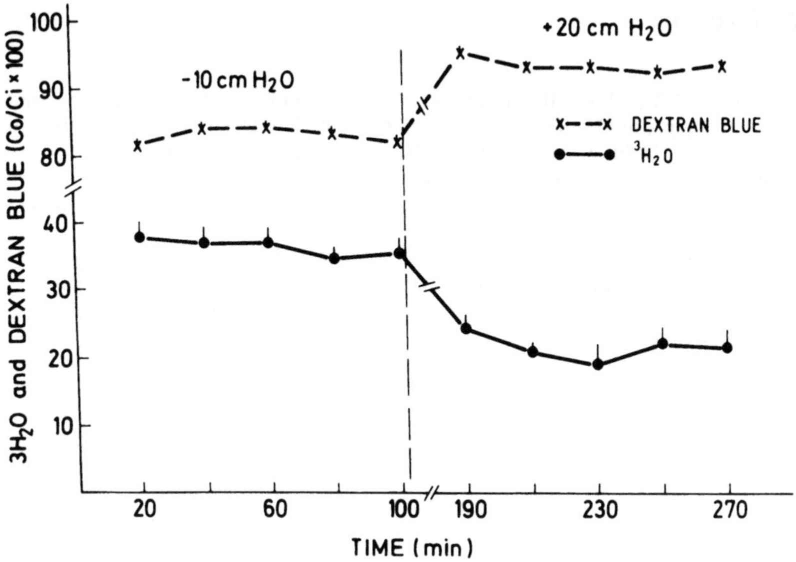

Fig. 1. The effect of intracranial pressure (−10 and +20 cm H_2O) on the percentage of outflow concentration (Co/Ci × 100) of Dextran Blue and ^3H_2O during ventriculocisternal perfusion (rate of perfusion: 92.44 μl/min). The broken line shows the percentage of outflow concentration of Dextran Blue, and the solid line represents the percentage of outflow concentration of ^3H_2O. The vertical broken line indicates the time when the pressure has been changed. Each point of the line is the mean value of three animals

Discussion

The present study shows that elevation of ICP decreases CSF formation (Vf; Table 1). These results obtained in the whole CSF system are in agreement with some previous results [1, 3, 5] and with recently published data obtained inside isolated brain ventricles [4]. The results presented suggest that Vf is a pressure dependent value as is Va, and that volume of CSF is regulated by hydrostatic pressure of CSF which influences the Vf as well as the Va.

The behaviour of ^3H_2O (Fig. 1) indicates also that the volume of CSF is pressure dependent. It appears that the rise of ICP forces water into surrounding tissue and blood vessels which is reflected as a reduction in outflow concentration of ^3H_2O (Fig. 1). However, if ^3H_2O disappears into the surrounding tissue, it is obvious that a part of increased outflow concentration of Dextran Blue is a consequence of water loss from the perfusate. Since Vf calculation is based on dilution of concentration of indicator by newly formed CSF, any other changes in concentration of indicator questions the validity of calculated Vf. It seems therefore, that Vf obtained in this way is erroneous, which discredits the perfusion method as a method for determination of this parameter.

References

1. Calhoun MC, Hurt HD, Eaton HD, et al. (1967) Rates of formation and absorption of cerebrospinal fluid in Hostein male calves. Bull Univ Conn Agri Expl Station 401:22–26
2. Heisey SR, Held D, Pappenheimer JR (1962) Bulk flow and diffusion of the cerebrospinal fluid system of the goat. Am J Physiol 203:775–781
3. Hochwald GM, Sahar A (1971) Effect of spinal fluid pressure on cerebrospinal fluid formation. Expl Neurol 32:30–40
4. Orešković D, Whitton PS, Lupret V (1991) Effect of intracranial pressure on cerebrospinal fluid formation in isolated brain ventricles. Neuroscience 41:773–777
5. Weiss MH, Wertman N (1978) Modulation of CSF production by alterations in cerebral perfusion pressure. Arch Neurol 35:527–529

Osmotic Force of the CSF and Intracranial Pressure in Health and Disease

M. KLARICA[1], B. GMAJNIČKI[2], D. OREŠKOVIĆ[3], and M. BULAT[1]

[1] Medical Faculty, University of Zagreb, [2] Institute of Immunology, and [3] Ruđer Bošković Institute, Zagreb, Croatia

Introduction

The role of the osmotic pressure of CSF in physiological and pathological conditions is unknown. In our preliminary experiments in cats we have observed that slow infusion of different hyperosmolal solutions in the lateral ventricle increases the ICP [1]. In the present experiments in dogs we have studied the effect of hyperosmolal sucrose solution and innoculum of Streptoccocus pneumoniae applied into the lateral ventricle on ICP and osmolality of CSF.

Methods and Results

Augmentation of CSF Osmolality and ICP. Mongrel dogs were anesthetized with alpha-chloralose (100 mg/kg i.p.). Two stainless steel cannulas were placed in the right lateral ventricle and one in the left lateral ventricle and the other one in the cisterna magna. ICP was measured simultaneously in the right ventricle and cisterna magna. Femoral artery was cannulated and blood pressure and $PaCO_2$ were controlled. A volume of 500 μl of solution was applied into right ventricle while simultaneously the same volume of CSF from the left ventricle was removed. When arteficial CSF was applied no significant changes of ICP were observed. However, when hyperosmolal sucrose (700 mOsm/kg) was applied the ICP was doubled during the next 15 min and thereafter the ICP returned towards control values at 30 min (Fig. 1). In three additional animals after application of sucrose, the samples of CSF from right ventricle were taken at 2, 7 and 20 min and measured osmolality was 380, 338 and 307 mOsm/kg respectively.

CSF Osmolality and ICP at the Beginning of Bacterial Meningitis. In both lateral ventricles chronic cannulas were implanted, one for recording ICP and another one for application of bacteria and sampling of CSF. In the control group of animals (n = 5), during 6 days, ICP and osmolality of ventricular CSF were stable. In another group of animals, 0.4 ml of ventricular CSF was removed and the same volume of innoculum of Streptoccocus pneumoniae (10^7 bacteria/ml) was applied into the ventricle at the third day after operation. Immediately before the innoculation ICP was recorded and samples of ven-

Table 1. ICP and CSF osmolality of lateral ventricle (LV) and cisterna magna (CM) immediately before and 8–19 hours after infection with Streptoccocus pneumoniae

Animal No.		Osmolality of CSF (mOsm/kg) 1	2	3	4		ICP ($cm\ H_2O$)
before infection	LV	291	294	290	280	289 ± 3[x]	12 ± 2[a]
after infection	LV	310	314	321	321	317 ± 3*	
" "	CM	300	302	304	---	302 ± 1**	30 ± 4**

[a] mean ± SEM
* $p < 0.001$ and ** $p < 0.01$ when compared to data before infection.

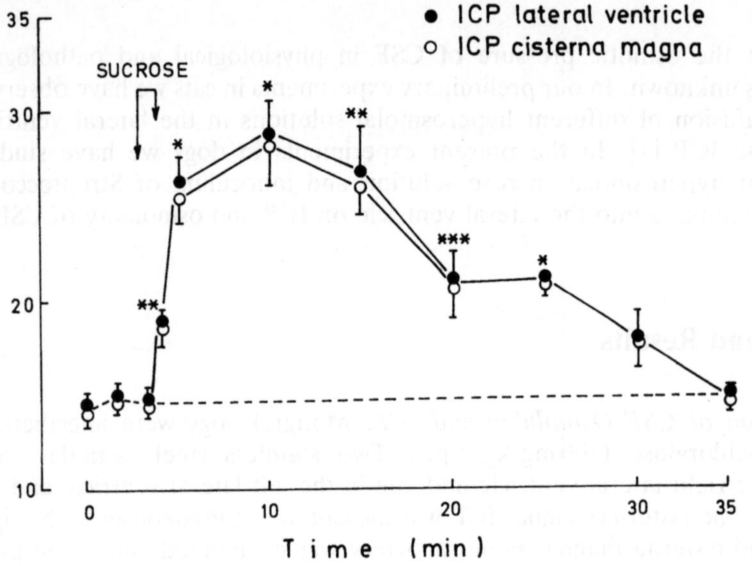

Fig. 1. ICP measured in lateral ventricle and cisterna magna before and after application of hyperosmolal sucrose into lateral ventricle. Values are means ± SEM (n = 4). Significant difference between mean values before and after application of sucrose: * $p < 0.001$; ** $p < 0.002$; *** $p < 0.01$

tricular CSF were taken (Table 1). Eight to 19 hours after infection, the ICP and osmolality of ventricular CSF were measured and thereafter samples of cisternal CSF were taken for analysis of osmolality. It can be seen (Table 1) that after infection both the osmolality in ventricular CSF and the ICP were enhanced. Increase of osmolality in ventricular CSF was higher than in cisternal CSF ($p < 0.01$).

Discussion and Conclusion

Application of hyperosmolal sucrose into the lateral ventricle is followed by an increase of CSF osmolality which causes an augmentation of ICP

(Fig. 1). Gradual fall of osmolality of ventricular CSF over time suggest that hyperosmolal CSF is diluted by osmotic arrival of water. This idea is supported by additional experiments which showed that after intravenous bolus injection of ^{3}H-water, concentration of ^{3}H-water in the ventricle with hyperosmolal sucrose was twice higher than in control ventricle. Eight to 19 hours after intraventricular application of innoculum of Streptoccocus pneumoniae osmolality of ventricular and cisternal CSF are increased accompanied by an augmentation of ICP (Table 1). Such animals develop over the next few days clinical symptoms of pronounced infection and biochemical changes in CSF characteristic of meningitis (increase of lactate and proteins and decrease of glucose). We assume that the increase of ICP observed after infection is due, at least partly, to the observed augmentation of CSF osmolality and osmotic arrival of water into CSF.

In conclusion, an increase of ICP is observed when CSF osmolality is enhanced either by experimental manipulation (Fig. 1) or by induction of a pathological process in the brain (Table 1). This suggests that CSF osmolality is an important factor in regulation of ICP in physiological and pathological conditions. We assume that various pathological processes in the brain (infection, ischemia, trauma etc.) may increase CSF osmolality, and consequently ICP, due to either damage of brain parenchyma and increased diffusion of some substances into CSF or damage of transport of some substances from CSF to bloodstream and accumulation of these substances in the CSF.

Acknowledgements. Supported by U.S.-Yugoslav Joint Board (JFP No. 721) and Ministry of Science and Technology of Republic Croatia.

References

1. Klarica M, Orešković D, Bulat M (1988) Effect of cerebrospinal fluid osmolality on the intracranial pressure. Iugoslav Physiol Pharmacol Acta 24 [Suppl 6]:189–190

CSF Outflow Resistance and Volume-Pressure Relationship

CSF Dynamics and Cerebral Hemodynamics in ATP-Induced Hypotension

A. Schettini and E.K. Walsh

Research Service, McGuire Veterans Administration Medical Center, Richmond, VA 23249, USA, and College of Engineering, University of Florida, Gainesville, FL 32611, USA

Introduction

Induced hypotension is frequently used in neurosurgery, particularly in operations involving cerebral aneurysms and vascular tumors. The hypotensive agent adenosine triphosphate (ATP) has been shown to produce controllable decreases in systemic arterial pressure (MAP) [4, 10]. ATP is converted to adenosine on the venous side of systemic circulation, and thus, its mode of action as a hypotensive agent is identical to adenosine.

The use of these agents is attractive since, first, adenosine is a normal intracellular component and one of the vasoactive compounds involved in regulating cerebral blood flow. Second, because of rapid cellular uptake, the recovery of near baseline arterial blood pressure following discontinuation is relatively fast. And third, adenosine has no direct CNS action, because the brain uptake index for nucleosides and purine bases is nearly negligible. As a result, adenosine (ATP) hypotension is due solely to its direct action on the vascular smooth muscle of systemic circulation.

However, as a vasodilator, adenosine may cause cerebral vascular expansion resulting in intracranial hypertension and possible cerebral ischemia. Indeed, moderate increases in intracranial pressure (ICP) due to ATP have been reported [9], but the degree of intracranial hypertension, in response to intracranial volume changes, cannot be predicted by the ICP alone, but requires a knowledge of intracranial compliance and CSF dynamics. The present study was designed to measure these functions, i.e. the compliance (C), which is obtained from the measured pressure-volume index (PVI), the outflow resistance (R_o), along with the cerebral perfusion pressure (CPP), cerebral vascular resistance (CVR), and local cerebral blood flow (lCBF) during ATP-induced hypotension in the normocarbic animal.

Materials and Methods

Fifteen dogs (18–24 kg) were chronically prepared for measurement of bifronto-occipital lCBF, ventricular cerebrospinal fluid (CSF) pressure (PvCSF), and CSF dynamics. The methods have been described elsewhere [8]. A femoral artery and vein were also cannulated for pressure recording, blood sampling, and drug administration.

Four days later each dog was anesthetized, intubated and mechanically ventilated. Body temperature and normocarbia were maintained. The tests involved the continuous monitoring of PvCSF and mean arterial pressure (MAP) using low-volume displacement transducers and an oscillograph tape recording system.

Following control measurements, the MAP was decreased in stepwise fashion to 70, 50, and 40 mmHg (referred to as *mild*, *moderate*, and *marked* hypotension) by increasing the infusion rate. The ATP dose, infused through the femoral vein, averaged to 2, 4, and 6 mg/kg/min, respectively. Each stage was held relatively constant for 30 min during which the variables under study were measured. The ATP infusion was then discontinued, the animals allowed to recover, and all measurements repeated at 20 min of recovery. In addition, CBF autoregulation was tested at MAP = 70 mmHg (n = 7) and at MAP = 50 mmHg (n = 6) by infusing angiotensin to raise the MAP to near baseline. The index for CBF pressure autoregulation was taken as the ratio (Δ%CPP/Δ%CVR) [6].

Statistical significance at each observation period was tested by univariate analysis of variance.

Results

The results for successive stages of hypotension are summarized in Figs. 1 and 2.

Mild hypotension: At a MAP of approximately 70 mmHg, PvCSF nearly doubled while CPP was reduced to 57% of baseline. Mean lCBF remained unchanged as CVR was reduced by 40%. The vasodilation affected the intracranial volume-pressure relation as the compliance (C) decreased by 31% and the outflow resistance (R_o) increased by 135%. Autoregulation was shown to be intact.

Moderate hypotension: At a MAP near 50 mmHg, the PvCSF reduced slightly (although still 64% above the baseline) and the CPP declined to 40% of baseline. At this point the lCBF had decreased by 33% and thus there was no additional change in CVR. With this further reduction in MAP, the compliance recovered to its baseline value, while the outflow resistance recovered somewhat, to a level 30% over the baseline value. Autoregulation was indicated as defective.

Marked hypotension: At a MAP near 40 mmHg, PvCSF did not change from the previous level and the CPP declined to 30% of baseline. The lCBF

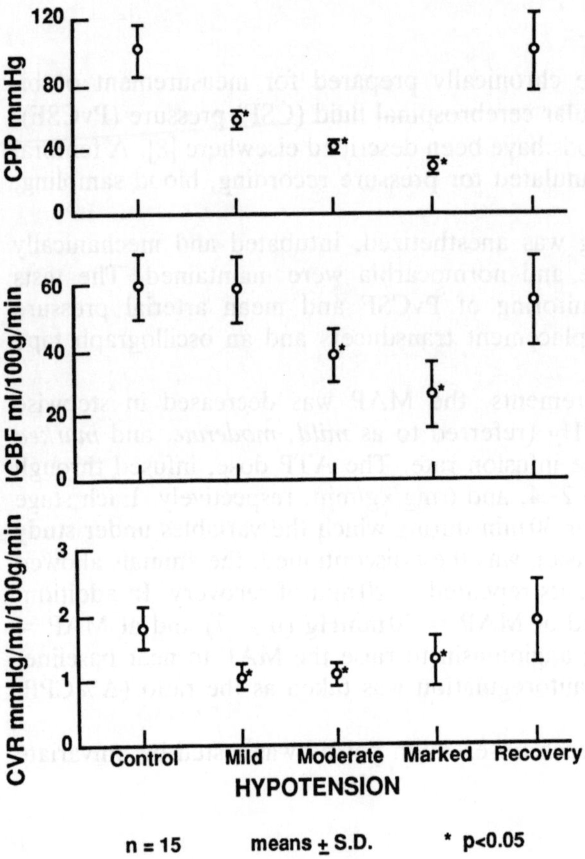

Fig. 1. Cerebral perfusion pressure (CPP), local cerebral blood flow (lCBF) and cerebral vascular resistance (CVR) at increasing stages of hypotension (means ± S.D., n = 15, * $p < 0.05$)

continued to decrease while the CVR did not change significantly. At this hypotensive stage there was no significant change in the values of the compliance or outflow resistance from those at moderate hypotension.

Recovery: At 20 min after terminating the ATP infusion, MAP, CPP and mean lCBF returned to baseline values. However, there remained evidence of cerebral vascular volume expansion in that the compliance was reduced by 35% and R_o was double the baseline value.

Discussion

With ATP induced mild hypotension, within the autoregulatory range, the cerebral resistance vessels dilated and flow remained constant. Intracranial compliance, however, decreased by one third while the resistance to CSF outflow (R_o) more than doubled, which represents an indication of cerebral vascular expansion. This inverse correlation between C and R_o implies that

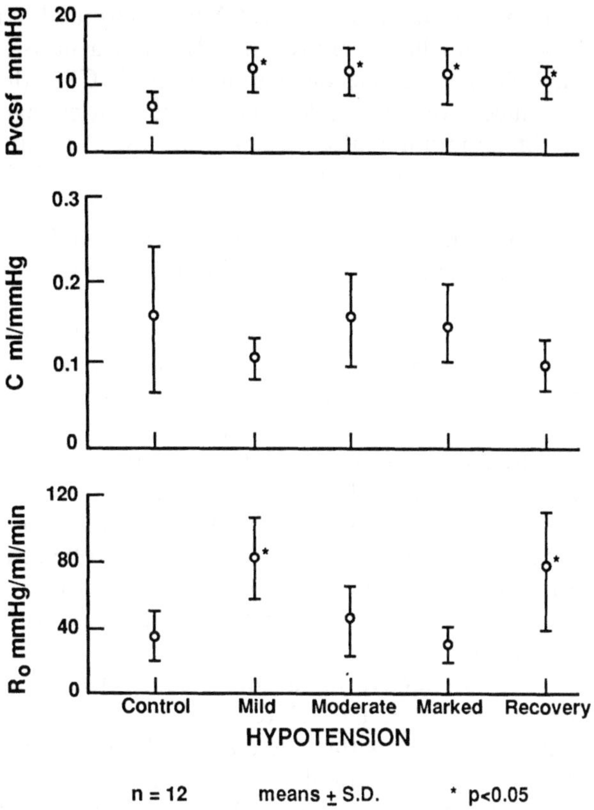

Fig. 2. Ventricular CSF pressure (PvCSF), compliance (C) and outflow resistance (R_o) at increasing stages of hypotension (means ± S.D., n = 12, * $p < 0.05$)

compliance and CSF dynamics become mutually dependent due to the intracranial volume change brought on by the ATP-induced increase in cerebral blood volume.

The increase in R_o does not imply that the impaired CSF dynamics had a significant role in the increase in ICP during ATP infusion. Studies of ICP dynamics indicate that the pressure level is determined by the sum of a pressure contribution related to the venous blood in the dural sinuses, P_v, and one obtained from the product of the CSF formation rate, I_f, and the outflow resistance, R_o; i.e. ($I_f \times R_o$) [3]. In our experiments this latter pressure contribution ranged from 25% at mild hypotension to 11% at marked hypotension. Thus, the major factor in the increase in ICP was due to an increase in the size of the cerebral venous pool.

With moderate hypotension (52 + 2 mmHg) both C and R_o returned to baseline. However, the volumetric buffering capacity of the craniospinal axis as measured by the PVI increased by 30%, reflecting, along with the increase in C, collapse of the vessels in the intracranial compartment and, most likely, a fall in cerebral blood volume. As a result of the further degree of hypotension, below the lower limit of autoregulation, a significant decrease in lCBF occurred with no additional change in CVR. Continued hypotension to MAP = 41 + 2 showed a further decrease in lCBF and a nonsignificant change in the CVR. The CSF dynamics as measured by the PvCSF, the compliance and the outflow resistance showed no additional significant change.

At 20 minutes after terminating the ATP infusion, the MAP returned to baseline as did the lCBF and CVR. The PVI, however, reduced to 75% of the baseline value and the compliance to 65% of baseline. Consistent with this, the outflow resistance increased to a level nearly double the baseline value, indicating impaired CSF circulation due to continued cerebral vascular expansion.

By regression analyses, several correlations between the CSF and hemodynamics parameters could be established. In particular, the PVI, a measure of the craniospinal buffering capacity, usually paralleled the changes in compliance, which is not surprising, since the compliance is calculated from the measured PVI. However, that calculation involves the base pressure at which the PVI is measured. Thus, any alteration in the ICP will influence the compliance. Nevertheless, looking at the sequence of stages of hypotension for the overall study, the trend was for the PVI to be sensitive to CPP with an inverse correlation ($r = -0.60$, $n = 12$). This is consistent with the results of Gray and Rosner [2] who reported that PVI increased with lowering of CPP below the autoregulatory range.

ATP is effective in causing a controlled reduction in MAP and CPP. The changes in lCBF and CVR are consistent with earlier studies [3, 7]; i.e., reduction of CPP within the autoregulatory range results in a lowering in CVR maintaining near normal lCBF, while further reduction leads to a lowering of lCBF with little change in CVR. Regarding the CSF dynamics, the increase in ICP and R_o along with a decrease in compliance with mild hypotension are consistent with cerebral vascular expansion. Further reductions in MAP and CPP leading to vascular collapse are evident in the return of C and R_o toward baseline. The ICP and R_o at recovery are somewhat above the baseline values indicating a residual vascular expansion. However, the CVR at recovery is at or slightly above the baseline value, which seems to be inconsistent with continued vascular expansion. It might be explained by a shift of the vascular resistance from the smaller pial vessels to the larger cerebral vessels [1]. Under such conditions, the CVR is increased due to constriction of larger cerebral arteries, while the CBF is also elevated due to continued vasodilatation in the microcirculation. The latter would imply that in the early recovery phase after ATP-induced hypotension, the brain would be more vulnerable to brief hypotensive insults, or small increases in CBV due to, e.g. pCO_2 fluctuations.

Acknowledgements. This research was supported by the VA Medical Research and the College of Engineering, University of Florida. We gratefully acknowledge helpful discussions with G. Bouma, M.D., and J.P. Muizelaar, M.D., of the Medical College of Virginia.

References

1. Faraci FM, Heistad DD (1990) Regulation of large cerebral arteries and cerebral microvascular pressure. Circ Res 66:8–17
2. Gray WJ, Rosner MJ (1987) Pressure-volume index as a function of cerebral perfusion pressure: Part 2: The effects of low cerebral perfusion pressure and autoregulation. J Neurosurg 67:377–380
3. Kassell NF, Boarini DJ, Olin JJ, Sprowell JA (1983) Cerebral and systemic circulatory effects of arterial hypotension induced by adenosine. J Neurosurg 58:69–76
4. Kontos HA, Wei EP, Navari RM, Levasseur JE, Rosenblum WI, Patterson JL (1978) Responses of cerebral arteries and arterioles to acute hypotension and hypertension. Am J Physiol 234(4):H371–H383
5. Marmarou A, Shulman K, LaMorgese J (1975) Compartmental analysis of compliance and outflow resistance of the cerebrospinal fluid system. J Neurosurg 43:523–534
6. Muizelaar JP, Ward JD, Marmarou A, Newlon PG, Wachi A (1989) Cerebral blood flow and metabolism in severely head-injured children: Part 2: Autoregulation. J Neurosurg 71:72–76
7. Newberg LA, Milde JH, Michenfelder JD (1985) Cerebral and systemic effects of hypotension induced by adenosine or ATP in dogs. Anaesth 62:429–436
8. Schettini A, Walsh EK (1991) Contribution of brain distortion and displacement to CSF dynamics in experimental brain compression. Am J Physiol 260:R172–R178
9. Van Aken H, Puchstein Ch, Anger C, Heinecke A, Lawin P (1984) Changes in intracranial pressure and compliance during adenosine triphosphate-induced hypotension in dogs. Anesth Analg 63:381–385
10. Van Aken H, Puchstein Ch, Fitch W, Graham DI (1984) Haemodynamic and cerebral effects of ATP-induced hypotension. Br J Anaesth 56:1409–1415

Computerized Infusion Test Compared to Conventional Lumbo-Ventricular Perfusion for Measurement of Resistance to CSF-Outflow

S.E. Børgesen[1], M. Albeck[1], F. Gjerris[1], M. Czosnyka[2], and P. Laniewski[3].

[1] University Clinic of Neurosurgery Rigshospitalet, Copenhagen, Denmark
[2] Institute of Electronic Fundamentals, University of Technology, Warsaw, Poland
[3] University Clinic of Anesthesiology, Child's Health Centre, Warsaw, Poland

Introduction

While it is generally agreed that measurement of resistance to outflow of CSF (R_{out}) is valuable in the diagnosis of diseases associated with disturbances in the CSF-dynamics, the invasive character and practical difficulties connected with steady state infusion or perfusion tests have limited their general use. A plain lumbar infusion at constant rate (the so-called Katzman test [7]) is easy to perform, but the interpretation of the results is difficult and the obtained values unreliable. With the introduction of computer analysis of the ICP-signal an exact filtration of artifacts in the pressure measurements is possible. Czosnyka et al. [4] have constructed a software program which makes it possible within a very short time to measure R_{out} together with other CSF dynamic parameters with an uncomplicated set-up. The purpose of the present study was to compare the values of R_{out} measured with this programme to a conventionally measured R_{out}. An acceptable correlation would render a lumbo-ventricular perfusion obsolete.

Method and Material

A conventional steady-pressure constant-infusion lumboventricular perfusion was performed, as previously described by Børgesen et al. [3], in 16 of the patients. Via a lumbar cannula Ringer lactate was infused at constant rate. Excess fluid was collected via an intraventricular catheter, through which also the ICP was measured. The height of the out-flow tube connected to the intraventricular catheter regulates the ICP making it possible to obtain several steady pressure levels at a steady infusion rate. R_{out} was calculated as the regression coefficient of the ICP/absorbed volume correlation. In the remaining five patients the R_{out} measurement was performed as a steady-pressure constant-infusion via a single lumbar cannula (patients no. 1, 2, and 7) or ventricular catheter (patients no. 11 and 16) connected to the pressure transducer and to the outflow tube.

After re-establishing a steady and normal ICP-level, lumbar (or in cases no. 11 and 16, ventricular) infusion was performed with a constant infusion rate and monitoring of the intraventricular or lumbar CSF-pressure. The analog pressure signal from the pressure amplifier was converted by an A-D converter and stored by the program, installed in a standard personal IBM computer. The ICP signal was processed by a spectral analysis, allowing for filtration of artifacts. From the baseline ICP (ICP_{bas}), the infusion rate (V_{inf}), and the end equilibrium-ICP (ICP_{end}), R_{out} is computed as:

$$R_{out} = (ICP_{end} - ICP_{bas})/V_{inf}.$$

If an end equilibrium steady pressure level is not obtained (for example due to vasomotor reactions) or if the infusion rate has to be changed, a dynamic method of computing R_{out} is employed. By this method the least square distance between the mean ICP rise and the theoretical curve describing a non-linear regression of the ICP/time relation is computed. Knowing R_{out}, the formation rate of CSF (FR) is calculated from the classical Davson equation:

$$ICP = FR \cdot R_{out} + P_{ss},$$

where P_{ss} (the pressure in the sagittal sinus) is estimated from the X-axis intercept of the regression line of ICP/pulse-wave amplitude relation. The results from the study, supplied with clinical data may be printed in a results protocol.

Assessment of correlation between the two methods was done by analysis of correlation and by analysis of the relation between differences and mean.

The material comprises 16 patients investigated by both methods. The patients represent a broad spectrum of CSF-disturbances, including normalcy (patients no. 1 and 2), normal pressure hydrocephalus (patients no. 3–5), syringomyelia (patient no. 6) benign intracranial hypertension (BIH) (patient no. 7), and the severe CSF disturbances associated with subarachnoid hemorrhage (SAH) (patients no. 8–10) or high pressure hydrocephalus (HPH-patients from 12 to 16) following operation for tumors in the posterior fossa. In Table 1 the age and the etiology (if present) are listed together with the results from the CSF investigations.

Results

R_{out} measured by the computerized infusion test proved to correlate very well with the R_{out} measured by lumbo-ventricular perfusion. The correlation coefficient was 0.98 ($p < 0.001$) and the regression coefficient was 0.93. For mathematical reasons, C_{out} rather than R_{out} was used to calculate the correlation in order to avoid extremely high values of R_{out}, as $R_{out} \rightarrow \infty$ when $C_{out} \rightarrow 0$. In Fig. 1 the respective values of conductance to out-flow ($1/R_{out}$) are plotted. The values obtained by the conventional perfusion are a little lower than those obtained by the computerized infusion test. After the insertion of the intraventricular drain a lumboventricular perfusion takes 1 to 2 hours to perform. In contrast, a computerized lumbar infusion may be finished in 30–40 minutes, including the lumbar puncture, calculations, etc.

No adverse reactions to any of the tests were observed in the present study.

Table 1. Clinical data and results from measurements

Pt. No.	Age Etiology	Perf-Cout (ml/min./mmHg)	Inf-Cout
1	24 normalcy	0.052	0.082
2	22 normalcy	0.14	0.161
3	33 NPH	0.079	0.079
4	71 NPH	0.066	0.08
5	70 NPH	0.15	0.152
6	60 Syring.	0.06	0.065
7	15 BIH	0.13	0.145
8	61 SAH	0.033	0.034
9	53 SAH	0.043	0.043
10	41 SAH	0.022	0.037
11	40 SAH	0.009	0.011
12	58 HPH	0.017	0.035
13	18 HPH	0.009	0.025
14	43 HPH	0.027	0.033
15	50 HPH	0.022	0.02
16	58 HPH	0.009	0.026

Perf-Cout, Cout measured by lumbo-ventricular perfusion; Inf-Cout, Cout measured by computerized lumbar infusion; NPH, normal pressure hydrocephalus; BIH, benign intracranial hypertension; SAH, subarachnoid haemorrhage; HPH, high pressure hydrocephalus.

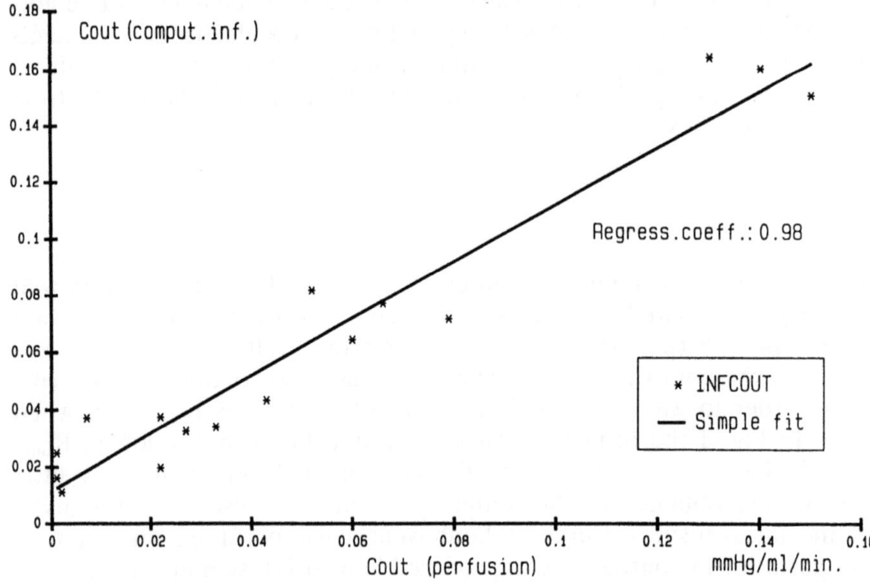

Fig. 1. Linear regression between conductance to CSF outflow measured during computerized lumbar infusion test (Y axis) versus conductance measured during perfusion study (X axis). Correlation coefficient $r = 0.98$, $p < 0.001$

Discussion

Measurement of resistance to outflow of CSF (R_{out}) has become established as the best diagnostic tool in conditions where disturbances in the CSF resorption are suspected. In a series of 333 patients with different disturbances of CSF dynamics, the steady pressure, steady infusion test has a diagnostic sensitivity of 100% if the upper normal level for R_{out} was placed at 12 mmHg/ml/min.

The steady pressure/steady infusion rate technique was developed to obtain a practical, clinical usable test with reliable, reproducible results [2]. It was important that the test was not too time-consuming. The interpretation of the pressure increase during the Katzman test with constant rate lumbar infusion is difficult and unreliable, while the exact steady state lumbar infusion developed by Portnoy [8] and by Ekstedt [5] is time-consuming and needs a sophisticated servo-controlled set-up for the infusion.

The lumbo-ventricular perfusion test, however, employs a ventricular drain inserted through a frontal burr hole. The advantage is the possibility of obtaining long-term intracranial pressure monitoring, but it increases the risk of complications. Czosnyka et al. [4] have developed a software program for measurement of R_{out} (and other parameters) by a simple lumbar constant rate infusion. The ICP analysis eliminates the influence from unwanted pressure fluctuations and artifacts, and permits calculation of R_{out} also when a steady pressure level is impossible to obtain. The calculations of R_{out} and PVI are based upon known relations between the parameters as given by the Davson equation, the monoexponential shape of the pressure/volume relationship, and the linear relation between the pulse wave amplitude and ICP. Various methods of computing R_{out} are offered by the software. In cases where a steady pressure level is not obtained or where great fluctuations in the ICP occurs during the infusion, or if the infusion rate has to be changed during the test, R_{out} may be computed by the least square distance of ICP from the theoretical ICP rise. These methods are hypothetical, dependent on the validity of the pressure-volume curve as a mono-exponential function, and also on a linear relationship between ICP and the amplitude of the pulse wave. It is left to the investigator using the software program to choose which method seems most appropriate for the computation of R_{out}.

In spite of these disputable presumptions, the correlation between the R_{out} measured by either method was remarkably good. The correlation coefficient was 0.98 ($p < 0.001$). In none of the 16 cases investigated did R_{out} differ unacceptably in the two tests. The good correlation was independent of the method of measurement; both lumbar and intraventricular measurements were assessed. This speaks in favour of using the computerized infusion test for measurement of R_{out}. The method is simple, quick to use and less invasive then perfusion tests. It is also much faster than the steady state servo-controlled infusion test. Information on CSF formation rate and on cranio-spinal elastivity may be obtained. The test may be performed through a ventricular or lumbar cannula as convenient.

We recommend that the computerized infusion test for measurement of R_{out} should be the investigation method of choice in patients where disturbances in CSF-dynamics are suspected.

References

1. Børgesen SE, Gjerris F, Schmidt J (1989) Measurement of resistance to CSF outflow by subarachnoid perfusion. In: Alfred Benzon Symposium 27. Gjerris F, Børgesen SE, Soelberg Sorensen P (eds) Munksgaard, Copenhagen, pp 121–129
2. Børgesen SE (1984) Conductance to outflow of CSF in normal pressure hydrocephalus. Acta Neurochir 71: 1–45
3. Børgesen SE, Gjerris F, and Sorensen SC (1978) The conductance to outflow of cerebrospinal fluid absorption in normal pressure hydrocephalus. Acta Neurol Scad 57: 88–96
4. Czosnyka M, Batorski L, et at. (1990) A computer system for the identification of the cerebrospinal compensatory model. Acta Neurochirurgica 105: 112–116
5. Ekstedt J, (1977) CSF hydrodynamic studies in man. Method of constant pressure infusion. J Neurosurg Neurol Psychiatry 40: 105–119
6. Gjerris G, Børgesen SE, Schmidt J, Soelberg Sorensen S (1989) Resistance to cerebrospinal fluid outflow in patients with normal pressure hydrocephalus. In: Alfred Benzon Symposium 27, Gjerris F, Børgesen SE, Sorensen PS (eds) Munksgaard, Copenhagen, pp 329-339
7. Katzman R, Hussey F (1970) A simple constant-infusion manometric test for measurement of CSF absorption. Neurology 20: 534–544
8. Portnoy HD, Croissant PD (1976) A practical method for measuring hydrodynamics of cerebrospinal fluid Surg Neurol 5: 237–277

Comparison of Lumbar and Ventricular Constant Flow and Bolus Infusions in Hydrocephalus

J.Th.J. Tans and D.C.J. Poortvliet

Department of Neurology and TNO Research Unit for Clinical Neurophysiology, Westeinde Hospital, Lijnbaan 32, 2512 VA The Hague, The Netherlands

Introduction

The ventricular catheter is considered to be the golden standard for the administration of constant flow and bolus infusions, but many investigators prefer the less invasive lumbar route. The question is whether the same resistance to outflow of CSF (Rout) and pressure-volume index (PVI) are obtained by perturbation and measurement in a different CSF space. We have, therefore, compared the results of lumbar and ventricular infusions and we have related these to ventricular size because CSF flow through CSF pathways might be influenced by ventricular dimensions.

Patients and Methods

Lumbar infusion tests were performed in over 200 adult chronic hydrocephalic patients during the past 10 years, referred to us because they were possible candidates for shunting. The same tests were repeated via a ventricular catheter within one month when there was uncertainty whether the hydrocephalus was communicating or noncommunicating or when there was a marked discrepancy between lumbar Rout on the one hand and the clinical and radiological findings on the other.

Following this regimen 16 patients with communicating hydrocephalus (CH) and 10 with noncommunicating hydrocephalus (NCH), all confirmed by contrast ventriculography on CT, were studied. They underwent one or more lumbar and ventricular constant flow infusions of 1.6 or 0.82 ml/min, yielding a lumbar and a ventricular R-out. They also received at least three 5 ml lumbar and ventricular bolus infusions from which one lumbar and one ventricular PVI was calculated [3, 4]. Administration and measurement were always carried out at the same site. Ventricular size was expressed as the Evans index on CT.

Results

All lumbar and ventricular baseline pressures were below 20 mmHg in CH and NCH. They agreed quite well, the difference between lumbar and ventricular

Table 1. Mean values of baseline pressure, Rout and PVI

	lumbar (l)[a]	ventricular (v)[a]	abs (v–l)
Communicating hydrocephalus, n = 16			
Mean baseline pressure	11.6 ± 3.0	12.3 ± 4.2	2.1 ± 1.3
Mean Rout	16.3 ± 8.5	18.5 ± 10.3	2.8 ± 2.2
Mean PVI	17.9 ± 5.5	15.4 ± 4.4	3.1 ± 2.8
Noncommunicating hydrocephalus, n = 10			
Mean baseline pressure	12.2 ± 3.0	13.1 ± 3.4	2.1 ± 1.2
Mean Rout	13.9 ± 4.7	17.5 ± 7.6	4.5 ± 4.2
Mean PVI	17.0 ± 4.9	13.4 ± 3.1	4.1 ± 3.8

[a] Both administration and measurement either lumbar or ventricular.

Table 2. Linear regression analysis of lumbar versus ventricular measurements[a]

	No of cases	Type of hydroc	Slope	Intercept	Cor coef	p
Baseline	16	CH	1.17	−1.38	0.83	0.0001
pressure	10	NCH	0.86	2.60	0.76	0.01
Rout	16	CH	1.18	−0.66	0.97	0.0000
	10	NCH	1.23	0.38	0.78	0.008
PVI	16	CH	0.63	4.14	0.80	0.0002
	10	NCH	0.32	7.88	0.54	0.1

[a] Both administration and measurement either lumbar or ventricular.

pressure never exceeding 4 mmHg. Ventricular pressures were slightly higher in most patients (Tables 1, 2).

The correlation between lumbar and ventricular Rout was excellent and their mean absolute difference was only 2.8 mmHg/ml/min in CH (Tables 1, 2). Ventricular Rout was higher, however, in 12 of the 16 patients. It is important to note that the whole series comprised patients with normal, mildly and markedly increased R-out. Ventricular and lumbar R-out agreed better than one might expect in NCH. Obviously ventricular Rout was higher, but not in all patients and in 6 of the 10 cases lumbar and ventricular Rout differed less than 3 mmHg/ml/min.

Regarding the PVI obtained from bolus infusions, lumbar and ventricular values correlated well in CH, but only moderately without reaching statistical significance in NCH (Tables 1, 2). Again, ventricular PVI's tended to be lower, the smallest differences occurring in patients with higher baseline pressure and higher R-out for both types of hydrocephalus.

Relating the Evans index to the absolute difference of ventricular and lumbar R-out, an inverse relationship emerged for CH as well as NCH (Table 3). In other words, the larger the ventricles, the better the agreement between ventricular and lumbar R-out. Such a relationship was not found for

Table 3. Linear regression analysis of Evans index versus absolute difference of lumbar and ventricular measurements[a]

	No of cases	Type of hydroc	Slope	Intercept	Cor coef	p
Rout	16	CH	−21.99	11.97	−0.67	0.005
	10	NCH	−48.28	26.69	−0.70	0.02
PVI	16	CH	−7.57	6.27	−0.18	0.5
	10	NCH	−1.28	4.69	−0.02	0.95

[a] Both administration and measurement either lumbar or ventricular.

the PVI. As in previous studies ventricular size did not correlate with Rout or PVI [3, 4].

Discussion

This study demonstrates that lumbar constant flow and bolus infusions provide a sufficiently reliable Rout and PVI in CH, when compared to ventricular perturbations. The somewhat higher ventricular Rout, obtained from constant flow infusion, might be contributed to small pressure gradients between the lateral ventricle and the CSF space at the convexity, particularly in patients with smaller ventricles. The best agreement between lumbar and ventricular Rout was found in patients with larger ventricles, suggesting unobstructed CSF flow in the ventricular system and the basal CSF spaces in these cases. Another explanation for the slightly, but consistently lower lumbar baseline pressure and Rout and the higher lumbar PVI is some leakage around the lumbar needle.

Regarding the faster bolus infusions, the question is whether the volume and pressure changes effect the whole CSF space in the same way or the effects are more pronounced close to the site of administration. In the latter case, lumbar and ventricular PVI could be different. In one study in cats, however, the ventricular PVI was somewhat lower, but not significantly different from the lumbar PVI. After increasing CSF pressure by saline loading, both PVI's became identical [2]. These results are confirmed by the present data in hydrocephalic patients.

Our findings in chronic NCH are interesting. Occasional observations of similar lumbar and ventricular baseline pressures were confirmed. Lumbar Rout was lower than ventricular Rout, but the difference was smaller in patients with larger ventricles, that apparently cause more compression of the cortical and basal arachnoid space leading to an increase of lumbar Rout. Lumbar Rout was indeed greater than 13 mmHg/ml/min in seven of the ten patients. Therefore, lumbar infusions can be useful in those patients suspected of NCH for whom the insertion of a ventricular catheter is not justified.

Not surprisingly, the lumbar and the ventricular PVI correlated less well in NCH. Yet, 7 of the 10 patients had a lumbar PVI below 18 ml, indicating reduced compliance in the spinal CSF space. The PVI of the isolated cranial and spinal compartment was studied by means of a reversible high cervical block in cats [1]. Contrary to our findings, the cranial PVI was twice as high as the spinal PVI. Of course, these acute experiments in nonhydrocephalic cats differ considerably from chronic adult NCH in which there are no two truly isolated CSF compartments. In some of these patients suffering from adult nontumoral aqueductal stenosis Rout was normal, indicating a compensated hydrocephalus, in others the obstruction at the level of the aqueduct was not complete.

In conclusion, the results of lumbar and ventricular constant flow and bolus infusions were remarkably similar in CH and closer than expected in NCH. Therefore, lumbar infusion tests are to be preferred in CH and they may be useful in selected cases of NCH.

References

1. Marmarou A, Shulman K, LaMorgese J (1975) Compartmental analysis of compliance and outflow resistance of the cerebrospinal fluid system. J Neurosurg 43:523–534
2. Takizawa H, Gabra-Sanders T, Miller JD (1986) Variations in pressure-volume index and CSF outflow resistance at different locations in the feline craniospinal axis. J Neurosurg 64:298–303
3. Tans JTJ, Poortvliet DCJ (1988) Reduction of ventricular size after shunting for normal pressure hydrocephalus related to CSF dynamics before shunting. J Neurol Neurosurg Psychiatry 51:521–525
4. Tans JTJ, Poortvliet DCJ (1989) Relationship between compliance and resistance to outflow of CSF in adult hydrocephalus. J Neurosurg 71:59–62

Normal CSF Dynamics in Man. Estimation of Pressure-Volume Index and Resistance to Outflow of CSF in Adults Without Intracranial Pathology

J. Sahuquillo[1], M.-A. Poca[1], A. Chasampi[1], T. Muxi[2], E. Campos[1], and E. Rubio[1]

[1] Department of Neurosurgery and [2] Department of Anesthesiology, Vall d'Hebron Hospital, Autonomous University of Barcelona, School of Medicine, Barcelona, Spain

Introduction

Cerebrospinal fluid (CSF) dynamics and intracranial pressure-volume relationships can be studied by a wide variety of procedures in clinical settings. Although infusion methods are considered to give better estimates of the resistance to outflow of the CSF (R_{out}), the technique described by Marmarou et al. [4] is attractive because it is relatively simple, fast and reliable. By the bolus test, we can, by a single procedure, calculate the pressure volume index (PVI), R_{out} and the compliance of the craniospinal axis (C_{csf}). Nevertheless, the value of this procedure in studying patients with suspected abnormal CSF hydrodynamics and especially in selecting patients for shunting in so-called "Normal pressure hydrocephalus" has been rather controversial. One of the problems when trying to define normal CSF dynamics is the lack of normal control values. The present study was undertaken to determine normal PVI, R_{out} and C_{csf} in adults without intracranial pathology.

Clinical Material and Methods

Thirty adults, 21 males and 9 females, aged 23 to 72 years (mean age 53.1 ± 12.1) were studied using Marmarou's bolus test while undergoing one of the following procedures: intrathecal morphine tests, baclofen tests or spinal reservoir implants for pain relief or spasticity. Informed consent was obtained for all studies. In all the patients intracranial mass or hydrocephalus was ruled out by a CT scan. All patients were awake during the study. Lumbar studies were performed with the patients in the left lateral recumbent position with a pillow under the head and the legs half flexed. A midline L3–L4 or L4–L5 lumbar puncture was made with a 18-gauge spinal needle. The cannula was connected to a transducer and to a paperchart recorder at a speed of 2 cm/min. All pressures were referenced to the same level as the lumbar cannula. A three-way stopcock was situated between the transducer and the cannula. A baseline measurement of the lumbar subarachnoid pressure was taken during 15 minutes. After a steady-state baseline was registered, bolus injections of 6 ml of normal saline were used at a rate of 1 ml per second. The ICP was allowed to return to baseline before the next bolus was injected. Pressure-volume index (PVI) was calculated by the following equation:

$$PVI = \frac{\Delta V}{LOG_{10}\frac{P_p}{P_0}}$$

where V is the volume injected, P_0 is the baseline pressure in the steady state and P_p the peak CSF pressure reached after the bolus injection of normal saline. All pressures were calculated using the mean pressure (diastolic + 1/3 pulse pressure). Resistance to CSF-outflow (R_{out}) was calculated by the following equation:

$$Rout = \frac{t \times P_0}{PVI \times \log\frac{P_t \times (P_p - P_0)}{P_p \times (P_t - P_0)}}$$

In this equation P_t is pressure on the return curve evaluated at time t in minutes. Rout was evaluated at 2 minutes after the P_p. Conductance to CSF outflow (Cout) was calculated as 1/Rout. Compliance (C_{csf}) was calculated by the following equation:

$$C_{CSF} = \frac{0.4343 \times PVI}{P_0}$$

At least two injections were done in every patient. Mean values were calculated for each study. Confidence intervals (CI) at 99% level were computed for each variable using the CIA program (supplied by British Medical Journal, London, Great Britain).

Results

In our study group, baseline pressure in the steady state (mean ± SD) was 8.3 ± 2.7 mmHg (CI 6.9 to 9.7). PVI was 20.3 ± 7.4 ml (CI 16.6 to 24.0). Resistance to outflow of the CSF calculated at 2 minutes was 3.4 ± 1.9 mmHg/ml/min (CI 2.50 to 4.38) while Compliance was 1.11 ± 0.62 (CI 0.80 to 1.42). Raw data are summarized in Table 1.

Discussion

Only a few studies have been directed to calculate normal hydrodynamic values in humans [1, 2, 5]. Normal reference data are important in order to evaluate patients in clinical settings and in research. The mean lumbar steady-state CSF pressure was 8.3 ± 2.7 mmHg in our study. In other studies, the normal ICP obtained in adults is around 10 mmHg, while the highest normal value falls within 11 and 12 mmHg [1–3, 5]. Shapiro et al. reported an estimated R_{out} of 2.40 ± 0.6 mmHg/ml/min determined by the bolus technique in 7 adults aged 19 to 55 years [5]. Our results gave a R_{out} of 3.4 ± 1.9. Although, in Shapiro's study, 1-minute post-injection time was used to compute

Table 1. CSF pressure and Hydrodynamic variables in the study group

	mean ± SD	99% CI[a]
Steady-state CSF pressure (mmHg)	8.3 ± 2.7	6.9 to 9.7
PVI (ml)	20.3 ± 7.4	16.6 to 24.0
R_{out} (mmHg/ml/min)	3.4 ± 1.9	2.5 to 4.4
C_{out} (ml/min/mmHg)	0.370 ± 0.20	0.269 to 0.471
C_{csf} (ml/mmHg)	1.1 ± 0.62	0.80 to 1.42

[a] Calculated 99% confidence intervals.

R_{out}, no statistically significant differences were found between Shapiro's and our results. We suggest that when using the bolus test, patients with R_{out} above 5 mmHg/ml/min should be considered to have an impaired CSF-reabsorption. PVI is defined as the calculated volume in milliliters necessary to raise the ICP by a factor of 10 [4]. Mean PVI in our 30 subjects was 20.3 ml with a lower 99% confidence limit of 16.6 and a higher of 24 ml. In adults without intracranial pathology, PVI was given as 26 ml in Shapiro's study with calculated 99% CI of 21.1 to 30.9 ml [5]. Although differences between our results and those of Shapiro are not statistically significant, the lower limit of PVI is clinically different. We suggest that in clinical settings only patients with a PVI below 16 ml should be considered to have a reduced volume buffering reserve.

References

1. Albeck MJ, Børgesen SE, Gjerris F, Schmidt JF, Sorensen PS (1991) Intracranial pressure and cerebrospinal fluid outflow conductance in healthy subjects. J Neurosurg 74:597–600
2. Ekstedt J (1978) CSF hydrodynamic studies in man 2. Normal hydrodynamic variables related to CSF pressure and flow. J Neurol Neurosurg and Psychiat 41:345–353
3. Gilland O, Tourtellotte WW, O'Tauma L, Henderson WG (1974) Normal cerebrospinal fluid pressure. J Neurosurg 40:587–593
4. Marmarou A, Shulman K, Rosende RM (1978) A nonlinear analysis of the cerebrospinal fluid system and intracranial pressure dynamics. J Neurosurg 48:332–344
5. Shapiro K, Marmarou A, Shulman K (1980) Characterization of clinical CSF dynamics and neural axis compliance using the pressure-volume index: I. The normal pressure-volume index. Ann Neurol 7:508–514

Intracranial Pressure and Cerebrospinal Fluid Dynamics in the Adult Chronic Hydrocephalus Syndrome

J. Sahuquillo, M.-A. Poca, A. Chasampi, F. Ramirez, E. Gabas, and E. Rubio

Department of Neurosurgery, Vall d'Hebron Hospital, Autonomous University of Barcelona, School of Medicine, Barcelona, Spain

Introduction

ICP monitoring and hydrodynamic studies have been widely reported in the adult chronic hydrocephalus syndrome (ACHS). Normal or low ICP, with high or low amplitude B waves and sometimes plateau waves, especially during REM sleep, have been reported as typical of this syndrome and clearly related to a good outcome [1]. Nevertheless, the value of long term ICP monitoring and/or CSF studies in order to select candidates for shunting is still controversial. The sensitivity, specificity and predictive value of ICP monitoring and CSF dynamics have not been defined yet. In general, a better knoweledge of the different forms of ACHS is still necessary to get a better understanding of the natural evolution, clinical symptoms and possible outcome in this important group of patients.

Clinical Material and Methods

Fifty-four shunt-respondent patients were selected from a prospective protocol directed to study patients with suspected ACHS, in which patients with gait disturbances, dementia, non-respondent L-Dopa parkinsonism, urinary or fecal incontinence and an Evans ratio above or equal to 0.30 on the CT scan were included. All patients underwent continuous intracranial pressure (ICP) monitoring using a fiberoptic extradural device (Ladd Research Industries, Inc., Burlington. Vermont) for at least 24 hours. Analysis of the ICP records were made following the method described by Børgesen [2]. The presence of high amplitude B-waves (1/2–2/minute ICP fluctuations more than 10 mmHg above base line and lasting at least ten minutes), were evaluated. A-waves were considered to be present in the case of constant pressure elevations at least 20 mmHg above the resting line with abrupt onset and end, and lasting at least 10 minutes. Plateau and B-Waves were expressed as a percentage of the first 24 hours period of the total recording time. In all patients resistance to outflow (R_{out}) was calculated using the bolus injection method through a lumbar cannula [4, 5]. According to the ICP recording, all patients were included in one of the following categories: 1) Active Hydrocephalus: mean ICP above 12 mmHg, 2) Compensated Hydrocephalus: mean ICP below or equal to 12 mmHg. Patients with compensated hydrocephalus were divided in Stable or Unstable if the ICP recording showed B-waves in less or more than 25% of the recording time.

Clinical Results

The age of the 54 patients considered as shunt responders was 64.9 ± 11 years (mean ± SD). Hydrocephalus secondary to subarachnoid hemorrhage and idiopathic communicating hydrocephalus were the most important groups (22 and 30% respectively). ICP and R_{out} data are summarized in Table 1. Twelve (22%) patients presented an elevated mean ICP (>12 mmHg) and were included in the Active Hydrocephalus group. Most of the cases (78%), were included in the Compensated group. Plateau waves were observed in 12 patients (22%). All patients with plateau waves were included in the Active Hydrocephalus (3 cases) or Unstable Compensated Hydrocephalus (9 cases) group. Patients included in the active hydrocephalus group had a mean R_{out} of 39.4 mmHg/ml/min, while the mean R_{out} was 20.8 mmHg/ml/min in the compensated group (student's t-test <0.05) (Table 1). Comparing resistance to outflow with the width of the cortical sulci and Sylvian cisterns in the CT scan, we found that R_{out} significanly increased when the width of the cortical sulci or Sylvian fissure was decreased in size.

Discussion

Two different problems should be distinguished in suspected ACHS. The first is how to find reliable diagnostic criteria of the syndrome and the second, to find and analyze those variables that influence or predict outcome from shunting. In our study, we have been able to show that patients with an ACHS are not homogeneous from an ICP point of view. The ICP profile is variable from cases in which mean ICP is continuously high to patients in whom resting ICP is normal, but who present more or less frequent intermittent fluctuations of the resting ICP (high amplitude B-Waves). B-waves represent an exaggerated response to physiological increases of cerebral blood volume in patients with abnormal CSF dynamics. Therefore, it seems rational to differentiate between

Table 1. Summary of ICP an Rout data

	n	Mean ICP (mmHg)	ICP (95% CI)	Rout (mean) (mmHg/ml/min)	Rout (95% CI)
Active hydrocephalus	12	22.0	16.3 to 27.7	39.4 [a]	33.6 to 45.2
Compensated hydrocephalus	42	8.9	8.2 to 9.6	20.8 [a]	17.0 to 26.8
Unstable	26	9.3	8.5 to 10.1	25.0 [a]	18.3 to 34.9
Stable	16	8.1	6.6 to 9.6	14.2 [a]	9.1 to 19.5

(95% CI): 95% confidence intervals. [a] Student's t-test < 0.05.

stable and unstable compensated hydrocephalus on the basis of B-waves. An important point in our study was that 70% of the patients with an ACHS presented continuous or intermittently raised ICP.

Although the etiology of the "normotensive hydrocephalus" is probably multifactorial, increased resistance to outflow of CSF has been the most constant abnormality reported by hydrodynamic studies [1, 2, 3]. Using the bolus test, we found that all the patients in our study had an increased Rout of CSF when compared with the normal values reported by Shapiro et al. [5]. Continuous measurement of the intracranial pressure, offers us one of the most reliable ways to study and select patients with a suspected ACHS. Controversial results in this field probably express differences in methods and lack of standardized evaluation of results rather than a true inability of ICP to distinguish patients with a normal or abnormal CSF dynamics. To clarify the ACHS, we need additional studies in which long term ICP monitoring should ideally be performed in all cases. When a clearer description of the population is defined, the specificity, sensitivity and predictive value of CSF dynamics in selecting patients for shunting will be possible. This should be the first stage, before conducting controlled studies to demonstrate the appropiate shunt (low pressure, high pressure, flow regulated etc.) for these patients.

References

1. Børgesen SE (1984) Conductance to outflow of CSF in Normal Pressure Hydrocephalus. Acta Neurochir (Wien) 71:1–45
2. Børgesen SE, Gjerris F, Sørensen SC (1979) Intracranial pressure and conductance to outflow of cerebrospinal fluid in normal-pressure hydrocephalus. J Neurosurg 50:489–493
3. Kosteljanetz M (1986) CSF dynamics and pressure-volume relationships in communicating hydrocephalus. J Neurosurg 64:45–52
4. Marmarou A, Shulman K, Rosende RM (1978) A nonlinear analysis of the cerebrospinal fluid system and intracranial pressure dynamics. J Neurosurg 48:332–344
5. Shapiro K, Marmarou A, Shulman K (1980) Characterization of clinical CSF dynamics and neural axis compliance using the pressure-volume index: I. The normal pressure-volume index. Ann Neurol 7:508–514

Plateau Waves and Cerebrospinal Fluid Circulation

M. Hayashi, Y. Handa, H. Kobayashi, H. Kawano, H. Ishii, and S. Hirose

Department of Neurosurgery, Fukui Medical School, Matsuoka, Fukui 910-11, Japan

Introduction

Plateau waves, as described by Lundberg [4], can often be observed in patients with increased intracranial pressure (ICP). The clinical significance as well as the pathophysiology of the plateau waves are still obscure despite so many studies concerning the pathogenesis. To clarify whether there is a relationship between the development of plateau waves and the dynamics of cerebrospinal fluid (CSF), we analyzed the correlation between the level and fluctuation pattern of ICP, the ventricular size, and the CSF flow and resistance to CSF absorption, in patients with intracranial hypertension.

Materials and Methods

We examined 94 patients with increased ICP, in whom continous ICP recording was carried out for more than 12 hours. The patients were divided into two groups on the basis of the ICP irregularities (plateau waves or rhythmic waves). Group I comprised 17 patients without plateau waves but with a high ICP and rhythmic waves. Group II consisted of 77 patients with plateau waves and high ICP. To evaluate the size of the ventricular system, the ventriculo-cranial ratio was measured on CT. Isotope cisternography was carried out to evaluate CSF flow and absorption. The intracranial isotope activity at 2, 6, 24, and 48 hr after the lumbar injection of isotope was calculated as a percentage of the maximum value. The conductance to CSF outflow was measured by the lumbo-ventricular perfusion method [1]. Physiological saline was infused through a lumbar cannula at rates (V_{in}) varying between 0.5 and 4.0 ml/min. The volume of outflow (V_{out}) from the ventricular catheter at the various levels of ICP, controlled by the height of the orifice of the ventricular catheter, was calculated. The CSF volume absorbed per minute (V_{abs}) was then calculated from the following formula: $V_{abs} = V_{in} + V_{csf} - V_{out}$ (V_{csf} = CSF formation rate). The V_{abs} was plotted against the different ICP values and the slope of the resulting regression line expressed the conductance to CSF outflow (normal value: more than 0.12 ml/min/mmHg).

Results

None of the patients in Group I had ventricular dilatation in spite of the high ICP, whereas 32 of 77 Group II patients showed hydrocephalus, resulting from meningitis carcinomatosa or communicating hydrocephalus after subarachnoid hemorrhage and the remaining 45 patients with brain tumors showed no hydrocephalus. The isotope cisternography in the Group I patients showed a normal pattern in six and a partial blocking of the subarachnoid pace in four. The head count rates of isotope showed maximum activity at 6 hrs followed by a gradual decrease in all patients. On the other hand, Group II patients with hydrocephalus showed a complete obstruction of the subarachnoid space, and patients without hydrocephalus showed a large accumulation of radioactivity over the cerebral convexities on the late images. In this group, peak isotope activity was not until 24 hr or 48 hr, indicating the sluggishness of the CSF circulation. The mean conductance to CSF outflow in the Group I patients was normal (0.143 ml/min/mmHg), while the conductance was markedly reduced in the Group II patients (0.041 ml/min/mmHg) (Table 1).

Discussion

Two major factors, which are essential for the development of plateau waves, have been proposed: a cerebral vasomotor reaction and a tight intracranial condition. As to the latter factor, it has been suggested that the intracranial CSF may play an important role in the development of the tight condition of the intracranial cavity [2, 3].

It has been reported that CSF circulation or absorption is markedly disturbed in patients with increased ICP, especially with papiledema resulting from brain tumors or benign intracranial hypertension. In the present study, the results obtained from isotope cisternography clearly demonstrated that delay of CSF circulation and absorption could not be observed in patients without plateau waves, whereas the patients with plateau waves showed marked sluggishness of CSF flow. The conductance to CSF outflow has been studied in various intracranial pathologies, and it was suggested that a conductance value below 0.10–0.12 ml/min/mmHg represents a significant CSF

Table 1. CSF formation rate and conductance to CSF outflow in two groups

	Estimated CSF formation rate (ml/min)	Conductance to CSF outflow (ml/min/mmHg)
Group I	0.36 ± 0.08 (n = 5)	0.143 ± 0.026 (n = 10)
Group II	0.39 ± 0.07 (n = 10)	0.041 ± 0.027* (n = 23)

CSF, cerebrospinal fluid; values are means ± S.D. *$p < 0.01$ compared between groups.

absorptive defect [1]. In the present study, the mean value of the conductance in patients without plateau waves was fairly normal. On the other hand, the mean value found in the patients with plateau waves was markedly reduced, indicating impairment of the CSF absorption capacity.

The rate of CSF formation was estimated in patients by measuring the time required for the return of the initial CSF pressure level following the removal of a certain amount of CSF [5]. Although it is suggested that the CSF formation is affected by the drainage, the technique of ventricular perfusion was introduced as a precise and physiological method [6]. Its results were fairly similar to the rate of 0.32 ml/min/mmHg obtained by Masserman [5]. In the present study, the CSF formation rate was estimated by the method of Masserman [5], which yielded values of 0.36 ml/min in the Group I and 0.39 ml/min in Group II. Both rates were similar to the 0.37 ml/min adult secretion rate reported by Rubin et al. [6]. These results indicate that there is no causal relationship between the ICP increase and the CSF production in the two groups.

The present observations demonstrated that the patients with both plateau waves and high ICP in the continuous ICP recording had a marked sluggishness of the CSF flow and a severe defect in the CSF absorption. It is suggested that the appearance of the plateau waves in continuous ICP recording is an important sign indicating impairment of CSF absorption capacities and a marked sluggishness in CSF flow.

References

1. Børgesen SE, Gjerris F, Sørensen SC (1978) The resistance to cerebrospinal fluid absorption in humans. Acta Neurol Scand 57:88–96
2. Hayashi M, Kobayashi H, Fujii H, Yamamoto S (1982) Ventricular size and isotope cisternography in patients with acute transient rises of intracranial pressure (plateau waves). J Neurosurg 57:797–803
3. Hayashi M, Kobayashi H, Kawano H, Handa Y, Kabuto M, Noguchi Y, Shirasaki N (1986) Isotope cisternography in patients with intracranial hypertension. J Nucl Med 27:471–477
4. Lundberg N (1960) Continuous recording and control of ventricular fluid pressure in neurosurgical practice. Acta Psychiat Neurol Scand 36, [Suppl 149]:1–193
5. Masserman JH (1934) Cerebrospinal hydrodynamics. Clinical experimental studies. Arch Neurol Psychiat (Chicago) 32:523–553
6. Rubin R, Henderson ES, Ommaya EK, Walker MD, Rall DP (1966) The production of cerebrospinal fluid in man and its modification by acetazolamide. J Neurosurg 25:430–436

Heart Rate Variability During Infusion Tests

D.J. Price, M. Czosnyka, Z. Czosnyka, H. Laniewska-Wollk, and M. Williamson

Pinderfields Hospital, Wakefield, UK
Warsaw University of Technology, Agricultural University, Warsaw, Poland

The measurement of outflow resistance to discriminate between patients with cerebral atrophy and Normal Pressure Hydrocephalus using variable infusion rates to procure a series of steady state levels is unfortunately rather time consuming [3]. After using the test for some 12 years in Yorkshire, we decided to consider an alternative method devised by Gjerris and Børgesen in Copenhagen [1]. This generates the data pairs for the same linear regression between flow rate and ICP but each ICP level is selected by changing the outlet height of an overflow tube and measuring the overall inflow of fluid by subtracting each outflow rate from each infusion rate. Before changing to this technique which we thought would expedite the measurement of outflow resistance, we compared the results of the two methods in a series of 37 patients. There was a surprising discrepancy in those patients with higher outflow resistances but as we now use 12 mmHg/ml/min as a threshold for advising a shunt, in only 4 patients would the difference in result make any difference to management (Fig. 1).

With the infusion technique, varying the infusion rate and measuring the ICP, 35% (40/115) had regression coefficients below 0.96 as compared with 32% (12/37) when the perfusion technique varying the ICP and measuring the overall flow was used. In 13/113 (11.5%) of the infusion tests and 3/36 (8.3%) of the perfusion tests, the poor regression was due to an unexpected elevated ICP at the maximum flow rate. The incidence of this phenomenon was not however related to the final ICP at the end of the test as the mean end-point ICP in those with the phenomenon was 41.6 ± 12 mmHg as compared with 38.4 ± 12 mmHg without.

During the tests, we noticed that in those with a higher than expected end-point in the ICP, the heart rate variability was more obvious and this encouraged us to accurately measure changes in heart rate during the test using software developed in Poland and already applied in head injury management for the previous two years. Meanwhile, as the time saved by using the perfusion test was only marginal, we continue with our original infusion technique which we choose to call the "gold standard" and are now comparing it with the computerised modelling techniques developed in Warsaw [2].

In a preliminary series of the next 5 infusion tests, we noted an overall increase in heart rate and in heart rate variability (expressed as the ratio between heart rate minus mean heart rate and the standard deviation of the heart rate).

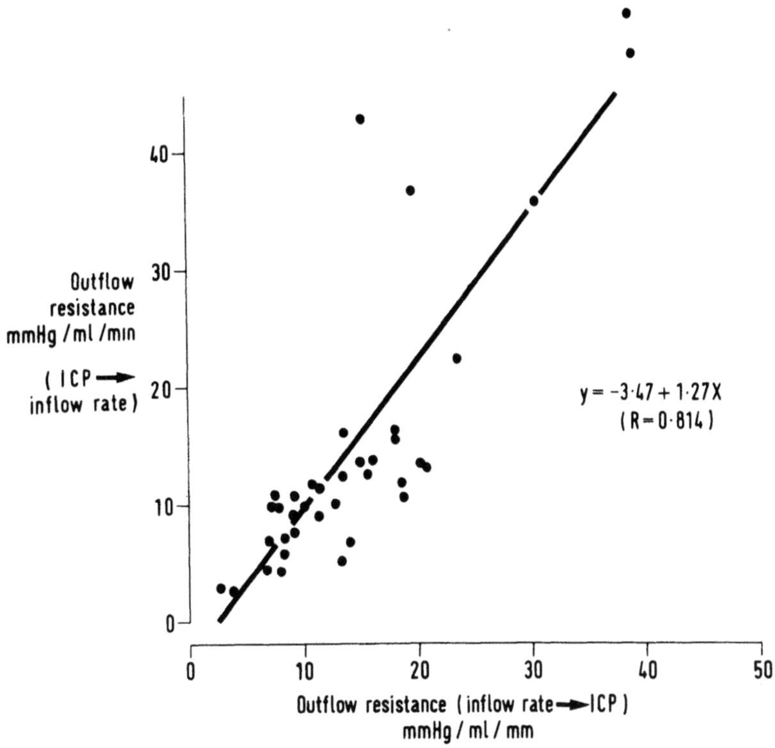

Fig. 1. A linear regression confirming the estimation of outflow resistance by infusion and perfusion methods. Most discrepancy occurred at the highest resistances – well above the threshold of 12 mmHg/ml/min used for shunting

Tape recordings of the analogue ICP signal from 53 tests carried out in Warsaw were then reanalysed by computer to examine the interdependence between the forced rise in ICP and heart rate changes. Forty of the patients were children. The heart rate response followed two patterns – one a gradual increase concurrent with the rise in ICP and secondly a more rapid increase associated with a sudden rise in ICP (Fig. 2).

Linear regressions of heart rate/ICP against an assortment of ICP and compensatory parameters was carried out. As expected, there was a correlation with the reciprocal of the initial cardiac amplitude, the increase in ICP during infusion and the formation rate of CSF (Table 1). When the same series of linear regressions was used with the heart-rate standard deviation against a similar assortment of parameters, the cardiac amplitude in both the initial pre-infusion recording and at steady state had the best correlation (Table 1).

If the infusion was at a very slow rate, an initial fall in heart rate was noted. Infusions in children were also associated with an initial bradycardia. With continuous infusions at higher rates, the heart rate invariably rose.

Table 1.

		Linear regression of Heart rate/ICP against ICP			Linear regression of heart rate standard deviation against ICP		
		Correlation coefficient	alpha	Slope	Correlation coefficient	alpha	Slope
Initial	Mean ICP	NS	NS	NS	0.33	$p < 0.05$	0.04
resting	Cardiac amplitude	−0.42	$p < 0.007$	−0.03	0.49	$p < 0.002$	0.17
Steady	Mean ICP	0.26	$p < 0.1$	0.005	0.29	$p < 0.06$	0.02
State	Cardiac amplitude	NS	NS	NS	0.45	$p < 0.003$	0.09
Plateau							
Increase in ICP during infusion		0.44	$p < 0.005$	0.1	NS	NS	NS
Outflow resistance		0.40	$p < 0.02$	0.01	NS	NS	NS
Pressure volume index		NS	NS	NS	NS	NS	NS
Slope of amplitude / mean		–	–	–	0.28	$p < 0.08$	1.5
Formation rate of CSF		−0.52	$p < 0.0007$	−0.11	–	–	–

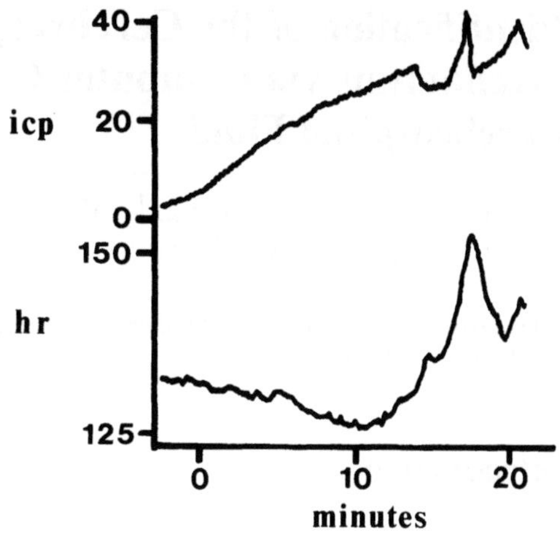

Fig. 2. During an infusion, the rise in ICP in this child is associated first with a small fall then a rapid rise in heart rate

Conclusion

We presume that a dramatic rise in heart-rate during an infusion test heralds cerebro-vascular vasodilatation. Careful monitoring of the heart rate may help avoid this by prompting earlier discontinuation of the infusion.

References

1. Børgesen SE, Gjerris F, Sørensen SC (1978) The conductance of outflow of cerebrospinal fluid absorption in normal pressure hydrocephalus. Acta Neurol Scand 57:88–96
2. Czosnyka M, Batorski L, Laniewski P, et al. (1990) A computer system for identification of the cerebrospinal compensatory model. Acta Neurochir (Wien) 105:112–116
3. Katzman R, Hussey F (1970) Simple constant infusion manometric test for measurement of CSF absorption 1. Rationale and method. Neurology (Minneap) 20:534–544

Identification of the Cerebrospinal Compensatory Mechanisms via Computer Controlled Drainage of Cerebrospinal Fluid

P. SMIELEWSKI[1], M. CZOSNYKA[1], W. MAKSYMOWICZ[2], W. KOSZEWSKI[2], P. LANIEWSKI[3], and A. WALENCIK[3]

[1] University of Technology, [2] Medical Academy, Warsaw, and [3] Children's Health Center, Miedzylesie, Poland

Introduction

The idea of the drainage test was born as an answer to the question: "How can an estimation of the cerebrospinal space compensatory parameters be obtained without actually provoking any vasomotor reactions?". In the classic infusion test, which seems so far to be the best way of estimating the resistance to cerebrospinal fluid outflow (Rcsf), the parameters are identified under the condition of raised Intracranial Pressure (ICP). This may provoke some uncontrolled changes in the cerebral blood volume by the mechanism of the vasomotor response, particularly when the initial ICP of the patient is already high. These changes are transmitted to the cerebrospinal fluid (CSF) compartment in the form of pressure waves, which in turn may cause strong disturbances in the pressure recordings [2], leading in the end to a faulty estimation of the compensatory parameters. Moreover, when the resting ICP of the patient is very high, it is dangerous, if not impossible, to perform the test. And if the test is performed in such circumstances, one must know that the parameters obtained may not correspond to the state of the patient's compensatory mechanisms. Firstly, because of the vasomotor reflexes mentioned above. And secondly, because under conditions of considerably raised ICP, resorption mechanisms may show some non-linear effects [1]. This may also have a significant influence on the parameters. Hence comes the question: Is it possible to perform the identification of the cerebrospinal compensatory model without disturbing the physiological conditions? The drainage test seems to be an interesting proposition here.

Methods

The main idea of the test is to measure the ICP and the amount of drained fluid at the same time. The data is then processed in a way very similar to the one used in the infusion test, giving the compensatory parameters of the CSF space as results. Such a method not only solves all the problems mentioned above (the test is carried out at a slightly decreased pressure level), but moreover:

- it doesn't need any external fluid addition;
- drainages may be repeated several times and by averaging the results it is possible to detect and exclude artifacts (the test can also be used as a technique for periodic examinations of compensatory mechanisms in long-term monitoring of ICP as in subarachnoid hemorrhage);
- the stages of drainage and pressure measurement are separated in time, making it possible to use only one needle.

Figure 1a shows the set-up of the measuring system. The instrumentation consists of an electromagnetically controlled clamp which can open or close the outlet of the lumbar drain under the computer control, the pressure monitor, and the standard electronic balance. All devices are connected to an IBM PC and controlled by the special software. The complete procedure of the test is presented on the basis of the ICP and the weight trends, which are shown in Figure 1b.

In Fig. 1b two curves are presented: time trends of the weight of the drained fluid and the mean intracranial pressure. They were recorded in the Children's Health Center in Miedzylesie during a drainage test performed on a 3-year old child suspected of hydrocephalus. Before the start of the test two levels of pressure, Pl and P2, must be set. They are usually fixed at: P1 = 1 mmHg lower than the resting pressure level, and P2 = from 2 to 4 mmHg below. The examination consists of two phases:

- The phase of controlled drainage, when the gradually decreasing pressure and the increasing weight are measured step by step. The phase ends when the mean ICP reaches the P2 level.
- The phase of spontaneous recovery, with the drain closed. When the mean ICP rises to the P1 level, the scale is reset and the phase is switched back to the controlled drainage.

These two phases may be repeated several times to allow for artifacts detection. The examination ends either when the physician who performs the test decides so, or automatically after a certain number of drainage/recovery cycles. This feature, along with the advantages of the test described above, requires the doctor to be present only at the beginning of the test. Subsequently it is only necessary to make sure that the patient lies still, a task easily done by a nurse. This seems to be particularly important in applying the test in cases with continuously monitored ICP. Switching to the software for drainage testing can be done once or twice a day, even automatically, and it doesn't need any extra maneuvers.

On the basis of the recorded data, the computer performs a full identification of the classic model of the cerebrospinal space.

Results

The drainage tests in patients with suspected hydrocephalus were first performed in the Neurosurgery Clinic of the Medical Academy Hospital in Warsaw and

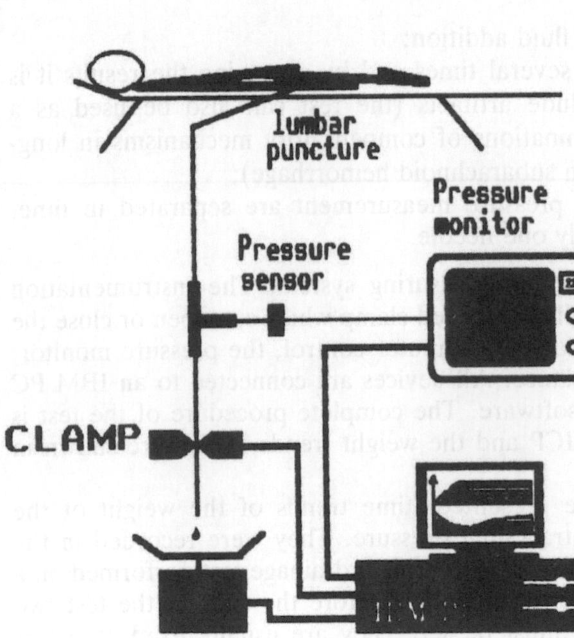

a

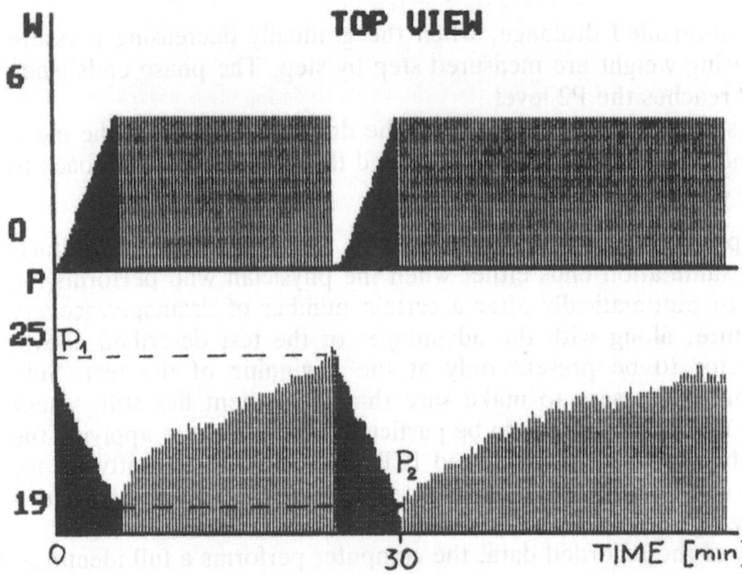

b

Fig. 1. **a** The set-up of the measuring system. **b** The recordings of the drainage test performed on a 3 years old child. P1 and P2 are given pressure limits

then also in the Children's Health Center in Miedzylesie. So far 15 patients were tested, out of whom 13 underwent the infusion test [2] just afterwards. The age of the patients varied between 14 months and 64 years (average 36 years). The distribution of etiology is given in Table 1. A correlation analysis

Table 1. Summary of etiological factors

Etiology	No. of cases
SAH	4
Meningitis	1
Trauma	2
Alcohol and barbiturates intoxication	1
Congenital	3
Unknown	4
Total	15

Table 2. Correlation coefficients of the resorption resistance obtained from the drainage and the infusion test

	Rcsf static	Rcsf dynamic
Correlation coefficient	0.775481	0.83761
Slope of the correl. line	0.592044	0.87159
Prob. level	0.00504	0.00130

between the results of the standard constant-rate infusion pressure-volume study and the drainage test was performed. The correlation coefficients for the resistance of CSF outflow are presented in Table 2. No significant correlation between the elastance coefficient from the infusion and the drainage test was found.

The statistical results show a strong correlation between the Rcsf obtained by the infusion and the drainage tests, but fail to show a significant correlation between the elastance coefficients from either test. This may be caused by the fact that the infusion test is based on a model of the cerebrospinal space with a constant P0 introduced into the pressure/volume characteristic.

The parameters obtained in two of the drainage tests differed so much from the results of the corresponding infusion test, that these cases had to be excluded from the regression analysis. The explanation is most probably as follows:

- In one case the test was disturbed by the high intensity of the pressure waves. The waves were so high that the real drainage/recovery curves were completely buried under the noise level. Hence the results from the approximation process did not correspond to the actual cerebrospinal compensatory parameters.
- The second case was a non-communicating hydrocephalus due to a Dandy-Walker malformation. This means that there was an obstruction in the pathway of the cerebrospinal fluid, and the resistance to CSF outflow measured by the infusion and drainage tests was in fact a serial combination of the resistance to CSF resorption (Rcsf) and the resistance of the obstruction. During the infusion test, an extra volume of fluid is forced into the CSF

space, which may cause the opening of the CSF outflow pathway and, therefore, the measured resistance is more or less equal to the real resorption resistance. However, during the drainage test, the withdrawal of fluid may even cause the narrowing of the outflow pathway, enlarging in this way the composite resistance to CSF outflow. Hence, the resistance measured in the drainage test can be much higher than the resistance to CSF reabsorption.

Conclusions

The results of the drainage tests performed on a group of 13 patients are quite satisfactory. The parameters calculated in the drainage test show a significant correlation with the results of the infusion test. Of course, the method needs further clinical verification (particularly with respect to the elastance coefficient) before it can be widely accepted as an alternative method for measuring the compensatory parameters of the cerebrospinal space. But considering all the advantages of the method it seems to have a fair chance of being introduced into the clinical practice.

References

1. Gjerris F, Børgesen SE, et al. (1989) Reproducibility and Reliability of Measurement of Resistance to CSF Outflow by Subarachnoid Perfusion. In: Hoff JT, Betz AL (eds). Intracronial pressure VII Springer, Berlin Heidelberg, New York London Paris Tokyo Hong Kong, pp 349–352
2. Price D, Czosnyka Z, et al. (1993) Heart rate variability in infusion test tests (this volume)

The Pressure-Volume Index (PVI) with Epidural Mass Expansion

E.K. Walsh and A. Schettini

College of Engineering, University of Florida, Gainesville, FL, 32611, USA
Research Service, McGuire Veterans Administration Medical Center, Richmond, VA, 23249, USA

Introduction

The pressure-volume index (PVI) is intended to provide a measure of the intracranial buffering capacity to be used in predicting the change in ICP course when the craniospinal system is subject to further volume increments. When an intraventricular bolus injection of volume ΔV is added, rapidly, to the intracranial system, it results in an increase in pressure from a baseline value, P_o, to a pressure $P_p > P_o$. It has been shown that the pressure-volume response of the system is nonlinear and can be characterized by a mono-exponential function [2]. In particular, $P = P_o \exp(k\Delta V)$, where $k = \ln 10/\text{PVI}$. It follows then that, for a single bolus injection, the value of the PVI is determined as $\text{PVI} = \Delta V/\log(P_p/P_o)$.

Any change resulting in an increase in the PVI would be interpreted as causing an increase in the buffering capacity of the system in that a greater volume would be required to cause the same pressure change, and similarly, a lowering of the PVI would indicate a less compliant system. The response of the craniospinal system is composed of a volume storage capacity determined by the elastic properties of the system and characterized by the volume-pressure response and a volume compensatory capacity controlled by the dynamics of CSF circulation [1]. Here we are concerned with the short time elastic compensatory behavior and the ability of the PVI to predict that behavior.

In a series of tests we found that variations in PVI may be a poor indicator of intracranial buffering capacity in the event of significant changes in the baseline pressure, P_o, which may occur, e.g., in the case of an intracranial mass expansion. In particular, during the incremental expansion of an epidural balloon, measurements were made to determine the PVI and then calculate the compliance, C, which is the slope dV/dP of the volume-pressure response. It is related to PVI by $C = (\log e)\text{PVI}/P_o$, when evaluated at the baseline pressure, P_o. As expected, the balloon expansion often caused a significant rise in the baseline pressure which resulted in a change in the PVI that was not consistent with the pressure rise resulting from the bolus injection or with the compliance. We found that the compliance, along with the pressure difference, $\Delta P = P_p - P_o$ (which, since ΔV is held constant throughout the test, is analogous to the VPR used by Miller et al. [3]), were more reliable indicators of intracranial buffering capacity than the PVI. Actually, in what follows, we report ΔP^{-1} in order to be consistent with C, which is dV/dP; the ΔV is the same at each stage of balloon inflation.

Materials and Methods

The experiments involved mongrel dogs (n = 10). Details of the method of preparation of the dogs and the methods of measurement of the CSF dynamics have been reported previously [4]. All relevant measurements were made under control conditions and then repeated at each 0.5 ml increment of inflation of an epidural balloon. The endpoint of balloon inflation was the onset of EEG delta activity or flat EEG.

Results

Figure 1 shows the changes (%) of PVI, C, and ΔP^{-1}, from their control values to a balloon volume of 4 or 5 ml for the ten dogs. Consider, e.g., dog 355. Over the range of balloon volume (BV) from 0 to 4.0 ml, the PVI

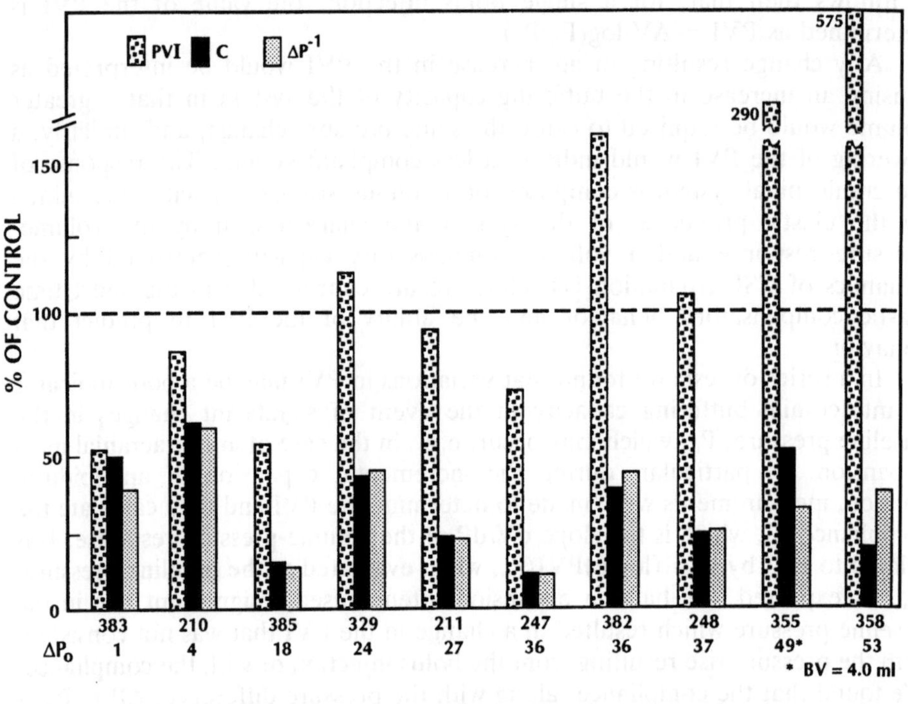

Fig. 1. Changes, in %, of the PVI, C, and ΔP^{-1} from the values at control to those at a balloon volume of 5 ml (4 ml for dog 355). Numbers at the bottom show the increase in baseline pressure, P_o, from control to 5 (4) ml balloon volume. For 5 of the 7 dogs with ΔP_o at or above 24 mmHg, the PVI and C gave conflicting predictions

indicated an upward trend, increasing from 1.78 to 5.16 ml, or nearly 300%, indicating that the system is becoming more compliant. However, the compliance, C, has decreased from 0.07 ml/mmHg at control to 0.037 ml/mmHg at BV = 4.0 ml, i.e., a decrease of 47%. Thus C indicates that the system is considerably less compliant than at control. At the same time ΔP shows an increase from 10 mmHg at control to 15 at BV = 4.0 ml, which indicates a decrease in ΔP^{-1} of 33%, again, an indication that the system is becoming more tight, or less compliant. For five of the seven dogs with a change in baseline pressure at or above 24 mmHg, the PVI and compliance gave conflicting predictions (Fig. 1).

Discussion

The reason for the apparent conflict is a result of the method of determination of the PVI from the results of a single bolus injection. Again, consider dog 355 and balloon volumes BV = 2.0 and 3.0 ml. The bolus injeections of 0.5 ml at these two stages resulted in pressure rises of 22 and 23 mmHg, respectively. This would seem to imply that the volume buffering capacity of the system was essentially unchanged. However, since the baseline pressure, P_o, had increased over that range from 15 to 42 mmHg, the logarithm of the ratio of P_p to P_o decreased, resulting in an increase in PVI by a factor of two. Meanwhile the compliance decreased from 0.037 to 0.027 ml/mmHg.

Ordinarily one would expect that epidural balloon inflation would result in a decrease in PVI and a consequent decrease in the compliance. Of course, for a fixed baseline pressure, any change in PVI will result in a similar change in C; the problem arises with significant changes in the baseline pressure. Thus, successive PVI measurements during a period which involves measurable changes in the baseline pressure, may give misleading indications. Under these circumstances, it appears that the compliance and ΔP (or ΔP^{-1}) are more reliable indicators of intracranial buffering capacity than the PVI; (we recognize that C and $\Delta V/\Delta P$ are nearly the same parameter; C representing the tangent, dV/dP, to the volume-pressure response, evaluated at P_o, and $\Delta V/\Delta P$ the secant to the response curve between P_o and P_p).

Acknowledgements. This study was supported by VA Medical Research and the College of Engineering of the University of Florida.

References

1. Avezaat CJJ, van Eijndhoven JHM (1986) How does the craniospinal system cope with a disturbance of its volume? In: Miller JD, Teasdale GM, Rowan JO, Galbraith SL, Mendelow AD (eds) Intracranial Pressure VI. Springer, Berlin Heidelberg New York Tokyo
2. Marmarou A, Shulman K, La Morgese J (1975) Compartmental analysis of compliance and outflow resistance of the cerebrospinal fluid system. J Neurosurg 43:523–534

3. Miller JD, Leech PJ, Pickard JD (1975) Volume-pressure response in various experimental and clinical conditions. In: Lundberg N, Ponten U, Brock M (eds) Intracranial Pressure II. Springer, Berlin Heidelberg New York Tokyo
4. Schettini A, Walsh EK (1988) Brain tissue elastic behavior and experimental brain compression. Am J Physiol 255:R799–R805

Relationship Between Pressure-Volume Index and Amp/ICP When the $PaCO_2$ is Changed

N. YASUI and H. NISHIMURA

Department of Surgical Neurology, Research Institute for Brain and Blood Vessels-AKITA, 6-10, Senshu-Kubota-machi, Akita, Japan

Introduction

A noninvasive and easy method to evaluate both the kinetics of the intracranial pressure (ICP), and the hydrodynamics of the cerebrospinal fluid (CSF) system, is needed. In one method, we could measure the ICP pulse wave in the CSF system because the arterial blood pressure indirectly transmits the pressure pulse through the vessel walls to the intracranial cavity, changing the CSF space. This pressure phenomenon is relevant to the CSF pressure-volume relationship. Generally, the curve of the pressure-volume relationship has a small gradient at low ICP (the pulse amplitude is small) and has a steep gradient at high ICP (the pulse amplitude is large). This curve looks like an exponential curve. In practice, the ICP pulse amplitude increases with the elevation of the ICP and is in direct proportion to the ICP. We speculate that the degree of the pressure buffer of the CSF system can be predicted by measuring the Amp/ICP (the ratio of the pressure pulse amplitude to the ICP level), because the ratio of Amp/ICP is small at a high level of the pressure buffer and is large at a low level of the pressure buffer. It should be noted that the pressure-volume index (PVI as proposed by Marmarou et al.) indicates the degree of the pressure buffer of the CSF system. The PVI is large at the higher level of the pressure buffer and small at the lower level. Therefore, we thought that the Amp/ICP of the patient must always be changing in inverse proportion to the PVI and that, in the clinical situation, the Amp/ICP can be used instead of the PVI. We next investigated the relation between PVI and Amp/ICP when the $PaCO_2$ changes.

Method

In five anesthetized patients who were mechanically ventilated and had undergone V-P shunt operations (where the shunt valve was closed before the examination), the PVI and Amp/ICP were measured using the bolus injection technique. For confirmation, the intraventricular and the spinal fluid pressure were simultaneously obtained using a computer measuring-system. Figure 1a shows an example of the trend of the arterial blood pressure, the end tidal volume, the intraventricular pressure, and the spinal fluid pressure. During the measurement, the arterial blood pressure of the patient remained constant, and the $PaCO_2$ was controlled at 40 mmHg and 30 mmHg, using CO_2 controller.

We used a new electrical circuit model (Fig. 1b) to approximate the hydrodynamics of the CSF system – which included the cerebrovascular system with two pressure buffers (the arterial and the venous pressure buffers) to simulate the clinical pressure kinetics of the CSF system. The mathematical equations of the model were computed for the PVI and Amp/ICP using a Macintosh II computer (Apple computer Inc.).

Result

When the $PaCO_2$ of the five patients was changed from 40 mmHg to 30 mmHg, PVI changed in direct proportion to Amp/ICP (Fig. 2a), but the direction of

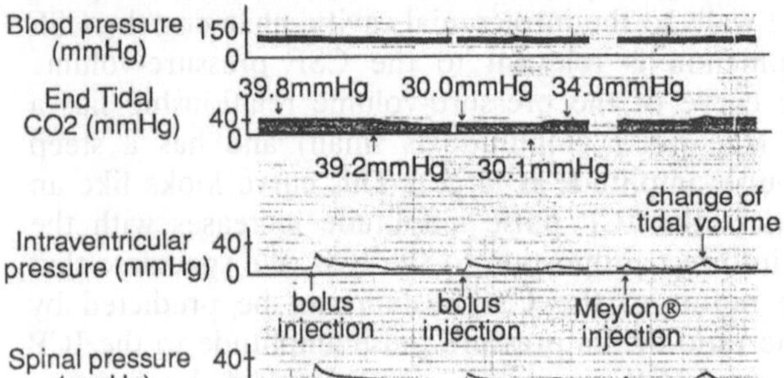

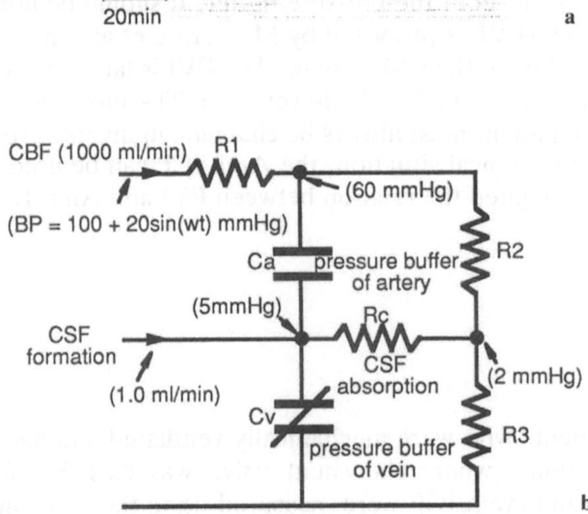

Fig. 1. Method **a** The trend of the arterial blood pressure, the end tidal CO_2, the intraventricular pressure and the spinal fluid pressure during the examination. **b** A new electrical circuit model of the CSF system that includes the cerebrovascular system with two pressure buffers (Ca: arterial pressure buffer, Cv: venous pressure buffer)

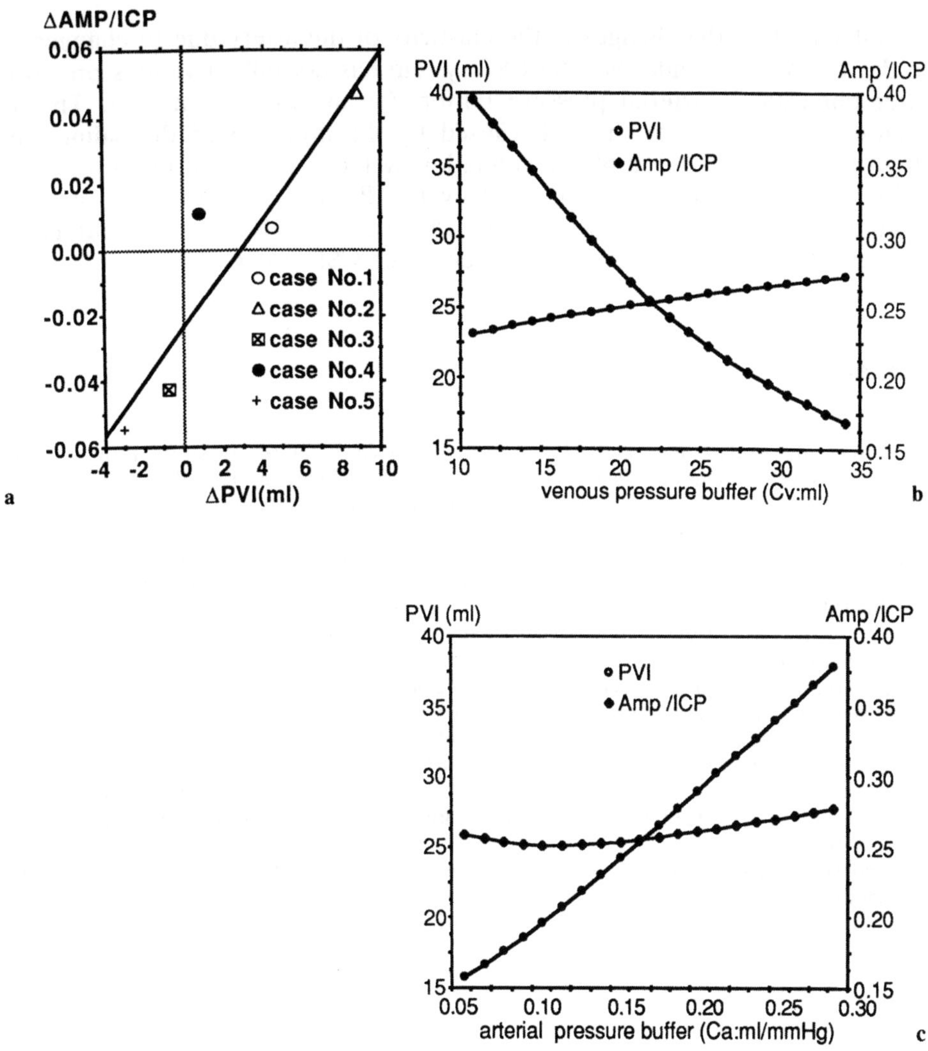

Fig. 2. Result **a** Relationship between ΔPVI and ΔAmp/ICP in five patients when the $PaCO_2$ was changed. **b** Computer simulation, showing the relationship of the PVI and the Amp/ICP during changes of the venous pressure buffer. **c** Computer simulation, showing the relationship of the PVI and the Amp/ICP during changes of the arterial pressure buffer

the change was uncertain. On computer simulation of the new model, the PVI was in inverse proportion to the Amp/ICP when the degree of venous pressure buffer was changed (Fig. 2b). The PVI was in direct proportion to the Amp/ICP when the degree of arterial pressure buffer was changed (Fig. 2c).

Conclusion

The results were not consistent with our speculation that the PVI changes in inverse proportion to the Amp/ICP. This means that the ICP pulse amplitude was influenced by the changes in the elasticity of the artery due to changes in the $PaCO_2$. We conclude that the CSF system has not only a venous pressure buffer but also an arterial pressure buffer, (as in our new model). This is because the elevation of the ICP caused by the injection of the saline can diffuse towards the arterial blood circulation system. Also the arterial pressure buffer and the ΔV will be influenced by the $PaCO_2$ more than the venous pressure buffer. Therefore, we believe that the Amp/ICP is an insufficient parameter to evaluate the pressure buffer of the CSF system.

References

1. Czosnyka M, Wollk-Laniewski P, Batorski L, Zaworski W (1988) Analisis of Intracranial Pressure Waveform During Infusion Test. Acta Neurochir (Wien) 93:140–145
2. Cardoso ER, Rowan JO, Galbraith S (1983) Analysis of the cerebrospinal fluid pulse wave in intracranial pressure. J Neurosurg 59:817–821
3. Hirai O, Handa H, Ishikawa M (1982) Intracranial pressure pulse waveform: Consideration about its origin and methods to estimating intracranial pressure dynamics. Brain Nerve (Tokyo) 34:1059–65
4. Kato Y, Auer LM (1989) Cerebrovascular Response to Elevation of Ventricular Pressure. Acta Neurochir (Wien) 98:184–188
5. Marmarou A, Shulman K, Rosende RM (1978) A nonlinear analysis of the cerebrospinal fluid system and intracranial pressure dynamics. J Neurosurg 48:332–344
6. Portnoy HD, Chopp M, Branch C (1983) Hydraulic model of myogenic autoregulation and the cerebrovascular bed: Effects of altering systemic arterial pressure. Neurosurgery 13(5):482–498
7. Takemae T, Kosugi Y, Ikebe J (1987) A Simulation Study of Intracranial Pressure Increment Using an Electrical Circuit Model of Cerebral Circulation. IEEE Trans Biomed Eng BME34, 12:958–962
8. Ursino M (1988) A Mathematical Study of human intracranial hydrodynamics. 1: The cerebrospinal fluid pulse pressure. Ann Biomedf Eng 16:379–401
9. Ursino M (1988) Mathematical Study of human intracranial hydrodynamics. 2: Simulation of Clinical Tests. Ann Biomedf Eng 16:379–401

Bulk Flow and To-and-Fro Flow of CSF Observed on MRI and CT Cisternography

S. OHARA[1], S. UMEMURA[1], M. MASE[2], H. NAGAI[2], and T. BANNO[3]

[1] Department of Neurosurgery, Gamagouri City Hospital, Aichi, Japan
[2] Department of Neurosurgery, Nagoya City University Medical School, Japan
[3] Department of Radiology, Nagoya City Rehabilitation and Sports Center, Japan

Introduction

The CSF flow comprises the slow flow forced out of the ventricles by the production of CSF itself, which is termed bulk flow, and the rapid movement of CSF propelled by the brain pulsations, which is termed to-and-fro flow. A disturbance of CSF circulation in the craniospinal cavity often results in hydrocephalus, the pathogenesis of which should be studied with an understanding of bulk flow and to-and-fro flow. In this study, the flow dynamics of CSF in patients suffering from communicating hydrocephalus were studied on MRI, and compared with the results obtained by CT cisternography.

Methods and Materials

MR Cine-Imaging

Superconductive MRI systems with a static magnet field of 0.5 T (Gyroscan S5, Philips, Netherlands) and 1.5 T (SMT150, Shimazu Medical, Japan) were used. On an ECG-triggered MRI, a pulsatile CSF flow was observed in the aqueduct. Ten to fifteen images in a cardiac cycle with a 15 msec phase delay from the R wave of the electrocardiogram (ECG) were obtained using the gradient echo technique with 50 or 80 msec of repetition time (Tr), 17 or 11 msec of echo time (Te), 7 or 25 degrees of flip angle and 7 mm of slice thickness on Gyroscan S5 or SMT150, respectively. Three groups of subjects were evaluated: 4 normal volunteers, 3 patients with (nonhydrocephalic) neurologic disease (controls), and 8 patients with hydrocephalus.

Results

Normal Volunteers and Neurologic Control Patients

In normal volunteers and neurologic control subjects, the signal intensity of the CSF in the aqueduct changed from a minimum of approximately 1000 to a maximum of 1700 (on Gyroscan S5). Because the range of the change in signal intensity was virtually the same in each group, the maximum CSF velocity was thought to be similar.

Patients with Hydrocephalus

The signal intensity of CSF in the aqueduct was measured in eight patients with communicating hydrocephalus secondary to subarachnoid hemorrhage, three of whom were examined with the Gyroscan S5 and the other five by SMT150. In patient 1 (41-year-old man), the signal intensity of CSF ranged between 580 and 1600. Because the minimum value of the signal intensity was the lowest of all the measurements taken, in both the volunteer and control groups, and also because the difference between the maximum and minimum value was the largest (Fig. 1), the maximum velocity of the CSF in this patient was thought to be the most rapid of all studied. CSF flow dynamics in this patient were classified as "high flow" on MRI. In patient 2 (69-year-old woman), the signal intensity of the CSF ranged from 1000 to 1500. Because the range of the signal intensity change resembled that of the volunteer and control groups, the maximum velocity of the CSF in the aqueduct of patient 2 was thought not to differ from the maximum velocity of the CSF in the volunteer and control groups (Fig. 1). CSF flow dynamics in patient 2 were classified as "medium flow" on MRI. In patient 3 (38-year-old man), the signal intensity ranged from 780 to 1100, the smallest range in the patients studied. Thus the velocity of the CSF in the aqueduct was thought to be the slowest studied concerning the maximum velocity and the change in the narrowest range as compared to other cases evaluated (Fig. 1). CSF flow dynamics in patient 3 were to be classified as "low flow" on MRI.

Thus, two of the eight hydrocephalic patients were classified as "high flow", two as "middle flow", and four as "low flow" on MRI (Fig. 2).

CT Cisternography

CT cisternography (CTC) was performed in eight patients suffering from hydrocephalus whose hydrodynamics were also examined with MRI, and the results were compared. A CT scan of the head was performed in these eight patients at 3, 6, 24, 48, and 72 hours following the intrathecal injection of a water-soluble contrast medium. The results were investigated and assessed with regard to whether the contrast medium refluxed into the ventricular system; when the reflux occurred; how long contrast medium remained in the ventricle

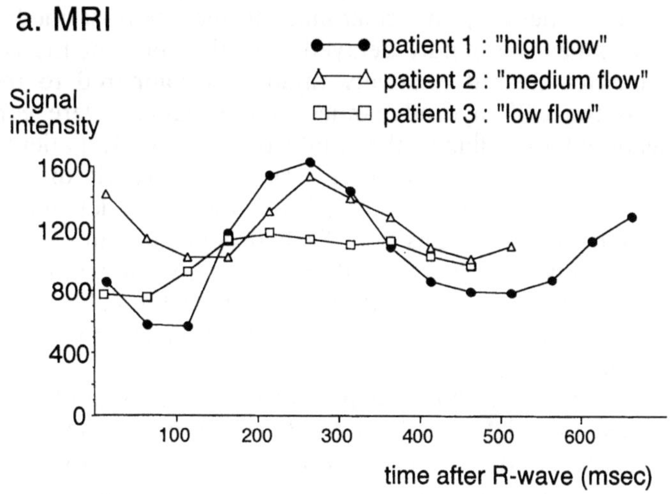

b. CTC

	patient 1	patient 2	patient 3
VENTRICULAR REFLUX ≤ 6HR	++	+	++
VENTRICULAR STASIS ≥ 24HR	+	+	+
VENTRICULAR STASIS ≥ 48HR	—	±	+
CONVEXITY STASIS ≥ 24HR	+	±	+
DISTURBANCE OF CSF CIRCULATION	MILD	MODERATE	SEVERE

Fig. 1. Grading of CSF flow on MRI and CTC in 3 hydrocephalic patients

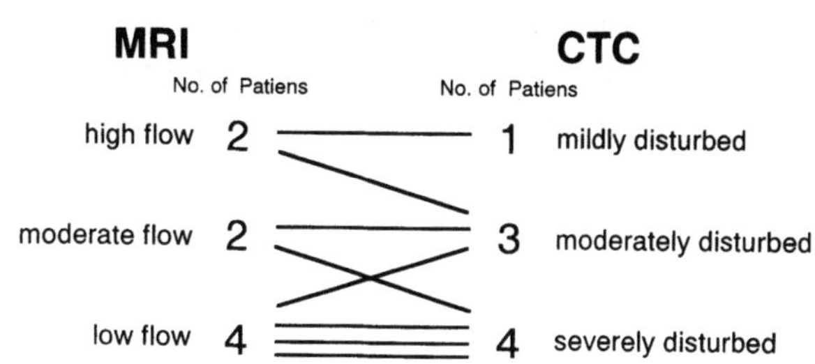

Fig. 2. Correlation of CSF flow grading on MRI and CTC

system, what amount of contrast medium was observed in the sulci of the cerebral convexities, and how long it remained. The hydrodynamics of CSF in each patient were then classified as "mildly", "moderately", or "severely" disturbed, according to Tamaki's classification.

In patient 1, the clearance of the contrast medium from the sulci of convexities was mildly delayed, and the stasis of the contrast medium in the ventricles cleared relatively rapidly as compared to the other two patients. Thus the CSF hydrodynamics in this patient were considered to be mildly disturbed according to the results of the CTC. In patient 2, the CSF circulation in the sulci of the convexities was more severely disturbed than in patient 1. The contrast medium refluxed into the ventricles and remained there longer than in patient 1. Thus the CSF hydrodynamics in patient 2 were thought to be moderately disturbed. In patient 3, the CSF flow in the sulci of the convexities was stagnant and the ventricular stasis of the contrast medium persisted for a longer period, indicating that the CSF circulation was severely disturbed in this patient (Fig. 1).

Considering that one patient classified as mildly disturbed on CTC was graded as "high flow" on MRI and three of the four patients classified as severely disturbed on CTC were graded as "low flow" on MRI, there appeared to be a good correlation between the results obtained on MRI and those on CTC (Fig. 2).

Discussion

The results of our study indicate that MRI may offer an alternative to CTC for studying the hydrodynamics of CSF (Fig. 2). In patient 1, the amplitude of CSF to-and-fro motion was large enough to stir the contrast medium with the CSF in the lateral ventricles. CSF bulk flow was mildly disturbed. As a result, contrast medium that reentered the lateral ventricles persisted for 24 hours after the injection, but was washed out within 48 hours on CTC. In patient 2, the amplitude of the to-and-fro motion of CSF flow was smaller than that in patient 1, but CSF bulk flow was maintained within normal limits. As a result, the ventricular reflux of the contrast medium into the lateral ventricles was not so severe as in patient 1. In patient 3, the to-and-fro motion of CSF flow and the bulk flow were restricted seriously. As a result, ventricular reflux was observed within 6 hours after the injection. This was thought to depend on the diffusion of the contrast medium in the mostly static CSF space. The stasis of the contrast medium in the ventricles and the sulci of the cerebral convexities were observed over 48 hours.

Conclusion

The concept that CSF flow is composed of two components, bulk flow and to-and-fro flow, is essential to the understanding of CSF hydrodynamics. Investigation of these two components on MRI may offer an alternative to CTC for studying the hydrodynamics of CSF, particularly if further investigation makes it possible to measure precisely not only the velocity but also the volume of CSF flow in the respective components, bulk flow and to-and-fro flow.

References

1. Njemanze PC, Beck OJ (1989) MR-gated intracranial CSF dynamics: evaluation of CSF pulsatile flow. AJNR 10:77–80
2. Ohara S, Nagai H, Matsumoto T (1988) MR imaging of CSF pulsatory flow and its relation to intracranial pressure. J Neurosurg 69:675–682
3. Tamaki N, Hujita K, Kusunoki T, et al. (1982) Computed tomography (CT) Cisternography in normal pressure hydrocephalus. Progress in Computerized Tomography 4:201–209

CSF Flow Analysis Using Cine MRI in Patients with Hydrocephalic States

T. Banno[1], H. Nagai[2], and S. Ohara[3]

[1] Departments of Diagnostic Imaging and [2] Neurosurgery, Nagoya City University Medical School and [3] Department of Neurosurgery, Gamagohri City Hospital, Aichi, Japan

Introduction

Recent advances in MRI techniques have enabled us to visualize the movements of craniospinal fluid using fast imaging with heart triggering. This is referred to as MRI Cine technique with multiphase imaging. Using this method, signal changes are observed in a heart cycle. We evaluated MRI signals in patients with enlarged ventricles and hydrocephalic states by plotting signal changes on MRI Cine images.

Materials and Methods

Fifteen patients, including 7 patients with post-subarachnoid hemorrhage (SAH) hydrocephalus and 8 patients suspected of brain atrophy with large ventricles were examined. The MRI unit used was SHIMAZU SMT150 with 1.5 Tesla high magnetic fields. The acquired sequence was the CINE sequence, the same as using a FLASH sequence with Gradient Echo. Imaging parameters were TR = 80 ms, TE = 11 ms, Number of excitation (NEX) = 2, and flip angle = 20 degrees. Imaging planes in the cine sequence were sagittal and coronal. The sagittal plane was aligned with the 3rd and 4th ventricles, and the aqueduct. The slice thickness was 7 mm. In this study, sagittal images were analyzed for plotting signal changes. Multiphase heart triggering acquisition was performed as in Fig. 1. Each pulse interval measured was 80 ms. The number of images acquired differed in each patient's heart cycle. The average number of images in each heart cycle was six. In the clinical situation, these cine sequential images were also recorded into a VTR recorder. The range of interest (ROI) was created on the cine image. Our MRI software enables us to plot 5 ROI's simultaneously. The ROIs were set on the lateral ventricle, the 3rd and 4th ventricles, and the brain parenchyma. Diameters of ROI were not fixed because there were small differences in anatomical details and among patients.

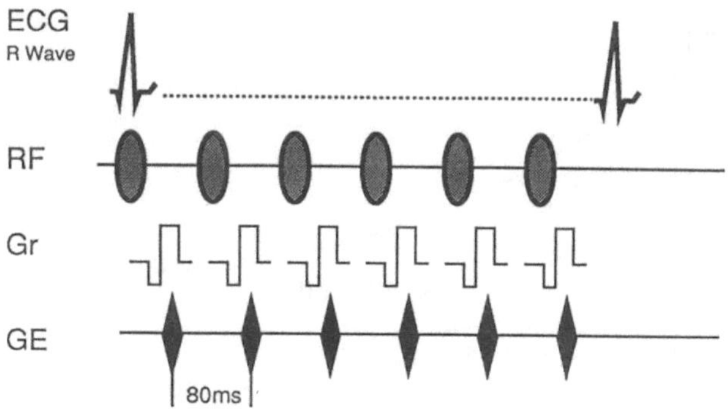

Fig. 1. Pulse sequence of Cine MRI

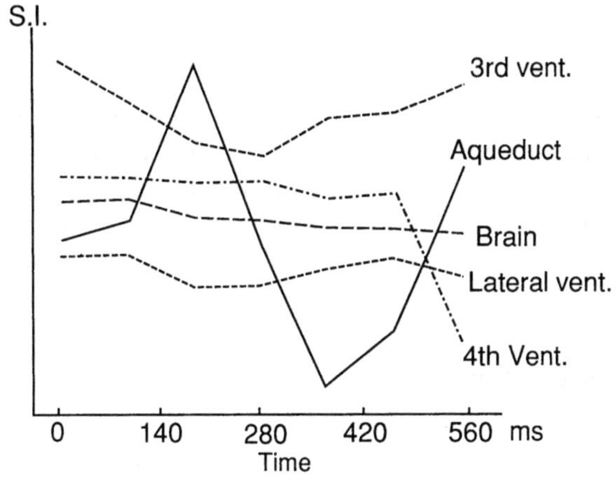

Fig. 2. Time intensity curves at each ROI point. Greater changes were recorded at the aqueduct

Case Presentation

A 66 year old male who was suspected of normal pressure hydrocephalus after a subarachnoid hemorrhage due to the rupture of an anterior communicating artery aneurysm. Time intensity curves of ROI points were plotted (Fig. 2). The 3rd curve line is a signal at the point of the acqueduct. Signal changes at the aqueduct are moderately large. A 40 year old female with cerebral palsy was studied, whose MRI showed an enlarged 4th ventricle. The MRI cine showed very few signal changes at each point (Fig. 3). Especially at the point of the aqueduct, there were no signal amplitude changes. We can see a gradual signal decrease after the beginning of the acquisition cycle. This is not a result of flow effect but of TR effect. For example, the signal curve of the brain parenchyma shows an almost linear decrease. Figure 4 shows plotted curves of signal changes at the aqueduct in each case. These signal changes may be

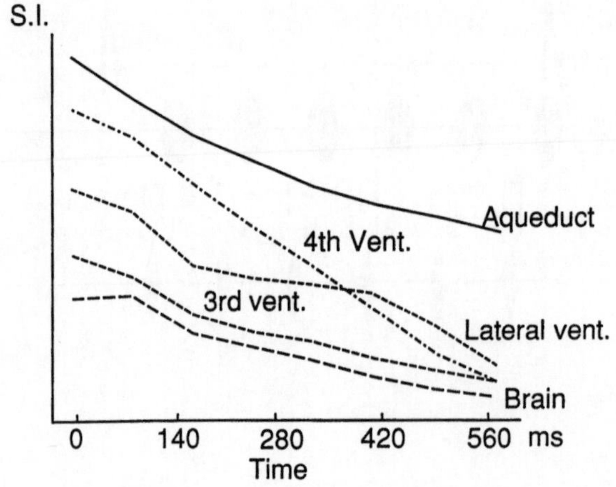

Fig. 3. Time intensity curves at each ROI point. Less signal changes were observed

classified into two general groups, one group of greater signal changes and another of less changes. In patients with hydrocephalus from hemorrhage, 4 out of 7 (57%), revealed greater signal changes, indicating a suspicion of normal pressure hydrocephalus. However, patients with enlarged ventricles due to atrophy have a tendency to present less signal changes.

Discussion

Research has been undertaken on CSF dynamics using magnetic resonance imaging. Sherman et al. [3] reported that signal decrease at the aqueduct of Sylvius was seen in retrospective observation by MRI. They suggested that the flow-void sign of CSF represents pulsatile CSF flow. Ohara et al. [2] reported pulsation and compliance of brain changes in each process of the disease; therefore, the signal of the 3rd and 4th ventricle show different patterns depending on the process. Mascalchi et al. [1] reported that the ratio of aqueductal and ventricular CSF signals in patients with NPH was larger than in normal patients or in patients with brain atrophy.

The aqueduct itself is a very narrow canal, and the high velocity of CSF flow in it may frequently show a flow void effect. However, CSF flow is not steady; it may have a pulsatile or a to-and-fro movement. This may complicate the linear correlation of CSF flow. However, there may be one parameter which indicates CSF flow dynamics in the ventricular cavity. Our results show the same tendency as that of Mascalchi et al. [1] who reported a higher ratio of aqueductal and ventricular signal in 18 cases. It is our opinion that cine MRI is not a definitive quantitative method, but that it may potentially be used to differentiate between pathological conditions such as NPH, and brain atrophy.

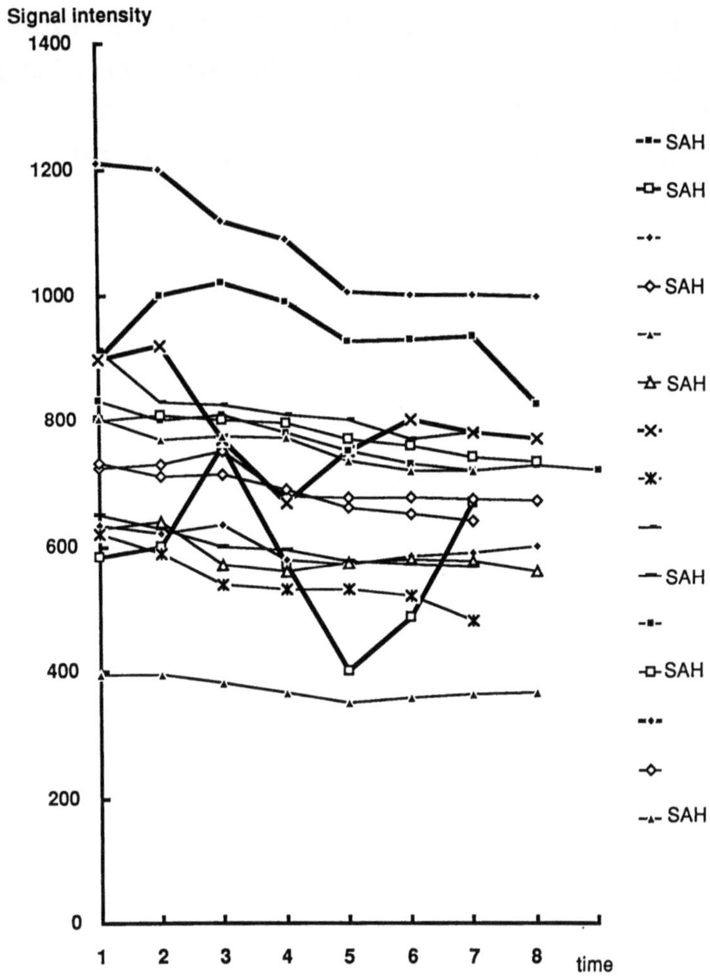

Fig. 4. Signal changes in the ROI at the aqueduct in each case. Bold lines show greater signal changes

References

1. Mascalchi M, Ciraolo L, Bucciolini M (1989) Fast multiphase MR imaging of aqueductal CSF flow in demented patients with hydrocephalus. Abstract of SMRM, pp 12
2. Ohara S, Nagai H, Matsumoto T (1988) MR imaging of CSF pulsatory flow and its relation to intracranial pressure. J Neurosurg 69:675–682
3. Sherman JL, Citrin CM (1986) Magnetic Resonance Demonstration of Normal CSF Flow. AJNR 7:3–6

Quantitative Analysis of CSF Pulsatile Flow in the Aqueduct with Dynamic MRI and Presaturation Bolus Tracking: The Flow Patterns and Clinical Aspects in Adults with Communicating Hydrocephalus

S. Nakajima, J. Haraoka, H. Itoh, and T. Miwa

Department of Neurosurgery, Tokyo Medical College, 6-7-1 Nishishinjuku, Shinjuku-ku, Tokyo, 160, Japan

Introduction

The various to-and-fro patterns of CSF flow in the aqueduct in adults with ventriculomegaly were studied and analyzed.

Clinical Cases and Methods

Ten normal adults, ten cases of secondary normal pressure hydrocephalus (NPH), and nine cases of idiopathic ventriculomegaly were examined by cine MRI with presaturation bolus tracking [2]. In this method, a presaturation pulse (PR) is added before the RF pulse of the gradient echo pulse sequence. Repeating it with cardiac gating, 5–9 frames are obtained in the ECG RR interval. In each image, the displacement (D) of the presaturated bolus in the aqueduct over the interval from PR to the echo (t) is observed. In addition, the average velocity (V) of the flowing CSF can be computed according to the formula; $V = D/2t$. The patients also underwent CT and RI-cisternography (RIc). In certain cases continuous ICP monitoring was also performed.

Results

Normal Adults

The direction of CSF flow changed at 25–30% and 75–80% through the cardiac cycle. In the early and late phases, the direction was rostral, and in the other phase it was caudal. The maximum velocity was 7.3 ± 1.7 mm/sec in the rostral direction, and 8.0 ± 2.4 mm/sec in the caudal direction.

Secondary NPH

The velocity of the CSF in the aqueduct was very fast, and the duration of the CSF flow in the caudal direction was longer than in the rostral. The points in which the CSF flow changed the direction was delayed (Figs. 1, 2). Among the 10 NPH cases, three showed dementia and gait disturbance, three showed the triad of NPH, and four demonstrated the apallic state. On CT, PVL was seen in nine cases. In these cases the larger the ventricular size was, the faster was the maximum velocity in both directions. On RIc, ventricular stasis was seen in all cases until 24 or 48 hours. The cases in whom maximum velocity in the caudal direction was less than 30 mm/sec showed peak accumulation of RI in the lateral ventricles at 24 hours, while the cases in whom maximum velocity in the caudal direction was more than 30 mm/sec showed a peak at 6 hours. ICP monitoring was performed in seven cases and pressure waves were recorded in all cases.

Idiopathic Ventriculomegaly

The CSF flow patterns in the aqueduct were classified into three types (Fig. 3).

Type I (Two Cases). The velocity was relatively fast, and the duration of the flow in the caudal direction was longer than in the rostral. These cases indicated the triad of NPH, and showed cortical atrophy and lacunar infarct with ventriculomegaly on CT and NPH pattern on RIc. Pressure waves were recorded in these cases.

Type II (Two Cases). The velocity was relatively fast, but the duration of the flow in the caudal direction was shorter than in the rostral. They were young and had only headache. CT demonstrated ventriculomegaly only. On RIc, Ventricular reflux was found but the clearance was relatively good. Pressure

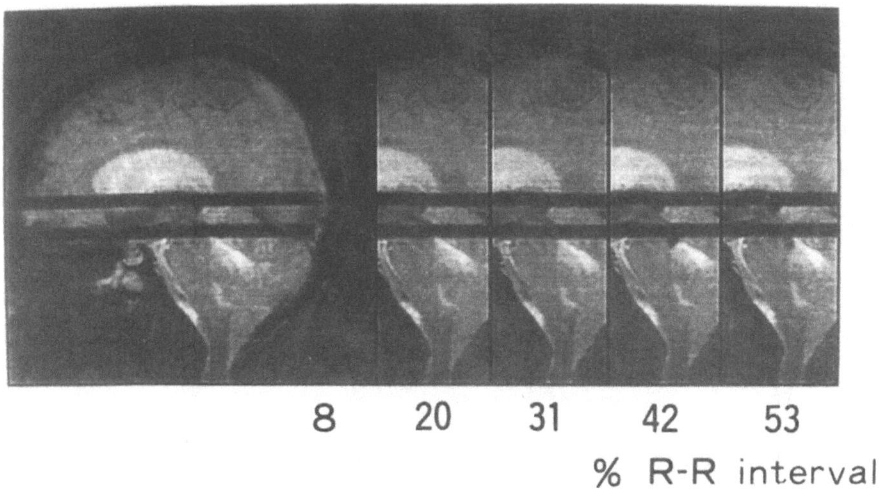

Fig. 1. Cine MRI with presaturation bolus tracking in a case with secondary NPH. The numbers below the images indicate the relative location in the cardiac cycle. The presaturated area appears dark. Note the presaturated bolus in the aqueduct moving in a to-and-fro manner

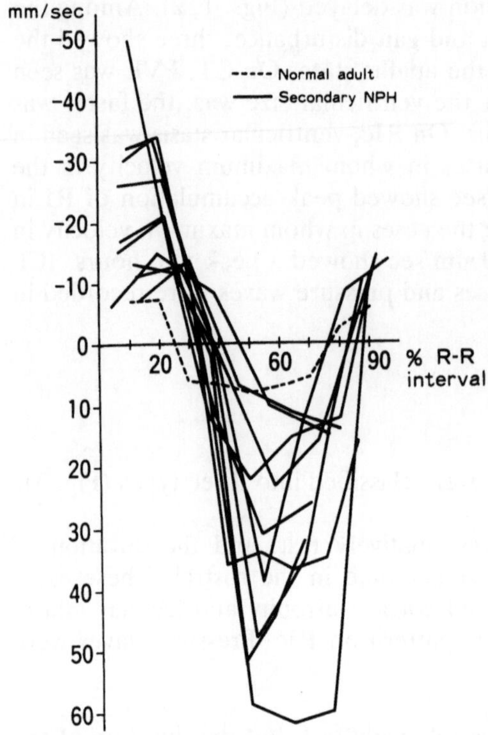

Fig. 2. Velocity of the CSF flow in the aqueduct (millimeters per second) versus relative location in the cardiac cycle (percent of RR interval). Negative numbers indicate caudocranial motion, while positive numbers show craniocaudal motion. The dotted curve indicates the mean value of normal adults, and solid curves indicate those of the patients with secondary NPH

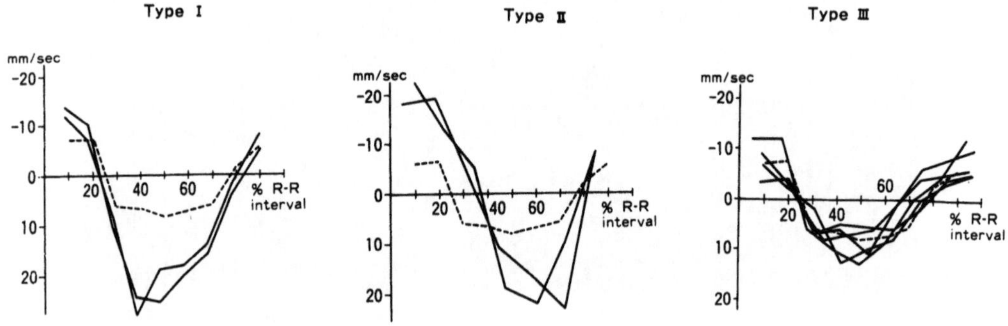

Fig. 3. Velocity of the CSF flow in the aqueduct (millimeters per second) versus relative location in the cardiac cycle (percent of RR interval). Negative numbers indicate caudocranial motion, while positive numbers show craniocaudal motion. The dotted curve indicates the mean value of normal adults. Solid curves indicate those of the patients with idiopathic ventriculomegaly, divided into three types

waves were not recorded but abnormal alteration of the baseline was found in one case.

Type III (Five Cases). The velocity was slow, and the duration of the flow in the caudal direction was shorter than in the rostral. These cases chiefly had dementia, and CT showed cortical atrophy and lacunar infarct with ventriculomegaly. RIc showed ventricular stasis and delayed clearance. No abnormal recordings were found on ICP monitoring.

Discussion

The CSF in the ventricular system flows toward the subarachnoid space of the brain and the spinal CSF space in a to-and-fro manner, responding to the pulsation of the brain parenchyma, as previously reported [1, 3–5]. In secondary NPH the amplitude of the flow was increased according to the degree of stagnation of the CSF in the subarachnoid space. in cases with idiopathic ventriculomegaly, three pulsatile flow patterns were confirmed. Type I was similar to secondary NPH, but the velocity of the CSF flow in the aqueduct was not very fast despite the ventriculomegaly. This finding is considered to result from the decrease in the driving force of the brain parenchyma due to atrophy. The Type II cases were young and showed no cortical atrophy on CT. We speculated that these cases may represent concordance of an arrested, perhaps congenital, hydrocephalus. Type III was similar to Type I on CT and RIc, but the CSF flow was very slow. This finding is considered to result from compensation for the hydrocephalic state of Type I.

References

1. Bradley WG, Whittemore AR, Kortman KE, Watanabe AS, Homyak M, Teresi LM, Davis SJ (1991) Marked cerebrospinal fluid void. Radiol 178:459–466
2. Edelman RR, Mattle HP, Kleefield J, Silver MS (1989) Quantification of blood flow with dynamic MRI and presaturation bolus tracking. Radiol 171:551–556
3. Enzmann DR, Pelc NJ (1991) Normal flow patterns of intracranial and spinal cerebrospinal fluid defined with phase-contrast cine MR Imaging. Radiol 178:467–474
4. Feinberg DA, Mark AS (1987) Human brain motion and cerebrospinal fluid circulation demonstrated with MR velocity imaging. Radiol 163:793–799
5. Thomsen C, Stahnlberg F (1990) Fourier analysis of cerebrospinal fluid flow velocities. Radiol 177:659–665

Aqueductal CSF Flow on MRI and its Relation to Intracranial Pressure Dynamics

J. MEIXENSBERGER[1], E. HOFMANN[2], A. BRAWANSKI[1], M. HOLZSCHUN[1], and W. ULLRICH[1]

[1]Department of Neurosurgery and [2]Neuroradiology University of Würzburg, 8700 Würzburg, Germany

Introduction

Since the introduction of cardiac gated gradient echo sequences in MRI, the noninvasive study of intracranial cerebrospinal fluid (CSF) pulsations became possible [2, 5]. Especially in hydrocephalic patients disturbances of CSF flow in the mesencephalic aqueduct may be of clinical importance in diagnosis and treatment. At the moment, invasive testing methods, like continous intracranial pressure monitoring and a spinal infusion test, are one of the best parameters for shunt indication. Therefore in our study we were interested in the following issues:

1. Is there a correlation between aqueductal CSF flow abnormalities and pathological ICP dynamics?
2. Is the noninvasive MRI analysis of aqueductal CSF flow a reliable indicator for shunting?

Patients and Methods

We studied 21 patients, 12 males, 9 females with suspected hydrocephalus on CT. Their age ranged from 18–74 years, with an average of 45.8 years. Clinical data of all patients were noted, especially unspecific symptoms (headaches and dizziness), mental deficits, gait disturbances and urinary incontinence. Every patient was examined by MRI. The "fast field echo" (FFE) sequence was applied to obtain sagittally orientated cardiac-gated images of the mesencephalic aqueduct (Fig. 1). This sequence is routinely installed on our Philips Gyroscan S15 scanner. A flip angle of 10° and echo time of 35 ms resulted in T2-weighted images. Slice thickness was 6 mm. The number of phases per cardiac cycle was

Fig. 1A,B. T2-weighted cardiac-gated sagittal gradient echo (FFE) images of the mesencephalic aqueduct. Four out of eight phases per heart-beat interval are shown. Both patients had the clinical triad of normal pressure hydrocephalus, an increase in B-waves and outflow resistance. In **A** no mesencephalic flow void indicates aqueduct stenosis, in **B** severely increased signal void is caused by increased CSF pulsations. Note superficial brainstem siderosis in **B** due to subarachnoid hemorrhage

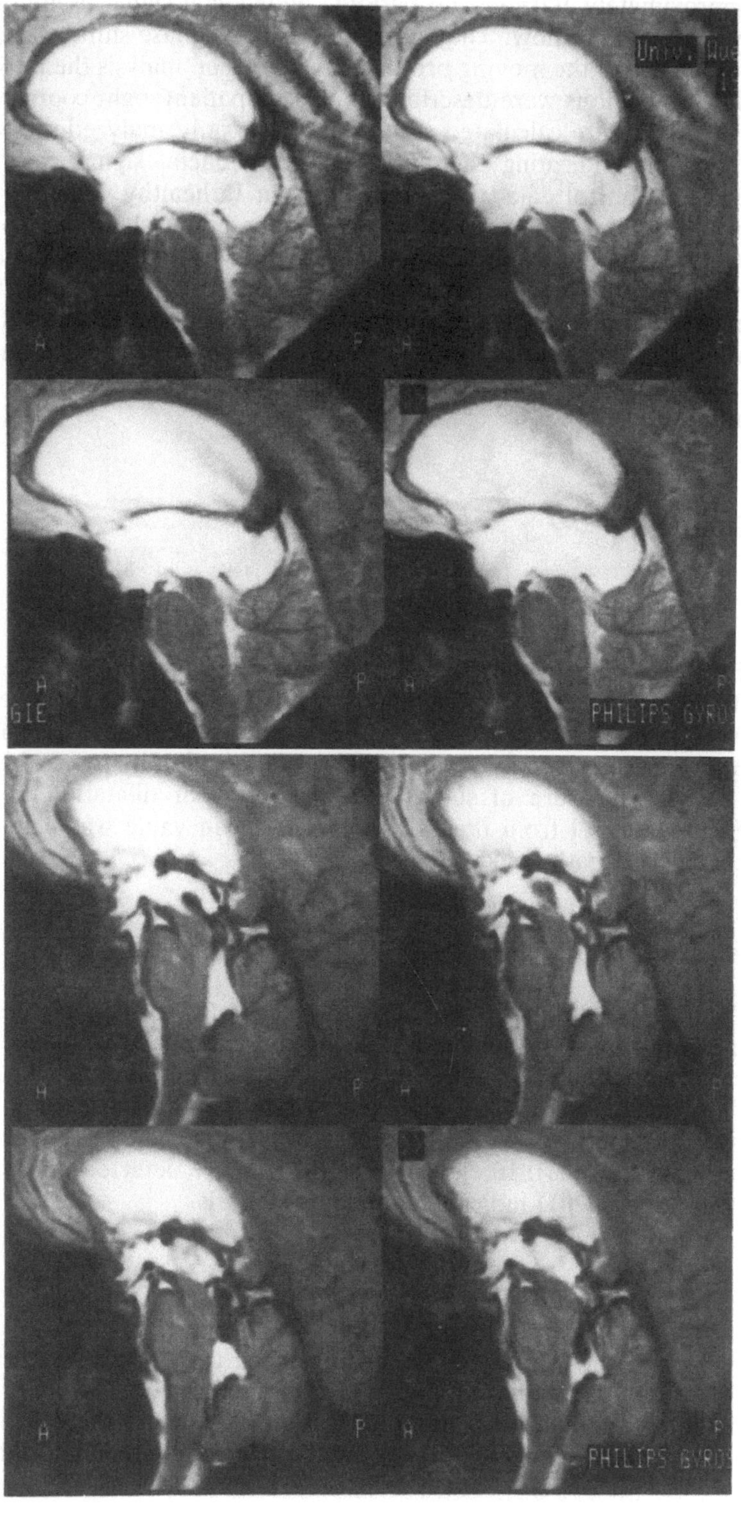

A

B

limited to the default minimum of 8. This corresponds to a time resolution of approximately 100 ms. The periodic aqueductal signal oscillations represented velocity of CSF flow. They were the result of phase shift, phase dispersion and turbulance of the moving protons. By a Fourier analysis the periodic aqueductal flow oscillations were described. For each patient eight coefficients (Ao to A4, B1 to B3) were calculated. In this study we only analyzed the most reliable Ao coefficient indicating the average of aqueductal signal void over the heart phases. Control data were obtained from 15 healthy volunteers. Additionally, in all patients we performed a continous epidural pressure monitoring. We analyzed the mean intracranial pressure (ICP) and the evidence of nightly B-waves. We defined as pathological a mean ICP greater than 15 mmHg and an increase of nightly B-waves more than 20%. The pressure volume index (PVI) after bolus injection (normal >20 ml) and the resistance to outflow after constant infusion (normal <12 mmHg/ml/min) were calculated after a spinal infusion test [3].

Results

Clinical and CT Characteristics

Eighty percent of our cases showed unspecific symptoms, like headaches and dizziness. We diagnosed mental deficits in 48% of our hydrocephalic patients, in 57% gait disturbances and in 33% urinary incontinence. The classical triad of normal pressure hydrocephalus was detected only in one third of our cases.

As a measure of supratentorial ventricular dilatation we calculated the Evans-ratio [1] from the CT scan. The mean value was 0.45 ± 0.14 SD and classified as pathological.

Aqueductal CSF Flow in MRI

Figure 2 summarizes the absolute values of the calculated Ao-coefficient measured by CSF flow studies in the mesencephalic aqueduct by MRI. In all cases we found Ao-coefficient values outside the normal range of the control data (mean 1088 ± 113 SD). Confirming the diagnosis of a communicating hydrocephalus we found an increase of the aqueductal CSF flow (Ao < 975) in ten cases (47.6%). In eleven cases (52.4%) we detected no flow-related signal void (Ao > 1201) indicating aqueduct stenosis.

Correlation of CSF Flow and Intracranial Pressure Dynamics

Analyzing the ICP values we distinguished two groups: one with pathological ICP values and one without. In eleven cases (52.4%) ICP dynamics were pathological indicating shunt operation. However, there were ten (47.6%) hydrocephalic patients with normal intracranial pressure values. Correlating

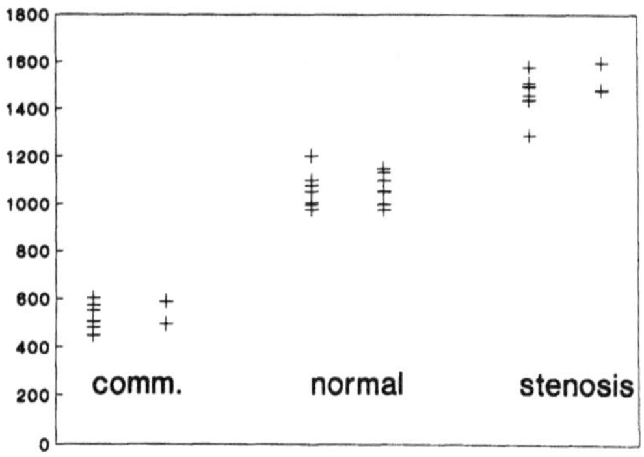

Fig. 2. Ao-Fourier coefficient in patients with suspected hydrocephalus (comm.: communicating hydrocephalus, n = 10, stenosis: aqueduct stenosis, n = 11) and normal healthy volunteers (normal, n = 15)

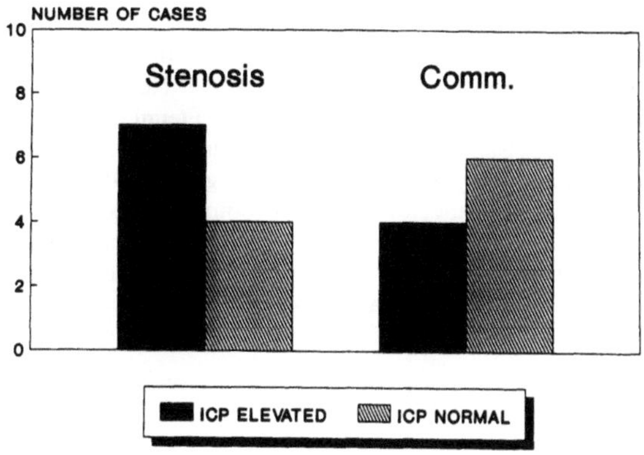

Fig. 3. Correlation of mesencephalic aqueductal CSF flow using fast field echo technique in MRI and intracranial pressure dynamics in hydrocephalic patients (stenosis: aqueduct stenosis, comm.: communicating hydrocephalus)

invasively measured ICP data with noninvasively calculated aqueductal CSF flow values (Fig. 3), the aqueduct stenosis group revealed pathological ICP in seven out of eleven cases. However, there were four cases with normal ICP and loss of signal void in the mesencephalic aqueduct stenosis. We found elevated ICP in only four out of ten cases with communicating hydrocephalus; six patients revealed normal intracranial pressure parameters.

Discussion

The FFE sequence in cardiac gated T2 weighted images in MRI allows the study of aqueductal CSF flow. For the first time the clinician is able, non-invasively, to get information on cerebrospinal fluid flow phenomena. This might be of major interest in hydrocephalic patients with suspected abnormalities of CSF production and secretion. Our results show that CSF flow studies using this method in MRI is a highly sensitive method to detect pathological pulsatility of CSF. We could clearly differentiate between patients with or without signal void in the mesencephalic aqueduct indicating communicating hydrocephalus or aqueduct stenosis (Fig. 1). However we could not confirm a reliable correlation between flow-related CSF abnormalities and invasive testing methods of intracranial pressure dynamics [4]. Therefore, this MRI method could not be a primary indicator for shunting alone. Perhaps in the future new developments in technology e.g. the quantitation of CSF flow volume in the mesencephalic aqueduct or elsewhere may provide a more precise estimation of intracranial pressure buffering capacity.

References

1. Gyldensted C (1977) Measurement of the normal ventricular system and hemispheric sulci of 100 adults with computed tomography. Neuroradiology 14:183–192
2. Klose U, Requardt H, Schroth G, Deimling M (1987) MR-tomographische Darstellung von Liquorpulsationen. Fortschr Röntgenstr 147:313–319
3. Marmarou A, Shulman L, LaMorgese J (1975) Compartmental analysis of compliance and outflow resistance of the cerebrospinal fluid system. J Neurosurg 43:523–534
4. Ohara S, Nagai H, Ueda Y (1989) CSF pulsatile flow on MRI and its relation to intracranial pressure. In: Hoff JT, Betz AL (eds) Intracranial Pressure VII. Springer, Berlin Heidelberg New York London Paris Tokyo Hong Kong
5. Sherman JL, Citrin CM (1986) Magnetic resonance demonstration of normal CSF flow. AJNR 7:3–6

Brain Edema Induced by Ventricular Puncture. A Study by Magnetic Resonance Imaging

C. Raftopoulos[1], C. Chaskis[1], L. Bidaut[2], F. Cantraine[3], D. Balériaux[4], C. Matos[4], F. Delecluse[5], and J. Brotchi[1]

[1] Departments of Neurosurgery [2] Medical Imaging [4] Neuroradiology and [5] Neurology of University Hospital Erasme and [3] Data Processing Department of Faculty of Medecine, Université Libre de Bruxelles, Brussels, Belgium

Introduction

The sensitivity of magnetic resonance imaging (MRI) in the detection of edema is well known [3]. We have reported that MRI clearly demonstrates "traumatic" brain edema surrounding the site of a ventricular catheter, whereas concomitant computed tomography (CT) demonstrates either no or only minimal changes [5]. The hyperdensity area surrounding a frontal chatheter appeared larger than that induced by puncture of the ventricular trigonum.

This last observation prompted the routine use of MRI after ventricular puncture in normal pressure hydrocephalic (NPH) patients to assess the hyperdensity signal surrounding the catheter track. Different groups of monitored and shunted patients were put together. For each group, we modified either the sequence of ventricular puncture, the catheter type, or the delay between puncture and MRI. The groups were compared in order to differentiate between the various mechanisms underlying the puncture induced brain edema.

Material and Method

Thirty-six consecutive NPH patients (i.e. lumbar pressure <20 cm H_2O and Evans' Index >0.30) were prospectively studied. The phase I group consisted of 8 males and 5 females. The age distribution ranged from 17 to 80 years with a mean age of 60 years. In the phase II group, there were: 16 males, 7 females, mean age: 63, range: 5 to 81 years.

In phase I, each patient was first subjected to a frontal ventricular catheterization with a Holter catheter for a 48 hours continuous intracranial pressure (ICP) monitoring. When the ICP monitoring was abnormal, a ventriculo-cardiac derivation by trigonal catheterization with a Pudenz-Schulte catheter was performed seven days later. Six days after each catheterization, MRI was performed on a 1.5 Tesla superconductor unit (Gyroscan S15) with a slice thickness of 5 mm. We used T2-weighted spin-echo images with a repetition time (TR) of 2050 ms and an echo time (TE) of 30 and 100 ms.

In phase II, the monitoring was performed by trigonal puncture and the MRI was made two days after the monitoring (catheter in place!) and then two days after shunting. Patients who were not shunted were also considered. The average hyperdensity signal width was calculated from digitized masks stored and processed by a Micro Vax (Digital Equipment Corporation) based high level multimodality display and processing system [2].

The groups were compared with each other. Statistical analysis was carried out using the SPSS (Statistical Package of Social Sciences) program. Both T and paired tests were used when relevant.

Results

The results, including statistical significance, are presented in Table 1.

Discussion

To explain the differences between the groups, six different hypothetical mechanisms, acting individually or together, are proposed.

Hypothesis 1

The frontal catheter is withdrawn after two days and the MRI is performed after six days, with the trigonal catheter permanently in place. The withdrawal could allow the CSF to seep into the disrupted parenchyma and produce CSF interstitial edema.

Hypothesis 2

The first MRI study, demonstrating the frontal brain edema, is necessarily performed when the patient is not yet permanently shunted, which is not the case for the second MRI study. The consequence of permanent shunting is the reduction of ICP [6]. This reduction lowers the pressure gradient and eventually reduces leakage of CSF into the brain through the ventricular wall disruption along the catheter, thereby causing less edema or no edema at all.

Hypothesis 3

The Holter catheter might be more traumatic than the flanged Pudenz-Schulte one, perhaps because of its larger external diameter (3.1 mm against 2.1 mm for the Pudenz-Schulte catheter).

Hypothesis 4

The frontal brain parenchyma might be more sensitive to puncture than the trigonal parenchyma. Perhaps in relation to this hypothesis, studies concerning

Table 1. Comparison of the Tranversal extension of the MRI hypersignal area around the ventricular catheterization track

	Pt	n°	Sx	Ag		Monitoring		Shunt		Statistical Analysis	
						Fr (H) A	Tr (H) B	Tr (P-S) C	Fr (P-S) D	Comparison of columns and phases	P
PHASE I	SAR	1	W	49		12.13	–	0	–		
	JAC	2	M	40	MRI	19.67	–	11.65	–		
	JEA	3	M	73	6 days	12.91	–	0	–		
	VAN	4	M	78	after the	11.7	–	12.85	–		
	TAC	5	W	19	puncture.	6.5	–	5.85	–		
	KEM	6	M	72		11.96	–	8	–		
	MAT	7	M	73	The drain is	6.44	–	0	–		
	VER	8	W	76	withdrawm	12.49	–	4.89	–		
	MAE	9	W	76	for column A	8.64	–	5.79	–		
	LOM	10	M	17		6.32	–	12.24	–		
	BOO	11	M	71		6.5	–	5.53	–		
	DEB	12	M	68		4.35	–	6.63	–		
	ROB	13	W	62		4.972	–	5.32	–		
	AVG			60		9.58	–	6.06	–		
	STADEV					4.35	–	4.40	–	I A with I C	0.044
PHASE II	NEF	1	M	80		–	6.12	–	4.93		
	HER	2	M	61		–	–	–	4.799		
	WIL	3	W	66		–	0	–	–		
	VAN	4	M	66		–	11.75	–	–		
	RIV	5	M	70		–	6.92	–	9.96		
	GYS	6	M	73		–	7.57	–	–		
	DEB	7	W	72		–	3.24	–	–		
	HAQ	8	M	81		–	0	–	–		
	NYS	9	M	59	MRI	–	9.469	–	0		
	FOR	10	W	77	2 days	–	6.69	–	–		
	DUP	11	M	76	after the	–	6.42	–	–		
	RAI	12	W	68	ventricular	–	0	–	–		
	GER	13	W	72	puncture	–	4.09	–	3.04		
	DEL	14	M	80	with	–	4.56	–	–		
	PUT	15	W	50	the catheter	–	0	–	–		
	HON	16	M	78	in place	–	–	–	4.87		
	ROB	17	M	5	for	–	0	–	–	Ph I with Ph II	0.004
	BEG	18	M	74	column A.	–	–	–	0		
	DER	19	W	75		–	0	–	–	II B with II D	0.051
	LAS	20	M	72		–	6.05	–	0		
	OUA	21	M	7		–	6	–	–	I A with II B	0.005
	BOU	22	M	44		–	12.1	–	5.75	I A with II D	0.001
	DET	23	M	68		–	7.77	–	0		
	AVG			63		–	4.94	–	3.33	I C with II B	0.46
	STADEV					–	3.95	–	3.36	IC with II D	0.107

Pt, patient; n°, number; Sx, sex; Ag, age; Fr, frontal; Tr, trigonal; (H), Holter catheter; (P-S), Pudenz-Schulte catheter; AVG, average; STDEV, standard deviation.

the frequency of post-shunt epilepsy showed that frontal catheterization was followed by a higher frequency of epilepsy than trigonal catheterization. Venes and Dauser [7] reported a 7.2% incidence of post frontal catheterization epilepsy, Albright et al. [1] a 30% rate and Dan and Wade [4] a 54.5% rate, in contrast to a post parietal catheterization epilepsy incidence of 6.6% reported by Dan and Wade [4]. The greater sensitivity of the frontal cortex might account for the more extensive frontal parenchyma edema observed in this study.

Hypothesis 5

On the other hand, the trigonal brain might be more sensitive to puncture than the frontal parenchyma.

Hypothesis 6

The traumatic lesion increases up to the sixth day. This means that either the edema is correlated with the vascular and cellular lesions induced by ventricular puncture, or a greater quantity of CSF seeps into the brain parenchyma through the catheter track.

Conclusions

Comparison of phase I and phase II suggests six hypotheses among which two notions seem particularly promising. First, the possibility of a variable traumatic effect depending on the catheter used, and secondly, a possible difference in the sensitivity of the brain parenchyma depending on the area punctured. In order to better separate the role of each one of these mechanisms, a phase III is actually in progress and a phase IV study is scheduled.

References

1. Albright AL, Haines SJ, Taylor FH (1988) Function of parietal and frontal shunts in childhood hydrocephalus. J Neurosurg 69:883–886
2. Bidaut L, Poncelet B (1990) A multi-modality display system and processing system: application to composite PET and MRI. Eur J Nucl Med 16(7):475
3. Bradley WG, Crooks B, Newton TH (1983) Physicals principles on NMR. In: Newton TH, Potts DG (eds) Modern Neuroradiology, vol. II: Advanced Imaging Techniques, Clavaled Press, San Francisco
4. Dan NG, Wade MJ (1986) The incidence of epilepsy after ventricular shunting procedures. J Neurosurg 65:19–21
5. Raftopoulos C, Balériaux D, Brotchi J, Voordecker Ph (1988) The traumatic aspect of ventricular catheterization demonstrated by Magnetic Resonance Imaging. Clin Neurol Neurosurg 90–1:47–52

6. Symon L, Dorsch Ph (1975) Use of long-term intracranial pressure measurement to assess hydrocephalic patients prior to shunt surgery. J Neurosurg 42:258–273
7. Venes JL, Dauser Ph (1987) Epilepsy following ventricular shunt placement. J Neurosurg 66:154–155

Session VIII: Hydrocephalus

Chairmen: H. Nagai and J. Ekstedt

Hydrocephalus – Analysis of 480 Infusion Tests

G. Costabile and Ch. Probst

Neurochirurgische Klinik, Kantonsspital Aarau, 5001 Aarau, Switzerland

Introduction

Since long term ventricular cerebrospinal fluid (CSF) drainage only increases the CSF outflow, it comes to aid of patients with communicating ventricular enlargement only if the pathological changes depend on a decrease of CSF outflow [1, 3, 6]. Therefore, measurement of CSF outflow is necessary before shunt operations.

If the CSF outflow is shown to be decreased, clinical improvement may occur after shunting. If not, the probability of a complication after this simple diversion procedure may well surpass that of a satisfactory response. By the same token, the investigations of CSF outflow should not carry the same risks as the shunt operations themselves. Moreover, the CSF outflow measurements should not cause discomfort or require too long a time, since most patients are not able to offer much co-operation [1, 5, 6]. Infusion procedures into the CSF space for the assessment of CSF outflow by measuring the inversely related CSF outflow resistance (R_{of}), are simple, not long lasting and relatively non-invasive tests, if they are carried out by lumbar puncture or – in shunted patients with or without occlusion of the proximal CSF pathways – by puncture with a ventricular catheter reservoir. The latter procedure allows the investigation of the failure of postoperative improvement, in which case the implanted shunt has failed to lower the R_{of} to values, which have been found to correlate with a postoperative clinical recovery.

Therefore, a CSF space infusion test (IT) is also necessary if the post-operative clinical outcome is unsatisfactory [1, 2]. In order to demonstrate the usefulness of the IT, this study was aimed at defining the pathological range of the preoperative R_{of}, as well as its postoperative normal range, correlating with clinical improvement after CSF diversion.

Clinical Material and Method

From 1979 to 1990, 480 infusion tests have been carried out in our department, 305 before and 175 after shunt operation, in 353 patients with symptomatic ventricular enlargement. Two-hundred and seventy-three CSF diversions have been carried out in the examined patients in the same period: 217 were first operations and 56 were revisions. The details of the patient group are listed in Table 1. The clinical outcome has been classified – after a follow-up time of 1 –145 months (mean: 54 months) – as improved if the preoperative symptoms, at least partially, had regressed. Only shunted patients have been evaluated. A reliable assessment of the clinical outcome was possible in 122 of them.

R_{of} was calculated as the difference between the steady-state CSF pressure during constant intrathecal infusion of Ringer's solution, and the opening CSF pressure divided by the infusion rate.

Of 480 IT 430 were performed by the lumbar and 50 by the ventricular route; 421 with an infusion rate of 2 ml/min, 22 with 1 ml/min and 36 with 2.1 and 0.5 ml/min.

In addition, in 40 patients measurement of the pressure-volume index (PVI) was carried out in order to assess the CSF space compliance [4], 33 by lumbar and 7 by ventricular reservoir puncture. The volume of the bolus injection varied from 2 to 5 ml with an injection rate of 1 ml/sec. Lastly, the CT-scans of 81 patients and the isotope cisternographic findings of 17 of them were evaluated, the former according to the ventricular enlargement classification of Vassilouthis [9] and the latter according to the classification of Yasargil [10].

Results

Of 122 shunted patients, 62 or 50.8% improved postoperatively and 60 or 49.2% did not show any regression of the preoperative symptoms. The R_{of} value was inversely related to the infusion rate. The R_{of} values at different infusion rates in relation to the postoperative outcome are shown in Table 2

Table 1. Clinical material

	Decade	1.	2.	3.+4.	5.+6.	7.	8.	9.
Age	M %	2.5	3.7	8.7	12.7	13.2	13.8	3.6
	f %	2.5	3.7	4.4	7	9.6	9.8	1.1
Etiology		idiop	traum	malform	hemor	postop	mening	occlus
	%	38	33	8	7	5	5	3
Symptoms		triad	gait+ POS	POS	gait	headache	ICP rise	prolong neurol deficit
	%	29.7	32	8.9	4.4	17.4	3.3	3.9

Table 2. Mean (SD) CSF outflow resistance (mmHg/ml/min) in various types of hydrocephalus at two different infusion rates: 2 ml/min (r = 2) and 1 ml/min (r = 1)

Hydrocephalus etiology	Outcome after shunt			
	Satisfactory r = 2	r = 1	Unsatisfactory r = 2	r = 1
Total material	17.9 (5.2)	23 (6.1)	11.5 (4.4)	20.2 (5.2)
Idiopathic	17.5		11	
Posttraumatic	19		11.5	
Malformative	10.5		13	
After surgery	8		5.5	
Postmeningitic	19.5		10	
Posthermorrhagic	16.5		15	

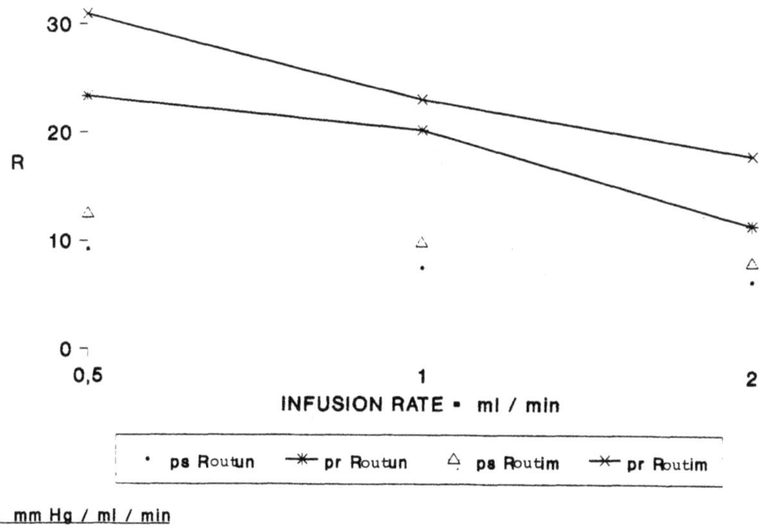

Fig. 1. Mean R_{of} values of hydrocephalic patients who improved after shunting: preoperative R_{of} ($prR_{of}im$) and postoperative R_{of} ($psR_{of}im$), and of hydrocephalic patients who did not improve after CSF diversion: preoperative R_{of} ($prR_{of}un$) and postoperative R_{of} ($psR_{of}un$).

and Fig. 1. The differences between the R_{of} of patients who postoperatively improved and those of patients with an unsatisfactory outcome were less evident at the infusion rate of 1 ml/min than at the rate of 2 ml/min. The postoperative R_{of} values of patients who did not improve after the first shunt, but did so after revision, amounted to 15.4, in contrast to the value of 8 mmHg/ml/min in patients who improved after just one shunt diversion (Fig. 2). After revision of the shunt, the R_{of} value of finally improved patients decreased from 15.4 to 7.8 mmHg/ml/min. The simple linear regression of the R_{of} values in dependence on age was: −15.5 mmHg/ml/min + 0.014, implying that the distribution of low and high R_{of} values is similar at every age. Table 2 shows an equal distribution of R_{of} among different etiologies of ventricular

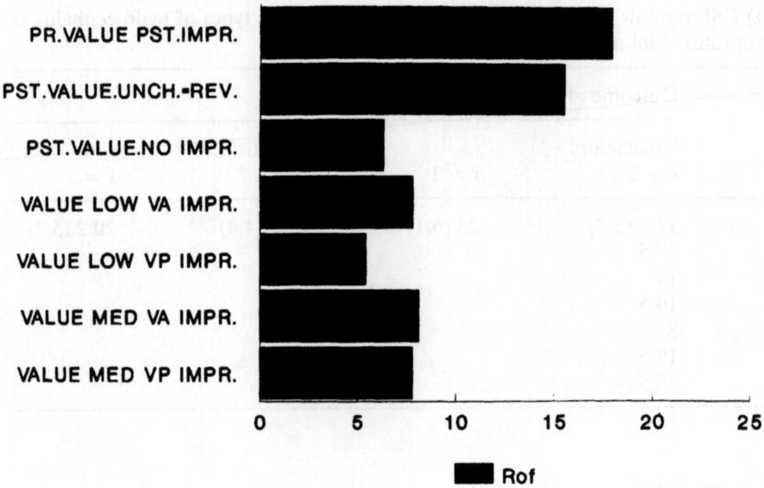

Fig. 2. Mean R_{of} values of patients who improved after shunting at the preoperative IT (PR.IMPR.), of patients who improved only after shunt revision at the IT before revision (PS.UNCH.=REV.), of improved patients after the first shunt of after revision operated on by ventriculoatrial low pressure (LOW VA IMPR.), medium pressure (MED VA IMPR.), ventriculo-peritoneal low pressure (LOW VP IMPR.) and medium pressure shunt (MED VP IMPR.).

enlargement. Exceptions are the malformative and postoperative ventricular enlargements with too low preoperative R_{of} values to warrant a postoperative improvement, as well as the posthemorrhagic ventricular dilatations with similar R_{of} values in patients who did and who did not improve after shunting. These exceptions might be explained by false negative or positive results due to the fact that aqueductal stenosis was the cause in most cases of malformative hydrocephalus and due to postsurgical CSF leaks or still present xanthochromy [8, 9].

The in-vitro evaluation of the function of some low pressure shunt devices also showed an increase in R_{of} in the presence of shunt stenosis or elevated protein content of the perfusion solution (Table 3).

The R_{of} values of patients operated on by different shunt systems are shown in Fig. 2.

The preoperative PVI values did not differ significantly between post-operatively improved and unchanged patients: 20 ml versus 19 ml respectively ($t = 0.3182$, $p = 0.7565$). The PVI increased postoperatively only in patients with a satisfactory outcome: 42 ml versus 18 ml in unchanged patients [7].

The preoperative CT-scans showed a similar ventricular size in patients with and without satisfactory outcome. The mean value of the ventriculocranial index (VCI) at the level of the foramina Monroi was 1/4.16 and 1/4 respectively. Obliteration of the sulci was observed in 60% of the postoperatively improved patients and in 40% of the unchanged patients. Postoperative CT control examinations showed a decrease of the ventricular size in 35% of favourable and in 50% of poor clinical outcome.

The ratio between highly abnormal isotope cisternographic findings (2nd and 3rd degree = intraventricular tracer for longer than 24 hours) and slightly

Table 3. Perfusion of low-pressure shunt devices in-vitro

Perfusion solution	Devices					
	Hakim		Sophy		Holter	
	p	s	p	s	p	s
Ringer	5	20	5	20	11	25
Ringer + 5% plasma proteins	7	28	5	26	14	38

perfusion rate, 2 ml/min; R = mm Hg/ml/min; p, pervious system; s, system stenosis 62%

abnormal findings (intraventricular tracer up to 6 hours after intrathecal application) was 4/1 in patients with satisfactory and 4/8 in patients with unsatisfactory outcome.

Discussion

Elevated R_{of} values do not guarantee postoperative improvement, as the symptoms in some patients have become irreversible. For example, patients with posthemorrhagic hydrocephalus and a R_{of} above 15 mmHg/ml/min improve after shunting, whereas with a R_{of} of 15 mmHg/ml/min or below they may not. Some of these patients have developed posthemorrhagic deficits, independent on the impaired CSF outflow, which will not improve after a shunt. Their R_{of} may be elevated up to a level which in other patients would be compatible with postoperative improvement.

Low R_{of} values may be compatible with postoperative good outcome if the hydrocephalus has a malformative etiology or has become evident soon after major intracranial surgery and if a CSF leak at the time of infusion test cannot be excluded [8].

Nevertheless, the analysis of the whole material shows a definite difference in R_{of} values between patients who do and who do not improve after shunting [1, 3, 6, 8]. Since the standard deviation of the preoperative R_{of} of improved patients, measured at the infusion rate of 2 ml/min, amounts to 5.2 mmHg/ml/min (Table 2), a favourable response after shunting can be expected, if the R_{of} value is at least 12.7 mmHg/ml/min. For the infusion rate of 1 ml/min this lower limit of R_{of} is 5 mmHg/ml/min higher. The higher infusion rate is preferable for reasons explained in the previous paragraph. Moreover, this rate is less discomforting, since it does not last longer than 30 minutes.

Only patients with postoperatively abnormal R_{of} values may benefit from a shunt revision.

The measurement of R_{of} is of value in selecting patients with hydrocephalus for a shunt operation. However, the possibility of the presence of irreversible symptoms should be taken into consideration. The postoperative R_{of} value, compatible with a good outcome depends on the implanted shunt device and amounts, with the most common non flow-regulated devices, to 8.5 mmHg/ml/min ± 2.5 SD.

References

1. Costabile G, Probst Ch, Schönholzer AM (1983) Further experiences with the intrathecal infusion test in the management of communicating hydrocephalus. In: Ishii S, Nagai H, Brock M (eds) Intracranial pressure V. Springer, Berlin Heidelberg New York Tokyo, pp 632–635
2. Costabile G, Probst Ch (1988) Intrathecal infusion test and decrease in shunt revision and infection. Neurochirurgia 31:134–135
3. Gjerris F, Børgesen SE, Schmidt J, Sørensen PS (1988) Resistance to cerebrospinal fluid outflow in patients with normal pressure hydrocephalus. In: Gjerris F, Børgesen SE, Sørensen PS (eds) Outflow of cerebrospinal fluid. Munksgaard, Copenhagen, pp 329–342
4. Marmarou A, Shulman K, LaMorgese J (1975) Compartmental analysis of compliance and outflow resistance of the cerebrospinal fluid system. J Neurosurg 43:523–534
5. Powell M, Crockard A, Brookes D (1988) Normal pressure hydrocephalus – ICP and PET scan studies before and after shunting. In: Gjerris F, Børgesen SE, Sørensen PS (eds) Outflow of cerebrospinal fluid. Munksgaard, Copenhagen pp, 377–389
6. Price DJ (1988) The clinical value of measurement of CSF outflow resistance. In: Gjerris F, Børgesen SE, Sørensen PS (eds) Outflow of cerebrospinal fluid. Munksgaard, Copenhagen, pp 390–401
7. Tans JThJ, Poortvliet DCJ (1988) Significance of compliance in adult hydrocephalus. In: Gjerris F, Børgesen SE, Sørensen PS (eds) Outflow of cerebrospinal fluid. Munksgaard, Copenhagen, pp 272–279
8. Trotter IL, Luzecky M, Siegel BA, Gado M (1974) Cerebrospinal fluid infusion test. Identification of artifacts and correlation with cisternography and pneumo-encephalography. Neurology (Minneap.) 24:181–186
9. Vassilouthis J, Richardson AE (1979) Ventricular dilatation and communicating hydrocephalus following spontaneous subarachnoid hemorrhage. J Neurosurg 51:341–351
10. Yasargil MG, Yonekawa Y, Zumstein B, Stahl H (1973) Hydrocephalus following spontaneous subarachnoid hemorrhage – Clinical features and treatment. J Neurosurg 39:474–479

Evaluation of Pressure Monitoring and CSF Conductance in NPH

J.C. GODERSKY[1] and N.R. GRAFF-RADFORD[2]

[1] Anchorage Neurosurgical Associates, 2841 DeBarr Road, Suite 34, Anchorage, AK 99508, USA
[2] Department of Neurology, Mayo Clinic Jacksonville, 4500 San Pablo Drive, Jacksonville, FL 32224, USA

Introduction

Predicting outcome following shunt placement in normal pressure hydrocephalus (NPH) remains problematic, especially for those individuals without a known cause for the hydrocephalus. A variety of tests have been devised to assess CSF absorption and intracranial dynamics and aid in patient selection. Some reports have also suggested improved results from monitoring intracranial pressure (ICP). We present our series of 45 patients evaluated prospectively for possible NPH, with specific reference to evaluation of CSF conductance and ICP monitoring in a group of patients with primarily idiopathic NPH.

Methods

All individuals had evidence of hydrocephalus on CT scan (Evans ratio >0.3), as well as dementia, an abnormal gait, and urinary symptoms (incontinence or urgency). A known etiology for the hydrocephalus was present in only 4 of the 45 individuals.

Surgical Methods

Medium Pressure Valves were utilized in all 38 shunted cases (ventrioculoperitoneal 35, ventriculoatrial 3). Shunt function was assessed by CT scanning or percutaneous testing of the shunt if the ventricular size was not smaller after surgery.

Evaluation of Outcome

All patients were assessed prior to surgery and at 2 and 6 months after shunt placement, utilizing 3 parameters:

1. Rating of gait was determined by review of video tapes;
2. Katz index of activities of daily living; and
3. a neuropsychological test battery.

In order to be classified as improved, they had to have sustained improvement at 6 months in 2 of the 3 indices.

ICP Monitoring

A right frontal ventriculostomy was inserted and ICP continuously recorded for 24 to 48 hours by paper print-out at a chart speed of 30 cm/hour. These tracings were then assessed for: 1) The percentage of time B waves were present; 2) The percentage of time the ICP exceeded 15 mmHg; 3) the percentage of time the ICP exceeded 20 mmHg.

CSF Conductance (C_{out})

A CSF conductance study was performed following the method of Børgesen [1]. This involves a lumboventricular perfusion at a constant rate but variable outflow pressures. Infusion periods of 5 minutes were used, 6 to 8 measures were made at outflow pressures of 7 to 33 mmHg. These data were then plotted and the conductance calculated.

Recommendations for Shunting

If the ICP monitoring demonstrated >50% B waves, or if the C_{out} was <0.10, we recommended shunt placement to the patient and family. In one individual a shunt was placed without ICP monitoring or CSF conductance having been done because of his clinical improvement following lumbar puncture.

Results

ICP monitoring was accomplished in 43 of the 45 patients. These consisted of 22 males and 21 females. Ages ranged from 51 to 86 years (mean of 72.5 years). The cause of the ventricular enlargement was unknown in 41/45 patients). Valid CSF conductance studies were completed in 28/45 individuals. Using the criteria above for shunt placement, 37 had shunts inserted. Improvement was noted in 30/37, or 81%. This included improvement in the neuropsychological test scores in 39%. The majority of those improving did so in the assessment of gait and the Katz index.

When those with B waves for more than 50% of the recording time were evaluated for improvement, 21/25 (84%) improved. When ICP exceeded 15 mmHg for more than 10% of the recording, 26/29 (90%) were improved. When ICP was greater than 20 mmHg for 5% of the tracing, 19/21 (90%) improved (Table 1).

Børgesen [1] has stated that a C_{out} of <0.08 is highly predictive of improvement. We elected to shunt all individuals with a C_{out} of <0.10, so as not to exclude potential responders. Of those with a C_{out} of <0.08, 14/18 improved. In those with a C_{out} >0.08 but <0.10, 3/4 improved. There were 6 in which C_{out} was >0.10 and none of these had shunt surgery (Table 2).

Complications included subdural fluid collections in three, one of these requiring surgery because of worsening symptoms. CSF pleocytosis occurred in three individuals after the conductance study. A shunt infection was present in one patient, requiring shunt removal.

Discussion

It remains an important goal to identify factors predictive of outcome in symptomatic adult hydrocephalus as the complication rate for shunt insertion in the elderly population remains significant [6]. A number of clinical factors help initiate this decision process [5]. These include onset of gait abnormality prior to onset of dementia; the duration the dementia has been present prior to the shunting; and impairment in visual naming on neuropsychological examinations.

Impaired CSF adsorption is cited by many authors in discussing the pathophysiology of NPH and forms the basis for a variety of invasive tests. However,

Table 1. Quantification of ICP vs. outcome

Status	B-Waves >50%	P > 15 mmHg for 10%	P > 20 mmHg for 5%
Improved	21/25 (84%)	26/29 (90%)	19/21 (90%)
Unimproved	4/25 (16%)	3/29 (10%)	2/21 (10%)

P, intracranial pressure

Table 2. Conductance vs. outcome

C_{out}	Improved	Unimproved
<0.08	14	4
>0.08 but <0.10	3	1

Table 3. Outcome vs. ICP monitoring

		Mean % of time (range)		
Status	N	B-Waves	P > 15 mmHg	P > 20 mmHg
Improved	30	63 (27–100)	47 (1–100)	24 (0–100)
Unimproved	7	47 (0–94)	29 (0–77)	10 (0–60)
Not shunted	6	16 (1–26)	10 (0–25)	0

N, Number of subjects; P, intracranial pressure.

the predictive role of these tests remains unclear [1, 2, 3, 9, 10]. The explanation for these differences could rest with the validity of the measurement tool for CSF adsorption or possibly be related to differences in patient population. It is generally agreed that those persons with a known cause for NPH fare much better than those with idiopathic NPH, suggesting a difference in the pathophysiology in these two groups. Our patient population is almost completely composed of those with idiopathic NPH. We found measurement of C_{out}, using a cut off of either 0.08 or 0.10, to be unreliable (Table 2). Although Børgesen strongly recommends this procedure, in his patients with an unknown cause for hydrocephalus this test was less predictive than in those with a known cause [2]. Using a conductance of 0.08 or less, 3/20 of his patients with an unknown cause for NPH failed to improve and one that would have improved would not have been recommended for shunting. We feel that the value of CSF conductance in predicting outcome in idiopathic NPH remains uncertain.

Intracranial pressure monitoring as a predictor of response to shunting has been utilized for a number of years [1, 8, 9]. Based on the data from our study, and literature review, we feel that this is a valuable indicator of response to shunting, when quantitatively analyzed. The frequency of B waves is important when they are present for more than 50% of the recording [1, 2, 6]. When ICP exceeds 15 or 20 mmHg for 10% or 5% of the tracing respectively, this is also prognostically important. When quantitation is not performed there is a measure of overlap in ICP recording between those individuals who improve and those who do not (Table 3). Utilizing parameters of B-waves >50% of the tracing, ICP >15 mmHg for 10% or >20 mmHg for 5% of the tracing, the predictive value improves (Table 1).

B waves are felt to be a normally occurring phenomenon and have been attributed to vasodilation occurring with variation in respiratory patterns and with rapid eye movement sleep. Experimental studies attribute B wave occurrence to sympathetic discharges from a brain stem vasomotor center [7]. Their occurrence in NPH with high frequency suggest a possible role in the pathogenesis of this disease. In individuals with impaired CSF absorption, this further increase in ICP associated with B-waves could result in brain dysfunction. Tanaka and Nishimura [10] have shown that B wave frequency and this maximal pressure are significantly reduced by shunting. A reduction in the frequency and height of B waves could eliminate further injury and allow recovery to take place.

References

1. Børgesen SE, Gjerris F (1982) The Predictive Value of Conductance to Outflow of CSF in Normal Pressure Hydrocephalus. Brain 105:65–86
2. Børgesen SE (1984) Conductance to Outflow of CSF in Normal Pressure Hydrocephalus. Acta Neurochirurgia 1:1–45
3. Delwel EJ, deJong DA, Avezaat CJJ, van Eijndhoven JHM, Korbee A (1989) CSF Dynamics in Patients with Suspected Normal Pressure Hydrocephalus. In: Hoff JT, Betz AL (eds) Intracranial Pressure VII. Springer New York London Paris Tokyo Hong Kong, Berlin Heidelberg, pp 379–382
4. Dirnagl U, Garner C, Haberl R, Mautner D, Schmiedek P, Einhäupl KM (1989) Correlation Between B-Waves and Intracranial Pressure-Volume Relationships. In: Hoff JT, Betz AL (eds) Intracranial Pressure VII. Springer New York London Paris Tokyo Hong Kong, Berlin Heidelberg, pp 213–216
5. Graff-Radford NR, Godersky JC, Jones MP (1989) Variables Predicting Sugical Outcome in Symptomatic Hydrocephalus in the Elderly. Neurology 39:1601–1604
6. Haan J, Thomeer RTWM (1988) Predictive Value of Temporary External Lumbar Drainage in Normal Pressure Hydrocephalus. Neurosurgery 22:388–391
7. Higashi S, Yamamoto S, Hashimoto M, Fujii H, Ito H, Kogure Y, Tokuda K (1989) The Role of Vasomotor Center and Adrenergic Pathways in B-Waves. In: Hoff JT, Betz AL (eds) Intracranial Pressure VII. Springer New York London Paris Tokyo Hong Kong, Berlin Heidelberg, pp 220–224
8. Symon L, Dorsch NWC (1975) Use of Long Term Intracranial Pressure Measurement to Assess Hydrocephalic Patients Prior to Shunt Surgery. J Neurosurg 42:258–273
9. Tanaka K, Nishimura S (1989) The Importance of Outflow Resistance of the Shunt System for Elimination of B-Waves. In: Hoff JT, Betz AL (eds) Intracranial Pressure VII. Springer New York London Paris Tokyo Hong Kong, Berlin Heidelberg, pp 368–373
10. Tans JTJ, Poortvliet DCJ (1984) Comparison of Ventricular Steady-state Infusion with Bolus Infusion and Pressure Recording for Differentiating arrested and non-arrested hydrocephalus. Acta Neurochirurgica 72:15–29

The Relative Prognostic Value of CSF Outflow Resistance Measurement in Shunting for Normal Pressure Hydrocephalus

E.J. DELWEL, D.A. DE JONG, and C.J.J. AVEZAAT

Department of Neurosurgery, University Hospital Rotterdam, Rotterdam, The Netherlands

Introduction

The diagnosis of normal pressure hyrocephalus is still subject of much controversy. Since the discovery of the syndrome by Hakim and Adams in 1965 [4], various diagnostic tools have been evaluated but none of them have been proven of decisive value.

In the present study the view was taken that the gold standard for the diagnosis of normal pressure hydrocephalus is improvement after shunting.

According to the literature, on average 60% of all patients suspected of NPH will improve as a result of a shunting procedure. This percentage is clearly influenced by the admission criteria to the study and these criteria should, therefore, always be mentioned.

Controversy concerning the predictive value of the CSF outflow resistance (Rout) led us to re-evaluate this parameter.

Patients and Methods

The admission criteria used in this study are shown in Fig. 1. The patients came from a population of 1,800,000 people comprising the city of Rotterdam and a large part of the South-West of Holland.

The patients referred to us had a variable clinical picture, not all of them showing the complete clinical triad.

Patients with a CSF outflow resistance lower than 8.0 mmHg/ml/min were not shunted for ethical reasons as values below this level are generally considered physiological and operative complications are not uncommon.

Improvement after shunting was concluded when consensus was reached between the neurosurgical attendant and the patient and/or his relatives about improvement of at least one feature of the clinical triad.

When the patient did not improve postoperatively and the ventricular size was not reduced, Rout measurement was repeated and the shunt revised if Rout was not significantly lower than the preoperative value.

The follow-up period after shunting was at least one year.

The following parameters were measured:

PATIENTS AND METHODS:

Admission criteria:

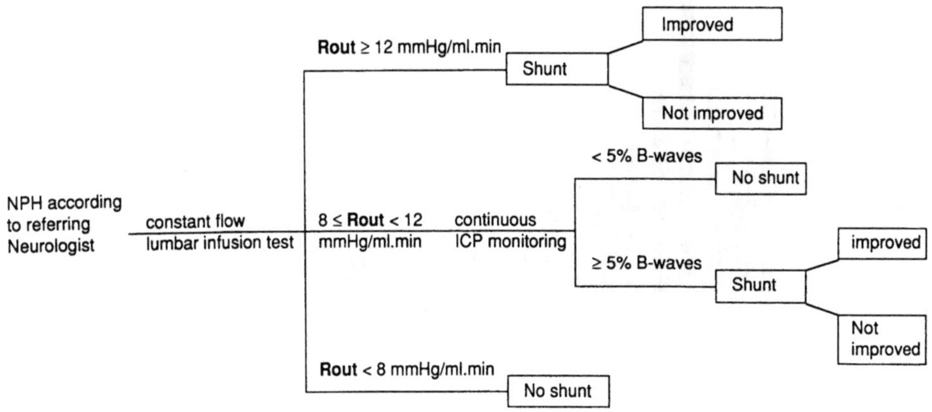

Fig. 1. Admission criteria to the study

Clinical Parameters

Duration of symptoms, mental slowness, loss of initiative, memory impairment, incontinence, slowness of gait and magnet effect.

CT Parameters

Evans ratio, temporal horn dilatation, third ventricle dilatation, periventricular lucency and peripheral atrophy.

Parameters of the CSF Dynamics

R_{out} as determined by the constant flow lumbar infusion test, the Elastance Coefficient (E_1, inversely related to the pressure-volume index) and the slope of the CSF pulse pressure versus ICP relationship. The last two parameters have been previously described [1, 3].

Results

Sixty-six patients were operated and 17 patients were rejected from the study. Thirty-nine operated patients improved and 27 of the operated patients did not improve. The overall results are thus comparable with most previous studies on this subject [2, 5, 6].

Figure 2a shows that the distribution of the CSF outflow resistance in the improved group did not significantly differ from the not-improved group of patients. There is even no cut-off point above which most patients do improve.

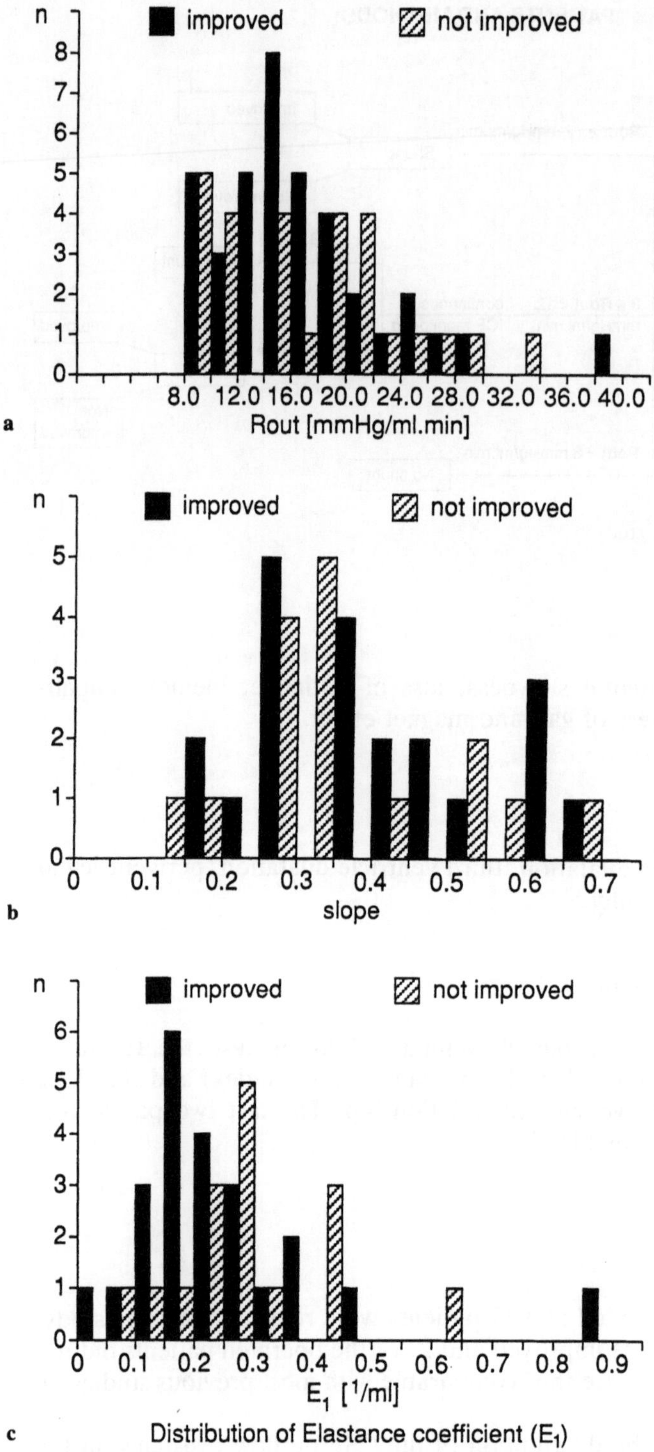

Fig. 2a–c. Distribution of the CSF outflow resistance (R_{out}). **b** Distribution of the slope of the linear regression of CSF pulse pressure versus ICP. **c** Distribution of the Elastance Coefficient (E_1)

Figure 2b shows the same pattern for the distribution of the slope of the CSF pulse pressure versus ICP relationship which parameter is considered to be related to the craniospinal pressure-volume relationship.

Figure 2c shows that the elastance coefficient was not significantly different in both groups.

However, various clinical and radiological criteria with a high predictive value concerning postoperative improvement could be identified (Table 1).

The complete clinical triad, mental slowness and loss of initiative in particular, certain aspects of hydrocephalus on CT-scan, such as dilatation of the temporal horns and third ventricle and absence of peripheral atrophy, and especially combinations of the above mentioned characteristics, and a short history of symptoms, are strong prognostic criteria. A unique finding is that for all the above mentioned criteria the predictive value is higher for men than for women.

In the group of 66 operated patients: 6 shunt infections and 11 subdural fluid collections were encountered.

Conclusions

Parameters of the CSF dynamics as measured by the constant flow lumbar infusiontest are of no use in the diagnosis of normal pressure hydrocephalus. Possible explanations for this conclusion are:

- failure of the constant flow lumbar infusion test in assessing a CSF absorption defect.
- failure of the pathophysiological concept of NPH in fully explaining the syndrome.

Table 1. Percentage of improved patients for each subgroup of patients with certain clinical characteristics

Subgroups	n	Predictive value		
		♂♀ (%)	♂ (%)	♀ (%)
Complete clinical triad	18	72	74	55
Mental slowness and loss of initiative	28	68	70	56
Third ventricle dilatation and absence of peripheral atrophy	15	80	91	67
Absence of peripheral atrophy	22	77	85	67
Temporal horn dilatation and absence of peripheral atrophy	21	76	80	67
Complete clinical triad and temporal horn and third ventricle dilatation and absence of peripheral atrophy	6	83	100	75
Male	43		65	
Female	23			48
Duration of symptoms <3 months	10	80	100	33

– the existence of a subgroup of patients with NPH who do not improve after shunting because of irreversible brain damage which subgroup, as yet, can not be identified.

Various clinical and radiological (CT scan) criteria are more useful in the diagnosis of NPH. The reason why men do better than women is unclear. Maybe NPH is in some way related to typically male-related diseases like hypertension and atherosclerosis.

Acknowledgements. We would like to thank Dr. A. Hoes and Dr. F.R. Rosendaal, clinical epidemiologists, for their help in preparing this manuscript.

References

1. Avezaat CJJ, van Eijndhoven JHM, Wyper DJ (1979) Cerebrospinal fluid pulse pressure and intracranial volume-pressure relationships. J Neurol Neurosurg Psychiat 42:687–700
2. Børgesen SE, Gjerris F (1982) The predictive value of conductance to outflow of cerebrospinal fluid in normal pressure hydrocephalus. Brain 105:65–86
3. Delwel EJ, de Jong DA, Avezaat CJJ, van Eijndhoven JHM, Korbee A (1989) CSF Dynamics in patients with suspected normal pressure hydrocephalus. In: Hoff JT, Betz AL (eds) Intracranial pressure VII. Springer, Berlin Heidelberg New York London Paris Tokyo Hong Kong, pp. 379–382
4. Hakim S, Adams RD (1965) The special clinical problem of symptomatic hydrocephalus with normal cerebrospinal fluid pressure. J Neurol Sci 2:307–327
5. Petersen RC, Mokri B, Laws ER Jr (1985) Surgical treatment of idiopathic hydrocephalus in elderly patients. Neurology 35:307–311
6. Vanneste JA (1991) Normal Pressure Hydrocephalus. Thesis, Radopi Press, Amsterdam

A Ventricular Infusion Technique for the Evaluation of Treated and Untreated Hydrocephalus

M.K. Morgan, I.H. Johnston, and P.J. Spittaler

Department of Surgery D06, The University of Sydney, Australia 2006

Introduction

In 1970 Katzmann and Hussey reported a CSF infusion study that allowed the evaluation of resistance to CSF flow in humans [5]. As many disorders of the CSF circulation involve abnormalities of resistance to CSF flow, this technique is of importance and has been found reliable [1]. However, in its original application by the lumbar route there is a limitation in utility because the abnormality in resistance may be within the ventricular system. The technique described in this study allows the repeated assessment of resistance to the flow of CSF from the ventricular system by performing the test through a permanently implanted subcutaneous Rickham reservoir in which the connected catheter has been placed in the lateral ventricle.

The aim of the study was to compare the reliability of the resistance to infusion with baseline ICP in the differentiation of the health of the CSF circulation.

Method

Patients considered for the study were prospectively and independently allocated into one of 6 categories utilizing clinical and CT scan guidelines. These were: "low probability of CSF circulation disorder" (LPCSF); "high probability of CSF circulation disorder" (HPCSF); indeterminate probability of CSF circulation disorder; "low probability of shunt malfunction" (LPSM); "high probability of shunt malfunction" (HPSM); and indeterminate probability of shunt malfunction. The clinical guidelines were based on a broad based grading system of clinical grade 1, in which there were no symptoms or signs suggesting raised ICP, clinical grade 3, clear cut signs and symptoms of raised ICP (e.g. abnormal increasing head circumference, headaches with altered level of consciousness), and clinical grade 2, in which symptoms and signs may be consistent with raised ICP but were not diagnostic. The CT scan classification was also graded according to broad based categories. These were: CT grade 1, normal ventricles; CT grade 3, uniformly dilated lateral ventricles; and CT grade 2, enlargement of a CSF space without their being uniform dilation of the lateral ventricles.

Patients were prospectively categorized prior to CSF infusion studies except where surgical exploration of shunts was performed immediately after the study allowing for operative assessment of shunt function. For patients with CSF shunts in-situ (Hakim and Orbis-Sigma shunts studied) a clinical grade of 1 was allocated to the LPSM group and a clinical grade of 3 was allocated to the HPSM group. For patients without shunts all patients in clinical grade 3 were considered to have a HPCSF as were patients with a CT grade 3 and a clinical grade 2. In patients with a normal CT scan a clinical grade 2 resulted in allocation to LPCSF and patients with a CT scan grade less than 3 and a clinical grade of 1 were also allocated to the LPCSF group. All other combinations were considered indeterminate and were not included in the study.

For the purposes of analysing the comparisons between the resistance to CSF flow and baseline ICP only 4 categories of patients were chosen. These are LPCSF ($n = 14$), HPCSF ($n = 10$), LPSM ($n = 14$) and HPSM ($n = 9$).

All patients in the study had a ventricular catheter inserted into a frontal horn of a lateral ventricle to which was connected a Rickham reservoir secured in a subgaleal location. In patients with shunts these two systems were independent. Postoperative CT scan was performed to confirm accurate location of the ventricular catheter.

The infusion study was carried out by placing 2 × 25G needles through the aseptically prepared skin into the Rickham reservoir of the conscious patient in a supine position. A transducer was connected to one needle and an infusion pump containing normal saline was connected to the other. A stable baseline ICP was obtained for 10 minutes after which constant ventricular infusion was commenced at 1 ml min^{-1}. The infusion was continued until a plateau in ICP was observed, neurological symptoms suggesting raised ICP occurred or ICP exceeded 40 mmHg. A Resistance Index was calculated by subtracting the baseline ICP from the plateau ICP (given as mmHg ml^{-1} min^{-1}) to allow for comparison with other studies.

Descriptive statistics for age, baseline ICP and resistance are given as mean ± standard deviation. Analysis of variance was applied to baseline ICP and the resistance index and group comparisons were made by Student's T-test with a Bonferroni correction for multiple comparisons. A $p < 0.05$ was considered significant.

Results

Forty-seven infusion studies were included in this evaluation. There were 14 in the LPCSF group, 10 in the HPCSF group, 14 in the LPSM group and 9 in the HPSM group. The baseline ICP for patients in the LPCSF group was 4.9 ± 4.2 mmHg, in the HPCSF group 8.4 ± 5.7 mmHg, LPSM group 1.9 ± 2.8 mmHg and in the HPSM group 15.2 ± 8.3 mmHg. Analysis of variance demonstrated a significant difference amongst the four groups ($p < 0.0001$) and Student's T-test (with Bonferroni correction) demonstrated a significant difference between LPSM and HPSM groups ($p < 0.01$). There was no significant difference in baseline ICP between the LPCSF and HPCSF groups.

The Resistance Index for the LPCSF group was 7.4 ± 2.5 mmHg ml^{-1} min^{-1} (highest reading 11 mmHg ml^{-1} min^{-1}) for the HPCSF group was 27.0 ± 8.6 mmHg ml^{-1} min^{-1} (lowest reading 16 mmHg ml^{-1} min^{-1}), for the LPSM group was 9.1 ± 6.1 mmHg ml^{-1} min^{-1} and for the HPSM group was 28.9 ± 8.7 mmHg ml^{-1} min^{-1} (lowest reading 13 mmHg ml^{-1} min^{-1}). In patients with Orbis-Sigma shunts who were grouped in the LPSM there was a tendency for the resistance to be higher. These shunts accounted for all 3 resistance index readings of greater than 12 mmHg ml^{-1} min^{-1} in this group of patients. Analysis of variance for these 4 groups demonstrated a significant difference in the resistance index ($p < 0.0001$) and Student's T-test (with Bonferroni correction) found a significant difference ($p < 0.01$) existed between the LPCSF group and the HPCSF group, the LPCSF group and the HPSM group and between the LPSM group and the HPSM group.

Discussion

The suggested normal resistance index in this study is less than 12 mmHg ml^{-1} min^{-1}. This is similar to that found by other investigators [1–4, 6, 7]. The results support the postulate that resistance in CSF absorption may be increased in hydrocephalus or in patients with blocked shunts. The functioning Orbis-Sigma shunts have a high resistance index presumably on the basis of their variable resistance function and therefore they are not assessable by this method. The conclusion drawn from these results is that the resistance index, as calculated by this methodology, is a more accurate method of assessing the health of the CSF circulation than baseline ICP.

References

1. Albeck MO, Børgesen SE, Gjerris F, Schmidt JF, Sørensen PS (1991) Intracranial pressure and cerebrospinal fluid outflow conductance in healthy subjects. J Neurosurg 74:597–600
2. Cutler RWP, Page L, Galicich J, Watters GV (1968) Formation and absorption of cerebrospinal fluid in man. Brain 91:707–720
3. Ekstedt J (1978) CSF hydrodynamic studies in man: 2.Normal hydrodynamic variables related to CSF pressure and flow. J Neurol Neurosurg Psychiatry 41:345–353
4. Janny P, Chazel J, Colnet G, Irthum B, Georget A-M (1980) Benign intracranial hypertension and disorders of CSF absorption. Surg Neurol 15:168–174
5. Katzmann R, Hussey F (1970) A simple constant infusion manometric test for measurement of CSF absorption. I. Rationale and method. Neurology 20:534–544
6. Philippon J, George B, Levante A, Thurel C, Visot A, Cophignon J (1976) Subarachnoid infusion test. Its value in the prognosis of shunted normal pressure hydrocephalus. In: Beks JWF, Bosch DA, Brock M (eds) Intracranial pressure III. Springer, Berlin Heidelberg New York, pp. 193–198
7. Sklar FH, Beyer CW, Ramanathan M, Cooper PR, Clark WK (1979) Cerebrospinal fluid dynamics in patients with pseudotumour cerebri. Neurosurgery 5:208–216

Quantitative Analysis of different Curves of Lumbar Repetitive Bolus Infusion Test in Patients with Ventriculomegaly

J. EELMÄE, M. KUKLANE, A. TIKK, and T. ASSER

Department of Neurology and Neurosurgery, 2 L. Puusepp Street, 202400, Tartu, Estonia

Introduction

Dilated cerebrospinal fluid (CSF) spaces can be found by computed tomography (CT), sonography and magnetic resonance imaging. The pathogenesis of ventriculomegaly should be defined in each patient in order to select the best treatment method. Patients with hydrocephalus due to atrophy can not improve after a shunting procedure.

Patients with ventriculomegaly caused by a disturbance of CSF circulation usually improve after restoration of the circulation. The result of a shunting procedure depends on the right time and indications of the operation. Of particular interest is the type of hydrocephalus in which the ventricular system is increasing without increase of ICP [1]. In the last 10–20 years many investigations have been published on successful shunting of patients with primary atrophic genesis of hydrocephalus. It is presumed that among these patients there were cases with concealed disturbance of CSF circulation [4, 5, 6].

For a successful treatment of hydrocephalus a complete investigation of both the CSF volume and the pressure-volume response compensation mechanisms in the craniospinal system must be performed by the measurement of the size of the ventricular system and by the quantitative analysis of CSF dynamics [3, 7, 8, 9].

Material and Method

This prospective study was carried out on 184 patients with various conditions. CT studies were performed on the "Delta-Scan-190" (Ohio Nuclears, USA), thickness of slices being 10 mm. To achieve maximum objectiveness a modified Evans' index (EI) was used in the evaluation of ventricular size. The patients were divided into four groups: hydrocephalus, EI > 0.3; encephalopathy, EI $= 0.2$–0.3; normal size ventricles, EI $= 0.1$–0.2 and brain edema, EI $<$ 0.1 [2].

The investigation of CSF dynamics by the repeated bolus injection technique was performed in the following way. After insertion of the spinal needle into the lumbar subarachnoid space the CSF pressure was measured

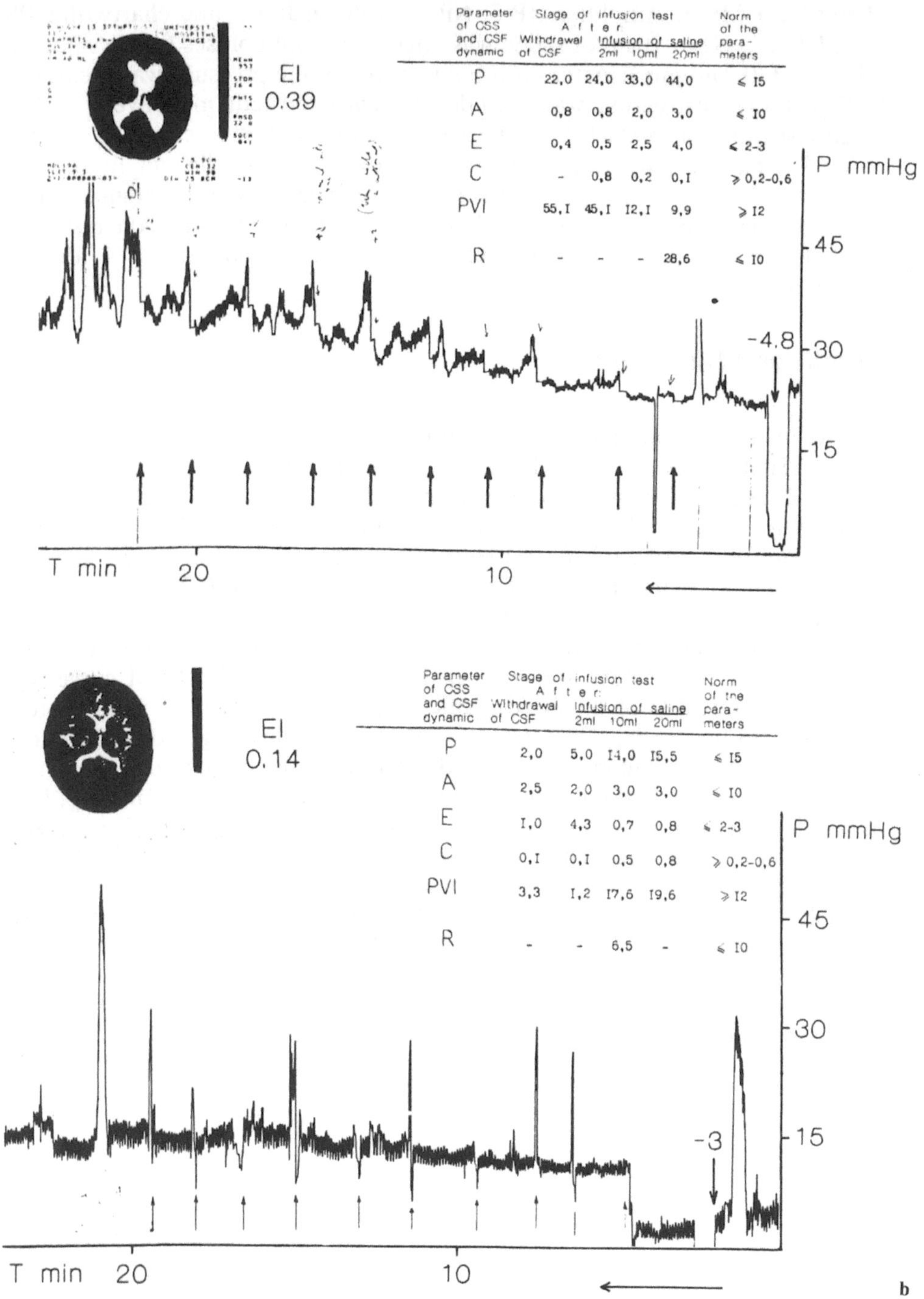

Parameter of CSS and CSF dynamic	Stage of infusion test After: Withdrawal of CSF	Infusion of saline 2ml	10ml	20ml	Norm of the parameters
P	22,0	24,0	33,0	44,0	≤ 15
A	0,8	0,8	2,0	3,0	≤ 10
E	0,4	0,5	2,5	4,0	≤ 2-3
C	-	0,8	0,2	0,1	≥ 0,2-0,6
PVI	55,1	45,1	12,1	9,9	≥ 12
R	-	-	-	28,6	≤ 10

Parameter of CSS and CSF dynamic	Stage of infusion test After: Withdrawal of CSF	Infusion of saline 2ml	10ml	20ml	Norm of the parameters
P	2,0	5,0	14,0	15,5	≤ 15
A	2,5	2,0	3,0	3,0	≤ 10
E	1,0	4,3	0,7	0,8	≤ 2-3
C	0,1	0,1	0,5	0,8	≥ 0,2-0,6
PVI	3,3	1,2	17,6	19,6	≥ 12
R	-	-	6,5	-	≤ 10

Fig. 1. a Preoperative, hypertensive type of pressure curve during infusion test and parameters of CSF dynamics in 39 years old patient with communicating hydrocephalus of unknown etiology. Evans' index 0.39. **b** Normal type of pressure curve during infusion test and parameters of CSF dynamics after shunting procedure in the same patient

(Transducer MP-4, Amplifier RP-3, Nihon-Kohden-Japan and chartwriter PS-1-02, USSR). Next, 20 ml of saline was injected in 2 ml boluses (mean injection rate: 1.7 ± 0.2 ml/min). After each bolus injection the pressure was measured. CSF pathway obstruction was excluded by Queckenstedt maneuver [2]. The mean test time was 24.0 ± 5.9 min. From the thus obtained curves a complex of CSF dynamics parameters was calculated: ICP, pulsatile amplitude (A), elastance (E), compliance (C), pressure-volume index (PVI), resistance to CSF absorption (R) and Ayala index (AI). The results of the infusion test were divided into five types: 1. atrophic, 2. normal, 3. compensated, 4. decompensated and 5. hypertensive [2].

Results and Discussion

The following normal values of the parameters of CSF dynamics were found: ICP < 15 mmHg, A < 10 mmHg, E = 2–3 mmHg/ml, C = 0.2–0.3 ml/mmHg, PVI > 12 ml, R < 10 mmHg/ml/min and AI > 2,3 mmHg. These data correspond to values published by other authors [7, 8, 9]. The preoperative parameters of a 34 years old patient with communicating hydrocephalus of unknown etiology are shown in Fig. 1a. He had an EI of 0.39, and a hypertensive type of infusion test. His ICP, E and R values were elevated, but PVI and C values were lower than normal. The postoperative infusion test and CSF dynamics parameters are given in Fig. 1b. A normal type of curve was found and the values of the visco-elastic properties of the craniospinal system were also normal. In Fig. 2a a correct indication for shunting is demonstrated. The curve was decompensated and CSF dynamics parameters had abnormal values after the last 2 ml bolus injection: ICP = 51 mmHg; A = 12 mmHg; E = 5.5 mmHg/ml; R = 25.5 mmHg/ml/min; C = 0.1 ml/mmHg, and PVI = 8.2 ml. After shunting the headache and gait disturbance disappeared and the EI decreased from 0.36 to 0.28. The compensated curve (Fig. 2b) of a patient with mental disorders and large ventricles on PEG did not justify shunting since five minutes after the last bolus injection ICP had decreased to normal values (16 mmHg).

In conclusion, by the infusion test we could exactly characterize the visco-elastic condition of the craniospinal compartment. The indications for shunting can be based on the type of the infusion test and the parameters of CSF dynamics.

Fig. 2. a Preoperative, decompensated type of pressure curve during infusion test and parameters of CSF dynamics in normal pressure hydrocephalus patient. Evans' index before and after operation was 0.36 and 0.28 respectively. **b** Compensated type of pressure curve during infusion test and parameters of CSF dynamics in a patient with mental disorders. Evans' index 0.34

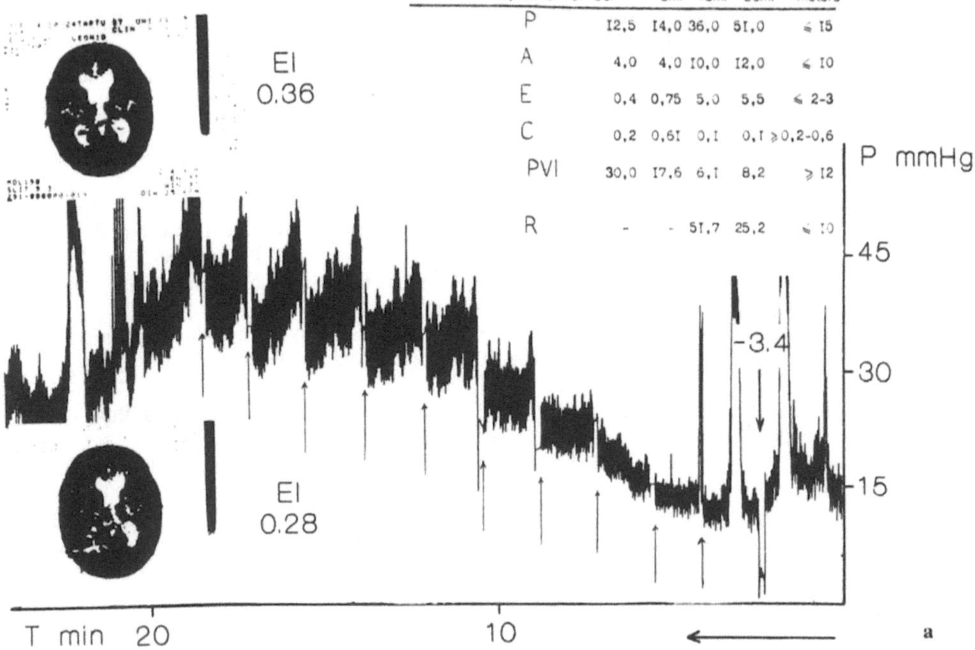

Parameter of CSS and CSF dynamic	Stage of infusion test After: Withdrawal of CSF	Infusion of saline 2ml	10ml	20ml	Norm of the parameters
P	I2,5	I4,0	36,0	5I,0	≤ I5
A	4,0	4,0	I0,0	I2,0	≤ I0
E	0,4	0,75	5,0	5,5	≤ 2-3
C	0,2	0,6I	0,I	0,I	≥ 0,2-0,6
PVI	30,0	I7,6	6,I	8,2	≥ I2
R	-	-	5I,7	25,2	≤ I0

a

Parameter of CSS and CSF dynamic	Stage of infusion test After: Withdrawal of CSF	Infusion of saline 2ml	10ml	20ml	Norm of the parameters
P	8,5	I0,0	I9,0	36,0	≤ I5
A	0,8	0,8	I,5	4,0	≤ I0
E	0,9	0,8	I,8	4,0	≤ 2-3
C	0,I	0,5	0,2	0,I	≥ 0,2-0,6
PVI	I0,9	I2,3	9,8	7,8	≥ I2
R	-	4,5	-	26,3	≤ I0

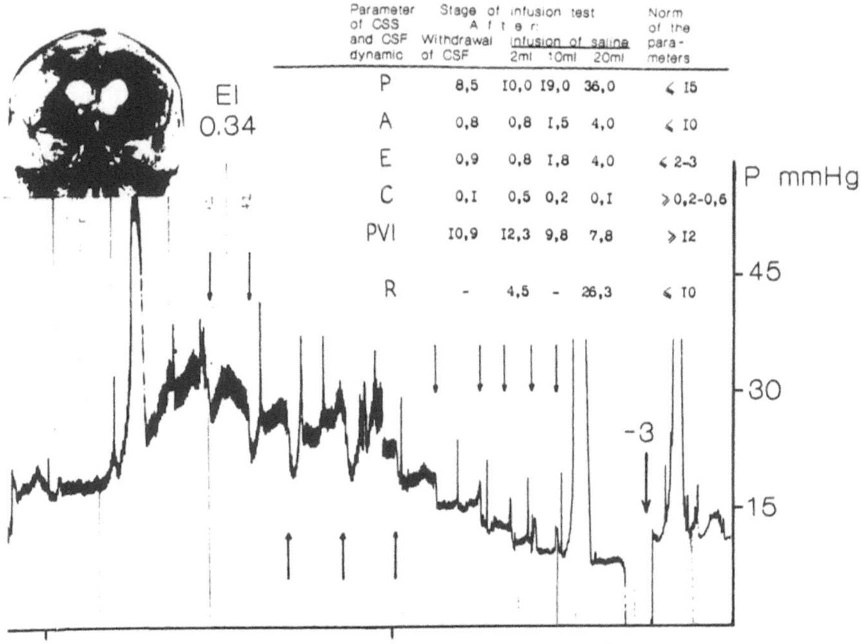

b

References

1. Arnold H, Laas R (1983) Extracellularraum und Liquorreabsorbtion. In: H. von Voght, Hydrocephalus im frühen Kindersalter. Stuttgart, pp 46–48
2. Eelmäe J (1988) Diagnostika izmenenii likvorodinamiki i vjazkouprugih svoistv mozga s ispolzovaniem nagruzocnogo testa bolusnoi techniki u bolnoh s gidrocefaliei raznogo geneza, Tartu pp 1–16
3. Ekstedt J (1977) CSF hydrodynamic studies in man: Method of constant pressure infusion. J Neurol Neurosurg Psychiat 41:105–119
4. Fox J, McCollough D, Green R (1973) Effects of cerebrospinal fluid shunts on intracranial pressure and cerebrospinal fluid dynamics. 2: A new technique of pressure measurement: Result and conception. 3. A concept of hydrocephalus. J Neurol Neurosurg Psychiat 36:211–216
5. Gado M, Patel J, Hughes C, Danziger W, Berg L (1983) Brain atrophy in dementia judged by CT scan ranking. Am J Neurol Radiol 4:699–702
6. Guidetti B, Galiardi F (1980) Dementia due to normal pressure hydrocephalus. In: Barbagallo-Songiorgi G, Exton-Smith AN, Aging brain: Neurological and mental disturbances. New York, pp 161–177
7. Marmarou A, Shulman K, Rosende R (1978) A nonlinear analysis of cerebrospinal fluid system and intracranial pressure dynamics. J Neurosurg 48:332–344
8. Sainte-Rose C, Hooven M, Hirsch J (1987) A new approach in treatment of hydrocephalus. J Neurosurg 66:213–226
9. Tans J, Poortvliet D (1985) CSF outflow resistance and pressure-volume index determined by steady-state and bolus infusion. Clin Neurol Neurosurg 87:159–165

Post-Shunting Improvement in Hydrocephalic Patients Described by Cerebrospinal Compensatory Parameters

W. Maksymowicz[1], M. Czosnyka[2], W. Koszewski[1], O. Szymanska[1], and W. Zabolotny[2]

[1] Neurosurgery Clinic-Medical Academy, [2] Warsaw University of Technology, Warsaw, Poland

Introduction

Many authors have studied the problem of predictive factors with regard to the post-shunting improvement in communicating hydrocephalus. There is still no agreement on the validity of such factors as the ventricular enlargement ratio seen on CT, clinical symptoms and parameters of the cerebrospinal volume compensation [1, 4]. This problem seems to be really important with respect to establishing the proper diagnostic protocol in hydrocephalus. There are many protocols, used in different centers, which seems to contrast with the current state of knowledge about this entity.

This work is aimed at a comparison between the predictive value of CT scan and pressure-volume study results in a group of hydrocephalic patients.

Material

The study was carried out in 21 patients with communicating hydrocephalus. The group consisted of 9 males and 12 females, aged from 20 to 70 years. The etiological factors are distributed as follows:

5 post SAH cases, 1 case of hydrocephalus after CNS infection, 2 after head injury, and 13 cases of unknown etiology. All the patients exhibited the symptoms of progressive dementia and 12 patients showed all the symptoms of the Hakim's triad. The remaining 8 had only the gait control disturbances (besides the dementia).

Method

The ventricular dilatation was estimated using CT. Ventriculo-cerebral bifrontal (BF) and bicaudal (BC) indices were calculated before and after shunting. For the purpose of further statistical analysis, the arithmetical mean of the BF and BC indices was calculated.

In each case a pressure-volume study using the computerized lumbar infusion test [3] was performed. The test was repeated for control purposes after shunting – later than 5 months after operation. The following compensatory factors were compared before and after shunting: resistance to CSF outflow, resting ICP level, cerebrospinal elasticity, and estimation of CSF formation rate [3]. The state after operation was assessed clinically on control examination and the following grading of post-shunting improvement was introduced: no improvement – 0, improvement observed only in psychological tests but not in behavioral functions – 1, improvement with slight influence on behavioral functions-2, and full recovery-3.

Results

Improvement in clinical status was observed in 16 patients. The entire group was subdivided into pairs of groups, taking into account the following factors:

- Subdivision no 1: division was made with respect to large (when (BF + BC)/2 < 40%) and smaller ventricles (BF + BC)/2 < 40%.
- Subdivision no 2: high resistance to CSF outflow (RCSF > 12 mmHg/ml/min) versus patients with the lower resistance (RCSF < 12 mmHg/ml/min),
- Subdivision no 3: high cerebrospinal elasticity (E > 0.2 l/ml) versus lower elasticity (E < 0.2 l/ml),
- Subdivision no 4: increased CSF production (I > 0.3 ml/min) and lower CSF production (I < 0.3 ml/min).
- Subdivision no 5: higher ICP level (ICP > 10 mmHg) versus cases with lower ICP level (ICP < 10 mmHg)

In each subdivision the mean values of the improvement coefficient were compared between both groups, using the Student T-test. The results of this comparison are shown in Table I. Additionally, in the subdivision no 2, the ventricular size ratio and the cerebrospinal compensatory parameters were compared before and after shunting. (The results are shown in Table 2.)

Table 1. Difference in the improvement coefficient between subdivisions made on the basis of the "lower" and "higher" values of the studied parameters

Subdivision made with respect to:	Improvement coeff. for lower values of parameter	Improvement coeff. for higher values of parameter	Significance level of difference in means
Resistance to CSF outflow	1.25	2.11	$p < 0.001$ signific.
(BF + BC)/2 ventricular size	1.53	1.75	$p < 0.35$ non. sign.
Formation rate of CSF	1.69	1.5	$p < 0.36$ non. sign.
Elasticity	1.46	1.87	$p < 0.18$ slightly significant
ICP resting level	1.6	1.8	$p < 0.35$ non. sign.

Table 2. Compensatory and CT parameters compared before and after shunting in two groups formed with respect to "low" and "high" resistance to CSF outflow

	Before	After	Statistical difference
RCSF > 12 mmHg/ml/min			
(BF + BC)/2	48%	38%	significant, $p < 0.05$
ICP resting [mmHg]	7.36	7.93	non signif.
RCSF [mmHg/ml/min]	17.8	7.8	signif., $p < 0.005$
Formation rate [ml/min]	0.22	0.62	signif., $p < 0.05$
Elasticity [l/ml]	0.23	0.19	slight signif. $p < 0.16$
RCSF < 12 mmHg/ml/min			
(BF + BC)/2	39%	31%	signif., $p < 0.01$
ICP resting	7.8	7.4	non signif.
RCSF	8.40	7.40	non signif.
Formation rate	0.49	0.54	non signif.
Elasticity	0.33	0.16	slightly signif. $p < 0.2$

Discussion

The only statistically significant difference between the improvement coefficients of two subgroups was found in the subdivision made on the basis of the criterion of the lower and higher resistance to CSF outflow. This suggests, that among the parameters considered, only the resistance to CSF outflow has a really predictive value with regard to post-shunting improvement. The improvement is independent of the ventricular enlargement seen before shunting. This means that the pressure-volume study, made in order to measure the resistance to CSF outflow, is the examination which cannot be substituted by CT scan. The remaining compensatory parameters have rather poor predictive values. The only exception seems to be the cerebrospinal elasticity having considerable, but not significant, probability level.

The comparison of compensatory and CT parameters, seen before and after shunting in the subgroup of high RCSF (>12 mmHg/ml/min), enables better interpretation of the mechanisms of improvement in compensatory ability: First of all, the shunt radically reduces the increased resistance to CSF outflow. It also reduces the elasticity and the size of the ventricles. The increased CSF production, seen after shunting in this group, may support the hypothesis that a lower CSF formation rate is due to a reduction in the cerebrospinal compensatory reserve [2].

In the subgroup with normal RCSF level (<12 mmHg/ml/min), only the ventricular reduction after shunting is significant.

If we take into account that clinical improvement is poorly correlated with the reduction of ventricular size, we should conclude that the decrease in the BF and BC indices is the general response to shunting and doesn't have predictive value.

Acknowledgements. Authors of all the papers prepared by the "Warsaw Group" wish to express their feeling of gratitude to Mr. Lee Moore for his linguistic corrections.

References

1. Børgesen SE, Gjernis F, Fedders O, Schmidt JF, Albeck MJ, Soelberg-Sørensen P (1989) Measurement of resistance to CSF outflow – Clinical experience in 333 cases. In: Hoff JT, Betz AL (eds) Intracranial pressure VII. Springer, Berlin Heidelberg New York London Paris Tokyo Hong Kong, 353–359
2. Børgesen SE, Gjernis F (1989) CSF production in patients with increased ICP. In: Hoff JT, Betz AL (eds) Intracranial pressure VII. Springer, Berlin Heidelberg New York London Paris Tokyo Hong Kong, 332–335
3. Czosnyka M, Batorski L, Laniewski P, Maksymowicz, Koszewski W, Zaworski W (1990) A computer system for the identification of the cerebrospinal compensatory model. Acta Neurochirurgica, 105:112–116
4. Kosteljanetz M, Westergaard L, Kaalund J, Neben AM (1989) The significance of outflow resistance measurements in the prediction of outcome after CSF-shunting in patients with NPH. In: Hoff JT, Betz AL (eds) Intracranial pressure VII. Springer, Berlin Heidelberg New York London Paris Tokyo Hong Kong, 383–385
5. Maksymowicz W, Czosnyka M, Koszewski W, Szymanska A, Traczewski W (1989) The role of cerebrospinal compensatory parameters in estimation of functioning of implanted shunt system in patients with communicating hydrocephalus. Acta Neurochirurgica 101:112–116

Diagnostic and Predictive Value of Axial and Coronal Spect with Technetium-99m Labelled D,L-Hexamethyl-Propylene Amine Oxime (^{99m}TC HM-PAO) in Patients with Normal Pressure Hydrocephalus Syndrome (NPH)

E.J. Delwel[1], D. Hasan[2], D.A. de Jong[1], E.P. Krenning[3], and C.J.J. Avezaat[1]

[1] Departments of Neurosurgery, [2] Neurology and [3] Nuclear Medicine, University Hospital Rotterdam, Rotterdam, The Netherlands

Introduction

The value of SPECT in dementia has been stressed by several authors [3, 5, 7]. Recently, several papers concerning SPECT in normal pressure hydrocephalus have been published [1, 4, 6]. Until now, a typical rCBF disturbance, as described in Alzheimers dementia, has not yet been identified.

Hasan et al. [2] described a typical pattern of rCBF impairment in the basal parts of the brain by means of SPECT using ^{99m}Tc HM-PAO in patients with acute hydrocephalus following subarachnoid hemorrhage.

Aim

It was investigated whether a typical distribution of rCBF disturbance exists in patients who are suspected of having a normal pressure hydrocephalus. In this respect, special attention was paid to the coronal slices aiming to visualize rCBF disturbances in the basal parts of the brain.

Patients and Methods

Fourteen patients (mean age 69 years) with clinical signs and CT findings of normal pressure hydrocephalus were studied. Ventriculo-peritoneal shunting was performed in twelve patients, who met the following criteria for shunting (Scheme 1).

The two remaining patients had a Rout <8 mmHg/ml/min but were nevertheless shunted because of strong clinical and CT evidence of normal pressure hydrocephalus.

SPECT scanning was performed in all patients before or at least 5 days after the lumbar infusion test and before operation and in four of these patients

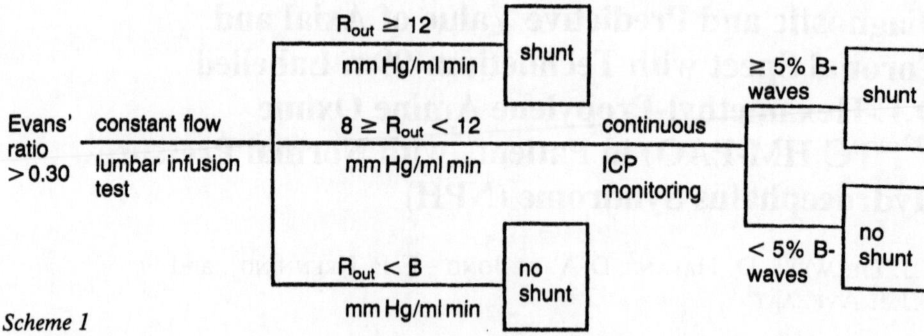

Scheme 1

Table 1A,B. Summary of clinical parameters, rCBF pattern on SPECT, CSF outflow resistance and CT parameters

Patient	Age	Sex	Basal rCBF disturbance on SPECT	Basal rCBF disturbance on postoperative SPECT	Improvement	R_{out} (mmHg/ml/min)	Incontinence
1	65	F	no		no	19.8	yes
2	80	M	yes		no	14.3	yes
3	66	F	no		no	10.2	yes
4	45	F	no		no	21.0	no
5	67	M	yes		yes	25.0	yes
6	74	M	no	diminished	yes	15.6	yes
7	69	F	yes		no	20.0	yes
8	74	M	yes		yes	17.5	yes
9	75	F	yes	diminished	yes	16.1	yes
10	61	F	yes		yes	20.4	yes
11	79	M	yes		yes	12.0	yes
12	69	F	no		no	8.3	yes
13	67	F	yes	diminished	yes	4.9	yes
14	74	F	yes	diminished	yes	7.2	yes

Patient	Temporal horn dilatation	Third ventricle dilatation	Peripheral atrophy	Mental slowness	Loss of initiative	Slowness of gait	Magnet effect
1	no	no	yes	yes	yes	yes	yes
2	yes	no	yes	yes	yes	yes	no
3	no	no	no	no	yes	yes	no
4	yes	yes	no	no	no	yes	no
5	no	no	yes	yes	no	no	no
6	no	yes	yes	no	yes	yes	yes
7	yes	yes	yes	no	no	yes	no
8	yes	yes	no	no	yes	yes	no
9	yes	yes	yes	no	yes	yes	yes
10	no	no	no	yes	no	yes	yes
11	yes	no	yes	yes	yes	yes	yes
12	yes	yes	yes	no	no	yes	no
13	yes	yes	no	no	yes	yes	no
14	yes	yes	no	yes	yes	yes	yes

SPECT scanning was repeated after shunting. SPECT scanning produced 15 serial axial slices and 15 serial coronal slices. Repeat CT scanning was performed and the clinical follow-up period was at least 6 months. If drain dysfunction was suspected, the lumbar infusion test was repeated. Drain revision was indicated when R_{out} was not significantly lower than the preshunt value.

Several other clinical and radiological parameters were recorded pre- and postoperatively (Table 1). Postshunting clinical improvement was based on the opinion of the treating neurosurgeon and the opinion of the patient and/or the patient's relatives.

Results

Preoperatively, nine of the 14 patients showed rCBF impairment predominantly in the basal parts of the brain, especially visible on the coronal slices. Eight of these 14 patients improved after shunting, seven patients with basal rCBF impairment and one without basal rCBF impairment (Table 1). Six of the 14 patients who underwent ventricular shunting did not improve, two with basal rCBF impairment and four without basal rCBF impairment. One of these two patients was suspected of drain dysfunction, but this patient refused further investigation.

The distribution of other clinical and CT parameters in relation to the rCBF pattern on SPECT scanning is shown in Table 2.

Clinical improvement and improvement of rCBF was seen in all four patients with a repeat SPECT scanning. Three of these patients had a preoperative rCBF impairment of the basal parts of the brain. As an example, Fig. 1 shows the SPECT studies in one of these patients (no. 14). An improvement of rCBF can be observed on the postoperative, coronal images.

Table 2. Distribution of clinical and CT parameters in relation to the rCBF pattern on SPECT

	SPECT	
	Basal rCBF disturbance (N = 9)	No basal rCBF disturbance (N = 5)
Incontinence	9	4
Temporal horn dilatation	7	2
Third ventricle dilatation	5	3
Peripheral atrophy	5	4
Mental slowness	5	1
Loss of initiative	6	3
Slowness of gait	8	5
Magnet effect	4	2

Before shunting

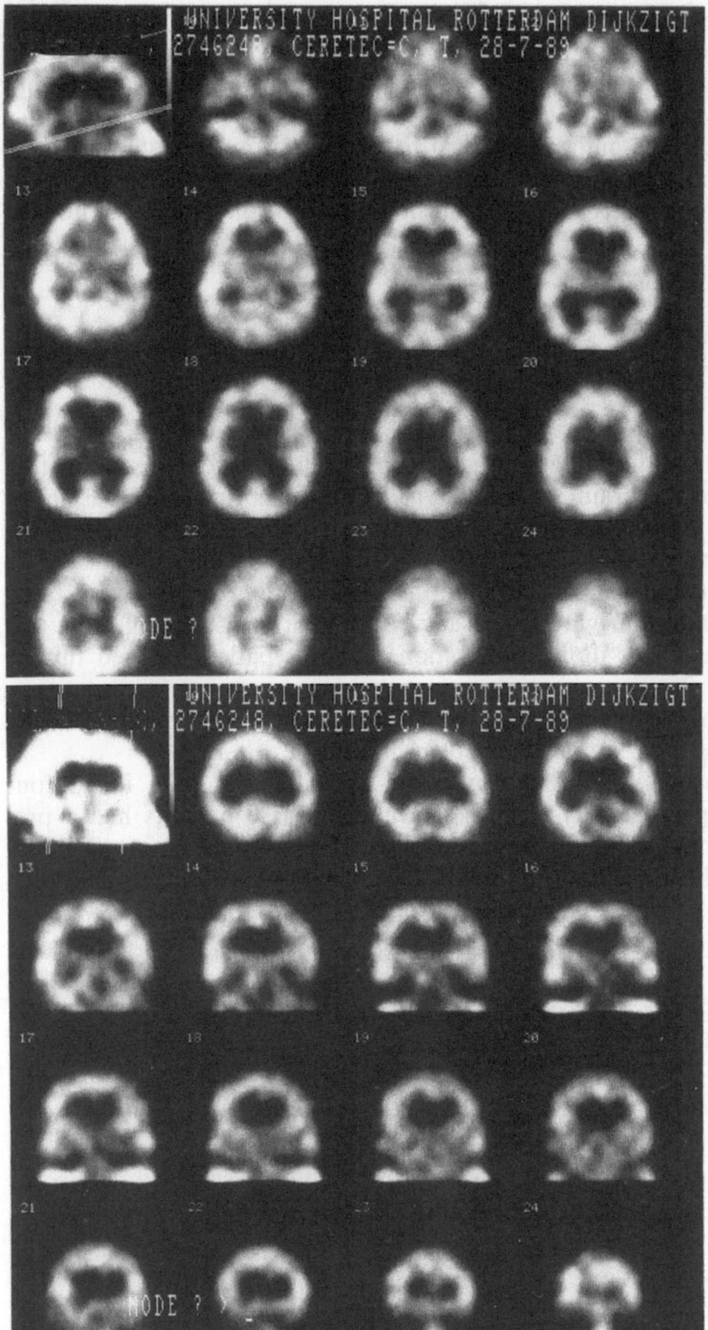

a

b

Fig. 1a–d. SPECT studies in patient no. 14: axial **a+c** and coronal **b+d** slices, before **a+b** and after **c+d** shunt operation. Note improvement of rCBF in the fronto-tempero-basal parts of the brain on the coronal images

After shunting

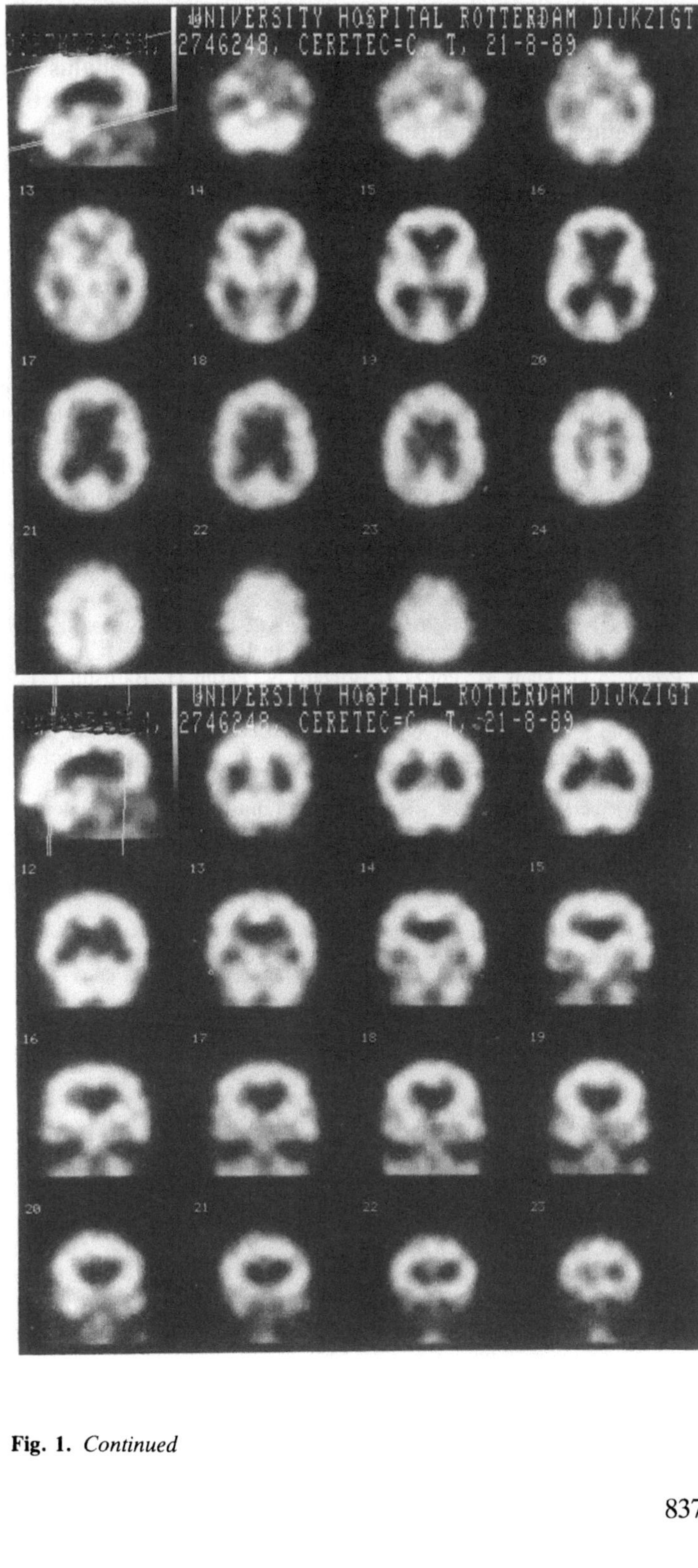

c

d

Fig. 1. *Continued*

Conclusion

With this study, we provide preliminary evidence that SPECT scanning is of value in the diagnosis of normal pressure hydrocephalus, especially the coronal slices. Moreover, SPECT scanning may have a predictive value for clinical improvement after shunting.

A study with a larger number of patients and with quantitative analysis of the changes in rCBF is required to confirm these findings.

References

1. Graff-Radford NR, Rezai K, Goderski JC, Eslinger P, Damasio H, Kirchner P (1987) Regional cerebral blood flow in normal pressure hydrocephalus. J Neurol Neurosurg Psychiatry 50:1589–1596
2. Hasan D, van Peski J, Loeve I, Krenning EP, Vermeulen M (1991) Single photon emission computed tomography in patients with acute hydrocephalus or with cerebral ischemia after subarachnoid hemorrhage. J Neurol Neurosurg Psychiatry, in press
3. Kuhl DE, Koeppe RA, Foster NL, Agranoff BW, Buchtel HA, Mountz JM (1989) Cerebral perfusion, metabolic, and transport relations in Alzheimer's and Parkinsonian dementia. J Cereb Blood Flow Metab 9:S525
4. Mamo HL, Philippe CM, Ponsin JC, Rey AC, Luft AG, Seylaz JA (1987) Cerebral Blood flow in normal pressure hydrocephalus. *Stroke* 18:1074–1080
5. Pizzolato G, Dam M, Ponza I, Borzato N, Ferlin G, Battistin L (1989) SPECT with ^{99m}Tc HM-PAO in the diagnosis and assessment of dementia. *J Cereb Blood Metab* 9:S516
6. Vorstrup S, Christensen J, Gjerris F, Sørensen S, Thomsen AM, Paulson OB (1987) Cerebral blood flow in patients with normal pressure hydrocephalus before and after shunting. J Neurosurg 66:379–387
7. Zilbovicius M, Raynaud C, Rancurel G, Tzourio N, Arzimanaglou A, Leder S, Bourguignon M, Syrota A (1989) Regional Cerebral Blood Flow measured by SPECT in Pick's disease. J Cereb Blood Flow Metab 9:S521

Hydrocephalus Following Aneurysmal Subarachnoid Hæmorrhage and Requiring Permanent Shunt

L. Sipos, O. Major, M. Horváth, and J. Vajda

National Institute of Neurosurgery, Budapest, Hungary

Introduction

A well known complication of subarachnoid hæmorrhage (SAH) is an altered circulation and absorption of the cerebrospinal fluid (CSF) which may lead to communicating hydrocephalus [1, 2, 5]. The incidence of hydrocephalus after SAH has been reported from 6 to 67% [2, 3]. The aim of our retrospective study was to analyse the various factors which may play a role in the development of hydrocephalus following aneurysmal SAH.

Clinial Material

From 1980 to 1989 1373 patients suffering aneurysmal SAH were operated on in our Institute. Shunt dependent hydrocephalus developed in 37 cases, which was 2.7% of all patients operated on for ruptured aneurysms. At the same time, this figure is 16.2% of all adult hydrocephalus cases who underwent surgery during the same period.

Shunt dependent hydrocephalus is more frequent among females of the fifth decade of age but this is also the age group most represented among cases harbouring ruptured aneurysms.

The diagnosis of SAH was established either by CT or LP or both.

Thirty-five percent of the patients were alert on admission, 43.2% were somnolent, almost one fifth were in sopor and 2.7% were comatose. Five somnolent patients and 4 in sopor and 1 comatose had two consecutive aneurysmal ruptures.

The grade of hydrocephalus was measured by using the bicaudate index which was calculated as the ratio of the width of the ventricles behind the frontal horns between the caudate nuclei to the width of the brain at the same level on the CT scan [4]. Another grading of the assumed intracranial hypertension was possible by observing periventricular lucency.

Acute hydrocephalus developed in 12 cases out of 37. In these cases the bicaudate index was greater than 0.25 on admission. There were 6 cases with intracerebral hæmatoma, intraventricular bleeding was in four patients and 1 subdural hæmatoma was also detected on CT done on admission.

In 14 cases the aneurysm was clipped within 48 hours, which is almost three percent of all patients operated on in the acute phase. In the remainder 23 cases the surgical repair of the aneurysm was performed later, which group constitutes 2.6% of all patients who underwent late operation.

In 11 cases SAH originated from an aneurysm of the internal carotid artery, in 13 cases from the anterior cerebral artery and its branches, in 4 cases from the middle cerebral artery, while in 9 patients the vertebro-basilar system was the origin of the aneurysms. The last group constitutes 15% of all operated aneurysms localized in the vertebro-basilar system. This differs significantly from the incidence of hydrocephalus in the other aneurysm localizations.

The indication for shunt insertion was based on both clinical and CT signs. Clinically, the development of a psycho-organic syndrome (disorientation, impaired memory, a decrease in mental and physical activity, lack of concentration), spastic gait and urinary incontinence were common. CT criteria were used as mentioned above.

In 2 cases the shunt operation were performed before the aneurysm surgery. In the remaining 35 cases the timing of shunt operation ranged from 14 to 419 days after the last rupture of the aneurysm.

Ventriculo-peritoneal (VP) shunts were inserted in 33 cases, while ventriculo-atrial (VA) shunts in 4 cases. Most of the patients improved after the shunt insertion. Eighty-one percent improved, 16.2% remained unchanged, and 1 patient deteriorated. In three cases late death occurred 6, 7 and 9 months after the aneurysm operation. Two among them suffered 2 SAH-s, were somnolent on admission and had vasospasm after the aneurysm surgery. The 3rd patient had severe intracerebral hæmatoma and was somnolent also.

In 6 cases the shunt system required a revision. In 2 cases out of 4 VA shunts the cardial drain was inserted into the peritoneal cavity.

At the last follow-up – at least two years after the shunt operation – 70% of the 30 patients are without complaints; the others have some restrictions in their everyday activity.

Conclusions

The level of consciousness on admission and the localization of the aneurysm significantly influenced the development of a shunt dependent hydrocephalus.

The greater the amount of blood in the subarachnoid cisterns after the rupture, the more likely it is that the red blood cell mass blocks the CSF circulation. This will raise the ICP which, in turn, may reduce cerebral blood flow and cause metabolic changes in the brain and consequently changes in the level of consciousness.

The least common source of bleeding was an aneurysm of the middle cerebral artery among patients in whom shunt dependent hydrocephalus developed later. On the other hand, among all localisations, shunt requiring hydrocephalus was observed most frequently in patients who underwent posterior fossa surgery for vertebral-PICA aneurysms, possibly due to either posthæmorrhagical or surgical interference with the subarachnoid spaces at the craniocervical junction.

The location of the aneurysm and its position in particular should obviously be significant factors, since those in direct communication with the subarachnoid spaces are most likely to bleed freely into the cisterns evoking greater meningeal reactions. Since these two factors, governing the development of hydrocephalus following an aneurysmal rupture, are equally present in cases of acute and late surgery, we feel that it is not surprising that the timing of the aneurysm operation did not play any role in the incidence of shunt dependent hydrocephalus in our cases.

When a hydrocephalus develops following aneurysmal SAH a VP shunt is the treatment of choice.

References

1. Dóczy T, Nemessányi Z, Szegváry Zs, Huszka E (1983) Disturbances of cerebral fluid circulation during the acute stage of subarachnoid hemorrhage. Neurosurgery 12:435–438
2. Graff-Radford NR, Torner J, Adams HP, Kassell NF (1989) Factors associated with hydrocephalus after subarachnoid hemorrhage. Arch Neurol 46:744–752
3. Hasan D, Vermeulen M, Wijdicks EFM, Hijdra A, van Gijn J (1989) Management problems in acute hydrocephalus after subarachnoid hemorrhage. Stroke 20:747–753
4. van Gijn J, Hijdra A, Wijdicks EFM, Vermeulen M, van Crevel H (1985) Acute hydrocephalus after aneurysmal subarachnoid hemorrhage. J Neurosurg 62:355–362
5. Yasargil MG, Yonekawa Y, Zumstein B, Stahl H-J (1973) Hydrocephalus following spontaneous subarachnoid hemorrhage. J Neurosurg 3:474–479

Idiopathic vs. Post-SAH Normal Pressure Hydrocephalus

O. Hirai, H. Kikuchi, and M. Ishikawa

Department of Neurosurgery, Faculty of Medicine, Kyoto University, 54-Shogoin Kawaharacho, Sakyo-ku, Kyoto 606, Japan

Introduction

Aneurysmal subarachnoid hemorrhage (SAH) is the most frequent cause of the normal pressure hydrocephalus (NPH) syndrome. However, it is suggested that post-SAH NPH differs from idiopathic NPH of unknown etiology in several aspects. The present study aimed at elucidating the characteristics of the two different types of NPH.

Materials and Methods

Twenty patients with idiopathic NPH (INPH) and 24 patients with NPH secondary to SAH (SNPH) were reviewed. In the SNPH group, cases with severe neurological deficits lasting from the ictus were excluded. The degree of ventricular dilatation on CT was evaluated by the bicaudate index. Cisternography (16 cases), continuous CSF pressure monitoring (31 cases), CBF measurement (23 cases) and CSF withdrawal test (14 cases) were employed as diagnostic tests for a CSF shunting operation. The postoperative mean follow-up period was 99 weeks.

Result

The mean age was not significantly different. The preoperative period was significantly longer in INPH. The main initial symptom was gait disturbance in INPH and mental dysfunction in SNPH. The preoperative clinical grade was generally poorer in SNPH. Ventricular dilatation and sulcal enlargement were significantly greater in INPH, while focal low density area on CT was more frequently seen in SNPH.

Continuous CSF pressure monitoring demonstrated that the pressure was elevated in most patients of the SNPH group, whereas only in 10 out of 18 cases in INPH. All cases had some low perfusion area on CBF images; the area dominated the frontal region in SNPH, whereas it was much more extensive in INPH.

Table 1. Comparison of clinical picture, CT findings and physiological data

		Idiopathic	Post-SAH	
No. of Cases		20	24	
Age (mean ± SE)		65.8 ± 1.9	60.9 ± 2.2	NS
Preoperative period (wks)		8–200 (med 39)	3–30 (med 4)	$p < 0.01$
Initial symptom				
gait disturbance		14	1	$p < 0.01$
mental dysfunction		5	22	
sphincter disturbance		1	1	
Ventricular dilatation bicaudate index (%) (mean ± SE)		28.4 ± 1.0	25.5 ± 0.8	$p < 0.05$
Sulcal enlargement	(+)	20	4	
	(−)	0	20	$p < 0.01$
Periventricular low density	(+)	14	14	
	(−)	6	10	NS
Focal low density area	(+)	4	12	
	(−)	16	12	$p < 0.05$
Cisternography	abnormal	11	1	
(n = 16)	normal	4	0	NS
Continuous CSF Pressure	low	8	2	
Monitoring (n = 31)	high	10	11	NS
Low Perfusion	frontal	1	7	
Area on CBF	periventricular	4	1	
Image (n = 23)	whole brain	7	3	$p < 0.02$
CSF Withdrawal	improved	4	7	
Test (n = 14)	unchanged	2	1	NS
Outcome				
Excellent + Good		7	18	
Fair + Poor		13	6	$p < 0.01$

Meaningful improvement following shunt operation was seen in only 7 of 20 cases in INPH, whereas it was noted in 75% of cases in SNPH. Furthermore, 4 patients in INPH deteriorated again several months after the initial improvement, while such recurrence of clinical symptoms was noted in 2 cases in SNPH. In each instance, however, the shunt system was proved to be functioning. Seven patients (INPH: 5, SNPH: 2) were not shunted on the basis of clinical and physiological findings, but subsequent clinical changes were not noted during follow-up period.

As for predictive factors, small or no visible sulci, elevated CSF pressure, and frontal-dominant CBF reduction were good predictors for shunt response with statistical significance.

Discussion

The present study demonstrated that there are distinct differences between both types of NPH. Diagnostic tests are necessary for INPH to predict shunt response, since NPH of unknown etiology is sometimes preceded by degenerative or ischemic parenchymal damage which will not be corrected by CSF diversion [1, 2, 3]. Elevated CSF pressure, and slight reduction of CBF dominating the frontal region are good predictors [2]. However, it should be kept in mind that postoperative improvement is limited.

In contrast, shunt operation should be recommended for most of the cases in NPH secondary to SAH, since clinical symptoms are mainly due to CSF circulatory impairment and resultant ventricular dilatation unless severe brain damage produced by SAH itself or a subsequent ischemic insult has occurred. Intricate diagnostic tests are not required and a typical clinical picture together with positive CT findings are sufficient indications for operation [4].

References

1. Hirai O, Handa H, Kikuchi H, Ishikawa M, Kinuta Y (1988) Continuous lumbar subarachnoid pressure monitoring as an indicator of shunt operation for so-called normal pressure hydrocephalus. Neurol Surg 16:1141–1147 (Tokyo)
2. Hirai O, Nishikawa M, Munaka M, Watanabe S, Kaneko T, Fukuma A, Handa H (1989) 123I-IMP-SPECT and lumbar subarachnoid pressure in adult hydrocephalus. In: Hoff JT, Betz AL (eds) Intracranial Pressure VII. Springer, Berlin Heidelberg New York London Paris Tokyo Hong Kong, pp 425–430
3. Hirai O, Kikuchi H, Ishikawa M (1991) Pathophysiology and surgical treatment of normal pressure hydrocephalus. Neurosurg Lett 1:17–30 (Kyoto)
4. Vassilouthis J, Richardson AE (1979) Ventricular dilatation and communicating hydrocephalus following spontaneous subarachnoid hemorrhage. J Neurosurg 51:341–351

Dynamics of Hydrocephalus Development After Spontaneous Subarachnoid Hemorrhage

W. Maksymowicz[1], M. Czosnyka[2], W. Koszewski[1], and W. Zabolotny[2]

[1] Department of Neurosurgery, Warsaw Medical Academy, and [2] Warsaw University of Technology, Warsaw, Poland

Introduction

In the early stage of the cerebrospinal compensatory disturbances seen after SAH, the ventricular system is not necessarily dilated [5]. ICP, however, is commonly increased immediately after SAH, but often recovers to a low or moderate level during vasospasm. A decrease in the blood flow velocity, which is considered to be a sign of recovery to the normal autoregulatory ability after vasospasm, is usually observed after the 3rd or 4th week [4, 5]. The further development of the high-(HPH) or normal-(NPH) pressure hydrocephalus has still an unknown nature.

While the opinion on the need of shunting in both NPH and HPH is obvious, it is still an open question when the decision on the operative treatment should be made. In some cases, even with dilated ventricles, spontaneous recovery to normal compensatory reserve can be observed (i.e. the shunting is not necessary). On the other hand, waiting too long may cause irreversible and substantial changes to the brain tissue which are very resistive to treatment. An attempt to study the dynamics of the hydrocephalus development after SAH, by estimates of cerebrospinal compensatory parameters, is presented in this work.

Material and Method

Twenty patients who had suffered spontaneous subarachnoid hemorrhage caused by aneurysmal rupture were studied in the Clinic of Neurosurgery at the Warsaw Medical Academy. Apart from a CT examination, a pressure-volume study was carried out in each case. The study was performed between the 3rd and 11th week after SAH. Intracranial pressure and cerebrospinal compensatory mechanisms were estimated by means of the constant rate lumbar infusion test, supported by computerized automatic analysis [1]. Two of the patients died in the posthemorrhagic course. In order to find the difference between the SAH group and all the patients examined because of dilated ventricles on CT, the averaged compensatory parameters after SAH were compared to the results of the examination of the whole group of patients studied in the Clinic. This group consists of 110 cases of adults with ventricular dilatation of miscellaneous etiology.

Results

All patients had a ventricular enlargement as shown on CT scan (ratio calculated as half of bifrontal and bicaudal indices was 36 ± 3.1) and specific periventricular lucency (all but two). Only in 4 cases was high pressure hydrocephalus (with the resting ICP higher than 13 mmHg) confirmed. Only in one case both ICP and resistance to CSF outflow were elevated – which are the symptoms of acute malresorptive hydrocephalus. Averaged results of the lumbar infusion pressure-volume study were summarized, and compared (if they differed significantly) to the whole hydrocephalus group studied (see Table 1). The correlation coefficient between the resistance to CSF outflow and the ICP resting level was low and non-significant ($r = 0.11$).

It differed significantly from the correlation coefficient between the resistance to CSF outflow and the end-equilibrium ICP level reached during the test:

$$RCSF = 0.408 \cdot ICPend + 0.91; \; r = 0.602, \; p < 0.005.$$

The dynamics of compensatory parameters (the resistance to CSF outflow, the pressure-volume index and the time- constant) are shown in Fig. 1a. Time histories of the resting pressure level, pulse wave amplitude and the slope of amplitude – pressure characteristic after SAH are presented in Fig. 1b.

The resting pressure level varied during the posthemorrhagic period from the third to the eleventh week within a range of 0 to 23 mmHg. The variations of the averaged value of ICP range from 8 to 12 mmHg, however, are not significant.

The increase in the pulse wave amplitude from 1.14 ± 0.7 mmHg in the third week to 1.9 ± 2.0 mmHg in the period from 4th to 6th week, was significant. It was correlated with the significant decrease in the slope of the amplitude-pressure characteristic: from 0.2 ± 0.12 in 3rd–4th week to 0.06 ± 0.08 in 5th–6th week.

The increase in the amplitude and the decrease in the amplitude-pressure slope may be formally explained by an increase in the pulsatile blood flow or an increase in the cerebrospinal elasticity (i.e. a decrease in the cerebrospinal

Table 1. Mean values and standard deviations of compensatory parameters after SAH and their comparison with the whole group of hydrocephalic patients studied

	SAH mean	S.dev.	Whole group (n = 110) (if differs significantly for level p < 0.05)
Resting pressure level [mmHg]	9.46	6.23	No difference
Resting pulse wave amplitude [mmHg]	1.57	1.41	No difference
Slope of amplitude-pressure line	0.16	0.10	0.23 ± 0.14
Pulsatile increase in CBV [ml]	0.712	0.31	1.01 ± 0.82
Resistance to CSF outflow [mmHg/ml/min]	19	13	10.1 ± 5
Pressure-volume index [ml]	12.4	11	No difference
Estimator of CSF formation [ml/min]	0.307	0.53	No difference
Cerebrospinal time-constant [min]	16.8	13	No difference

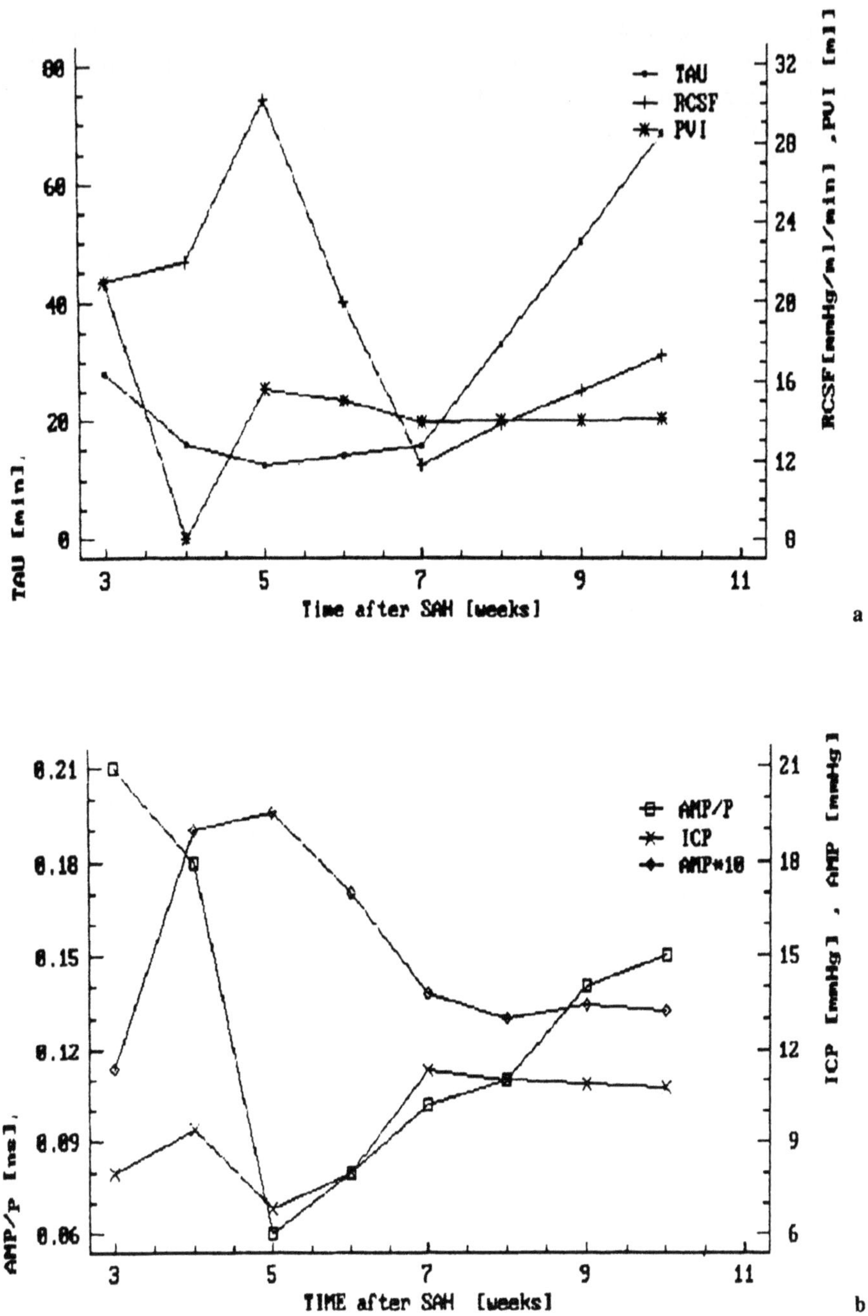

Fig. 1. a Dynamics of cerebrospinal compensatory parameters: cerebrospinal time-contstant (points – left axis), resistance to CSF outflow (crosses-right axis) and pressure volume index (asterisks-right axis) versus weeks after SAH. **b** Dynamics of ICP parameters: slope of amplitude-pressure characteristic (left axis-squares), mean ICP (stars-right axis) and mean pulse wave amplitude (multiplied 10 times – diamonds, right axis) versus weeks after SAH.

volume-compensation reserve). In fact, the decrease in the pressure-volume index could be observed in the fourth week (it decreased significantly, relative to the third week, and then started to increase). This short decrease in PVI preceded the decrease in the resistance to CSF outflow, observed in 6th–7th week (however, in most cases it was still elevated above the critical level of 13 mmHg/ml/min).

The cerebrospinal time constant started to decrease after the 3rd week and a secondary increase could be observed after the seventh week.

The time trend of the ventricular dilatation ratio did not show any significant changes.

Discussion

The dynamics of the changes in the cerebrospinal compliance and the resistance to CSF outflow may be interpreted as a specific course in the development of posthemorrhagic hydrocephalus. In fact, we did not observe any significant elevations in ICP after the third week in the post-SAH period (which seems to be in agreement with [4]).

The resistance to CSF outflow was elevated, which may suggest that the deficit in the CSF resorptive reserve is still remarkable. The low ICP with the high resistance to CSF outflow may support the hypothesis, proposed by Kosteljanetz [3], on the possibility of a reduction of the rate of CSF formation after SAH. Indeed: the low ICP indicates satisfactory volume reserve at this stage; however, the mechanism of CSF outflow is disturbed. There is also a second explanation possible:

The increase in the pulse wave amplitude and the decrease in the pressure-volume index within the period of the fourth–fifth week, may be interpreted as a sign of the recovery to the normal autoregulation ability after the period of cerebrovascular vasospasm (the timing seems to be in agreement with TCD studies, reported in [2, 4]). The recovery to the normal control of the vascular wall tension may provoke the observed increase in the pulse wave amplitude, the temporary decrease in the pressure-volume index (due to an increase in the cerebral blood volume), and a decrease in the slope of the amplitude pressure-characteristic.

The presented material seems to indicate that, the evidence of recovery from the vasospasm stage precedes the decrease in the resistance to the CSF outflow seen between the 5th and 7th week after SAH. It is also remarkable that apart from its significant decrease, the resistance still remains elevated pointing out that in the majority of cases pathological compensation, as we can name the phase of normal pressure hydrocephalus, usually takes place.

These results enable us to frame a hypothesis on the dynamic course in the compensation of post – hemorrhagic hydrocephalus. The increased resistance to CSF outflow, seen from the very beginning after SAH, may not evoke an increase in ICP, if the cerebral blood volume is reduced due to vasospasm or suppression of the CSF formation rate. After the period of the increased resistance to CSF absorption (statistically until the 7th week) it remains elevated or returns to the normal value (no deficit in the compensatory reserve). In this period the decision on shunting should be made. All the cases of NPH, determined on the basis of the pressure-volume study, should be shunted. If the symptoms of increased ICP are observed earlier, shunting or external drainage should be considered.

The presented material supports the hypothesis that cerebral vasospasm should be considered as a factor, which may help in the cerebrospinal volume compensation at an early stage of the posthemorrhagic course. This may mask the results of the examination of the cerebrospinal compensatory reserve. The decision on shunting should be made on the basis of the pressure-volume study 6–7 weeks after SAH. In this period only the resistance to CSF outflow decides on the compensatory reserve.

References

1. Czosnyka M, Maksymowicz W, Koszewski W (1990) A computer system for the identification of the cerebrospinal compensatory model. Acta Nerochirurgica 105:112–116
2. Harders A, Gilsbach (1988) Haemodynamic Effectiveness of Nimodipine on Spastic Brain Vessels after Subarachnoid Haemorrhage Evaluated by the Transcranial Doppler Method. A review of Clinical Studies. Acta Neurochirurgica, Suppl 45:21–28
3. Kosteljanetz M (1988) Cerebrospinal Fluid Production in Subarachnoid Hemorrhage. British Journal of Neurosurgery 2:161–168
4. Richard KE, Sanker P, Alcantra M (1989) Intracranial Pressure and Cerebral Blood Flow in Patients with Subarachnoid Hemorrhage Under Treatment with Nimodipine. In: Hoff JT, Betz AL (eds) Springer, Intracranial pressure VII. Berlin Heidelberg New York London Paris Tokyo Hong Kong, 72–73
5. Stoiber H-P, Castel J-P, Dabadie P, Loiseau H (1989) ICP in the Diagnosis of Acute Hydrocephalus after Aneurysmal Subarachnoid Hemorrhage. In: Hoff JT, Betz AL, (eds) Springer, Intractranial pressure VII, Berlin Heidelberg New York London Paris Tokyo Hong Kong, 732–735

Management Problems in Acute Hydrocephalus After Subarachnoid Hemorrhage

D. Hasan

Department of Neurology, University Hospital Rotterdam, Rotterdam, The Netherlands

Introduction

Acute hydrocephalus is not an uncommon complication after subarachnoid hemorrhage [3, 4]. Reports on its frequency of occurrence range from 9% [7] to 67% [1], mainly because of varying definitions. The decision to treat acute hydrocephalus may be difficult for several reasons. First, impaired consciousness on admission may result from the initial bleeding or from hydrocephalus. Second, when the decision to perform ventricular drainage has been made, the question rises whether this should be done by external CSF drainage or by internal shunting. Third, it has been suggested that early ventricular drainage may precipitate rebleeding. In this study we report on the management problems of 102 patients with hydrocephalus after subarachnoid hemorrhage, from a consecutive series of 473 patients.

Patients and Methods

During a period of 9½ years (from November 1977 until May 1987) we prospectively studied 473 consecutive patients admitted to the Department of Neurology of the University Hospital Rotterdam within 72 hours of subarachnoid hemorrhage. Cerebral angiography and aneurysm surgery were performed depending on the patients' clinical condition. In the majority of patients delayed aneurysm surgery was planned around day 12. During various parts of the study period patients were treated with long term, or short term tranexamic acid [10]. In the first part of the study period (until December 1982) daily fluid intake was between 1.5 and 2 liters, being further restricted in cases of hyponatremia. From January 1983 onward this policy was considered incorrect and daily fluid intake was maintained at least three liters; fluid restriction and diuretic medication were avoided. When signs of cerebral ischaemia had developed, extra fluid was administered.

The causes of deterioration occurring in these patients were analysed and defined as:

- probable delayed cerebral ischaemia
- definite delayed cerebral ischaemia
- probable rebleeding

- definite rebleeding
- acute hydrocephalus
- deterioration from hydrocephalus.

Acute hydrocephalus was defined as the bicaudate index, measured on the initial CT or on a repeat CT within one week after the initial subarachoid hemorrhage, exceeding the upper normal limit (95th percentile) corrected for age [3, 4]. Deterioration from hydrocephalus was defined as deterioration of the level of consciousness with no detectable causes other than hydrocephalus [4]. In patients with acute hydrocephalus ventricular drainage was carried out if the Glasgow Coma Scale was ≤13 on admission and the impairment of the level of consciousness was thought to be caused by hydrocephalus. In all other patients and in patients with unumpaired (GCS 15), or slightly impaired (GCS 14), consciousness on admission ventricular drainage was performed only if deterioration from acute hydrocephalus occurred.

Outcome of the survivors was assessed at three months according to the 5-point Glasgow Outcome Scale. The influence of hydrocephalus and its treatment on causes of secondary deterioration and outcome were analysed with the Yates' corrected chi-square test. If the expected number in any cell was <5, the two-sided Fisher's exact probability test was applied.

Results

Frequency of Acute Hydrocephalus

Acute hydrocephalus was measured on the initial CT in 91 (19%) of the 473 patients. Of these 91 patients 25 (27%) had no impairment of consciousness on admission, 13 (14%) had a GCS of 14 and in the remaining 53 (58%) the GCS was <14. The degree of ventricular enlargement was not clearly different among these groups. In another 11 patients ventricular enlargement was found on a repeat CT after clinical deterioration had developed within one week after the initial hemorrhage. Angiography was negative in nine (10%) of the 91 patients with acute hydrocephalus on admission, in one of the 11 patients who developed acute hydrocephalus within one week, and in 36 of the remaining 371 patients. The proportion of ventricular enlargement on the initial CT in patients with a negative angiogram was similar to that of the whole study group.

Ventricular Drainage

Of the 102 patients with acute hydrocephalus, 32 underwent ventricular drainage. Eight patients received a primary internal shunt and 24 patients external CSF drainage. The decision to treat hydrocephalus by external drainage or by internal shunting was influenced mainly by the interval after the initial bleeding. In nine of the 24 patients with external CSF drainage, an internal shunting procedure was later performed.

Twenty-five (78%) of the 32 drained patients showed an initial improvement of consciousness after CSF drainage. In the remaining seven patients CSF drainage had no such favourable effect. This absence of effect was caused by other events leading to secondary deterioration or due to complications of the CSF drainage in five patients: two patients developed definite cerebral ischaemia; one patient rebled one day after the insertion of the ventricular catheter; and two patients deteriorated secondary to infection of the ventricular catheter.

Complications After Treatment of Acute Hydrocephalus

Twelve (50%) of the 24 externally drained patients, but none of the eight internally drained patients developed ventriculitis, especially if drainage was maintained for more than three days. In one patient ventriculitis was followed by a lethal septic shock. Two other patients had a nonfatal deterioration.

Among patients not treated with long-term tranexamic acid, the rebleeding rate of those with ventricular drainage was significantly higher than that of patients without acute hydrocephalus (10 of 23 patients, 43%, versus 53 of 265 patients, 20%, $p = 0.019$) and higher than that of patients with acute hydrocephalus without ventricular drainage (10 of 23 patients, 43%, versus eight of 52 patients, 15%, $p = 0.02$). The effect of long-term tranexamic acid treatment in patients with subarachnoid hemorrhage, who also had ventricular drainage could not be assessed because the number of patients with rebleeding was too small for statistical analysis.

Delayed cerebral ischaemia developed in eight (26%) of the 31 hydrocephalic patients with ventricular drainage, in 18 (30%) of the 61 hydrocephalic patients without ventricular drainage, and in 63 (19%) of the 335 patients without acute hydrocephalus. Statistical analysis showed an increased tendency for occurrence of delayed cerebral ischaemia in patients with acute hydrocephalus versus patients without acute hydrocephalus ($p = 0.067$).

Outcome After Three Months

Outcome after three months in the 427 patients with aneurysmal subarachnoid hemorrhage is shown in Table 1. The proportion of patients who were independent three months after subarachnoid hemorrhage was significantly lower in patients with acute hydrocephalus with or without ventricular drainage than in those without acute hydrocephalus ($p = 0.031$). The higher proportion of patients without drainage dying from the initial hemorrhage was offset by the higher proportion of patients dying of complications after ventricular drainage.

Discussion

In our unselected consecutive series of 473 patients admitted to the Department of Neurology within 72 hours after subarachnoid hemorrhage, CT showed

Table 1. Outcome 3 months after subarachnoid hemorrhage in relation to acute hydrocephalus in 427 patients with aneurysmal subarachnoid hemorrhage

Outcome	Acute hydrocephalus					
	Yes				No	
	Ventricular drainage					
	Yes no.	%	No no.	%		
Dead	17	55	37	60	158	47
Initial SAH	0	0[a]	8	22[a]	35	22[a]
Rebleeding	7	41[a]	12	32[a]	61	38[a]
Cerebral ischemia	3	18[a]	7	19[a]	22	14[a]
Hydrocephalus	5[b]	29[a]	2[b]	5[a]	4[c]	3[a]
Other	2	12[a]	8	22[a]	36	23[a]
Dependent	6	19	4	7	31	9
Independent	8	26	20	33	146	44[d]
Total	31		61		335	

Percentages, % of total, except [a] % of dead patients.
[b] Includes patients who died of ventriculitis or drain removal following ventriculitis.
[c] Hydrocephalus that developed >1 week after subarachnoid hemorrhage
[d] $p < 0.05$ different from acute hydrocephalus

hydrocephalus on admission in 19%. The same frequency of acute hydrocephalus was found in a subgroup of 46 patients with clinical signs and symptoms of subarachnoid hemorrhage and blood in the basal cisterns, but with a negative angiogram. In these 46 patients acute hydrocephalus was the only cerebral complication.

The risk of deterioration from hydrocephalus between three days and one week after subarachnoid hemorrhage in patients without ventricular enlargement on admission is low (3%). Acute hydrocephalus was not symptomatic in all 91 patients with enlarged ventricles on admission. The level of consciousness was unimpaired in 27%, slightly impaired in 14% and moderately to severely impaired in 58%. There was no relation between the level of consciousness and the degree of enlargement of the ventricles. The majority of the patients with an unimpaired or a slightly impaired level of consciousness did not subsequently deteriorate from acute hydrocephalus. Ventricular drainage in the patients with acute hydrocephalus resulted in clinical improvement in 78%, but the outcome after three months remained poor. The most frequent adverse events after ventricular drainage were rebleeding and infection. The risk of rebleeding was significantly increased after ventricular drainage, and the infection rate in the externally drained patients was high.

The frequency of acute hydrocephalus in our series is in accordance with the findings of one other study, but is different from those of many others [1, 2,

5, 6, 7, 9, 12]. These differences can be explained by differences in diagnostic criteria, by patient selection, and by timing of the investigations.

What Can be Done to Improve the Outcome of Patients with Acute Hydrocephalus?

Although the risk of rebleeding can be diminished by long-term antifibrinolytic treatment, the benefit is negated by an increased frequency of delayed cerebral ischaemia. In a previous report on the initial study period of this series, the frequency of delayed cerebral ischaemia was very high in patients with ventricular drainage [3]. In this extended series, the frequency and mortality due to delayed cerebral ischaemia in patients with acute hydrocephalus was still higher, but no longer significantly so. Probably this is caused by the fact that fluid restriction was no longer applied in patients with hyponatremia. To improve outcome, it might be necessary to combine antifibrinolytic agents with plasma volume expansion or calcium antagonists. An alternative could be to have treatment of hydrocephalus by ventricular drainage soon followed by or simultaneously performed with clipping of the aneurysm. Such a policy will improve outcome only if early surgery is not accompanied by increased mortality and morbidity.

It has been suggested that rebleeding after ventricular drainage can be prevented if the CSF pressure does not fall below 15 to 25 mmHg [6]. We could not confirm this, since the CSF pressures after drainage in our series were within this "safe" range. Infection was a frequent complication in the externally drained patients, especially if drainage was maintained for more than three days. This complication should have been preventable. It has been suggested that ventriculitis can be prevented by using a long subcutaneous tunnel [5]; others prefer antibiotic prophylaxis and a short duration of external drainage [8, 11]. Another possibility might be to treat hydrocephalic patients with serial lumbar punctures, provided the CSF blockage is in the subarachnoid space and not in the ventricular system and provided there is no hematoma with a mass effect [4]. The risk of infection with this procedure is small [4], and the fall in CSF pressure is probably more gradual.

References

1. Black PM (1986) Hydrocephalus and vasospasm after subarachnoid hemorrhage from ruptured intracranial aneurysms. Neurosurgery 18:12–16
2. Graff-Radford NR, Torner J, Adams HP, Kassell NF (1987) Factors associated with hydrocephalus in subarachnoid hemorrhage (abstract). Ann Neurol 22:137
3. Van Gijn J, Hijdra A, Wijdicks EFM, Vermeulen M, van Crevel H (1985) Acute hydrocephalus after aneurysmal subarachnoid hemorrhage. J Neurosurg 63:355–362
4. Hasan D, Lindsay KW, Vermeulen M (1991) Treatment of acute hydrocephalus after subarachnoid hemorrhage with lumbar puncture. Stroke 22:190–194
5. Milhorat TH (1987) Acute hydrocephalus after aneurysmal subarachnoid hemorrhage. Neurosurgery 20:15–20
6. Pickard JD (1984) Early posthemorrhagic hydrocephalus. Br Med J 289:569–570

7. Spallone A, Gagliardi FM (1983) Hydrocephalus following aneurysmal subarachnoid hemorrhage. Zentralbl Neurochir 44:141–150
8. Smith RW, Alksne JF (1986) Infections complicating the use of external ventricular drainage. J Neurosurg 44:567–570
9. Steinke D, Weir B, Disney L (1987) Hydrocephalus following aneurysmal subarachnoid hemorrhage. Neurol Res 9:3–9
10. Vermeulen M, Lindsay KW, Murray GD, Cheah F, Hijdra A, Muizelaar JP, Schannong M, Teasdale GM, van Crevel H, van Gijn J (1984) Antifibrinolytic treatment in subarachnoid hemorrhage. N Engl J Med 311:432–437
11. Wyler AR, Kelly WA (1972) Use of antibiotics with external ventriculostomies. J Neurosurg 37:185–188
12. Yasargil MG, Yonekawa Y, Zumstein B, Stahl HJ (1973) Hydrocephalus following spontaneous subarachnoid hemorrhage. J Neurosurg 39:474–479

Continous Intraventricular Pressure and Simultaneous Cerebral Blood Flow Velocity (CBFV) Measurements During Sleep in Hydrocephalic Children*

D. Goh[1], R.A. Minns[1], S.D. Pye[2], and A.J.W. Steers[3]

[1] Dept. of Paediatric Neurology, Royal Hospital for Sick Children, Edinburgh, Scotland
[2] Dept. of Medical Physics, Western General Hospital, Edinburgh, Scotland
[3] Dept. of Surgical Neurology, Western General Hospital, Edinburgh, Scotland

Introduction

The clinical importance of episodic elevations of ICP during sleep is not entirely clear. A major concern is the secondary ischaemic insult which may occur during sustained elevation in ICP. This study aims to assess the cerebral haemodynamic response to ICP increases during sleep in hydrocephalic children by noninvasive mesurement of cerebral blood flow velocity (CBFV) using transcranial Doppler ultrasonography (TCD) with simultaneous ICP monitoring.

Patients and Methods

Eight sleep studies were performed in seven patients (5 males, 2 females), age range 12–118 months. All but one patient had pre-existing CSF shunts. Three patients were symptomatic and four patients were clinically asymptomatic but had persistent or increasing ventricular dilatation.

Direct intraventricular pressure was measured via a Rickham reservoir in all patients using a non-displacement pressure transducer (Gaeltec Ltd). Maximum mean ICP levels during stable and unstable epochs and the type of pressure elevations i.e. A/plateau, B or C waves were characterised. Blood pressure was measured by an oscillometric method (Dinamap). CBFV was measured in the middle cerebral artery using a 2 MHz pulsed-wave probe attached to a Doppler unit (Decoder–Doptek Ltd.) which performs real-time spectral analysis on the ultrasound signal. Doppler signals were recorded on an audio cassette deck. CBFV measurements were made at 10–15 minute

* We are grateful to the Earl of Elgin and Kincardine and the Trustees Savings Bank Foundation, Scotland for supporting research into Hydrocephalus at the Royal Hospital for Sick Children, Edinburgh, U.K.

intervals while ICP was stable and more frequently during unstable ICP states from a constant optimal position and depth throughout each study. Values of the Pourcelot Resistance Index, RI = (S-D)/S, an index of cerebrovascular resistance; time-averaged mean flow velocity (MFV- a reliable index of mean flow assuming a constant vessel diameter[2]); peak systolic (S), end-diastolic (D) velocities were obtained. Each calculated value was obtained from the mean of at least 5–10 consecutive cardiac cycles of good quality. Graphical plots of simultaneous ICP, CPP and CBFV change over time were made for each individual study.

Results

Table 1 summarises the results of mean ICP during stable and unstable periods, and correlations between ICP with MFV and RI in each sleep recording. There were two main patterns of MFV response observed in association with episodic increased ICP.

Ischaemic-Type CBFV Response

In four studies increased ICP was associated with a progressive decrease in MFV (overall correlation: $r = -0.44$, $p < 0.001$) and increase in RI ($r = +0.64$, $p < 0.001$) which we have termed an 'ischaemic-type' CBFV response. MFV descreased as CPP decreased (correlation: $r = +0.44$, $p < 0.001$). In three of these patients who were symptomatic, chronic CSF overdrainage with slit-ventricle syndrome was suspected. Figure 1 shows a sleep recording which illustrates the "ischaemic-type" CBFV response. Plateau/A and B waves were recorded in these three patients. The fourth patient had gradually deteriorating shunt function.

Table 1. Mean basal and unstable ICP levels and correlation with Doppler indices in individual studies

Case No.	Mean basal ICP (mmHg)	Mean max. unstable ICP (mmHg)	ICP/MFV r	p	ICP/RI r	p
1.	4.4	33.4	−0.64	<0.001	+0.89	<0.001
2.	9.0	32.3	−0.46	<0.05	+0.7	<0.001
3. (pre)	17.5	33.5	−0.24	ns	+0.61	<0.001
3. (post)	16.7	24.3	+0.58	<0.001	+0.03	ns
4.	14.7	31.3	−0.13	ns	+0.41	<0.01
5.	10.5	21.5	+0.37	<0.01	+0.69	<0.001
6.	16.4	24.0	+0.64	<0.001	+0.13	ns
7.	15.2	31.2	+0.63	<0.001	−0.8	<0.001

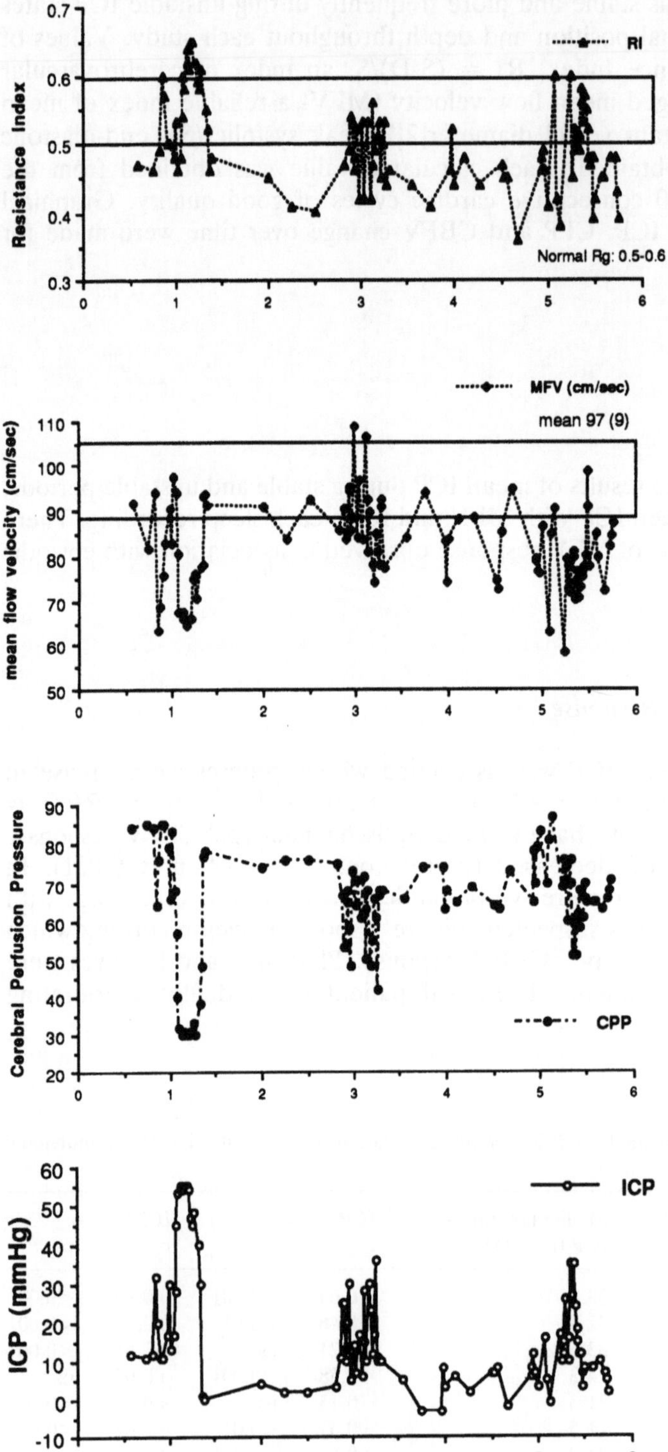
RI
Resistance Index
Normal Rg: 0.5-0.6
MFV (cm/sec)
mean 97 (9)
mean flow velocity (cm/sec)
Cerebral Perfusion Pressure
CPP
ICP
ICP (mmHg)
TIME (HRS)

Hyperaemic-type CBFV Response

Another pattern of increased MFV when ICP increased (overall correlation: $r = +0.65$, $p < 0.001$) which we have termed a "hyperaemic-type" CBFV response was observed in 4 studies. There was an overall increase in MFV as CPP decreased ($n = 3$, $r = -0.46$, $p < 0.001$). Figure 2 shows a sleep study which illustrates the "hyperaemic-type" CBFV response. In three of these studies increased ICP was associated with increase in RI while in one patient, RI decreased as ICP increased. None of these studies had sustained plateau or B waves recorded; the maximum were elevations of 10–20 minutes duration rising to a mean maximum pressure of 20–30 mmHg. A repeat study performed in one patient showed improvement with reduction in mean ICP levels and a change to a "hyperaemic-type" response following a skull morcellation procedure.

Discussion

It has been well established that cerebral blood flow increases during REM sleep, probably mediated by vasodilatation, but in patients with reduced intracranial compliance the resulting increase in intracranial blood volume is inadequately buffered thus producing a greater rise in ICP. In an experimental model [1] significant pial arterial dilatation occured when ICP was increased from 13 to 45 mmHg by ventricular infusion of mock CSF but with further rise of ICP no further dilatation occurred. Thus maximum cerebrovascular compensatory response has already occurred and further increase in ICP will by likely to result in reduced perfusion. In our study the "ischaemic-type" CBFV response suggests that inadequate haemodynamic compensation to raised ICP may be more likely to occur in those with reduced intracranial compliance. During plateau/A and B waves a clear "ischaemic-type" response suggests that circulatory reserve may be critical during these episodes.

Our results suggest that in hydrocephalic children with a "hyperaemic-type" CBFV response, appropriate cerebrovascular response, probably through distal pial arterial dilatation, occurs with moderately increased ICP to maintain an adequate cerebral perfusion. Evaluation of calculated CPP change alone does not reliably predict those with adequate haemodynamic compensation.

In conclusion, simultaneous monitoring of CBFV and ICP change during sleep may help to identify those patients with limited circulatory reserve who are at greater risk of ischaemic insult ("ischaemic-type" response) from episodic increases in ICP.

←

Fig. 1. Graphical plot of simultaneous ICP, cerebral perfusion pressure, mean flow velocity (*MFV*) and resistance index (*RI*) during sleep study in case no. 1. It illustrates an "ischaemic-type" response with decreased MFV and decreased CPP as ICP increased. The horizontal bands represent the reported mean (±standard deviation) range of MFV and RI for the patient's age.

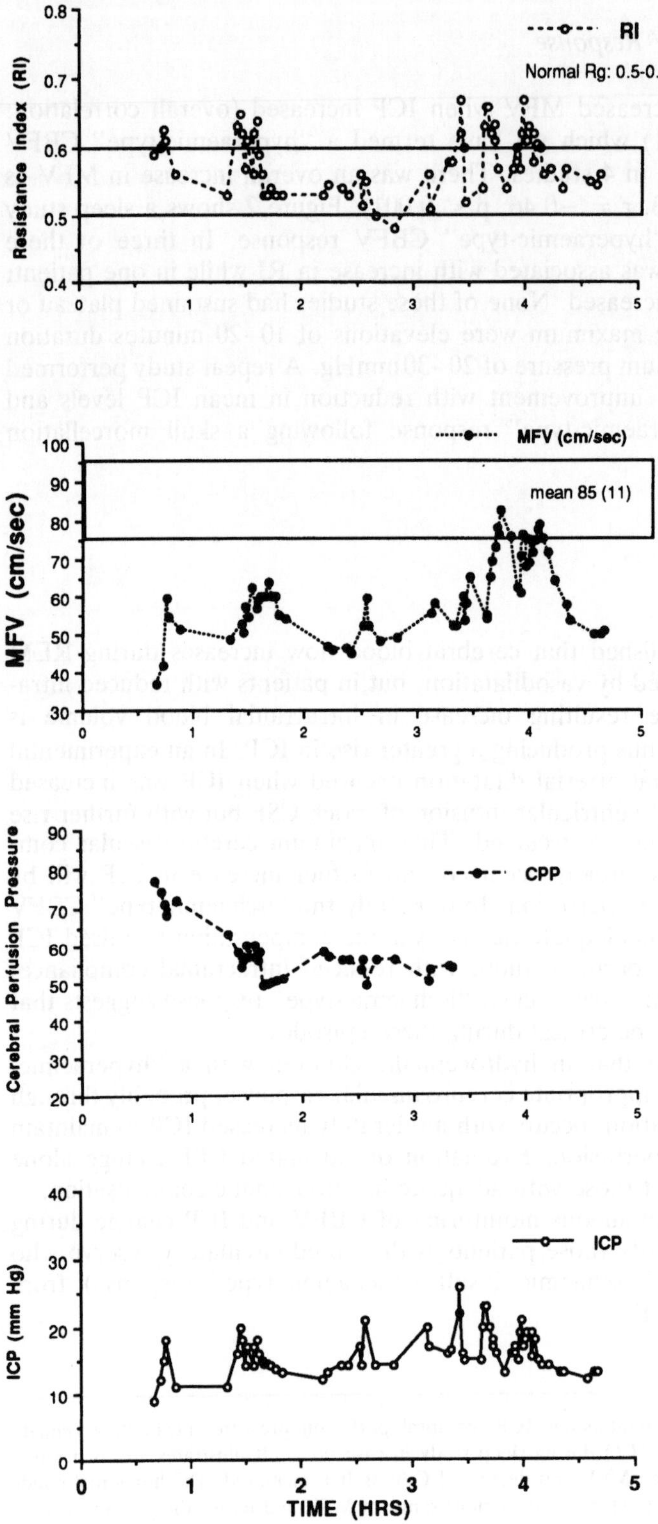
RI
Normal Rg: 0.5-0.6
Resistance Index (RI)
MFV (cm/sec)
mean 85 (11)
MFV (cm/sec)
CPP
Cerebral Perfusion Pressure
ICP
ICP (mm Hg)
TIME (HRS)

References

1. Kato Y, Auer LM (1989) Cerebrovascular response to elevation of ventricular pressure. Acta Neurochir (Wien) 98:184–188
2. Kirkham FJ, Padayachee TS, Parsons S, et al. (1986) Transcranial measurements of blood velocities in the basal cerebral arteries using pulsed Doppler ultrasound: velocity as an index of flow. Ultrasound in Med & Biol 12:15–21

Fig. 2. Simultaneous ICP, cerebral perfusion pressure, mean flow velocity (*MFV*) and resistance index (*RI*) from sleep study in case no. 5. This illustrates a "hyperaemic-type" response with increased MFV and increased RI as ICP increased. The horizontal bands represent the mean (±standard deviation) range of MFV and RI for the patient's age.

A Volume-Blood Flow Velocity (VFR) Relationship Derived From CSF Compartment Challenge as an Index of Progression of Infantile Hydrocephalus*

R. A. Minns[1], D. Goh[1], S.D. Pye[2], A.J.W. Steers[1], and R.A. Elton[3]

[1] Dept of Paediatric Neurology, Royal Hospital for Sick Children Edinburgh, Scotland
[2] Dept of Medical Physics, Western General Hospital, Edinburgh, Scotland
[3] Medical Computing and Statistics Unit, University of Edinburgh, Edinburgh, Scotland

Introduction

It is important to differentiate infants with progressive hydrocephalus (with secondary ischaemic damage from raised ICP) from those cases which will spontaneously arrest. In this preliminary series we have used ventricular CSF manipulation and noninvasive transcranial Doppler ultrasound (TCD) measurement of cerebral blood flow velocity (CBFV) to define a volume-flow velocity response (VFR), before an ischaemic point is reached. Sequential challenge may indicate if the volume buffering capacity is increasing (i.e. arrest) or decreasing (decompensating).

Patients and Methods

Fifty-six ventricular taps were performed on 16 patients (8 males, 8 females) with hydrocephalus of varying aetiology. Group I consisted of 10 neonatal patients and Group II of 6 children (aged 1–14 years). Four patients in Group II had existing ventricular peritoneal shunts in-situ. Indications for CSF taps were signs or symptoms of raised ICP and imaging evidence of increasing ventricular dilatation. ICP was measured directly from a CSF access device by a non-displacement strain gauge pressure transducer (Gaeltec Ltd). CSF was drained in 1 ml increments with repeated ICP and CBFV measurements until ICP was within normal range for age. CBFV in the middle cerebral artery was recorded throughout the tap using pulsed-wave Doppler (Decoder–Doptek Ltd) with a 2 or 4 MHz probe. Doppler signals were recorded onto audiotape. Values of the peak systolic (S), end-diastolic (D) velocities, Pourcelot Resistance Index, RI = (S-D/S), and MFV (time averaged mean of maximum velocity envelope) were obtained from a mean of at least 10 cardiac cycles. As a ratio, the RI minimises error due to variability in angle of insonation.

Pre- and post-tap Doppler indices were compared by paired t-test. Plots of RI (y) against volume CSF (x) drained were fitted to an exponential curve $y = a + be^{cx}$ (a = equilibrium RI (RIe), a + b = initial RI (RIo), b = change in RI

* We are grateful to the Earl of Elgin and Kincardine and the Trustee's Savings Bank Foundation, Scotland for supporting research into hydrocephalus at the Royal Hospital for Sick Children, Edinburgh, U.K.

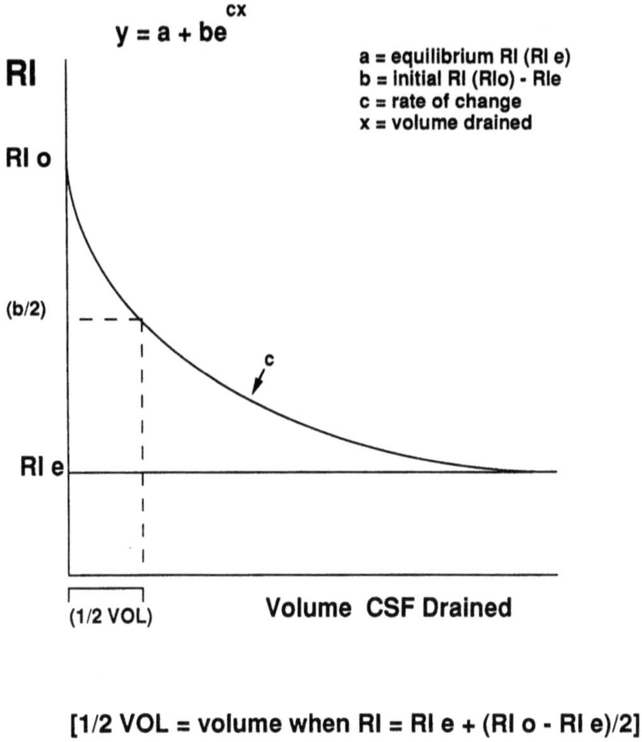

Fig. 1. shows a predicted exponential curve fit, $y = a + be^{cx}$ for serial observed RI (Resistance Index) Decay with volume depletion during CSF taps. Half-volume = −0.70/c, i.e. the volume drained when 1/2 change in RI i.e. (RIo-RIe)/2 has occurred

(RIo-RIe), and c = rate of exponential decay), see Fig. 1. A half-volume when half the change in RI had occurred was obtained by calculation i.e. half-volume = −0.7/c.

Results

In Group I and II patients there was a statistically significant decrease in ICP ($p < 0.01$) and RI ($p < 0.001$) after volume withdrawal. Increase in D was also statistically significant ($p < 0.03$) in all but increase in S was only significant in the neonatal group, thus the decrease in RI was mainly due to improved diastolic flow. Increase in MFV was statistically significant only in Group I ($p < 0.001$). There was a significant overall positive correlation of RI to ICP ($r = +0.70$, $p < 0.02$) in Group II patients. In the neonatal group, overall correlation between RI and ICP was poor for the whole group but in individual neonates who had repeated studies, there was a significant correlation ($p < 0.001$) in their individual measurements.

Fifty-six serial RI and volume plots were fitted to the exponential equation as described and only 6 did not fit the predicted curve. Serial taps were

Table 1. Results of volume-flow velocity response studies

Patient groups	Initial RIe	Final RIe	Initial d RI (RIo-RIe)	Final d RI (RIo-RIe)	Initial half-volume (mls)	Final half-volume (mls)
Neonates eventually shunted						
no. 1 (LF)	0.64	0.69	0.09	0.07	0.87	0.30
no. 2 (RA)	0.73	0.71	0.07	0.13	3.23	0.67
no. 3 (MR)	0.63	0.64	0.09	0.11	2.65	0.53
no. 4 (CM)	0.68	0.70	0.16	0.13	5.28	1.85
4 patients (single taps), mean:	0.64 (0.03)		0.07 (0.03)		1.21 (1.0)	
neonates unshunted (2 patients)	0.72 (0.1)		0.13 (0.05)		1.97 (2.4)	
Children with blocked VP-shunt (4 patients)	0.48 (0.1)		0.13 (0.03)		2.13 (1.0)	
children: ventricular dilatation, not shunted						
no. 5 (CMcM)	0.48		0.15		11.9	
no. 6 (VH)	0.58		0.04		2.2	

performed on 4 neonatal patients who progressed and required shunting. Table 1 shows the values of VFR plots from initial and final taps in those with repeated studies and also summarises the mean values of other Group I and II patients who only had single taps. Plots of serial "half-volumes" in the 4 neonatal patients showed a fluctuating trend in 2 but all had final reduced predicted "half-volumes" which suggests that there was reduced volume buffering capacity with progression of hydrocephalus. Figure 2 shows a plot of observed and predicted RI with volume depletion in a neonatal patient requiring shunting which illustrates the exponential change in RI as CSF is withdrawn. One child (aged 17 months) with long-standing nonprogressive ventricular dilatation had a much larger predicted "half-volume" compared to other patient groups suggesting a greater volume-buffering reserve in this patient. There was little difference in the predicted "half-volumes" of other neonatal and older shunted patients (Table 1).

Discussion

In hydrocephalus, progressive ventricular dilatation and raised ICP can cause secondary ischaemic damage. The exponential relationship between intracranial volume-ICP has been characterised by the Pressure-Volume Index [2] and Volume-Pressure Response [1] using volume challenge techniques. Compliance estimation, however, does not directly relate perfusion response at various stages of the hydrocephalic process. Change in cerebral perfusion pressure is assumed whenever ICP is altered.

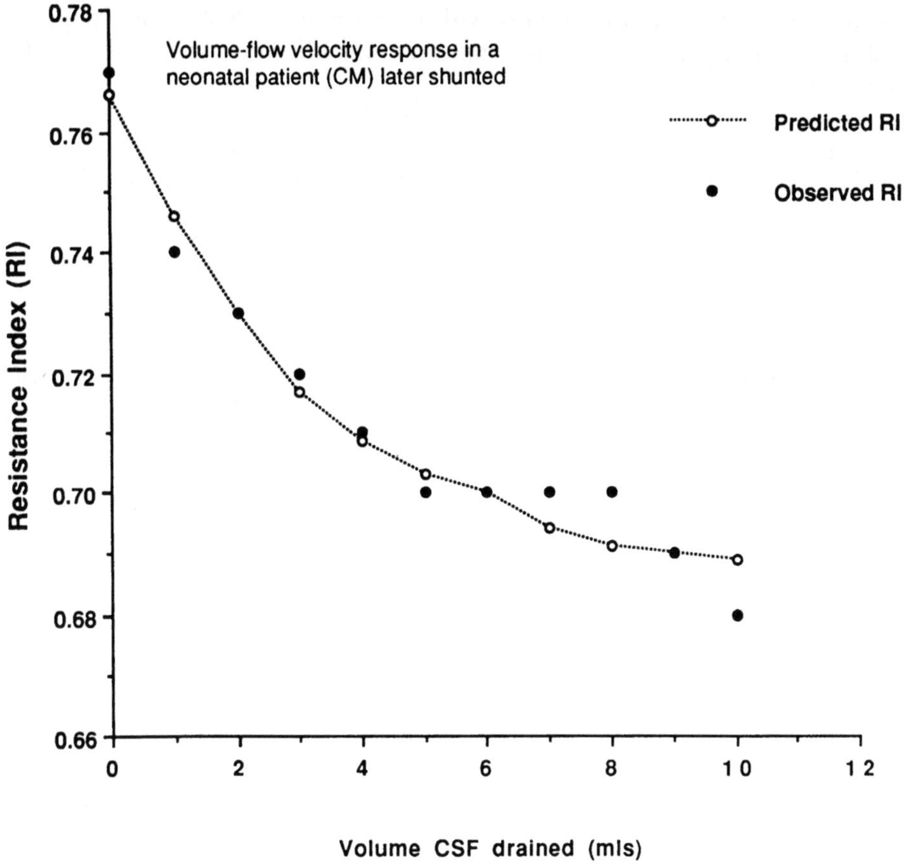

Fig. 2. Plot of predicted RI (*open circles*) and observed RI (*closed circles*) against CSF volume drained in a neonatal patient requiring shunting which illustrates a rapid exponential decay in RI

Our results suggest that the change in RI can be a reliable index of change in distal cerebrovascular resistance as RI decreases significantly due to increase in diastolic flow after CSF drainage and correlates significantly with ICP. We have shown that decrease in RI with volume depletion generally followed an exponential curve similar to the ICP/volume relationship suggesting that there is similarly a "critical" volume buffered before blood flow response is significantly altered. Thus by assessing serial change in RI with volume manipulation (VFR) we may be able to directly assess change in volume buffering available for individual patients before significant ischaemia occurs.

In neonates and young infants single ICP measurements do not predict those who require shunting. If RI remains elevated compared to normal range for age and serial VFRs show deterioration or no change with time, surgical intervention would be indicated as there is no development of natural arrest. Repeated RI measurements showing an improvement towards normal values for age and serial VFRs suggesting increased volume buffering reserve would encourage non-interventional management. Ventricular dilatation per se without cerebral perfusion compromise should not be shunted if there is adequate volume buffering as most patients with CSF shunts become shunt-dependant and thus remain at risk from long-term complications such as infection, blockage and overdrainage.

Noninvasive TCD monitoring of cerebrohaemodynamic change in hydrocephalus, in particular serial flow velocity change with volume manipulation, (VFR) may help to select more precisely those who require intervention.

References

1. Miller JD, Garibi J, Pickard JD (1973) Induced changes of cerebrospinal fluid volume. Effects during continous monitoring of ventricular fluid pressure. Arch Neurol 28:2652
2. Shulman K, Marmarou A (1971) Pressure volume considerations in infantile hydrocephalus. Dev Med Child Neurol 13:90

Non-Invasive ICP-Monitoring in Childhood Hydrocephalus: A Comparison Between Anterior Fontanelle Pressure and Transcranial Doppler

P.W. Hanlo[1], K.P.J. Braun[1], R.H.J.M. Gooskens[1], W.C.G. Overweg-Plandsoen[4], A.C. van Huffelen[3], J. Willemse[1], and C.A.F. Tulleken[2]

[1] Departments of Child-Neurology, [2] Neurosurgery and [3] Clinical Neurophysiology of the University Hospital Utrecht, Heidelberglaan 100, 3584 CX Utrecht, The Netherlands
[4] Department of Child-Neurology of the Academical Medical Centre, Meibergdreef 9, 1105 AZ Amsterdam, The Netherlands.

Introduction

The ability to discriminate between ventriculomegaly and progressive hydrocephalus often relies on clinical assesment of increasing head circumference, developmental deficits and a change in ventricular size and configuration. Some patients with slowly progressive hydrocephalus cannot be detected adequately with the methods currently in use for monitoring hydrocephalus. Previous studies have demonstrated that the resistance index [1] (RI) or pulsatility index [2] (PI) are useful indicators of increased intracranial pressure (ICP) and the need for a shunt. Shunt dysfunction was correlated with elevated RI's [3]. In none of these studies the variables were related to the actual ICP.

This study was designed to investigate the value of non-invasive techniques for detecting patients with progressive hydrocephalus at an early stage, in order to establish the most appropriate treatment at the right moment and thus prevent secondary brain damage. For ICP-monitoring we used anterior fontanelle pressure (AFP) and transcranial Doppler (TCD) measurements.

Aim of the Study

To study the relationship between transcranial Doppler and anterior fontanelle pressure measurements, aiming at the use of TCD for monitoring ICP non-invasively after closure of the fontanelle, in the follow-up of patients with hydrocephalus.

Methods

We examined 25 patients with hydrocephalus under the age of two years. For AFP measurements, we used the Rotterdam Teletransducer, a telemetric device [4]. With this apparatus, the externally exerted pressure does not interfere with the actual ICP monitoring. AFP measurements were carried out over a longer period of time, mostly overnight. For TCD examinations, we used the EME TC 2-64B. The hematocrit was also determined and whenever the child cried or was restless the examination was interrupted. Pre- and post-operative measurements were performed. When TCD could not be performed during the course of AFP measurements, the mean AFP was correlated with the TCD parameters (Fig. 1). In simultaneous AFP/TCD measurements, the actual AFP was correlated with the corresponding TCD parameters (Fig. 2) and the results were evaluated for each patient individually.

Results

Pre- and postoperative AFP and TCD measurements as well as measurements in cases of shunt dysfunction were carried out. Consecutive AFP/TCD measurements show that the pulsatility index of the right middle cerebral artery (PI/ACMR) correlates reasonably well with the AFP values. When investigated intra-individually, the PI tends to increase or decrease together with the AFP value (Fig. 1). Several patients with very mild clinical signs of increased ICP were detected as having raised AFP values (with periodical A-waves) and increased PI, as compared with an earlier examination.

To test the correlation between AFP and PI, simultaneous AFP/TCD measurements were performed. With increasing AFP, we found an increasing average PI [Fig. 2; compared with AFP-values: 1. below 20 mmHg the mean PI was 0.81 (95% confidence interval: 0.77–0.84); 2. between 20–30 mmHg the mean PI was 0.88 (95% confidence interval: 0.85–0.91); 3. between 30–40 mmHg the mean PI was 0.96 (95% confidence interval: 0.92–0.99)].

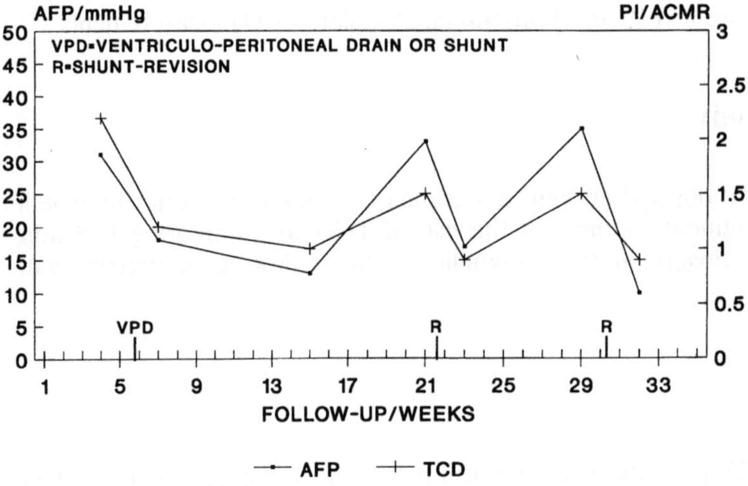

Fig. 1. Childhood hydrocephalus consecutive AFP/TCD measurements. Non-invasive ICP-monitoring case study

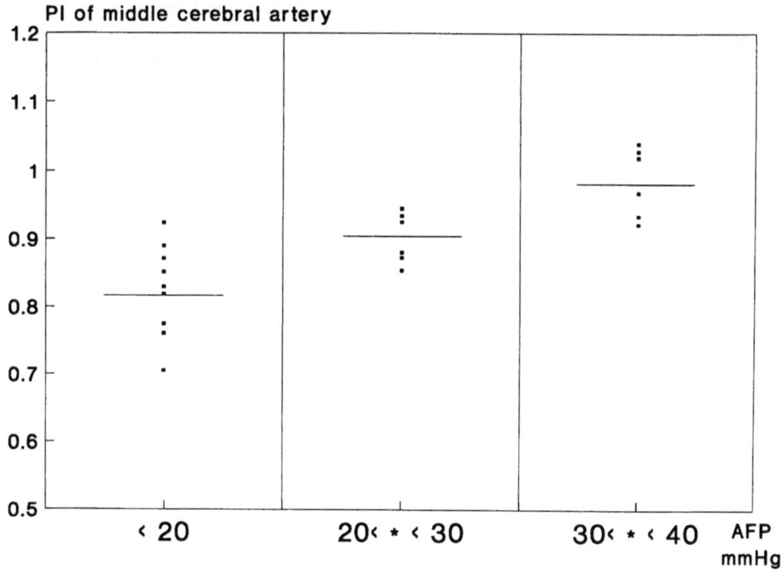

Fig. 2. Childhood hydrocephalus simultaneous AFP/TCD measurements

Non-invasive ICP-monitoring in childhood hydrocephalus, by means of AFP and TCD measurements, can therefore be of great value in detecting progressive hydrocephalus, even when clinically dubious.

Conclusions

This study shows a relationship between AFP and TCD. With increasing ICP (progressive hydrocephalus and shunt dysfunction) the pulsatility index tends to increase. TCD measurements can, therefore, be used in monitoring ICP in childhood hydrocephalus. Better indications for shunt implantation and early detection of shunt dysfunction can thus be achieved. In our view, TCD might also prove to be a useful instrument in the follow-up of patients after closure of the fontanelle.

Acknowledgements. We would like to thank M. Musbach for her expertise in performing the Doppler studies; W.P. Vandertop and C.J.J. Avezaat, neurosurgeons, for their critical advice and cooperation; Y. van der Graaf and J.S.M. Uytewaal for their assistance in the data-processing.

References

1. Chadduck WM, Seibert JJ, Adametz J, Glasier CM, Crabtree M, Stansell CA (1989) Cranial Doppler ultrasonography correlates with criteria for ventriculoperitoneal shunting. Surg Neurol 31:122–128

2. Norelle A, Fischer AQ, Flannery AM (1989) Transcranial Doppler: a noninvasive method to monitor hydrocephalus. J Child Neurol Suppl 4:87–90
3. Chadduck WM, Crabtree HM, Blankenship JB, Adametz J (1991) Transcranial Doppler ultrasonography for the evaluation of shunt malfunction in pediatric patients. Child's Nerv Syst 7:27–30
4. Plandsoen WCG, De Jong DA, Maas AIR, Stroink H, Avezaat CJJ (1987) Fontanelle pressure monitoring in infants with the Rotterdam Teletransducer: a reliable technique. Med Progr Technol 13:21–27

ICP and TCD Guided Treatment of Slit Ventricle Syndrome

K.E. RICHARD and P. SANKER

Neurochirurgische Klinik der Universität zu Köln, Joseph-Stelzmann-Str. 9, 5000 Köln 41, Germany

Introduction

The slit ventricle syndrome (SVS) is still one of the most difficult therapeutic problems of shunts complications [2].

Before the mode of treatment of a post-shunt SVS can be selected, the following questions have to be clarified:

- Is there a hypertensive or a hypotensive SVS, i.e. is the ICP elevated or not?
- Does an open craniospinal CSF communication exist or not?

As ICP-measurement is an invasive method, we also investigated the question, how far transcranial Doppler sonography (TCD) is useful for the assessment of the intracranial dynamic situation.

Pratients and Methods

In 1989/90 7 patients with symptomatic slit ventricles were treated. In all 7 patients ICP- and TCD-measurements were combined perioperatively.

ICP was monitored epidurally with a fiberoptic LADD system or with a Spiegelberg probe.

Equipment used for TCD-monitoring included a TC 2000 S (EME Company) and a TC-Trak module. The transtemporal starting frequency was 2 MHz. Blood flow velocity (BFV) was measured transtemporally in the basal arteries and the pulsatility index (PI) was computed from the values of the systolic, diastolic and median BFV:

$$\frac{Vs - Vd}{Vm}$$

Results

The results are shown in Table 1. In all patients, the SVS syndrome developed during the growth period, in 5 of them after numerous revisions of the shunt.

Table 1. Data of patients with a slit ventricle syndrome

No	Pat	Age. yrs	Sex f	Sex m	Primary Shunt VA/VP		Multiple Revisions yes	Multiple Revisions no	Slit ventricles unilat./bilat.		Develop. during growth yes	Develop. during growth no	Open CSF-communic. yes	Open CSF-communic. no	ICP mm Hg	BFV cm/s	PI	Operat. Procedure	Reexpansion of ventricles yes	Reexpansion of ventricles no
1	H.C.	17	+			VP	+		+		+		+		38	20	2.7	LP-SH	+	
2	B.S.	7		+	VA		+		+		+		+		65	30	2.9	Adj.V.	+	
3	S.C.	15		+	VA		+		+		+		+		60	30	1.8	LP-Sh	+	
4	R.J.	6		+	VA		+			+	+		+		85	30	1.3	LP-Sh	+	
5	K.C.	19		+	VA		+			+	+			+	8	31	0.7	Adj.V.	+	
6	L.F.	18		+	VA			–		+	+			+	10	45	0.6	Adj.V.		–
7	C.M.	9		+		VP	+			+	+			+	15	38	0.5	–		

Complaints, such as headaches, nausea, vomiting and diplopia in upright and horizontal position, high ICP and PI values and a pathologically low BFV were typical parameters of the *hypertensive slit ventricle syndrome*. Four out of our 7 cases belonged to this group. Selection of the operative procedure could be reliably based on an *intraoperative ICP- and/or TCD-measurement*: If during lumbar puncture, ICP and/or the PI dropped immediately below normal values and the BFV increased significantly, an open craniospinal CSF-communication was assumed (Fig. 1). In all 4 patients with hypertensive SVS, results of this test indicated an open CSF communication. In 3 of them, the syndrome could be treated successfully by implantation of a *lumboperito neal shunt* [1]. Some days after implantation, CT and/or MRI of the now symptom-free patients showed a reexpansion of the slit ventricles and a restoration of ventricular symmetry.

In one patient, on account of abdominal adhesions after peritonitis, LP-shunt was not possible. After stereotactical positioning of a new ventricular catheter, the Neurone valve was replaced by an 8-step magnetically adjustable valve (Sophysa).

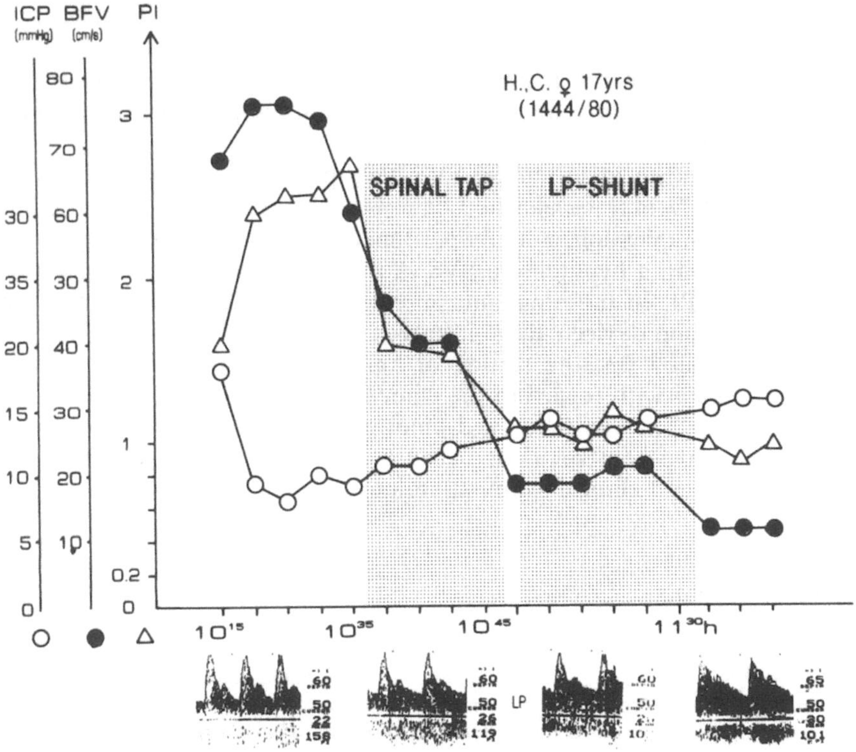

Fig. 1. Intraoperative simultaneous measurement of epidural pressure (*EDP*), blood flow velocity (*BFV*) and pulsatility index (*PI*). The parallel drop of EDP and PI and the increase of BFV values after lumbar puncture indicate an open craniospinal CSF-communication. Therefore, an LP-shunt can be implanted

Headaches, nausea, vomiting and diplopia in up-right position, BFV-values distinctly or slightly below the age-dependent normal range together with a normal PI and a normal ICP were the pathognomic parameters of 3 patients with a *hypotensive slit ventricle syndrome*. CT showed bilateral slit ventricles. The intraoperative test of an open craniospinal CSF-communication was negative. Therefore, the overdraining shunt valve was replaced by a modern shunt valve with electromagnetic adjustable steps of resistance (Medos-Hakim).

For the assessment of intracranial dynamics in shunted SVS patients, TCD-measurement proved to be of great value, not only in the immediate postoperative period, but also in the follow-up phase.

Indications for a new adjustement of the valve with variable resistances or for an operative revision could be based reliably on symptoms and TCD-values during dynamic tests, such as varying the patient's position or compression of jugular veins.

Conclusion

1. For the treatment of a slit ventricle syndrome (SVS), TCD-measurements of blood flow velocity (BFV) and pulsatility index (PI) are helpful to differentiate between the hypertensive and the hypotensive form, to select the operative procedure and to assess the efficacy postoperatively and during follow-up.
2. Patients with a hypertensive SVS have pathologically elevated ICP and PI values; BFV may be elevated or lowered. In cases of an open craniospinal CSF-communication, a lumboperitoneal shunt should be implanted.
3. Patients with a hypotensive SVS show subnormal ICP and BFV values and a normal PI. In these patients an electromagnetically adjustable valve with an antisiphon device can be inserted.
4. During follow-up, the setting of an adjustable valve can be based upon TCD-values with regard to the clinical findings.
5. The term "slit ventricle syndrome" should include both the hypertensive and the hypotensive SVS, because both forms are characterized by slit ventricles and clinical symptomatology.

References

1. Richard KE, Heimann G (1983) Lumboperitonealer Shunt beim sog. Schlitzventrikelsyndrom. In: Voth D (ed) Hydrocephalus im frühen Kindesalter. Enke, Stuttgart, pp 250–254
2. Sott RM (1991): Shunt complications. In: Wilkins RH, Rengachary SS (eds) Neurosurgery update II, McGraw Inc, New York, pp 309–319

Cerebrospinal Compensation in Hydrocephalic Children

M. Czosnyka[1], L. Batorski[2], Z. Czosnyka[3], J. Tomaszewski[2], J. Wocjan[2], A. Walencik[2], and W. Zabolotny[1]

[1] Warsaw University of Technology, [2] Clinic of Neurosurgery, Children's Health Center, and [3] Main School of Farming, Agricultural University, Warsaw, Poland

Introduction

Hydrocephalus in children is often still difficult to diagnose and difficult to decide on the optimal treatment.

Works dealing with characteristics of hydrocephalus take into account cerebrospinal compensatory parameters – the resistance to cerebrospinal fluid outflow (RCSF) and the pressure volume index (PVI) – and discuss their role in the development, course, and prognosis of this disease [1, 3, 4].

Although certain general features of the cerebrospinal compensation in children's hydrocephalus have been considered, some characteristic patterns specific to different types of this disease can be found. They seem to improve the understanding of the pathophysiology of this entity and help in the selection of the proper kind of treatment.

Material and Method

A group of 117 children, with ventricular enlargement confirmed on a CT scan and other symptoms of hydrocephalus was examined at the Clinic of Neurosurgery, Children's Health Center.

Etiological factors, results of clinical examination, psychometric test, funduscopic findings, and compensatory parameters investigated by means of the computerized lumbar infusion test [2] were compared with each other in four groups. The groups were formed, taking into consideration the resistance to CSF outflow and the resting ICP level measured during the initial phase of the test. Although this way of differentiation of hydrocephalus seems to be artificial, it characterizes well the current stage of the disease with respect to the conditions of the CSF circulation within the cerebrospinal fluid compartments.

Group I: ICP < 8 mmHg, RCSF < 8 mmHg/ml/min; $n = 9$.

Only enlarged ventricles show that pathological changes in the brain are advanced. Because of the normal compensation, they have a rather atrophic character.

Group II ICP < 10 mmHg, RCSF > 12 mmHg/ml/min; $n = 18$.

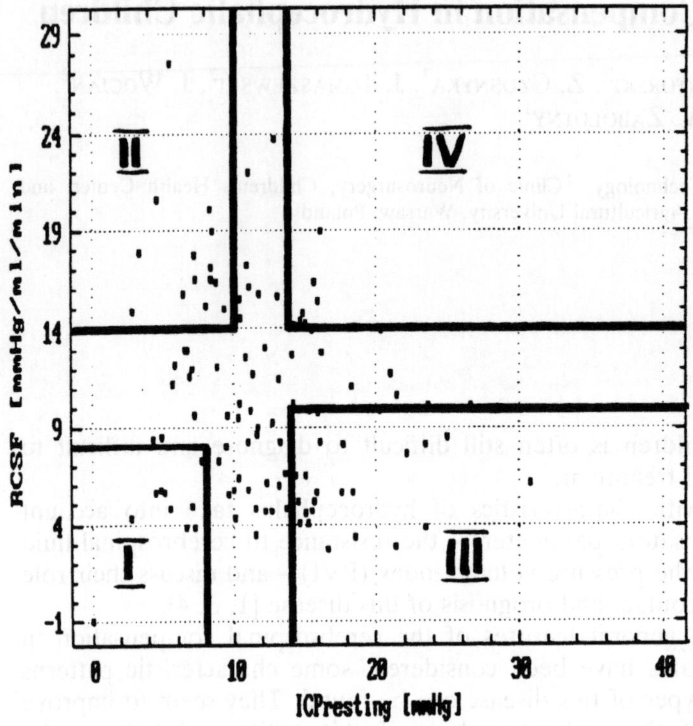

Fig. 1. 117 cases of hydrocephalus in children, expressed as points on a resistance to CSF outflow (y-axis) vs ICP resting level (x-axis) plane. The four groups: *I* atrophy or normalcy, *II* normal pressure hydrocephalus, *III* obturative hydrocephalus, *IV* acute or malresorptive hydrocephalus are indicated on the plot

Normal pressure hydrocephalus; low ICP level with an increased resistance to CSF outflow.

Group III: ICP > 14 mmHg, RCSF < 10 mmHg/ml/min; n = 28.

Normal resistance to CSF outflow with an increased ICP in the lumbar subarachnoid space needs some comments. Almost all the confirmed cases of hydrocephalus caused by obstacles in pathways of the CSF circulation are present here (Dandy Walker syndrome, aqueductal stenosis, arachnoid cyst etc.). These can be named "non-communicating" or "obturative" types of hydrocephalus. A high ICP in the lumbar subarachnoid space can be explained by the considerably high transmantle pressure gradient, which causes a narrowing of the CSF flow routes at the brain convexity, which in turn increases the ICP in the subarachnoid space by an introduction of additional nonlinear resistance to the CSF flow. This resistance is rapidly diminished during the lumbar infusion due to the provoked decrease in the transmantle gradient. Hence, normal RCSF is still measured in this group.

Group IV: ICP > 14 mmHg, RCSF > 14 mmHg/ml/min; n = 7.

This group is named "Acute" because of increased ICP and RCSF – i.e. malresorptive hydrocephalus in its uncompensated stage.

There are several cases (n = 55) lying within the border zone. The formal aim of further considerations is to find criteria to classify these "uncertain" cases. The distribution of etiological factors in the discussed groups is given in Table 1.

Results

The results of the clinical, psychometric, funduscopic examinations and the results of the pressure-volume study are given in Table 2. A correlation between the resting pressure level and the resistance to CSF outflow was found only in the fourth group (acute hydrocephalus): r = 0.81, RCSF = 2.85*ICP-24.32; $p < 0.026$.

In the remaining three groups, a significant correlation was found between the resistance and end-equilibrium ICP reached during the infusion test. There was no correlation between RCSF and cerebrospinal elasticity in any of the groups.

Table 1. The distribution of etiological factors in the four patient groups

	Group 1	Group 2	Group 3	Group 4
Congenital malformation	33%	22%	25%	14%
Birth trauma	66%	44%	32%	0%
CNS infection	11%	11%	7%	71%
Epilepsy	22%	27%	57%	14%
Head injury	0%	11%	0%	0%

Table 2. Results of pressure-volume study, clinical, CT and funduscopic findings in the 4 groups of hydrocephalus (mean/standard deviation)

	Group 1	Group 2	Group 3	Group 4
Resting ICP (mmHg)	5.7/1.6	7.0/1.9	18.1/4.1	15.3/2.5
Resting pulse wave amplitude-AMP (mmHg)	3.8/3.6	2.2/1.1	5.3/3.3	3.5/1.5
Slope of AMP/ICP regression line (n.s.)	0.43/0.29	0.32/0.15	0.36/0.17	0.4/0.18
Resist. to CSF outflow (mmHg/ml/min)	5.1/1.1	16.7/3.6	6.4/2.3	15.5/1.7
Pressure-volume index PVI (ml)	19.4/13	20.3/16	41.3/41	16.2/6
Estimator of CSF formation (ml/min)	1.07/0.64	0.37/0.18	2.41/1.5	0.54/0.4
Time constant TAU (min)	18.6/21	38/34	6.53/4	24/9
ICP*AMP (mmHg*mmHg)	24.2/27	16.5/9	99/75	54/9
RMS distance between real and predicted ICP	0.438/0.43	0.89/0.38	0.97/1.22	1.69/2
Age (months)	42/41	24/17	47/51	51/63
Head circumference (% deviation from 50 percentile of norm)	7/7.6	8.2/6	7.4/6.5	7.9/6.8
Evans' ratio	0.58/0.18	0.52/0.1	0.47/0.17	0.60/0.13
Psychomotor development (Brunet-Lezine test)	5.1/0.9	4.2/1.1	4.9/1.3	5/1
Funduscopic picture	1.5/0.25	2.25/1.8	2.1/1.6	2.1/1.4

1, no changes; 2, stasis; 3, oedema; 4, atrophy

Discussion

The first group can be considered as a norm – without a remarkable deficit in the compensatory reserve. The only pathological symptom here is the enlargement of the ventricles and an accelerated head growth. Both funduscopic and psychometric results are normal. As for compensatory parameters, several significant features of this group can be listed:

- there is a significantly lower mean ICP to pulse wave amplitude ratio;
- there is the lowest root mean square distance between the real and theoretical trends of ICP. It may reflect the commonly observed phenomenon that the pressure trend in atrophic patients is almost perfectly smooth-without any vasomotor artifacts and disturbances.

The second group (NPH) is specific with respect to:

- the lowest level of the resting pulse wave amplitude,
- the lowest (and the nearest to the physiological norm) level of the estimator of the cerebrospinal fluid formation (with the exception of the lack of a significant difference with the acute hydrocephalus group),
- the longest time-constant,
- the highest RCSF to resting pulse wave amplitude ratio.

The third group is specific with respect to:

- the highest level of the pulse wave amplitude,
- the highest value of the CSF formation rate estimator,
- the shortest time-constant,
- the highest value of the pressure-volume index,
- the highest level of the pulse wave amplitude and mean ICP product.

The fourth group of the acute hydrocephalus is specific with respect to:

- the same level of CSF formation rate estimator as in the NPH group, significantly higher than in the first and third groups,
- the highest level of the mean square distance between the real ICP and theoretical trends.

There are differences between this group and the NPH group – i.e. the lower time-constant and higher pulse wave amplitude. The differentiation between this group and NPH can be made, taking into account its significantly lower pressure volume index and longer time-constant.

The Evans' ratio and psychomotor development do not differ significantly between the groups (however, the largest Evans' ratio is in the fourth group). The funduscopic changes are slightly advanced in the three "active" groups relative to the first "atrophic" group. The highest head circumference was found in the NPH group (however not significant).

The above results show that in addition to ICP and the resistance to CSF outflow, the remaining cerebrospinal compensatory parameters can be helpful in the differentiation between the types of hydrocephalus. NPH can be considered as the compensated stage of acute hydrocephalus. Thus, this group differs only in parameters, showing a better buffering capacity than in acute stages (i.e. lower ICP level, pulse wave amplitude, and longer cerebrospinal time-constant). Acute hydrocephalus is undoubtedly the stage where the increased RCSF is responsible for the increased resting ICP. Therefore, the highest correlation between RCSF and ICP was found in this group. It is also specific to the highest rate of vasomotor disturbances during the infusion test, demonstrating low cerebrospinal compensatory reserve.

Group III, which contains several types of obturative hydrocephalus, is characterized by good compensatory ability – manifested by the highest PVI, the highest pulse wave amplitude and ICP*AMP product, and the shortest time-constant. This may support the dynamic compensation hypothesis by the shifts of the brain mantle, due to the changes in ventriculo-subarachnoid pressure gradient.

The differentiation between these three groups of "active" hydrocephalus and the atrophic (No 1) group is not difficult if we take into account other compensatory parameters. The most important problem of finding the difference between this and the NPH group can be solved taking into consideration such parameters as pulse wave amplitude and CSF formation estimator.

References

1. Børgesen SE, Gjerris F, Fedders O, Schmidt JF, Albeck MJ, Scelberg-Sørensen P (1989) Measurement of Resistance to CSF outflow-clinical experiences in 333 patients. In: Hoff JT, Betz AL (eds), Intracranial Pressure VII, Springer, Berlin Heidelberg New York London Paris Tokyo Hong Kong, pp 353–355
2. Czosnyka M, Batorski L, Laniewski P, Maksymowicz W, Koszewski W, Zawcrski W (1990) A computer system for the identification of cerebrospinal compensatory model. Acta Neurochirurgica (Wien), 105:112–116
3. Shapiro K, Fried A, Marmarou A (1985) Biomechanical and hydrodynamic characterization of the hydrocephalic infant, J. Neurosurg 63:69–75
4. Tans JTJ, Poortvliet DCJ (1989) Does Compliance Predict Ventricular Reduction After Shunting for Normal Pressure Hydrocephalus. In: Hoff JT, Betz AL (eds), Springer, Berlin Heidelberg New York London Paris Tokyo Hong Kong, pp 386–389

Surgical Vs. Non Surgical Treatment of Neonatal Intraventricular Hemorrhage

F.W. GAMACHE, JR., and M. BILSKY

The New York Hospital-Cornell Medical Center, Department of Neurological Surgery, 525 East 68th Street, New York, NY 10021, USA

Introduction

The advent of the neonatal intensive care unit has brought improved survival for all neonates, particularly those suffering from what has been recognized as a common problem: neonatal intraventricular hemorrhage. Neonatal intensivists have become very familiar with the complications of neonatal intraventricular hemorrhage, and the associated problems with intracranial pressure management. From their experience at The New York Hospital-Cornell Medical Center, the authors have made an effort to identify similarities and differences between babies whose elevated intracranial pressure was successfully managed medically as opposed to those for whom diversion of ventricular fluid was necessary.

Material and Methods

The charts of 130 neonates treated nonsurgically for neonatal intraventricular hemorrhage were randomly chosen for review for the treatment period of 1984–1989.

Results

Sixty-eight of the 130 babies had hemorrhage outside the ventricle in addition to having intraventricular hemorrhage. Seventy-nine of the 130 babies were judged radiographically to have mild or moderate hydrocephalus; no baby had severe hydrocephalus. One hundred eighteen babies experienced respiratory distress syndrome requiring prolonged periods of assisted ventilation. Cardiac abnormalities requiring pediatric cardiology attention, episodes of documented generalized sepsis, and necrotizing enterocolitis were frequently encountered as well. Of interest, a history of maternal drug abuse during pregnancy was elicited in 10% of cases. Seizures occurred in approximately 25% of babies experiencing intracranial intraventricular hemorrhage who were managed medically.

Follow-up was available for 77 babies. Evaluations were performed by pediatricians employing simple evaluation forms. Thirty-two babies were judged to be developmentally normal, 45 were judged to be developmentally abnormal. There were 26 deaths among the 130 babies due in decreasing frequency to refractory cardiac problems, pulmonary failure, sepsis, and multi systems failure.

During the same interval 54 babies were treated with ventricular diversion procedures because of elevated intracranial pressure and expanding ventricular volume. This occurred despite serial lumbar punctures or ventricular taps. Mean gestation, apgar scores, and mean birth weights were not significantly different compared to the non surgical group. Twenty-five of the 54 babies had extraventricular hemorrhage in addition to the intraventricular hemorrhage. Hydrocephalus, however, was judged radiographically as being severe in 22 of the 54 babies and moderate to severe in 29 of the babies. None of the babies had mild hydrocephalus. The initial ventricular diversion procedure generally occurred eight weeks after birth. Forty-one babies underwent a single shunt revision, 11 a second revision, and 3 a third revision. Ventricular catheter obstruction accounted for 14 revisions and distal catheter obstruction for 11. Nineteen of the 25 obstructions were associated with prior ventriculitis or peritonitis. Thirteen revisions resulted because of system colonization from generalized sepsis. Five shunts were revised because of hardware distraction. Sixty % of the shunted babies experienced seizures.

Forty babies were available for follow-up. Eight of these were judged as normal and 32 as abnormal by examining pediatricians. Eleven deaths occurred in the surgical group. These occurred between 4 and 39 weeks following surgery. Deaths occurred because of refractory cardiopulmonary failure.

Discussion

While the incidence of periventricular and intraventricular hemorrhage has decreased in recent years, the management of neonatal intraventricular hemorrhage remains controversial. Diversion of ventricular fluid for a baby who has failed with conservative measures (in controlling expanding head size), is generally considered reasonable and appropriate. A good review of the management of hydrocephalus secondary to intracranial hemorrhage in the newborn has been provided by James, et al. [2]. Lumbar punctures, ventricular punctures, ventricular reservoirs, and ventriculostomies have been used at this institution as recommended by others. Ventriculo-peritoneal shunts were used when repeated drainage over a prolonged period of time appeared necessary to maintain ventricular and head size. The most obvious difference between the medically managed versus the surgically managed patients is suggested by the fact that medically managed patient's had mild to moderate hydrocephalus, while the majority of the surgical patients had either frankly severe or moderate to severe hydrocephalus. A remarkable difference between the two groups is also suggested by the difference in the incidence of seizures: 25% (medical) vs. 75% (surgical). This likely reflects the greater degree of brain injury (i.e. more devastating hemorrhage) rather than simple hydrocephalus. This is also reflected in the developmental evaluations i.e. just under half of the medically managed babies were judged to be developmentally normal, where as about 20% of those babies requiring ventricular diversion was judged to be developmentally normal. Similar findings have been observed by other neonatologists [1]. Death rates were approximately the same for the two groups.

Of particular interest to the surgical community is the high number of reoperations in neonates undergoing VP-shunts. Approximately half of the reoperations were associated with either proximal or distal obstructions and 1/3 were due to sepsis during the course of neonatal intensive care stay.

Management of intracranial hypertension remains a challenge for the pediatric intensive care physician as well as the neurosurgeon. Generalized infection in the form of sepsis complicates the integrity of the ventriculo-peritoneal shunting hardware and exposes the system to either blockage (because of the development of inflammatory tissue) or colonization requiring shunt removal and replacement. Since sepsis occurs frequently in these high risk neonates it provides a constant problem for ventricular fluid diversion devices.

References

1. Boynton BR, Boyton CA, Merritt TA, Vaucher YE, James HE, Bejar RF (1986) Ventricular Peritoneal Shunts in Low Birth Weight Infants with Intracranial Hemorrhage: Neuro-development Outcome. Neurosurgery 18:141–145
2. James HE, Bejar R, Merritt TA, Gluck L, Coen R, Mannino F (1984) Management of Hydrocephalus Secondary to Intracranial Hemorrhage in the High Risk Newborn. Neurosurgery 14:612–618

CSF Shunts

The Effect of Body Position on Cerebral Blood Flow in Normal Subjects and Subjects with Shunts

S. Higashi[1], J. Yamashita[1], H. Matsuda[2], M. Hashimoto[1], K. Futami[1], and M. Hasegawa[1]

[1] Departments of Neurosurgery and [2] Nuclear Medicine, School of Medicine, Kanazawa University, Kanazawa

Introduction

The introduction of shunt systems with differential-pressure valves has proven to be a definite advance in the treatment of hydrocephalus. However, some problems still remain unsolved. The variety of valves available on the market today is partly related to them. These problems include extracerebral fluid collection, subdural hematoma, overdrainage syndrome, slit ventricle syndrome, trapped ventricle syndrome, post-shunt craniosynostosis, spinal canal stenosis, and spontaneous pneumocephalus. Complications due to overdrainage are directly related to the hydrodynamic characteristics of valves. The negative pressure associated with CSF shunts has been cited as a cause of subdural hematoma after placement of the shunt. It may also be manifested as postural headache, nausea, lassitude, and diplopia; overdrainage syndrome or orthostatic intracranial hypotension [2]. This troublesome problem has stimulated considerable effort to design new valves and other shunt devices to resolve it [6]. Currently a new shunt system with a variable-resistance valve, operating as a flow regulator, was developed by Sainte-Rose et al. [7].

Recent studies have shown that, when the head is elevated, normal subjects have ventricular fluid pressure (VFP) near atmospheric pressure in the supine position or upright position, and those who have shunts with differential-pressure valves develop significantly negative VFP [1]. Although many authors have investigated the effect of body position on VFP in subjects having a variety of shunt types, they disregard the dynamic changes in cerebral perfusion pressure (CPP) as well as cerebral blood flow (CBF). In this report, we describe these dynamic changes and pathogenesis of the overdrainage syndrome.

Materials and Methods

This series included 30 hydrocephalic patients of various causes and 5 normal subjects. They were divided into 4 subgroups: 12 subjects who received shunts with differential-pressure valves, 8 who received shunts with variable-resistance valves, 10 with hydrocephalus who had not received shunts, and 5 normal subjects.

CBF measurements were performed using technetium-99m hexamethylpropyleneamine oxime (^{99m}Tc HM-PAO). Single photon emission computerized tomographic (SPECT) images were obtained both in the sitting position and supine position using the following subtraction technique. For the first step, 20 mCi of ^{99m}Tc HM-PAO was injected intravenously with the patient in the sitting position. Five minutes after the injection, acquisition of projection data was started with the patient lying supine to obtain SPECT images of sitting position. For the second step, without any change in the patient's head position, the additional dose of 20 mCi of HM-PAO was injected. Five minutes after the injection, the second data acquisition was started in the same manner as in the first. After reconstruction, the tomographic images in the first step were subtracted from the images in the second step to obtain those of supine position. Regions of interest (ROIs) were drawn over the frontal, temporal, and parietal cortex of transaxial tomographic images. Activity counts of ROIs of sitting position images were compared with those of supine position images, then the percent change of regional CBF in the sitting position (regional %ΔCBF) was calculated in each ROI as follows:

$$\text{regional } \%\Delta CBF = 100(CBF_{sit} - CBF_{sup})/CBF_{sup},$$

where CBF_{sit} and CBF_{sup} are the activity counts of each ROI of sitting and supine position images, respectively. The percent change of mean CBF in the sitting position (mean %ΔCBF) was taken as the average value of regional %ΔCBF.

Results

Mean %ΔCBF was 24.9 ± 14.9% (mean ± SD) ($p < 0.05$) in the differential-pressure group, 5.0 ± 10.3% in the variable-resistance group, 3.6 ± 7.0% in the hydrocephalus group, and 4.5 ± 5.0% in the normal group (Fig. 1). In either normal or hydrocephalic subjects, there was no significant difference in mean CBF between supine and sitting position. The %ΔCBFs in the subjects with variable-resistance valves were similar to those in normal subjects. In contrast, significant augmentation of ΔCBF occurred in subjects with differential-pressure valves. With regard to regional %ΔCBF, there was no significant regional difference in all subgroups.

Only four of the 12 patients with differential-pressure valves developed symptoms of headache, nausea, and lethargy after shunt placement, which were affected by posture and were quickly relieved by recumbency. The mean %ΔCBFs of these 4 patients were significantly larger; 51, 46, 40, and 38%, respectively. None of the 8 patients with variable-resistance valves had posture-related symptoms.

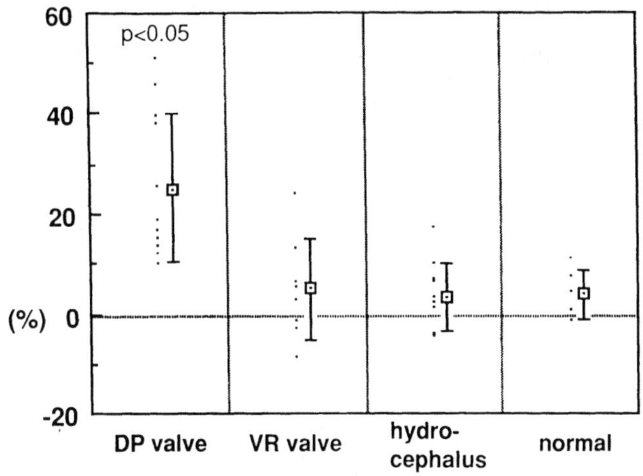

Fig. 1. Percent changes of mean CBF in the sitting position (mean ΔCBF) were as follows: differential-pressure group, 24.9 ± 14.9% ($p < 0.05$); variable-resistance group, 5.0 ± 10.3%; hydrocephalus group, 3.6 ± 7.0%; and normal group, 4.5 ± 5.0% (mean ± SD)

Discussion

A number of investigators have examined the problem of postural intracranial pressure changes by direct ventricular cannulation [3]. Recently, Chapman et al. reported the relationship between VFP and body position in normal subjects and subjects with shunts using a chronically implanted telemetric pressure sensor [1]. Review of these reports makes it clear that people who have shunts with a differential-pressure valve develop significantly negative VFP in the upright position. Although the effect of body position on VFP has been investigated in subjects having a variety of shunt types, it disregards the dynamic changes in cerebral perfusion pressure (CPP) as well as cerebral blood flow (CBF).

Currently we have investigated the effects of body position on cerebral perfusion pressure (CPP) in subjects having shunts with differential-pressure valves or variable-resistance valves, and in subjects without shunts (Fig. 2). CPP was taken as the difference between systemic arterial pressure (SAP) and VFP. The pressure values were referenced to the level of the foramen of Monro. In subjects without shunt (n = 3), as head elevation progressed, there was a gradual decrement in SAP from 87 mmHg in the supine position to 70 mmHg in the sitting position. The VFP similarly declined from 8.8 to 0 mmHg for the same head elevation. Because SAP declined faster than VFP, there was a net decrement in CPP; the average drop was from 79 to 70 mmHg). In subjects with variable-resistance valves (n = 6), posture-related changes in VFP and CPP were similar to those in subjects without shunts. In contrast, subjects with differential-pressure valves (n = 9) developed a significantly negative VFP of −17 mmHg in the sitting position. The CPP showed non-physiological augmentation from 86 to 94 mmHg. Although the effect of body

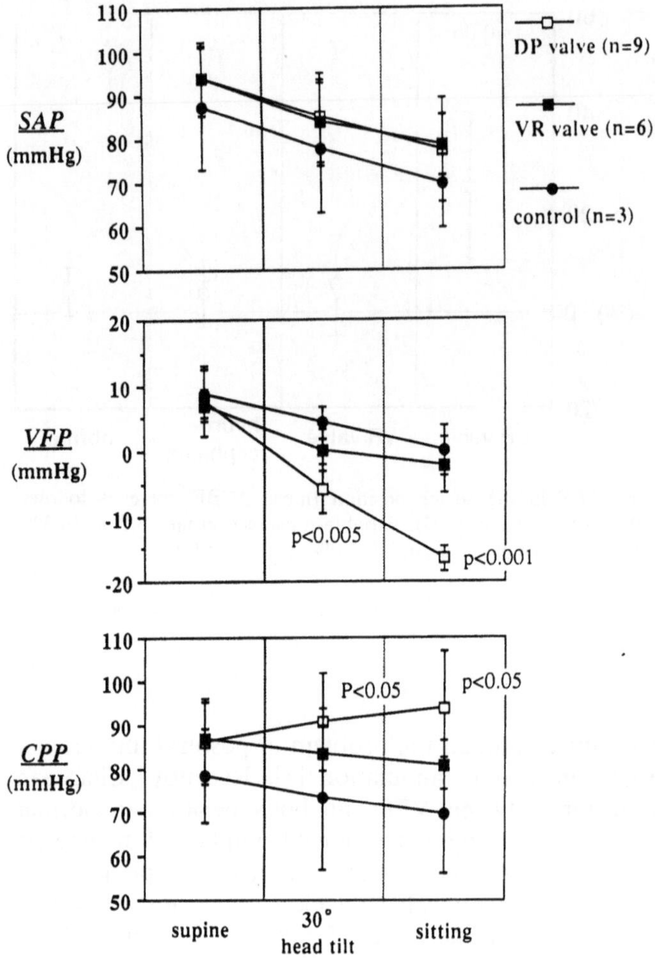

Fig. 2. The effects of body position on systemic arterial pressure (*SAP*), ventricular fluid pressure (*VFP*), and cerebral perfusion pressure (*CPP*), respectively, in subjects having shunts with a differential-pressure valve or a variable-resistance valve, and in subjects who have normal VFP without shunt

position on CPP has been demonstrated by this study, its effects on CBF remains unknown. Our purpose in this report was to measure the effect of body position on CBF in subjects having a variety of shunt types. These results were compared with similar observations in groups of subjects without shunts.

^{99m}Tc HM-PAO has the specific property of excellent retention at steady state. Its distribution pattern in brain tissue is determined in a short period and kept for a long time after intravenous injection. This property is quite useful for evaluating perfusion changes during interventional studies of short duration [5]. We applied this property to investigate perfusion changes during the sitting position. Regional CBF was measured in the cortex of whole lobes except the occipital lobe, because CBF of the occipital cortex may be influenced by visual activation.

To the best of our knowledge, this is the first report of postural changes of CBF in hydrocephalic patients with or without shunts and in normal subjects. Significant augmentation of CBF on sitting up occurred only in patients with differential-pressure valves. In other subgroups, there was no significant difference between mean CBF in the supine and sitting position. In addition, only 4 patients with differential-pressure valves developed an overdrainage syndrome, and their mean ΔCBFs in the sitting position were the largest four of all.

Postural overdrainage syndrome has been attributed to a negative ICP secondary of overdrainage of CSF [2]. While most of shunted patients have a significantly negative VFP, symptomatic overdrainage is not present in the majority of those patients. The explanation for this is not clear. Our results provide sound evidence that augmentation of CBF as well as negative VFP on head elevation may be closely related to the postural symptoms. Similar symptoms due to an increase in CBF have been reported in other situations such as hyperperfusion or luxury perfusion syndrome after carotid endarterectomy or extracranial to intracranial bypass surgery [4, 8].

The explanation for this non-physiological increase in CBF on sitting up in shunted patients having differential-pressure valves is not clear. It may be related to disturbed cerebral autoregulation. As emphasized by Portnoy et al., the conventional shunt valves function on the basis of a pressure differential across the device [6]. Conventional shunts with differential-pressure valves create a simple hydrostatic system, once the opening pressure of the valve has been exceeded. This typically occurs on head elevation greater than 30°. As a result, the valve will only close when the VFP is sufficiently negative to offset the hydrostatic pressure difference. As mentioned above, non-physiological augmentation of CPP occurs in such a situation. When CPP elevation occurs under intact cerebral autoregulation, vasoconstriction of arterioles will follow to prevent non-physiological augmentation of CBF. If autoregulation of the cerebral vessels is disturbed, extraordinary increase of CBF, or luxury perfusion, may occur [4, 8]. In contrast, patients having variable-resistance valves did not develop negative VFP on head elevation. Therefore, postural changes of CBF and CPP in patients having this kind of valves were similar to those in normal subjects. As a result, patients with this type of valves do not develop the overdrainage syndrome. The variable-resistance valve appears to be more physiological than differential-pressure valve.

References

1. Chapman PH, Cosman ER, Arnold MA (1990) The relationship between ventricular fluid pressure and body position in normal subjects and subjects with shunts: A telemetric study. Neurosurgery 26:181–189
2. Foltz EL, Blanks JP (1988) Symptomatic low intracranial pressure in shunted hydrocephalus. J Neurosurg 68:401–408
3. Fox JL, McCullough DC, Green RC (1973) Effect of cerebrospinal fluid shunts on intracranial pressure and on cerebrospinal fluid dynamics. 2. A new technique of pressure measurements: Results and concepts. 3. A concept of hydrocephalus. J Neurol Neurosurg Psychiatry 36:302–312

4. Higashi S, Matsuda H, Fujii H, et al. (1989) Luxury perfusion syndrome confirmed by sequential studies of regional cerebral blood flow and volume after extracranial to intracranial bypass surgery: Case report. Neurosurgery 25:85–89
5. Matsuda H, Higashi S, Asli IN, et al. (1988) Evaluation of cerebral collateral circulation by technetium-99m HM-PAO brain SPECT during Matas test: Report of three cases.
6. Portnoy HD, Schulte RR, Fox JL, et al. (1973) Antisiphon and reversible occlusion valves for shunting in hydrocephalus and preventing post-shunt subdural hematoma. J Neurosurg 38:729–738
7. Sainte-Rose C, Hooven MD, Hirsch JF (1987) A new approach to the treatment of hydrocephalus. J Neurosurg 66:213–226
8. Sundt TM, Jr. (1983) The ischemic tolerance of neural tissue and the need for monitoring and selective shunting during carotid endarterectomy. Stroke 14:93–98

Chronologic Changes in Intraventricular Pressure and Ventricular Size After Ventriculo-Peritoneal Shunt – Telemetric Measurement Using Osaka Telesensor (NS-20)

T. Ohta, H. Miyake, S. Nagasawa, Y. Nagano, and H. Tanabe

Department of Neurosurgery, Osaka Medical School, Osaka, Japan

Introduction

The indication for shunt procedures in normal pressure hydrocephalus (NPH) has been extensively investigated, including RI cisternography using ^{131}I-RIHSA, CSF absorption using artificial CSF, clinical improvement after CSF withdrawal, cerebral blood flow (CBF), and continuous intraventricular pressure (IVP) monitoring. However, there are only few reports on chronologic changes in the intracranial compartment after a shunt procedure. Shunt function has been evaluated by clinical symptomatology, ventricular size, continuous IVP monitoring, and shunt flow measurement, among which the continuous IVP monitoring is regarded as the most reliable method. In addition to the telemetric IVP sensor (Osaka Telesensor [8, 9] (NS-20); Nagano Keiki Seisakusyo Co. Ltd., Dow Cornig K.K.), our standard ventriculo-peritoneal (V-P) shunt method consisted of a Sophy's programmable hydrostatic pressure valve (Sophy valve) and an on-off flushing reservoir (on-off valve). The chronologic changes in IVP and ventricular size following V-P shunt operation, especially their relation to the postural IVP change, are reported.

Operative Procedure

The operative procedure is basically the same as with the conventional V-P shunt, except for the right anterior horn puncture. A right frontal semicircular scalp incision is made and the Osaka telesensor is placed into the right frontal burr hole. Although the Osaka telesensor is small enough to be placed into a burr hole of the usual size, the outer table around the burr hole is enlarged in order to reduce the protrusion of the sensor. Also in this way, the abdominal catheter is not injured at the connection site of the Osaka Telesensor. The circumferential bony spur at the bottom of the burr hole should be removed. An on-off valve and a Sophy valve are placed on the chest wall. These valves are implanted as superficially as possible.

Materials and Methods

Thirty-nine hydrocephalic patients underwent the V-P shunt operation as described above at the department of neurosurgery, Osaka Medical School hospital between March 1988 and May 1991. The etiology of the hydrocephalus was as follows: ruptured cerebral aneurysm in 19, ruptured cerebral AVM in 3, brain tumor in 6, brain abscess in 2, idiopathic in 5, and other in 4 cases.

Chronologic Changes in IVP and Ventricular Size After V-P Shunt Placement

Chronologic changes in IVP and ventricular size after V-P shunt placement were investigated in 28 cases who showed clinical improvement after the shunt operation. IVP was measured daily for about an hour until the IVP had been stabilized. The condition 24 hours after shunt surgery with the on-off valve closed was regarded as control (equivalents of pre-operative condition). The initial pressure setting of the Sophy valve was decided depending on the control value as follows; the Sophy was set in "high(H)" at IVP $\geqslant$ 13 mmHg, "medium(M)" at 9 mmHg $\leqslant$ IVP $<$ 13 mmHg, and "low(L)" at IVP $<$ 9 mmHg. Pressure setting of the Sophy valve was corrected in some cases after considering the CT findings, IVP value, and clinical symptoms. Ventricular size was described as the bicaudate cranio-ventricular index (CVI) on CT scan. Clinical symptoms were evaluated by the level of consciousness (JCS: Japan Coma Scale [7]), urinary incontinence and gait disturbance.

Postural IVP Changes

Postural IVP changes were measured in the most recent 7 cases. Posture was changed from supine (0°) to upright position (90°). The postural IVP changes were investigated with regard two opening and closing of the on-off valve, control and post-operation, and among the three different pressure settings of the Sophy valve.

Results

Chronologic Changes in IVP and Ventricular Size After V-P Shunt

Three patterns of chronologic changes in IVP and ventricular size were observed after V-P shunt placement (Table 1). Type I: Both IVP and ventricular size decreased. Nineteen cases (ruptured cerebral aneurysm in 10, ruptured cerebral AVM in 3, brain tumor in 4, others in 2) belonged to this type. The average age of the patients with this type was 45.2 ± 20.1 years old. The average control IVP in type I was 18.6 ± 5.9 mmHg. Type II: Only IVP decreased after V-P shunt but not ventricular size. Seven cases (ruptured

Table 1. Summary of chronologic changes in IVP and ventricular size and the number of patients in each type

Type	Definition		Etiology					Total	Age (Mean ± SD)
	ICP	Ventricular Size	SAH	AVM	Tumor	Idiopathic	Others		
I	↘	↘	10	3	4		2	19	45.2 ± 20.1]*
II	↘	→	2		2	2	1	7	66.7 ± 8.9]*
III	→	↘	1				1	2	51.5

* $P < 0.05$

cerebral aneurysm in 2, brain tumor in 2, idiopathic in 2, other in 1) belonged to this type. The average age in this type was 66.7 ± 8.9 years old. The average control IVP value in this type was 13.3 ± 6.7 mmHg. Type III: Only ventricular size decreased after V-P shunt but not IVP. Two cases (ruptured cerebral aneurysm and brain abscess) belonged to this type. Statistical analysis could not be completed because of the small numbers. A typical case in Type I and II is presented.

Case 1 (Fig. 1a)

This was a 41 year-old male with NPH after subarachnoid hemorrhage. The bicaudate CVI was 35% on pre-operative CT scan, which decreased to 24% in two days and 20% in nine days after operation. Control IVP in the supine position was 21 mmHg decreasing to 15 mmHg and 7 mmHg; clinical symptoms also improved. The initial pressure setting of the Sophy valve was "high" and it remained unchanged. This is a typical case of type I exhibiting a parallel decrease in both IVP and ventricular size.

Case 2 (Fig. 1b)

This was a 53 year-old female with NPH after subarachnoid hemorrhage. At first, both IVP and ventricular size did not change with the Sophy valve in the "high" setting. Three weeks after changing the pressure setting of the Sophy valve to "medium", only IVP decreased to 8 mmHg while the bicaudate CVI remained almost the same value.

Postural IVP Change

IVP fell with elevation of the bed. The slope of the IVP decrease was steep until around 30–45 degrees but became progressively less or even rose slightly beyond this degree. The initial IVP decline was steeper with the "on" setting of the on-off valve than with the "off" position. The initial IVP decline was

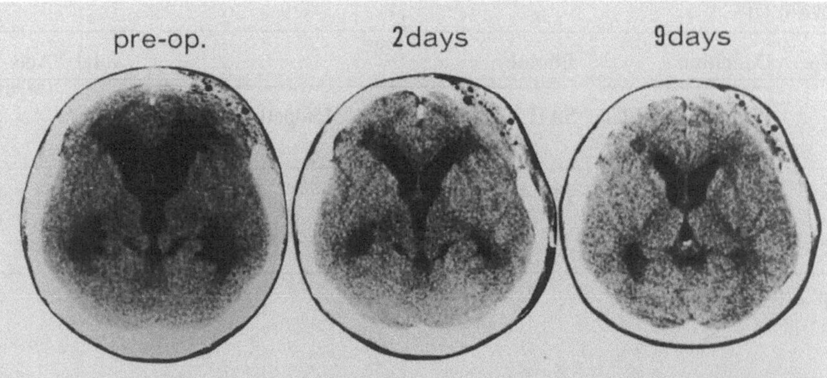

	pre-op.	2days	9days
BCI (%)	35	24	20
IVP (mmHg)	21	20	7
Sophy		(High)	(High)
JCS	1	1	0

a

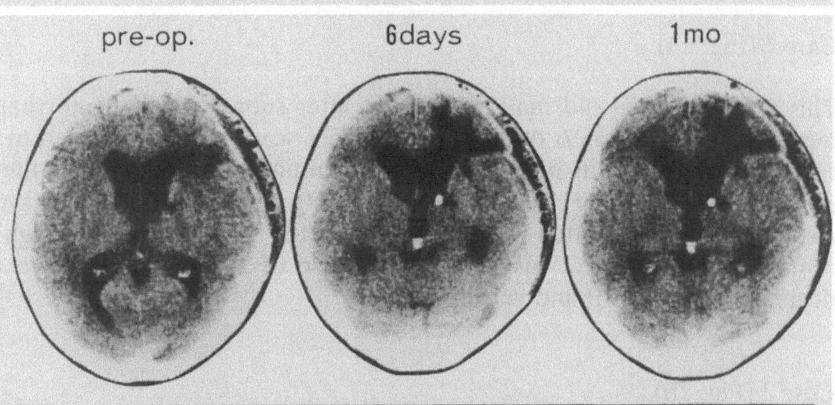

	pre-op.	6days	1mo
BCI (%)	25	28	26
IVP (mmHg)	15	15	8
Sophy		(High)	(Medium)
JCS	2	2	1

b

Fig. 1. **a** Chronologic changes in IVP, ventricular size and clinical findings in a Type 1 case. Both IVP and ventricular size decreased after shunt operation. JCS = Japan Coma Scale **b** Chronologic changes in IVP, ventricular size and clinical findings in a Type 2 case. IVP decreased after changing the pressure setting of the Sophy valve, from high to medium, but ventricular size remained unchanged

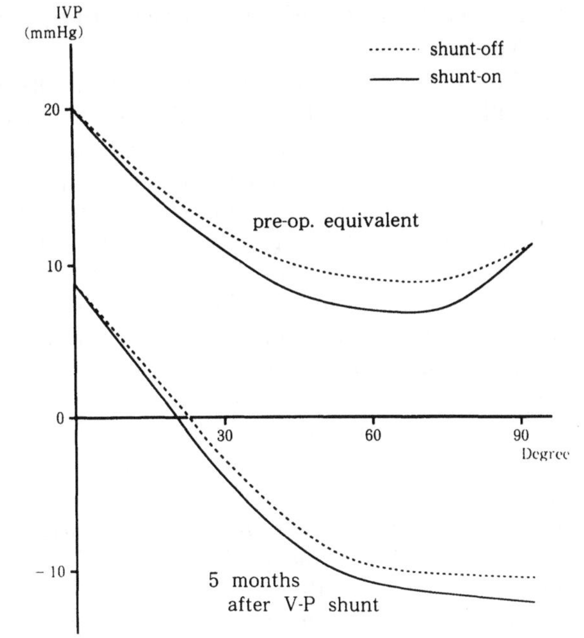

Fig. 2. Postural IVP changes in shunt-on and shunt-off positions, pre- and postoperatively

steeper in the post-operative than in the control condition. This was true even in the measurements with the on-off valve in the "off" position (Fig. 2). The IVP after shunt operation in the upright position was usually negative at a mean value of -10.7 mmHg ranging from -0.5 to -21 mmHg. The lower the pressure setting of the Sophy valve, the steeper the initial IVP declines.

Discussion

Few reports exist concerning the intracranial conditions after V-P shunt placement, because of the difficulty of long term ICP monitoring. The NS-20 makes this possible. Gücer, et al. [2] reported that eight out of seventeen hydrocephalic patients had stabilized in ICP after shunt operation. Yamaguchi, et al. [10] using the Osaka Telesensor, reported a decrease in IVP and disappearance of B waves after shunt operation. They also reported two types of IVP decline, one immediate and the other gradual; most of their cases belonged to the latter type. As reported previously, both CSF circulatory disturbances and organic brain damage should be considered in the pathophysiology of hydrocephalus [6]. It was found in our series that IVP and ventricular size did not always decrease simultaneously, demonstrating the complicated relationship between these two factors. We believe that in Type I, a CSF circulatory disturbance was the main cause of hydrocephalus and that the brain itself retains adequate plasticity. On the other hand, brain parenchymal damage as well as CSF circulatory disturbances are considered to be responsible for the hydrocephalus in Type II.

Postural IVP changes have been investigated by several authors. McCullough and Fox [5] reported that a negative IVP of around $-251\,mmH_2O$ could be produced by an upright position after the V-P shunt operation. This may cause a subdural hematoma as a complication of the V-P shunt. Magnaes [3, 4] reported on the effect of postural changes on lumbar CSF pressure. They proposed the concept of a "hydrostatic indifferent point", which means the "neutral point" with regard to the postural ICP change, and they concluded that this point shifted caudally after the shunt operation. Chapman et al. [1] reported the relationship between IVP and body position, using their telemetric pressure sensor. They found that a rapid decline in IVP occurred within the first 30 to 45 degrees during a postural change from supine to upright. They also concluded that the major contribution to postural regulation of ICP was the venous system. The initial slope with the "on" setting of the on-off valve became steeper just after turning the on-off valve to "on". This is believed to indicate that the shunt increased the intracranial compliance by expanding the buffering space of the CSF to the abdominal cavity. Comparing the initial slopes of the reduction curves, recorded in the control and post-operative conditions in the same patient who had exhibited clinical improvement, the slope in the latter condition was steeper, not only with the shunt open but also with the shunt closed. This may indicate that the brain compliance itself also improves after V-P shunt placement. Although there are some experimental reports, no clinical study of the Sophy valve has been performed in these intracranial pressure problems. The initial slope of IVP with postural change was found to differ depending on its preset pressure. This interesting finding requires further investigation.

References

1. Chapman PH, Cosman ER, Arnold MA (1990) The Relationship between Ventricular Fluid Pressure and Body Position in Normal Subjects and Subjects with Shunts: A Telemetric Study. Neurosurg 26:181–189
2. Gücer G, Viernstein L, Walker AE (1980) Continuous intracranial pressure recording in adult hydrocephalus. Surg Neurol 13:323–328
3. Magnaes B (1976) Body position and cerebrospinal fluid pressure. Part 1: Clinical studies on the effect of rapid postural changes. J Neurosurg 44:687–697
4. Magnaes B (1976) Body position and cerebrospinal fluid pressure. Part 2: Clinical studies on orthostatic pressure and the hydrostatic indifferent point. J Neurosurg 44:698–705
5. McCullough DC, Fox JL (1974) Negative intracranial pressure hydrocephalus in adults with shunts and its relationship to the production of subdural hematoma. J Neurosurg 40:372–375
6. Nakamura S, Koga N, Tsubokawa T, et al. (1980) Cerebral and Ventricular Changes after the Shunts Operation of the Hydrocephalus. Progress in CT 2:45–51
7. Ohta T, Kikuchi H, Hashi K, et al. (1986) Nizofenone administration in the acute stage following subarachnoid hemorrhage. Results of a multi-center controlled double blind clinical study. J Neurosurg 64:420–426
8. Ohta T, Yamashita M, Miyake H, et al. (1989) Detection of the site of V-P shunt malfunction using a telemetric IVP sensor. In: Hoff JT, Betz AL (eds), Intracranial Pressure VII, Springer, Berlin Heiderberg New York London Paris Tokyo Hong Kong, pp. 137–141

9. Osaka K, Murata T, Okamoto S, et al. (1981) Development of a New Completely Implantable Intraventricular Pressure Meter and Preliminary Report of Its Clinical Experience. Neurol Med Chir (Tokyo) 21:1051–1060
10. Yamaguchi Y, Yamaguchi T, Yanaki T, et al. (1990) The Changes of Intracranial Pressure after Shunt Surgery: Measurements of Pre- and postshunt ventricular fluid pressure with an implanted telemetric ICP sensor. Neurol Surg 18:175–182

Changes of ICP After Shunt Surgery for Hydrocephalus – Long Time Evaluation by Telemetric Sensors

J. Haraoka, S. Nakajima, Y. Takeda, T. Miki, and T. Miwa

Department of Neurosurgery, Tokyo Medical College 6-7-1 Nishishinjuku, Shinjuku-ku, Tokyo, 160, Japan

Introduction

It can be assumed that ICP in a patient with hydrocephalus, treated with a CSF shunt, is influenced in a complicated manner by his daily behavior and by the opening pressure of the shunt system.

However, the actual condition of post-shunt ICP is still obscure. Therefore, the authors conducted a clinical trial of monitoring post-shunt ICP by an implantable telemetric sensor for hydrocephalic patients, from the early to the late stage after operation. Some experiments on ICP monitoring were also performed employing a model simulating the post-operative state following shunt surgery, based on the data obtained by the above, implanted sensors.

Materials and Methods

Clinical Study

Eleven cases of non-hypertensive hydrocephalic patients (NPH) (8 cases: secondary to ruptured aneurysm, 2 cases: post-operative state of brain tumor, 1 case: idiopathic NPH) were included in this study. They were treated with a Pudenz type valve system (Heyer-Schulte, Chicago, USA) (5 cases, 4 of them with on-off valves), and with a programmable shunt system (S-3, SOPHY, Besançon, France). Telemetric ICP sensors (NS-50, Nagano Keiki, Tokyo, Japan) were implanted and connected with those systems. The ICP was monitored for a considerable time after operation (0–25 months). Even after all patients were discharged from the hospital and returned to their usual life, their ICP continued to be monitored.

ICP changes caused by alteration of posture from a recumbent to sitting position, were monitored in the chronic stage after operation for the 5 cases treated with the Pudenz type valve.

The examinations were carried out when the system was "on" (system, open) and "off" (system, closed) for the patients with an on-off valve.

The ICP of the 6 patients treated with the programmable valve were evaluated in the same manner as mentioned above. In these cases, ICP changes caused by alteration of the program modes, from low (opening pressure: 50 mmH_2O), medium (100 mmH_2O) to high (160 mmH_2O) were also analyzed.

Experimental Study

An experimental model simulating a CSF shunt with a programmable valve system, using the pump-injection method, was made to evaluate the pressure-flow curves in this system.

The model consists of a proximal chamber filled with water, by pump injection simulating the ventricular system, a ventricular tube connected with the ICP sensor and programmable valve, and a peritoneal tube draining into a distal chamber simulating the abdominal cavity.

Changes of ICP and out-flow volume caused by the tilt of the models from 0–90° and by the change of the program modes were monitored.

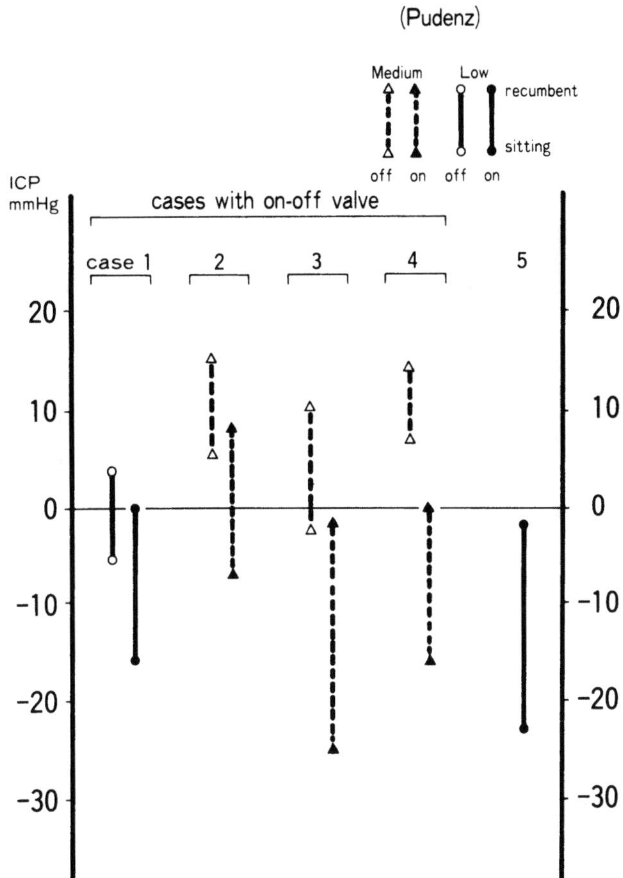

Fig. 1. Posture-related changes in ICP in 5 cases treated with Pudenz type valves (4 cases with on-off valves), monitored in 5 to 25 months after surgery

Results

Clinical Study

Serial monitoring of ICP after shunting, performed from the early to late stage after surgery, showed that the ICP became low, falling to zero and a negative value by 1 or 2 months after surgery and becoming fixed at the same level thereafter.

We monitored ICP changes caused by alteration of the posture of the 4 patients treated with a Pudenz type (with on-off) valve from a recumbent to sitting position, when the shunt systems were "off". ICP decreased by 7–12 mmHg (mean: 10.5 mmHg) by the alteration of posture.

However, when the shunt systems were set "on", the range of decrease in ICP became wide: 16–22 mmHg (mean: 18.3 mmHg) (Fig. 1).

The same maneuvers were performed in 6 patients with programmable valves, and ICP changes with alteration of program modes, from high to low, were also examined.

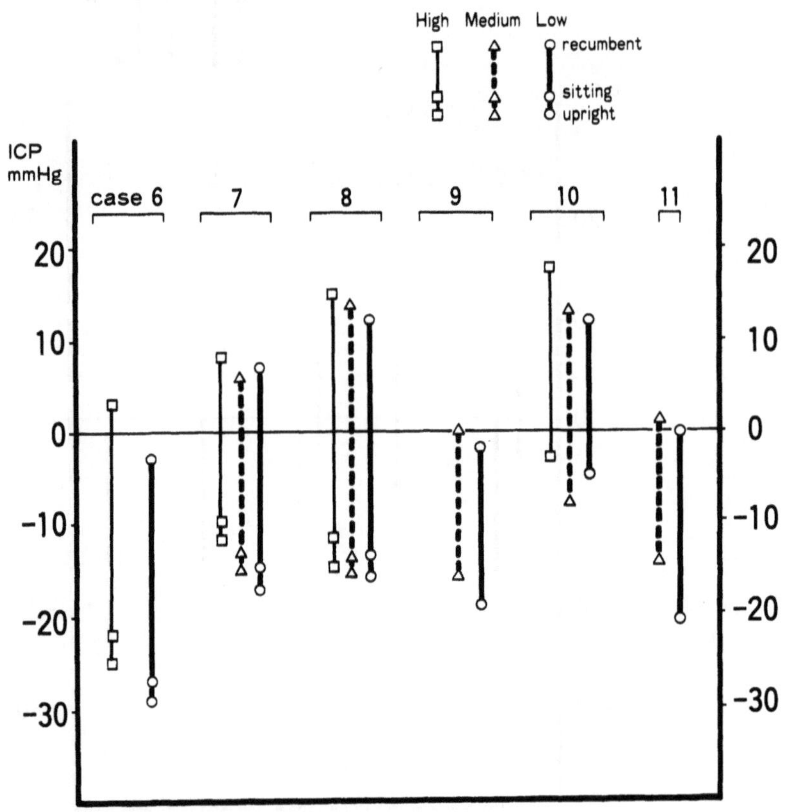

Fig. 2. Posture-related changes in ICP in 6 cases treated with programmable valves, monitored in 4 to 18 months following shunt surgery

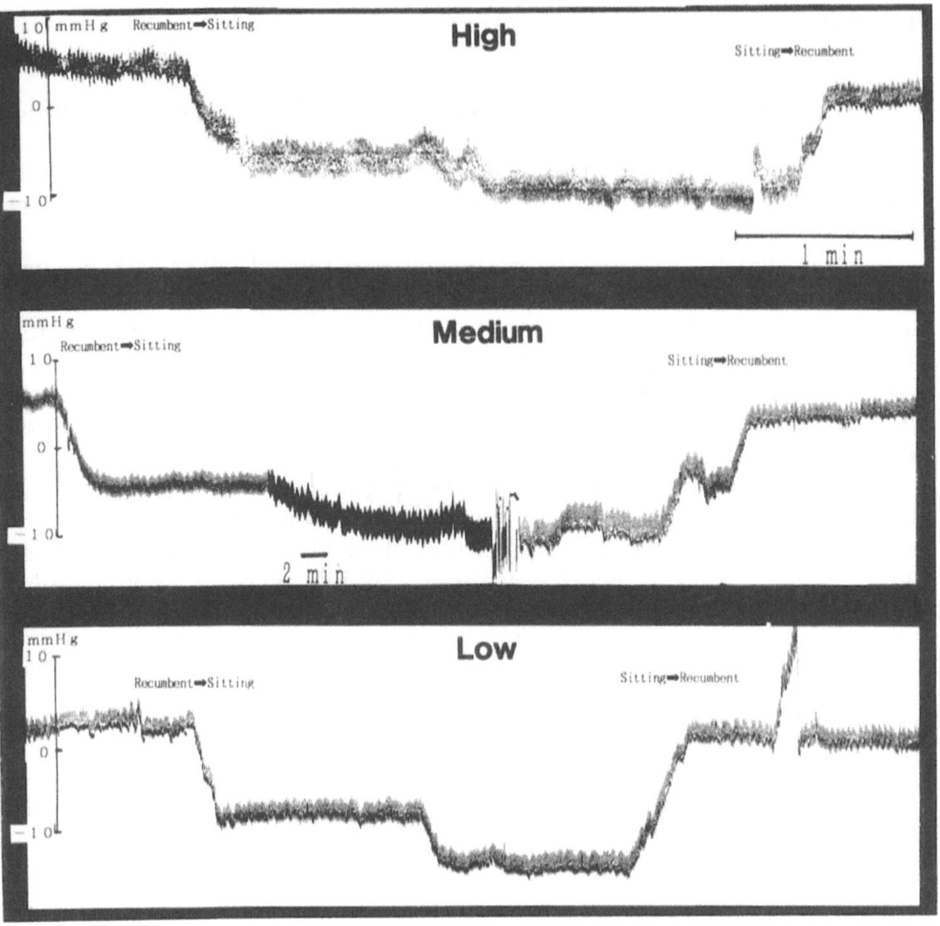

Fig. 3. Posture-related changes in ICP in case 7, 12 months after shunt surgery with programmable valve

Although a mean decrease in ICP of 20 mmHg was observed with alteration of posture, no significant drop caused by changes of the program mode, from high to low, was observed (Figs. 2, 3).

Experimental Model

When the system was set horizontally, adequate pressure-flow curves varying from 0.1 to 1.5 ml/min, were observed, corresponding with the pressure of the proximal chamber.

By tilting the system, ICP decreased, showing negative values. Pressure-flow curves were obtained in the same manner, even when ICP values were extremely low.

Discussion

ICP changes caused by the alteration of posture have been reported by various investigators [1, 2, 4, 5].

They reported that the ICP decrease was in the range of approximately 10 mmHg with a posture change from recumbent to sitting when the shunt system was "off".

In some studies [1, 3, 6], the posture change-related fall in ICP became more marked (18 to 27 mmHg) in the patients treated with ventriculo-peritoneal shunt (in our study: shunt system "on"), and their ICP values were significantly low, being as low as zero or even showing negative pressure.

It is believed that the hydrostatic pressure gradient between the ventricle and the abdominal cavity, caused by the alteration of posture, acts as a force to open the shunt valve even if the ICP itself is controlled at a low level.

The actual condition of ICP of the patients treated with shunt surgery is clearly demonstrated by this study. It is hoped that these methods will prove useful in preventing complications caused by the hydrostatic pressure gradient following surgery, such as low ICP syndrome, slit-like ventricle syndrome, and subdural hygroma.

References

1. Chapman PH, Cosman ER, Arnold MA (1990) The relationship between ventricular fluid pressure and body position in normal subjects and subjects with shunts: A telemetric study. Neurosurg. 26:181–189
2. Fox JL, McCullough DC, Green RC (1973) Effect of cerebrospinal fluid shunts on intracranial pressure and on cerebrospinal fluid dynamics. 2. A new technique of pressure measurements: Results and concepts. 3. A concept of hydrocephalus. J Neurol Neurosurg Psychiatry 36:302–312
3. McCullough DC, Fox JL (1974) Negative intracranial pressure hydrocephalus in adults with shunts and its relationship to the production of subdural hematoma. J Neurosurg 40:372–375
4. Lopman J, Myerson A, Goldman D (1935) Effect of alterations in posture on the cerebrospinal fluid pressure. Arch Neurol Psychiatry 33:1279–1295
5. Utsugi O (1990) Comparative study of intracranial environment before and after cranioplasty in decompressive craniectomized cases in chronic stage. J Tokyo Med Coll 48:584–597 (In Japanese)
6. Yamaguchi Y, Yamaguchi T, Yanaki T, Masuzawa N (1990) The changes of intracranial pressure after shunt surgery: Mesurements of pre- and postshunt ventricular fluid pressure with an implanted telemetric ICP sensor. Neurol Surg 18:175–182 (In Japanese)

Long Term in Vitro Test Results of Various New and Explanted Hydrocephalus Shunt Valves

H.A. Trost[1], G. Claussen[2], H.E. Heissler[2], and M.R. Gaab[2]

[1] Neurosurgical Department, University - GHS, 4300 Essen, Germany
[2] Neurosurgical Department, Medical School Hannover, Konstanty-Gutschow-Str. 8, 3000 Hannover 61, Germany

Introduction

Implantation of shunting devices for treatment of hydrocephalus has become a routine operation in most neurosurgical departments. Various shunting systems are available, some simple and some very sophisticated types. However, there is no consensus on which specifications a shunting device has to meet, which valve is the most physiological one, and how to control the function of an implanted device.

We, therefore, began routine testing of all explanted shunt valves and of samples of various new hydrocephalus shunt devices to get comparable pressure/flow diagrams and long term characteristics.

Materials and Methods

Thirty-two hydrocephalus shunt valves have been tested (Table 1). We test all valves explanted at our clinic in case of malfunction or infection and we have also tested various samples of new valves.

As test method we use a modified ASTM test [1]. The valves are perfused for 2 weeks with a) Ringer-Lactate and Ringer-Lactate with 5 g/l albumen. The resistive properties of a valve are determined by measuring the differential pressure at various flow rates (5, 10, 20, 40, 50 ml/h), perfusing for 1 hour at each flow rate, followed by an overnight perfusion (16 hours) at 20 ml/h. After perfusion of the valve under low flow for 1 week, the test is repeated a second time, and a third time after perfusing for another week. The first and second test are done with Ringer-Lactate, the third with Ringer-Lactate and 5 g/l albumen.

Results

The resulting pressure/flow characteristics and the results of the long term perfusion tests are given in Table 2.

Table 1.

Type of valve		Number of tested valves	
Codman	Holter medium	2 explanted	
Cordis	Hakim high	1 explanted	
	Hakim low	1 explanted	
	Orbis Sigma	1 explanted	2 new
Denver	Denver low		2 new
Holter-Hausner	normal	2 explanted	
	medium	5 explanted	
	low	1 explanted	
	very low	1 explanted	1 new
Medos Hakim	programmable 80 mmHg		1 new
	140 mmHg		
Neurone	Neurone medium		1 new
PS medical	medium + ASD		1 new
	medium	3 explanted	
	low	2 explanted	
Sophysa	Sophy SU 8 high		1 new
	Sophy SU 8 medium		1 new
	Sophy SU 8 low		1 new
Total		19 explanted	13 new

Conclusions

Manufacturers still have problems producing shunt valves with reliable pressure/flow characteristics. The best results, e.g. findings similar to the specifications of the manufacturer, were found in diaphragm valves (PS medical) and ball-spring valves (Cordis Hakim, Medos Hakim). These tests, however, are only suitable for simple pressure/flow relations. Hydrodynamic stress on hydrocephalus shunting devices during postural changes can only be covered by new test methods, simulating physiological conditions of cerebrospinal fluid [2, 5]. We, therefore, developed a model of cerebrospinal compartments, allowing the testing of hydrocephalus shunt devices under hydrodynamic pressure changes according to physiological relations [3, 4]. All available shunt valves without anti-siphon device will open in the upright body position (differential pressure head-abdomen up to 60 cm H_2O) and will be flushed at maximum flow dependent on the type of valve, thus clearing adhesions and obstructions. Maximum flow reaches values of more than 400 ml/h in low pressure ball and spring valves, thus leading to a steep fall in intracranial pressure. Slit and diaphragm valves have lower maximum flow

Table 2.

Valve type	Pressure/flow relation	Long-time reliability
Slit valves		
Codman Holter slit valve	inconstant deviation ± 100%	unstable adhesions
Neurone slit valve	extremely high deviation 200–800%	stable at too high pressure
Holter-Hausner cruciform slit valve	inconstant deviation 10–250%	mostly stable, some adhesions
Denver	deviation 200–400% sensitive to albumine	unstable, rise in pressure
Ball and spring valves		
Cordis Hakim	deviation <50%	stable
Programmable ball and spring valves		
Sophysa SU 8	deviation <100% sensitive to protein	unstable
Medos Hakim programmable	excellent values	stable
Diaphragm valves		
PS medical contoured	most values according manufacturer's specifications	stable
Selfadjusting diaphragm valves		
Cordis Orbis Sigma	"Sigma" shifted: critical range 20–30 ml/h	unstable under perfusion at 20–30 ml/h

values, thus leading to a markedly delayed fall in intracranial pressure. Antisiphon devices do prevent negative intracranial pressure even in the upright position, the selfregulating diaphragm valve almost simulates physiological cerebrospinal fluid pressure relations [4].

Acknowledgements. [1]We gratefully acknowledge the donation of valve samples by Codman (Codman GmbH, Am Hehsel 38/40, D-2000 Hamburg 63), Cordis (Cordis Deutschland GmbH, Max-Planck-Str. 20/22, D-4006 Erkrath) and Sophysa (Rehaforum Medical GmbH, Auf der Kaiserbitz 20, D-5000 Köln 90). The authors like to thank Mrs. Swanhild Fischer for her patience and competent support in preparing this paper.

References

1. American Society for Testing Materials (1980) Standard Practics for Evaluating and Specificying Implantable Shunt Assemblies for Neurosurgical Application. Annual Book of ASTM Standards. American National Standards Institute, New York, part 46, F 647
2. Keith HD, Watts C (1983) Testing of cerebrospinal fluid shunt systems under dynamics flow conditions. Medical Instrumentation 17:297–302
3. Trost HA, Heissler HE, Vokmann P, Gaab MR (1991) A new method for in vitro testing of hydrocephalus shunt systems. Poster presented at First European Conference on Biomedical Engineering, Nice, France, February 17–20, 1991

4. Trost HA, Heissler HE, Gaab MR (1991) Hydrocephalus shunt valves: clinical value of bench tests. Advances in Neurosurgery, in press
5. Yamada S, Ducker TB, Perot PL (1975) Dynamic changes of cerebrospinal fluid in upright and recumbent shunted experimental animals. Child's Brain 1:187–192

Flow-Regulating Devices Vs. Differential Pressure Valves in the Treatment of Triventricular Hydrocephalus

P.M. Rampini[1], M. Egidi[1], M.L. Zavanone[1], E.P. Sganzerla[1], A. Parma[2], and M. Farabola[3]

[1] Neurosurgery Institute, University of Milan; [2] Department of Anesthesiology and Intensive Care, and [3] Department of Neuroradiology, "Policlinico" Hospital of Milan, Milan, Italy

Introduction

A recent retrospective study of shunt failures in hydrocephalic patients proved that the percentage of failures is significantly higher in cases with slit ventricles [4]. In this respect, overdrainage seems to be responsible for either shunt obstruction or phenomena like shunt dependency, slit ventricle syndrome [5], subdural hematoma [2], and post-shunt craniostenosis.

The most important characteristic shared by all the conventional valves is that they offer a fixed preset resistance dependent on the differential pressure between the proximal end and the distal end of the shunt (differential pressure valves). With this type of valves, overdrainage can be considered constantly in standing patients, since in that position the draining capacity of the shunt exceeds the CSF secretion rate [3].

To obviate this problem a new type of shunt, which is able to operate as a "flow regulator" within certain differential pressure values, has been proposed.

To ascertain the effectiveness of this flow regulating valve in the treatment of hydrocephalus we implanted the shunt in a group of patients affected with chronic triventricular hydrocephalus (which is, in our opinion, the form of hydrocephalus more susceptible to overdrainage complications) and compared the results with a homogeneous group of patients treated with conventional shunt devices during the same period.

Patients and Methods

From January 1988 to December 1990 32 patients (study group) suffering from triventricular hydrocephalus under-went ventricular shunting with a flow regulating valve (Orbis-Sigma valve manufactured by Cordis). The patients were from 1 month to 77 years old (mean age 29.9 ± 25.5, median 23.5) and were affected with triventricular hydrocephalus due to different etiologies: the majority of them (14 cases) was non-tumoral aqueductal stenosis; in 9 cases the etiology was a tumor-related aqueductal stenosis, in 6 cases the hydrocephalus was associated with developmental anomalies and in 3 cases it had various etiologies.

All patients were clinically controlled for a follow-up period ranging from 6 months to 3 years (mean 13.7 ± 8.9, median 10.0). Control CT examinations were possible in 29 out of 32 patients. In these cases, using the Cella Media Index (CMI) as indicator [1], the preoperative and postoperative ventricular sizes were calculated. According to Gyldensted's data we used the 95th percentile (CMI = 6.8) as upper limit of normality. These values were obtained from the preoperative and postoperative CT scans performed at different times after the implant.

During the same period, 52 patients (control group) were treated for triventricular hydrocephalus with a conventional device (differential pressure valve). The clinical follow-up data were available for all cases, while preoperative and postoperative CT scan examinations were possible in 28 out of 52 patients.

Both groups (study group and control group) were analyzed as far as post-shunt complications and ventricular size modifications were concerned. Initial homogeneity of the study group versus the control group was statistically proven for sex, age, first implantation of a shunt device, etiology, preoperative CMI and follow-up period.

Statistical analysis of the data was performed according to SPSS/PC+ (Statistical Package for Social Sciences). Significance ($p < 0.05$) was tested by the Chi-Square Test and the Fisher Exact Test for categorical variables, and with parametric tests (T-Test for pairs and independent samples) and non-parametric tests (Mann-Whitney U Test, Median Test, Wilcoxon Matched-Pairs Signed-Ranks Test) for continuous variables. Parametric tests were utilized only if the examined data were normally distributed according to the One-sample Kolmogorow-Smirnow Test.

Results

Overdrainage

One out of the 32 study group patients (3.1%) developed an ex vacuo subdural hematoma 6 months after the shunt implant. In the control group 6 out of 52 patient (11.5%) presented symptoms due to overdrainage (3 cases of slit syndrome, 2 cases of subdural hematoma, 1 case of extradural hematoma). The etiology and the type of shunt for each patient are shown in Table 1.

Shunt Failure

Shunt malfunction occurred in 3 out of the 32 study group patients (9.4%), due to ventricular catheter obstruction in 2 cases and undetermined in the third one. In the control group shunt failure was observed in 5 out of 52 cases (9.6%); it was caused by distal slit valve obstruction in 3 cases and by ventricular catheter obstruction in 2 patients.

The overall frequency of post-shunt complications was 21.1% in the conventional valve group versus 12.5% in the flow-regulating valve group. In all

Table 1. Hydrocephalus etiology and type of valve in cases of overdrainage

Complication	Etiology	Valve
Slit syndrome	Aqued. stenosis	Pudenz middle p.
Slit syndrome	Aqued. stenosis	Raimondi middle p.
Slit syndrome	Posthemorrhagic	Raimondi middle p.
Extradural hematoma	Tum. aq. sten.	Raimondi middle p.
Subdural hematoma	Aqued. stenosis	Pudenz middle p.
Subdural hematoma	Aqued. stenosis	Sophy high p.
Subdural hematoma	Aqued. stenosis	Orbis-Sigma

Table 2. CMI measurements and percentage of change before and after shunt in the study group vs control group

	CMI pre (mean ± SD) (range) (median)	*CMI post* (mean ± SD) (range) (median)	*% of change* (mean ± SD) (range) (median)
Study group	3.4 ± 0.7	5.1 ± 1.5	54.1 ± 41.3
(n = 29)	1.6–4.8	1.8–8.0	9.1–160
	3.4	5.0	50.0
Control group	3.3 ± 0.7	5.7 ± 3.3	65.4 ± 69.2
(n = 28)	1.7–4.6	2.0–20.0	5.6–350
	3.3	5.1	47.0
Significance	N.S.	N.S.	N.S.

the other cases the preoperative symptomatology was satisfactorily controlled, independently of the type of implanted valve.

Ventricular Size Evaluation

The results of morphometric analysis are summarized in Table 2. Considering the ventricular size evaluated by CMI, 25 out of 29 patients in the study group (86.2%) and 25 out of 28 patients in the control group (89.3%) presented preoperatively enlarged or severely enlarged ventricles (CMI < 4.2). Post-operative CT scans showed a normalization of the ventricular sizes (CMI ranging from 4.2 to 6.8) in 16/29 study group patients (55.2%) and in 15/28 control group patients (53.6%).

Large ventricles (CMI < 4.2) on the postoperative control CT scans were observed in 8/29 (27.6%) patients of the study group and in 8/28 (28.6) patients of the control group. Slit ventricles (CMI > 6.8) occurred in 5/29 patients of the study group (17.2%) and in 5/28 cases of the control group (17.9%). Slit ventricles were associated with the clinical syndrome only in 3 cases of the control group. None of the observed morphometric differences were statistically significant.

Discussion and Conclusions

Initial homogeneity and comparability between the study group and the control group were statistically assessed; nevertheless, this is not a randomized study and a bias might be introduced because of the prevalent assignment to the study group of patients considered to be at a higher risk of overdrainage complications.

Post-shunt overdrainage occurred more frequently in the conventional valve group (11.5%) compared with the flow-regulating valve group (3.1%), suggesting a protective effect of the flow-regulating device against this complication. This difference, although not statistically significant, acquires much more value in consideration of the possible initial bias.

In contrast, the frequency of shunt failures was found to be quite similar in both groups (9.4% study group versus 9.6% control group).

The quantitative analysis of the postoperative ventricular size reduction showed no statistically significant differences between the study group and the control group. In particular, very small ventricles (CMI > 6.8) occurred in 5/28 control group patients (17.9%) compared to 5/29 study group patients (17.2%); however, only patients treated with conventional valves developed a relevant clinical slit ventricle syndrome (3 out of 5 with very small ventricles in this group), whereas no patient treated with flow-regulating devices suffered from overdrainage related symptoms in spite of a high ventricular size reduction (Fisher Exact Test: $p = 0.08$).

These data seem to suggest that the development of symptomatic post-shunt overdrainage phenomena (ex vacuo hematoma, slit ventricle syndrome) is related to the intrinsic valve working modality (differential pressure versus flow regulation) more than to post-shunt ventricular sizes.

On the basis of this study we believe that flow regulating valves may actually represent an effective and safe method for the treatment of triventricular hydrocephalus and that a reduction of post-shunt overdrainage complications can be expected with their clinical use.

References

1. Gyldensted C (1977) Measurements of the normal ventricular system and hemispheric sulci of 100 adults with computed tomography. Neuroradiology 14:183–192
2. Portnoy HD, Schulte RR, Fox JL, Croissant PD, Tripp L (1973) Anti-siphon and reversible occlusion valves for shunting in hydrocephalus and preventing post-shunt subdural hematomas. J Neurosurg 38:729–738
3. Sainte-Rose C, Hoffman MD, Hirsch JF (1987) A new approach in the treatment of hydrocephalus. J Neurosurg 66:213–226
4. Sainte-Rose C, Hoffman HJ, Hirsch JF (1989) Shunt failure. In: Marlin AE (ed) Concepts in Pediatric Neurosurgery, vol 9. Basel, Karger, pp 7–20
5. Serlo W, Saukkonen AL, Heikkinen E, Wendt L (1989) The incidence and management of the slit ventricle syndrome. Acta Neurochir (Wien) 99:113–116

Non-Invasive Quantification of CSF Flow in Shunts

J. RYDER[1], R.A. ZAPPULLA[1], C. DROST[2], A. DRAUDT[2], and A.M. ARON[1]

[1] Mt. Sinai Medical Center, Department of Neurosurgery, 1 Gustav Levy Place, New York, NY 10029, USA and [2] Transonics Systems Inc. Warren Road Business Park, 34 Dutch Mill Rd. Ithaca, NY 14850, USA

Introduction

The primary risk for patients with indwelling shunts is an acute failure of the system to relieve intracranial pressure (ICP) due to obstruction of cerebrospinal fluid (CSF) flow within the shunt tube. Cerebral hemodynamics provides for a certain amount of compliance and elasticity; however, a significant increase in the ICP can have catastrophic consequences for the patient. Shunt failure can be due to obstruction of the valves or occlusion of either the proximal or distal parts. The reported incidence of shunt failure which required revision, has varied among studies, in part due to the duration of the studies, with the lowest frequency being about 28% and the highest at 77% [2, 3, 5].

Determining the rate of CSF flow in a shunt is the best indicator of its function. Flow rates have been most accurately measured with externalized shunts. Recently, Drake et al. [1] monitored CSF output on nine children with ventriculostomies in whom they found a mean flow rate of 6.33 ml/hr with a range of 0.08 to 22.2ml/hr. Other studies report comparable findings, with CSF flow rates ranging from 0.6 to 115 ml/hr [4, 6]. The methods used to measure these exceedingly slow flow rates (an average of about 0.15 ml/min) have been based on indirect estimates of flow which could only be made periodically. The ideal flow device would offer a safe, accurate means to directly measure CSF flow for long periods of time and do so non-invasively. This report describes a new instrument that can quantify and monitor flow of CSF as low as 0.03 ml/min from outside the shunt tube. This technique does not require penetration of the tube, hence it can measure flow non-invasively, however, a tiny transducer and inductive coil would have to be implanted subcutaneously to allow measurement. The clinical utility of this system is discussed and compared to other existing measurement techniques.

Methods and Materials

A series of experiments was performed using a Transonics T106 Flowmeter and the 1R perivascular transducer (Transonic Systems Inc, Ithaca, NY) which utilize ultrasound techniques to quantify flow data. The 1R probe contains two transducers that bounce signals off a flat steel reflector which is attached

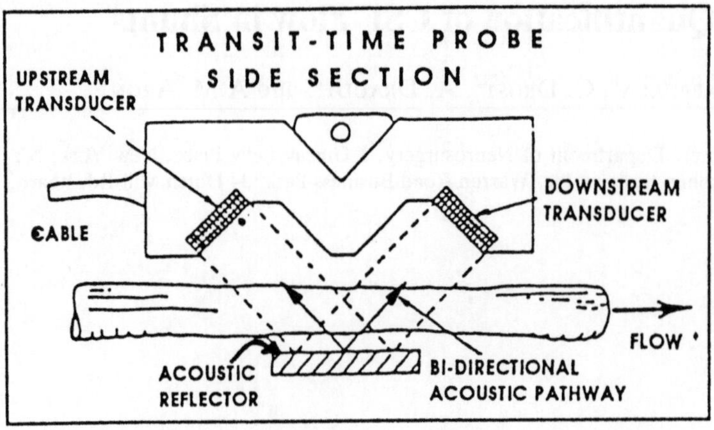

Fig. 1. This is a diagram of the Transonics 1R transducer, actual size is 6 mm × 6 mm × 3 mm. The acoustic reflector acts as a brace to hold the tube up against the probe.

around any shunt tube (Fig. 1). The flow rate is calculated by measuring the phase difference of the two acoustic signals as they travel across the tube and bounce back. This method is called "transit-time". The two transducers are placed against the wall of a tube at a 90 degree angle to each other so that when the acoustic signals bounce back there will be a difference between the "upstream" and "downstream" signals; that difference is used to calculate the flow rate. The T106 has several filter settings to decrease artifacts, all tests were performed with the 0.1 Hz filter.

In laboratory testing, we studied the performance of this flow meter using mock CSF (saline) with various shunt tubes manufactured by Cordis (Cordis Corp. Miami, Fl) and Codman (Codman & Shurtleff Inc., Randolph, Ma). Each 20 cm shunt tube was tested by placing the 1R probe around the center of the tube which was either submerged inside a small plastic bath filled with water or they were surrounded with Acusonic 100 ultrasound conductive medium (Parker Labs, Orange, NJ) which eliminated any air between the tube and probe interface. The mock CSF was pumped through the shunts using a Sage Infusion Instrument 351 (Orion Research Inc, Cambridge, Ma). The fluid was collected in a small graduated cylinder in order to quantify the flow rate independently. Various flow rates were evaluated by a minimum of two ten minute runs which were averaged to measure the meter's performance at each flow rate and with each shunt.

The flow probe was attached to the meter through a pair of inductive coils (1 cm in diameter 0.5 cm apart) which are embedded in silicone. One pair of coils could potentially be implanted with the transducer subcutaneously to enable transcutaneous measurement. During testing a 4 mm thick sponge soaked in saline served as artificial skin separating the inductive coils. Before testing, adequate transmission could be checked with a special function on the flow meter. During testing the flow was periodically turned off to calibrate baseline zero. To test effects of obstruction either finger pressure or a hemostat clamp was applied to the shunt tube 6 to 10 cm from the probe. The data was recorded on a single channel strip chart recorder, Fisher Series 500 (Houston Instruments, Austin, TX).

Results

The Transonics Flow meter's resolution proved to be adequate to easily identify changes in flow of 0.03 ml/min or greater. Upon testing different shunt tubes there were no significant differences in the performance of the system between various samples. The comparisons were made at a constant flow of 0.25 ml/min.

The flow rate displayed on the meter corresponded very closely to the volume collected in the graduated cylinder; the differences were proportional to the rate of flow with the error not exceeding ten percent. Fluctuations seen in the flow may either reflect artifact and noise in the system or the pulsatile movements of the infusion pump. With higher flow rates (0.80 ml/min) the fluctuations decreased significantly. The displayed flow rates did drift if the recording period was extended more than ten minutes, however, when flow was interrupted the zero point increased in proportion to the drift.

Figure 2 displays a flow rate of 0.04 ml/min through a 2.2 mm OD Cordis shunt tube, beginning with a zero baseline and continuing for ten minutes. The

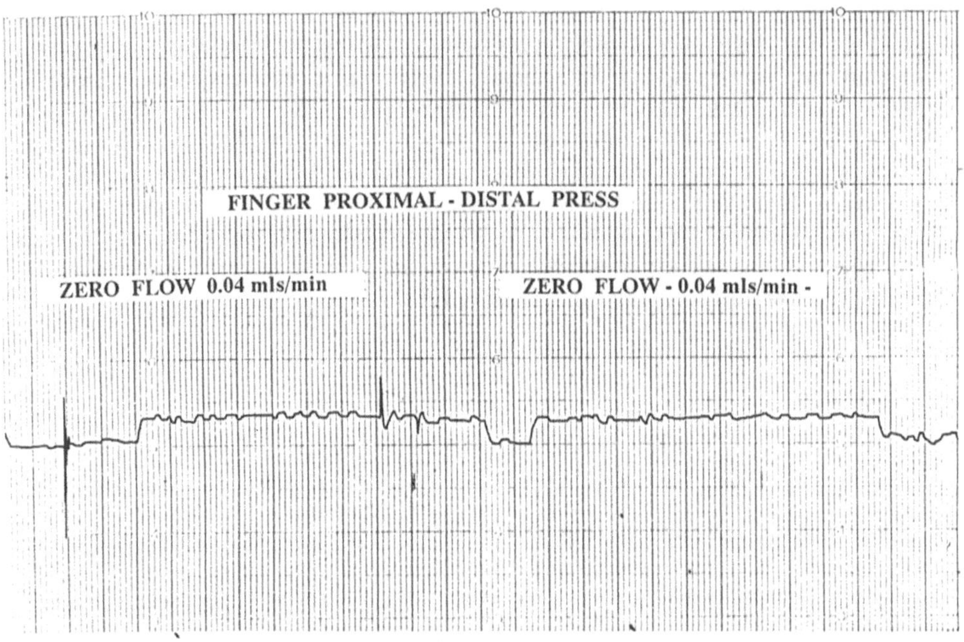

Fig. 2. This graph represents a ten minute recording of mock CSF flow through a Cordis shunt. First, zero baseline is recorded after which fluid was infused at a rate of 0.04 ml/min. The two sharp waves are a proximal and distal compression of the shunt with brief finger pressure. The flow was interruped mid way to check zero point and at the end.

two sharp waves represent two brief finger compressions of the shunt: the first proximally between the pump and probe, the second, distally between the probe and exit port. After turning off the infusion pump, the flow rate rapidly returns to zero baseline which is demonstrated in the middle and end of the recording.

Higher flow rates (above 0.25 ml/min) appeared to be more stable than the lowest rates closer to the threshold of the instrument's sensitivity. However, regardless of the flow rate, any perturbation of the shunt tube, pump, or transducer would be visible on the recording. When testing the Cordis valve during low flow or zero flow one would observe a rapid and large increase of flow followed by a brief decrease or period of negative flow after compressing the reservoir.

Discussion

The flow of CSF through the shunt is a critical indicator of normal function. The need for an effective telemetric system to evaluate CSF flow in indwelling shunts has been sought for many years. Previous reports have described methods to estimate the flow, however, each system contains certain drawbacks that limit their clinical utility or pose some degree of risk to the patient. For those patients who repeatedly experience problems with their shunts or are at risk for shunt failure, a system that could provide a detailed record of their flow rates and CSF output, non-invasively, could be an important advance in their care and management. The results of this work offer a simple, accurate, efficient technique to directly quantify and monitor CSF flow for long periods of time. This preliminary evaluation, at least, demonstrates that this instrument can measure CSF flow rates in shunts in the range that have been previously reported in vivo. With further experience it is likely that this system will also be able to determine the location of an obstruction if one exists within the shunt tube. Although more testing is necessary, this technique may prove to become the method of choice in the near future.

References

1. Drake JM, Sainte-Rose C, DaSilva M, Hirsch JF (1991) Cerebrospinal fluid flow dynamics in children with external ventricular drains. Neurosurg 28:242–250
2. Hayden PW, Shurtleff DB, Stunz TJ (1983) A longitudinal study of shunt function in 360 patients with hydroceph. Dev Med Child Neurol 25:334–337
3. Hoffman H, Smith M (1986) The use of shunting devices for cerebrospinal fluid in Canada. Can J Neurol Sci 13:81–87
4. Martin AJ, Drake JM, Lemaire C, Hankelman RM (1989) CSF shunts: Flow measurement with MR imaging. Rad 173:243–247
5. Milhorat TH (1978) Pediatric Neurosurgery. Davis Co. Phil
6. Numoto M, Hara M, Sakai T, Kadowaki C, Takeuchi K (1984) A non-invasive CSF flowmeter. J Med Eng Tech 8:218–220

Application of Digital Subtraction Angiography for Quantitative Estimation of Shunt Function

Y. Okada, T. Shima, S. Matsumura, M. Nishida, T. Yamada, K. Yamane, S. Okita, and H. Sato

Departmennt of Neurosurgery, Chugoku Rousai Hospital , Kure 7370-1 Japan

Introduction

CSF shunt systems have been widely applied in the treatment of hydrocephalus patients whose prognosis would be strictly dependent on shunt function. Although many shunt function tests have been introduced, no simple and quantitative method is available [1, 2]. In this study, the authors introduced a new method using digital subtraction angiography (DSA) as CSF shunt function test and evaluated its clinical applicability.

Materials and Methods

Twenty-nine patients who underwent a shunt operation were subjected to this study. This group consisted of 23 adults with normal pressure hydrocephalus following subarachnoid hemorrhage, three with obstructive hydrocephalus due to tumor, and three infants with communicating hydrocephalus.

Preliminary an experimental open shunt system was prepared to investigate how the infused metrizamide flowed in the chamber. A shunt system was connected to a tube filled with physiologic saline solution. The height of saline was fixed at 10 cm from the tip of the shunt system. Then 0.5 ml of metrizamide was injected into the chamber and DSA was made to obtain a shuntgraphy in the following way. In the chamber changes in density were measured. The regression curve (RC) was calculated by the method of least squares and the respective gradient coefficient was obtained. Three kinds of tubes with low, medium or high pressure valves were examined.

In patients, shunt function test was performed by shuntgraphy in sitting and supine position. The chamber was punctured with a 27 gauge needle to slowly drain 0.5 ml of CSF, followed by the formation of mask image. Then 0.5 ml of metrizamide in a concentration of 170 mg/ml was slowly infused into the chamber for about 12–14 seconds to make a subtraction with real-time of 20 seconds using a DSA instrument (DF-X, Toshiba). Next the patient was put in the sitting position and DSA shuntgraphy was repeated in the same way. After the DSA was performed, a region of interest (ROI) was set up within the center of the chamber to continually measure the density from which the regression curve in the supine and sitting position were calculated by the least square method. The ratio of the gradient coefficient in the sitting position to that in the supine position was obtained in each case.

Results and Conclusions

The gradient coefficient of the regression curve in vitro studies for low, medium and high pressure tubes were −15.4, −9.98 and −7.5 respectively. These results might suggest that our DSA method could be applied as CSF shunt function test.

Figure 1 shows a shuntgraphy in a 54-year-old male who presented with normal pressure hydrocephalus and recovered completely after shunt operation. The gradient coefficients in the supine and sitting position were −6.90 and −9.36 respectively and the ratio was calculated as 1.36.

Figure 2 presents the shuntgraphies in a 72-year-old female who suffered from obstructive hydrocephalus caused by a cerebellopontine angle tumor. The tumor was partially excised and a V-P shunt operation was performed using a medium pressure valve. Although she had a good postoperative course, she exhibited gait disturbances and urinary incontinence about six months later. Her shuntgraphies demonstrated gradient coefficients of −3.72 and −1.16 in the supine and sitting position respectively, and the ratio was 0.43. This result suggested dysfunction of the shunt system and at surgery ventricular obstruction was revealed.

The mean gradient coefficients in the supine and sitting position were −2.4 and −7.4, in the low pressure tube group, −2.4 and −5.6 in the medium

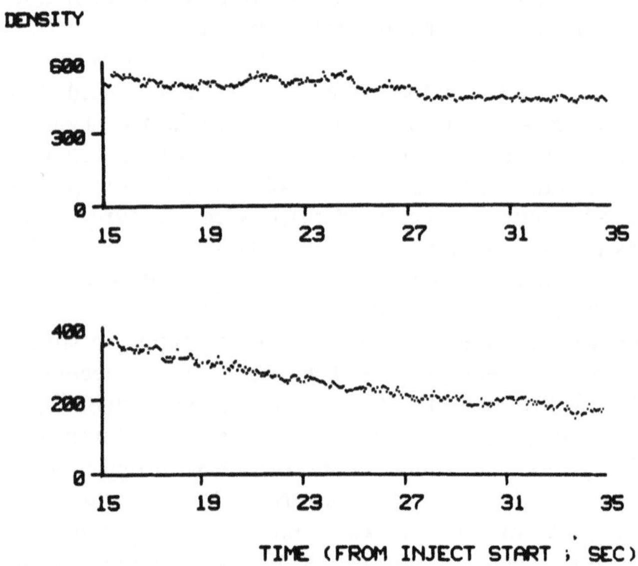

Fig. 1. Shuntgraphies in the supine (*upper*) and sitting position (*lower*) in normal pressure hydrocephalus

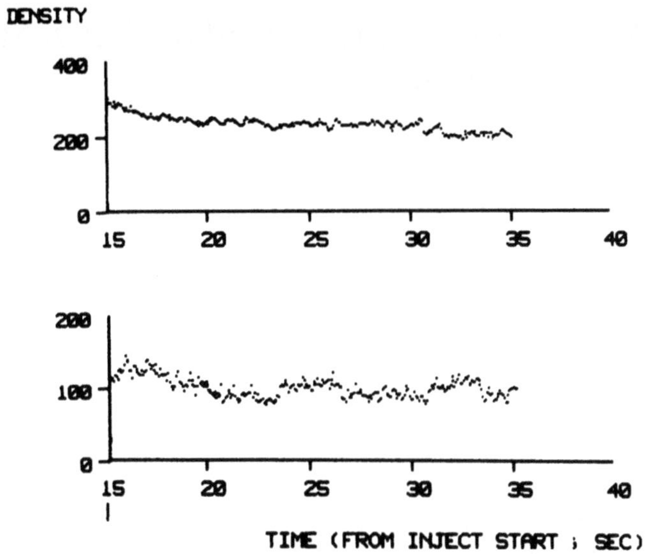

Fig. 2. Shuntgraphies in the supine (*upper*) and sitting position (*lower*) in obstructive hydrocephalus

pressure tube group, and −4.8 and −6.8 in the high pressure tube group. No significant differences among the gradient coefficients could be found in the low, medium and high pressure group. The ratio was 3.2 on the average ranging from 1.3 to 25.7. The cases presenting dysfunction of the shunt demonstrated a ratio of less than 1.00. It is suggested that DSA shuntgraphy can be applied to evaluate the CSF shunt function easily and quantitatively.

References

1. Brisman R, Schneider S, Carter S (1973) Subarachnoid infusion and shunt function Technical note. J Neurosurg 38:379–381
2. Graham P, Howman-Giles R, Johnston I, Besser M (1982) Evaluation of CSF shunt patency by means of Technetium-99m DTPA. J Neurosurg 57:262–266

Non-Invasive Measurement of ICP in Shunt System by Collapse Technique

T. Hashimoto, N. Nakamura, H. Shimazu, M. Gondoh, and T. Tamai

Department of Neurosurgery, Jikei University School of Medicine, Tokyo, Department of Physiology, Kyorin University School of Medicine, Tokyo, and Japan MDM Ltd., Tokyo, Japan

Introduction

A new non-invasive method for regulation of cerebrospinal fluid flow and measurement of intracranial pressure (ICP) in a ventriculo-peritoneal shunt system has been developed. The device consists of two major parts: A flow control device and a pressure device (Fig. 1). The size of the flow control device is 18 × 17.5 × 6 mm with two slit valves and two titanium balls. One of the slit valves is with high resistance and the other is with low resistance. The flow rate is regulated through the valves with four settings: off, low, medium and high, by the location of two titanium balls which can be moved by the neurosurgeon percutaneously. Because of its material, this flow regulatory device is compatible with MRI.

The pressure device, a 0.4 mm thick silicon reservoir, is 17 mm in diameter and 6 mm in height. It is connected between the ventricular port and the flow control device and allows non-invasive measurement of ICP percutaneously. It consists of two elements: a) a reservoir made of a thin silicone dome, and b) a detector which has a pusher dome via the skin.

The detector with the pusher dome at the front end is placed exactly over the reservoir underneath the skin. By increasing and decreasing external pressure, collapse of the pressure dome occurs, when external pressure exceeds pressure inside the device, and restoration occurs in the reverse process. This restoration point and collapse point reflects ICP (Fig. 2). A small error may be caused by material characteristics: shape resistance etc. may be needed to be compensated. However, this may be done automatically by introducing an error factor.

The newly designed monitoring system can automatically control the measuring sequence and indicate the pressure on a display. The calculated ICP values and its average can also be printed. The flow control device and pressure device can be used separately and they are compatible with other types of shunt systems.

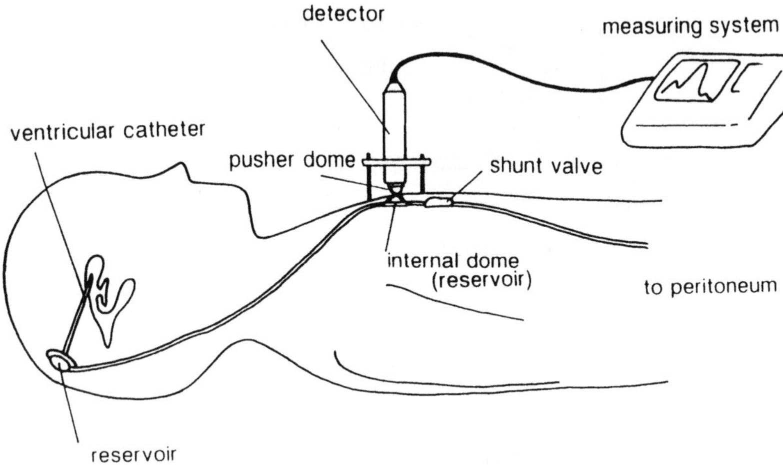

Fig. 1. Schematic drawing of the system for measurement of intracranial pressure

Results

Animal Studies

Experiments were done on 21 dogs under anesthetized conditions. 650 Pairs of recordings were obtained. The pressure device was implanted in subcutaneous tissue at the thoracic wall of each dog. Actual measurement was performed every two weeks and carried out for six months. The results indicated that there was a good correlation in a range of 0 to 40 mm H_2O. The linear regression equation and correlation coefficient were $Y = 1.087X + 2.636$ and $r = 0.995$, respectively. The actual pressure was obtained within ± 3 cm H_2O error range (Fig. 3).

Clinical Application

The flow control device has not been used clinically. The pressure device was used in 10 cases with a Sophy pressure programmable shunt system. The system was implanted at the thoracic wall of each patient. Pressure measurement can be done immediately after the shunt operation and measuring can be repeatedly performed non-invasively. In these studies, one patient with Dandy Walker syndrome treated by Sophy shunt system with its pressure control set to medium, still showed symptoms of increased ICP, even though reduction of ventricular size was seen on CT-scan. The ICP of the patient was 8.8 cm H_2O. After changing the pressure controle to low pressure, the clinical symptoms disappeared. ICP was measured again, and it was 1.7 cm H_2O. The pressure of Sophy shunt system was changed in four cases on the basis of ICP monitoring, CT-scan and clinical condition.

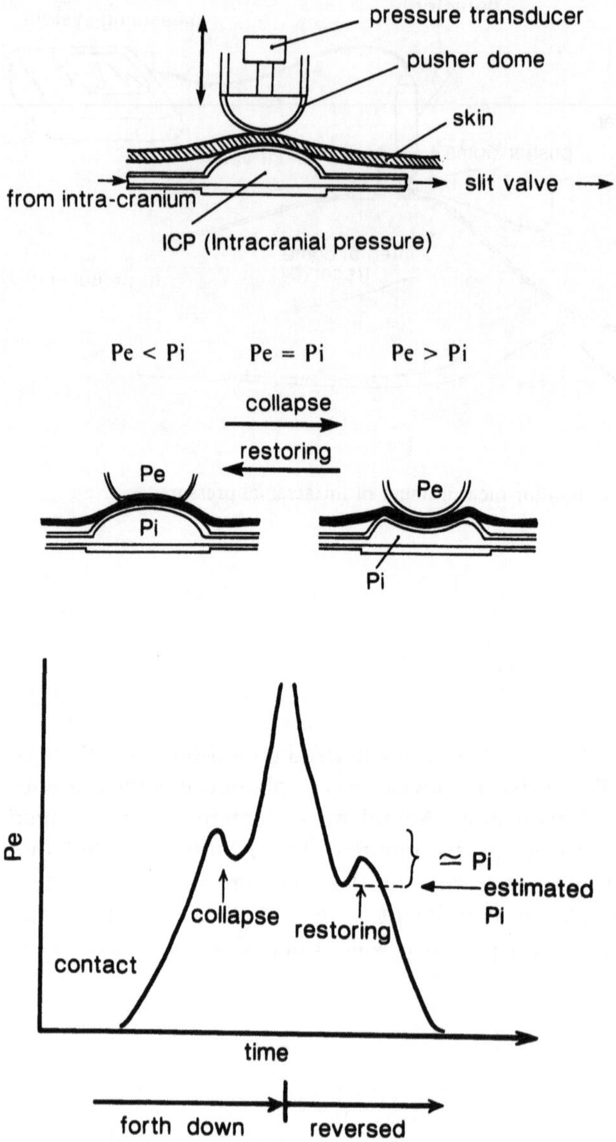

Fig. 2. Schematic drawing of indirect measurement of pressure non-invasively. Collapse and restoration of the dome occurs by the pressure difference between internal and external dome. The recording shows collapse and restoration of the dome using pressure transducer. Restoring point indicates ICP

Discussion

Shunt function has been studied using isotope, contrast medium, Doppler method, Camereonprint, thermography, and quantitative measurement of pressure in the shunt system. However, most of these methods have not been

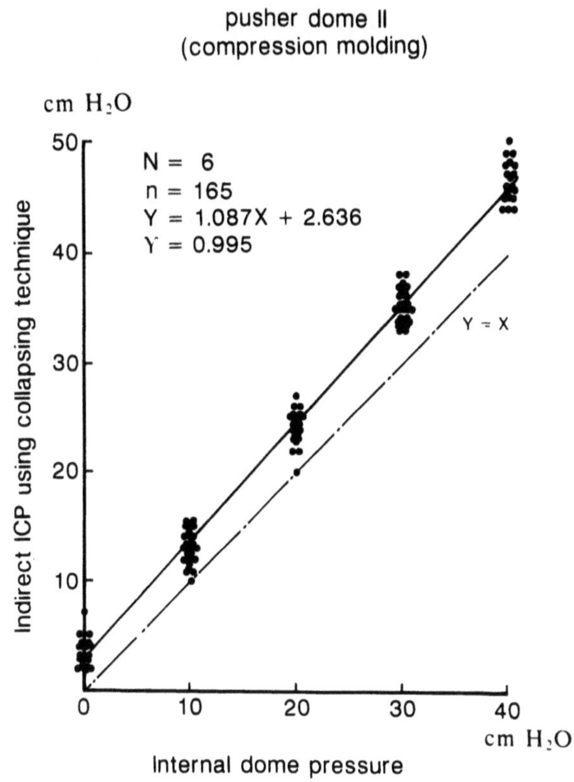

Fig. 3. Correlation of indirectly estimated pressure and direct pressure of the internal dome subcutaneously implanted in a dog

Table 1. Summary of programmable pressure valve and. pressure measurement. The pressure of Sophy shunt system should be changed in 4 cases by pressure monitoring an clinical status

Case	Age	Sex	Cause of Hydrocephalus	PPV Pressure	Pressure meas. cmH_2O	Complication
1	62	M	SAH	Medium	12.4	None
2	56	F	Obstructive	Medium → Low	8.5 → 1.7	Hypofunction → None
3	51	F	SAH	Medium	11.8	
4	67	F	SAH	Medium	15.6	None
5	40	M	SAH	High → Low	→ 7.2	Hypofunction → None
6	42	M	Tumor	Medium	14.0	None
7	36	F	Tumor	Medium	Collapse	Slit Vent. None
8	19	M	Trauma	Medium → Low	22.3 → 13.2	Hypofunction → None
9	54	F	SAH	Medium Low	21.3	Obstruction
10	27	M	Tumor	High	Collapse	Slit Vent. None

used routinely for management of hydrocephalus because they are complicated and non-invasive.

The theory of measurement of ICP in the multipurpose shunt system is a modification of the coplanar method and is called collapsing technique.

Measurement of ICP can be done non-invasively and repeatedly. The function of the shunt system can be estimated by periodical measurement, and the obtained data indicates the error is within ±3 cm H_2O compared to actual ICP.

The authors have experienced several cases with discrepancy between ICP and the clinical condition. The results suggested that the optimal ICP may be different in individual patients with hydrocephalus. Therefore, a flow regulatory device with pressure monitoring device is useful in the treatment of hydrocephalus.

References

1. Hashimoto T, Nakamura N, Kanki T, Shimazyu H, Yamakoshi K, Gondo M, Tamai T (1990) A new shunt system with non-invasive flow rate regulation and pressure measurement. In: Proceeding of international symposium on hydrocephalus (in press)
2. Numoto M, Hara M, Kadowaki K (1984) A non-invasive CSF flowmeter. J of Med Eng and Technol 8:218–220

Complications and Malfunctions of Derivative Surgery for Hydrocephalus

P. Buoncristiani, M. Nardi, G. Ghetti, and A. Casotto

Department of Neurotraumatology, General Hospital of Perugia, Perugia, Italy

Introduction

"The history of ventricular shunting for hydrocephalus is largely a history of efforts to prevent the complications of shunting" [1].

The aim of this retrospective study is to delineate the real incidence, type and severity of the principal complications of the CSF shunting system for hydrocephalus, trying to put them in relationship with the types of valve used. For this purpose, we have re-evaluated all the shunting operations for hydrocephalus performed at our Department during the last two decades.

Material and Methods

During the years between 1972 and 1989 a total of 803 operations for hydrocephalus were performed (with a medium of 46 oper./year) at our Department on 538 patients (294 male; 244 female; average age 47 years), approximately 1.49 operations per patient.

The most frequent age classes were 0–10 years (98 patients) and 61–70 years (113 patients).

The types of shunt used in the first operation were ventricular-atrial (V-A) in 512 cases and ventricular-peritoneal (V-P) in 26 cases.

The type of valve used for the operations during the years 1972–1980 was the Heyer-Schulte (H-S) continuous flow valve (cardiac and peritoneal catheters with a variable resistance: low, 2–5 cm H20; medium, 6–9 cm H20; high, 10–14 cm H20; according to the desired pressure gradient for each case).

During the years 1981–1986 the Pudenz-Schulte (P-S) valve was used, characterized by a low, medium, high pressure flow-control with a cut-off system (universal type of cardiac and peritoneal catheters without pressure regulation) and, finally, during years 1986–1989 the P-S valves were used in 70% of the cases and H-S in the remaining 30%.

The etiology of hydrocephalus in our patients is shown in Table 1:

In the present study the following aspects were examined:

- the causes of malfunction of the shunting systems globally and in relation to the type of shunting system;
- the time interval between the first operation and the first revision;

Table 1. Causes of hydrocephalus

Etiology	No. cases	%
Neoplastic	187	34.7
Malformative	116	21.5
Normal press. elderly	110	20.4
Post hemorr.	60	11.1
Post traumatic	27	5.0
Sec. to meningoenceph.	26	4.8
Sec. to surgery	12	2.2

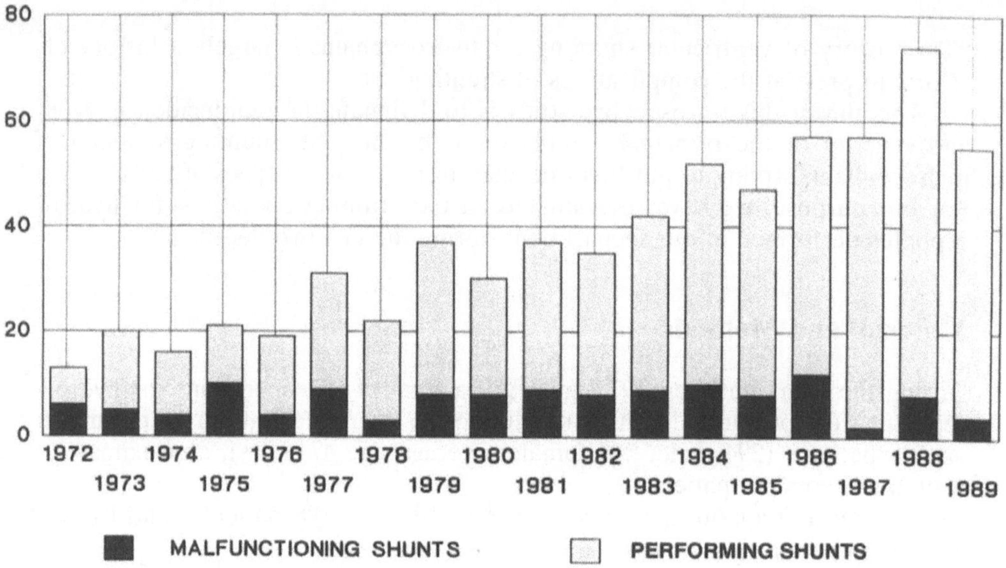

Fig. 1. Malfunctioning/performing shunts ratio years 1972–1989

- the number of operations performed on each patient;
- the number and percentage of malfunctioning shunts with regard to the years in which the first operation was performed and the type of shunting system inserted;
- the number of malfunctioning shunts in relation to age and etiology;
- the mortality in relationship to surgical procedures and to the malfunctioning of shunt systems.

Results

A total of 127 patients needed surgical revision of the initial shunt and were submitted to 265 reoperations.

Table 2. Malfunctioning-performing shunts ratio according to type of valve used

Type of valve	Shunts performing	Shunts malfunctioning	
Heyer-Schulte 1972–80	152	67	37%
Pudenz-Schulte 1981–86	214	56	26%
Mixed 1987–89	172	14	8%

These patients represent 24% of the total population operated for hydrocephalus since 1972 to 1989. Figure 1 shows the shunt operations performed in each year and the number of shunts of that year requiring surgical revision during the observed period until now.

The percentage of malfunctioning shunts in the three groups mentioned above, are presented in Table 2. Figure 2 shows the varius complications responsible for reoperations. Figure 3 shows the number of reoperations per patient related to age. Only few cases were operated more than three times; in 53% of patients one revision was sufficient. Table 3 presents the number of reoperations.

Discussion and Conclusions

During the period 1972/1989 the percentage of malfunctioning shunts was reduced from 86% to 8%.

Many factors influenced these results, the most evident being the progress in surgical technique and experience, followed by the diagnostic facilities allowing the precise knowledge of the pathology and the proper choice of the shunt's pressure level. Regarding the results obtained with two different types of shunt, Heyer-Schulte versus Pudenz-Schulte, the different percentage of malfunction (37.5/26.1) is probably secondary to the general improvement and not to the shunt type properties. Actually, in the last period 1987–1989 the malfunctioning shunts further decreased to 8.1%, while using either the H.-S. or the P.-S. valves.

The overall complication rate of 24% appears rather low, considering the wide time span of the study. Evaluating the type of complications, we did not observe true hypersensitive immune reaction to the foreign body [2]. The most common complication was proximal ventricular catheter obstruction (44.1%) in spite of the constant research of a proper position of the catheter tip cephalad to the Monro foramen [3]. Other important complications were global malfunction (including overdrainage and subdural collections), valve rupture and detachment, and distal catheter obstruction.

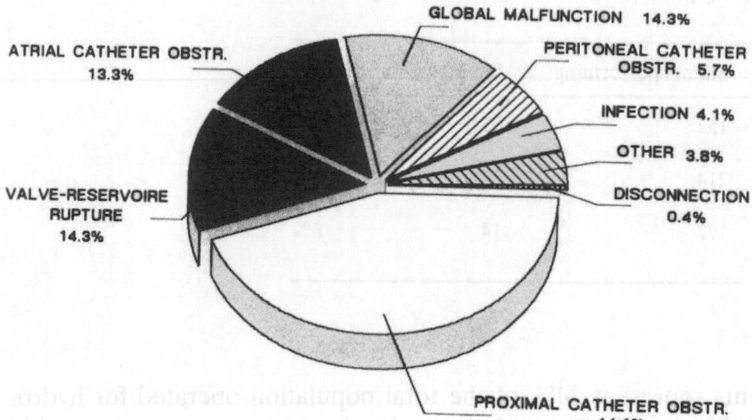

Fig. 2. Types of complications: all cases years 1972–1989

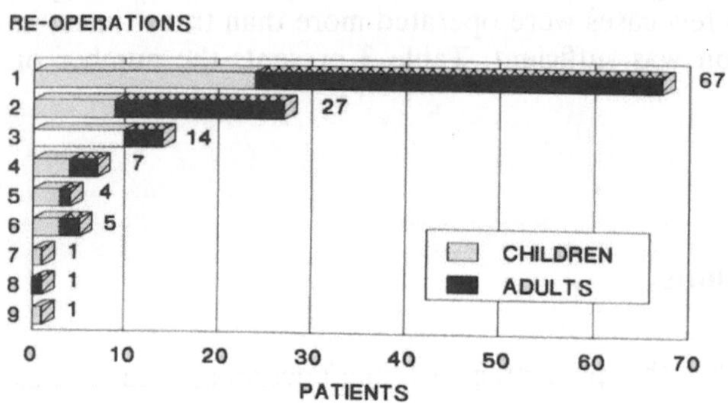

Fig. 3. Number of re-operations and children/adults ratio

Table 3. Re-operations ratio children/adults

Age of patients	Total patients	Re-operated patients	(%)	Number of re-operations
Pediatric age				
0–10 years	98	46	(47)	115 (2,5/pt.)
11–15 years	23	9	(39)	19 (2,1/pt.)
	121	55	(45)	134 (2,4/pt.)
Adult age				
16–80 years	417	72	(17)	131 (1,8/pt.)
Total	538	127	(24)	265 (2/pt.)

Infection was responsible for 4.1% of all the complications, occurring just in 2% of all shunted patients. This is very favourably compared to the 10% of Raimondi [4], the 20% of Walters [5] and the 19.5% of Pui [6].

Our policy was based on common surgical antiseptic principles with particular attention to the position of the reservoir and to the perioperative antibiotic profylaxis.

The first re-operation had to be done within the first year in 79% of patients and within the second year in 87%, confirming the general experience.

We observed a clear influence of age in shunt malfunctions with 45% in 121 childrens compared to 17% in 417 adults. Di Rocco had 47% complications [7]. The shunt failure related deaths were 11 (2%). Fifty-nine patients died for causes unrelated to shunt function, mostly in neoplastic cases.

New materials and new shunt types are still required in order to further improve the shunting surgery of hydrocephalus with respect to mechanical complications, changing pressure conditions, and the duration of the system.[8]

References

1. Mc Laurin RL (1982) Shunt Complications. Pediatric Neurosurgery; Surgery of the developing Nervous System, Grune & Stratton, New York, pp 243–253
2. Gower DJ, Lewis JC, Kelly DL (1984) Sterile shunt malfunction: a scanning electron-microscopic perspective. J Neurosurg 61:1079
3. Becker DP, Nulsen FE (1968) Control of Hydrocephalus by valve-regulated venous shunt: avoidance of complications in prolonged shunt maintenance. J Neurosurg 28:215
4. Raimondi AJ, Robinson JS, Kjwamura K (1977) Complications of ventriculo-peritoneal shunting and a critical comparison of the three-piece and one-piece systems. Child's Brain 3321
5. Walters BC, Hoffman HJ, Hendrich EB, et al. (1984) Cerebrospinal shunt fluid infection: influences on initial management and subsequent outcome. J Neurosurg 60:1014.
6. Pui CH, Ch. Ien LT, Vanderzwaag R (1981) Shunt-associated bacterial infections in Hydrocephalic children. Ala J Sci 18:134
7. Di Rocco C, Iannelli A (1987) Complications of CSF shunting in the treatment of infantile Hydrocephalus, Ed. CRC Press Inc
8. Portnoy HD (1982) Treatment of hydrocephalus. Pediatric Neurosurgery, Grune & Stratton, New York 2:211

Panel 4
CSF Dynamics and Hydrocephalus

Moderator: A. Marmarou

Members: M. Czosnyka, J. Ekstedt, S. Higashi, D.J. Price, J.T.J. Tans

On the subject of theoretical models FRIDEN emphasized that the vascular bed should be incorporated in the models. He referred to the study by Heissler et al in which attention was drawn to the unwanted secondary vascular reactions to fast and large bolus infusions. They had used "diamox" stimulation to estimate the extent of vascular interference. CZOSNYKA said that transcranial doppler offers, for the first time, the opportunity of studying the dynamics of cerebral blood flow together with the ICP dynamics. He mentioned the model of Gulioni and Ursino that takes into account both the vascular changes and the CSF dynamics. In the future, continuous monitoring of cerebral perfusion pressure and cerebral blood flow may be replaced by a more important parameter like the cerebral vascular resistance. MARMAROU remarked that with the increasing use of fiberoptic devices not placed in the CSF, we need models in which vascular changes can be introduced and their influence on compliance and outflow resistance measured. He questioned the concept of Bulat that there is no flow of CSF between the various CSF spaces and that the volume of CSF is determined by osmotic and hydrostatic forces operating between CSF and the vascular bed.

EKSTEDT stressed the advantages of performing infusion tests with the patient in the supine position. He uses the constant pressure method. The constant flow infusion can be shortened by starting with a higher infusion rate to load the system with fluid, after which the pressure can be allowed to stabilize from a higher value to the plateau. DELWEL remarked that, with higher infusion rates, he had frequently observed B-waves as a result of secondary vascular reactions. In order to prevent vasomotor responses SMIELEWSKI employs a computer controlled drainage that provides the same data as constant pressure or constant flow infusion.

The studies on normal pressure hydrocephalus (NPH) were evaluated by TANS. The predictive value of Rout for the outcome of shunting varied from almost 100% to as low as 55%. He considered patient selection the major issue here. If patients with different types of hydrocephalus, including cerebral atrophy, are investigated Rout alone seems unable to identify shunt responders with sufficient reliability. Therefore, infusion tests should be used primarily to select for shunting patients with a clinical diagnosis of NPH and not to differentiate NPH from other conditions with enlarged ventricles. The second point raised by TANS was that some investigators were of the opinion that the higher Rout the better the outcome of shunting, whereas others, like Delwel, had not find such a relationship. The level of Rout above which patients were shunted varied between 8 and 18 mmHg/ml/min. MARMAROU commented that most authors seem to favor a threshold of 10 to 12 mmHg/ml/min. According to ANILE the primary cause of NPH is not an increased Rout, but a change of intracranial elastance. Therefore, elastance is the main criterion for shunting.

PRICE summarized some posters on benign intracranial hypertension. Mangiola had found a good correlation between optic nerve diameter variations measured by echography of the orbit and ICP changes induced by infusion tests. ROSNER reported that sodium intake in these patients was high. Signs and symptoms of benign intracranial hypertension, including ICP, improved markedly on a 2 gram sodium diet. Supposedly, the sodium is responsible for brain swelling, upon which MILLER commented that a low sodium may cause brain swelling as well.

Discussing the contributions on shunt function, HIGASHI remarked that the best shunt system is the one that is the most physiological. To prevent overdrainage flow regulating valves are better than differential pressure valves, because with flow regulating valves changes in body position cause changes in ICP, cerebral perfusion pressure and cerebral blood flow that are similar to those in normal subjects. TANS amplified that ventriculo-peritoneal shunts with a membrane or spring ball valve are the best choice for the treatment of NPH. The experience with programmable valves is limited but they seem to offer a number of advantages. HIGASHI mentioned some new non-invasive methods to investigate shunt function like infrared imaging, ultrasonic flow measurement and pressure measurement in the shunt. RYDER emphasized that all shunt systems should have the telemetric ability to give both flow and pressure. RICHARD noted that transcranial doppler is helpful in differentiating between the hypotensive and the hypertensive form of the slit ventricle syndrome.

MARMAROU closed the session by observing that not much material had been presented regarding the etiology of NPH. We have available the techniques that can identify the degree of the absorptive deficit but their success in predicting the results of shunting depend on what criteria are adopted at each institution. As the population grows older, the number of patients with NPH seems to increase. So, there is enough work to do for the young investigators both in the understanding of NPH and in its management.

Subject Index

Springer-Verlag and the Environment

We at Springer-Verlag firmly believe that an international science publisher has a special obligation to the environment, and our corporate policies consistently reflect this conviction.

We also expect our business partners – paper mills, printers, packaging manufacturers, etc. – to commit themselves to using environmentally friendly materials and production processes.

The paper in this book is made from low- or no-chlorine pulp and is acid free, in conformance with international standards for paper permanency.

MIX
Papier aus verantwortungsvollen Quellen
Paper from responsible sources
FSC® C105338

If you have any concerns about our products,
you can contact us on
ProductSafety@springernature.com

In case Publisher is established outside the EU,
the EU authorized representative is:
Springer Nature Customer Service Center GmbH
Europaplatz 3, 69115 Heidelberg, Germany

Printed by Libri Plureos GmbH
in Hamburg, Germany